DIAGNOSTIC PATHOLOGY

Hospital Autopsy

FYFE | MILLER

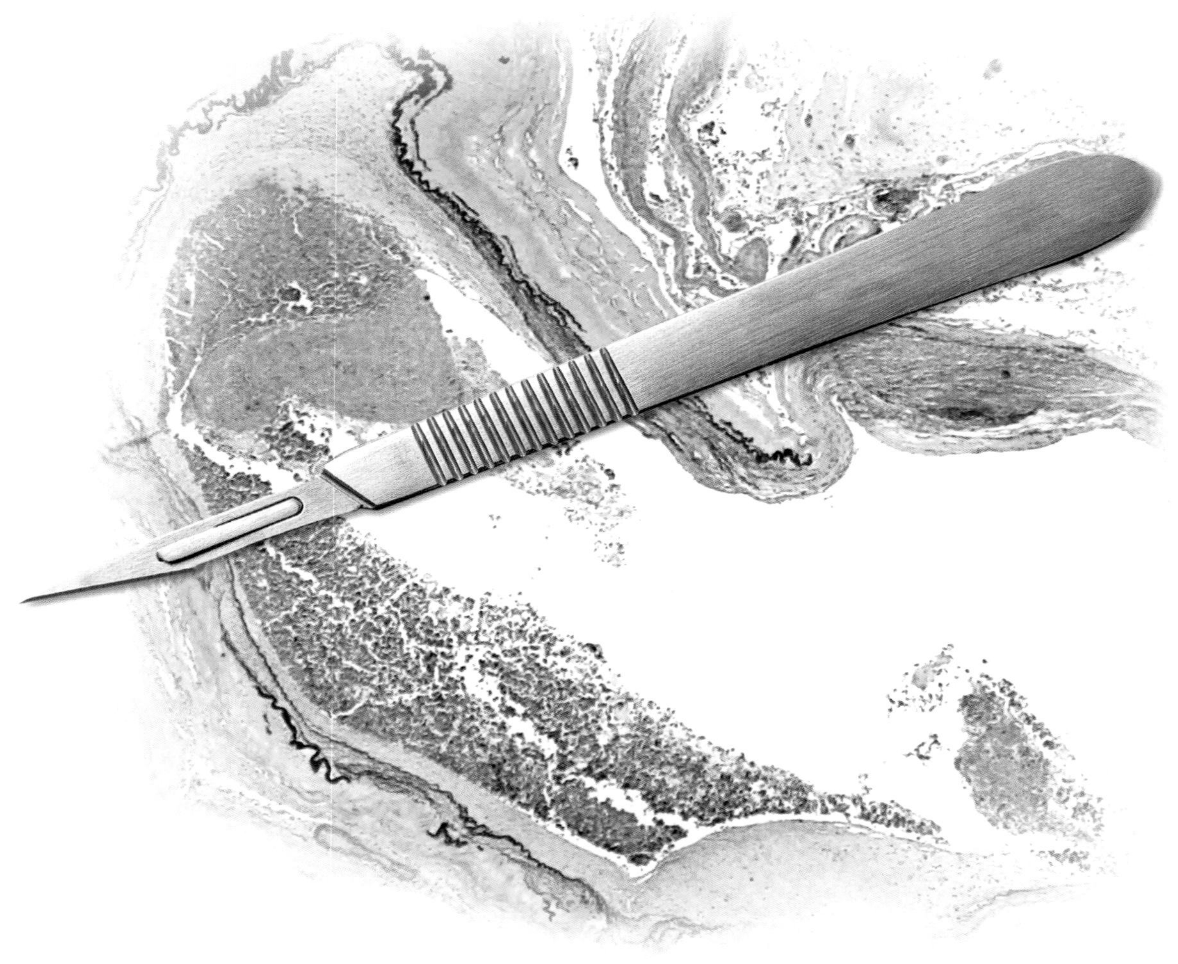

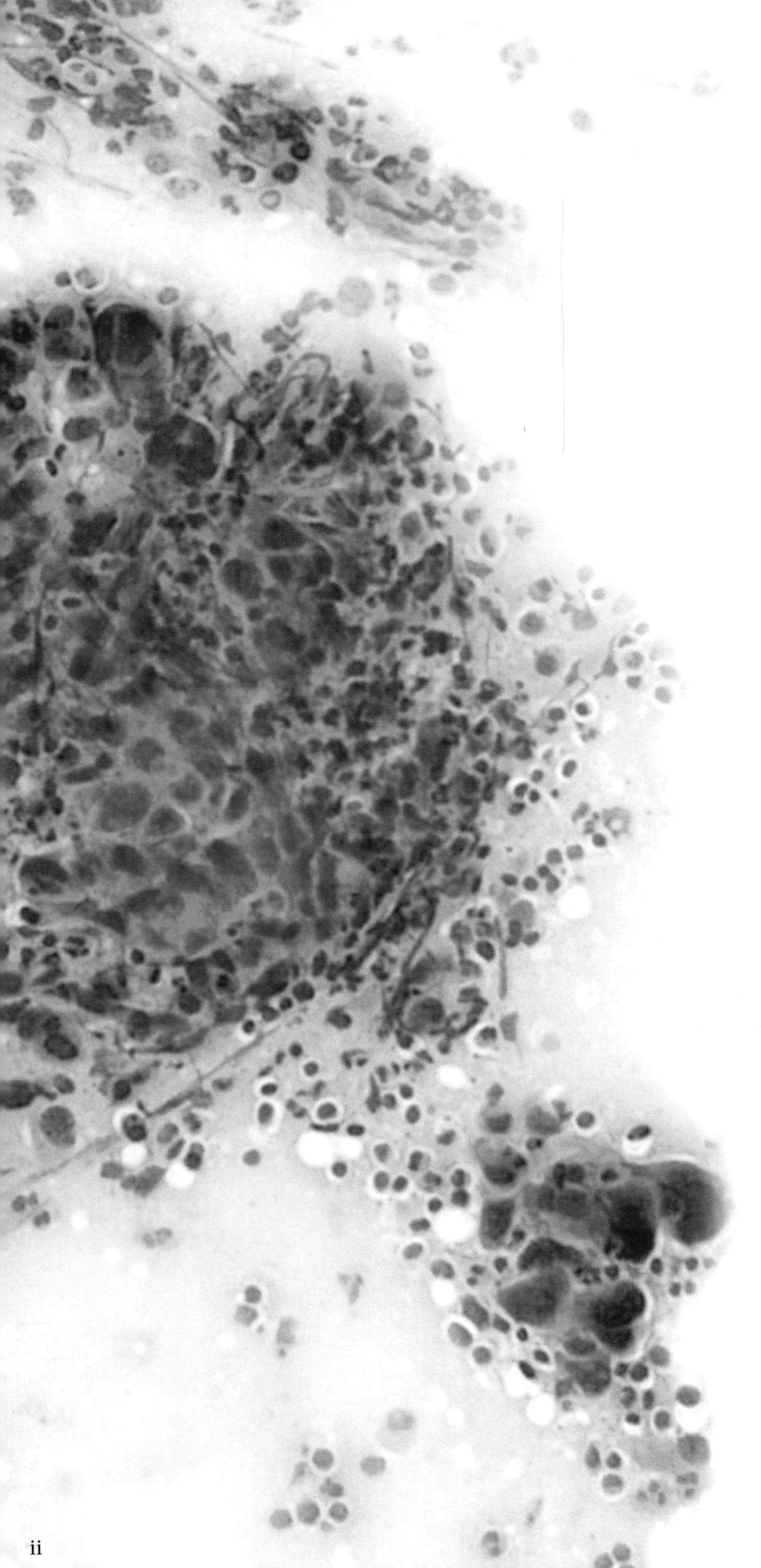

DIAGNOSTIC PATHOLOGY

Hospital Autopsy

Billie Fyfe, MD
Professor of Pathology
Rutgers Robert Wood Johnson Medical School
New Brunswick, New Jersey

Dylan V. Miller, MD
Clinical Associate Professor of Pathology
University of Utah School of Medicine
Director of Electron Microscopy and Immunostains
Intermountain Central Laboratory
Salt Lake City, Utah

ELSEVIER

1600 John F. Kennedy Blvd.
Ste 1800
Philadelphia, PA 19103-2899

DIAGNOSTIC PATHOLOGY: HOSPITAL AUTOPSY

ISBN: **978-0-323-37676-1**

Notices

Knowledge and best practice in this field are constantly changing. As new research and experience broaden our understanding, changes in research methods, professional practices, or medical treatment may become necessary.

Practitioners and researchers must always rely on their own experience and knowledge in evaluating and using any information, methods, compounds, or experiments described herein. In using such information or methods they should be mindful of their own safety and the safety of others, including parties for whom they have a professional responsibility.

With respect to any drug or pharmaceutical products identified, readers are advised to check the most current information provided (i) on procedures featured or (ii) by the manufacturer of each product to be administered, to verify the recommended dose or formula, the method and duration of administration, and contraindications. It is the responsibility of practitioners, relying on their own experience and knowledge of their patients, to make diagnoses, to determine dosages and the best treatment for each individual patient, and to take all appropriate safety precautions.

To the fullest extent of the law, neither the Publisher nor the authors, contributors, or editors, assume any liability for any injury and/or damage to persons or property as a matter of products liability, negligence or otherwise, or from any use or operation of any methods, products, instructions, or ideas contained in the material herein.

Publisher Cataloging-in-Publication Data

Diagnostic pathology. Hospital autopsy / [edited by] Billie Fyfe and Dylan V. Miller.
pages ; cm
Hospital autopsy
Includes bibliographical references and index.
ISBN 978-0-323-37676-1 (hardback)
1. Autopsy--Handbooks, manuals, etc. 2. Autopsy--Methods--Handbooks, manuals, etc.
I. Fyfe, Billie. II. Miller, Dylan V. III. Title: Hospital autopsy.
[DNLM: 1. Autopsy--methods--Atlases. QZ 35]
RB57 .I434 2015
616.07/59--dc23

International Standard Book Number: 978-0-323-37676-1

Cover Designer: Tom M. Olson, BA

Printed in Canada by Friesens, Altona, Manitoba, Canada

Last digit is the print number: 9 8 7 6 5 4 3 2 1

Dedications

To the giants who patiently mentored me at Mayo Clinic (Drs. Edwards, Parisi, Holly, Aubry, Smyrk, and Pfeifer) and the amazing support staff of the old Baldwin basement and later Stabile 9. To Drs. Collins and Sinard and many colleagues on the CAP Autopsy Resource Committee for opening my eyes to a wider world of pathology practice. To the many able minds who helped conceive, gestate, and deliver the book's content and whose names dignify its pages. To Dave, Angie, and Kellie at Amirsys/Elsevier for their patience and trust. And most of all to Tonya, for her undying tolerance and support.

DVM

This book is dedicated with gratitude to my mentors, who gave me the courage and opportunity to pursue autopsy pathology, and to my mentorees, who make the work so rewarding. This project would not have been possible without the forward vision of the Amirsys/Elsevier team, especially Angela Terry, who supported this unique addition to their pathology collection, and the tremendous expertise shared by Dylan Miller and all of the authors. As always, I must thank my sons, Justin and Alexander, who make everything worthwhile, and my parents, who encouraged me from the beginning.

BF

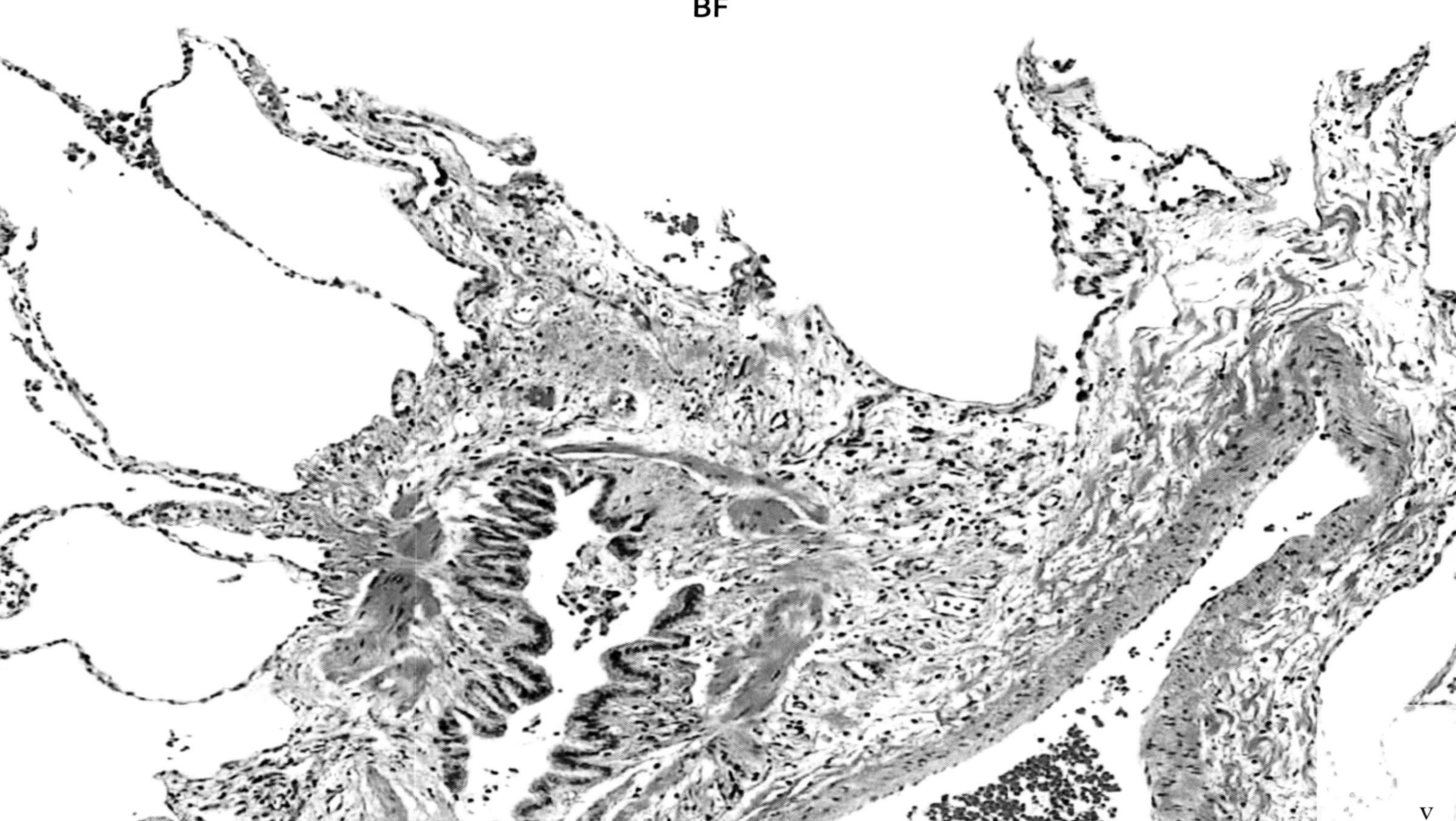

Contributing Authors

Brandon T. Larsen, MD, PhD
Assistant Professor of Pathology
Department of Pathology
Banner – University Medical Center
University of Arizona College of Medicine
Tucson, Arizona

Monica P. Revelo, MD, PhD
Professor of Pathology
Department of Pathology
University of Utah School of Medicine
Salt Lake City, Utah

Rebecca A. Irvine, MD, FRCPA
Senior Staff Specialist, Forensic Pathology
Department of Forensic Medicine, Sydney
NSW Forensic and Analytical Science Service
Glebe, NSW, Australia

George P. Batsides, MD
Assistant Professor of Surgery
Chief, Section of Cardiac Surgery
Surgical Director, Mechanical Circulatory Support
Division of Cardiac Surgery
Rutgers Robert Wood Johnson Medical School
New Brunswick, New Jersey

Jeanine Chiaffarano, DO
Anatomic and Clinical Pathology Resident
Department of Pathology
Rutgers Robert Wood Johnson Medical School
New Brunswick, New Jersey

Christine Minerowicz, MD
Resident of Pathology
Department of Laboratory Medicine and Pathology
Rutgers Robert Wood Johnson Medical School
New Brunswick, New Jersey

Leslie A. Litzky, MD
Professor, Department of Pathology and
Laboratory Medicine
Perelman School of Medicine
University of Pennsylvania
Chief, Section of Medical Pathology,
Hospital of the University of Pennsylvania
Subspecialty Director, Thoracic Pathology,
Section of Surgical Pathology
Philadelphia, Pennsylvania

Harold Sanchez, MD, FCAP
Associate Chief of Pathology
Department of Pathology
Hospital of Central Connecticut
New Britain, Connecticut

Roy H. Rhodes, MD, PhD
Professor
Director, Neuropathology
Medical Director, RWJUH EM Services
Department of Pathology
Rutgers Robert Wood Johnson Medical School
New Brunswick, New Jersey

Paisit Paueksakon, MD
Associate Professor
Associate Director
Division of Renal Pathology/Electron Microscopy
and Renal Pathology Fellowship
Department of Pathology, Microbiology, and Immunology
Vanderbilt University Medical Center
Nashville, Tennessee

Hasini Reddy, MD, DPhil
Department of Pathology, Dalhousie University
Director of Neuropathology
The Moncton Hospital
Moncton, New Brunswick, Canada

Rachel Hudacko, MD
Medical Director, Department of Pathology/Laboratory
St. Anthony Community Hospital
Warwick, New York
Clinical Instructor, Department of Pathology
Rutgers Robert Wood Johnson Medical School
New Brunswick, New Jersey

Patrick Lento, MD
Professor of Clinical Pathology and Medicine
New York Medical College
Valhalla, New York

Corinne L. Fligner, MD
Professor, Department of Pathology
Adjunct Professor, Department of Laboratory Medicine
Director, Autopsy and After Death Services, UW Pathology
University of Washington
Seattle, Washington

Vidhya Nair, MBBS, MD, FRCPC
Associate Professor
Department of Pathology and Molecular Medicine
McMaster University
Cardiovascular Pathologist, Hamilton Health Sciences
Hamilton, Ontario, Canada

Elizabeth H. Hammond, MD
Professor of Pathology and Adjunct Professor of Medicine (Cardiology)
University of Utah School of Medicine
Pathology Consultant
Intermountain Healthcare
Salt Lake City, Utah

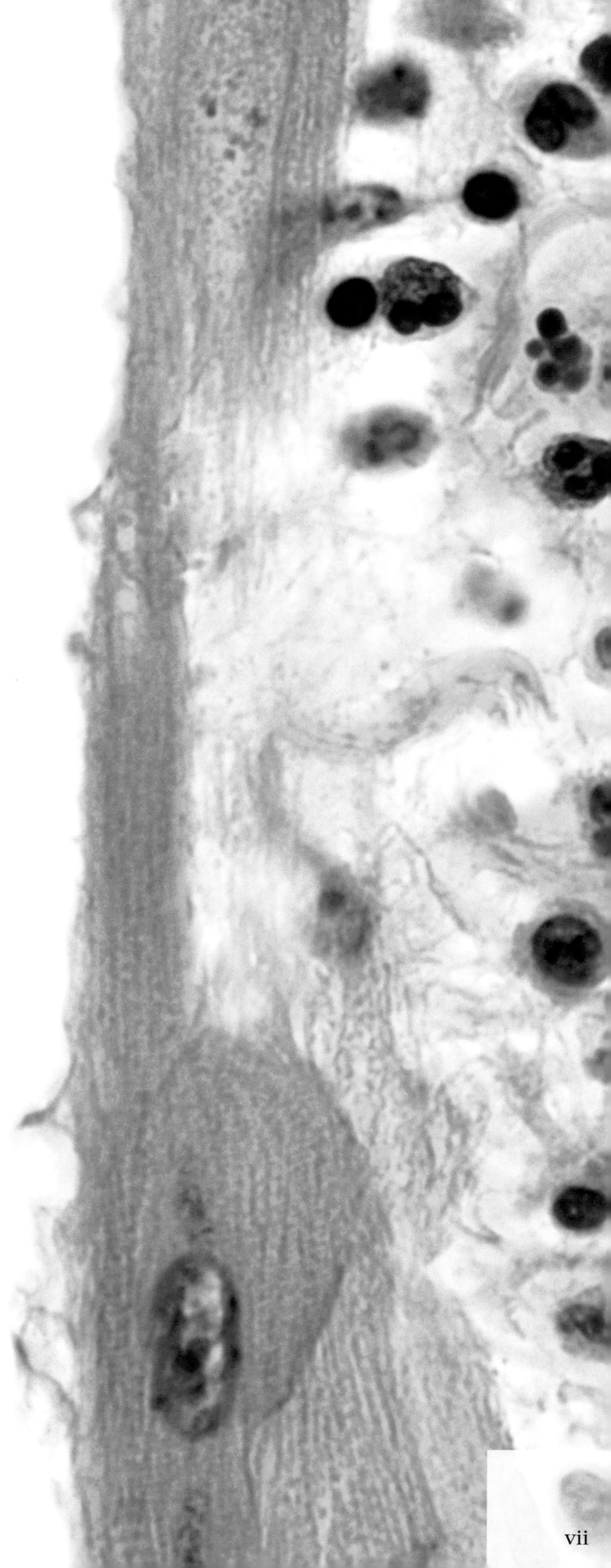

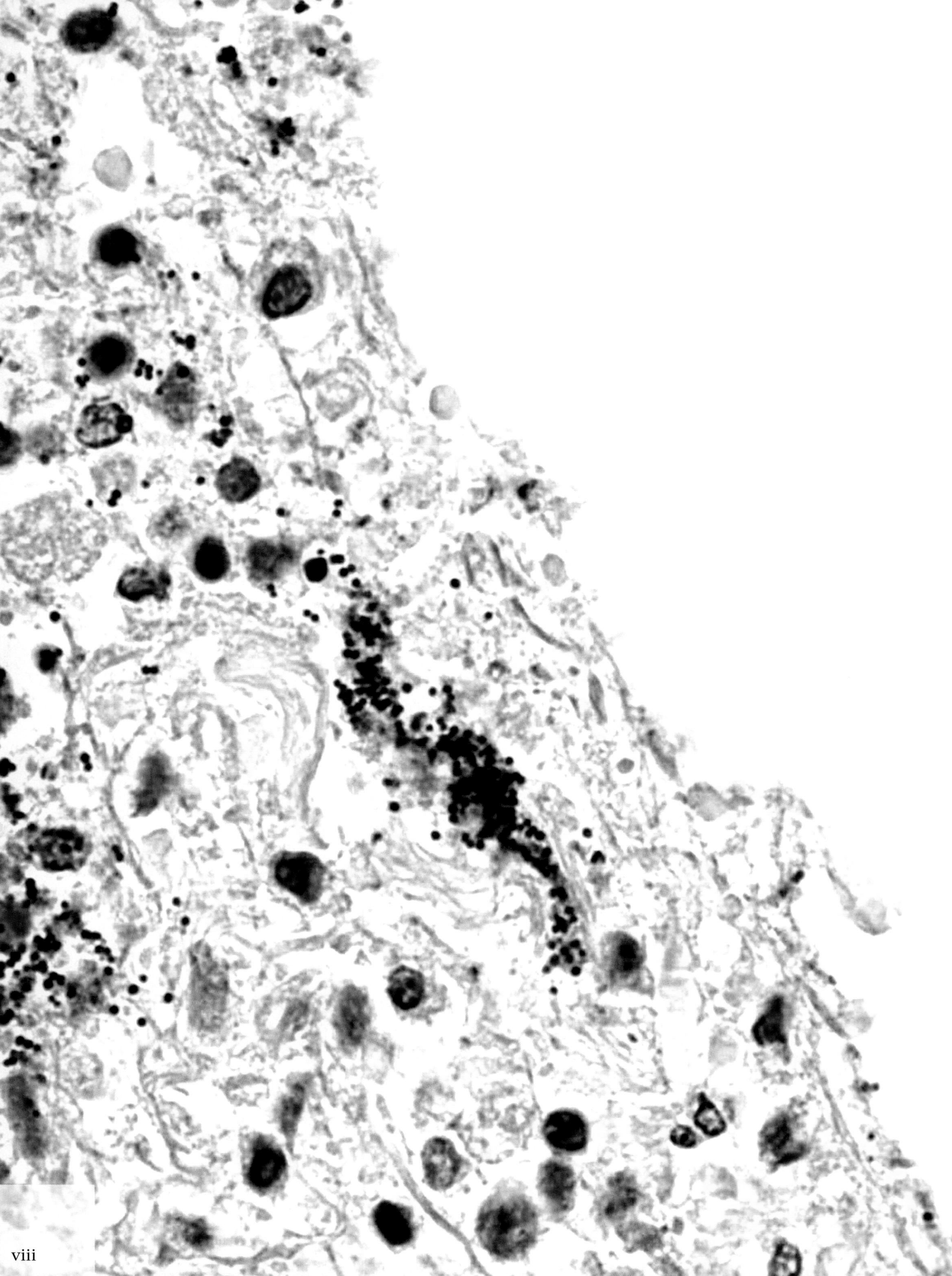

Preface

Declining rates of hospital autopsies have not diminished the enthusiasm of those of us who practice this field of pathology. This multi-author text that combines the talents of many experts in this field is a witness to this.

Engaging young pathologists in autopsy is vital to preserving what is arguably the bedrock of all pathology knowledge. This volume aims to present the hospital autopsy as it is really practiced — with real case presentations, approaches to dissection, chart review focusing, and reporting suggestions. This is, in part, intended to assist in the training and just-in-time preparation for trainees and new pathologists, as well as those who unfortunately don't get the chance to perform autopsies routinely.

The format follows other volumes related to surgical pathology in the *Diagnostic Pathology* series. At first, fitting an autopsy text into such a format was challenging but ultimately made sense as a way to emphasize the role that autopsy plays in modern medicine. Making diagnoses at autopsy and correlating them clinically is not fundamentally different from the diagnostic processes in surgical pathology.

One key distinction between autopsy and surgical pathology is the number of stakeholders affected by the autopsy diagnosis: first and foremost the next of kin, then caregivers, health care systems, and the community. It is our hope that this text will improve the quality of hospital autopsies, impact families and communities through the answers that the autopsy can provide, and help pathologists enjoy the diagnostic journey.

Billie Fyfe, MD
Professor of Pathology
Rutgers Robert Wood Johnson Medical School
New Brunswick, New Jersey

Dylan V. Miller, MD
Clinical Associate Professor of Pathology
University of Utah School of Medicine
Director of Electron Microscopy and Immunostains
Intermountain Central Laboratory
Salt Lake City, Utah

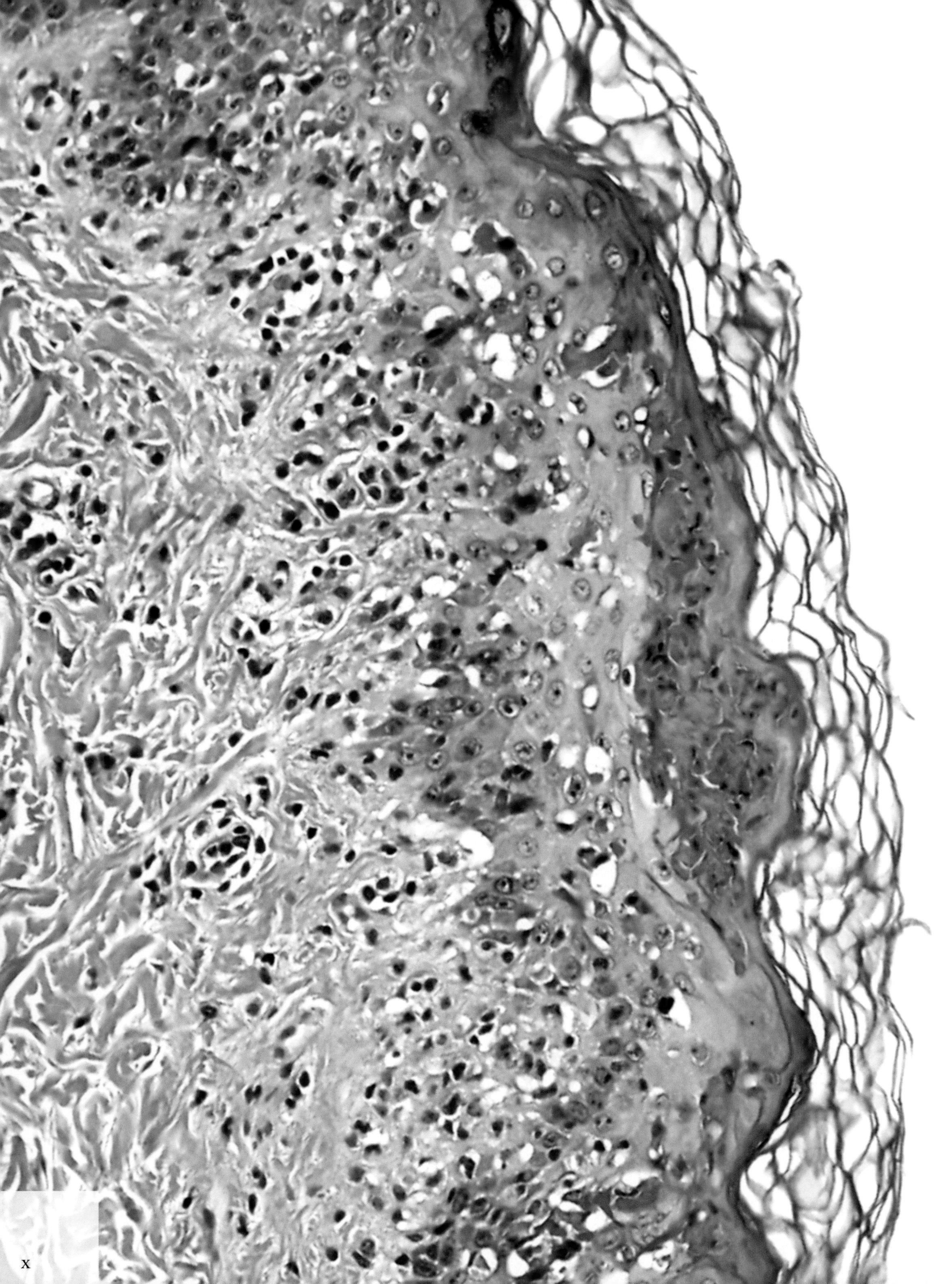
x

Acknowledgments

Text Editors

Dave L. Chance, MA, ELS
Arthur G. Gelsinger, MA
Nina I. Bennett, BA
Sarah J. Connor, BA
Tricia L. Cannon, BA
Terry W. Ferrell, MS
Lisa A. Gervais, BS

Image Editors

Jeffrey J. Marmorstone, BS
Lisa A. M. Steadman, BS

Medical Editor

Michael B. Ward, MD

Illustrations

Lane R. Bennion, MS
Laura C. Sesto, MA
Richard Coombs, MS

Art Direction and Design

Tom M. Olson, BA
Laura C. Sesto, MA

Lead Editor

Angela M.G. Terry, BA

Production Coordinators

Angela M.G. Terry, BA
Rebecca L. Hutchinson, BA

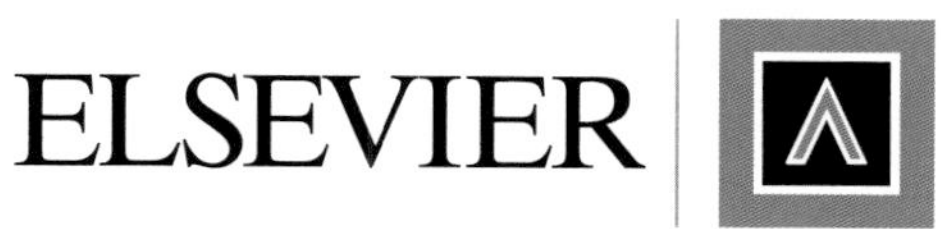

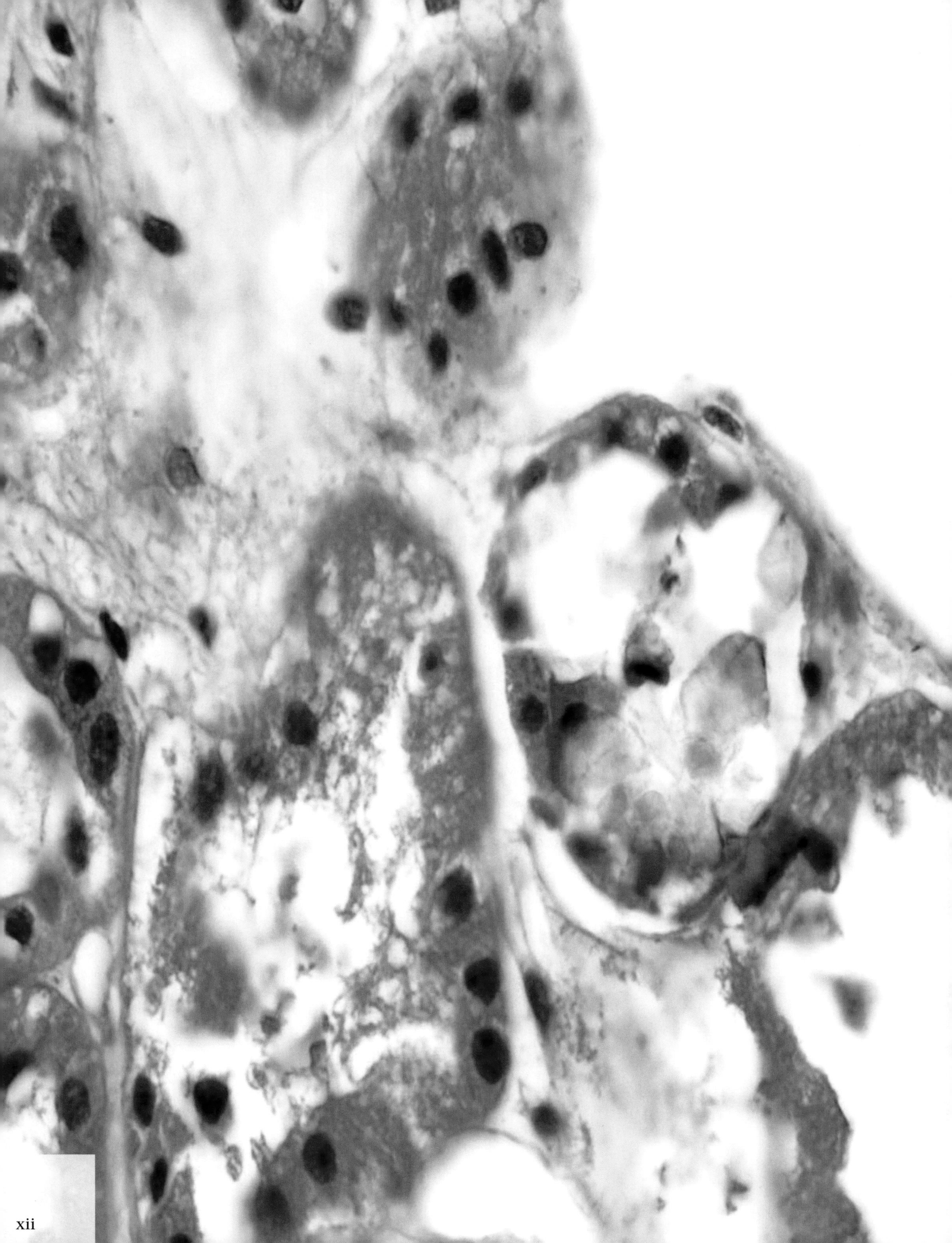

Sections

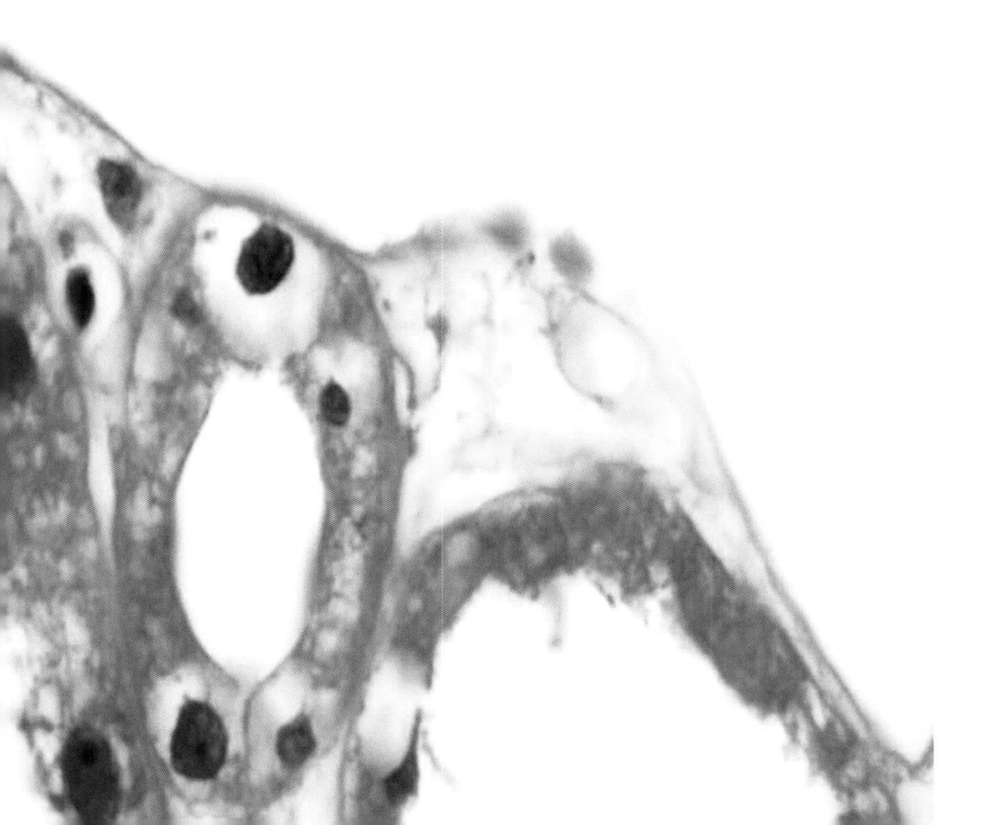

TABLE OF CONTENTS

PART I
Autopsy Fundamentals

PART II
Organ System Approach to Autopsy

SECTION 1
Sudden and Unexpected Death

Cardiovascular

Respiratory

Gastrointestinal

Hepatobiliary

Genitourinary

Endocrine

CNS

SECTION 2
Postoperative/Post-Interventional Death

Iatrogenic

Cardiovascular

Gastrointestinal and Hepatobiliary

CNS

PART III
Disease Process Approach to Autopsy

SECTION 1 Transplantation

SECTION 2 Infection-Related Death

Systemic Infection/Sepsis Overview

Organ System Infection

SECTION 3 Neoplasia-Associated Death

SECTION 4 Other Common Hospital Death

DIAGNOSTIC PATHOLOGY

Hospital Autopsy

FYFE | MILLER

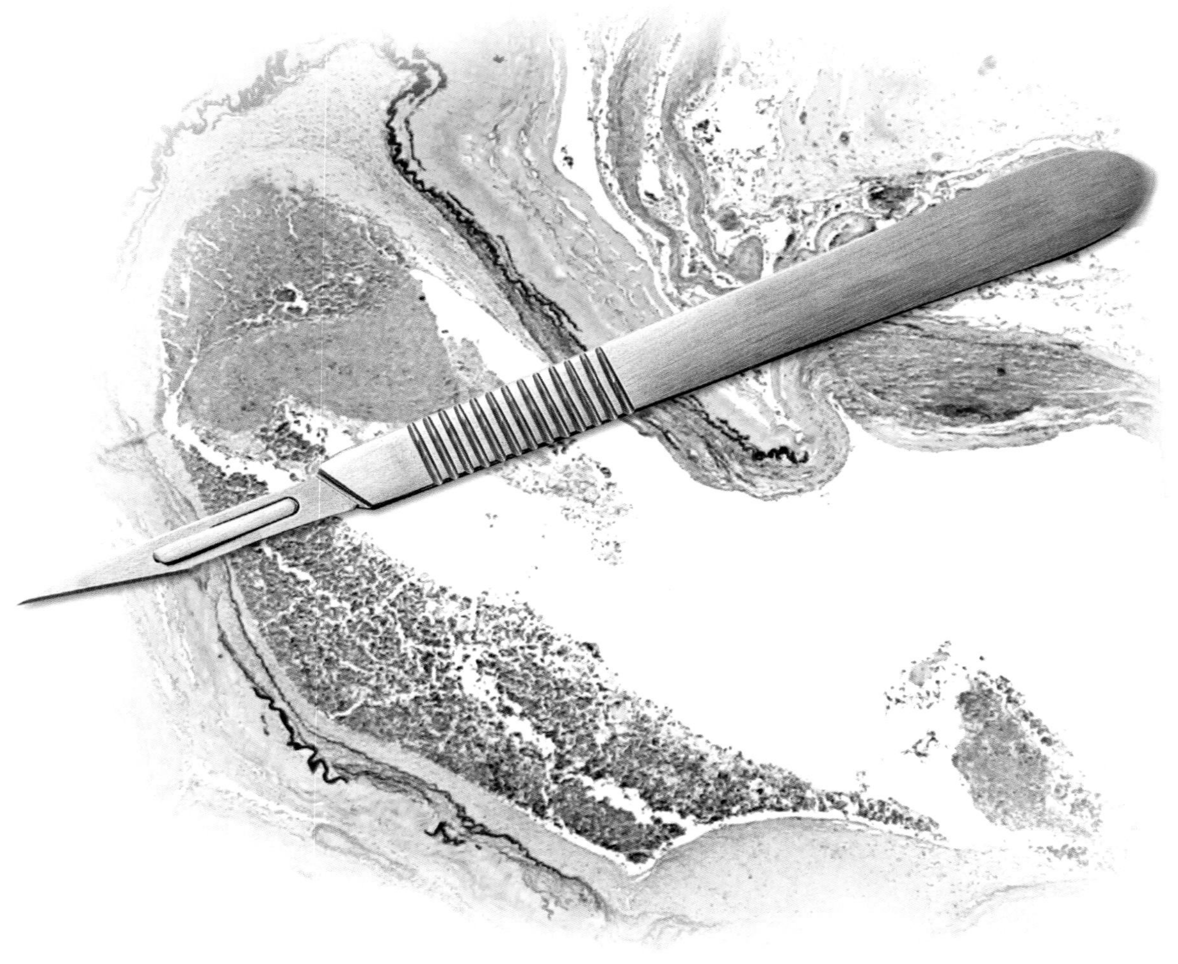

SECTION 1

Introduction

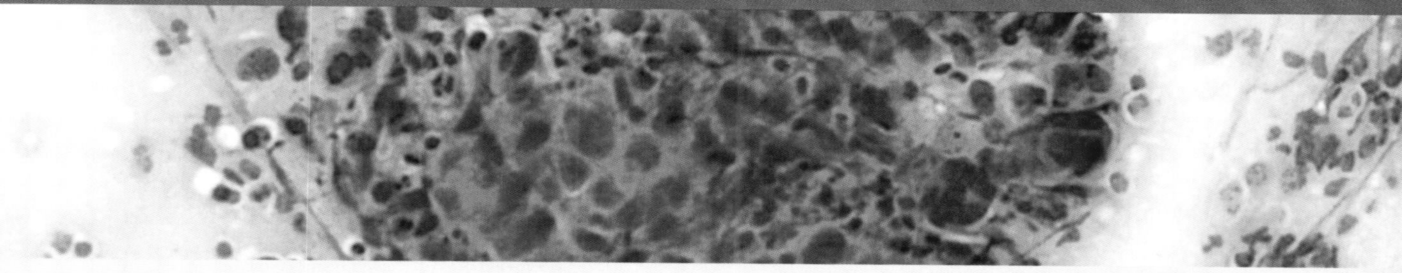

HISTORY OF AUTOPSY

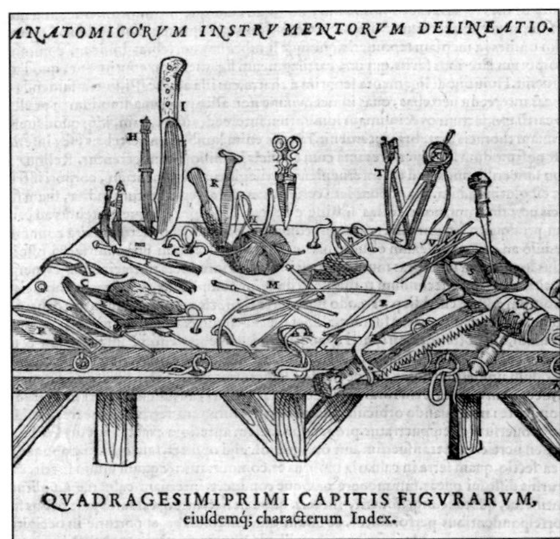

Published in 1543, De Humani Corporis Fabrica was unprecedented for the accuracy of its descriptions, the beauty of its illustrations, and its bold emphasis on observation rather than tradition.

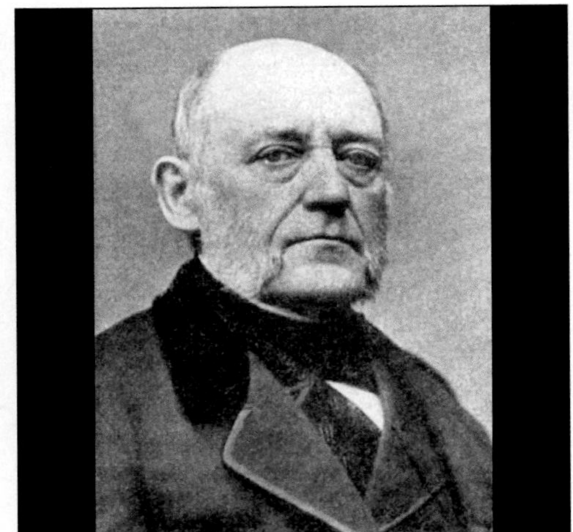

Carl von Rokitansky (1804-1878), was a phenomenally prolific prosector and author who helped establish pathology as a separate medical specialty and helped make Vienna the medical capital of the world.

ANCIENT SOCIETY, DEATH REMAINS, AND MEDICINE

Societal Attitudes Toward Human Remains

- Prehistoric societies may have had funeral rituals
- All known societies have rules for handling of the dead
  - Universal prohibitions against desecration of the dead
  - No systematic study of internal anatomy in antiquity
- Advances in normal and pathologic anatomy occur in societies that promote and fund arts and sciences
  - Governmental support is crucial
  - No suspension of religious and societal customs possible without governmental support

Medicine in Antiquity

- Prior to Greece: Health and disease depend on forces outside of nature
  - Healing intimately associated with religion
  - Clinical examination and surface anatomy highly developed
    - **Knowledge of internal anatomy unimportant**
  - Biblical description (Hebrew tradition)
    - Intimate knowledge of animal anatomy; sacrificial rites
    - Cadavers "unclean"
    - Obese King Eglon stabbed in abdomen "and the dirt came out" suggests some working knowledge, possible comparative to animals
    - Frequent mention of flesh, sinews, bone, and marrow
- Greece and Hippocrates
  - Medicine as natural science, not religious function
    - Superb clinical observations, diagnosis, prognostication
    - Good surface anatomy
    - Virtually no human dissection; anatomy extrapolated from animal dissections
    - Corpses ritually unclean; human dissection prohibited
  - Humoral theory: Health depends on balance of 4 humors (blood, phlegm, black bile, yellow bile)
    - Internal organs produce and circulate humors
    - Knowledge of organ function largely speculative and somewhat fanciful
- Galen
  - Expands and elaborates on humoral theory
  - Anatomy based on dissections of pigs and Barbary apes
  - **Galen's medical and anatomic works: Final authority for > 1,000 years**
    - Roman and Arabic physicians elaborate and comment on Galen without any thought of criticism
- **Alexandria: Only exception to prohibition of human dissection in ancient world** (300 BCE)
  - Ptolemaic king establishes world's largest library and museum; invites scholars
  - Physicians permitted to dissect
  - Physicians Herodotus and Erasistratus make remarkable advances in anatomy
    - Lasted only a generation

ADVANCES TOWARD MODERN AUTOPSY PRACTICE

Europe in Middle Ages

- 1213 CE: Holy Roman Emperor Frederick II permits dissection on executed criminals in Salerno Medical School
- Students come to Salerno from across Europe
- Anatomy spread to schools in Italy (Padua, Bologna) and France (Montpellier)

HISTORY OF AUTOPSY

- When observed anatomy contradicted Galen's anatomy, observation was largely ignored
- **1st European autopsies performed in 14th century**
  - Deaths in epidemics
  - Questions of foul play (often in cases of suspected poisoning)
  - Investigations into sainthood (search for miraculous findings, e.g., postmortem clots that resemble religious symbols)
- Role of coroner
  - Established in 12th century England (Articles of Eyre)
  - Duty to "keep the pleas of the crown" (protect financial interest of royalty in criminal proceedings)
  - Role also defined in the Magna Carta
  - Those who find deceased persons in suspicious circumstances must raise "hue and cry" to notify coroner

The Enlightenment

- Andreas Vesalius: Professor of anatomy in Padua
  - De Humani Corporis Fabrica (1543): 1st book of human anatomy based on observation
    - Errors of Galenic anatomy challenged; knowledge of normal anatomy improved
    - Galenic humoral medicine continues uncontested
- Autopsies become more common
  - High profile autopsies of monarchs (Henry II of France) and popes (Alexander V)
  - Gradual increase in knowledge of pathologic anatomy
- Published collections of cases try to correlate clinical symptoms and pathological anatomy
  - De Abditis (1507) by Antonio Benivieni: Hundreds of clinical cases, 20 autopsies
  - De Sepulchretum (1679) by Theophilus Bonetus: 3,000 autopsy cases
- Giovanni Battista Morgagni
  - De Sedibus (1761): Product of a lifetime of clinical practice and autopsies
    - 646 cases with clinical records and autopsies organized by organ system; **birth of clinical pathological correlation (CPC)**
    - Perhaps 1st pathology text

Paris School

- French Revolution of 1790
  - Radical restructuring of French medical system
  - Enormous public hospitals in Paris, Strasbourg, and Montpellier
    - Huge numbers of patients concentrated in few places
    - Physicians permitted to autopsy all charity patients dying in hospital
    - **Autopsy and clinical pathological correlation on unprecedented scale**
    - Foreigners from USA and across Europe study in Paris medical schools

2nd Vienna School

- Holy Roman Emperor Joseph II provides funds for Allgemeines Krankenhaus (1784)
  - Law required all military, forensic, and hospital autopsies to be performed there (1818)
  - Astronomical numbers of autopsies
    - Karl Rokitansky: Performs 30,000 cases, supervises another 60,000
    - **Apotheosis of autopsy gross pathology**
- Autopsy and clinical pathological correlation at heart of academic medicine
- Rudolf Virchow and development of microscopy and cellular pathology
- Foreigners from USA and across Europe study in Vienna

Autopsy in USA

- 1910: Richard Cabot promotes case-based teaching with autopsy review
  - Case records of Massachusetts General Hospital in New England Journal of Medicine
  - Landmark paper on clinical diagnostic pitfalls revealed in 3,000 autopsy cases (1912)
- 1910 Flexner Report on American Medical Education
  - Scathing indictment of American medical schools → closure of 1/2 of existing schools
  - Remaining schools adopt European model
    - Scientific approach to medicine with autopsy/CPC as its centerpiece
- Academic clinicians and their teams expected to attend autopsy reviews
- Academic clinicians promote autopsy
- Hospital autopsy rate seen as measure of commitment to quality care
  - By 1950s, average USA hospital rate ~ 50%; many hospitals with much higher rates

Decline of Hospital Autopsy

- Post World War II: Federal funding for medical basic science research increases dramatically
  - Academic pathologists focus on obtaining grants for research
  - Autopsy not seen as way to further academic career
- Rise of surgical pathology and laboratory medicine
  - Both pursuits are more time sensitive and more remunerative than autopsy pathology
- 1971: Joint Commission eliminates requirement for minimum hospital autopsy rate for accredited hospitals
- High rates of medical malpractice litigation
  - Concern that autopsy findings could lead to lawsuits
- Improved imaging modalities: ↑ ability to detect pathological anatomy without autopsy
  - 1974: 1st clinical CT scanner
  - 1980: 1st clinically useful MR images
- 1986: Federal government eliminates direct reimbursement for autopsies
  - Reimbursement for autopsy included in administrative budget
    - Same part A reimbursement for 1 autopsy as for 100
    - **Financial incentive to do fewer autopsies**
- Average USA hospital autopsy rates estimated to be as low as 5-10%

HISTORY OF AUTOPSY

- Many community hospitals do few if any

Notable Autopsies in Medical History

- 1533: 1st autopsy in New World
  - Hispaniola: Conjoined twins survived 8 days
  - Autopsy performed to determine if there were 1 or 2 children (and souls)
- 1724: Herman Boerhaave's masterpiece of clinical pathological correlation
  - Boerhaave attends gravely ill Admiral of Dutch fleet
    - Meticulous case notes (including detailed inventory of preceding extraordinarily intemperate meal)
    - Vomiting, pain, collapse
  - Boerhaave's autopsy findings: Esophageal rupture and mediastinitis
- 1859: Discovery of parathyroid glands
  - Rhinoceros at London zoo dies after a week of vomiting
  - Richard Owen performs autopsy
    - Finds rib fractures with lung puncture
    - Describes pea-sized gland attached to thyroid gland
  - Ivar Sandstrom finds same glands in humans in 1880
- 1847: Pathologist Jacob Kolletschka dies of sepsis
  - Cut himself during autopsy of woman with puerperal sepsis
  - Obstetrician Ignaz Semmelweis notes similarities in autopsy findings in Kolletschka and women dying of puerperal sepsis
  - Semmelweis realizes he and colleagues spread infection from morgue to obstetric patients
    - Institutes 1st program of handwashing
- Clandestine autopsies
  - About 1883: William Osler attends patient with Addison disease
    - Family denies permission for autopsy
    - Osler uses transanal approach to obtain adrenals
  - 1910: Harvey Cushing attends patient with acromegaly
    - Family denies permission for autopsy
    - Cushing's assistants bribe funeral director
    - Harvest brain with pituitary gland moments before funeral ceremony

CHALLENGES AND ALTERNATIVES

Current State of Autopsy

- Autopsy rates ↓ despite literature demonstration of continued effectiveness
  - Autopsies still find significant diagnostic discrepancies
    - Repeatedly documented in reports from Cabot in 1912 to Shojania and Burton in 2003 and beyond
    - True even in cases with sophisticated laboratory and diagnostic imaging work-ups
  - Death certification and vital records improve with higher autopsy rates
- Fewer autopsies → loss of expertise
  - Fewer pathologists with experience to teach
  - Fewer cases for residents to learn from
- Compelling financial and professional disincentives unlikely to change soon

Proposed Alternatives to Traditional Hospital Autopsy Approach

- Regional autopsy centers
  - Single facility performs all medical autopsies for hospitals in large geographic region
  - Concentrates numbers of cases and expertise
    - Programs already exist at several medical examiners' offices and academic hospitals
  - Issues: Reimbursement, logistics, lack of interaction with clinical staff at originating hospital
- Radiographic or virtual autopsy (virtopsy)
  - Pioneered in Switzerland
  - Whole body CT or MR scan replaces traditional autopsy
    - Allows excellent visualization of hard-to-dissect areas
    - Overcomes religious objections to dissection
  - Issues: Expense, availability, logistics, lack of histologic confirmation

SELECTED REFERENCES

1. Hurren ET: Remaking the medico-legal scene: a social history of the late-Victorian coroner in Oxford. J Hist Med Allied Sci. 65(2):207-52, 2010
2. Pendleton C et al: The autopsy was conducted "Under most inauspicious circumstances:" John Turner, Harvey Cushing's case XXXII, and his unwitting contributions to the early understanding of acromegaly. Pituitary. 13(4):324-8, 2010
3. Wright JR Jr: Sins of our fathers: two of The Four Doctors and their roles in the development of techniques to permit covert autopsies. Arch Pathol Lab Med. 133(12):1969-74, 2009
4. Hirt M et al: History of forensic medicine-the second part. The autopsy in the Middle Age and the Renaissance. Soud Lek. 50(3):32-7, 2005
5. Fu LK: Sung Tz'u (1186-1249) and medical jurisprudence in ancient China. J Med Biogr. 12(2):95-104, 2004
6. Shojania KG et al: Changes in rates of autopsy-detected diagnostic errors over time: a systematic review. JAMA. 289(21):2849-56, 2003
7. Mant AK: Forensic medicine in Great Britain. II. The origins of the British medicolegal system and some historic cases. Am J Forensic Med Pathol. 8(4):354-61, 1987
8. Goldman L et al: The value of the autopsy in three medical eras. N Engl J Med. 308(17):1000-5, 1983
9. King LS et al: A history of the autopsy. A review. Am J Pathol. 73(2):514-44, 1973

Evolution of the Autopsy

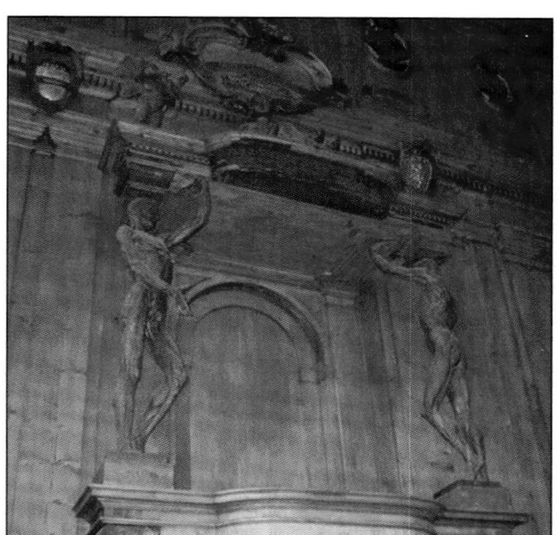

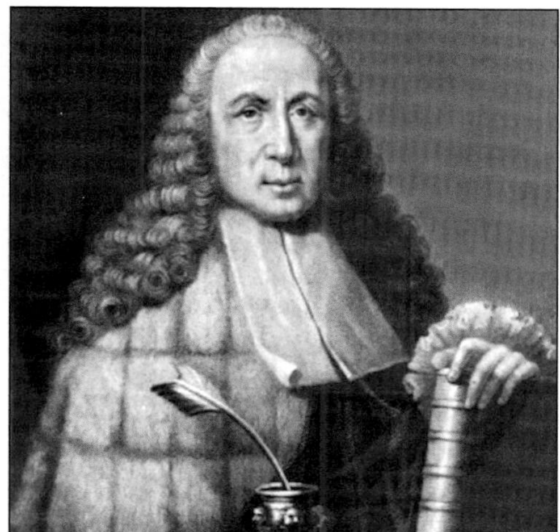

(Left) *Lecturer's chair in the anatomic theater in Bologna: Prior to 1543, the professor of anatomy would sit above the dissection and read from a Galenic text while a prosector dissected. For centuries, discrepancies between the descriptions in the text and the structures in the body were simply ignored.* ***(Right)*** *Giovanni Battista Morgagni (1682-1771) helped establish derangements in normal anatomy as the cause of disease and put an end to centuries of medicine based on humoral theory.*

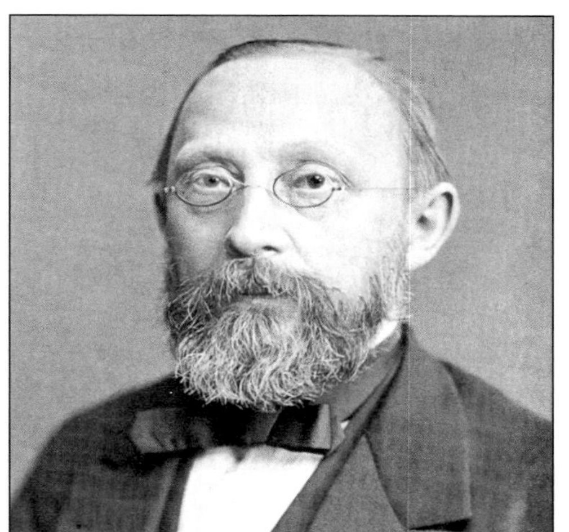

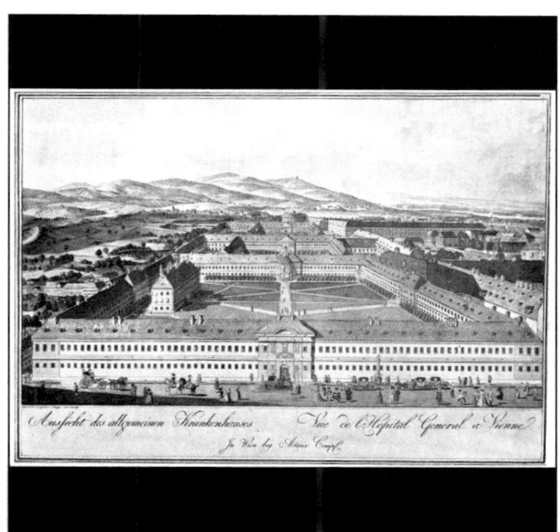

(Left) *Rudolf Virchow (1821-1902) brought microscopy into mainstream practice of pathology, and his Cellular Pathology (published in 1858) helped establish the cellular basis of pathology.* ***(Right)*** *The Allgemeines Krankenhaus in Vienna, home to some of the greatest figures in pathology & clinical medicine in Europe, attracted students from around the world and disseminated the use of clinical pathologic correlation as the cornerstone of medical education and practice.*

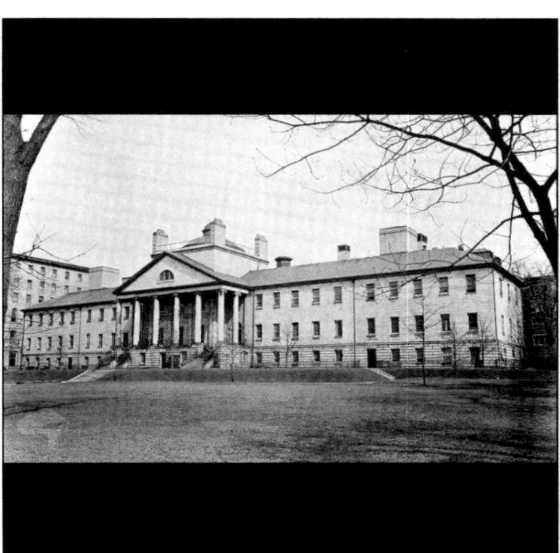

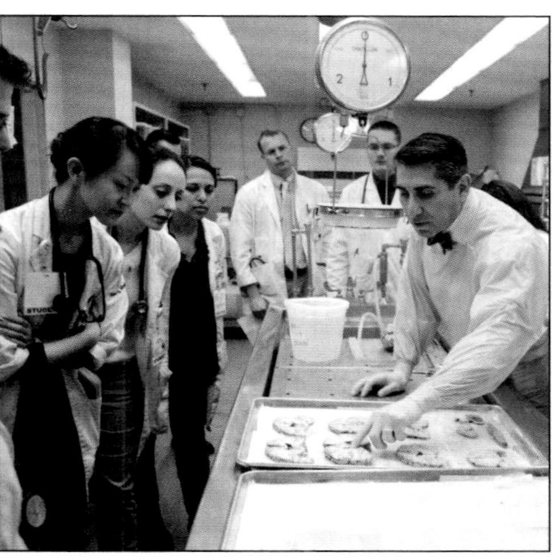

(Left) *The Bullfinch Building, Massachusetts General Hospital: After the 1910 Flexner Report, pathology assumed a central role in USA medical education. The Case Records of the MGH are an illustration of the continued educational power of the clinical pathological correlation.* ***(Right)*** *The autopsy remains a highly effective (if drastically underutilized) method for teaching medicine, improving the quality of patient care, and providing answers to family members.*

AUTOPSY SAFETY

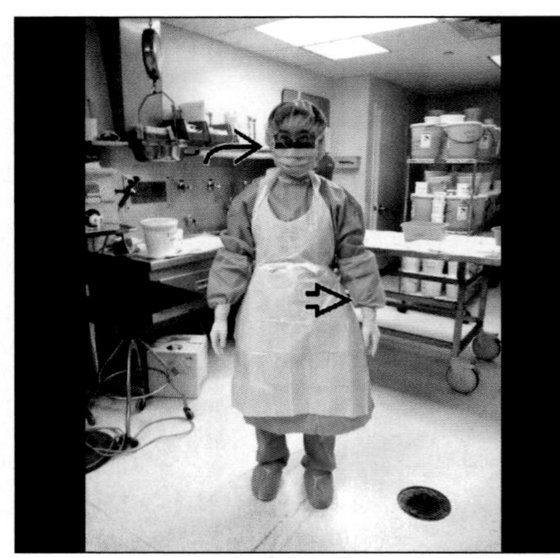

The resident in this photo is demonstrating the use of personal protective equipment with all body parts covered with waterproof apron and sleeves ⮚ and eye and face protection ⮚.

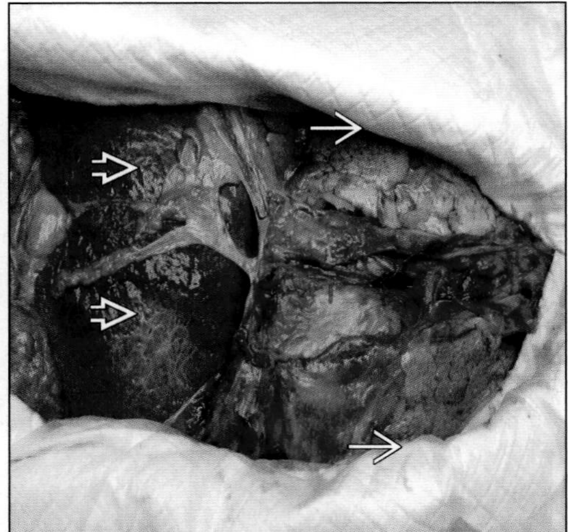

Note the use of chucks ⮚ as a protective barrier over the cut ends of the ribs. The nodular cirrhotic liver ⮚ makes use of universal precautions mandatory.

TERMINOLOGY

Definitions

- Autopsy safety: Actions taken to protect prosectors and those present during the process of performing autopsy
  - Involves being aware of pathogens, hazards, and risk
- Hazard: Potential source of harm or adverse health effect
  - Types of autopsy hazards (Wetli): Mechanical, sharp force injury, electrical, chemical, radiation, infection
- Risk: Likelihood a person suffers adverse health effect if exposed to hazard
- High-risk autopsy: Autopsy where there is a high risk of transmission of disease to prosectors; most often confers risk of pathogen acquisition
- Pathogen: Any disease-producing agent, particularly virus, bacteria, parasite, or infectious particle (prion)
  - Exposure to pathogen may be via blood/body fluid; inhalation; ingestion; direct inoculation; through mucous membranes of eyes, nose, and throat; and through breaks in skin barrier

SAFE AUTOPSY PRACTICES: REDUCING RISK

Mechanical Risk Reduction

- Risk includes injury from physical efforts such as lifting
- Adequate staffing and equipment in autopsy suite to transport and transfer decedents helps reduce this risk

Sharp Force Risk Reduction

- Risk includes injury from sharp tools or sharp edges at autopsy (scalpels, cut ends of ribs)
- Reduction starts with sharps awareness: Monitoring number of sharps being used at any time
  - Stop dissection if sharp (scalpel blade, saw blade, large or small knife, sharp tip scissors, sharp tip probe) is missing
- Scalpel blade removal: Use of hands-free devices instead of hands, forceps, or hemostats
- Prosector precautions
  - Potential sharp hazards in body: Sharp rib edges or skull after sawing, edges of calcified vessels, wire sutures and meshes, and cut ends of metallic device leads
    - Incising ribs through costochondral junction leads to naturally smooth surface, ↓ sharps risk

Electrical Shock Risk Reduction

- Risk includes injury from electrical devices implanted in body such as automatic implantable cardioverter defibrillators
  - Beware of implanted electrical devices within decedent, check chart, check externally for incisions over generator pockets, call device manufacturer (or local device) to deactivate implantable cardioverter defibrillators

Chemical Risk Reduction

- Risk is potential injury from exposure to chemicals used during autopsy
  - Formaldehyde/formalin is greatest risk
  - Formaldehyde is mixture of formaldehyde gas and water
    - Formaldehyde solution with 10-15% methyl alcohol = formalin
  - Acute exposure effects include irritation to nose and eyes and mucous membranes
  - Controversial carcinogenic effects of prolonged exposure
- Follow formaldehyde exposure monitoring policies of institution
- Use chemical hood for pouring large quantities of formaldehyde

- Have access to chemical spill kit for formaldehyde spills

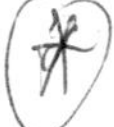

Radiation Risk Reduction

- Risk is potential injury related to exposure to radiation from devices implanted in body
  - Review chart for implanted radioactive devices (seeds): Type, distribution, duration (↑ duration ↓ radiation risk)
  - If chart unclear but suspicion for presence of seeds, postmortem radiograph may reveal presence
    - Seeds are radiopaque, ~ 4 x 8 mm
  - Seeds may migrate from initial site (lungs, heart, etc.)
- Contact radiation safety officer for advice in cases of acute seed implantation or if other questions

Infection Risk Reduction

- Risk is potential injury related to exposure to pathogens
  - Use impervious barriers (personal protective equipment) and universal precautions meant to decrease risk of pathogen permeation through normal barriers such as skin, nasal membranes, eye and mucous membranes, and inhalation
  - Universal precautions treat all body fluids as potentially infectious
- Personal protective equipment (PPE)
  - Personal body coverings including gowns, masks or respirators, goggles, aprons, gloves, arm sleeves, and shoe covers meant to form a barrier against contamination in autopsy room
  - Masks are a protective physical barrier meant to protect wearer from hazards such as splashes of blood and body fluids
    - Keeps contaminated hands and fingers away from mouth and nose
  - Respirators are protective equipment designed to decrease a prosector's risk from airborne pathogen
    - Prosector must be fitted to a respirator NIOSH (National Institute for Occupational Safety and Health) certified and used as part of comprehensive occupational health program
    - Most often used in autopsies with risk of mycobacterial or influenza infection

High-Risk Autopsy Examples

- *Mycobacterium tuberculosis*
  - Occupational infection is usually pulmonary (90%) or cutaneous infection from inoculation (10%)
  - Emergence of multidrug-resistant strains keeps *M. tuberculosis* an important pathogen to consider at autopsy

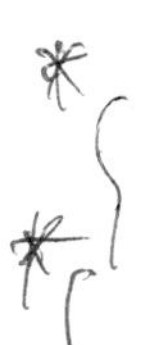

  - Risk of tuberculosis to pathologists performing active tuberculosis autopsies is ~ 10%, ↑ from that of nonpathologist physicians
  - Tubercle bacilli can be located from autopsy suite even 24 hours after postmortem examination
  - Use of respirator (not mask) mandatory in cases of suspected *M. tuberculosis*
  - Use of postmortem tissue culture or PCR to confirm diagnosis in suspect cases
- Human immunodeficiency virus
  - Blood-borne pathogen with low seroconversion rate (0-0.42%) after occupational exposure
  - Rate of HIV seroconversion after single percutaneous exposure with (1 μL): 0.1-0.36%
  - Mucocutaneous seroconversion rate: 0.04-0.63%
  - Seroconversion risk relates to viral load in decedent, volume/nature of exposure, and underlying health of prosector and use of post-exposure prophylaxis
  - Viral titers in patients expiring from terminal HIV are generally high
  - Viral particles do not survive in blood exposed to environment outside body; they are inactivated by desiccation and disinfectants
  - Blood and saliva testing has been shown to be reliable in postmortem setting but may require separate consent, so consultation with risk/legal services of institution advisable prior to testing
- Hepatitis virus
  - Hepatitis B is very contagious, but preexposure vaccination has ↓ risk of occupational infection
  - Hepatitis C is less contagious than hepatitis B, but there is no preexposure vaccination so risk of occupational infection is 2.7-10%
- Creutzfeldt-Jakob Disease (transmissible spongiform encephalopathy)
  - Fatal human prion disease; can be acquired, but transmission to health care workers is rare
  - Most institutions refer possible CJD autopsies to specialty centers
  - Transmission by infected tissues and equipment (infected neurosurgical instruments and contaminated tissue implants/products)
  - Most highly infectious tissue: Brain, dura mater, pituitary gland, spinal cord, posterior segment of eye, cranial and dorsal root ganglia, olfactory epithelium
  - Prevention of aerosolization during brain removal is mandatory (wet cloth over saw, vacuum system, etc.)
  - All higher infectivity tissue should be treated as such and appropriately labeled
  - CJD resistant to alcohols and formols
    - Fix infectious tissue in formaldehyde followed by formic acid for 1 hour
    - Wash tissue again in formaldehyde prior to machine processing
    - Instruments used for CJD autopsies should preferably be disposed of or dedicated to CJD cases with separate sterilization

SELECTED REFERENCES

1. Nine JS et al: Universal precautions and high-risk autopsies. Medscape. 2012
2. Flavin RJ et al: Mycobacterium tuberculosis at autopsy--exposure and protection: an old adversary revisited. J Clin Pathol. 60(5):487-91, 2007
3. Singleton M et al: The radioactive autopsy: safe working practices. Histopathology. 51(3):289-304, 2007
4. Burton JL: Health and safety at necropsy. J Clin Pathol. 56(4):254-60, 2003

SECTION 2

Autopsy Performance

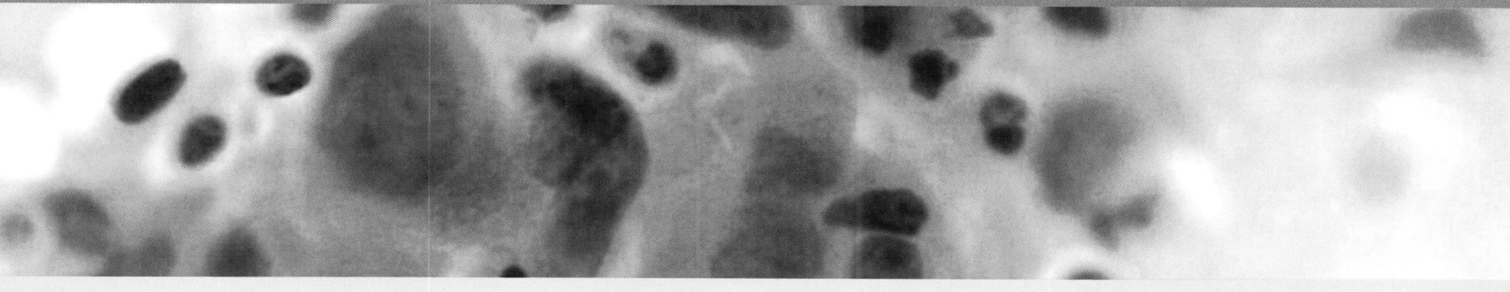

External Examination

Internal Examination

Laboratory Testing

Postmortem Imaging

MEDICAL INTERVENTION

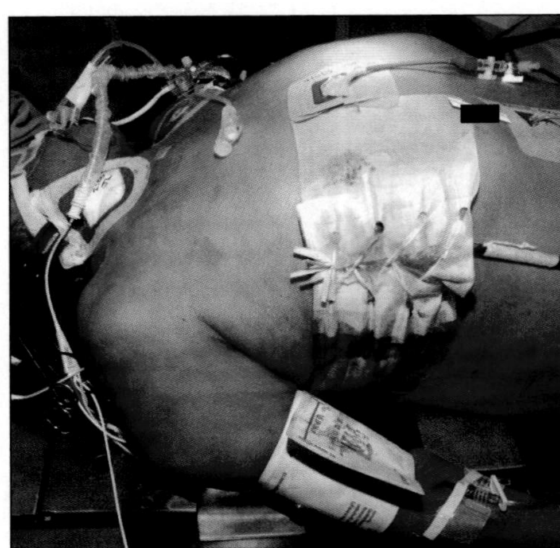

A systematic approach to autopsy external examination is essential to avoid accidental omission of findings, particularly in complex disease processes when medical devices are numerous.

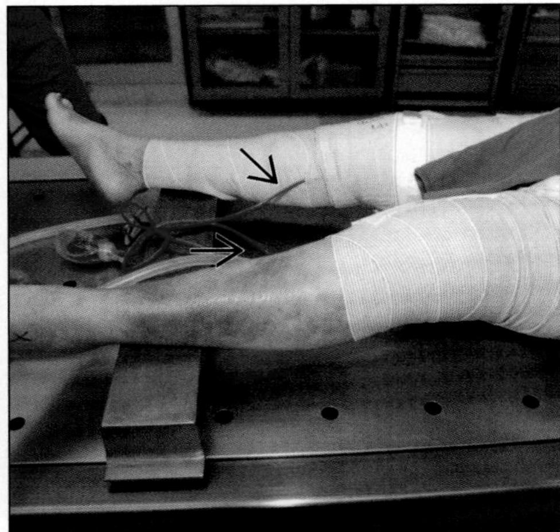

External examination provides clues to underlying diseases. Bandages and drains ➔ on legs suggest ischemic heart disease and saphenous vein harvesting for coronary artery bypass grafting.

TERMINOLOGY

Definitions

- Medical interventions relevant to hospital autopsy external examination include all forms of health care intervention, regardless of
  - Time when provided (recent or old)
  - Timing relative to death (antemortem or postmortem)
  - Site where provided (in hospital or elsewhere)
  - Status of caregiver (physician, nurse, emergency medical technician, layperson, or otherwise)
  - Type of intervention (noninvasive, invasive, or otherwise)
- Categories of medical intervention
  - Recent vs. old
  - Noninvasive vs. invasive
  - ± indwelling device
  - Antemortem vs. postmortem (organ and tissue procurement)

CLINICAL IMPLICATIONS

General Considerations

- Institutional policies and legal considerations
  - All medical care items must be left on decedent's body, and should not be removed prior to transfer of body to autopsy suite
  - Deaths within 24 hours of admission to hospital fall under medical examiner's jurisdiction in some states
  - Deaths in emergency room, operating room, postoperative recovery room, &/or maternity ward also fall under medical examiner's jurisdiction in some states
  - Authorization for performance of autopsy ("autopsy permit") must be obtained and documented prior to performing autopsy
- Preparation for autopsy
  - Review decedent's medical records in detail
    - Past medical history
    - Past surgical history
    - Nonsurgical interventions
    - Imaging findings
    - Laboratory findings
    - Events leading up to death
  - Communicate with treating clinicians and surgeons
    - Clarify intraoperative findings or complications
    - Clarify specific questions to be answered
- Approach to external examination
  - Systematic approach is essential to prevent accidental omissions
    - "Clockface" approach: Begin by examining head (12:00), then proceed around table in a circle, examining left arm (3:00), left leg (5:00), right leg (7:00), right arm (9:00), and then finish by examining chest, abdomen, and back
    - "Head to toe" approach: Begin by examining head, followed by arms, torso and back, and then finish by examining legs

Documentation of Findings

- Document all interventions in detail
  - Monitoring pads or automated defibrillator pads
    - Appropriate placement, shaving of body hair
  - Recent surgical incisions
    - Location, length, appearance, and adequacy of closure
  - Old healed surgical incisions/scars
    - Location, length, and appearance
  - Indwelling tubes, catheters, and other devices
    - Location, type, appropriate placement (to be confirmed upon internal examination)
    - After documenting, external portions may be cut off if absolutely necessary, but internal portions should be left in place to facilitate evaluation of correct placement during internal examination
- Utilize a body diagram

  - If findings will be dictated later, write detailed notes
  - Draw pictures of interventions
- Photography
  - Essential for medical, legal, and educational purposes
  - Usually best achieved with handheld, high-quality digital SLR camera
  - Ensure adequate lighting; use flash or proper overhead lighting
  - Include ruler and identifiers of decedent/case number in photograph
  - Avoid distractions
    - Obscure nonessential elements with drapes or blue towels
    - Keep retracting hands and instruments out of photograph
    - Frame shot close enough to visualize finding well, but far enough away that anatomic location and relationships are clearly discernible
    - Clean away blood and body fluids
  - Have a low threshold for photographing medical interventions: When in doubt, photograph!
- Reporting
  - Utilize templates to prevent omissions
  - Dictate external findings as soon as possible before details are forgotten
  - After preliminary report is transcribed, review for accuracy as soon as possible

MACROSCOPIC FINDINGS

General External Examination

- Standard measurements in adults
  - Height
  - Weight
  - Pupillary diameters
- Additional standard measurements in infants and young children
  - Crown-heel length
  - Crown-rump length
  - Head circumference
  - Chest circumference (at level of nipples)
  - Foot length
  - Interpupillary distance
- Head and neck findings
  - Appearance relative to documented age
  - Hair color and distribution
  - Color of irides and sclerae
  - Status of dentition (normal vs. partially or completely edentulous)
  - In infants: Position of ears (low-set vs. normal), appearance of face (presence of abnormal facies), status of palate (clefted vs. normal)
  - Any other abnormalities
- Other external findings
  - Tattoos and distinctive piercings
  - Abnormal skin coloration (e.g., cyanosis, jaundice)
  - Ecchymosis
  - Decubitus ulcers
  - In infants: Appearance of limbs (normal vs. dysmorphic), patency of anus, presence of Mongolian spot
  - Any other abnormalities

External Evidence of Common Antemortem Interventions

- Noninvasive interventions
  - Bandages
  - Electrocardiogram monitoring pads
  - Automated defibrillator pads and burns
  - Compression stockings/pneumatic compression devices
- Invasive interventions without indwelling device
  - Venipuncture sites
  - Surgical incisions (recent and old)
  - Colostomy site (with colostomy bag)
  - Amputations
- Invasive interventions with indwelling device
  - Vascular access devices
    - Intravenous catheters
    - Arterial catheters
    - Central venous catheters
    - Intraosseous vascular access devices
    - Extracorporeal membrane oxygenation (ECMO) cannulae
  - Intracranial pressure monitoring catheter
  - Nasogastric/orogastric tube
  - Endotracheal/tracheostomy tube
  - Pacemaker/defibrillator (AICD)
  - Chest tubes
  - Gastrostomy/jejunostomy tubes
  - Surgical drains (e.g., Jackson-Pratt drain)
  - Suprapubic catheter
  - Foley catheter
  - Epidural catheter

External Evidence of Postmortem Interventions (Organ and Tissue Procurement)

- Internal organs
  - May include heart, lungs, liver, kidneys, pancreas, &/or intestines
  - Surgical incision with simple crude closure
- Musculoskeletal tissues
  - Bones often replaced with plastic rods
  - Crudely closed surgical incision, with distortion of limbs (e.g., feet externally or internally rotated)
- Eyes (corneal tissue)
- Skin

SELECTED REFERENCES

1. Rutty GN: The external examination. In: Burton JL et al: The Hospital Autopsy : A Manual of Fundamental Autopsy Practice. Boca Raton: CRC Press. 90-103, 2010
2. Finkbeiner WE et al: Basic postmortem examination. In: Autopsy Pathology: A Manual and Atlas. Philadelphia: Saunders Elsevier. 35-56, 2009
3. Waters BL: Ensuring quality in the hospital autopsy. In: Handbook of Autopsy Practice. New York City: Humana Press. 3-10, 2009

MEDICAL INTERVENTION

External Examination of Interventions

*(**Left**) Institutional policy should ensure that no medical devices are removed from the decedent prior to arrival in the autopsy suite, regardless of their nature or number. A systematic approach to external examination is essential to avoid accidental omission of findings and medical devices. (**Right**) Medical devices are common in the head and neck. Note nasogastric tube ➔, tracheostomy tube ➔, and multiple central vascular access catheters ➔. Also note median sternotomy ➔.*

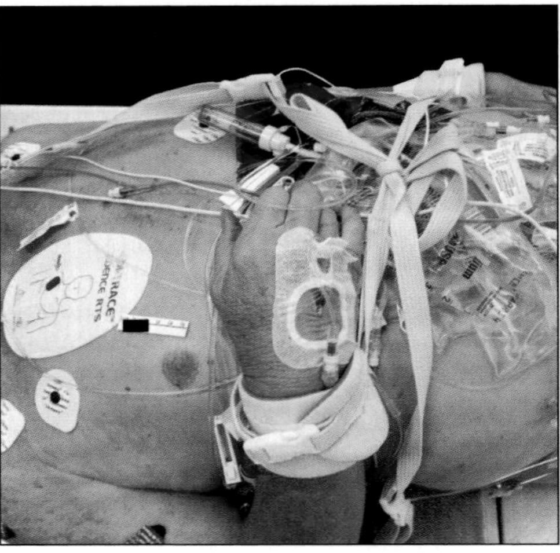

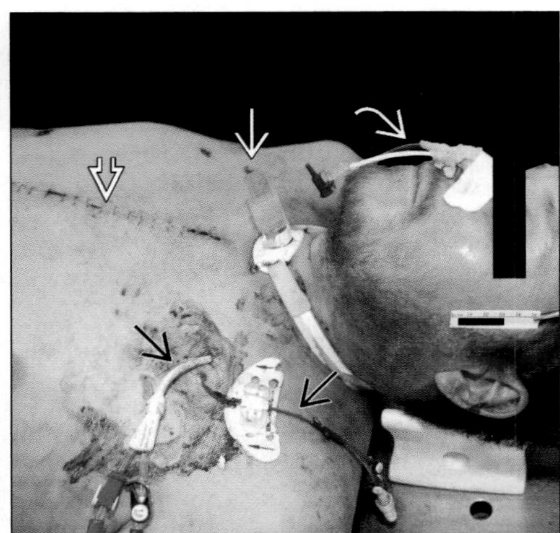

*(**Left**) Old scars provide important clues. Note median sternotomy scar ➔, suggestive of remote cardiac surgery (ascending aortic aneurysm repair). This decedent died of a dissecting aneurysm with fatal rupture 2 days after blunt force trauma to the abdomen (note contusions ➔). (**Right**) A large incision ➔ in the groin with ecchymosis ➔ suggests recent cannulation of femoral vessels with large-bore cannulae, as in this case of fatal H1N1 influenza requiring ECMO support.*

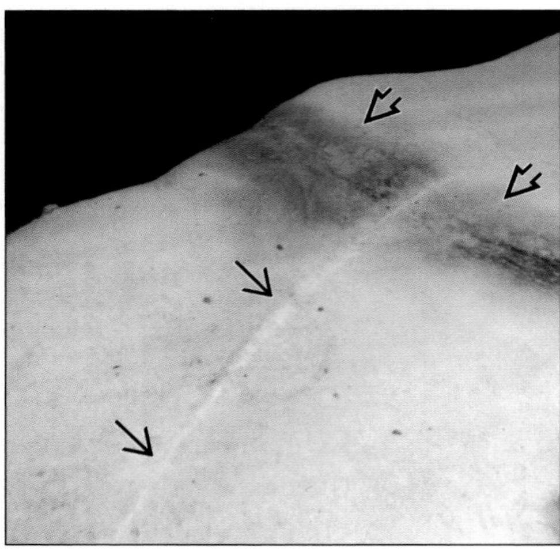

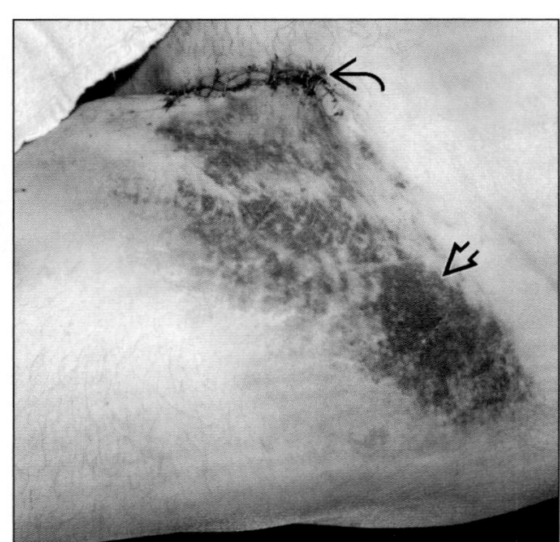

*(**Left**) The presence of a vacuum-assisted wound closure device ("wound vac") ➔ surrounded by erythema ➔ suggests the possibility of infection with sepsis. (**Right**) After removal of the wound vac, a large chest wall defect ➔ is visible, repaired internally with a membrane. The defect is surrounded by purulence ➔, further suggesting infection. This patient died of bacteremia and sepsis 1 month after undergoing a chest wall resection for sarcoma.*

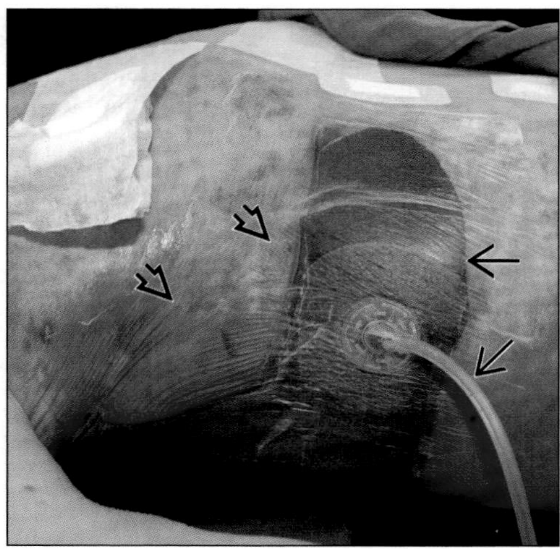

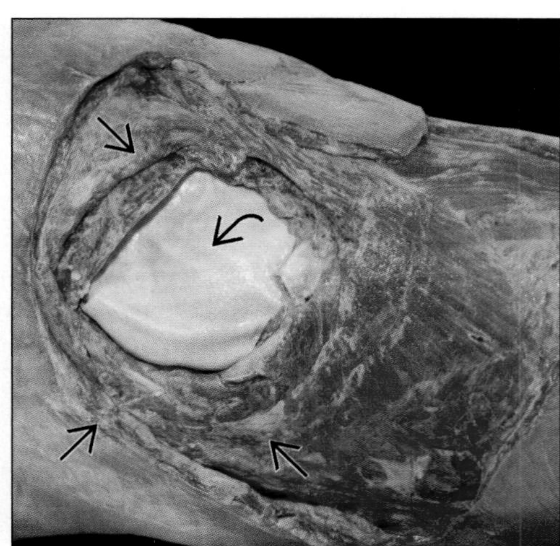

External Examination of Interventions

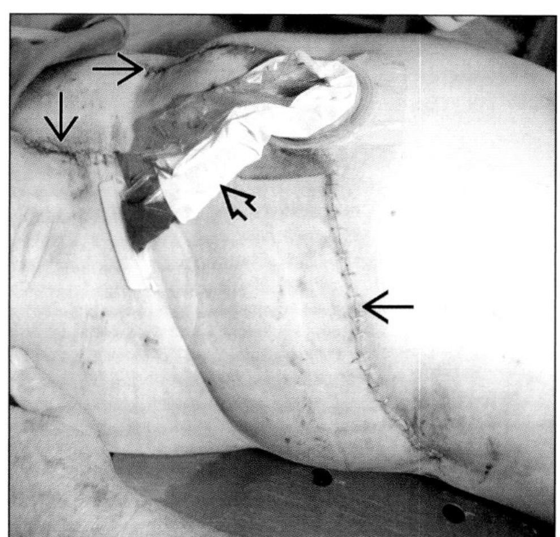

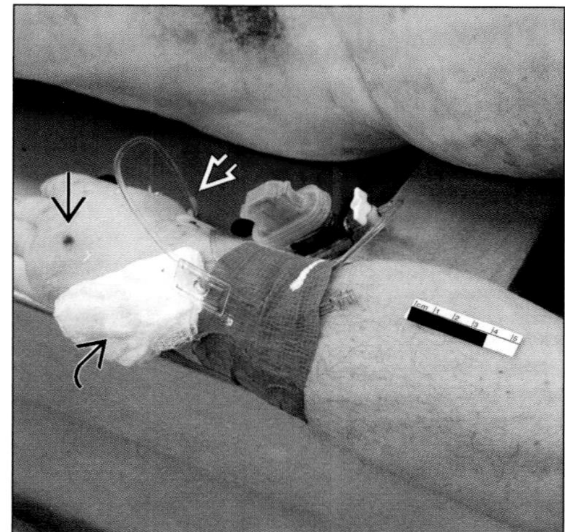

(Left) *This patient died after repair of a thoracoabdominal aortic aneurysm; clues regarding complications thereof are evident externally. Note colostomy bag ⇨, consistent with hemicolectomy due to bowel ischemia. Also note numerous recent, stapled surgical incisions →.* ***(Right)*** *All evidence of intervention should be documented, regardless of perceived importance. Here, note arterial line ⇨, bandage ↷, and puncture wound → consistent with previous vascular access site.*

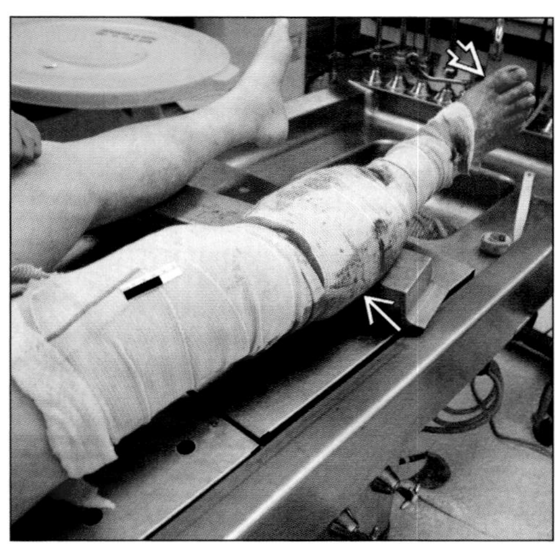

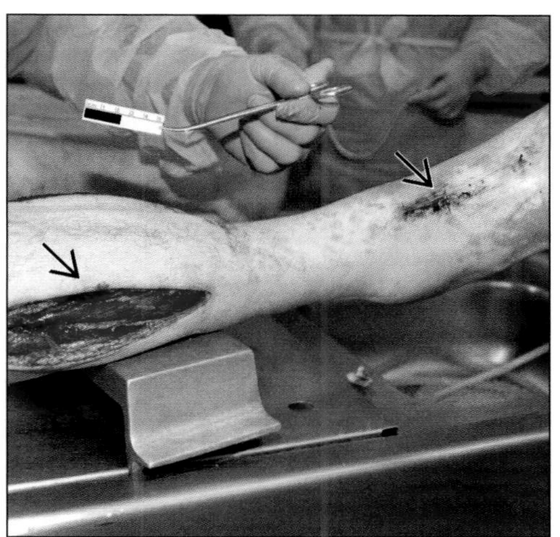

(Left) *In some cases, external findings strongly suggest a disease process, even when details of the clinical history are unavailable. This patient developed leg ischemia (note red foot ⇨) following repair of an abdominal aortic aneurysm, necessitating fasciotomy. Note blood-soaked bandage wrapping right leg ➔.* ***(Right)*** *All bandages should be removed to expose tissues underneath. Here, 2 fasciotomy sites → are readily identified, corresponding to blood-soaked areas on bandages.*

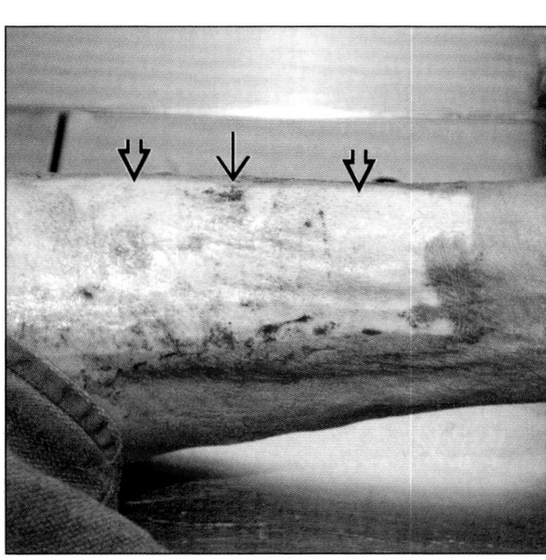

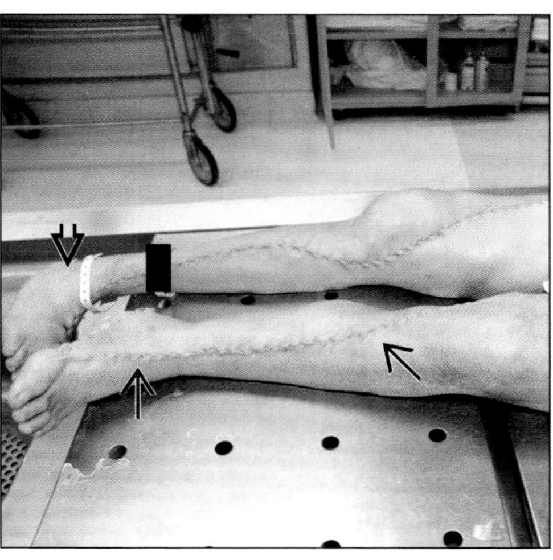

(Left) *Skin removal ⇨ is apparent on the lower arm of this decedent who required skin grafts elsewhere. Postmortem harvesting of skin would appear similar, but would lack bleeding →.* ***(Right)*** *Postmortem interventions largely consist of organ/tissue harvesting for transplantation. Evidence thereof is readily apparent externally, as in this case where leg bones were harvested and replaced with plastic rods. Note crude closures → and internally rotated right foot ⇨.*

POSTMORTEM CHANGES AND EXTERNAL EXAMINATION

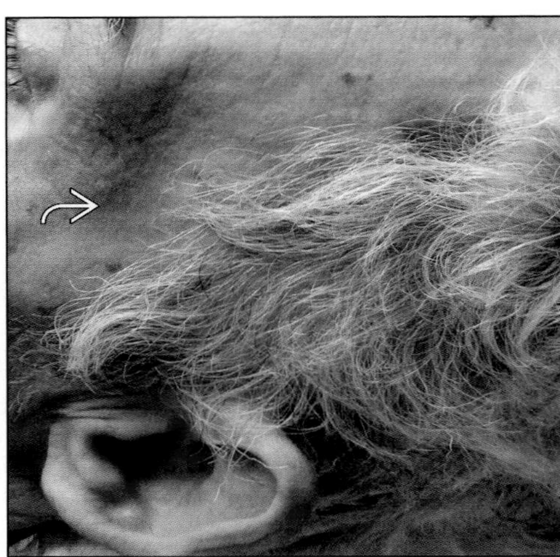

Loss of temporal muscle mass (bitemporal wasting) ➔ is a sign of marked wasting (cachexia) and may indicate underlying malignancy or chronic illness causing a malnourished state.

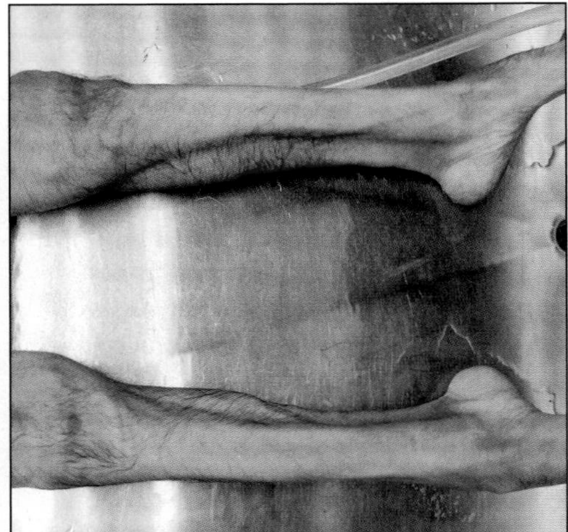

Loss of muscle mass in the lower extremities also supports a diagnosis of cachexia. External examination can give important clues to underlying diseases, such as malignancy in this case.

TERMINOLOGY

Chapter Overview

- This chapter will cover aspects of external examination of body and changes that happen in postmortem state
- Traumatic and marked decomposition changes are not discussed as they are more relevant to forensic autopsies

Definitions

- Postmortem interval: Time from death to start of postmortem examination
  - Has important implications for degree of autolysis and ability to perform ancillary testing such as microbiologic and molecular studies

EXTERNAL EXAMINATION PROCESS

Identification and Consent

- Prior to autopsy, decedent identity must be confirmed, usually via wrist band, toe tag
  - If question of identity, clarify before autopsy
- Consent must be reviewed prior to autopsy for accuracy and extent of examination

Postmortem Physical Exam (Inspection and Palpation)

- Head and neck
  - Hair distribution (alopecia, male pattern baldness), length, and color
  - Eyes: Iris color, pupil size and symmetry, sclera color (jaundice), conjunctival petechiae or pallor, edema, protuberant (thyroid ophthalmopathy), sunken (dehydration)
    - Petechiae indicate hypoxia; pallor indicates anemia
    - Asymmetric pupils, markedly dilated may indicate CNS abnormality, drug effect, etc. (normal pupils: 1-8 mm)
  - Nose: Discharge, ulcers, erosions
  - Oral cavity
    - Contents (gastric contents suggest terminal aspiration, blood), ulcers, erosions, masses
    - Tongue size and appearance (e.g., thrush, atrophic glossitis, enlargement with amyloidosis)
    - Tongue laceration (potential seizure disorder)
    - Presence or absence of teeth and oral hygiene
  - Face: Hirsutism, rashes, swelling and plethora (congestion), muscle wasting (bitemporal wasting), cachexia
    - Marked facial swelling and plethora may indicate SVC syndrome; hirsutism may indicate Cushing syndrome
  - Neck: Tracheal deviation, palpable adenopathy, enlarged thyroid
- Chest
  - Shape: Barrel chested (emphysema), concave chest wall (pectus excavatum)
  - Breasts: Shape, nipple appearance/discharge, palpable masses (include breast examination in male decedents)
    - Gynecomastia in men: Consider age, chronic ETOH or marijuana exposure, antiandrogen, and other medications
- Abdomen
  - Shape: Protuberant, concave
    - If protuberant, check for fluid wave of ascites (place hands in a line along midline of abdomen, assistant taps 1 flank and checks for vibration on other flank)
  - Striae
    - If large purple striae with central obesity, consider Cushing syndrome
- Extremities

- Edema, cyanosis, venous stasis, ischemic changes, ulcers, nail color and length and onychomycosis, muscular atrophy, myxedema
  - Ischemic changes include thin shiny skin, hair loss, muscle loss; isolated ischemia to distal extremity digit may be embolic in origin (blue toe syndrome)
  - Venous stasis changes include brown discoloration of skin and thickening of skin as well as mild edema
  - Myxedema: Thickening of skin and subcutaneous tissue of lower extremities that is nonpitting and may be seen in thyroid disease
  - Lower extremity edema is common and multifactorial; upper extremity edema usually in severe edema (anasarca) and isolated upper extremity edema may indicate SVC syndrome

- Back: Examination of the back is part of complete autopsy and must be performed
  - Spine anatomy (scoliosis), decubitus ulcers, skin lesions, scars
  - Anal area (warts, fissures, ulcers)
- Genitalia
  - Male: Examine penis for lesions, discharge; scrotum for swelling, hernia, presence of testes
  - Female: Vulva hair distribution, lesions (warts, ulcers), labia (warts, ulcers), vaginal discharge, ulcers/warts

General

- Height and weight must be recorded
- Skin elasticity, lesions, color, tattoos should be noted

Medical Intervention

- Ideally, all medical devices/lines are left in situ when autopsy is to be performed and left intact after external examination to determine internal location
  - If devices/lines have been removed prior to autopsy examination, it should be stated in the report
- Record location and placement of all devices (examples)
  - Endotracheal tube (ETT): Length, how secured, associated trauma, placement, balloon inflation
  - Intravenous/intraosseous lines: Note location and any associated erythema or swelling
  - Central lines
    - Location (chest, neck, groin), number of ports, any erythema, internal location of tip (radiograph may be warranted if question regarding central line placement)
  - Pacer and AICD generators
    - Note location of subcutaneous generator pockets and note skin erythema, evidence of infection
    - If AICD generator is noted, prepare to deactivate device prior to internal examination (strong magnet overlying generator); contact institutional cath lab for specific information
  - Nasogastric tube: Note location within nose
  - Gastrostomy tube: Location, associated erythema around ostium, and location after internal examination
  - Foley catheter
    - Note any urine within reservoir (may be used for urinalysis; not good source for urine culture postmortem), any associated urethral edema or erythema
    - Remember to deflate balloon prior to removal of catheter
  - Chest tubes
    - Examine location (note intercostal space from external exam, confirm on internal examination), any discharge
- Resuscitation-related changes
  - These changes related to ACLS with defibrillation and CPR are almost ubiquitous in hospital autopsy practice
  - Sternal bruising, palpable fractured ribs, and skin burning from defibrillator
- Surgical interventions
  - Record incisions, extent of healing, implanted surgical devices, complications, etc.

Postmortem Changes

- General
  - Usually little decomposition in hospital autopsy practice; if body seems markedly autolyzed with appropriate temperature storage, consider sepsis
  - Livor: Purple discoloration of dependent tissues due to pooling of blood in small vessels when circulation stops
    - Portions of the body that rest against firm surfaces do not develop livor
    - Develops within 30 minutes to 2 hours and becomes fixed (does not blanch when pressure is applied) at ~ 12 hours
    - Tardieu spots are small petechiae that develop in areas of dependency
  - Rigor: Tightening of muscles seen postmortem due to depletion of ATP; begins ~ 2-6 hours postmortem and begins in face and neck, affected by size of decedent and muscle mass, begins to pass within ~ 24 hours
    - Rigor of erector pilae may led to postmortem goose bumps
  - Decomposition: Describes process of autolysis of the body after death
    - Green discoloration of right lower quadrant skin is early sign
  - Purge fluid: Decomposition fluid that exudes from nasal and oral cavities

SELECTED REFERENCES

1. Zhou C et al: Factors and processes causing accelerated decomposition in human cadavers - An overview. J Forensic Leg Med. 18(1):6-9, 2011
2. Sauvageau A et al: Postmortem changes mistaken for traumatic lesions: a highly prevalent reason for coroner's autopsy request. Am J Forensic Med Pathol. 29(2):145-7, 2008

External Examination and Postmortem Changes

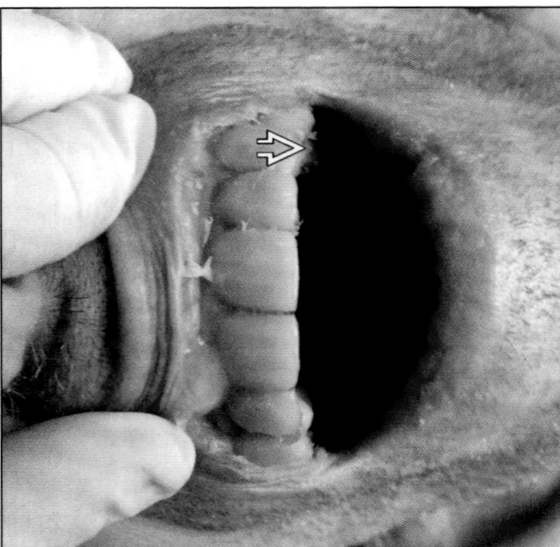

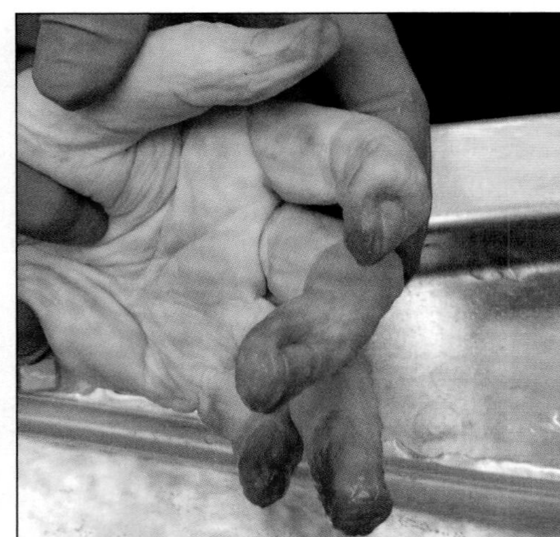

(Left) *Examination of the oral cavity is important at autopsy. This patient had dentures, and there was some gastric content within the mouth focally adhering to the dentures ➩. Terminal aspiration is frequently noted at autopsy.* ***(Right)*** *The red-blue discoloration of these distal digits is due to ischemia and gives a clue to shock as a potential cause of death.*

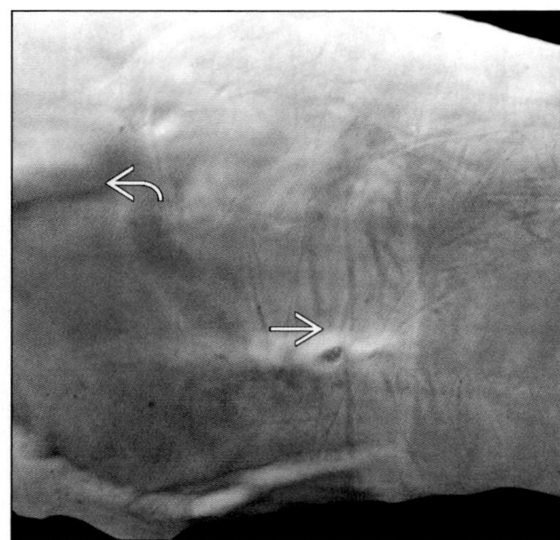

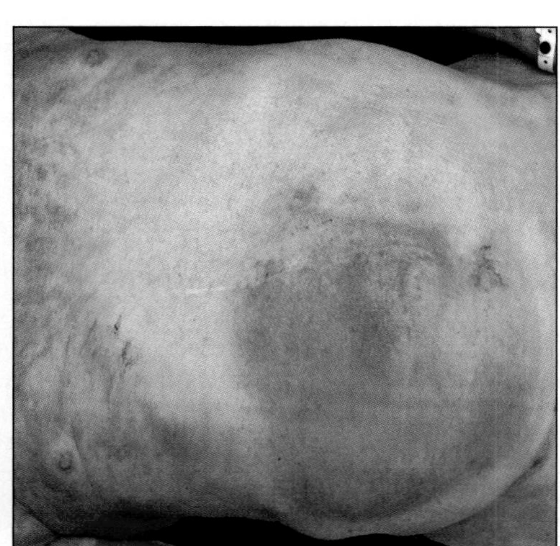

(Left) *Livor mortis is purple discoloration ➔ due to the pooling of blood in dependent small vessels when circulation stops. Areas that are against a firm surface do not develop livor as noted by the pale area ➔ on the back of this decedent.* ***(Right)*** *This large area of green discoloration extending from the right lower quadrant is evidence of decomposition. This decomposition generally starts in the right lower quadrant due to the bacterial content in the cecum.*

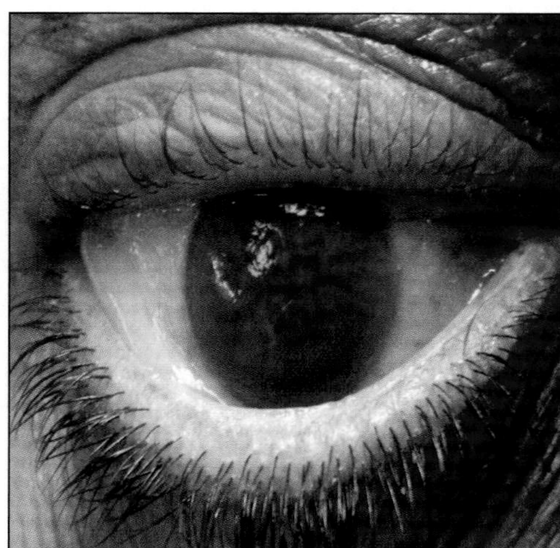

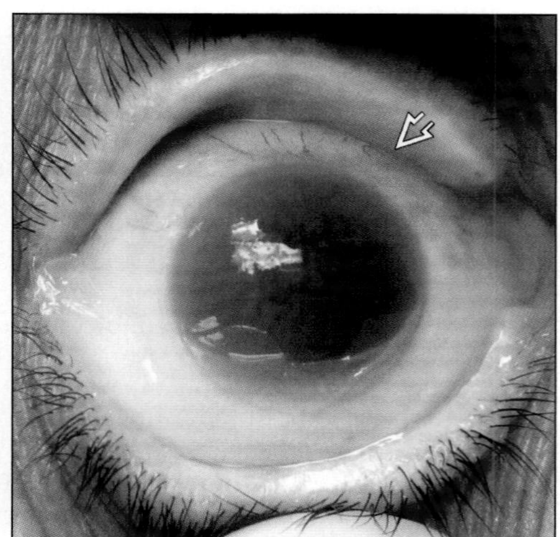

(Left) *Corneal drying and clouding as demonstrated here are a common postmortem finding.* ***(Right)*** *There is marked pallor of the conjunctiva ➩ in this decedent related to marked anemia related to hemorrhagic shock.*

Postmortem External Features

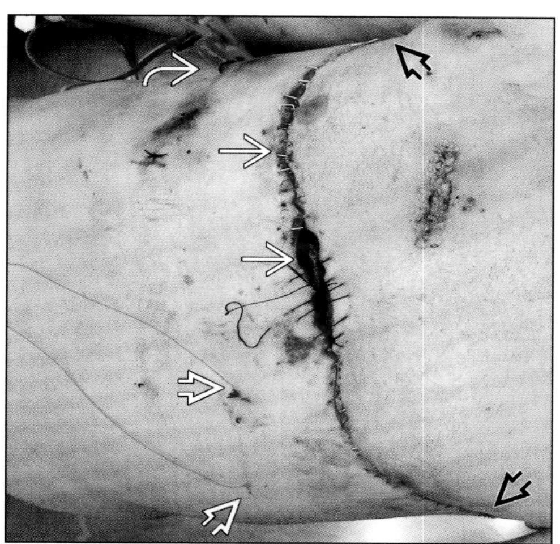

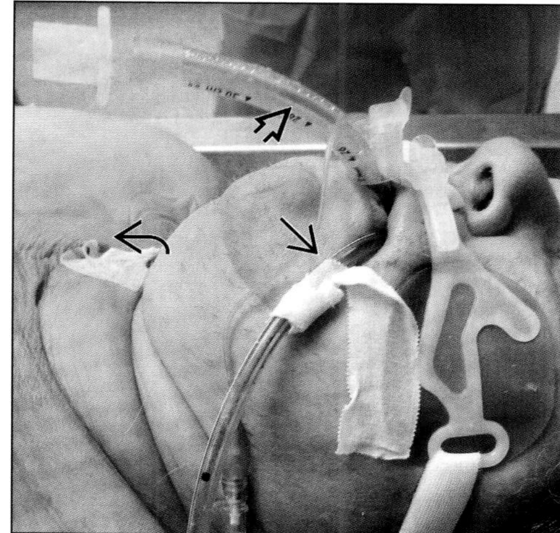

(Left) *Postoperative cases, as demonstrated here, show evidence of multiple medical interventions. There is a recent large clamshell incision from axilla to axilla, a chest tube, and epicardial pacer lead wires.* ***(Right)*** *Another postoperative case demonstrates an endotracheal tube, orogastric tube, and central line. The length of endotracheal tube should be recorded as it exits the mouth (cm markings are on tube).*

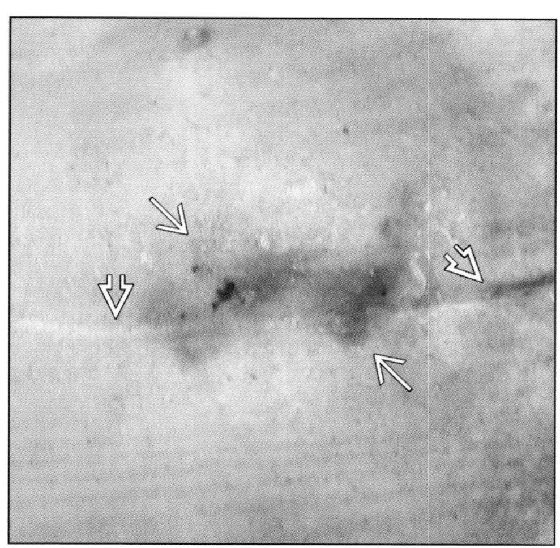

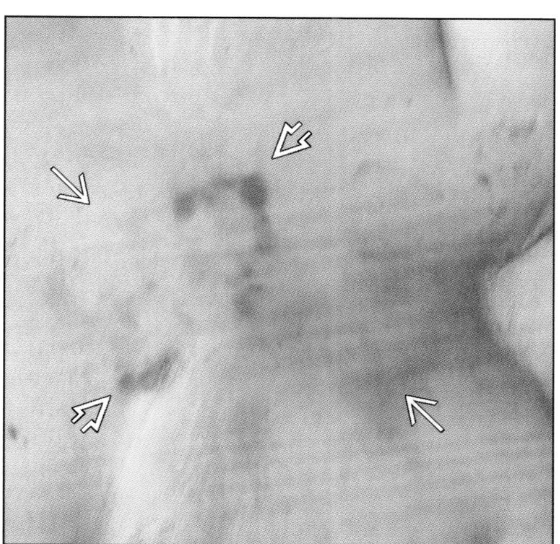

(Left) *There is a large sternal bruise present due to resuscitation attempts in this patient who also has evidence of a prior sternotomy scar.* ***(Right)*** *This decedent has a larger area of hematoma from resuscitation and an abrasion related to defibrillation.*

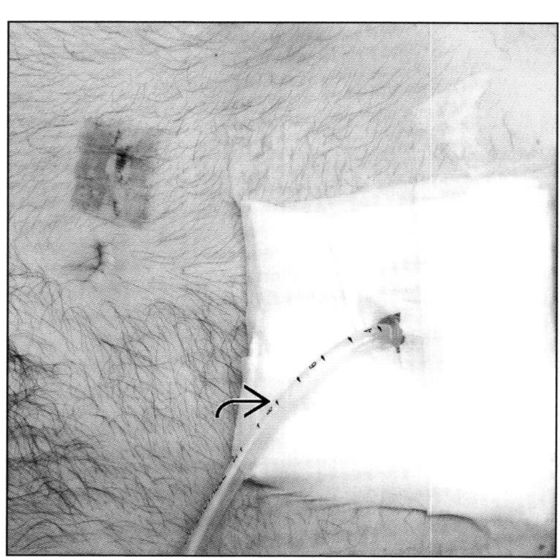

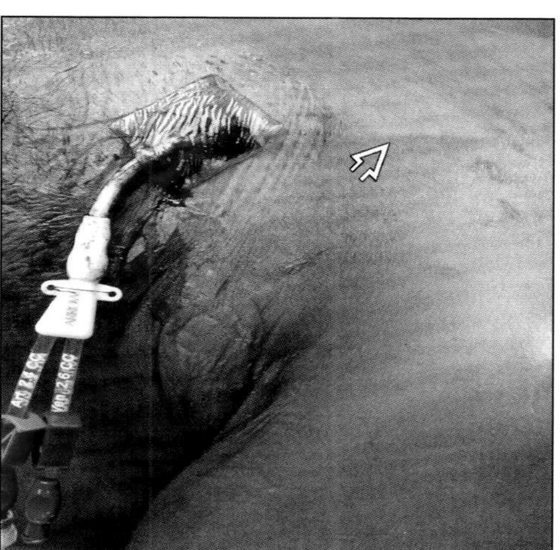

(Left) *All interventions should be noted. This patient had a gastrostomy tube present in the left upper quadrant. Removal of all bandages at external examination should be performed to be able to identify device insertions, wounds, etc.* ***(Right)*** *This PICC line is tunneled under the skin into the left subclavian vein. If there are questions regarding placement of PICC lines, radiography should be performed prior to internal examination.*

BODY CAVITIES

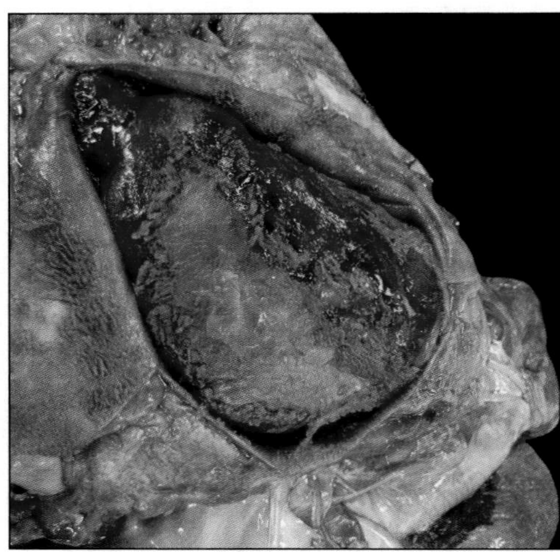

The pericardial sac and epicardial surface from this patient with chronic renal failure show a characteristic, dull fibrinous "bread and butter" pericarditis.

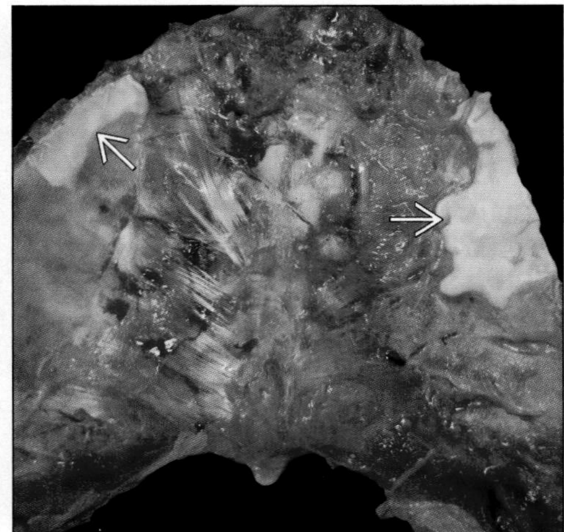

Fibrous pleural plaques ➡ are shown on the parietal pleural surface. These are benign pleural lesions that have been associated with exposure to asbestos.

TERMINOLOGY

Definitions

- Pericardial cavity
  - Normally ~ 50 mL of serous fluid
- Pleural cavities
  - Estimated at up to 0.13 mL/kg of body weight
  - Normally no more than 10 mL of serous fluid per pleural cavity
- Peritoneal cavity
  - Normally 20 mL or less of serous fluid
  - Divided into greater and lesser sacs
  - May communicate with inguinal canal

EPIDEMIOLOGY

Incidence

- ~ 1.5 million cases of pleural effusion/year in USA

Gender

- 2/3 of malignant pleural effusions occur in women
  - Particularly associated with breast and gynecologic tumors

ETIOLOGY/PATHOGENESIS

Effusions

- Imbalances in vascular function, fluid dynamics
  - Changes in permeability of mesothelial lining: Inflammation, malignancy
  - Increased capillary hydrostatic pressure: Congestive heart failure (CHF)
  - Decreased plasma oncotic pressure: Hypoalbuminemia, cirrhosis
  - Capillary disruption: Trauma, malignancy, inflammation
  - Blocked lymphatic drainage: Malignancy, trauma
- Transudates: Extracellular fluid with low protein content and low specific gravity; serous fluid
  - CHF
  - Cirrhosis
  - Atelectasis
  - Hypoalbuminemia
  - Renal failure
- Exudates: Extracellular fluid rich in protein with high specific gravity
  - Infections: Purulent pericarditis, empyema, bacterial peritonitis
  - Inflammation: Asbestosis, pancreatitis, collagen vascular disease
  - Malignancy
  - Lymphatic abnormalities

CLINICAL IMPLICATIONS

Acute Life-Threatening Compartment Syndromes

- All body cavities have more or less rigid boundaries
- Rapid accumulation of fluid, blood, air → compromise of organ function and death
  - Both volume and rate of accumulation influence outcome
- Pleural cavity
  - Tension pneumothorax
- Pericardial cavity
  - Pericardial tamponade
- Peritoneal cavity
  - Abdominal compartment syndrome

Ascites

- Ambulatory patients with cirrhotic ascites: 50% 3-year mortality
- Patients with refractory ascites: < 50% 1-year survival

MACROSCOPIC FINDINGS

General Comments

- Consider checking for pneumothorax before opening the chest (potential causes: COPD, asthma, recently placed central line)
  - Reflect the chest flaps (skin and subcutaneous tissue) laterally without entering pleural cavity
  - Fill the pocket between flap and chest wall with water
  - Create stab wound into pleura below the water level; look for bubbles or foam
- Fluid collections
  - Measure and describe
    - Opacity: Clear, cloudy, turbid, purulent
    - Color: Straw colored, hemorrhagic, milky
  - Ascites + right pleural effusion + benign ovarian tumor = Meigs syndrome
- Frank blood and clot
  - Exclude artifact associated with autopsy procedure
  - Try to identify source
    - If obscure, consider en bloc (Rokitansky) evisceration
- Adhesions
  - Describe: Fibrinous, fibrous, dense
  - Correlate with clinical history and surgical absences

Pericardial Cavity

- Serous effusions
  - Post myocardial infarction or myocardial trauma
  - Collagen vascular disease
    - Accompanied by other changes of underlying illness (rash, arthropathy, etc.)
- Hemopericardium
  - Transmural myocardial infarction with rupture
  - Aortic dissection/rupture
  - Coronary artery dissection/rupture
  - Trauma
- Pericardial rupture
  - Traumatic; may be accompanied by other traumatic injuries
  - Appropriately sized defects allow for cardiac herniation
- Pericarditis
  - Infectious
  - Fibrinous: Chronic renal failure ("bread and butter" pericarditis)

Pleural Cavity

- Serous effusions
  - CHF
    - Pulmonary edema with heavy, congested lungs, dilated ventricles, pedal edema
- Parapneumonic
  - Adjacent consolidated lung
- Malignant: ~ 40% of symptomatic pleural effusions
  - Especially lung cancer, breast, lymphoma
  - Primary effusion lymphoma in HIV/AIDS patients
- Hemothorax
  - Chest wall trauma: Rib fractures, intercostal vascular disruption, aortic rupture
  - Aortic dissection, aneurysm
  - Iatrogenic (i.e., central line placement)
- Pneumothorax
  - Spontaneous: Pulmonary blebs and changes of emphysema; changes associated with smoking
  - Traumatic: Blunt or penetrating
  - Catamenial: Secondary to pleural endometriosis
    - Exclusively in women
    - May have endometriotic implants in pelvis and abdomen
  - Lymphangioleiomyomatosis
    - Emphysema-like changes with cyst formation
    - Usually in reproductive-age women
- Chylothorax
  - Milky white, triglyceride-rich fluid
  - Disruption or obstruction of thoracic duct or tributaries
    - Malignancy: Especially lymphoma
    - CHF: Accompanied by other signs of congestive failure
    - Developmental anomalies (e.g., Down syndrome)
- Empyema
  - Purulent exudate in pleural space
    - Complication of pneumonia: Pneumonic changes in adjacent lung tissue
    - Esophageal rupture (Boerhaave syndrome): Food and esophageal contents in pleural cavity, usually left sided
- Pleural plaques
  - Tan white, firm, fibrotic plaques
  - Especially near vertebrae, near lung bases, dome of diaphragm
  - Associated with asbestos exposure
- Mesothelioma
  - Tumor studding of pleural surfaces or continuous, plaque-like tumor covering pleural surfaces
  - May be difficult to distinguish from lung cancer grossly
  - Often associated with history of asbestos exposure

Peritoneal Cavity

- Ascites
  - Benign
    - May be associated with signs of cirrhosis (esophageal varices, splenomegaly)
  - Malignant (e.g., associated with ovarian cancer or mesothelioma)
    - Consider cytologic evaluation
- Peritonitis
  - Infectious
    - Associated with perforation in gastrointestinal tract
    - Tuberculous: Numerous millimeter-sized nodules studding the peritoneum; usually part of disseminated infection
    - Spontaneous bacterial peritonitis: Usually associated with cirrhosis and ascites; usually enteric bacteria
  - Noninfectious
    - Pancreatitis
    - Extravasated urine (e.g., secondary to trauma)
    - Ruptured dermoid cyst
    - Collagen vascular disease

BODY CAVITIES

- Chylous ascites: Milky white, triglyceride-rich fluid
  - May be associated with abdominal trauma, tumors, cirrhosis, radiation therapy
- Hemoperitoneum
  - Trauma: Blunt or penetrating
  - Arterial aneurysm/rupture: Aorta, splenic artery
  - Perforation/rupture of other structures: Gastric ulcer, intestinal tumor, hepatic tumor, ectopic pregnancy, corpus luteum
- Endometriosis
  - Red-blue, "powder burn" lesions on peritoneal surfaces, especially pelvic peritoneum
  - Lesions of intestinal serosa may → fibrosis and obstruction
  - Fibrotic lesions may mimic metastatic nodules
- Mesothelial cysts
  - Often multiple, thin-walled, clear fluid-filled cysts
- Mesothelioma
  - Tumor studding or diffuse plaques of tumor
- Pseudomyxoma peritonei
  - Accumulation of mucinous fluid in peritoneum
  - Associated with mucinous tumors of appendix and ovaries
- Hernias
  - Protrusion of viscera and peritoneum beyond normal confines of abdominal cavity
  - Common types
    - Hiatal
    - Abdominal wall: Ventral, postsurgical
    - Inguinal, femoral
  - Note presence or absence of incarcerated or infarcted bowel
- Internal hernia
  - Protrusion of viscera through opening in peritoneum or mesentery within normal confines of abdominal cavity
    - Loops of bowel may become incarcerated/ infarcted
    - Through foramen of Winslow, paraduodenal, transomental; through cecal or sigmoid mesocolon
  - Much less common than standard hernias
- Peritoneal carcinomatosis: Especially associated with ovarian cancer
- Primary peritoneal carcinoma
  - Peritoneal carcinomatosis without identifiable primary source
  - Histologically identical to ovarian serous carcinoma
    - Ovaries uninvolved, minimally involved, or absent
- Peritoneal loose bodies (a.k.a. peritoneal MICE)
  - Oval, 0.5-2.5 cm calcified
  - Found free floating in abdominal cavity
  - Thought to originate from torsed, detached appendix epiploica

MICROSCOPIC FINDINGS

Normal Mesothelium

- Lines all body cavities and produces scant serous fluid
- Single layer of mesothelial cells on basement membrane
  - Basement membrane with stomata that connect to lymphatics
  - Allows passage of fluids, small and large molecules

Reactive Mesothelium

- Mesothelial cell response to inflammation, infection, other insults
- Increased size of nuclei, nucleoli, mitoses, vacuolated cytoplasm
  - Features may mimic malignancy (particularly in fluid cytology)
- Features favoring malignancy: Gross nodule formation, necrosis, stromal invasion

Mesothelioma

- May be difficult to distinguish from metastatic carcinoma histologically
- Types
  - Epithelioid: May mimic adenocarcinoma
  - Sarcomatoid: Spindle cell tumor, may mimic sarcoma
  - Biphasic: Epithelioid and sarcomatoid areas
- Immunoperoxidase stains are usually necessary for definitive diagnosis
  - Positive in most mesotheliomas: CK 5/6, calretinin, WT1
  - Positive in most adenocarcinomas: Ber-Ep4, MOC-31, CEA
- Electron microscopy of mesothelioma
  - Epithelioid tumors: Long, narrow, branching microvilli
- Lungs may show evidence of asbestosis
  - Interstitial fibrosis
  - Ferruginous bodies

Other Histologic Findings

- Endometriosis
  - Benign endometrial glands, endometrial stroma, hemosiderin
- Peritoneal cysts
  - Thin-walled cysts with simple mesothelial lining
- Tuberculous pleuritis/peritonitis
  - Characteristic granulomas with central caseous necrosis
  - Acid-fast organisms on special stain
- Pseudomyxoma peritonei
  - Rare islands of malignant cells floating in mucin

SELECTED REFERENCES

1. Visouli AN et al: Catamenial pneumothorax. J Thorac Dis. 6(Suppl 4):S448-60, 2014
2. Dubeau L et al: Coming into focus: the nonovarian origins of ovarian cancer. Ann Oncol. 24 Suppl 8:viii28-viii35, 2013
3. Fede G et al: Renal failure and cirrhosis: a systematic review of mortality and prognosis. J Hepatol. 56(4):810-8, 2012
4. Noppen M: Normal volume and cellular contents of pleural fluid. Curr Opin Pulm Med. 7(4):180-2, 2001

Gross Features

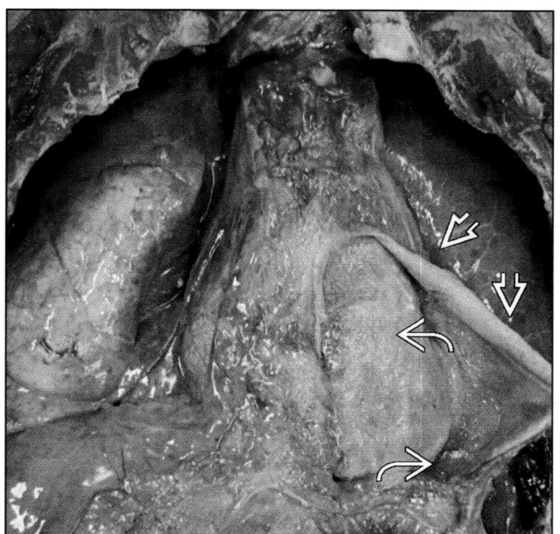

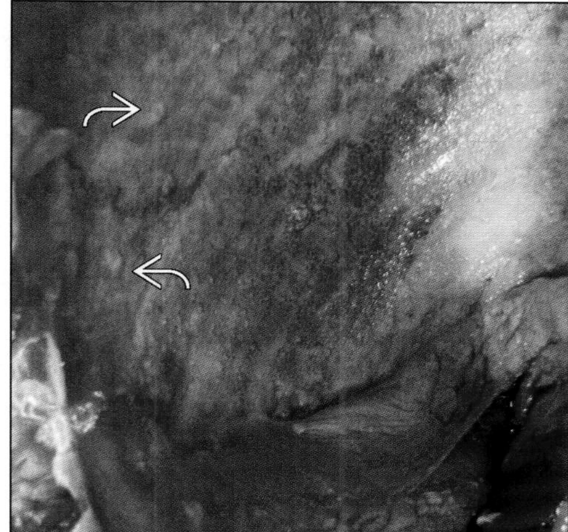

(Left) *This in situ photograph shows the pericardium folded back ➭ from the epicardium to reveal a green-yellow purulent pericarditis ➭. These are most often bacterial and originate from either infections in contiguous structures or bloodstream infections.* ***(Right)*** *The parietal pleural surface is completely covered by tiny tan-white nodules ➭, a characteristic appearance for tuberculous pleuritis. The nodules are often below the resolution of imaging techniques.*

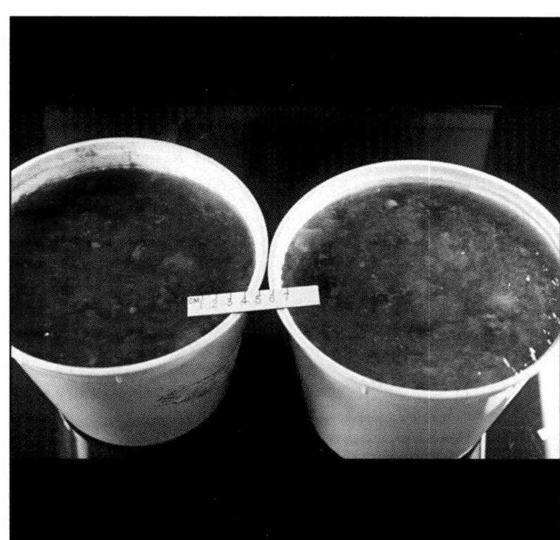

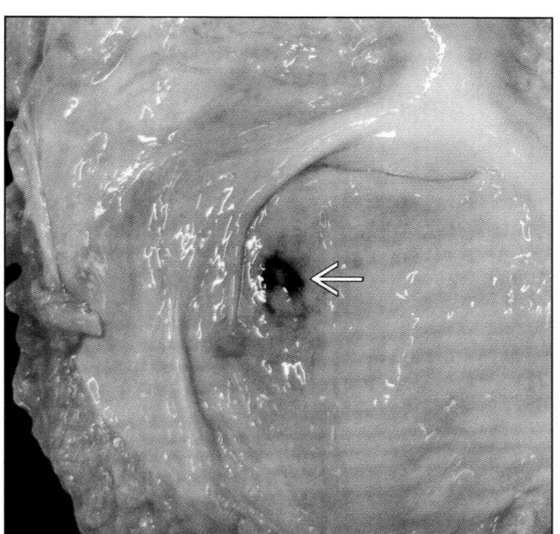

(Left) *The abdominal cavity normally has 20 mL or less of serous fluid. These containers hold the mucoid contents from the peritoneal cavity of a patient with a mucinous ovarian tumor, a condition know as pseudomyxoma peritonei.* ***(Right)*** *This segment of peritoneum shows a dark gray-black, "powder burn" discoloration, characteristic of peritoneal endometriosis ➭.*

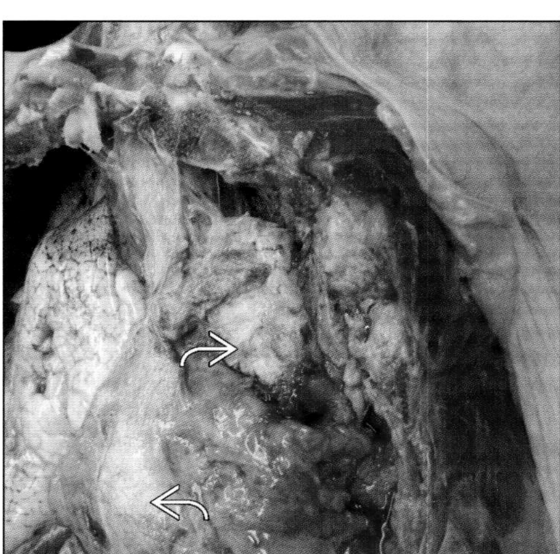

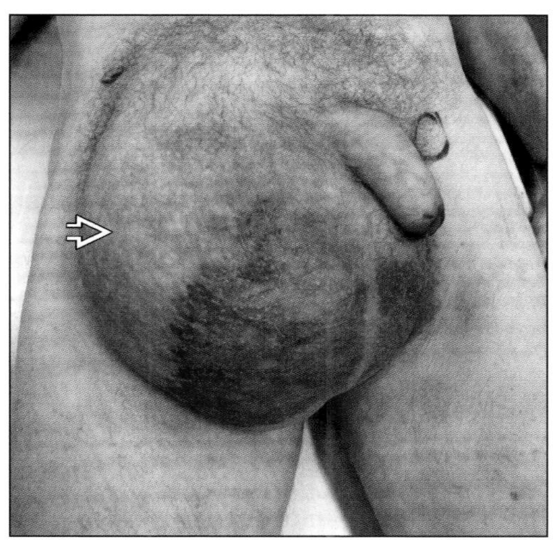

(Left) *This in situ photograph shows a thick, tan-white pleural-based tumor ➭ that covers much of the exposed parietal pleura. Microscopy with immunoperoxidase was diagnostic of mesothelioma.* ***(Right)*** *This external photograph shows a massive inguinal hernia ➭. Such hernias may contain most of the small and large bowel as well as omentum. They are associated with impaired mobility, possible bowel obstruction, and scrotal ulceration.*

CARDIOVASCULAR SYSTEM

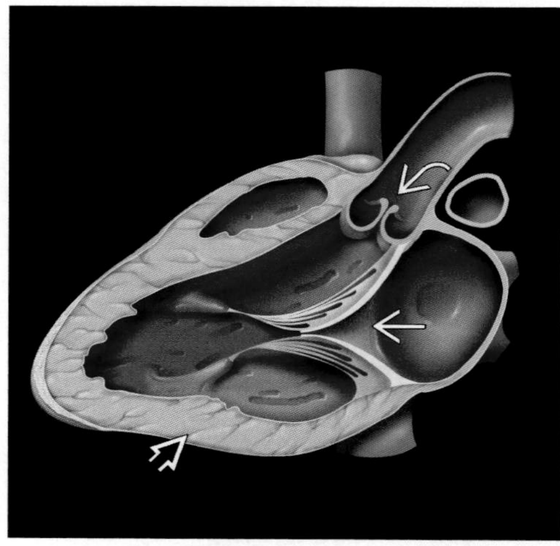

This illustration shows cardiac anatomy in the (parasternal) long axis view. The mitral valve ➡ and aortic valve ➡ are seen in this plane, as is the left ventricular myocardium ➡.

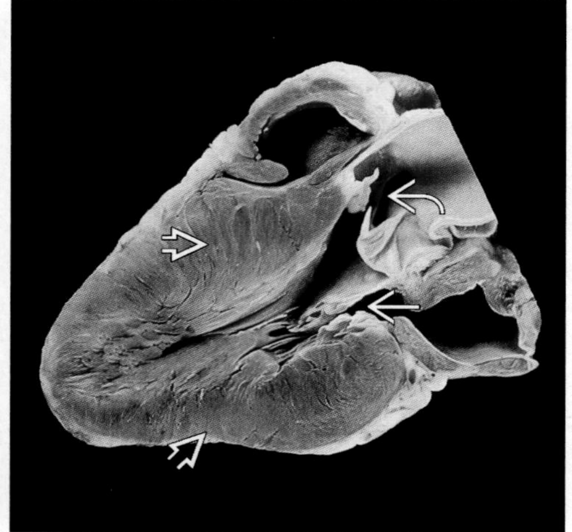

This corresponding gross photograph of an autopsy heart cut in long axis shows the mitral leaflets ➡ and aortic valve ➡. The left ventricle is hypertrophied ➡.

MACROSCOPIC FINDINGS

External Examination

- Accurate body height and weight important for calculating expected heart weight
- Surgical scars
  - Median sternotomy or other thoracotomy
  - Midline abdomen (abdominal aortic aneurysm repair)
  - Vein harvesting sites
  - Dialysis fistula (hypertension)
  - Pacemaker pocket, other implantable devices
- Edema, ascites (congestive heart failure)

General Features

- Prosection
  - Removed en bloc with lungs
    - Remove chest plate, taking care to preserve any internal mammary artery grafts
    - Just below thoracic inlet, cut through trachea, esophagus, and aortic arch vessels
    - Using caudal traction on trachea, cut through posterior pleural reflections, following along vertebral bodies, to diaphragm
    - Lift heart from diaphragm where IVC enters right atrium
    - Cut IVC and remaining attachments tethering thoracic organ block
    - Follow piecemeal instructions below
  - Removed piecemeal
    - Open pericardium and measure fluid (normal ~ 50 cc), note any adhesions
    - Open main pulmonary artery for saddle embolus inspection (optional)
    - Cut great arteries (aorta and pulmonary artery) 2 cm above ventricles
    - Lift apex of heart, putting tension on pulmonary veins
    - Cut through pulmonary veins on both sides, taking care not to disrupt left atrium
    - Cut through any remaining pericardial attachments to free heart specimen
  - Heart
    - Remove/strip parietal pericardium
    - Note position and patency of proximal coronary arteries, any vein grafts
    - Section each coronary artery at 5 mm intervals and estimate cross-sectional area stenosis
    - Coronary arteries may be examined in situ or after removing by dissection (decalcification may be needed, stented segments may need special processing)
  - Combined short-axis and inflow-outflow technique
    - Cut 3 or 4 slices (1 cm thick) in short axis through ventricles (parallel to posterior/inferior coronary groove, stopping at mid papillary muscle level)
    - Inspect ventricular myocardium for mottling, scars, rupture, etc.
    - Using scissors, incise right atrium from IVC to tip of appendage
    - Inspect right atrium for patent oval foramen, coronary sinus ostial obstruction, etc.
    - Using long blade, cut through atrium, tricuspid anulus, and ventricle, along posterior septum
    - Unfold ventricle to inspect tricuspid valve and measure its circumference
    - Using scissors, cut right ventricle anteriorly out through pulmonary valve
    - Unfold ventricle in this plane to inspect pulmonary valve and measure its circumference
    - Using scissors, incise left atrial appendage tip and cut along left atrium just above mitral annulus
    - Inspect left appendage for clot
    - Using long blade, cut through left atrium, mitral anulus, and ventricle, in between papillary muscles

- Unfold ventricle to inspect mitral valve and measure its circumference
- Cut through left ventricle anteriorly through outflow tract and aorta
- Unfold ventricle in this plane to inspect aortic valve and measure its circumference
  - Four-chamber
    - This view shows relation of atria, ventricles, and atrioventricular valves
    - Best performed with long, sharp knife
    - Begin at cardiac apex
    - Proceed along plane defined by: 1) apex, 2) acute margin of right ventricle, and 3) inferior/posterior obtuse margin of left ventricle; pins may be placed to mark this plane
    - Extend cut into mitral and tricuspid valves and through atria
    - Knife should end 1 cm posterior to roots of great arteries
  - Long-axis method
    - This view shows anterior mitral leaflet-aortic continuity with mitral inflow and aortic outflow tracts on either side
    - Best performed with long, sharp knife
    - Begin at cardiac apex
    - Proceed along plane defined by: 1) apex, 2) right aortic sinus of Valsalva, and 3) mitral valve annulus midway between right and left pulmonary veins; pins may be placed to mark this plane
    - Extend cut through right ventricular outflow tract (in cross section) and aorta (in longitudinal section)
- Thoracic aorta
  - Beginning at proximal arch, cut posteriorly along line ~ 1 cm posterior to arch branches
  - Continue to descending thoracic end
  - Inspect for atherosclerosis (assess % surface area and note any calcification or ulceration) or dissection
  - Open each arch vessel and visually inspect intercostal branch ostia
- Abdominal aorta
  - Beginning proximally, cut along line posteriorly, just to one side of intercostal branches
  - Continue through one of the iliac branches to end; then, starting at bifurcation, cut through other iliac
  - Inspect renal arteries, celiac axis, superior and inferior mesenteric and other branches
    - Inspect renal artery stenosis or fibromuscular dysplasia
  - Inspect for atherosclerosis (assess % surface area and note any calcification or ulceration) or aneurysm

COMMON CARDIOVASCULAR DISEASES AT AUTOPSY

Ischemic Heart Disease

- Segmental evaluation of short-axis ventricle sections, according to coronary territory
  - Antero-septo-lateral (LAD)
  - Lateral (LCX)
  - Infero-septal and right ventricle (posterior descending)
    - Right dominant (RCA), left dominant (LCX)
- Careful evaluation of entire coronary tree in cross section
  - In situ or after dissecting free from heart
  - Decalcification may be necessary
- Document interventions (stents, bypasses)

Idiopathic Dilated Cardiomyopathy

- Left ventricle internal short-axis diameter > 5.0 cm
- Mitral annular circumference often > 10.5 cm
- Right ventricle may be secondarily enlarged
- Exclude ischemic disease
- Clinically exclude
  - Chronic ethanol abuse
  - Hemochromatosis
  - Familial

Sudden Cardiac Death

- Determine if heart is "structurally normal"
- Exclude conditions associated with acute arrhythmia
  - Arrhythmogenic cardiomyopathy
  - Hypertrophic cardiomyopathy
  - Coronary artery obstruction
  - Myocardial scarring (ischemia, old myocarditis)
  - Myxomatous mitral valve disease (mitral valve prolapse)
  - Acute myocarditis
  - Coronary artery anomalies
- Consider examination of conduction system

SPECIAL STUDIES

Tetrazolium Chloride Incubation for Detection of Acute Myocardial Infarction

- 2 common tetrazolium salts used: Nitro blue (BBT) and triphenyl tetrazolium (TTC)
  - Viable tissue with intact dehydrogenase activity reduces solution to colored formazan salt: NBT blue and TTC red
  - Results: Infarct unstained, viable tissue blue (NBT) or red (TTC), scar white
  - Technique includes dilution of tetrazolium salt in buffered solution and incubation of fresh slides myocardium at 37° C; usually 30 min until color develops
  - Fix myocardial slice in formalin to aid contrast between viable and infarcted tissue

SELECTED REFERENCES

1. Kakimoto Y et al: The effectiveness and limitations of triphenyltetrazolium chloride to detect acute myocardial infarction at forensic autopsy. Am J Forensic Med Pathol. 34(3):242-7, 2013
2. Basso C et al: Guidelines for autopsy investigation of sudden cardiac death. Virchows Arch. 452(1):11-8, 2008
3. Edwards WD. Cardiac anatomy and examination of cardiac specimens. In: Damjanov et al. Anderson's Pathology, 10th ed. CRC Press: Kansas City. 80-117, 1995

CARDIOVASCULAR SYSTEM

Gross Features

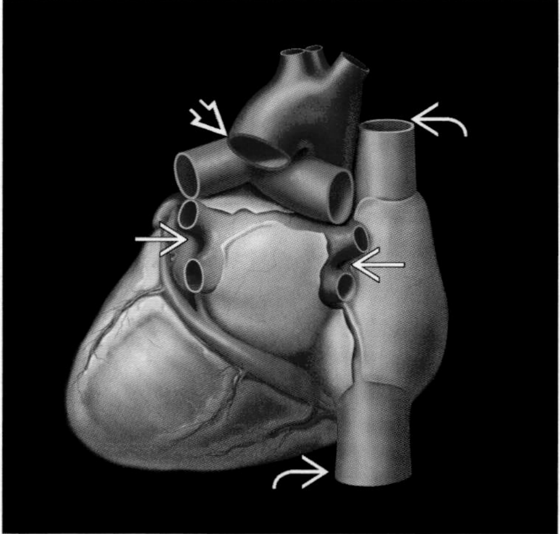

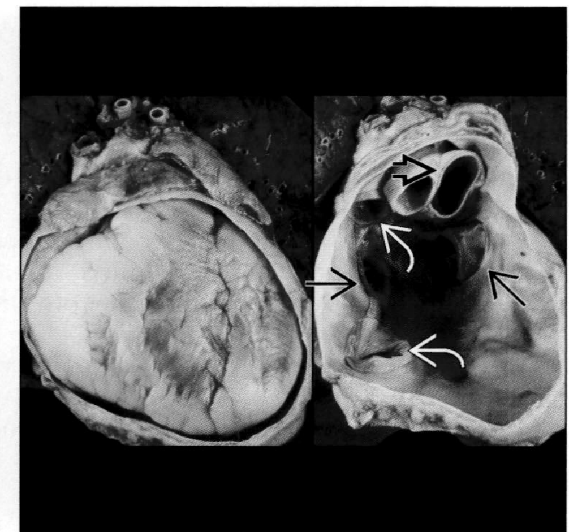

(Left) *Illustration shows the heart viewed posteriorly. From this perspective, all of the attachments that must be cut during prosection can be viewed, including the inferior and superior vena cava ➲, the pulmonary veins ➔, and great arteries ➲.* ***(Right)*** *Gross photograph of the pericardial sac after heart removal also shows the connections: Vena cava ➲, pulmonary veins ➔, and great arteries ➲. (Courtesy W.D. Edwards, MD.)*

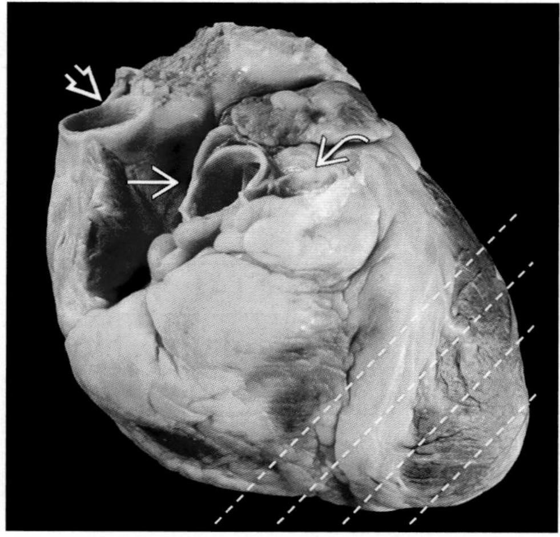

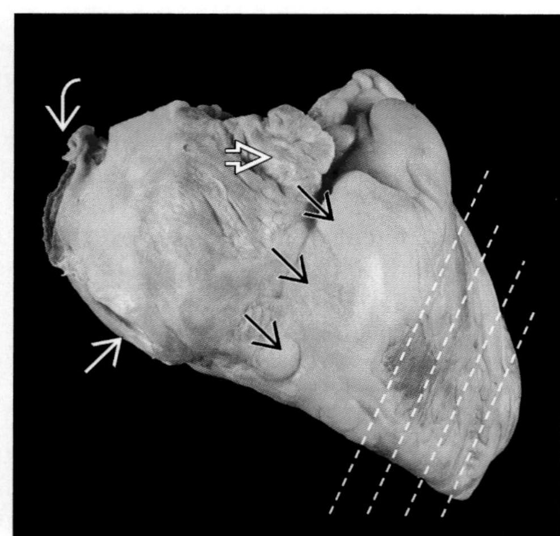

(Left) *Heart removed at autopsy is viewed anteriorly, with the superior vena cava ➲, aorta ➔, and pulmonary artery ➲ serving as landmarks. Short-axis ventricle sections should be cut, roughly along the dashed lines; running parallel to the coronary (atrioventricular) groove.* ***(Right)*** *This right lateral view of the heart (with superior ➲ and inferior ➔ vena cava, and right atrial appendage ➲) shows how short-axis sections should be cut parallel to the coronary groove ➔.*

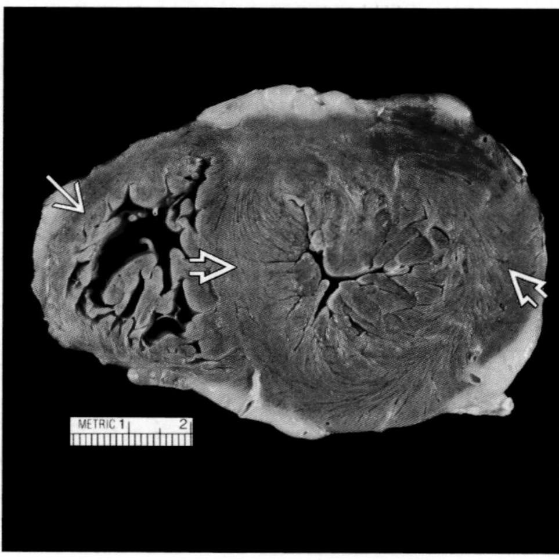

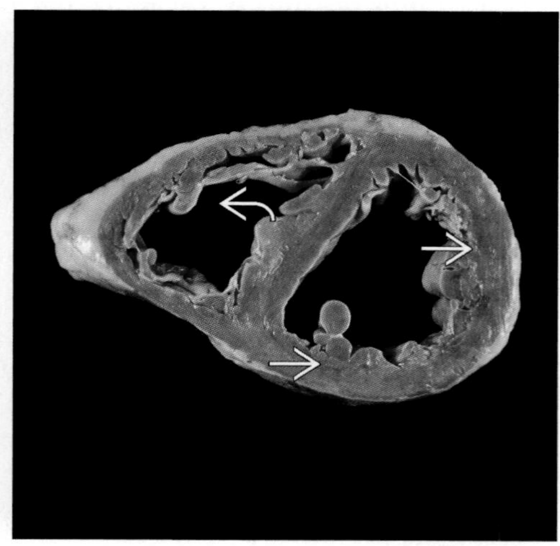

(Left) *Short-axis section of an autopsy heart shows marked concentric left ventricular hypertrophy ➲. The right ventricle ➔ size and wall thickness is relatively normal.* ***(Right)*** *Short-axis view of an autopsy heart shows features of dilated cardiomyopathy. The left ventricle wall thickness ➔ is relatively normal, but the left ventricular chamber is dilated (diameter > 5 cm). There are no scars to suggest an ischemic etiology. The right ventricle ➲ is dilated as well.*

Gross Features

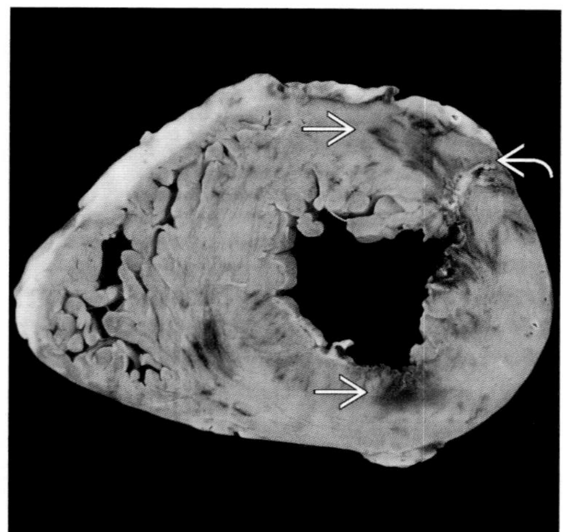

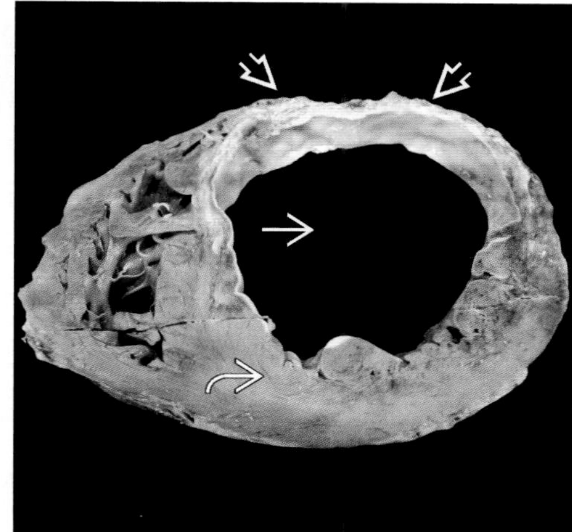

(Left) *This autopsy heart, viewed in short axis, shows acute myocardial infarction with myocardial mottling* → *. A fibrin-lined rupture tract* → *is also visible in the free wall.* ***(Right)*** *This short-axis ventricular section is from an autopsy of a patient with longstanding ischemic cardiomyopathy. A large anterior wall old infarction* → *is seen. There has been extensive remodeling, with dilatation* → *and wall thinning. There is also compensatory hypertrophy in the viable myocardium* → *.*

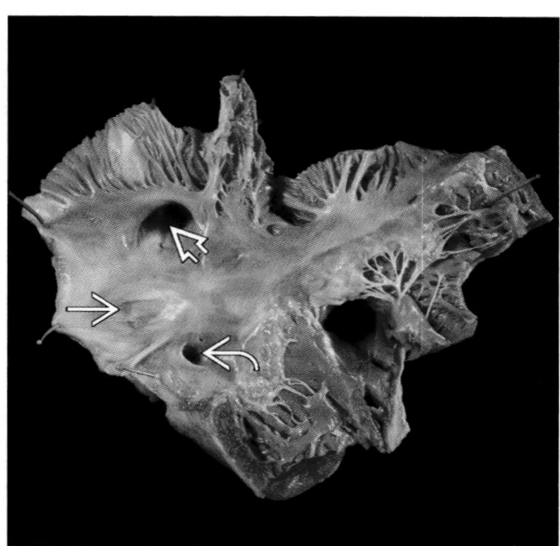

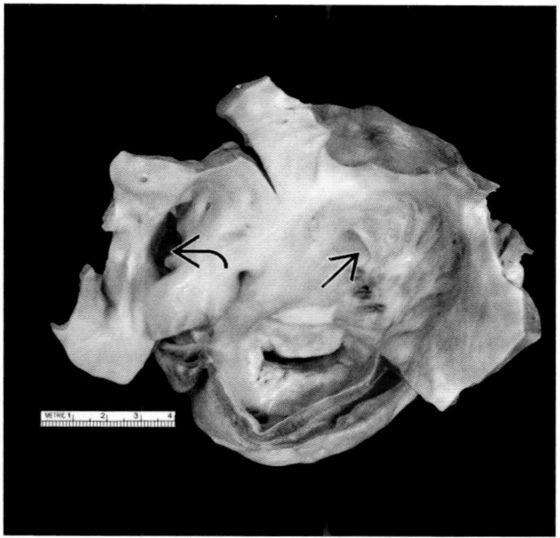

(Left) *The right atrial structures can easily be examined after short-axis ventricle sections are cut. This view with the tricuspid valve annulus opened shows the oval fossa* → *, superior vena cava* → *, and coronary sinus ostium* → *.* ***(Right)*** *The left atrial structures are also easily viewed in this dissection method, as in this autopsy heart specimen from a patient with rheumatic mitral valve disease. The limbus remnant of the oval fossa* → *and pulmonary vein orifices* → *are shown.*

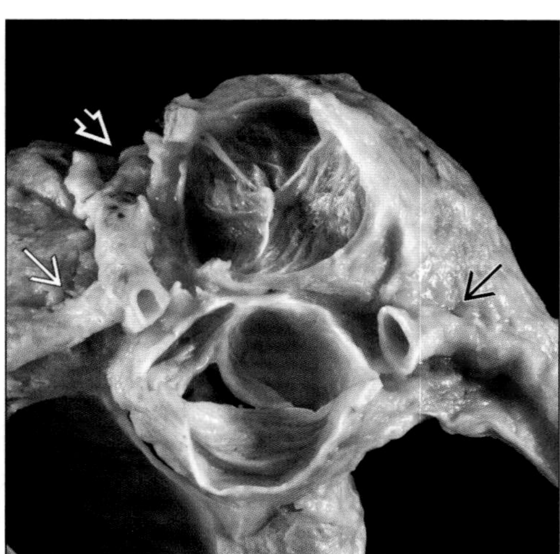

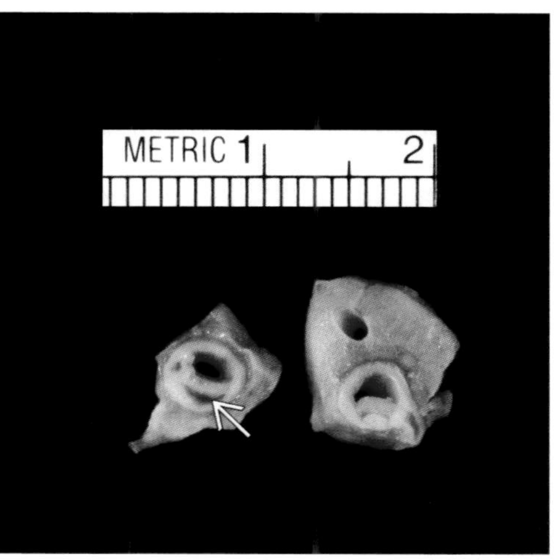

(Left) *The origin and course of the coronary arteries should be documented at autopsy. These include the right* → *, left anterior descending* → *, and left circumflex* → *coronary arteries.* ***(Right)*** *The coronary arteries are best evaluated in cross section, either in situ or after removal from the heart. In this cross section of the left anterior descending artery, there is is significant luminal obstruction as well as gross evidence of intraplaque hemorrhage* → *.*

RESPIRATORY SYSTEM

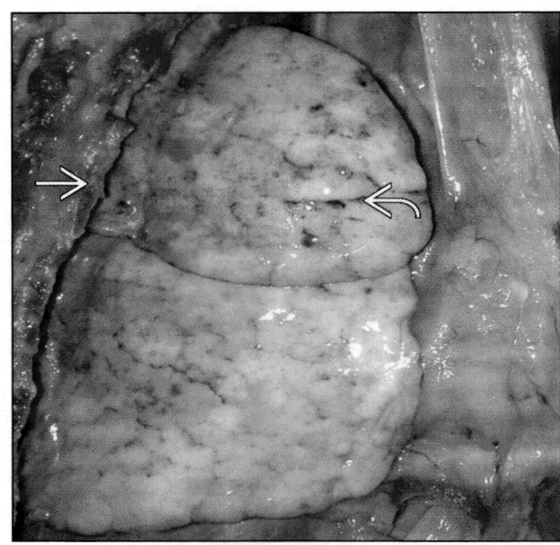

This is a normal and appropriately expanded right lung that adequately fills the thoracic cavity (chest wall ➡). The pleural surface is glistening, and a small amount of anthracotic pigment ➡ is noted.

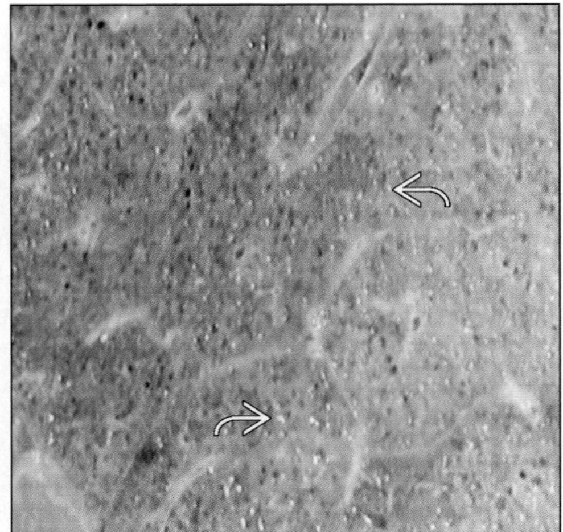

The cut section shows grossly normal lung parenchyma with alveolar spaces ➡ imparting a spongy appearance to the parenchyma.

MACROSCOPIC FINDINGS

General Features

- Right lung consists of 3 lobes: Right upper, right middle, and right lower
  - Horizontal fissure (or minor fissure) separates right upper and right middle lobes
  - Oblique fissure (or major fissure) separates right middle and lower lobes
- Left lung consists of 2 lobes: Left upper and left lower, plus lingula, which is rudimentary appendage that arises from left upper lobe
  - Oblique fissure (or major fissure) separates left upper and lower lobes
- Each lobe is further divided into bronchopulmonary segments, each supplied by its own segmental bronchus
- Segments are further divided into lobules
  - Lobule consists of multiple pulmonary acini, bound by connective tissue (interlobular septa)
  - Each lobule is 1-2 cm in diameter and can be identified on high-resolution CT scans
  - Lobules are also grossly visible from pleural surface of lung or on cut surface because of their septal demarcation
    - A number of pathologic processes may accentuate lobular architecture, including fibrosis, inflammation, or blood accumulation
- Lung has dual blood supply
  - Bronchial arteries are derived from systemic circulation, most often from thoracic aorta
    - Supply blood to airways to level of respiratory bronchioles and to connective tissues of lung
    - However, there is variation, particularly on right side
  - Pulmonary arterial circulation receives deoxygenated blood via right ventricle where it is oxygenated at level of alveolar microvasculature and returned to left atrium
  - Main pulmonary artery divides in front of left mainstem bronchus into right and left pulmonary arteries
  - Right superior, right inferior, left superior, and left inferior pulmonary veins drain into left atrium
- Mediastinal, hilar, and intrapulmonary lymph nodes are easily identified by presence of anthracotic pigment deposition
  - Some anthracotic pigment deposition is typical of most urban/suburban populations
  - Marked anthracotic pigment deposition is seen in smokers, recreational inhalation drug users (especially crack cocaine), industrial/mining occupations, and in regions where cooking over open fire (particularly in a closed space) is customary
- Slightly enlarged subcarinal lymph nodes are common finding at autopsy and usually of no significance

Specimen Handling

- Cutting lungs in a fresh state enhances appreciation of some pathologic processes (e.g., pulmonary edema) and may be appropriate in some circumstances
  - Formalin perfusion of lung and fixation allows for better overall appreciation of many other pathologic processes such as infection, parenchymal disease, and malignancy, many of which coexist in hospital autopsy population
    - Formalin perfusion is therefore recommended
- Sequence of evaluation is extremely important
  - External examination of thorax for lines, chest tubes, surgical sites, symmetry, tracheal deviation, muscular/bone abnormalities, and skin lesions
  - Following standard Y-shaped incision and reflection of skin and subcutaneous tissue from bony thorax, test for pneumothorax if clinically appropriate
  - Following removal of chest plate, assessment should continue with

- Presence, quantity, and character of fluid in pleural space
- Presence of adhesions and other parietal/visceral pleural lesions
- Thoracic surface of diaphragm and its appropriate position should be included

- **Description of lung volumes**
  - Common terms used to characterize deviation from normal lung volumes
    - Hyperinflation (lungs may meet in midline of anterior mediastinum)
    - Compression atelectasis (partial/complete, unilateral/bilateral) due to fluid, air, or tumor
    - Contraction atelectasis due to pulmonary or pleural fibrosis
    - Decrease in size due to hypoplasia (most commonly seen in neonatal and pediatric populations)
  - Procurement of fresh tissue for microbiology cultures or other special studies
  - Assessment for saddle embolism prior to separation of right and left pulmonary arteries from main pulmonary artery and heart
  - Complete gross inspection of surfaces of lungs and palpation following removal from thoracic cavity and detachment from heart and mediastinal structures
    - Obtain lung weights prior to formalin perfusion
  - Formalin perfusion either through mainstem bronchi or trachea with attached lungs, depending on circumstances
    - Although rarely used in daily practice, it is possible to perfuse lungs through pulmonary arterial system
- Following removal of thoracic organs, chest wall and parietal pleura should be reinspected (plaques, adhesions, etc.)
- Sectioning of lungs following perfusion and fixation
  - Fixed lung is firm and easy to slice thinly for optimal gross examination
  - In any plane of sectioning, slices should be no thicker than 2 cm, and all larger airways and vessels should be opened with scissors if incompletely cut
    - Even with these thin sections, one must palpate lung slices thoroughly in order to identify and localize radiographic abnormalities (normally visualized radiographically down to ~ 0.5 cm) or smaller unsuspected lesions
  - Parasagittal (slab) sectioning demonstrates lung from apex to base; lobar demarcations are well seen
  - Lung is serially sectioned with lateral pleural surface down on cutting board and hilar region facing up, thus distinguishing more central regions from periphery
    - Important, as many pathologic processes in lung are characterized by preferential distribution of upper lobe predominant vs. lower lobe predominant or central vs. peripheral
  - Transverse sectioning is useful if close CT correlation is indicated
  - Liebow bronchial probe technique is alternative method when, for example, clinical history suggests a primary pulmonary malignancy
    - Probes are passed down airways and used as a guide for slicing
    - Resulting cuts are in neither sagittal nor coronal plane, but technique is excellent for demonstrating relationship of tumor to airway
- Mediastinal and hilar/intrapulmonary lymph nodes sections are generally recommended depending on clinical circumstances and pulmonary findings

Anatomic Features

- Some normal anatomic variations and common clinically insignificant abnormalities may be identified, particularly in older patients
  - Apical fibrosis, often bilateral (a.k.a. apical cap)
    - Previously believed that this apical fibrosis represented healed tuberculosis
    - Now thought to represent a localized scarring of subpleural parenchyma due to relative underperfusion of apices
  - Focal scarring and chronic inflammation are also common at lobar tips, particularly in middle and lower lobes

MICROSCOPIC FINDINGS

General Features

- Bronchi are cartilaginous airways, usually > 1 mm in diameter
  - Bronchi conduct air, and presence of cartilage in their walls helps to prevent airway collapse
  - Cartilaginous plates (both in bronchi and trachea) may calcify with aging
    - Normal finding in older patients
  - Bronchial mucosa consists of surface epithelium, which rests on a basement membrane and elastin-rich layer of connective tissue below it
  - Submucosa is beneath mucosa and includes submucosal glands, cartilage, nerves, ganglia, and branches of bronchial artery
  - Boundary between mucosa and submucosa is not well defined histologically
    - Beyond submucosa, there is loose peribronchial connective tissue that is contiguous with pulmonary artery
  - Pseudostratified columnar epithelium includes numerous ciliated columnar cells with less frequent interspersed mucous (goblet) cells, as well as scattered and often inconspicuous neuroendocrine and basal cells
    - Goblet cell metaplasia (generally but not precisely defined as ~ 10 or more goblet cells in a row) is very common finding in smokers and in other patients with chronic airway diseases
  - As airways become smaller, there is progression from pseudostratified ciliated columnar epithelium to a more cuboidal epithelium

- Bronchioles are membranous airways without cartilage in their walls and are usually < 1 mm in diameter
  - Terminal bronchioles are nonrespiratory bronchioles just proximal to respiratory bronchioles
  - Respiratory bronchioles have alveoli budding from their walls
  - Lambert canals are direct communications between nonrespiratory bronchioles and alveoli
    - Inconspicuous under normal conditions but become more prominent in scarred airways when surrounded by metaplastic bronchiolar epithelium (a.k.a. peribronchiolar metaplasia, lambertosis, or bronchiolarization)
    - Peribronchiolar metaplasia is not a normal finding and can be seen in a number of diffuse lung diseases
- Acinus is functional unit of gas exchange
  - One definition of acinus is a single terminal bronchiole and pulmonary parenchyma distal to it
  - Others define acinus as a single respiratory bronchiole and all alveolar ducts and sacs distal to it
- Alveoli have thin walls containing rich capillary network (pulmonary microvasculature)
  - Many nuclei that appear most obvious on routine microscopic sections of alveoli are endothelial cell nuclei
  - Alveoli are lined by flat squamous type I pneumocytes
  - Cuboidal type II pneumocytes, which produce surfactant, are fewer in number
    - Although not specific to etiology, type II pneumocyte hyperplasia indicates reparative response to alveolar injury
- A few scattered intraalveolar macrophages are normal in lung
  - Pigmented pulmonary macrophages are greatly increased in smokers (respiratory bronchiolitis) as are Langerhans-type macrophages (S100, CD1a positive)
  - Although not specific to etiology, hemosiderin-laden macrophages indicate prior presence of blood within alveolar spaces; etiologies include
    - Chronic outflow obstruction (most commonly due to cardiac disease and quite rarely due to pulmonary venoocclusive disease)
    - Diffuse alveolar hemorrhage
    - Localized alveolar hemorrhage secondary to any number of causes such as infection, infarction, vasculitis, and malignancy
- Large pulmonary arteries are elastic arteries
  - Elastic fibers are relatively prominent until level of bronchi branching into bronchioles
  - At level of bronchioles, pulmonary arteries become primarily muscular arteries with well-defined internal and external elastic lamina
    - As pulmonary arteries become smaller, double elastic lamina is replaced by single elastic lamina, making a distinction from venules more difficult
  - Pulmonary veins have single lamellated elastic lamina
    - Small intraacinar pulmonary veins merge into larger pulmonary veins within interlobular septa
- Identification of pulmonary vasculature under normal and pathologic conditions rests on these defining microscopic features and vessel location, with location being more reliable of the 2 criteria under certain conditions, such as pulmonary hypertension
  - Some degree of pulmonary arteriole hyalinization, as well as pulmonary arterial and venous intimal thickening, is seen in aging individuals
- Visceral pleura is composed of outer mesothelial layer (which is easily denuded by mechanical manipulation and autolysis) with underlying connective tissue layered between 2 elastic lamina layers, and connective tissue layered at interface with alveolated parenchyma
  - In some instances, these elastic layers are distinct, and in other instances, elastic fibers are less well organized
  - Although common and not always specific to etiology, any thickening beyond these 5 layers indicates reactive response to injury
- There is lymphoid tissue associated with airways (bronchial-associated lymphoid tissue [BALT])
  - Otherwise, lymphoid tissue should be sparse or inconspicuous under normal conditions
  - Lymphatics run within bronchovascular bundles and pulmonary veins within septa and pleura
  - There are no lymphatics within alveolar walls

COMMON RESPIRATORY SYSTEM PATHOLOGY AT AUTOPSY

Bronchopneumonia

- Lungs are consolidated usually in patchy distribution and heavy with polymorphonuclear leukocytes and fibrin within airways and alveoli

Diffuse Alveolar Damage

- Diffusely consolidated and firm heavy lungs with intraalveolar hyaline membranes with variable organization

Pulmonary Edema

- May be noncardiogenic (diffuse alveolar damage) or more commonly cardiogenic at autopsy
  - Cardiogenic pulmonary edema with increased weight, congestion, and often frothy fluid in airways and microscopic alveolar capillary congestion and intraalveolar, pink-appearing edema fluid

SELECTED REFERENCES

1. Leslie KO et al: Lungs. In Mills S: Histology for Pathologists. 4th ed. Philadelphia: Lippincott Williams & Wilkins. 505-39, 2012
2. Murali R et al: The pleura in health and disease. Semin Respir Crit Care Med. 31(6):649-73, 2010
3. Van Der Spuy JC: The surgical anatomy of the pulmonary vessels. Thorax. 8(3):189-94, 1953

Lung Dissection Technique

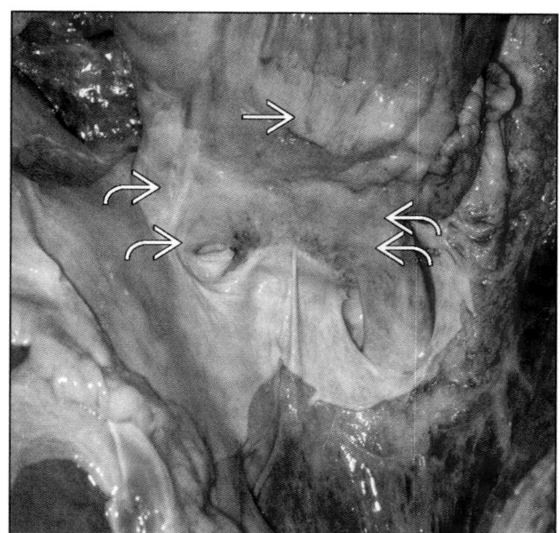

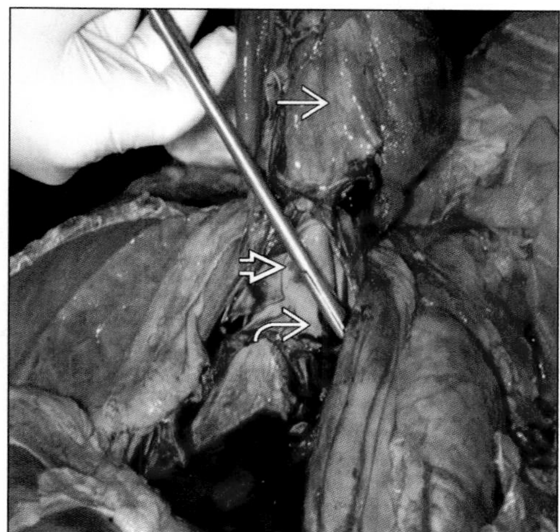

(Left) *The pericardial sac is open, and the heart ➡ is lifted up to reveal the pulmonary veins ➡ as they empty into the left atrium.* ***(Right)*** *The pericardial sac is open, the heart is lifted up ➡, and the pulmonary veins have been cut to expose the pulmonary artery. The main pulmonary artery has been opened ➡ and is being checked for a pulmonary embolus in the left pulmonary artery ➡.*

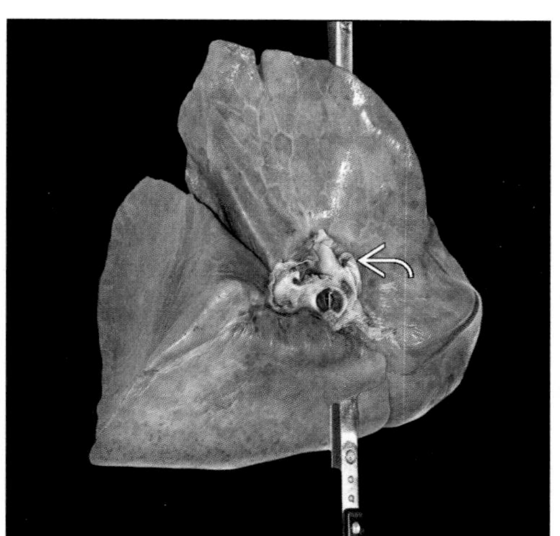

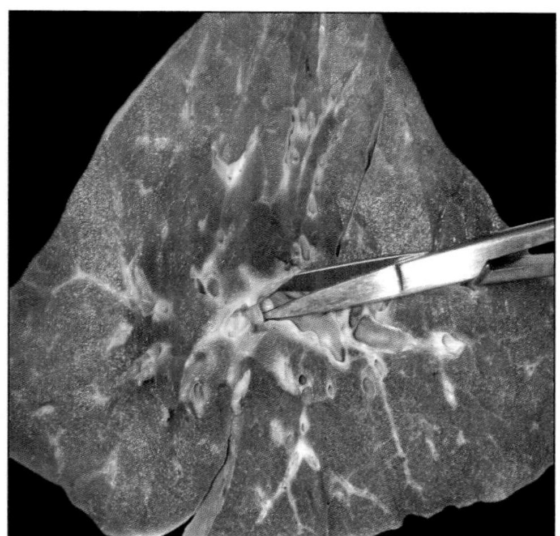

(Left) *The slab method of whole lung sectioning is illustrated here. The hilar region is facing up ➡, and the knife is used to cut a full parasagittal section from apex to base. The slices should be ≤ 2 cm in thickness.* ***(Right)*** *The next step in the slab method of whole lung sectioning is illustrated here. After the initial cuts, scissors must be used to open up partially cut airways and vessels for a complete examination.*

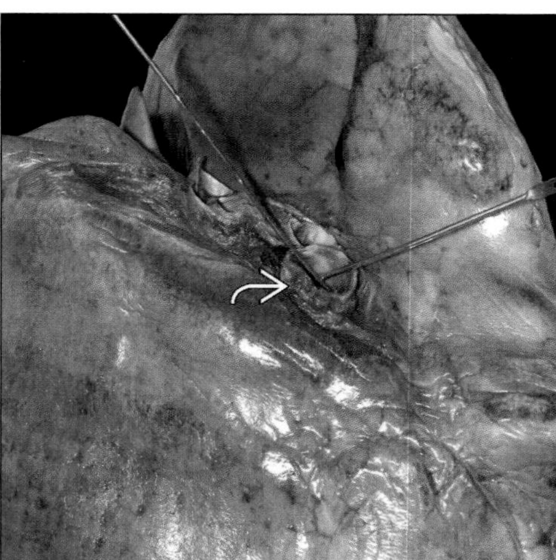

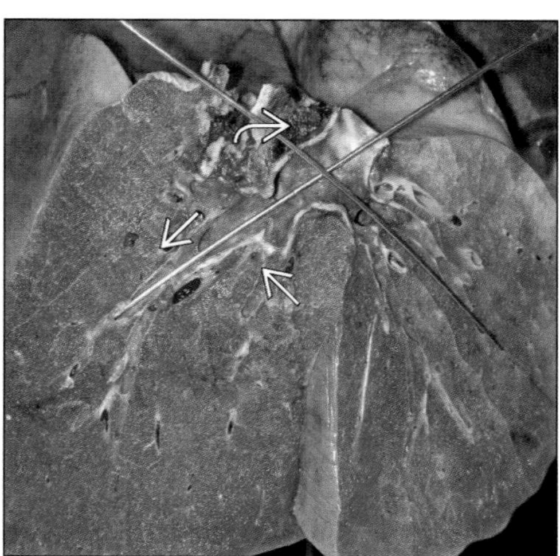

(Left) *The bronchial probe technique for sectioning the lung is demonstrated. Two probes have been inserted into the mainstem bronchus and used as a guide for sectioning ➡.* ***(Right)*** *The post probe section shows the bronchial anatomy ➡. Also note how well a hilar lymph node is exposed ➡.*

HEMATOPOIETIC SYSTEM

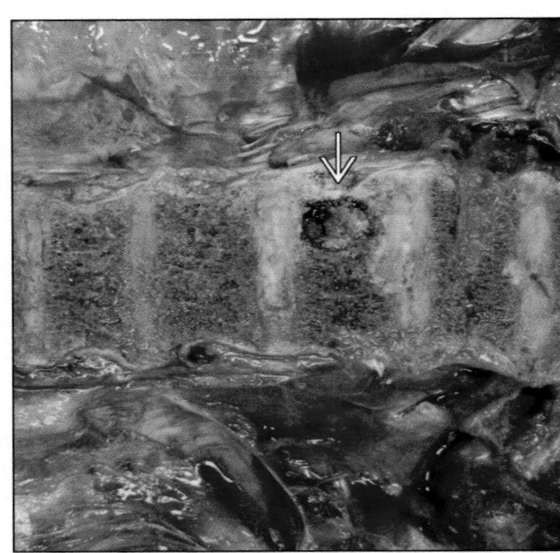

Metastasis to bone ➡ is a common complication of epithelial tumors, especially breast, prostate, and lung. This in situ image shows the lumbar vertebral column with the anterior 1/2 removed.

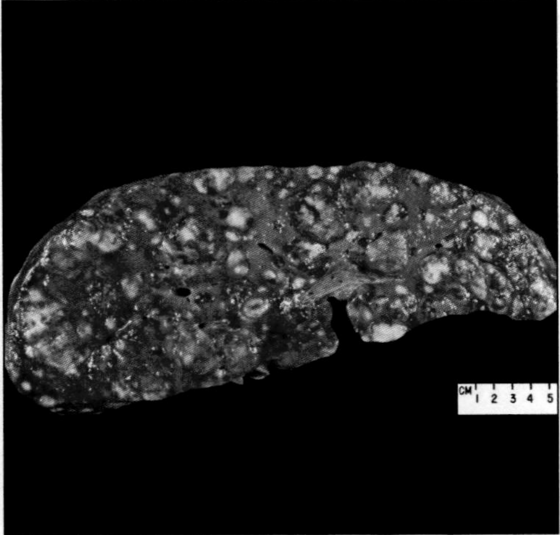

Splenomegaly may be caused by a wide variety of causes (portal hypertension, infection, hematologic disorders). Shown here is a spleen largely replaced by metastatic lung cancer.

DEFINITIONS

Hematolymphoid Tissue

- Lymph nodes
  - Normally discrete, < 1 cm greatest dimension
- Extranodal hematolymphoid tissue
  - Upper aerodigestive tract: Waldeyer ring
    - Tonsils: Pharyngeal, palatine, tubal, and lingual
    - Typically inaccessible during standard autopsy
  - Thymus
    - Located in anterior mediastinum
    - Readily identified in infants and young children
    - Usually regresses afterwards; not typically found in adults
  - Bronchial-associated lymphoid tissue (BALT)
  - Gut-associated lymphoid tissue (GALT)
    - Intraepithelial lymphocytes: Predominantly T-cells
    - Intramucosal lymphoid aggregates
    - Peyer patches
    - Mesenteric lymph nodes
  - Spleen
    - Normal weight approximately 150 grams; 10-11 cm in greatest dimension
- Bone marrow
  - Red marrow: Relatively more hematopoietic tissue, less fat
    - Confined to axial skeleton in adults
    - Found in all bones in infants
  - Yellow marrow: Relatively less hematopoietic tissue, more fat
- Peripheral blood
  - Examine smears of premortem samples retrieved from hospital laboratory if available

DISSECTION

Lymph Nodes

- Note presence and distribution of any lymphadenopathy
  - Palpate for superficial (cervical, supraclavicular, axillary, inguinal) adenopathy
- Sample any enlarged or otherwise grossly abnormal nodes
  - Consider touch prep cytology/frozen section to guide work-up
    - Suspicious for lymphoma: Save fresh tissue in appropriate cell culture medium for flow cytometry
    - Suspicious for infection: Submit tissue for culture

Spleen

- Note appearance of capsule, color, size, weight
  - Massive splenomegaly: Spleen tip extends across midline, into left lower quadrant, or into pelvis
- Take culture in cases of suspected sepsis
- Serially section, note appearance of cut surfaces
- Submit section of normal spleen and other sections as needed

Bone Marrow

- After evisceration, use saw to cut off anterior aspect of lumbar vertebrae
- Note color of bone marrow, presence or absence of masses
- Shave off a thin slice from exposed marrow, fix, decalcify, and submit a section for histology
  - Alternatively, end of rib can be squeezed with pliers; expressed marrow can be fixed, lightly decalcified, and submitted for histology; consider bone marrow smear in cases of suspect hematolymphoid malignancy involving bone marrow

    - Smears and bone marrow biopsies can be performed from posterior superior iliac spine as in living patients using bone marrow biopsy needle

Special Procedures

- Note: Complete hematopathologic evaluation may not be possible
  - Some procedures require viable cells
  - Cost of some procedures may be a barrier in autopsy setting
- Immunoperoxidase
  - Usually readily available
  - Tissue should be well preserved but need not be viable
  - Along with histology and clinical picture, often enough to establish diagnosis
- Flow cytometry: Unlikely to work on postmortem tissue unless postmortem interval is short
  - In some cases (e.g., suspected leukemia), peripheral blood flow cytometry is useful
  - Obtain premortem blood from clinical laboratory if available
- Cytogenetics: Requires viable cells; unlikely to yield results on autopsy tissue

MACROSCOPIC FINDINGS

External Examination

- Body habitus: Weight loss associated with a variety of hematologic conditions
- Skin
  - Pallor associated with anemia
  - Rashes associated with cutaneous lymphomas
  - Petechiae associated with thrombocytopenia
- Oral cavity: Gingival hyperplasia in acute monocytic leukemia

Lymph Nodes, Nonneoplastic Conditions

- Lymphadenitis
  - Typically confined to single nodal group draining a lesion
  - Some etiologic agents associated with grossly necrotizing inflammation
    - Tuberculosis: Caseating lung focus + draining bronchial nodes = Ghon complex
    - Cat scratch disease
- Infectious agents
  - EBV: Adenopathy (particularly cervical), splenomegaly, fever
  - Granulomas: Tuberculosis, some fungi, *Brucella*
    - All are dangerous respiratory pathogens
    - All pose substantial risk to autopsy personnel, use N95 particulate respirator
  - Geographic necrosis: Cat scratch (*Bartonella*)
- Chronic reactive changes
  - Preserved nodal architecture, patent sinuses
  - Follicular hyperplasia with prominent germinal centers and tingible body macrophages
  - Lots of variability in size and shape of lymphoid follicles
- Sarcoidosis
  - Epithelioid granulomas (typically without necrosis)
  - Granulomas may extensively replace nodes
  - Typically in mediastinal and peribronchial nodes
- Rheumatologic diseases
  - May be associated with lymphadenopathy
  - Other signs of connective tissue disorder often present (e.g., rash in systemic lupus erythematosus, arthritic changes in rheumatoid arthritis)

Lymph Nodes, Selected Neoplastic Conditions

- Note: Definitive diagnosis in some cases may require clinical data, gross and histologic findings, immunoperoxidase, flow cytometry, cytogenetics, and molecular testing
  - Definitive diagnosis may not be possible on autopsy material
  - Refer to appropriate references and consider consultation with hematopathologist
- Classic gross appearance of lymphoma: Enlarged nodes with tan-white, homogeneous, "fish flesh" cut surface
- Non-Hodgkin lymphoma
  - Has extranodal forms (MALT lymphoma), nodal form, and splenic form
  - B cell: Selected diagnoses
    - Diffuse large cell lymphoma: Most common B-cell lymphoma; usually rapidly growing nodes
    - Chronic lymphocytic lymphoma/small lymphocytic lymphoma: Early on, lymphocytosis; later on, lymphadenopathy, splenomegaly, anemia
    - Hairy cell leukemia: Potentially massive splenomegaly, marrow involvement with cytopenias, abdominal but not peripheral adenopathy
    - Lymphoplasmacytic lymphoma (Waldenstrom macroglobulinemia): IgM spike; 30-40% splenomegaly and lymphadenopathy
    - Follicular lymphoma: Nodes may have a grossly nodular cut surface
    - Mantle cell lymphoma: Often adenopathy, splenomegaly, and bone marrow involvement; may involve GI tract (lymphomatous polyposis coli); may have fever, weight loss
    - Burkitt lymphoma: Fastest growing tumor known
  - T cell: Selected diagnoses
    - Adult T-cell leukemia/lymphoma: Visceral involvement, skin lesions, osteolytic bone lesions, hypercalcemia
    - Enteropathy associated T-cell lymphoma: GI lymphoma; arises in background of celiac disease; can present as weight loss and diarrhea or obstruction/perforation
    - Mycosis fungoides/Sezary syndrome: Cutaneous lymphoma; variety of skin lesions; erythematous rash, plaques with adenopathy, mass lesions, erythroderma, circulating Sezary cells
    - Angioimmunoblastic T-cell lymphoma: Fever and generalized adenopathy early on; later, hepatosplenomegaly and hemolytic anemia

- Anaplastic large cell lymphoma: Adenopathy and extranodal involvement with weight loss and fever
- Hodgkin lymphoma
  - Classic Hodgkin lymphoma: Some subtypes have characteristic gross findings
    - Nodular sclerosis: Thickened fibrotic capsule and radiating bands of fibrosis; grossly nodular cut surface; typically mediastinal
    - Mixed cellularity: Often involves abdominal nodes and spleen
- Metastasis
  - Microscopic metastases often found in subcapsular sinuses first
  - Diffuse replacement by metastasis and extracapsular extension can lead to matted lymph nodes

Spleen

- Splenic Infarction
  - Wedge-shaped pale areas with base at capsular surface
  - Multiple infarcts suggest embolic cause
  - Look for other evidence of bacterial endocarditis
    - Valve vegetations, embolic infarcts in kidneys, brain
- Splenomegaly
  - Portal hypertension: May be associated with cirrhosis, ascites, esophageal varices
  - Hematolymphoid disorders
    - Splenic marginal zone lymphoma: Splenomegaly, adenopathy confined to splenic hilum; bone marrow involvement; circulating villous lymphocytes
    - Myeloproliferative disorders: Potentially massive splenomegaly, marrow abnormalities, teardrop red cells
    - Hodgkin lymphoma
  - Thalassemia major: Potentially massive splenomegaly from massive extramedullary hematopoiesis (EMH)
    - Skull and other bone deformities: Result of massive chronic EMH
    - Skin ulcerations
    - Hepatomegaly
    - Bilirubin gallstones
    - Changes 2° to transfusion-related iron overload
  - Amyloidosis: Firm, abnormally pale, waxy cut surfaces
    - Follicular deposition of amyloid: Sago spleen
    - Diffuse deposition of amyloid: Lardaceous spleen
    - Other organs may be involved
  - Storage diseases
    - Gaucher disease: Diffusely fine granular cut surface
    - Glycogen storage disorders
  - Infectious diseases
    - Visceral leishmaniasis (kala-azar)
    - Schistosomiasis when associated with portal hypertension
  - Rheumatologic conditions
    - Felty syndrome: Rheumatoid arthritis, splenomegaly, neutropenia
- Splenic atrophy and autosplenectomy associated with sickle cell anemia
  - Splenomegaly may occur early in course of disease
  - Increases risk for infections especially with encapsulated bacteria
- Splenic lacerations
  - Often associated with fractures of left lower ribs
  - Can be seen associated with EBV (mononucleosis)

Bone Marrow

- Multiple myeloma
  - Pallor secondary to anemia
  - Findings related to thrombocytopenia: Ecchymoses and purpura
  - Plasmacytomas: Soft tissue masses composed of plasma cells; can occur anywhere
  - Lytic bone lesions and pathologic bone fractures, particularly axial skeleton
  - Paraprotein-related renal disease: Myeloma cast nephropathy, amyloidosis, light chain deposition disease, consider immunofluorescence and ultrastructural studies on renal tissue
  - Changes secondary to amyloidosis: Skin and shoulder joint nodules, macroglossia, peripalpebral purpura ("raccoon eyes")
- Leukemia
  - Marrow: Often no gross abnormalities; histologic evaluation is essential
  - Visibly thickened buffy coat layer in tubes of peripheral blood
  - Pallor from anemia
  - Ecchymoses and purpura from thrombocytopenia
  - Infectious complications secondary neutropenia
- Metastasis: Often thoracolumbar
  - 3rd most common site of epithelial metastasis (after lungs and liver)
  - 73% of patients dying of breast cancer and 68% dying of prostate cancer have bony metastases
  - Lung, thyroid, and renal tumors also frequently metastasize to bone

Thymus

- Thymoma
  - May be associated with myasthenia gravis
  - Tan-pink cut surface; cystic changes common
- Thymic hyperplasia: Enlargement of thymus due to lymphoid infiltration (lymphoid hyperplasia, enlargement without inflammatory infiltration: True thymic hyperplasia)
  - Lymphoid hyperplasia has increased numbers of germinal centers and is most frequently associated with myasthenia gravis but may be seen in other autoimmune diseases
  - True thymic hyperplasia has normal-appearing thymus histologically: May be associated with endocrine abnormalities (Graves disease), sarcoidosis, and Beckwith Wiedemann syndrome or can be rebound after stress such as steroid therapy or chemotherapy

GALT

- Hyperplastic Peyer patches

- Seen with variety of infections; classically described with *Salmonella typhi*
- In infants and young children, can serve as lead point for intussusception

- Extranodal marginal zone lymphoma (MALToma)
  - Fleshy mass lesion
    - May perforate or cause obstruction
  - Most commonly gastric

MICROSCOPIC FINDINGS

Lymph Nodes

- Non-Hodgkin lymphoma: General comments
  - In most cases, normal nodal architecture completely effaced by infiltrate of malignant lymphocytes
    - Loss of subcapsular sinuses and germinal centers
- Hodgkin lymphoma: General comments
  - Diagnosis rests on identification of Reed-Sternberg (RS) cells and variants
    - Classic RS cell: Large, atypical cell, binucleated with prominent ("owl eyes") nucleoli; positive with immunoperoxidase for CD15 and CD30
    - RS cells are rare (a few percent); background of benign mixed inflammatory cells
  - Subtypes
    - Nodular sclerosing: RS and lacunar cells on inflammatory background; node divided by fibrotic bands (60-80% of cases)
    - Mixed cellularity: Diffuse mixed inflammatory infiltrate and classic RS cells (15-30%)
    - Lymphocyte-rich: RS or lacunar cells on predominantly lymphocytic background (5%)
    - Lymphocyte-depleted: Scant background, many RS cells and bizarre variants readily identifiable (< 1%)
    - Nodular lymphocyte-predominant: Rare or absent RS cells; lymphocytic and histiocytic cells CD20(+), CD15(-), CD30(-)

Marrow

- Leukemia
  - Acute leukemias: Requires > 20% blasts in marrow aspirate
    - Blasts are CD34(+)
  - Acute myelogenous leukemia
    - Decreased/absent mature granulocytes
    - Myeloblasts: Cytoplasmic granules, Auer rods; CD33(+), CD13(+)
  - Acute lymphoblastic lymphoma
    - Blasts usually lack granules
    - Lymphoblasts: TdT(+), pax-5(+), CD22(+)
- Multiple myeloma
  - > 30% plasma cells in bone marrow aspirate; CD138(+)
  - Immature/atypical plasma cells often present
  - May be accompanied by paraprotein in blood/urine
- Myeloproliferative disorders
  - Polycythemia vera: ↑ erythroid precursors, ↑ hematocrit, splenomegaly, *JAK2* mutation
  - Essential thrombocytosis: ↑ megakaryocytes, ↑ platelet count
  - Chronic myelogenous leukemia (CML): Increase in immature red and white cell precursors, splenomegaly, Philadelphia chromosome
  - Agnogenic myeloid metaplasia: Marrow fibrosis, teardrop red cells

Thymus

- Thymoma: Biphasic tumor composed of epithelial cells (plump or spindle shaped) and nonneoplastic lymphocytes

Peripheral Blood

- Red cell abnormalities
  - Sickle cell anemia: Sickle-shaped red cells, commonly in areas of low oxygen tension
  - Thalassemia major: Target cells
  - Parasites
    - Malaria: Intraerythrocytic ring-shaped trophozoites; extracellular forms
    - *Babesia*: Intraerythrocytic ring trophozoites
    - Trypanosomes: *Trypanosoma cruzi*, *Trypanosoma brucei*
    - Worms: *Brugia malayi*, *Wuchereria bancrofti*, *Loa loa*
- White cell abnormalities
  - Leukemia: Circulating immature forms
    - Acute leukemias: Decreased mature forms and circulating blasts
    - CML: Erythroid and white cell precursors of every stage of maturity ("circulating marrow")
  - Sezary syndrome: Circulating medium to large T cells with cerebriform nuclei

SELECTED REFERENCES

1. Podduturi V et al: A case series of clinically undiagnosed hematopoietic neoplasms discovered at autopsy. Am J Clin Pathol. 143(6):854-60, 2015
2. Podduturi V et al: Sickle cell trait as a contributory cause of death in natural disease. J Forensic Sci. 60(3):807-11, 2015
3. Al-Salem AH: Splenic complications of sickle cell anemia and the role of splenectomy. ISRN Hematol. 2011:864257, 2011
4. Sens MA et al: Unexpected neoplasia in autopsies: potential implications for tissue and organ safety. Arch Pathol Lab Med. 133(12):1923-31, 2009
5. Coleman RE: Clinical features of metastatic bone disease and risk of skeletal morbidity. Clin Cancer Res. 12(20 Pt 2):6243s-6249s, 2006

Gross and Microscopic Features

*(**Left**) This image shows the cut surface of a thymoma taken from a patient with myasthenia gravis. The thymus is not typically grossly visible in adults, but remnants may be found in the adipose tissue in anterior mediastinum. (**Right**) Many conditions can cause splenomegaly. The differential diagnosis for massive splenomegaly is more limited. Massive splenomegaly (spleen tip in LLQ or pelvis or across midline) is most often seen in myeloproliferative disorders, certain lymphomas, thalassemia major, Gaucher disease, and kala-azar.*

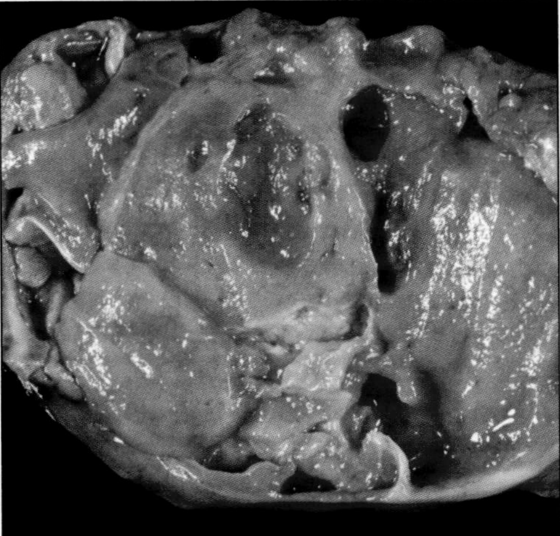

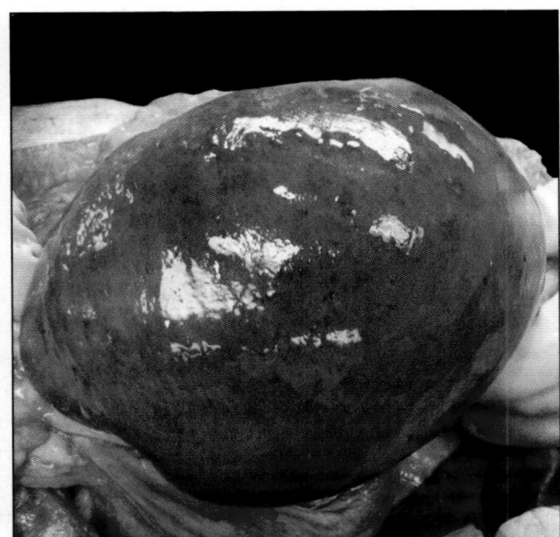

*(**Left**) This cluster of enlarged, matted, lymph nodes ➡ was found in a patient with a high-grade B-cell lymphoma. Note the tan-pink, homogeneous, "fish flesh" appearance. (**Right**) This section of a lymph node with follicular lymphoma shows replacement of the normal nodal architecture by follicles ➡ that lack the germinal centers and tingible macrophages seen in benign follicular hyperplasia.*

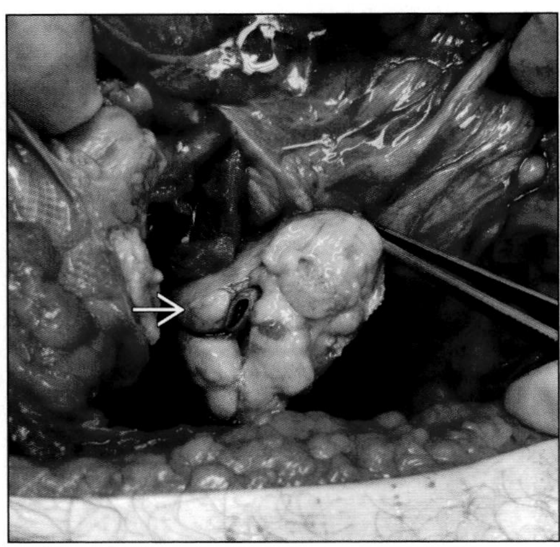

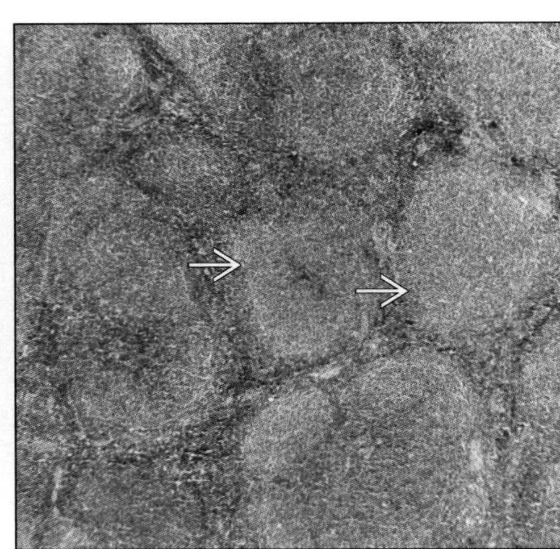

*(**Left**) Lymph nodes involved in sarcoidosis typically show diffuse involvement by epithelioid granulomas ➡ without central necrosis, although necrosis can occasionally be seen. (**Right**) Classic Hodgkin lymphoma is most typically characterized by large, atypical, binucleate Reed-Sternberg cells ➡ with prominent eosinophilic nucleoli (and variants thereof) on a background of benign mixed inflammatory cells.*

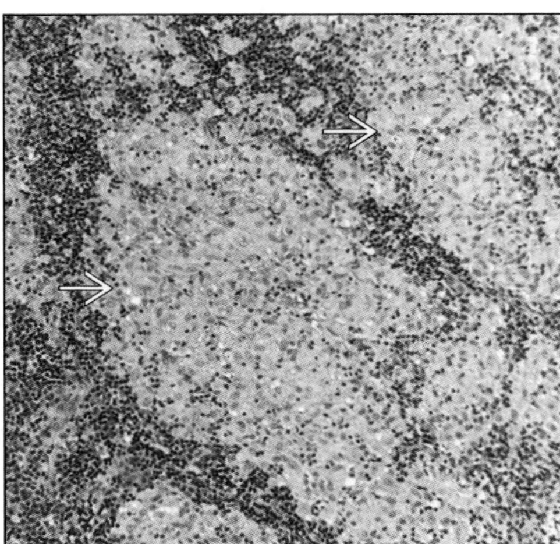

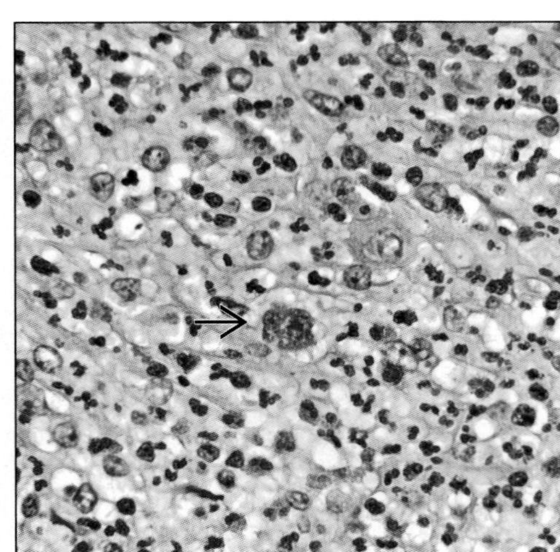

Bone Marrow Examination

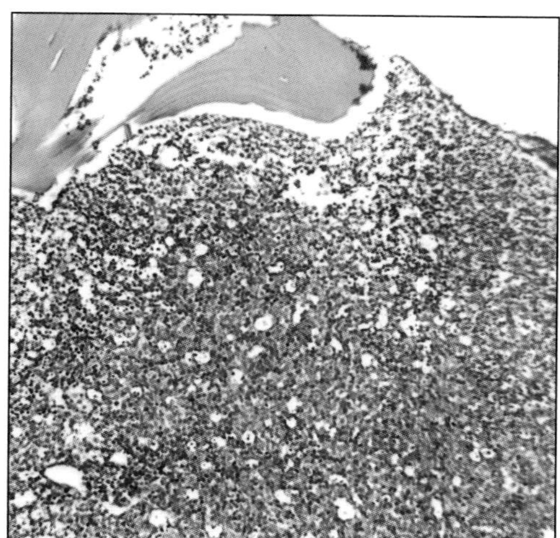

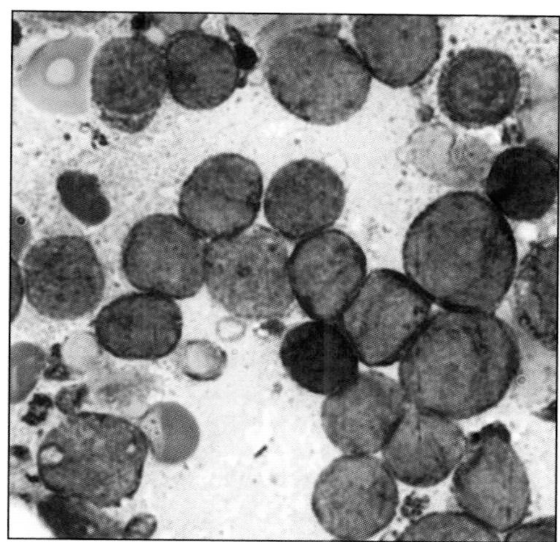

(Left) *Acute leukemia is typically characterized by a hypercellular bone marrow (note the near complete lack of fat), decrease or absence of mature forms, and increase in blasts.* ***(Right)*** *This high-power field shows monotonous blast cells with a remarkably increased nucleus:cytoplasm ratio (just a thin rim of cytoplasm is visible) and "cookie cutter" nucleoli. Note that no mature leukocytes are visible. A definitive distinction between AML and ALL often requires special testing.*

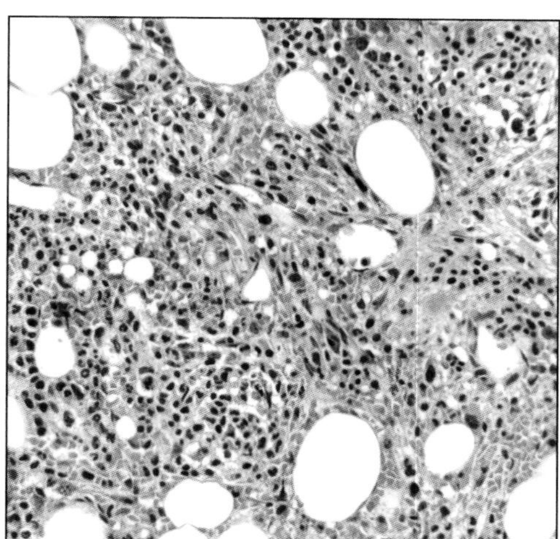

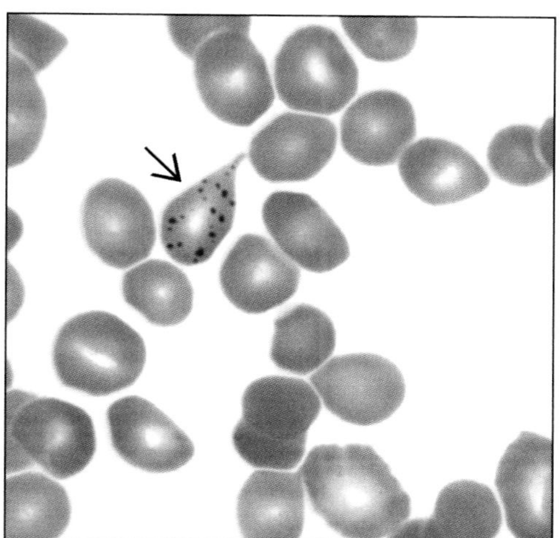

(Left) *This marrow was taken from a patient with agnogenic myeloid metaplasia (a.k.a. myelofibrosis). Note the marrow fibrosis. Most patients also have splenomegaly, sometimes massive splenomegaly.* ***(Right)*** *This Wright-Giemsa-stained smear of peripheral blood from a patient with agnogenic myeloid metaplasia shows a teardrop-shaped red cell ⇨. Teardrop cells (or dacrocytes) can also be seen in other disorders that replace the marrow.*

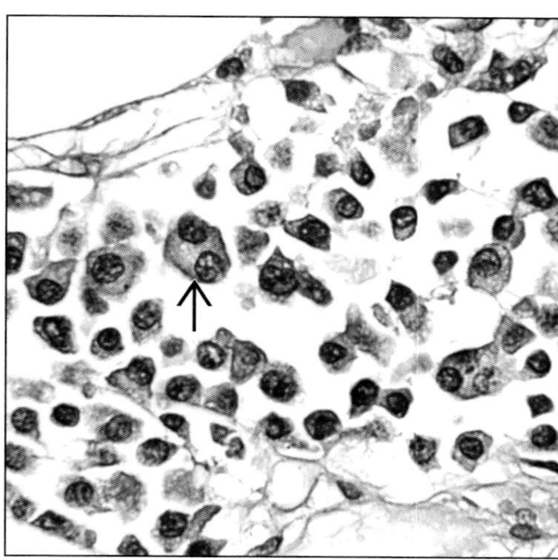

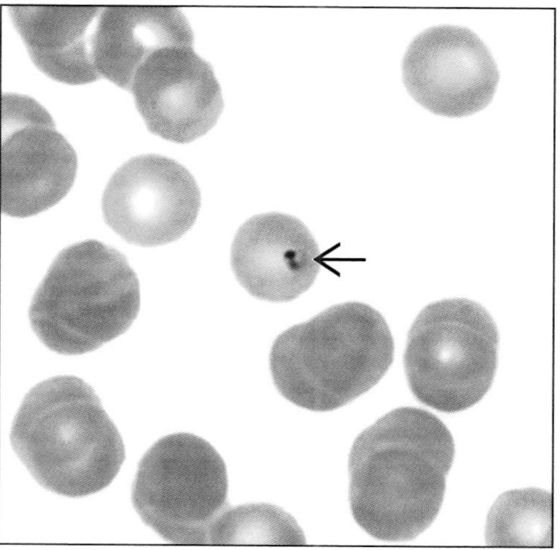

(Left) *This section of bone marrow from a patient who died with multiple myeloma shows near complete replacement of normal marrow elements by plasma cells including a binucleate plasma cell ⇨.* ***(Right)*** *This Wright-stained peripheral blood smear shows an intraerythrocytic ring-shaped trophozoite ⇨. In the absence of extracellular parasitic forms, it may be hard to distinguish between Babesia and malaria. Travel history is essential.*

GASTROINTESTINAL SYSTEM

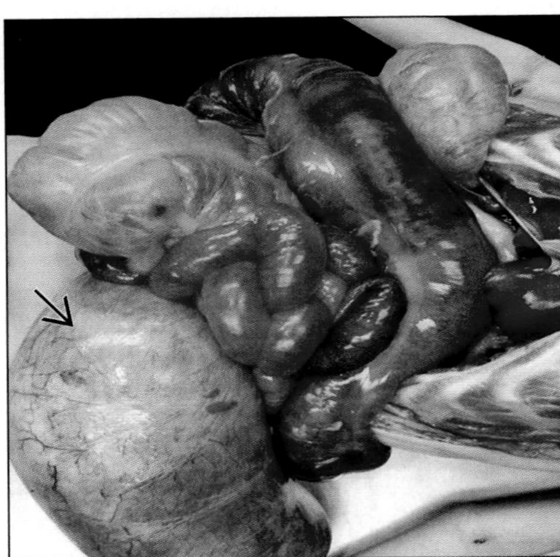

Colonic dilatation > 12 cm ⇒ that is not caused by mechanical obstruction is often referred to as megacolon. The abdomen is typically distended and tympanitic.

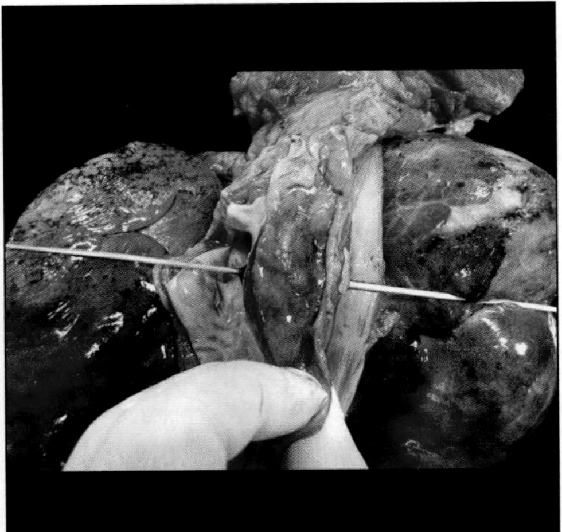

Aortoesophageal fistula (demonstrated with the probe) is a rare, often fatal cause of upper gastrointestinal hemorrhage. It usually arises in the setting of aortic pathology such as an aortic aneurysm.

TERMINOLOGY

Definitions

- Upper gastrointestinal (GI) tract: From lips to ligament of Treitz
  - Esophagus, stomach, duodenum, pancreas, extrahepatic biliary tree
- Lower gastrointestinal tract: From ligament of Treitz to anus
  - Jejunum, ileum, ascending colon, transverse colon, descending colon, sigmoid colon, rectum

DISSECTION OF GASTROINTESTINAL TRACT

Handling of Gastrointestinal Tract

- If taking cultures, do so **before** manipulating GI tract
- Open, rinse, and examine entire GI tract
  - Rinse in cold water
  - Do not rub mucosae
- Fix thoroughly; autolysis occurs soon after death

Dissection of Lower GI Tract

- Retract greater omentum and transverse colon upward and displace small bowel to right
  - Ligament of Treitz is visible where small bowel emerges from retroperitoneum
- Place 2 ties around proximal jejunum and transect jejunum between them
- Free jejunum and rest of small bowel from mesentery
  - 1st alternative
    - Hold cut end of jejunum in nondominant hand to apply traction
    - Use scalpel with a violin bow motion to cut mesentery near its attachment to bowel
  - 2nd alternative
    - Use scissors to cut through mesentery near its attachment to small bowel
- Free colon from its mesenteries and attachments to body wall
  - Use scissors, scalpel, or blunt dissection
  - Expect resistance at cecum and gastrocolic ligament
- Place 2 ties around distal sigmoid colon and transect between them
- Open intestines using an enterotome (scissors with a blunt leading blade)
  - Insert blunt end into bowel lumen; do not snip
  - Hold enterotome open (~ 45°) and pull antimesenteric side downward onto hinge

Dissection of Upper GI Tract

- Use scissors or scalpel to free gallbladder from hepatic bed
- Cut hepatic duct, portal vessels, inferior and superior vena cava
- Remove liver from upper GI tract
- Free esophagus from laryngopharynx, posterior trachea, and aorta
- Leaving biliary tract and pancreas attached to duodenum, free stomach and duodenum from aorta
- Open esophagus along posterior midline
- Continue cut along greater curvature of stomach
- Continue cut to open duodenum, taking care to preserve ampulla of Vater

Dissection of Biliary Tree

- Gently squeeze gallbladder and look for appearance of bile at ampulla of Vater
- Probe common bile duct into ampulla of Vater
- Open gallbladder, hepatic duct, and common bile duct

Dissection of Pancreas

- 1st alternative
  - Transect tail of pancreas to identify pancreatic duct
  - Insert a fine probe into pancreatic duct
  - Use probe as a guide and bisect pancreas lengthwise along duct

- Leave half of pancreas with exposed duct attached to duodenum
  - Probe proximal pancreatic duct into ampulla of Vater
- 2nd alternative
  - Serially cross section tail and body of pancreas
  - Probe proximal pancreatic duct into ampulla of Vater

Special Procedures

- Eversion of esophagus (to identify esophageal varices)
  - Use a forceps to thread a string down proximal end of unopened esophagus and into stomach
  - Tie opposite end around proximal end of esophagus
  - Open stomach along greater curvature
  - Grasp free end of string and pull to evert esophagus
- Inflation of gastrointestinal segment
  - Clamp one end of specimen closed
  - Rinse with cold water to remove contents
  - Fill specimen with formalin and clamp open end
  - Fix overnight
  - Use scissors to open fixed specimen

Sections for Microscopy

- Sample any grossly abnormal tissues
- Sections of grossly normal tissue will vary according to local practice
- Suggested sections of normal tissue
  - Section of gastroesophageal junction
  - Section of small bowel
  - Section of colon
  - Section of pancreas

MACROSCOPIC FINDINGS

External Examination

- Body habitus
  - Cachexia
- Mouth, nose, anus
  - Evidence of frank blood, melena, "coffee ground" emesis
- Skin
  - Surgical scars
  - Pallor of skin, possibly due to mucous membranes, could indicate anemia and GI hemorrhage
  - Jaundice
    - Association with portal hypertension, cirrhosis, ascites
    - Risk of GI hemorrhage
    - Consider everting esophagus to demonstrate varices
  - Umbilical (Sister Mary Joseph) nodule
    - 50% associated with GI malignancy
  - Ostomies: GI diversion
- Taut abdominal distension
  - Peritonitis, ruptured viscus, toxic megacolon

In Situ Examination of Organs

- Inspect any anastomoses (especially recent)
- If evidence of peritonitis, attempt to locate source
- Intraluminal blood is often visible through walls of bowel
- Note presence, characteristics (fibrinous, fibrous, dense, fine) of adhesions
- Note presence, characteristics (location, contents, incarceration) of any hernias
- Endometriosis
  - Serosal-based implants/lesions with variable appearance
  - Red, bluish, powder burn black, white and fibrous
  - May cause fibrosis and kinking of involved bowel segments

Esophagus

- Structural
  - Zenker diverticulum: Outpocketing of posterior pharyngeal wall just above esophagus
  - Mallory-Weiss tears: Linear, longitudinal tears in mucosa, usually distal
  - Rupture (Boerhaave syndrome): Usually in left lower esophagus
- Infectious: More common in immunosuppressed patients
  - Candida: White plaques
  - Herpes: Blisters early on, followed by ulcers
  - CMV: Single or multiple ulcers, especially in distal esophagus
- Inflammatory
  - Reflux esophagitis: Most common cause of symptomatic esophagitis
    - Erythema in distal esophagus ± ulceration
  - Barrett esophagus
    - Velvety tan-red mucosa in distal esophagus/GEJ
  - Eosinophilic esophagitis
    - "Corrugated" esophagus with concentric mucosal rings
  - Chemical esophagitis
- Neoplastic
  - Squamous cell carcinoma
  - Adenocarcinoma
    - Typically in distal esophagus
    - May arise in setting of Barrett esophagus with dysplasia
- Miscellaneous
  - Esophageal varices
    - Dilated esophageal submucosal veins in patients with portal hypertension
    - May see associated cirrhosis, ascites, splenomegaly
    - May collapse postmortem; consider everting esophagus to demonstrate them
  - Acute esophageal necrosis ("black esophagus")
    - Friable black distal mucosa; stops abruptly at GE junction
  - Aortoesophageal fistula

Stomach

- Infectious/inflammatory
  - Acute gastritis
    - Associated with aspirin, ethanol, smoking, shock, chemical irritation
    - Hyperemia ± erosions, hemorrhages
  - Chronic gastritis
    - Associations: Ethanol, smoking, *Helicobacter pylori*, pernicious anemia

        - Mucosal hyperemia and mucosal flattening
    - Peptic ulcer disease
        - Sharply punched-out gastric or duodenal ulcers without raised edges
        - May be associated with *H. pylori*
        - Multiple ulcers &/or ulcers in unusual locations should suggest Zollinger-Ellison syndrome
    - Stress ulcers
        - Typical lesions: Punctate, scattered areas of dark red discoloration and mucosal hemorrhage
        - Seen in patients with severe acute illnesses: Trauma, burns, sepsis, shock, increased intracranial pressure
    - Wischnewski ulcers
        - Multiple submucosal hemorrhages ("leopard spots")
        - Associated with hypothermia
- Hypertrophic gastropathy: Giant cerebriform rugal folds
    - Menetrier disease
        - Excessive mucus production, protein loss, decreased acid
    - Gastric gland hyperplasia secondary to Zollinger-Ellison syndrome
        - Gastrin producing pancreatic tumor → increased acid production
        - Increased acid, associated with multiple refractory peptic ulcers
        - **Almost 25% of patients with multiple gastrinomas will have multiple endocrine neoplasia type I; examine pituitary and parathyroids**
    - Hypertrophic-hypersecretory gastropathy
        - Hyperplasia of parietal and chief cells
        - Increased acid, associated with multiple refractory peptic ulcers
- Neoplastic
    - Gastric polyps
        - Fundic gland polyps
        - Hyperplastic polyps
    - Adenocarcinoma
        - Intestinal type: Raised, sometimes ulcerated masses
        - Diffuse type (a.k.a. signet ring cell type, leather bottle stomach, linitis plastica): Diffuse infiltration of gastric wall without obvious mass
    - Lymphoma: Usually extranodal marginal B-cell lymphoma
        - Homogeneous, tan-white, "fish flesh" cut surface
        - May be associated with chronic *H. pylori* infection
    - Gastrointestinal stromal tumor (GIST): Typically exophytic subserosal masses
- Miscellaneous
    - Bezoar: Mass of undigested material
        - Vegetable material (most common), hair, medications, etc.

Small Intestine

- Structural/mechanical
    - Hernias
    - Meckel diverticulum: Vitelline duct remnant
        - 2-3 feet proximal to cecum
        - May contain heterotopic gastric or pancreatic tissue
    - Volvulus
        - Twisting of bowel along its mesentery
        - Dilation and hyperemia proximal to obstruction
- Infectious/inflammatory
    - Celiac disease
        - Flattening of mucosal villi; increased intraepithelial lymphocytes
        - May be associated with weight loss and diarrhea
        - Laboratory testing: Antigliadin and anti-tissue transglutaminase antibodies, HLADQ2 and DQ8
    - Inflammatory bowel disease (IBD)
        - Chronic active inflammatory process
        - Ulcerative colitis: Involves rectum and can extend proximally; no skip areas; inflammation confined to mucosa and submucosa, does not involve upper GI
        - Crohn disease: Usually focused in lower GI, but can involve any portion of GI tract; can show skip areas, transmural inflammation with wall thickening
- Ischemia
    - Affected segment: Dusky, dark red-purple, congested; may progress to black color and necrosis
    - Examine mesenteric vessels
- Neoplastic
    - Neuroendocrine (carcinoid) tumors: Most common primary tumor of small bowel
        - If metastatic to liver, may be associated with carcinoid syndrome
    - Adenocarcinoma: Much less common than colonic adenocarcinoma
    - GIST
    - Lymphoma
        - Usually extranodal marginal zone B-cell lymphoma
        - T-cell lymphomas may arise in setting of celiac disease

Colon and Rectum

- Structural
    - Diverticular disease
        - At mesenteric border, near point of penetration of small vessels
        - May be associated with abscess formation and fistula formation
    - Volvulus: Can lead to ischemia and necrosis
        - Sigmoid is most common location, especially older patients; associated with constipation
        - Cecum 2nd most common location
- Infectious/inflammatory
    - Bacterial, viral infections
    - Antibiotic-associated (*Clostridium difficile*) colitis
        - Characteristic adherent yellow plaques (pseudomembranes)
    - IBD
        - Ulcerative colitis and Crohn disease
        - Crohn disease may be associated with fistula formation, sinus tracts
- Ischemia

  - Affected segments dusky dark red-purple; can progress to black and necrotic
  - May be result of low flow or vascular occlusion (e.g., by thromboemboli)
  - Watershed areas (splenic flexure and rectosigmoid junction) are particularly vulnerable
- Neoplastic
  - Hyperplastic and serrated polyps
  - Juvenile polyps
  - Neuroendocrine tumors (carcinoid tumors)
    - Submucosal, yellowish mass
    - Especially common in rectum and tip of appendix
  - Adenomas
    - Tubular, villous, tubulovillous
    - 30% of adults at autopsy
    - ↑ risk of carcinoma if numerous polyps, family history, > 1 cm size
  - Leiomyomas
  - GIST
  - Adenocarcinoma
    - 98% of colonic malignancies
  - Neuroendocrine (carcinoid) tumors
- Miscellaneous
  - Megacolon
    - Diameter > 12 cm (varies)
    - Congenital or acquired
  - Stercoral ulcers
    - Abrasions from hard stool
    - Commonly seen in debilitated patients

Appendix

- Inflammation/infection
  - Appendicitis
    - Idiopathic
    - Obstructive: Fecalith, tumor, lymphoid hyperplasia, *Enterobius vermicularis*
    - *Yersinia enterocolitica*: granulomatous appendicitis
  - IBD
- Neoplasms
  - Adenoma
  - Adenocarcinoma
  - Mucinous adenocarcinoma
    - May be associated with pseudomyxoma peritonei
  - Neuroendocrine tumors (carcinoids)

MICROSCOPIC FINDINGS

Some Characteristic Microscopic Findings

- Eosinophilic esophagitis
  - Eosinophilic infiltrate, often patchy, with foci showing > 15 eosinophils per high-power field
  - Epithelial hyperplasia
- Reflux esophagitis
  - Elongated epithelial pegs and mild eosinophilic infiltrate
- Barrett esophagus
  - Intestinal metaplasia of gastric mucosa at gastroesophageal junction
  - Dysplasia in Barrett associated with ↑ risk of adenocarcinoma
- Gastric adenocarcinoma
  - Intestinal type: Infiltrating malignant glands
  - Diffuse type: Infiltrate of signet ring cells without obvious mass
    - Signet ring cells may be mistaken for inflammatory cells
    - Tumor cells will stain for keratin and intracytoplasmic mucin
    - Will be negative for E-cadherin
- Neuroendocrine (carcinoid) tumor
  - Cords and trabeculae of monotonous cells
  - Nuclei with fine chromatin
- GIST
  - Arise from interstitial cells of Cajal in intramuscular neural plexus
  - May be spindle celled or epithelioid
- Inflammatory bowel disease
  - Features common to ulcerative colitis and Crohn disease
    - Acute changes: Neutrophils, cryptitis, crypt abscess
    - Chronic changes: Regenerative changes with branched crypts, ↑ lymphocytes in lamina propria
  - Ulcerative colitis
    - Typically limited to mucosa; no thickening of bowel wall
    - No granulomas
  - Crohn disease
    - May involve full thickness of bowel wall
    - May be associated with sinus and fistula formation
    - Granulomas may be seen

SELECTED REFERENCES

1. Epelboym I et al: Zollinger-Ellison syndrome: classical considerations and current controversies. Oncologist. 19(1):44-50, 2014
2. Ishida M et al: Intravascular gas distribution in the upper abdomen of non-traumatic in-hospital death cases on postmortem computed tomography. Leg Med (Tokyo). 13(4):174-9, 2011
3. Finkbeiner WE et al. Autopsy Pathology: A Manual and Atlas. Philadelphia: Saunders/Elsevier, 2009
4. Rose AG.Atlas of gross Pathology with Histologic Correlation. New York: Cambridge University Press, 2008
5. Ludwig J. Current Methods of Autopsy Practice. 2nd ed. Philadelphia: W.B. Saunders, 1979

Removal of Gastrointestinal Tract

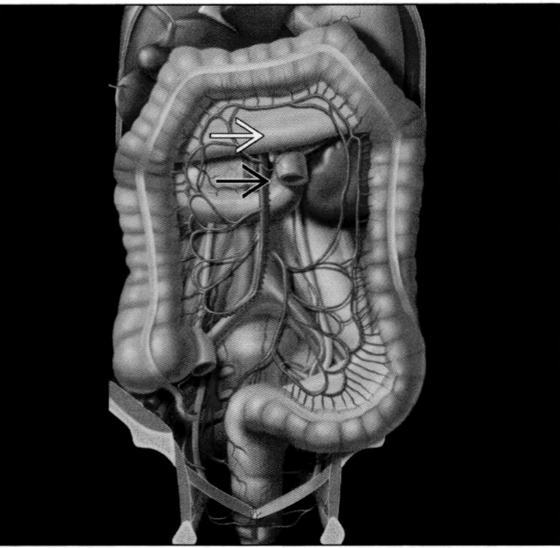
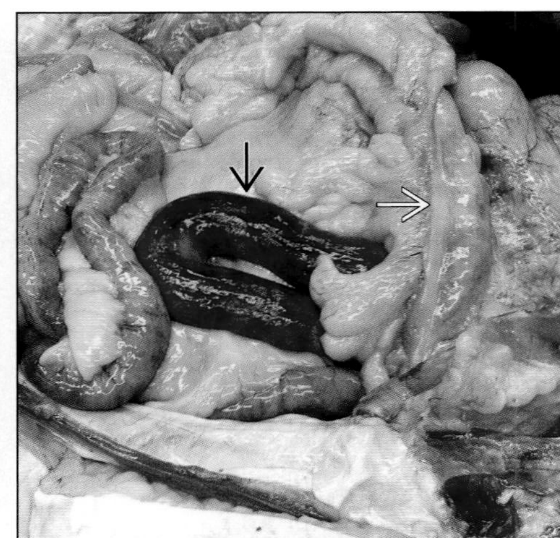

(Left) *The ligament of Treitz separates the distal duodenum from the jejunum. It can be located by lifting the transverse colon with the attached gastrocolic ligament ➡ and pushing the small bowel (previously removed in this diagram) to the right. The proximal jejunum ➡ can be seen emerging from the retroperitoneum to the left of the midline.* ***(Right)*** *The congested jejunum ➡ can be seen emerging from the retroperitoneum below the transverse colon ➡.*

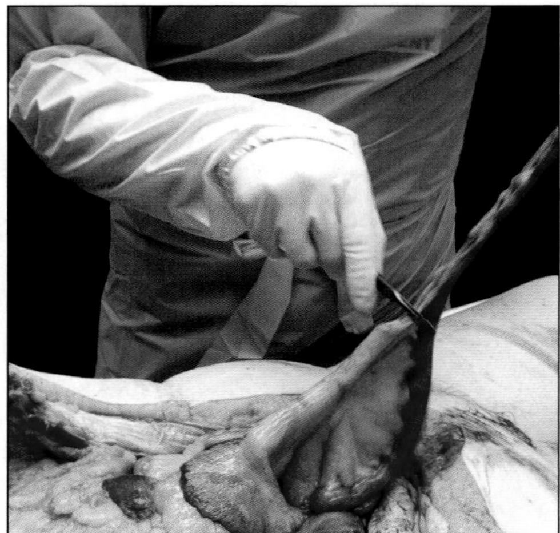
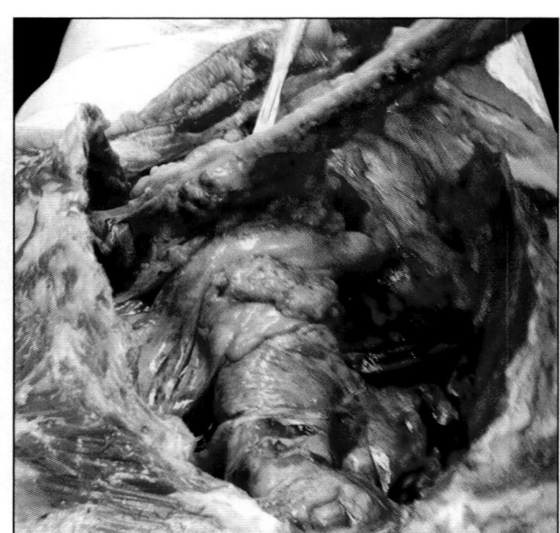

(Left) *To remove the small bowel, the free end is held in the nondominant hand and traction is applied to render the attachment to the mesentery taut. A scalpel is used in a violin bow motion to progressively free the small bowel near its attachment to the mesentery.* ***(Right)*** *The colon can be freed from its attachments to its mesenteries and the body wall by using a scalpel (shown), scissors, or by blunt dissection.*

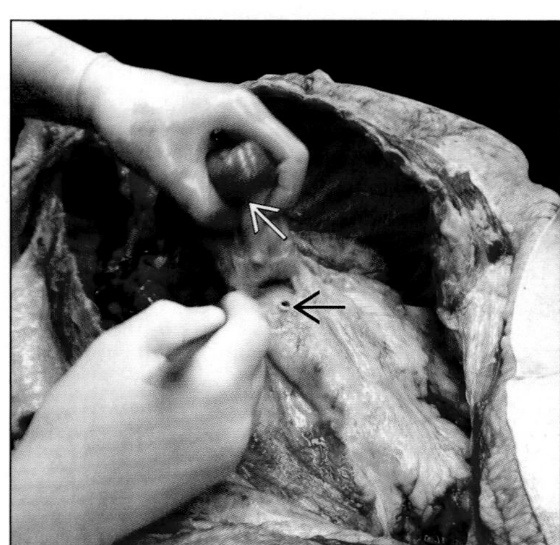
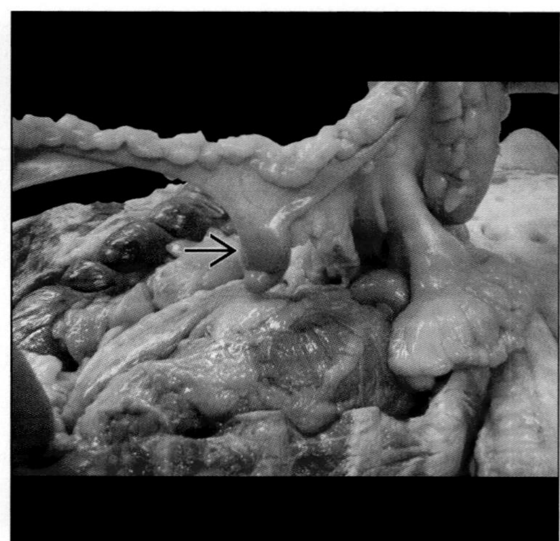

(Left) *Here the duodenum ➡ is being freed from its vascular attachments. The cut end of the superior mesenteric artery ➡ can be seen.* ***(Right)*** *Meckel diverticulum is shown ➡, a remnant of the embryonic vitelline duct. It typically arises 2-3 feet from the cecum and may contain ectopic gastric or pancreatic tissue.*

Esophagus and Stomach

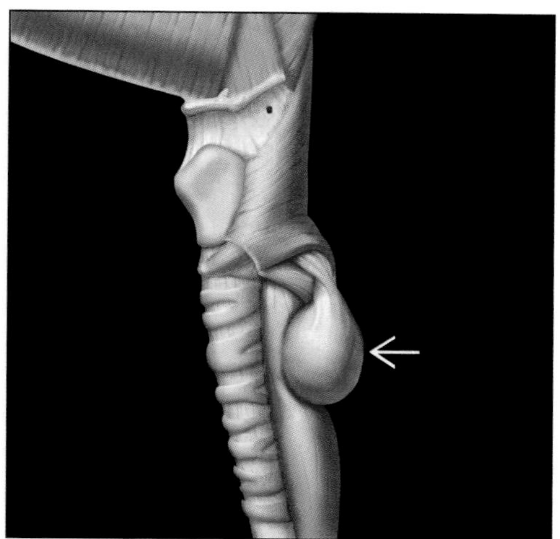

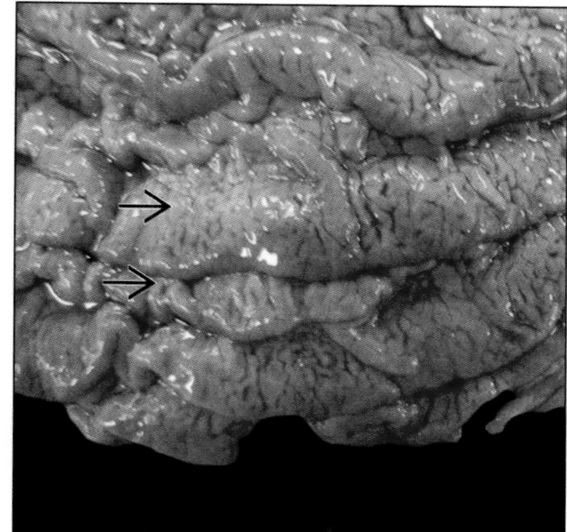

(Left) Zenker diverticulum ➡ is an outpocketing of the mucosa and submucosa of the pharynx that arises immediately above the upper esophageal sphincter. *(Right)* The mucosal surface of this stomach shows the thickened, cerebriform mucosal folds ➡ that characterize hypertrophic gastropathy. This was a case of hypertrophic-hypersecretory gastropathy, Menetrier syndrome, and Zollinger syndrome may appear similar.

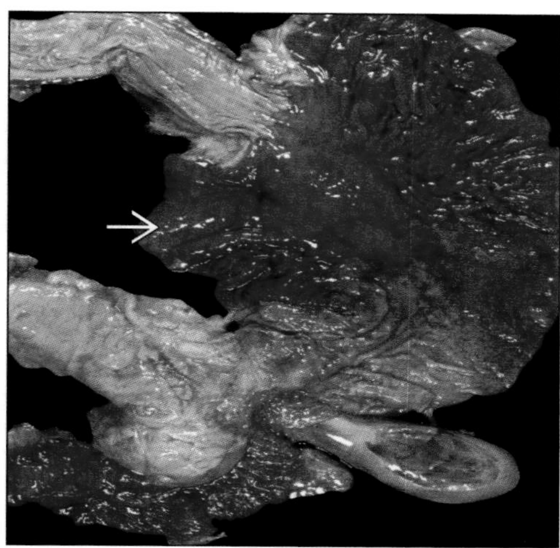

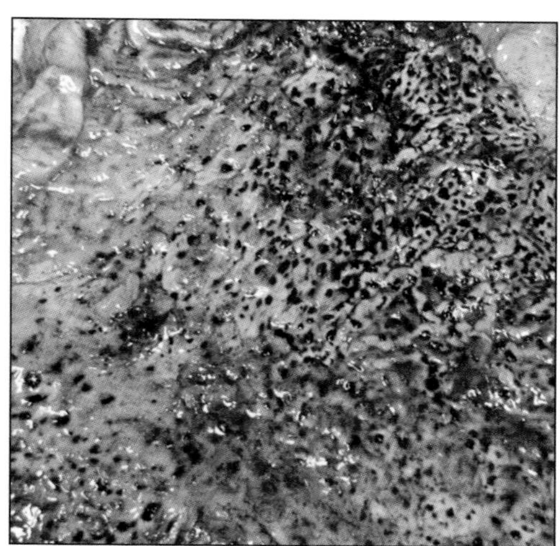

(Left) The gastric mucosa ➡ is diffusely and strikingly hyperemic in this case of acute gastritis. Causes include aspirin, ethanol, shock, and chemical irritants. *(Right)* This close-up image of the gastric mucosa from a patient who died of hypothermia shows diffuse, punctate, submucosal hemorrhages in a leopard spot pattern. Known as Wischnewski ulcers, these lesions, though present in 40-90% of cases of hypothermia, are not specific for any single etiology.

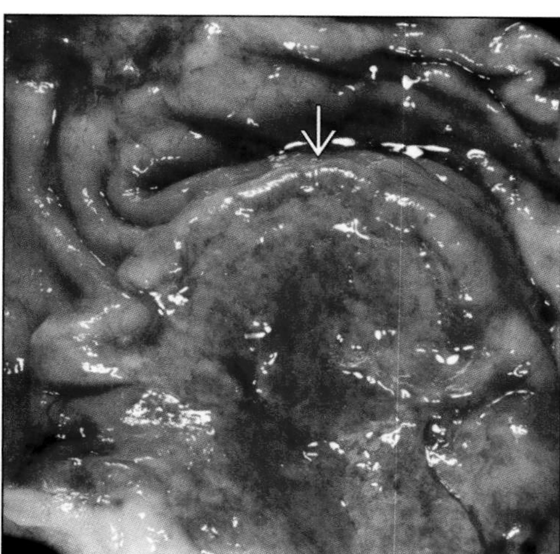

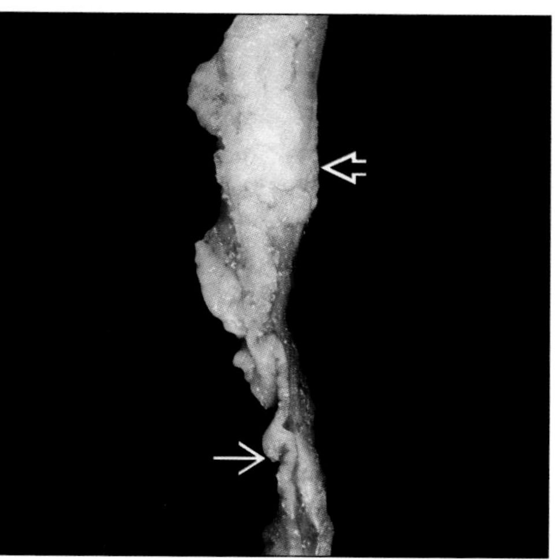

(Left) Intestinal-type gastric adenocarcinoma ➡ characteristically presents as a mass that rises above the surrounding gastric mucosa. Central ulceration is common. For unknown reasons, there has been a marked decrease in the worldwide incidence of gastric cancer. *(Right)* Shown here is a section of gastric wall from a patient with diffuse (signet ring cell) -type gastric adenocarcinoma. Contrast the involved wall ➡ with the adjacent normal wall ➡.

Small Bowel

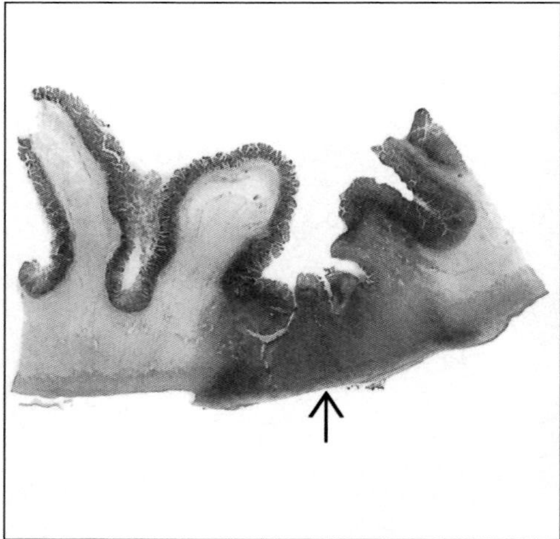

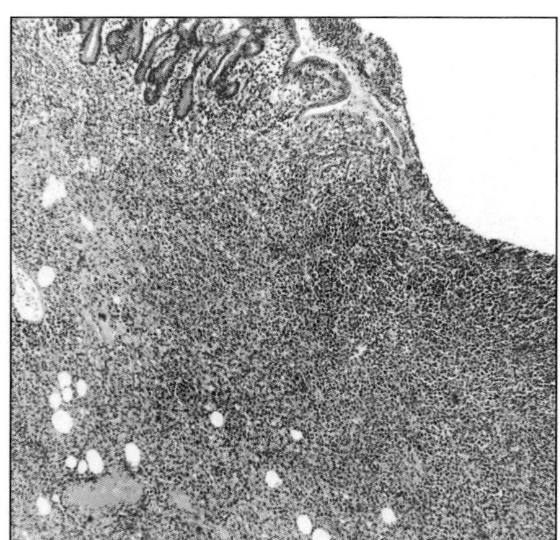

(Left) *This whole-mount image of a section of small bowel involved with lymphoma shows a transmural infiltrate* ⮕ *that replaces the full thickness of the bowel wall. This patient presented with an acute abdomen and perforated jejunum.* ***(Right)*** *A higher power view of the small bowel shows effacement of normal structures by a diffuse infiltrate of lymphocytes. Most GI lymphomas are extranodal marginal zone B-cell lymphomas or diffuse B-cell lymphomas. T-cell lymphoma is unusual.*

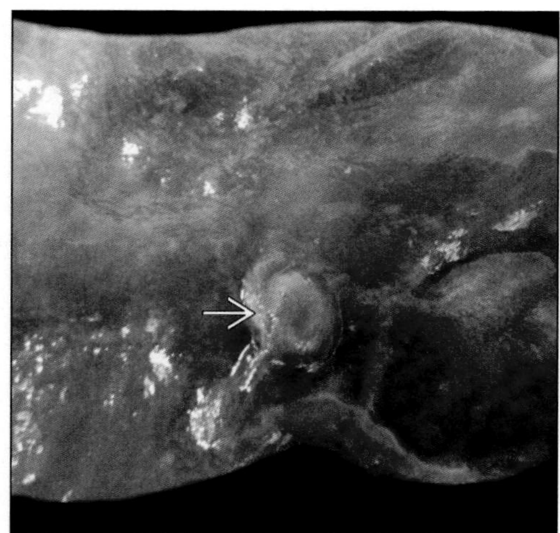

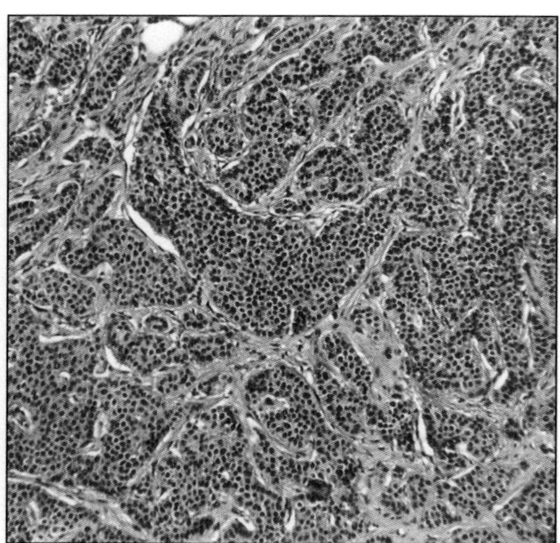

(Left) *This close-up image of bowel mucosa shows a slightly raised submucosal nodule* ➡*. The appearance is typical of a neuroendocrine tumor or carcinoid tumor. The cut surface of such tumors is often yellow.* ***(Right)*** *This H&E section of a neuroendocrine tumor shows islands and trabeculae of monotonous cells with fine nuclear chromatin. Immunoperoxidase stains for synaptophysin and chromogranin were positive.*

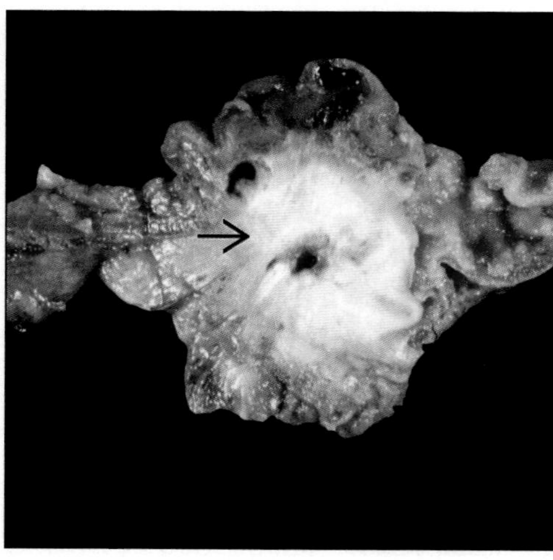

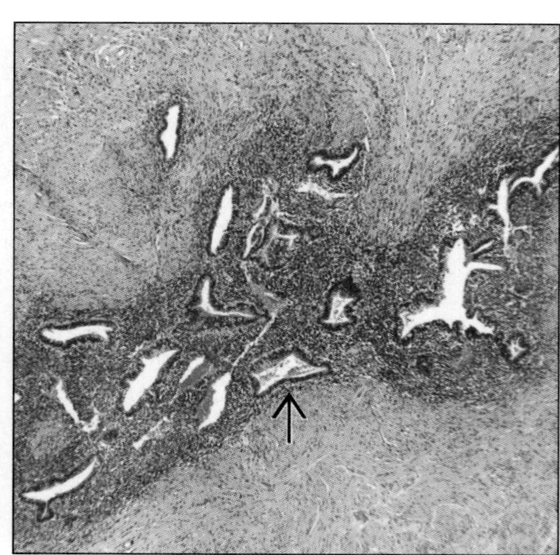

(Left) *This image is an example of GI involvement by endometriosis. The arrow* ⮕ *indicates a fibrous mass that involves the serosa and muscularis of this segment of small bowel. The overlying mucosa is unremarkable. Lesions like this may be mistaken for primary or metastatic malignancies.* ***(Right)*** *This H&E-stained section shows endometriosis involving the muscularis of the small bowel. Benign endometrial glands and stroma* ⮕ *can be seen.*

Colon

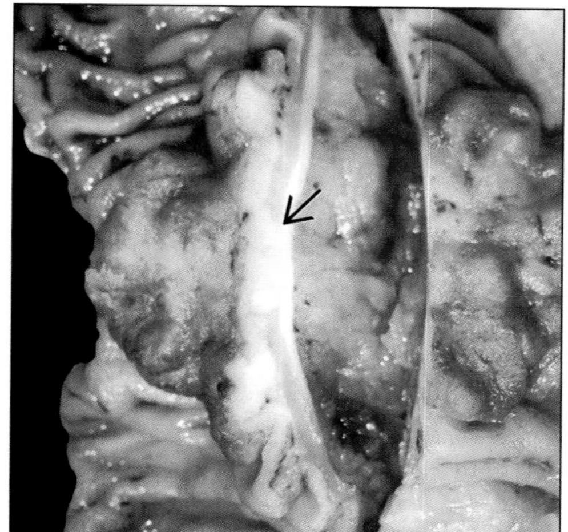

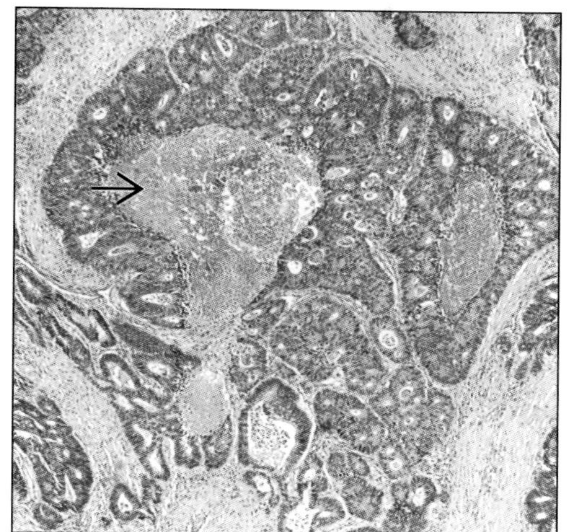

(Left) *This close-up image of a colonic adenocarcinoma shows a polypoid tumor rising above the surrounding uninvolved mucosa. The cut surface shows the tan-white tumor ⇒ infiltrating into the muscularis propria.* ***(Right)*** *Typical colonic adenocarcinoma is composed of malignant glands with cribriformed architecture made up of markedly dysplastic cells. There is loss of normal nuclear polarity and mucin production. Areas of "dirty" necrosis ⇒ are particularly characteristic.*

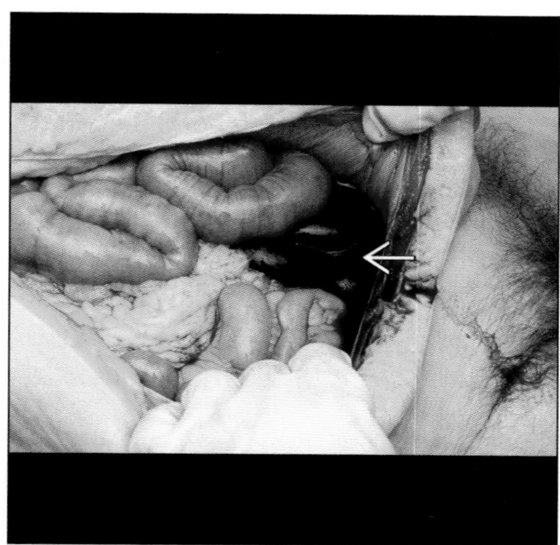

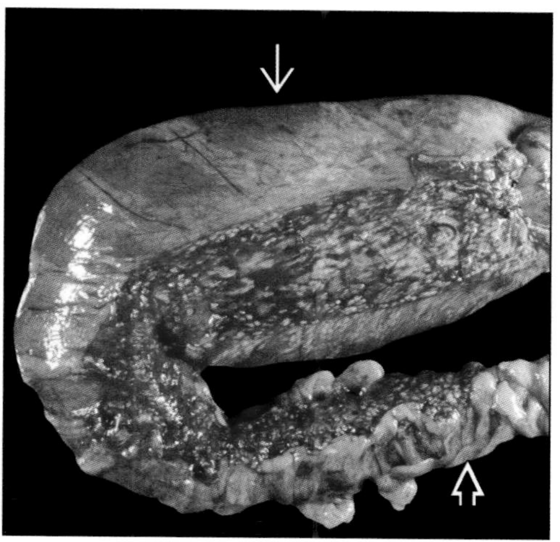

(Left) *Loops of black, dusky, ischemic small bowel are indicated ➡. Contrast the appearance of the adjacent tan-pink, normal small bowel with smooth glistening serosal surfaces.* ***(Right)*** *Volvulus is the result of a segment of bowel twisting on its mesentery. This congested segment of sigmoid colon shows a normal-diameter portion ➡ nearer the twist, and a dilated distal portion ➡ more distally. The sigmoid colon is the most commonly involved segment of the GI tract.*

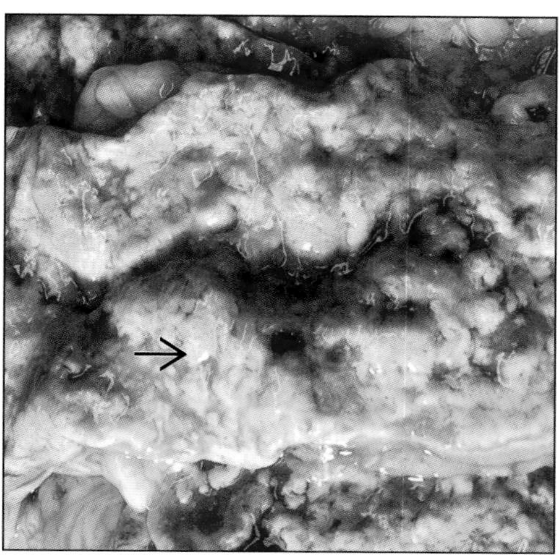

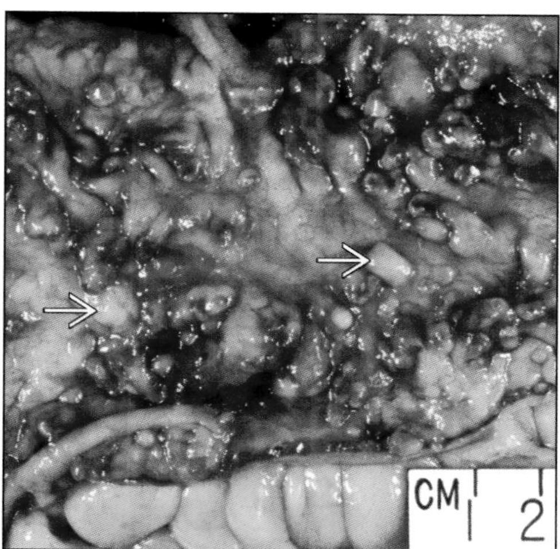

(Left) *Antibiotic-associated colitis results from selective overgrowth of toxin-producing strains of Clostridium difficile following antibiotic therapy. The mucosal surface shows hyperemia and tan-yellow plaques ⇒ or pseudomembranes.* ***(Right)*** *The mucosal surface of this segment of colon involved by inflammatory bowel disease shows pseudopolyp ➡ formation and a characteristic cobblestone appearance.*

HEPATOBILIARY SYSTEM

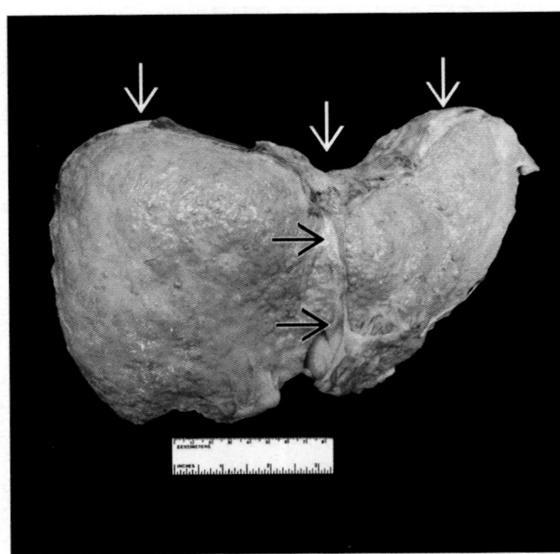

This cirrhotic liver has a pale yellow appearance due to fatty liver disease. The falciform ligament ⇨ separates right and left lobes. The coronary ligament ➡ attaches to the diaphragm.

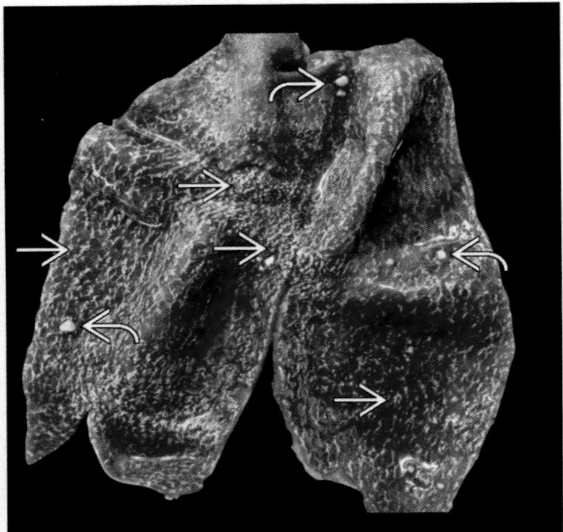

The gallbladder mucosa is normally green-brown. Scattered yellow specks ➡ represent cholesterolosis. Few small yellow cholesterol stones ➦ are also present.

TERMINOLOGY

Definitions

- Includes liver, extrahepatic bile ducts, gallbladder, and exocrine pancreas

MACROSCOPIC FINDINGS

External Examination

- Findings suggesting hepatobiliary disease
  - Jaundice (indicates bilirubin of at least 2.5-3 mg, seen with many hepatobiliary diseases)
  - Ascites (chronic/acute liver disease, malignancy, pancreatitis)
  - Muscle wasting/cachexia (malnutrition: Chronic liver failure, chronic pancreatitis, malignancy)
  - Palpable periumbilical lymph node (metastatic pancreatic carcinoma)
  - Periumbilical edema/hematoma (Cullen sign: Hemorrhagic pancreatitis)
  - Flank bruising (Grey Turner sign, indicates intra-/retroperitoneal hematoma: Hemorrhagic pancreatitis)

General Features

- Liver
  - Located mainly in right upper quadrant beneath 7th-11th ribs, inferior to diaphragm
  - Same dissection for either Rokitansky or Virchow methods
    - Open portal vein, vena cava, and hepatic veins into hilum
    - Hepatic arteries can be opened or examined by transverse sectioning
    - Remove liver by freeing attachments to diaphragm, falciform and coronary ligaments, stomach, and duodenum
- Extrahepatic bile ducts
  - Right and left hepatic ducts join to form common hepatic duct in liver hilum; common hepatic duct joins cystic duct from gallbladder to form common bile duct (CBD)
    - CBD is most anterior structure in porta hepatis; portal vein lies posteriorly and to left of CBD; hepatic artery and nerves lie most posteriorly
    - CBD passes posterior to 1st portion of duodenum into head of pancreas
    - In situ evaluation of continuity of ductal system: Open 1st and 2nd portions of duodenum to expose ampulla, squeeze gallbladder to express bile through extrahepatic ducts and out of ampulla
- Gallbladder
  - Hollow sac inferior to right lobe of liver
  - Remove with liver by transecting CBD or free it from liver bed and open in continuity with ductal system
- Exocrine pancreas
  - Identify pancreas in retroperitoneum posterior to stomach extending between duodenum and spleen
  - Main pancreatic duct runs length of organ and drains into ampulla ± accessory duct, which drains into minor papilla
  - Intrapancreatic portion of CBD runs inferiorly through pancreatic head and empties into ampulla (usually joins main pancreatic duct proximal to ampulla)
  - Can keep in continuity with extrahepatic bile ducts (if ductal pathology is suspected) or separate from duodenum and spleen

Specimen Handling

- Liver
  - Dissect from diaphragmatic attachments, serially section in horizontal plane at 1 cm intervals
  - Normal parenchyma red-brown, normal weight 1,400-1,600 g

- Sample right/left lobes, hilum, any gross pathology
- Extrahepatic bile ducts
  - Cannulate CBD and open retrograde into pancreas
  - Note presence of stones and lesions, section any gross pathology
- Gallbladder
  - Open CBD into cystic duct or open gallbladder from fundus if cystic duct is too small
  - Normal size 7-10 cm, wall thickness 1-3 mm
  - Record quantity and quality of bile and presence, color, and shape of stones
  - Normal mucosa is green and velvety
  - Mucosa autolyzes quickly due to bile (sample early in autopsy procedure if pathology suspected)
  - Representative sections of entire thickness of gallbladder wall and any gross pathology
- Exocrine pancreas
  - Normal size and weight 15 cm, 60-140 g
  - Best dissection method to probe CBD and pancreatic duct from ampulla and bisect organ along that plane
    - May serially section if difficult to probe
    - If cystic lesion is present, note relationship to ductal system
  - Section head and tail of pancreas and any gross pathology

MICROSCOPIC FINDINGS

General Features

- Liver
  - Polygonal hepatocytes with eosinophilic, sometimes granular cytoplasm and well-defined borders with prominent nucleolus, arranged in cords 1, sometimes 2 cells thick
    - ↑ variation in size, number of nuclei, and lipofuscin pigment deposition with age
  - Plates/cords separated by sinusoids lined by specialized endothelial cells (negative for CD31 and CD34)
    - Kupffer cells (specialized hepatic macrophages) and occasional lymphocytes lie in sinusoids
  - Space of Disse located between sinusoids and hepatocytes
    - Contains hepatic stellate cells (involved in fibrogenesis) and extracellular matrix including reticulin network
  - Parenchyma divided into 3 zones with decreasing tissue oxygenation
    - Zone 1 (periportal), zone 2 (midzonal), and zone 3 (centrilobular/perivenular)
  - Portal tracts contain interlobular bile duct, portal venule, hepatic arteriole, lymphatics and occasional lymphocytes embedded in fibrous stroma
    - ↑ collagen density and number of mononuclear inflammatory cells with age
  - Interlobular bile ducts lined by cuboidal or low columnar epithelium ([+] for CK7 and CK19), which drain into larger septal ducts lined by tall columnar epithelium
    - Bile canaliculi located between hepatocytes, not seen on H&E stain, highlighted by polyclonal carcinoembryonic antigen (CEA)
    - Bile flow: Hepatocytes → bile canaliculi → canals of Hering → bile ductules at periphery of portal tracts → interlobular ducts → septal ducts toward hilum; bile not seen on H&E stain in normal liver
- Extrahepatic bile ducts
  - Lined by tall columnar cells with unevenly distributed peribiliary mucous glands, muscle layer present in distal 1/3 of ductal system
- Gallbladder
  - Lined by simple columnar epithelium arranged in branching folds; no discrete muscularis mucosa or submucosa
  - Muscularis propria and perimuscular connective tissue/adventitia, lined by peritoneum except where attached to liver
  - Rokitansky-Aschoff sinuses: Outpouching of mucosa that penetrate muscle wall
  - Ducts of Luschka: Lobular aggregates of ductules lined by cuboidal epithelium deep in wall adjacent to liver
- Exocrine pancreas
  - Acini: 80% of parenchyma, basophilic/amphophilic pyramid-shaped to columnar cells with apical zymogen granules, oriented radially within acinus, scant stroma
  - Centroacinar cells: Located in center of acinus, pale cytoplasm, single or in clusters
  - Intercalated ducts (cuboidal epithelium) → intralobular ducts (cuboidal epithelium) → interlobular ducts (cuboidal-columnar epithelium) → main pancreatic duct (simple columnar mucinous epithelium)

CLINICAL CORRELATES

Pertinent Antemortem Labs

- Hepatobiliary: Aspartate transaminase (AST), alanine transaminase (ALT), alkaline phosphatase, bilirubin, gamma-glutamyl transferase (GGT)
- Liver: Viral hepatitis serologies, autoimmune markers (e.g., anti-smooth muscle and antimitochondrial antibodies), α-fetoprotein, ceruloplasmin, α-1-antitrypsin (A1AT), iron studies
- Exocrine pancreas: Amylase, lipase

FREQUENT AUTOPSY FINDINGS

Liver

- Shock changes
  - Gross: "Nutmeg" liver with variegated cut surface due to zone 3 hemorrhagic necrosis and preserved portal areas; larger areas of necrosis/infarction are pale and soft
  - Microscopic: Centrilobular congestion ± hepatocellular coagulative necrosis, periportal areas usually preserved (except with massive necrosis/ infarction)

HEPATOBILIARY SYSTEM

- Sepsis changes
  - Gross: Green discoloration of parenchyma (cholestasis), ± abscesses, ulcers/erosions ± thickening of bile ducts (cholangitis)
  - Microscopic: Canalicular cholestasis, ductular cholestasis ± associated neutrophils, neutrophils within walls and lumina of bile ducts (acute cholangitis)
- Cirrhosis
  - Gross: Nodules surrounded by fibrous tissue, micronodular (≤ 3 mm), macronodular, or mixed
  - Microscopic: Regenerative nodules of hepatocytes surrounded by fibrous bands **without** central veins
- Tumors
  - Benign: Hemangioma (most common primary tumor), focal nodular hyperplasia, hepatocellular adenoma, cysts, bile duct adenoma
  - Malignant: Metastasis (most common), hepatocellular carcinoma, cholangiocarcinoma

Extrahepatic Bile Ducts

- Choledocholithiasis: Usually in CBD, may involve intrahepatic ducts
  - Complications include ascending cholangitis ± abscesses, pancreatitis, ileus
- Cholangiocarcinoma, "Klatskin tumor" when present at confluence of right and left hepatic ducts

Gallbladder

- Cholelithiasis
  - Cholesterol: Pure or mixed with calcium, phosphate, or bile, yellow to green, smooth, hard and round to oval, sometimes popcorn-like
  - Pigment: Unconjugated bilirubin and calcium salts, chronic hemolysis (black stones), and infection (brown stones) are risk factors; may be spiculated
- Cholesterolosis: Due to bile supersaturation with cholesterol, yellow specks on mucosa, foamy macrophages in lamina propria, ± cholesterol polyps
- Acute cholecystitis
  - Gross: Enlarged, red-green-black discoloration, serosal fibrinopurulent exudate, thickened edematous wall, fibrinous/purulent contents, mucosal erythema/ulcers
  - Microscopic: Acute inflammation, mural edema with myofibroblastic proliferation, congestion, ulcers, abscesses, gangrene
- Chronic cholecystitis
  - Gross: May appear normal, serosal fibrosis, variably thickened wall, mucosa usually normal or ulcerated under impacted stones
  - Microscopic: Mucosal chronic inflammation, thickened wall with Rokitansky-Aschoff sinuses, pyloric and intestinal metaplasia
- Adenomyoma (localized mass-like diverticulum)
  - Gross: Polypoid nodule in wall of fundus with cystic cut surface, ± overlying mucosal dimple
  - Microscopic: Mucosal herniation with cystically dilated glands lined by normal epithelium and prominent smooth muscle hypertrophy
- Tumors: Adenomas, cysts, adenocarcinoma

Exocrine Pancreas

- Acute pancreatitis
  - Gross: Edematous, pale, indurated parenchyma, fat necrosis (yellow nodules ± calcification), ± hemorrhage/necrosis, pseudocysts, abscesses
  - Microscopic: Acute inflammation, edema, fibrinous exudate, ± hemorrhage and necrosis of all parenchymal components, fat necrosis, calcification
- Chronic pancreatitis
  - Gross: Focal, segmental, or diffuse involvement by fibrosis, indurated ± mass-like, irregular ductal dilatation ± calculi, atrophy
  - Microscopic: Irregular loss of acinar/ductal tissue, chronic inflammation/fibrosis with preservation of lobular architecture, duct ectasia ± inspissated secretions, ductal metaplasia, islets usually preserved
- Cystic neoplasms
  - Communication with ductal system: Intraductal papillary mucinous neoplasm and variants
  - No communication with ductal system: Serous cystadenoma (most common cystic neoplasm), mucinous cystic neoplasm, acinar cell cystadenoma
- Malignant tumors
  - Adenocarcinoma (pancreatic duct, ampulla, or CBD), pancreatic endocrine neoplasm, solid pseudopapillary neoplasm, acinar cell carcinoma

ANCILLARY TESTS

Serum

- AST, ALT, amylase and lipase ↑ rapidly postmortem, not useful
- GGT data varies, can possibly be used in evaluation of biliary disease postmortem
- Bile ↑ slightly postmortem, accurate if markedly ↑
- Antibodies for viral hepatitis B and C are reliable
- PCR for hepatitis B DNA and hepatitis C RNA are reliable

Urine

- Bile and urobilinogen not normally present in urine; detection postmortem is accurate

SELECTED REFERENCES

1. Palmiere C et al: Postmortem chemistry update part II. Int J Legal Med. 126(2):199-215, 2012
2. Weedn, VW et al: Postmortem Chemistry. In Sapse D et al: Forensic Science Advances and Their Application in the Judiciary System. Boca Raton: CRC Press. 235-54, 2011
3. Eriksen MB et al: Postmortem detection of hepatitis B, C, and human immunodeficiency virus genomes in blood samples from drug-related deaths in Denmark*. J Forensic Sci. 54(5):1085-8, 2009

In Situ and Excised Organs

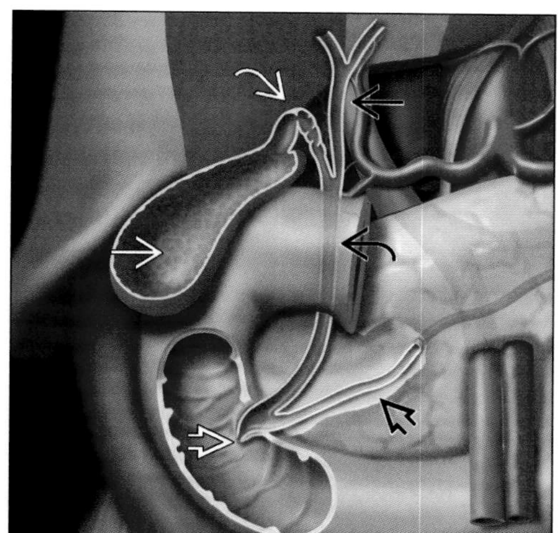

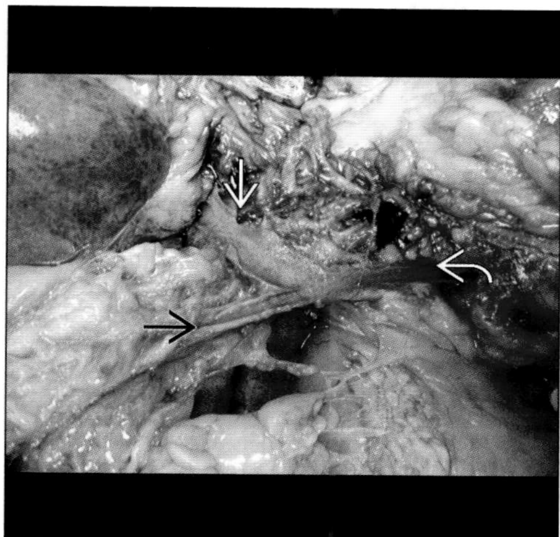

(Left) *The gallbladder empties bile via the cystic duct. The cystic duct joins the common hepatic duct as it exits the liver to form the common bile duct. This empties into the duodenum after traversing the pancreatic head and joining the main pancreatic duct at the ampulla.* **(Right)** *The extrahepatic bile duct system is opened to show the cystic duct joining the common hepatic duct as it exits the liver to form the common bile duct.*

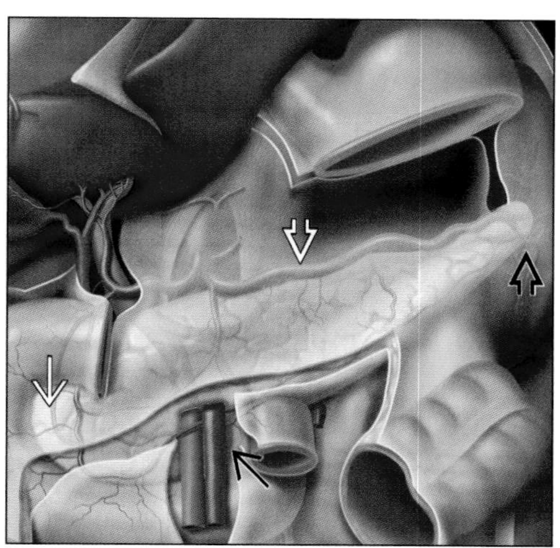

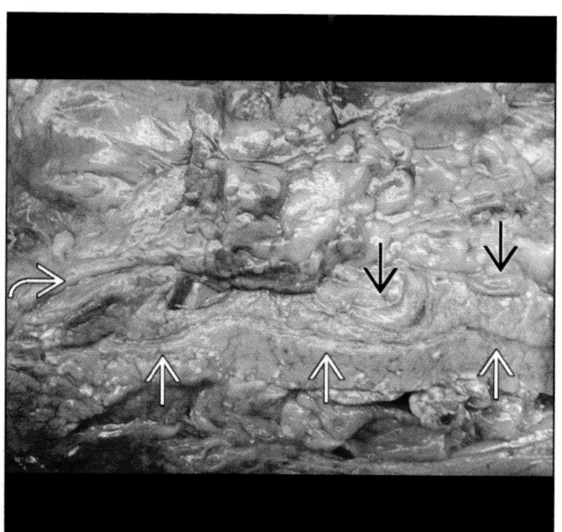

(Left) *The head of the pancreas rests in the C-shaped 2nd and 3rd portion of the duodenum. The uncinate process extends medially from the head and posterior to the superior mesenteric vein and artery. The tail of the pancreas extends to the hilum of the spleen. The splenic artery lies superior to the pancreatic body.* **(Right)** *The pancreas is bisected along the pancreatic duct. The common bile duct traverses the pancreatic head (splenic artery).*

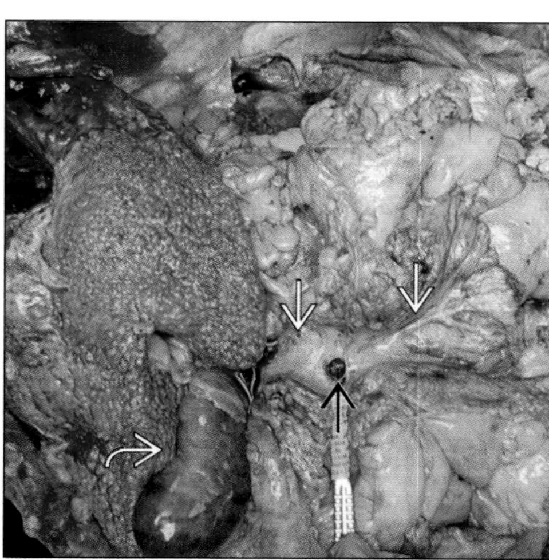

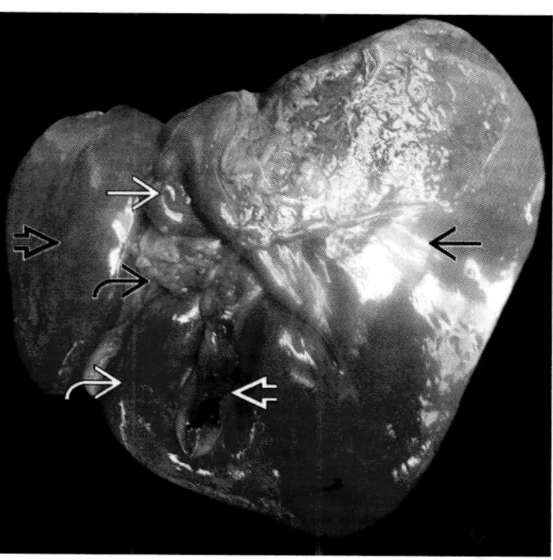

(Left) *The portal vein is opened as it exits the liver to show a small thrombus. The gallbladder extends inferiorly from this cirrhotic liver.* **(Right)** *The caudate and quadrate lobes can be viewed from the posterior surface of the liver. The gallbladder is located to the right of the quadrate lobe and inferior to the porta hepatis, which contains the hepatic portal vein, hepatic artery, and common hepatic bile duct (right and left lobes).*

Normal Histology

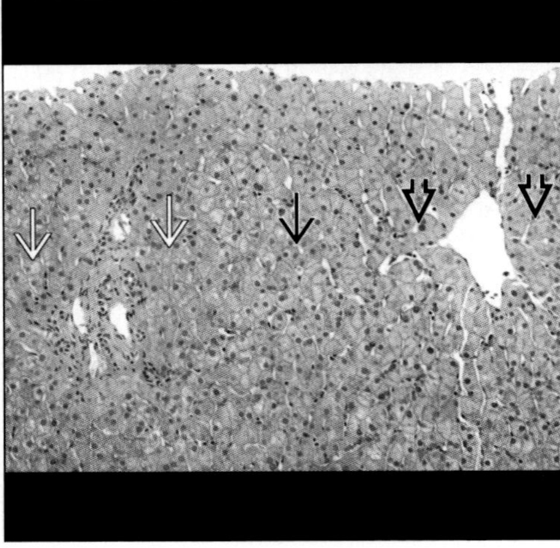

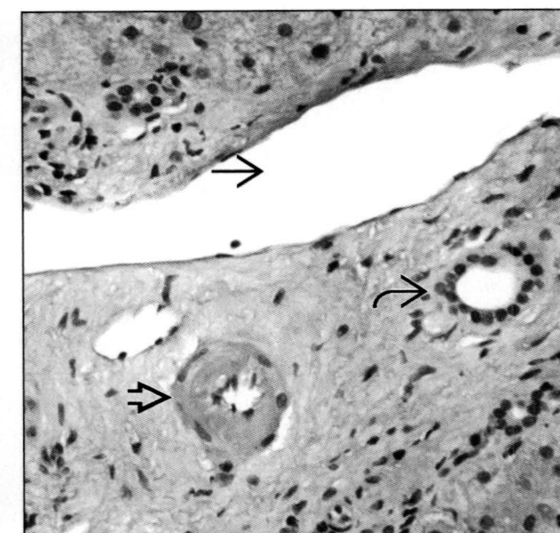

(Left) The liver parenchyma can be divided into 3 zones of hepatocytes: (1) Periportal ➡, (2) mid zonal ➡, and (3) perivenular/centrilobular ➡. **(Right)** The portal tract is composed of an interlobular bile duct ➡, hepatic arteriole ➡, and portal venule ➡ embedded in a fibrous stroma with scant mononuclear inflammatory cells.

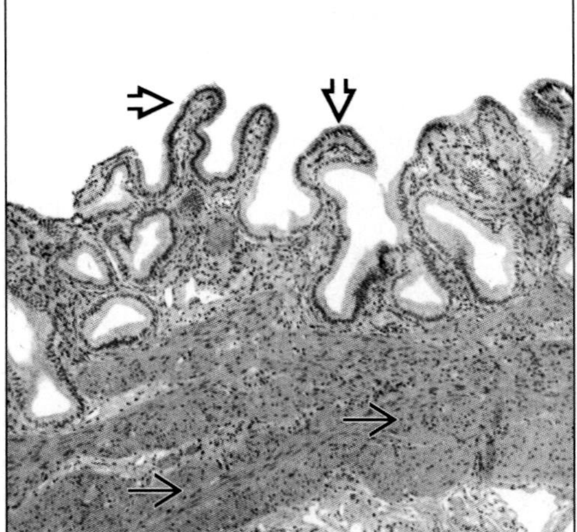

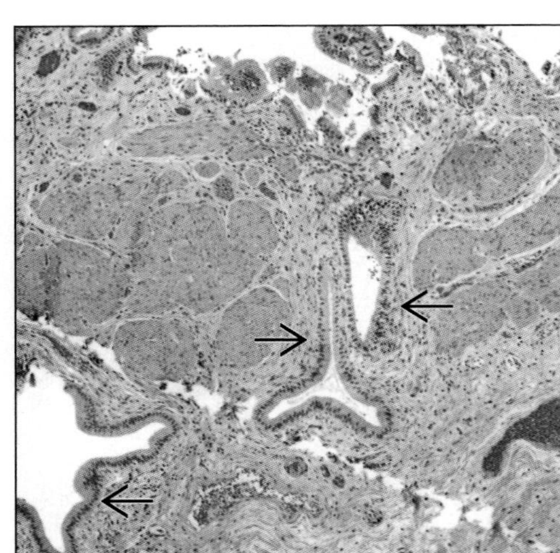

(Left) The gallbladder mucosa is arranged in branching folds ➡ lined by simple columnar epithelium without a discrete muscularis mucosa or submucosa. The muscularis propria ➡ lies beneath the mucosal folds. **(Right)** Mucosal herniations through the gallbladder wall are known as Rokitansky-Aschoff sinuses ➡. These irregularly shaped tubular structures are lined by simple columnar or cuboidal epithelium and are often present in gallbladders with chronic cholecystitis.

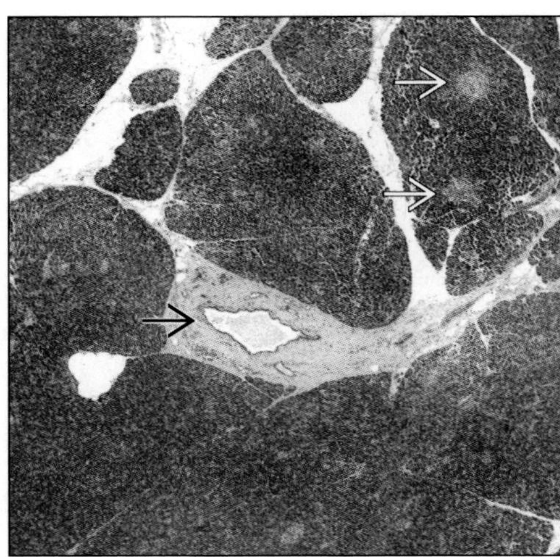

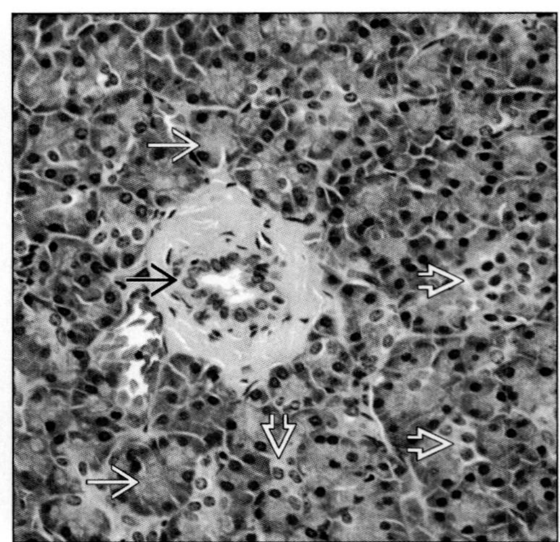

(Left) This low-power view of the pancreas shows its lobular parenchyma composed of acinar cells with interspersed islets ➡ and scant stroma. Interlobular ducts ➡ are lined by cuboidal-columnar epithelium. **(Right)** The intralobular ducts ➡ are lined by cuboidal epithelium. The exocrine acinar cells have basophilic to amphophilic cytoplasm with apical eosinophilic zymogen granules ➡. Centroacinar cells are small and round with pale cytoplasm ➡.

Frequent Autopsy Findings

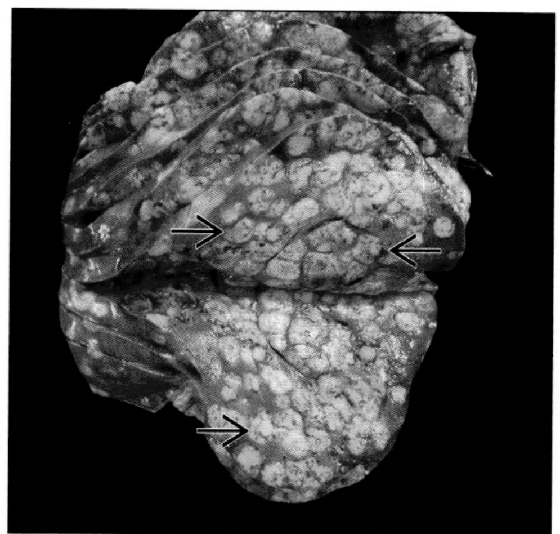

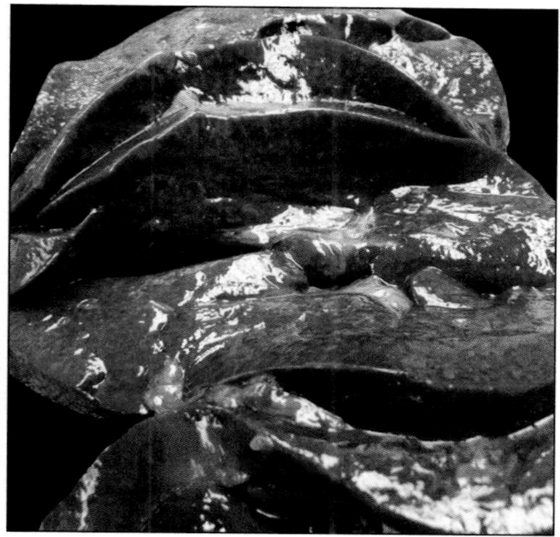

(Left) *The cut surface of this liver shows innumerable metastatic deposits ➔ with patchy necrosis in a patient with breast cancer.* ***(Right)*** *The cut surface of this liver shows diffuse green discoloration due to cholestasis in a patient on total parenteral nutrition.*

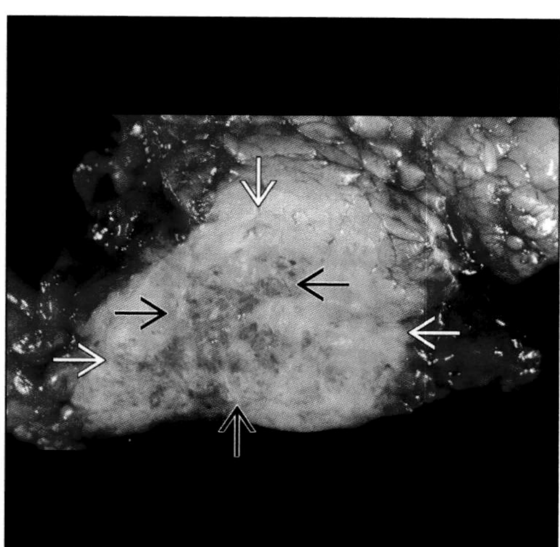

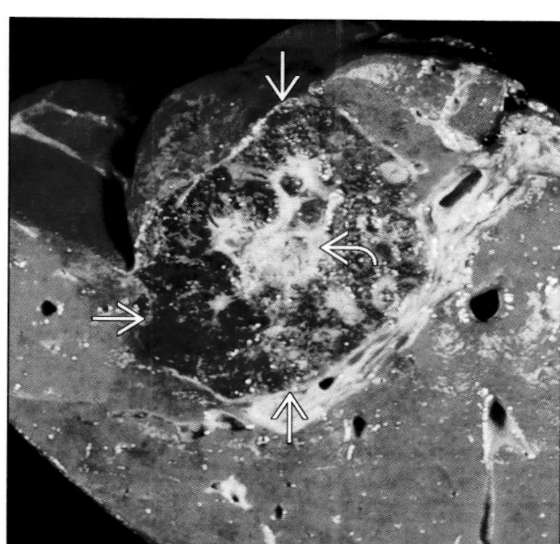

(Left) *The cut surface of this pancreas shows a mass-like area of fibrosis ➔ with patchy necrosis ➔ due to chronic pancreatitis. (Courtesy D. Rubin, MD.)* ***(Right)*** *Hemangiomas are the most common benign tumor of the liver. The cut surface is red and spongy ➔ with fibrotic foci ➔. Thrombosis and calcification were present microscopically in these areas. (Courtesy D. Rubin, MD.)*

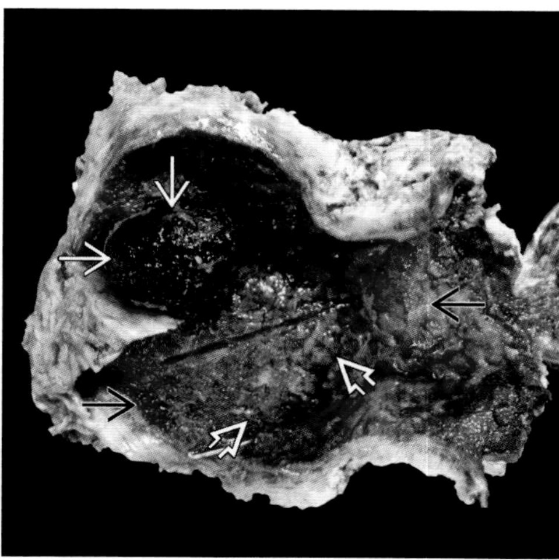

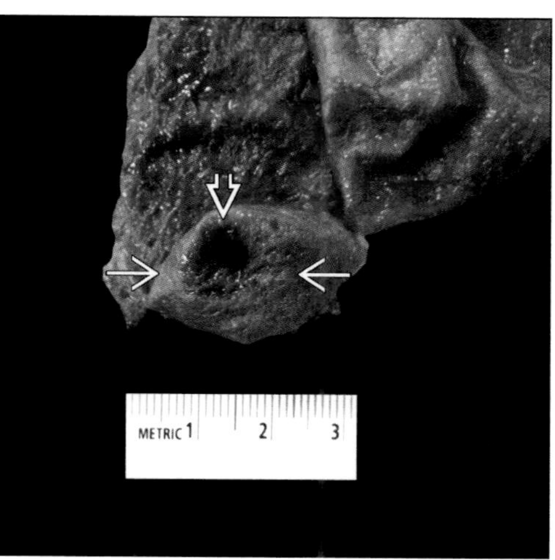

(Left) *A large black pigmented stone ➔ was present in this gallbladder with acute and chronic cholecystitis. The mucosa is erythematous and ulcerated ➔ with a green purulent exudate ➔, and the wall is markedly thickened.* ***(Right)*** *Adenomyoma of the gallbladder fundus (a.k.a. adenomyomatous hyperplasia, diverticulum) is a submucosal nodule ➔, often with an overlying mucosal outpouching or "dimple" ➔. The cut surface may appear multicystic.*

GENITOURINARY SYSTEM

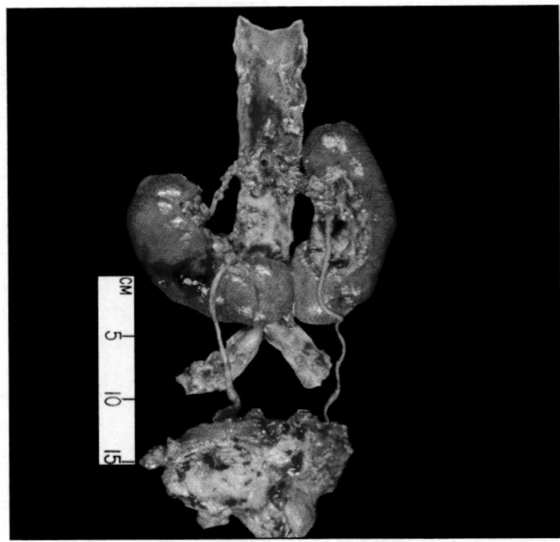

Horseshoe kidney is the congenital and usually asymptomatic fusion of the inferior poles of the kidneys. The isthmus of the fused kidneys is usually found just below the inferior mesenteric artery.

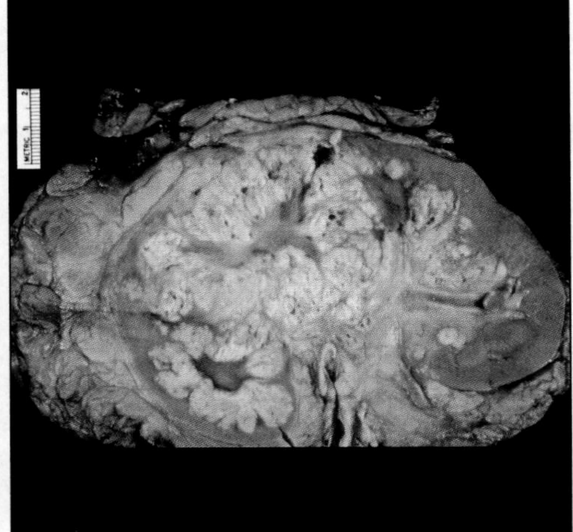

Urothelial carcinoma can arise in the calyces, pelvis, ureters, and bladder. It is often papillary and may be multifocal.

DEFINITIONS

Normal Anatomy

- Urinary tract: Kidneys, ureters, bladder, urethra
- Female genital tract: Vagina, cervix, uterus, fallopian tubes, ovaries
- Male genital tract: Prostate, seminal vesicles, vas deferens, testes

DISSECTION

Virchow (Piecemeal) Evisceration

- Aorta exposed after abdominal organs removed
  - Kidneys and adrenals located in perirenal fat on either side of abdominal aorta
- Remove left adrenal gland
  - Located in perinephric fat at superomedial pole of kidney, applied closely to lateral aspect of aorta
  - Incise perinephric fat adjacent to aorta at level between celiac and superior mesenteric artery (SMA) to expose adrenal
    - Adrenal will have tan-pink lobulated appearance
  - Dissect adrenal from surrounding kidney and fat
- Remove right adrenal gland
  - Located in perinephric fat at superomedial pole of kidney, at level of SMA, tucked behind inferior vena cava (IVC)
  - Transect IVC, insert finger into lumen, and rotate it laterally
  - Incise perinephric fat in IVC bed at level of SMA to expose adrenal
  - Dissect adrenal from surrounding kidney and perinephric fat
- Expose kidneys
  - Incise lateral aspect of perinephric fat to expose dark red renal cortex covered by renal capsule
  - Incise renal capsule along lateral aspect of kidney
  - Use fingers or forceps to strip perinephric fat and renal capsule medially toward renal hilum
  - Continue to strip medially to expose renal vessels and ureter
  - Follow ureter inferiorly
- Dissection of pelvic organs
  - Insert nondominant hand into retropubic space
  - Work hand down into pelvis
    - Palm of hand is now anterior to bladder
  - Encircle pelvic organs with fingers
    - Fingers should sit against coccyx and behind rectum
  - Use upward and anterior traction to remove pelvic organs from pelvic walls
    - This motion will be accompanied by a sucking sound
  - Pull pelvic organs upwards and posteriorly to create a space behind pubic bone
  - While maintaining traction on pelvic organs, use dominant hand to insert scalpel into retropubic space as inferiorly as possible (below cervix/prostate)
  - Carefully cut across inferior attachments of pelvic organs (urethra, vagina, rectum)
    - Scalpel blade will not be visible
    - Take care to keep nondominant hand clear of scalpel blade
- Transect right and left common iliac arteries
- Kidneys and rest of genitourinary tract can now be removed en bloc or piecemeal
- Testes are removed through inguinal canal

Rokitansky Evisceration (en Bloc) Technique

- Dissect heart, respiratory tract, liver, and gastrointestinal tract away from organ block
- Remove adrenal glands as described above under Virchow technique
- Place organ block on cutting board, anterior surface down, posterior surface facing you

- Incise perinephric fat along its lateral aspect until reaching dark red renal cortex
- Incise renal capsule over lateral aspect of kidney
- Use forceps or fingers to strip perinephric fat and renal capsule medially toward hilum
- Continue to strip fat to reveal renal vessels and ureters
- Follow ureters to bladder
- Dissect rectum ± gynecologic tract from bladder
  - Alternatively in males, leave rectum attached and open it longitudinally
- Kidneys can be dissected from left attached to aorta and bladder

Dissection of Kidneys, Ureters, and Bladder (2 Alternatives)

- 1st alternative: Intact urinary tract attached to aorta and bladder
  - Open aorta along its posterior aspect from superior to inferior
  - Insert scissors into renal artery ostium and open renal artery into renal hilum
  - Bisect kidneys in coronal plane leaving 1/2 attached to renal artery and ureter
  - Using fine scissors, open ureter to its junction with bladder
  - Open urethra and bladder anteriorly; probe distal ureter into bladder
  - Make serial sections through detached 1/2 of kidney parallel to original cut
  - Make similar sections in attached 1/2 of kidney, taking care to leave a section attached to renal artery and ureter
  - Advantages: Preserves normal anatomic relationships (for presentation to clinicians or photography)
  - Disadvantages: More labor intensive; makes accurate weighing of kidneys more difficult
    - Some weigh detached 1/2 of kidney and double weight
    - Some dangle attached kidney onto weighing pan
- 2nd alternative: Piecemeal dissection
  - Transect renal artery close to renal hilum
  - Transect right ureter close to renal hilum and left ureter a few cm from hilum
    - Allows for identification ("left is long")
  - Open ureters with fine scissors
  - Open urethra and bladder anteriorly
  - Probe ureters into bladder
  - Advantages: Faster; allows for accurate kidney weights
  - Disadvantages: Disrupts normal anatomic relationships

Dissection of Gynecologic Tract

- Detach gynecologic tract (vaginal cuff, cervix, uterus, fallopian tubes, ovaries) from bladder and rectum
- Open vaginal cuff along its right and left lateral aspects to expose cervix
- Open cervix and uterus
  - 1st alternative
    - Bisect cervix and uterine corpus along right and left lateral aspects into anterior and posterior halves
  - 2nd alternative
    - Open cervix and uterus anteriorly with Y-shaped incision
    - Insert scissors into cervical canal and open cervix anteriorly
    - Open endometrial cavity by extending cervical incision toward right and left cornua
- Serially section ovaries

Dissection of Male Urogenital Tract

- Remove rectum from posterior aspect of bladder and prostate
- Open prostatic urethra anteriorly into bladder
- Dissect adherent soft tissue from posterior aspect of prostate to expose seminal vesicles and vas deferens
- Bisect seminal vesicles into anterior and posterior halves
- Serially section prostate from inferior to superior
- Serially section testes

Sections for Histology

- The following are suggestions for sections of grossly normal organs
  - Some authors suggest fewer or no sections of grossly normal organs; others suggest more sections
    - Local preferences will dictate number of histologic sections submitted for histology
  - Always take additional sections of gross abnormalities as indicated by individual case
- Kidneys
  - 1 section from each kidney to include renal cortex and medulla
- Adrenals
  - Complete cross section to include cortex and medulla
- Bladder: 1 full thickness section
- Prostate: 1 representative section
- Testes: 1 representative section
- Gynecologic tract
  - 1 section of cervix
  - 1 section of cervix to include squamocolumnar junction
  - 1 section of uterus including endo- and myometrium
  - Representative section of ovary and fallopian tube in 1 cassette

PATHOLOGIC FINDINGS

External Examination

- General
  - Chronic renal failure (CRF)
    - Muscle wasting
    - Dry, brittle hair
    - Sallow, gray-yellow skin
    - Dialysis catheter, fistula
  - Abdominal distension and ascites in ovarian malignancy
- Skin

GENITOURINARY SYSTEM

- Malar rash of systemic lupus erythematosus
- Petechial hemorrhages associated with microangiopathy (DIC, TTP, HUS)
- Ulcerations associated with calciphylaxis
- Pallor associated with anemia

- External genitalia
  - Male
    - Penis: Inflammation, masses
    - Scrotum: Testes (undescended?), masses, fluid accumulations
  - Female
    - Vulva: Inflammation, masses

Internal Examination

- Body cavities
  - Ascites and peritoneal nodules in ovarian malignancy
- Cardiovascular
  - Fibrinous ("bread and butter") pericarditis and pericardial effusion in CRF
  - Hypertensive nephrosclerosis
    - Cardiomegaly and left ventricular hypertrophy
  - Renal arterial changes (atherosclerosis, fibromuscular dysplasia)
- Lungs: Pulmonary edema and congestion in renal failure
- Kidneys
  - Horseshoe kidney: Inferior poles of kidneys connected; 1 in 400-800 births; usually asymptomatic
  - Renal cysts
    - Few, small: Common and clinically insignificant
    - Diffuse replacement: Adult polycystic kidney disease (enlarged kidneys with large cysts); dialysis kidney (normal-sized kidneys, cysts < 0.5 cm)
  - Hypertensive nephrosclerosis
    - Finely granular cortical surface
    - Infarcts: Wedge-shaped depressed cortical lesions, often embolic
  - Ischemic injury
    - Pale, usually patchy cortical areas, congested medullae, ± petechiae
  - Nephrolithiasis: Common cause of obstruction in young adults
  - Hydronephrosis: Dilated pelvis and calyces ± thinned renal cortex
  - Abscesses: Tan-yellow cortical lesions with hyperemic borders
  - Renal tumors
    - Metastatic tumors: Most common malignant renal tumors found at autopsy; especially from lung and breast; often bilateral
    - Renal cell carcinomas: Cortical, tan-yellow, variegated, hemorrhagic, may be large
    - Angiomyolipomas: Fatty yellow tumors; can be associated with tuberous sclerosis
    - Renomedullary interstitial cell tumors (a.k.a. medullary fibromas): Gray-white, small
- Ureters and pelvis
  - Bifid or duplicated ureters
  - Hydroureter: Dilated, sometimes tortuous ureters; secondary to obstruction
  - Tumors: Predominantly urothelial carcinomas
- Bladder
  - Urachal remnants/cysts: At apex of bladder
  - Cystitis: Hyperemic mucosa
  - Obstructive changes: Distended trabeculated bladder
  - Stones
  - Tumors
    - Urothelial carcinoma: Most common; typically gray-white and papillary; may be multifocal
    - Less commonly: Squamous cell carcinoma, small cell carcinoma
- Prostate
  - Hyperplasia
    - Enlarged, classically symmetrical gland with bulging cut surface
    - Common cause of urethral obstruction and obstructive changes in bladder
  - Tumors
    - Almost exclusively adenocarcinoma
    - Typically minimal gross changes in prostate gland
    - Metastases (bone, lymph nodes) usually easier to see
- Urethra
  - Posterior urethral valves: Can be associated with hydroureter and hydronephrosis
- Gynecologic tract
  - Pelvic inflammatory disease
  - Endometriosis
  - Benign tumors
    - Cervical and endometrial polyps
    - Uterine leiomyomas
    - Ovarian cystadenomas, cystadenofibromas, mature teratomas
  - Malignant tumors
    - Cervix: Squamous cell, adenocarcinoma
    - Endometrium: Adenocarcinoma, carcinosarcoma
    - Myometrium: Leiomyosarcoma
    - Ovaries: Surface epithelial tumors, germ cell tumors, stromal tumors
- Testes
  - Cryptorchidism
  - Hydrocele
  - Orchitis
  - Tumors
    - Germ cell tumors: Seminoma, nonseminomatous, mixed
    - Lymphoma: Especially in patients older than 60
- Hepatobiliary
  - Hepatic cysts common in patients with polycystic kidney disease

SELECTED REFERENCES

1. Lim AKh: Diabetic nephropathy - complications and treatment. Int J Nephrol Renovasc Dis. 7:361-81, 2014
2. Roy A et al: Common and uncommon bilateral adult renal masses. Cancer Imaging. 12:205-11, 2012
3. Winterberg PD et al: Acute kidney injury: the beginning of the end of the dark ages. Am J Med Sci. 344(4):318-25, 2012
4. Levin A: Clinical epidemiology of cardiovascular disease in chronic kidney disease prior to dialysis. Semin Dial. 16(2):101-5, 2003

Dissection of the Genitourinary Tract

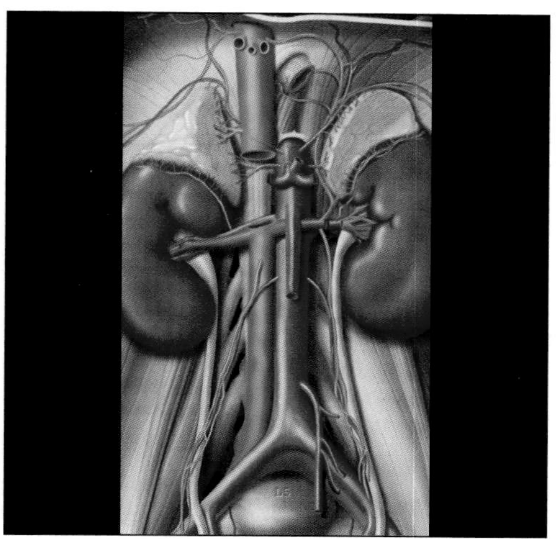

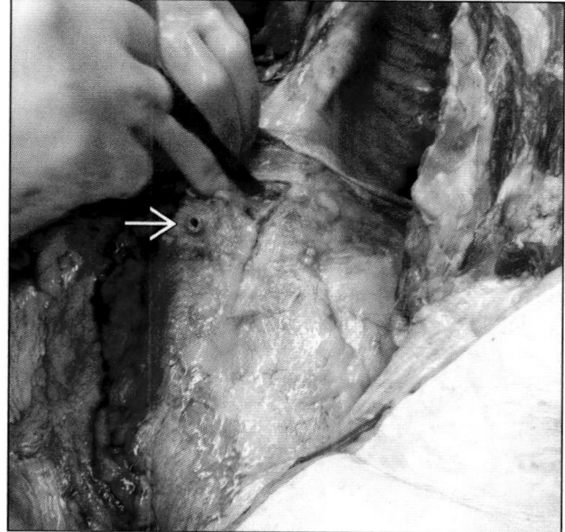

(Left) *The adrenal glands, buried in perinephric fat, can be difficult to locate. They sit at the superomedial aspect of the kidneys. Their medial borders abut the inferior vena cava (right) and aorta (left) around the level of the celiac and superior mesenteric arteries.* ***(Right)*** *The left perinephric fat is incised near the superomedial aspect of the kidney, adjacent to the aorta, and at the level of the superior mesenteric artery ➡ to expose the left adrenal.*

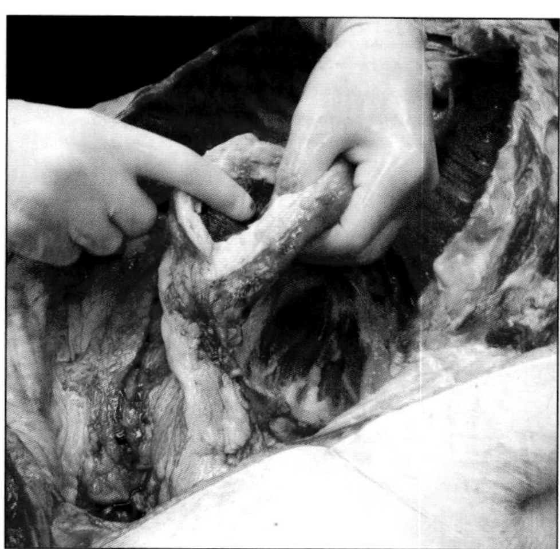

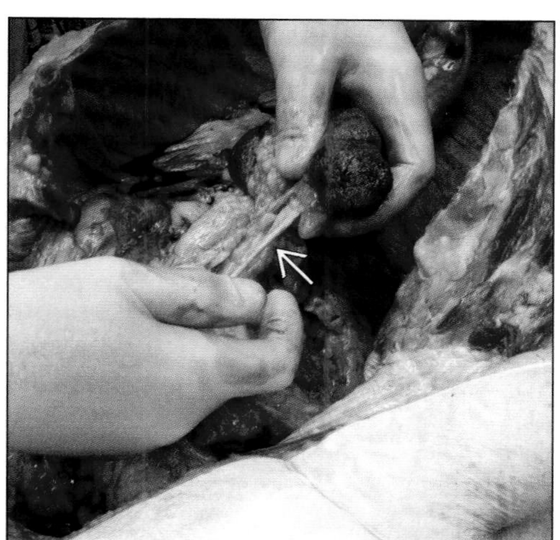

(Left) *The perinephric fat has been freed from the body wall. The lateral aspect of the perinephric fat is incised to expose the dark red renal cortex. The renal capsule is lightly incised over a few cm. Use your fingers to strip the capsule and renal fat from the kidney.* ***(Right)*** *The perinephric fat and renal capsule have been stripped away from the kidney and proximal ureter ➡. The ureter will be exposed down to its insertion into the bladder.*

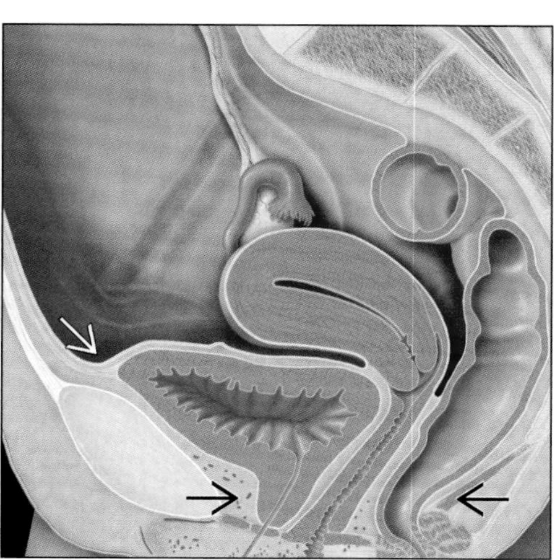

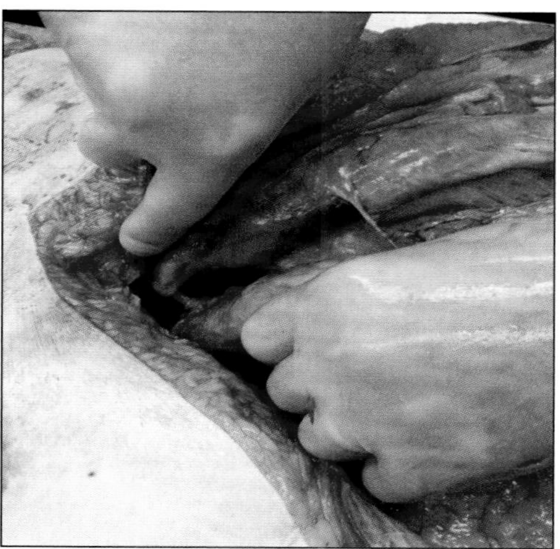

(Left) *Removal of the pelvic organs cannot be done entirely under direct visual inspection. The nondominant hand must be introduced into the retropubic space ➡. The thumb and fingers should then encircle the pelvic organs ⇨.* ***(Right)*** *Upward traction is applied to the pelvic organs. This is accompanied by a sucking sound. While maintaining traction, use the scalpel to (blindly) transect the inferior attachments of the pelvic organs below the cervix/prostate.*

Urinary Tract Gross Pathology

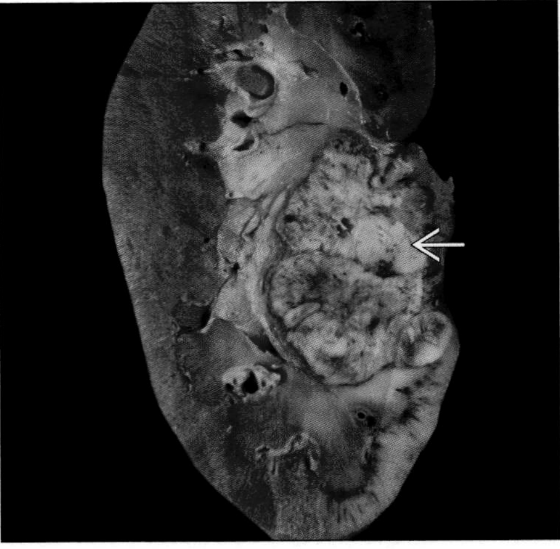

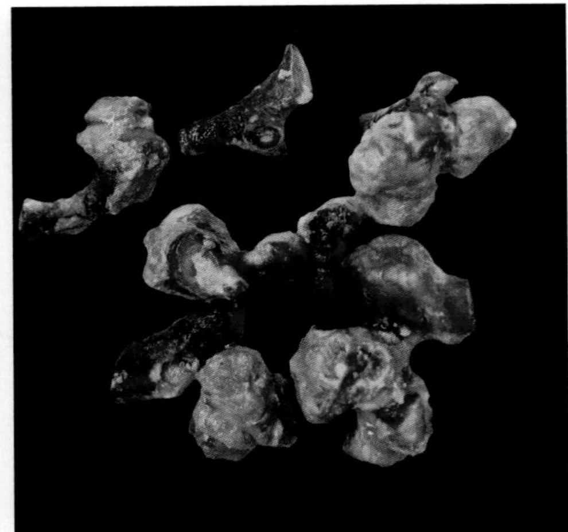

(Left) *Renal cell carcinoma, the most common renal malignancy, arises in renal cortex and has a variegated yellow cut surface, often with evidence of hemorrhage and necrosis ➡. It has a propensity for bony metastases.* ***(Right)*** *Urease-producing bacteria, such as Proteus, form ammonia and hydroxide from urea, alkalinize the urine, and promote the formation of large magnesium ammonium phosphate or struvite calculi, so-called staghorn calculi.*

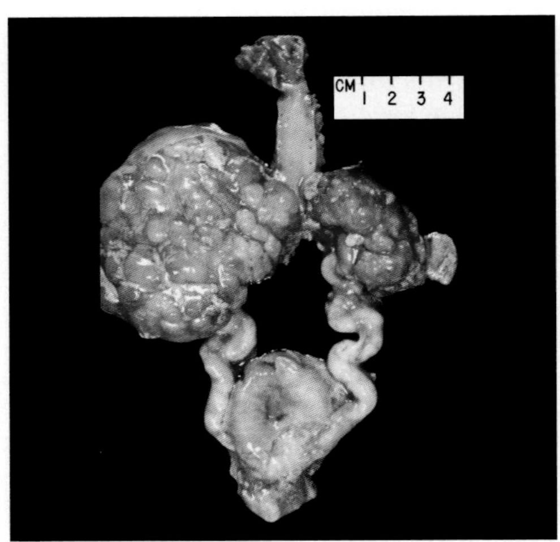

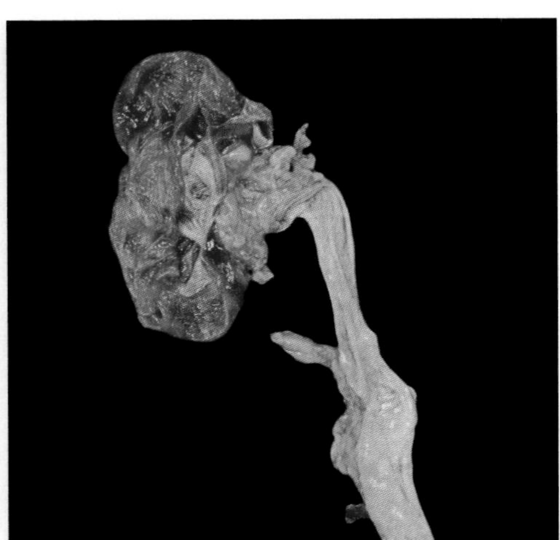

(Left) *This specimen from a fetal autopsy shows cystic kidneys and bilateral hydronephrosis caused by posterior urethral valves. Posterior urethral valves occur exclusively in males, and approximately 1/3 of children born with this condition progress to end-stage renal disease.* ***(Right)*** *Chronic ureteral obstruction leads to hydroureter and hydronephrosis. In this case, renal cortex has been reduced to a membranous sac.*

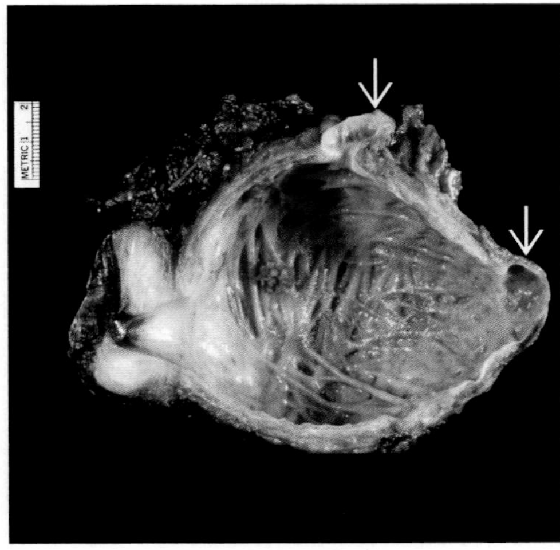

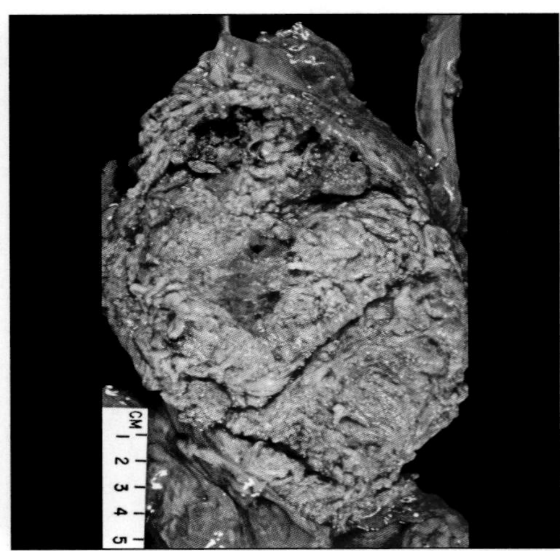

(Left) *This bisected prostate and bladder shows the results of chronic urinary obstruction by prostatic hyperplasia and increased intravesical pressure. Note the trabeculations and bladder diverticula ➡.* ***(Right)*** *Squamous cell carcinoma of the bladder is much less common than urothelial carcinoma and often arises in the the setting of chronic inflammation (chronic catheterization, urinary retention, lithiasis, schistosomiasis). Unlike urothelial carcinoma, it is more common in women.*

Genital Tract

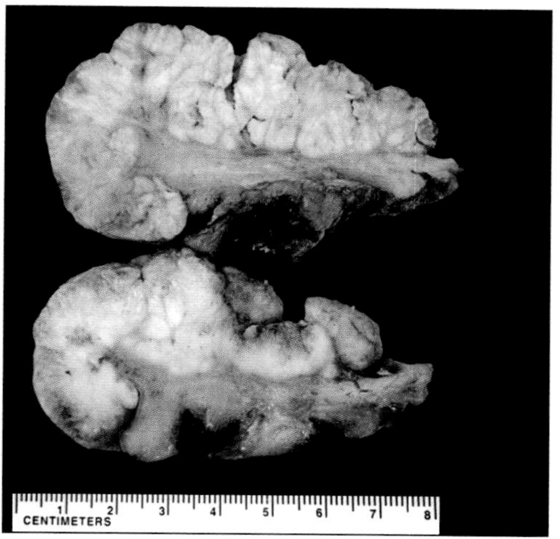

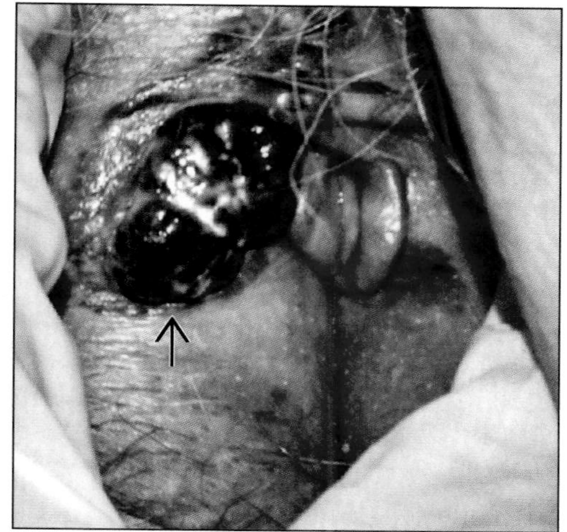

(Left) *Shown are sections of a polypoid vulvar squamous cell carcinoma. These tumors typically arise in women older than 65 and account for over 80% of vulvar malignancies. Some may be related to HPV infection.* ***(Right)*** *Melanoma is the second most common vulvar malignancy and represents 5% of malignant vulvar tumors. Genital melanomas comprise approximately 3% of all melanomas. This example is nodular and darkly pigmented ➔, but they may be amelanotic as well.*

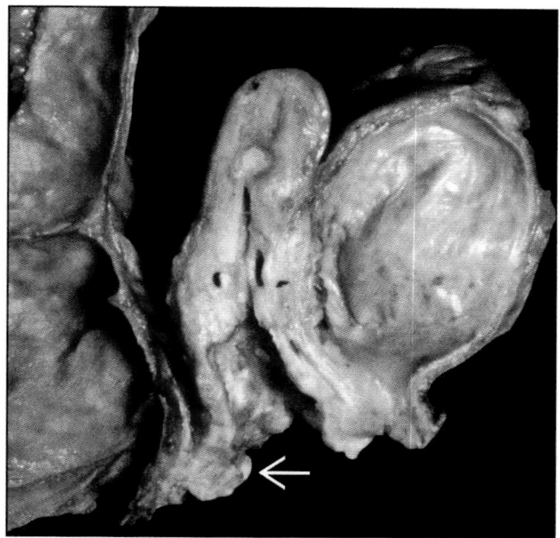

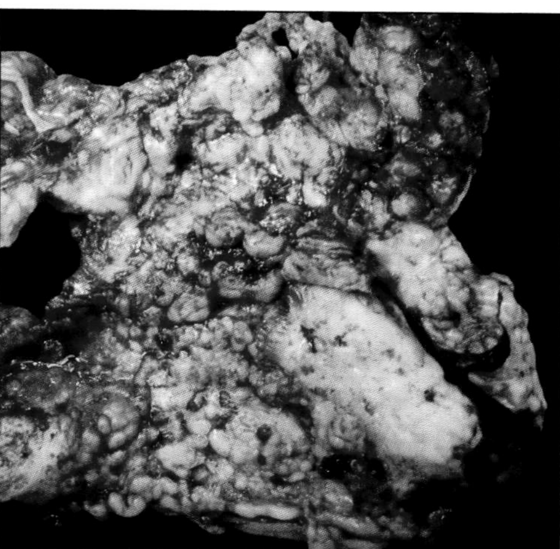

(Left) *Squamous cell carcinoma of the cervix ➔ is the most common malignant tumor of the cervix, and the vast majority are the result of infection with high-risk HPV. As shown here, cervical squamous cell carcinoma can invade adjacent structures.* ***(Right)*** *This omentum is extensively replaced by ovarian carcinoma, a phenomenon referred to as omental cake. Ovarian carcinomas often involve the peritoneal surfaces of the abdomen.*

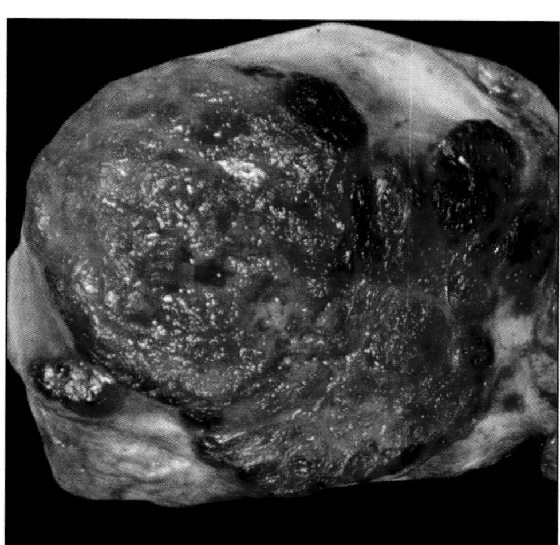

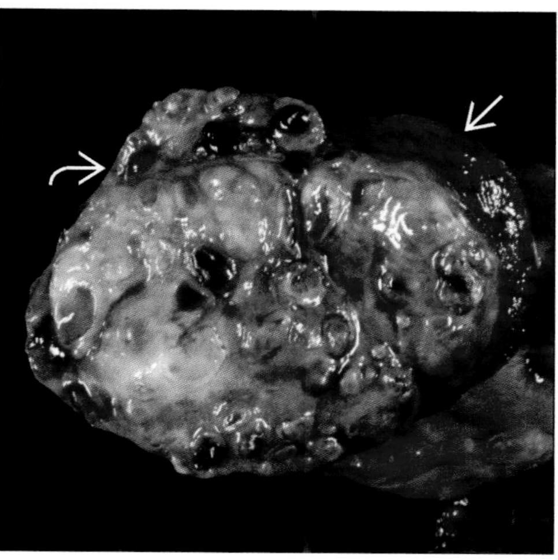

(Left) *This bisected testis has been extensively replaced by a dark red hemorrhagic tumor, which histologically proved to be choriocarcinoma. Choriocarcinoma often metastasizes widely and the primary testicular tumor may regress.* ***(Right)*** *This bisected testis is extensively replaced by mature cystic teratoma ➔, which has a variegated solid and cystic cut surface. There is a thin rim of residual uninvolved tissue ➔.*

ENDOCRINE SYSTEM

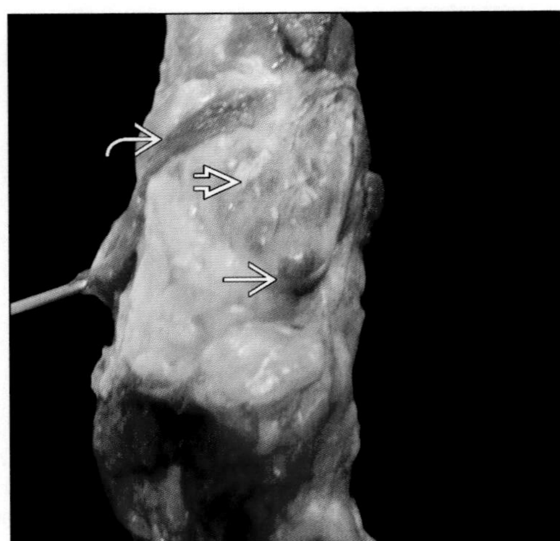

The sternothyroid muscle is being reflected to reveal the underlying thyroid gland and a parathyroid gland.

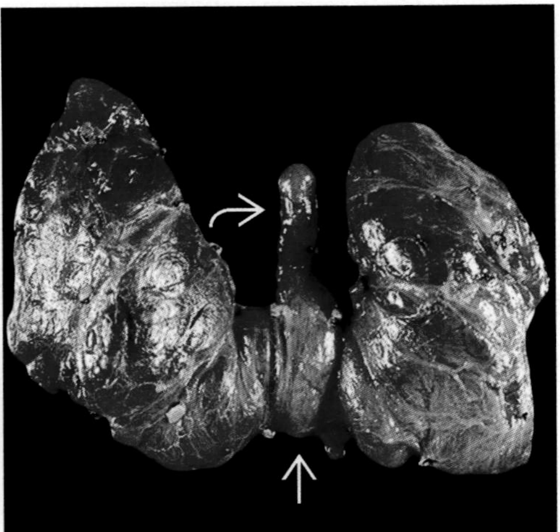

The bilobed thyroid consists of 2 lobes connected by an isthmus. A pyramidal lobe is seen in 40%, considered a vestige of the thyroglossal duct. (From DP: Normal Histology.)

TERMINOLOGY

Definitions

- Includes adrenal, thyroid, parathyroid, endocrine pancreas, and pituitary

CLINICAL CORRELATES

Clinical Diagnosis of Endocrine Disorder

- e.g,. Cushing disease, thyroid storm, hyperparathyroidism, diabetes, acromegaly

Pertinent Antemortem Labs

- Thyroid: TSH, T3, T4, TSI (Graves), antimicrosomal Ab (Hashimoto)
- Adrenal: Electrolytes, urine/serum catecholamines, 24-hour cortisol, dexamethasone suppression test
- Pituitary: Electrolytes, ACTH, GH, prolactin
- Endocrine pancreas: Glucose and electrolytes, ketones

DISSECTION TECHNIQUES

Parathyroid and Thyroid

- Removed together with neck organ block
  - Remove sternohyoid and sternothyroid muscles to expose thyroid
  - Parathyroids appear tan-brown
- Inferior parathyroids often visible even without dissecting thyroid from trachea
  - Inferior to thyroid along anterolateral trachea
    - Precarious in position: Anterior lower pole of thyroid, posterior lower pole of thyroid, or anywhere in anterior cervical fat, extending into mediastinum
- Superior parathyroids often within superior tracheal fat pad
  - Posterior medial portion of mid thyroid
  - May become visible as thyroid removed
- Thyroid
  - Removed by incising fascia along posterior aspect (from either upper or lower pole), dissecting free from trachea

Adrenals

- Paired; retroperitoneal, anteromedial to kidneys
- Identified by careful dissection through retroperitoneal fat until golden-yellow cortex is visualized
  - Right gland inferior to liver
    - En masse (Rokitansky): Approach liver from lateral aspect and reflect to reveal adrenal
    - Piecemeal (Virchow): Easily viewed in retroperitoneal fat as right lobe liver reflected (or deep to porta hepatis as portal structures are cut)
  - Left gland between left kidney and aorta
    - En masse (Rokitansky): Approach from left, posterolaterally from aorta, ~ 2 cm above left renal artery
    - Piecemeal (Virchow): Dissect retroperitoneal fat medial to superior pole of left kidney and inferior to tail of pancreas/splenic artery

Endocrine Pancreas

- Identify pancreas inferior to stomach extending between duodenum and spleen
- Islets are contained within head, body, and tail of pancreas

Pituitary

- Within sella turcica of sphenoid bone, infundibular stalk connects pituitary gland to hypothalamus
  - After brain removal, incise dura overlying pituitary gland
  - Grasping infundibular stalk with forceps, apply gentle traction while freeing gland from sella using sharp dissection

GROSS EVALUATION/SECTIONING

Parathyroids

- Record size and weight (normal: 4-6 mm, 25-40 mg; varies with age, race, illness)
- Cut surface is tan to yellow (depending on fat content)
- Submit intact or bisect larger glands

Thyroid

- Right and left lobes connected by isthmus
  - Pointed superior and blunt inferior pole of lobes
- Midline pyramidal lobe (vestige of thyroglossal duct) may be present (40%)
- Record size and weight (normal: 15-25 g; varies with age, gender, iodine intake, hormonal status, body habitus)
- Sample right and left lobes, isthmus, any gross pathology

Adrenals

- Right gland pyramidal and left crescentic in shape
- Record size and weight (normal: 4-6 g each; varies with age, gender, stress)
  - Remove surrounding fat for accurate weight
- Section perpendicular (4 mm slices) to long axis
  - Adrenal cortex normally golden yellow
  - Adrenal medulla: Gray brown, ellipsoid; ~ 10% of adult adrenal gland
  - Submit 2 sections per gland, any gross pathology

Endocrine Pancreas

- Islets are contained within head, body, and tail of pancreas and are seen in those sections

Pituitary

- Record size and weight (normal: 0.4-0.6 g; varies with pregnancy, multiparity
- Ovoid; larger anterior, smaller posterior lobe
- Bisect gland sagittally through infundibulum, submit both halves

NORMAL HISTOLOGY

Parathyroids

- Parenchymal cells: Chief, oxyphil, clear (rare) cells
  - Chief: Small, amphophilic vacuolated cytoplasm, central nucleus, in nests and cords with rich capillary network
  - Oxyphil: Larger, abundant eosinophilic granular cytoplasm, in small clusters, ↑ with age
  - Clear: Vacuolated cytoplasm due to abundant glycogen, uncommon
- Stroma adipose tissue and fibrovascular network
  - Adipose ↑ with age ↓ in hyperactive gland
    - Adult gland 20-40% adipose tissue

Thyroid

- Follicles containing central colloid; lined by monolayer of epithelial cells
  - Capillary network surrounds follicle
  - Follicular cells change shape with activity
    - Flat is inactive; cuboidal is secreting; columnar is resorbing colloid

Adrenals

- Cortex organized into 3 zones: Glomerulosa, fasciculata, and reticularis
  - Glomerulosa: Thin, discontinuous, subcapsular; small cells with scant eosinophilic to amphophilic cytoplasm
  - Fasciculata: Thickest, middle layer; larger cells with finely vacuolated lipid-laden cytoplasm
  - Reticularis: Inner layer, abuts medulla; cells with eosinophilic cytoplasm, arranged in cords
- Medulla
  - Cells with abundant basophilic granular cytoplasm, vesicular nuclei with clumped chromatin, occasional central nucleoli

Endocrine Pancreas

- Islets throughout gland, ~ 1-2% of adult gland
- Islands of cells with small amount of amphophilic to basophilic cytoplasm, demarcated from surrounding tissue and with rich capillary network

Pituitary

- Anterior (adenohypophysis)
  - Comprises 80% of adult gland
  - Cells in nests/acini rimmed by sustentacular cells
    - Mixed population of different cell types
  - Reticulin network rich in capillaries
- Posterior (neurohypophysis)
  - 20% of adult gland
  - Modified glial cells (pituicytes) and neuropil (network of unmyelinated axons)

COMMON AUTOPSY FINDINGS

Parathyroid

- Adenoma
  - Asymmetrically enlarged gland with nodular monotonous cell population without fat
- Hyperplasia
  - All glands enlarged; common in chronic renal failure; malabsorption (↓ vitamin D)

Thyroid

- Multinodular goiter
  - Enlarged thyroid containing multiple nodules
    - Weight may reach or exceed 2 kg
    - Nodules may be hemorrhagic, cystic, calcified, &/or associated with fibrosis
- Colloid nodule
  - Well-circumscribed glassy-appearing nodule

Adrenals

- Cortical adenoma
  - Well-circumscribed yellow nodule within adrenal cortex
    - Size usually < 5 cm and weight usually < 50 g
    - Most arise from zona fasciculata
- Metastatic carcinoma

External Examination Clues to Endocrine Disease

Area Examined	Findings	Endocrine Disease Association
Head and integument	Alopecia (scalp and lateral eyebrows)	Hypothyroidism, hypopituitarism (decreased TSH)
	Dry, brittle hair	Hypothyroidism, hypopituitarism (decreased TSH)
	Hirsutism	Adrenal excess (hypercortisolism)
	Exophthalmos	Hyperthyroidism (Grave disease)
	Periorbital puffiness	Hypothyroidism, hypopituitarism (decreased TSH)
	Coarse facial features	Hypothyroidism, hyperpituitarism (increase GH), hypopituitarism (decreased TSH)
	Frontal bossing	Hyperpituitarism (increased GH)
	Prognathism	Hyperpituitarism (increased GH)
	Rounded (moon) face	Adrenal excess (hypercortisolism)
	Acne	Adrenal excess (hypercortisolism)
	Hyperpigmentation of sun-exposed skin	Adrenal insufficiency, pituitary insufficiency (ACTH deficiency)
	Hypopigmentation	Pituitary insufficiency (decreased MSH)
	Thin skin with bruising	Adrenal excess (hypercortisolism)
Neck	Palpable anterior thyroid	Hyperthyroidism (Grave disease), goiter, adenoma, carcinoma
	Palpable lateral neck mass(es)	Parathyroid adenoma, hyperplasia
Breasts	Galactorrhea	Pituitary excess (prolactin) (women)
	Darkened areola	Adrenal insufficiency, pituitary insufficiency (ACTH deficiency)
Abdomen	Striae	Adrenal excess (hypercortisolism)
	Central obesity	Adrenal excess (hypercortisolism), endocrine pancreas insufficiency (diabetes mellitus, especially type 2)
	Necrolytic migratory erythema (often involves perineum and buttocks)	Endocrine pancreas excess (glucagon)
Genitalia	Testicular atrophy and softening	Hyperpituitarism (prolactin)
Extremities	Pretibial myxedema	Hypo-/hyperthyroidism
	Necrobiosis lipoidica diabeticorum (usually pretibial)	Endocrine pancreas insufficiency (diabetes) (rare complication, usually women)
	Large hands and feet	Hyperpituitarism
	Clubbing of fingers and toes	Hyperthyroidism (rare)
	Foot ulcers	Endocrine pancreas insufficiency (diabetes)
	Gangrene	Endocrine pancreas insufficiency (diabetes)

- Metastatic tumor deposits are grossly distinct from surrounding adrenal but are usually well circumscribed

Endocrine Pancreas

- Amyloid in islets of type 2 diabetics (islet amyloid polypeptide amylin)

Pituitary

- Micro- (< 10 mm) and macroadenomas
  - Soft, well-circumscribed tan nodule
  - May be confined to sella or extend out (suprasellar)
  - Micro: Uniform polygonal cells without reticulin network
  - May be composed primarily of acidophilic, basophilic, or chromophobic cells
- Rathke cleft cysts (30% of pituitary glands)
  - Usually only seen microscopically; occur in adenohypophysis
  - Cyst lined by ciliated cuboidal cells, occasional goblet cells and anterior pituitary cells
- Salivary gland rests in posterior pituitary may be seen at junction with infundibulum

ANCILLARY TESTS

Serum

- Hormone assays
  - TSH shown to be stable post mortem
  - Mostly specific forensic use, not routine
- Glucose
  - Spuriously low (postmortem glycolysis)

Vitreous and CSF

- More stable for glucose and electrolytes

Urine

- Urine glucose and protein relatively stable post mortem

SELECTED REFERENCES

1. Palmiere C et al: Postmortem chemistry update part I. Int J Legal Med. 126(2):187-98, 2012
2. Elias AN et al: Pathology of endocrine organs in chronic renal failure--an autopsy analysis of 66 patients. Int J Artif Organs. 7(5):251-6, 1984

In Situ, Excised Endocrine Organs

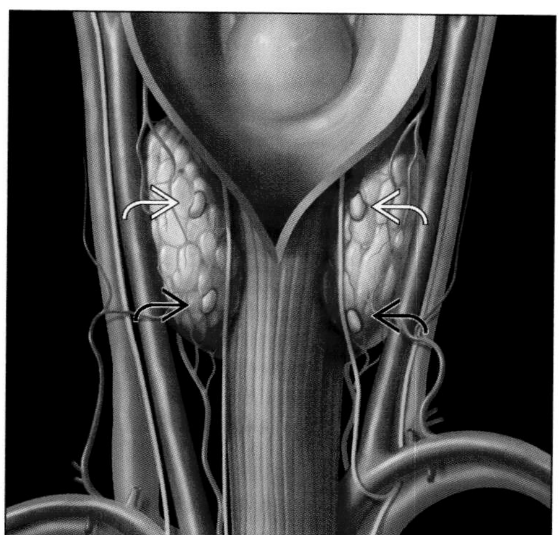

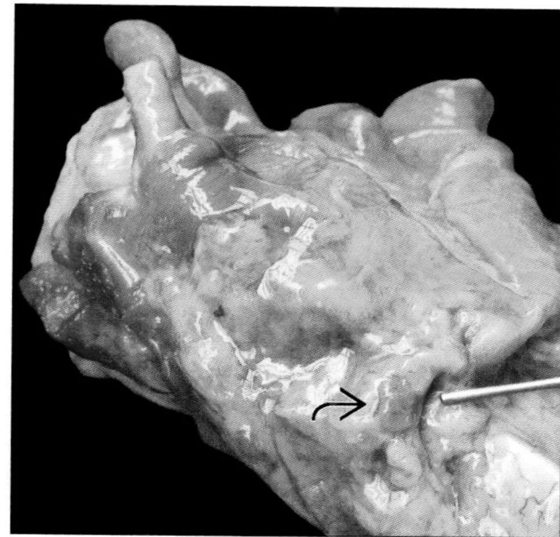

***(Left)** This illustration shows the positioning of the parathyroid glands along the posterior surface of the thyroid gland. The superior glands are more uniform in location than the inferior glands. **(Right)** Right inferior parathyroid gland embedded within adipose tissue shows a normal tan-brown appearance. Note that this gland is located somewhat lateral to the thyroid, not along the posterior surface. Inferior parathyroid glands can be variable in position.*

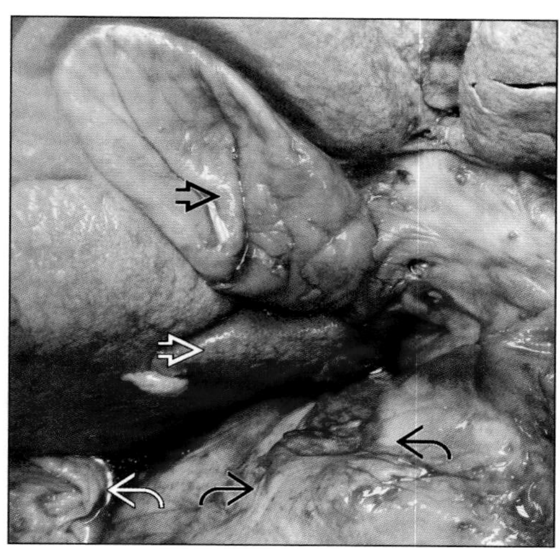

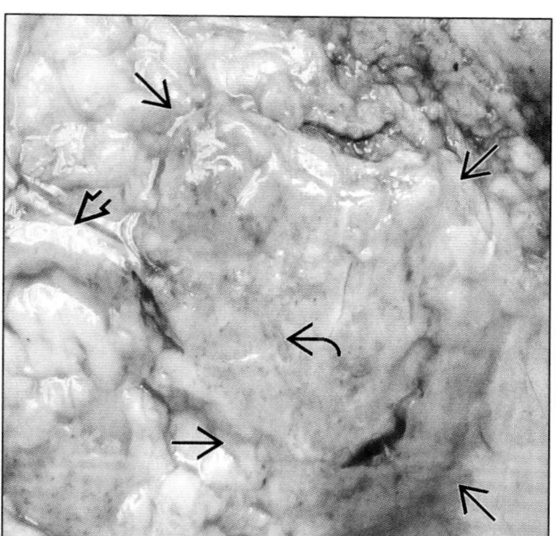

***(Left)** This is an in situ view of the right adrenal gland. It is located beneath the right lobe of the liver, slightly lateral to the liver hilum (note gallbladder) and inferior to the diaphragm. **(Right)** The left adrenal gland is superomedial to the left kidney and inferior to the pancreas. The left adrenal vein is visualized as it courses towards the left renal vein. The tan-white tissue surrounding the adrenal is the adrenal capsule.*

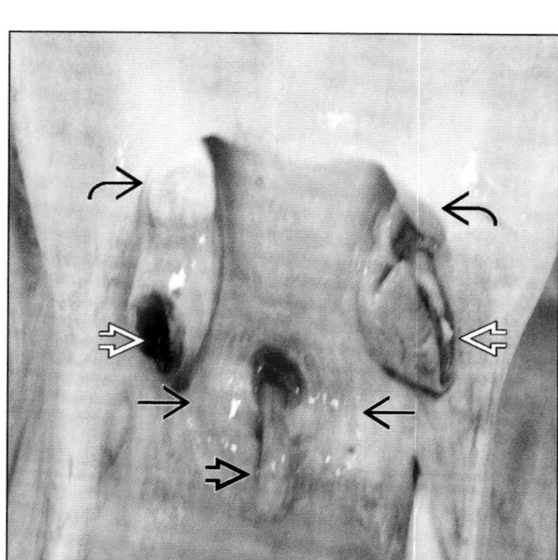

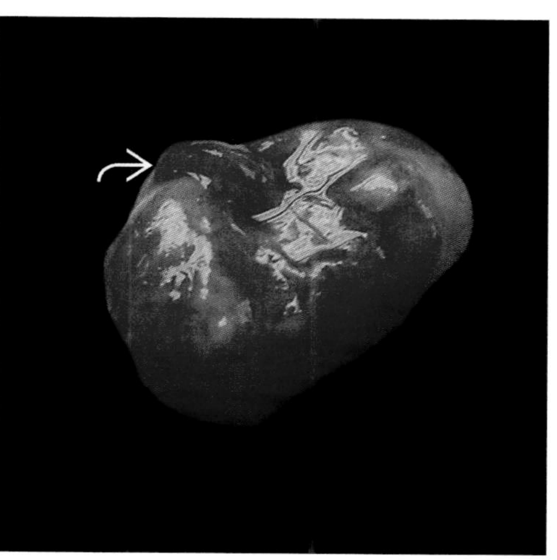

***(Left)** The pituitary gland sits in the base of the skull. The infundibulum (stalk) protrudes through the dura overlying the sella turcica. The cut ends of the optic chiasm and the internal carotid arteries demonstrate the proximity of these important structures to the pituitary. (Courtesy R. Rhodes, MD.) **(Right)** This gross image of a normal pituitary gland demonstrates its ovoid shape and the attached stalk. The normal pituitary weighs between 0.4-0.6 gms.*

Normal Histology

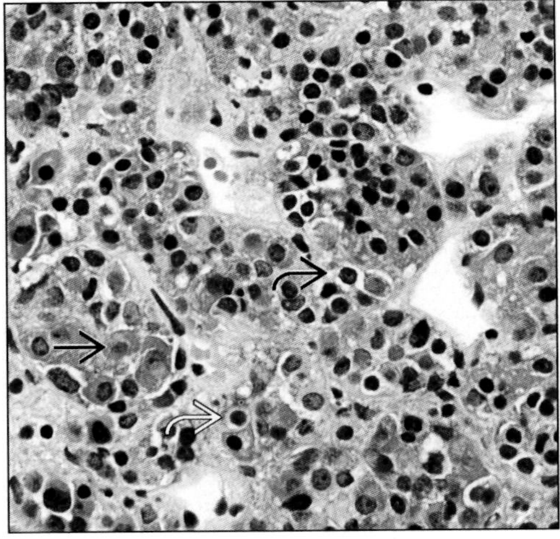

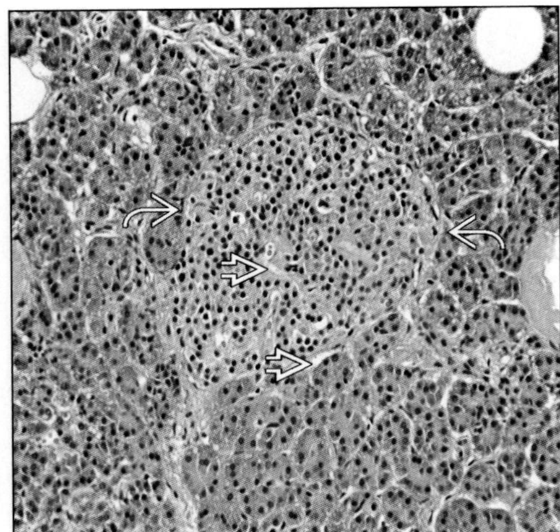

(Left) The adenohypophysis has eosinophilic ⮕, basophilic ⮕, chromophobe ⮕, and sustentacular cells with surrounding capillaries. Hormone secretion can be determined by immunohistochemistry. (From DP: Normal Histology.) ***(Right)*** *The pancreas has ~ 1 million islets ⮕, which are distinct cell clusters with a rich vascular network ⮕. They contain β, α, δ, and PP cells producing insulin, glucagon, somatostatin, and pancreatic polypeptide, respectively. β cells are the most numerous.*

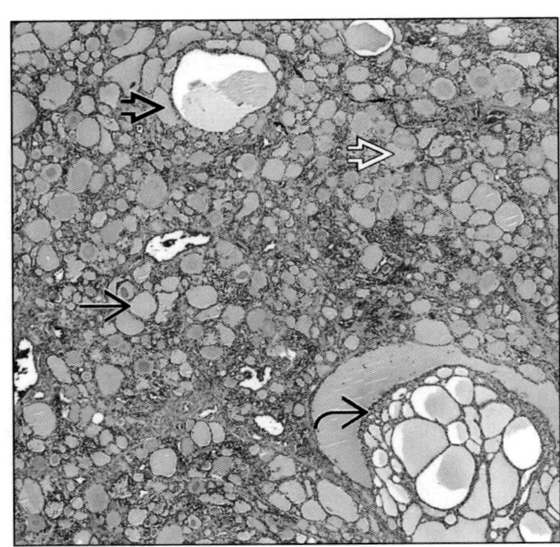

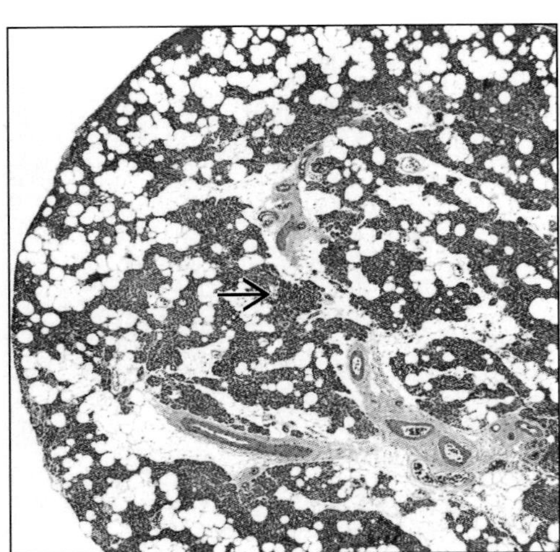

(Left) *Follicles ⮕ are the functional thyroid unit and comprise a single layer of follicular cells around colloid ⮕. There is a microscopic nodule ⮕ and a small colloid nodule ⮕ present. (From DP: Normal Histology.)* ***(Right)*** *The parenchymal cell of the parathyroid is the chief cell ⮕. Adipose tissue and fibrovascular tissue comprise the stroma. Fat increases with age and decreases with activity of the gland. (From DP: Normal Histology.)*

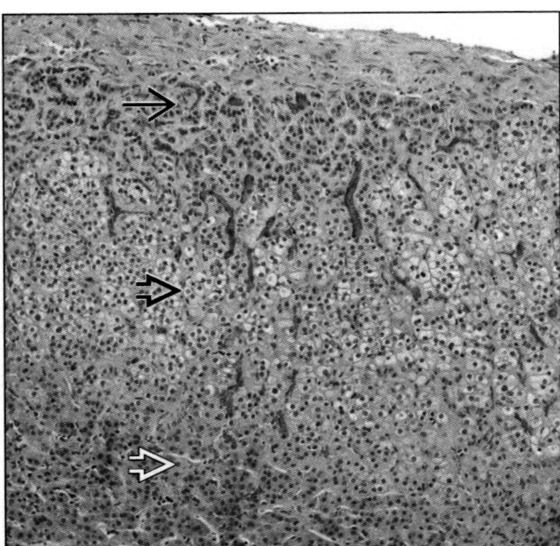

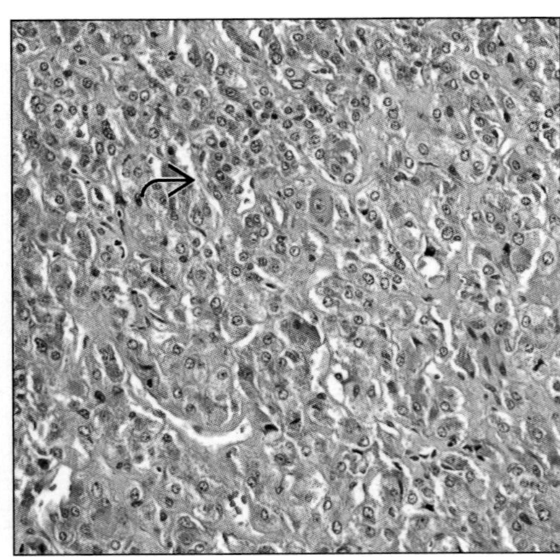

(Left) *The adrenal cortex is organized into 3 layers from the capsule toward the medulla: The glomerulosa ⮕, fasciculata ⮕, and reticularis ⮕. The fasciculata comprises the majority of the cortex, and the cells contain abundant lipid that imparts the yellow color to the adrenal gland macroscopically. (From DP: Normal Histology.)* ***(Right)*** *The adrenal medulla is composed of large polygonal cells with abundant basophilic cytoplasm ⮕. (From DP: Normal Histology.)*

Frequent Autopsy Findings

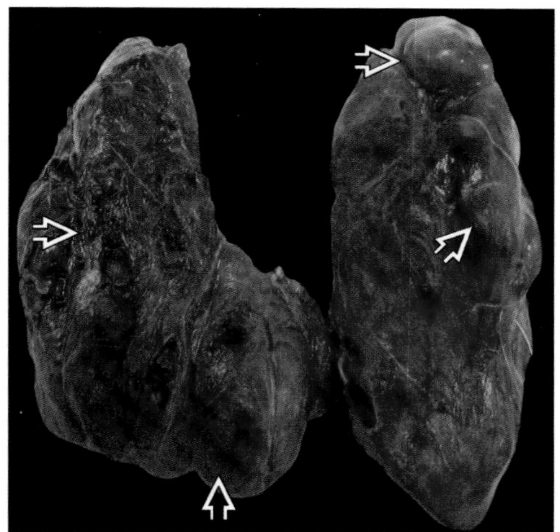

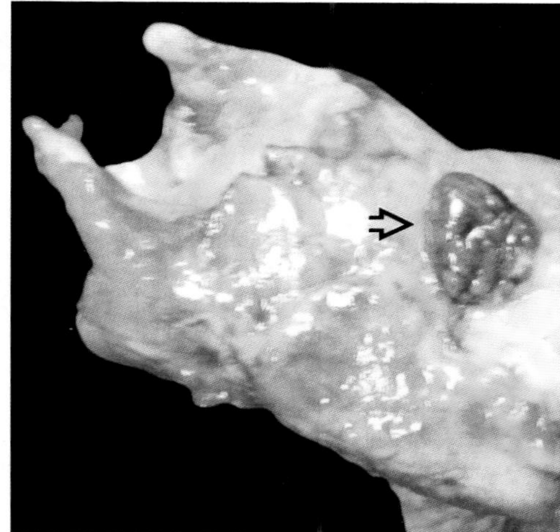

(Left) *This asymmetrically enlarged and multinodular ➡ thyroid represents a multinodular goiter. An enlarged gland without nodules is a simple goiter. Multinodular goiter can reach marked sizes ≥ 2 kg.* ***(Right)*** *This enlarged parathyroid gland ➡ (1.5 cm) was the only enlarged gland identified and represents a small adenoma.*

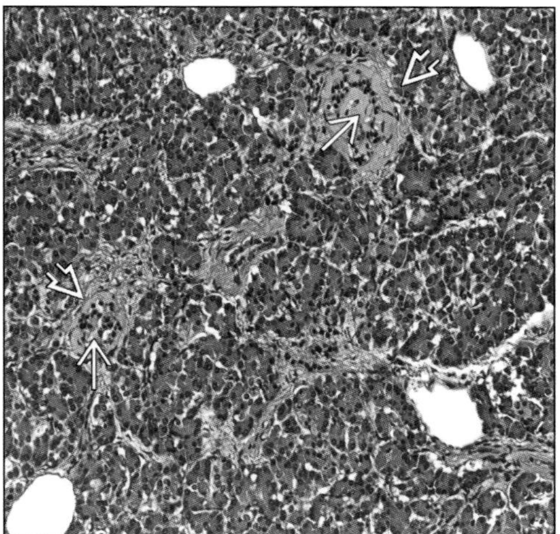

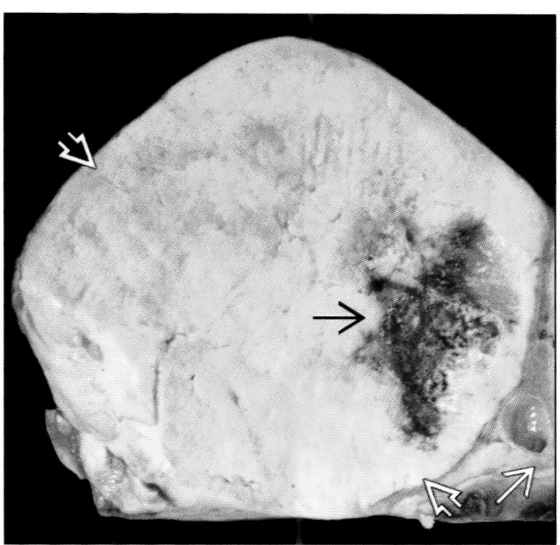

(Left) *These islets ➡ of a type 2 diabetic contain hyaline-appearing amyloid ➡. The amyloid protein is islet amyloid polypeptide (amylin). The cells can be obscured when large amounts of amyloid are deposited.* ***(Right)*** *This well-circumscribed yellow nodule ➡ within the adrenal gland (residual cortex ➡) represents an adenoma. Although slightly larger than most identified at autopsy, this adenoma demonstrates a classic appearance, except for the small focus of hemorrhage ➡.*

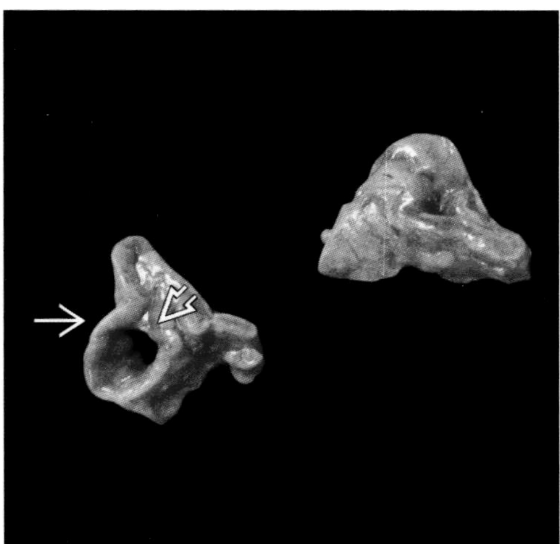

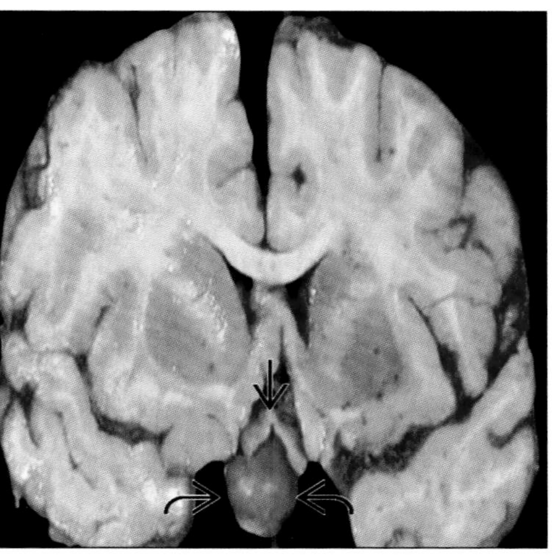

(Left) *The adrenal glands are often autolyzed at autopsy, as demonstrated here. The autolysis affects the adrenal medulla before the cortex, often leaving a space ➡ surrounded by the residual adrenal cortical tissue ➡.* ***(Right)*** *This coronal section of the brain reveals a large, brown-appearing pituitary adenoma ➡ attached to the optic chiasm ➡. This proximity to the optic chiasm accounts for the visual disturbances caused by adenomas.*

CENTRAL NERVOUS SYSTEM

Inferior view of a brain shows all the cranial nerves that were cut during removal, except the olfactory. The internal carotid arteries are also seen. There is a collection of blood over the left inferior cerebellum.

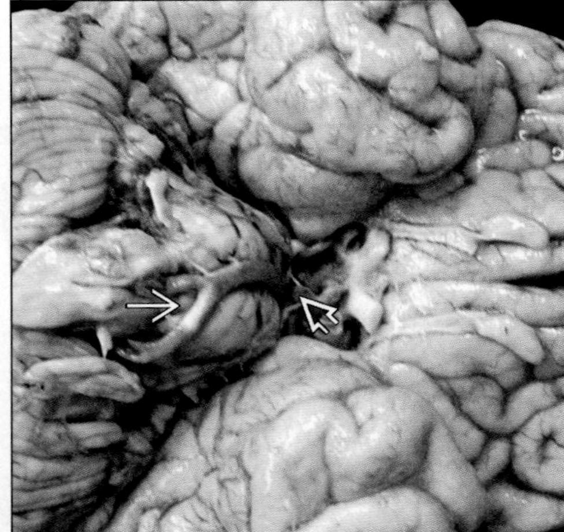

Atherosclerosis of the left vertebral artery is apparent from this inferior view of the brain. The mamillary bodies are also seen (a landmark for coronally sectioning the brain).

TERMINOLOGY

Definitions

- Brain and spinal cord

Abbreviations

- Central nervous system (CNS)

MACROSCOPIC FINDINGS

External Examination

- Trauma (pattern of injury)
  - Bruising, lacerations
  - Fractures
    - Bruising around eyes (raccoon sign), mastoid: Basal skull fracture
- Limb musculature
  - Asymmetry, atrophy: Stroke, demyelination, neurodegenerative disease
- Deformities
  - Facial dysmorphism
  - Skin abnormalities (e.g., café au lait spots in neurofibromatosis type 1)
  - Cleft lip/palate: Septo-optic dysplasia
- Debilitation
  - Feeding tube
  - Decubitus ulcers
- Anoxia
  - Evidence of resuscitation (rib fractures, automated external defibrillator [AED] pads, etc.)
  - Survival for at least 6-12 hours needed for microscopic evidence

Prosection

- Brain
  - Block between shoulder blades helps position skull
  - Bitemporal skin incision from pinna to pinna across vertex scalp
    - Peel skin forward to just above brow anteriorly and below occiput posteriorly
  - Divide temporalis muscle on each side along line connecting pinna and eyebrow
    - Scrape clean path for saw pass-through (exposing underlying bone)
  - Remove skull cap using vibrating saw cutting in semicircle from temporal to frontal, then from temporal to occiput
    - Triangular notch ensures fit after autopsy
  - With hand support posteriorly, incise falx, vessels, and cranial nerves (except olfactory) to release brain from vault
  - Transect upper cervical cord and remove from body
  - Strip dura from skull base (examine for fractures) and calvaria (examine dural sinuses)
  - Remove pituitary by unroofing (fracturing) the dorsum sellae, incising around diaphragm
- Fixation
  - 10-20% formalin for 7-10 days before sectioning
    - Hang by string under basilar artery
  - Dehydrate blocked sections 24 hours in 70% ethanol, then 24 hours in 95% ethanol before routine processing and embedding
- Brain cutting
  - Remove cerebellum by transecting midbrain horizontally at level of cerebellar peduncles
  - Section cerebellum and pons axially in 5 mm sections
  - Divide brain into anterior and posterior halves for coronal sectioning
    - Hemispheres facing down on cutting board
    - Initial cut through mamillary bodies
    - Aim for symmetry using temporal lobe horns as a guide
    - Incise midbrain on 1 side to help with orientation
  - Section each half coronally in 1 cm sections
    - Lay out sections serially

- Invert each section from one of the halves to maintain right-left orientation in serial sections

- Spinal cord
  - Removed en bloc from cervical to cauda equina, using either anterior or posterior approach
  - Anterior approach (most common, allows ganglia and nerve roots to be removed)
    - Place body supine with block between shoulders
    - Dissect paraspinal muscles away from all vertebral pedicles
    - Use vibrating saw to cut line connecting pedicles to body; adjust angle of cut as vertebra change shape
    - Use wedge hammer to pry vertebral bodies up and expose canal
  - Posterior approach (for craniocervical anomalies, neck injuries, and meningoceles)
    - Place body prone with block under sternum
    - Incise skin along line of spinous processes
    - Dissect muscle and soft tissue to expose vertebral laminae
    - Use vibrating saw to cut line at laminae, lift posterior bony plate to expose canal
    - Use saw/rongeurs to expose roots and ganglia at each level
  - Cord removal
    - Incise dura lengthwise from neck to sacrum
    - Cut dura circumferentially at level high in neck
    - Gently tug high cord down through high neck
    - Continue caudally, freeing cord and dura from canal
    - "Bread-loaf" section entire cord at 5 mm intervals
- Vertebral artery
  - Should be examined in traumatic deaths (may also be spontaneous)
  - Blood in cisterna magna may be seen with vertebral artery injury
  - Travels in transverse foramina of cervical vertebrae (expose using rongeurs)
  - Enters foramen magnum
- Fetal CNS
  - Incise along fontanelles and sutures and expose skull in butterfly fashion
  - Removal similar to adult, but tissue is extremely soft
  - Use posterior spine approach in Dandy-Walker cyst, occipital encephalocele, craniocervical abnormalities

General Features

- Surface
  - Hemisphere symmetry: Stroke, degenerative disease
  - Gyral effacement, sulcal prominence
  - Cerebellar vermis atrophy: Chronic alcohol abuse
  - Tonsillar, uncal herniation
  - Meninges
    - Opaque, purulent: Meningitis
- Cut sections
  - Grey-white junction: Focally indistinct in ischemia, demyelination, dysplasias
    - Site of subtle metastatic tumor, emboli, thrombi
  - Ventricle enlargement and hippocampal atrophy: Neurodegenerative, seizure
  - Basal ganglia, pons, and cerebellum
    - Common locations for lacunar infarcts
    - Lentiform nuclei atrophy, discoloration: Neurodegenerative, toxic
    - Caudate atrophy: Huntington disease
  - Midbrain substantia nigra and locus ceruleus
    - Loss of pigmentation in Parkinson disease and multisystem atrophy
  - Pediatric
    - Congenital malformations
    - Choroid plexus/germinal matrix hemorrhage
    - Periventricular white matter discoloration/ cavitation
  - Cerebral vasculature
    - Carotid atherosclerosis
    - Circle of Willis (atherosclerosis, aneurysm)
    - Vertebrobasilar system (atherosclerosis, dissection)
- Spinal cord
  - Softening/darkening may indicate hemorrhage, ischemia
    - Watershed between anterior 2/3 and posterior 1/3 of each cross section
    - Craniocaudal watersheds at T1-T4 and L1-2 (few collaterals)
  - White matter discoloration: Demyelinating disease
  - Atrophic anterior roots: Amyotrophic lateral sclerosis, polio
  - Traumatic laceration, contusions, or old cavitation (syrinx)
- Sections to be submitted
  - Sample any suspected lesions; corresponding sections from other side may be taken for comparison
  - Routine sections
    - Cortex and white matter (frontal, temporal, parietal, occipital), e.g., superior midfrontal gyrus
    - "Watershed" areas (frontotemporal-anterior/ middle cerebral arteries, parietooccipital-middle/ posterior cerebral arteries)
    - Basal ganglia, thalamus, mamillary bodies
    - Hippocampus
    - Midbrain
    - Pons (locus ceruleus)
    - Cerebellum with vermis &/or deep nuclei
    - Cervical, thoracic, and lumbar cord (with ganglia, if possible)
    - Pituitary gland, bisected along long axis and submitted en face
  - Neurodegenerative disease (in addition to routine)
    - Cingulate, insula
    - Amygdala
    - Nucleus basalis
    - Medulla (inferior olivary nucleus)
    - Motor cortex
  - Staining
    - Routine sections through brain are stained with H&E alone or also stained with Luxol fast blue (LFB) to highlight myelin; these H&E/LFB sections show gray matter as pink and white matter as blue
    - Sections without expected white matter, such as pituitary gland, can be stained with H&E alone

- In patients > 65 years of age, even without clinical history of dementia, routine sections through frontal and temporal cortex and hippocampus can be stained with Bielschowsky silver stain to screen for age-related amyloid plaques and neurofibrillary tangles

MICROSCOPIC FINDINGS

General Features

- 6-layered cortex and underlying white matter with normal myelination
  - Pediatric brains: Cortical maturation, myelination matched for age
- Basal ganglia: Evidence of arteriosclerosis or Alzheimer type II astrocytosis (metabolic encephalopathy)
- Loss of neurons (or "red" neurons) in susceptible areas: Cerebral hypoxia
  - CA1 region of hippocampus
  - Cerebellar Purkinje cells
- Increased cellularity indicating neoplasia or gliosis
- Intraneuronal or intraglial inclusions
  - Neurodegenerative
  - Inflammatory
  - Metabolic
- Areas of necrosis: Infarction or neoplasia

CLINICAL CORRELATES

Neurologic History

- Handedness, neurological disease, risk factors or trauma, swallowing difficulty/aspiration (neurodegenerative)

Systemic Disease

- Diabetes, atherosclerotic risk factors (cerebrovascular disease)
- Atrial fibrillation, coagulopathy, endocarditis (stroke)
- Hepatic, renal failure (encephalopathy)
- Drugs (anticonvulsant, immunosuppression)
- Shock, volume loss (watershed ischemia)
- Vasculitis, sarcoid, etc.

SPECIAL PRECAUTIONS

Suspected Prion Disease

- Incidence and transmission risk is extremely low
- Universal precautions (mask, eye protection, disposable gown, and double gloves)
- Extra precautions
  - Dedicated room
  - Dedicated or disposable instruments
  - Isolation tent to collect bone dust
  - PAPR, HEPA filter breathing apparatus
  - Disposable pads to prevent cuts, punctures
- Tared container (weighed before and after brain submerged)
  - Formic acid formalin fixation
- Cleaning instruments and surfaces
  - NaOCl (bleach) solution of 20,000 ppm
  - 1 normal NaOH
  - Autoclave (121° C gravity displacement of 134° C porous load)
- Rapid triage process sample from frontal lobe
  - 100% formic acid for 1 hour, formalin for 48 hours, then processed
  - If spongiform encephalopathy, then continue precautions for brain cutting

ANCILLARY TESTS

Lumbar Puncture

- Increased WBC count, abnormal protein or glucose, indicating infection
- CSF cultures for bacteria, fungi, acid-fast bacilli, PCR for viruses
- CSF may show malignant cells in carcinomatous meningitis or ventricular tumors

EEG

- Premortem EEG may indicate seizure disorder, focal lesion, prion disease

CT/MR

- Mass lesions, skull fractures (CT), meningeal enhancement, infarcts/hemorrhages

Angiography

- Conventional or CT angiogram/MR angiogram (vasculitis, vascular malformations)

EMG/Nerve Conduction Studies

- Denervation may indicate peripheral or central (cord or roots) nervous system disease

SELECTED REFERENCES

1. Center for Disease Control and Prevention Guidelines: Creutzfeldt-Jakob Disease Infection-Control Practices. http://www.cdc.gov/ncidod/dvrd/cjd/qa_cjd_infection_control.htm. Published August 23, 2010. Accessed May 12, 2014
2. Finkbeiner W et al: Autopsy Pathology: A Manual and Atlas. 2nd Ed. Philadelphia: Saunders Elsevier, 2009
3. Waters B: Handbook of Autopsy Practice. 4th Ed. Totowa: Humana Press, 2009
4. Love S: Post mortem sampling of the brain and other tissues in neurodegenerative disease. Histopathology. 44(4):309-17, 2004
5. Gilles FH: Perinatal neuropathology. In: Davis RL et al: Textbook of Neuropathology. Baltimore: Williams & Wilkins. 331-85, 1997
6. Budka H et al: Tissue handling in suspected Creutzfeldt-Jakob disease (CJD) and other human spongiform encephalopathies (prion diseases). Brain Pathol. 5(3):319-22, 1995
7. Adams VI: Autopsy technique for neck examination. II. Vertebral column and posterior compartment. Pathol Annu. 26 Pt 1:211-26, 1991

Brain Removal and Prosection

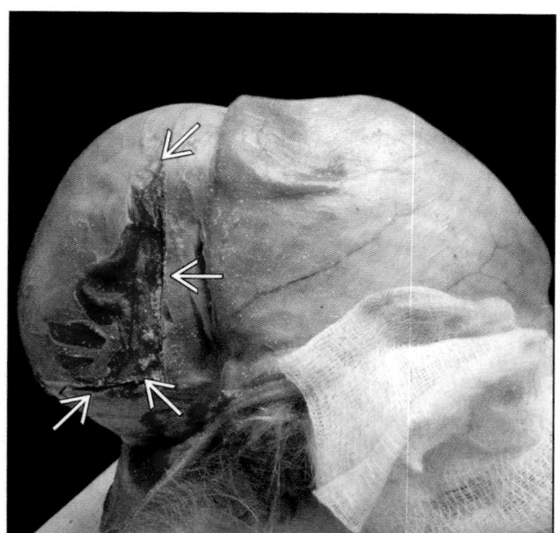

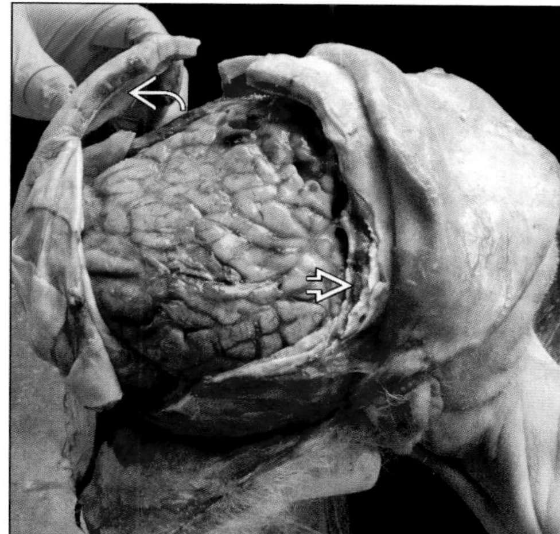

(Left) *Gross picture at autopsy shows the scalp incised and reflected to expose the skull and dissected temporalis muscle creating a path for the vibrating saw. The saw lines ➔ can also be seen.* ***(Right)*** *This image demonstrates removal of the skull cap ➔ and cutting through any dural attachments. A large defect ➔ is also seen from prior craniectomy.*

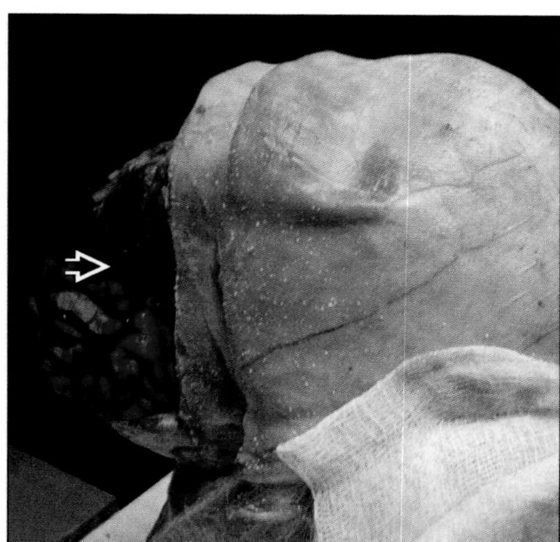

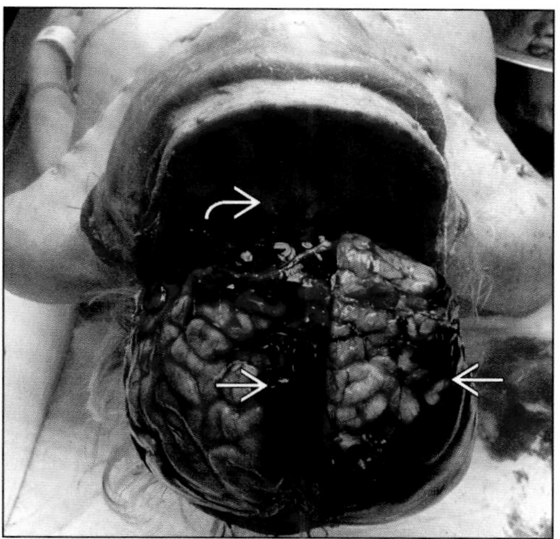

(Left) *Gross photo viewed from the right side shows the appearance of the brain after removal of the skull cap and dura. Note diffuse subarachnoid hemorrhage ➔.* ***(Right)*** *Anterior attachments, including olfactory tracts, infundibulum, and optic chiasm ➔ have been cut. Attachments at the middle cranial fossa and posterior dural attachments can now be cut. Note the bilateral subarachnoid hemorrhages ➔.*

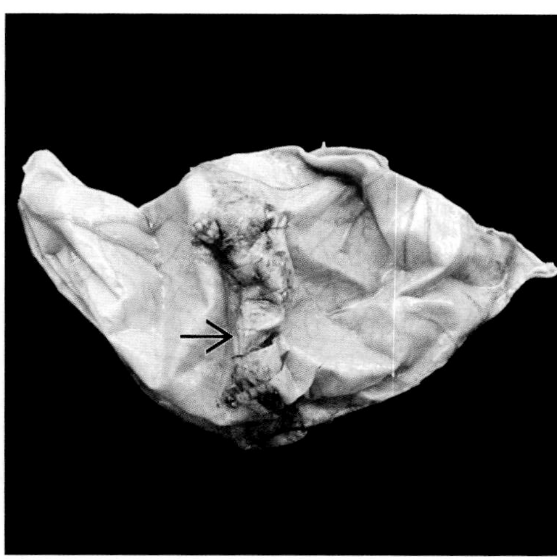

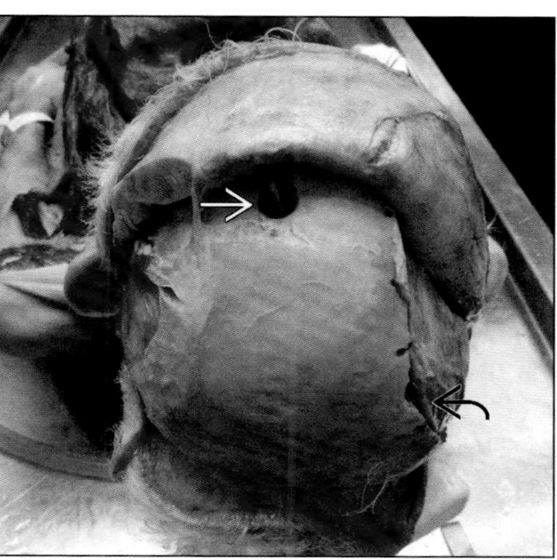

(Left) *This portion of dura, peeled from the skull cap, shows serial cuts ➔ through the superior sagittal sinus to assess patency and presence of clots.* ***(Right)*** *This patient with previous craniectomy ➔ and drain placement ➔ presents more of a challenge for brain removal. The standard approach to removal should still be followed as closely as possible, cutting around or through any surgical incisions.*

CENTRAL NERVOUS SYSTEM

Brain Cutting

*(**Left**) This superior view of the brain after stripping the meninges allows better assessment of landmarks. Note the omega (Ω) shape of the hand area of the motor (precentral) gyrus ➙. (**Right**) Right lateral view shows fixed autopsy brain with meninges stripped. This gyral pattern is normal (in comparison to the gyral atrophy and widened sulci seen in dementia, especially in the frontal and temporal lobes in frontotemporal dementia). The cerebellum ➙ has not yet been removed.*

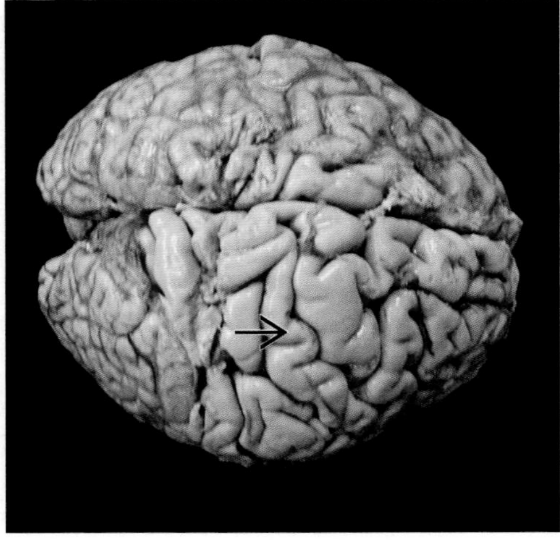

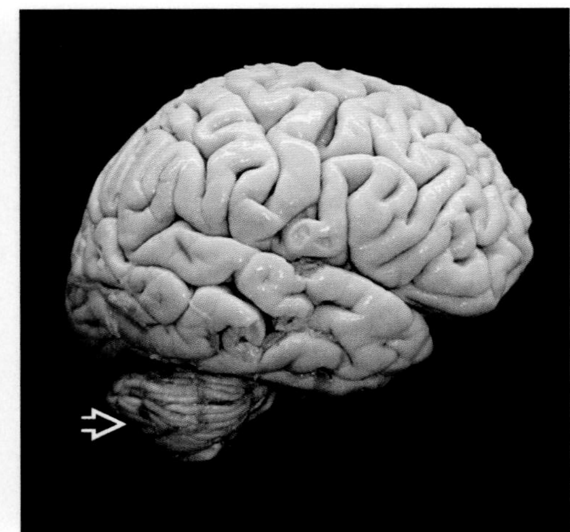

*(**Left**) Lifting the brainstem away from the cerebrum, the cerebellum can be removed by a horizontal midbrain incision ➙ through the cerebellar peduncles. (**Right**) The 1st step in brain cutting is to coronally separate the anterior and posterior halves of the cerebrum. A coronal cut is made directly downward through the mamillary bodies ➙. The anterior temporal lobes ➙ can be used as a guide to ensure a symmetric cut.*

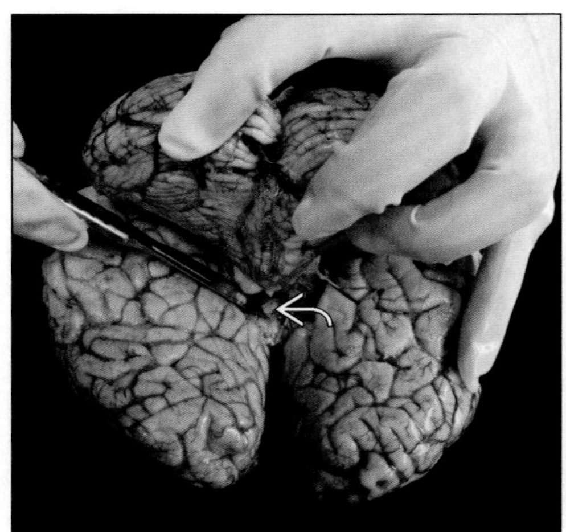

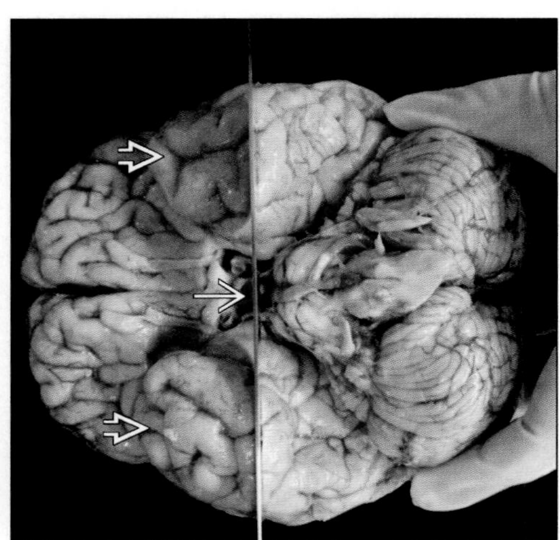

*(**Left**) Scoring ➙ either the right or left side of the brainstem can be performed so that laterality can be established on microscopic sections. (**Right**) Alternatively, the cerebellum can be removed after the coronal cut through the hemispheres. Using a scalpel, a straight horizontal incision is made caudal to the mamillary bodies ➙, through the midbrain (cerebellar peduncles).*

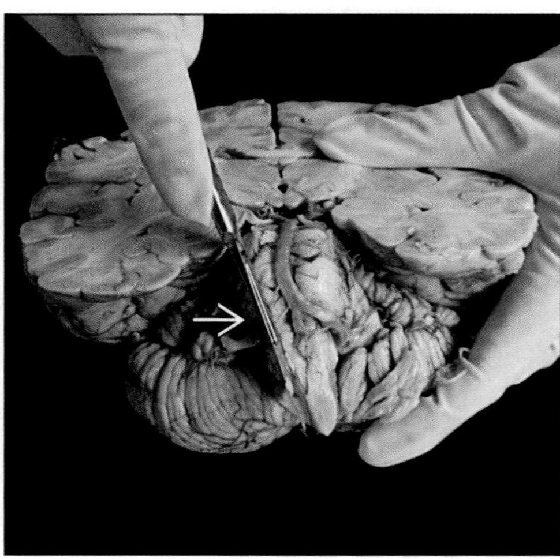

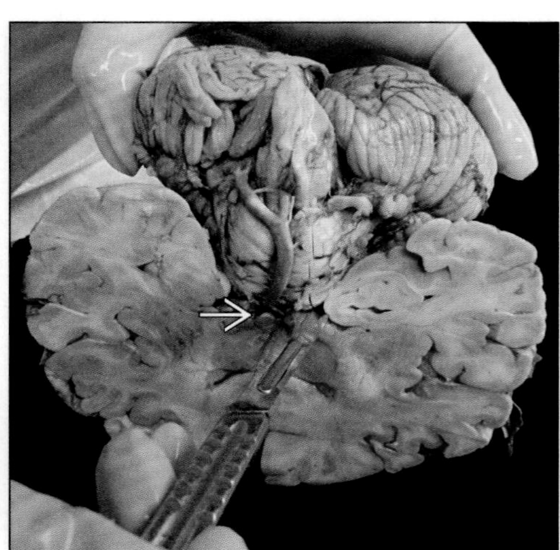

Brain Cutting

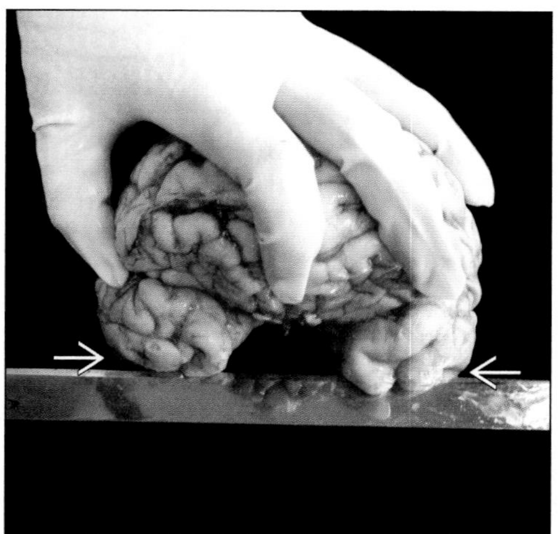

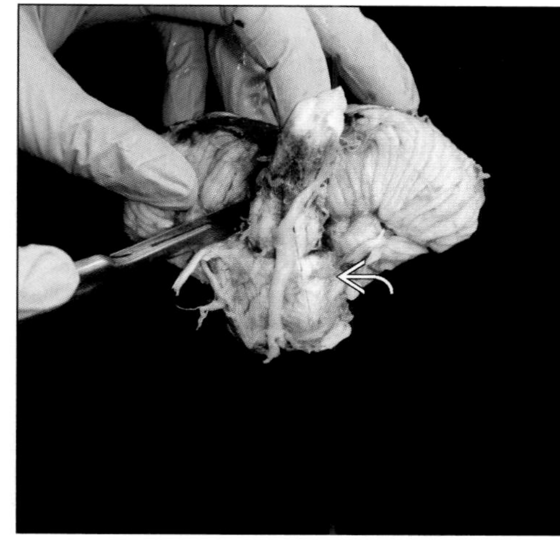

(Left) *After the brain is divided in half, each half is sectioned coronally ➡ with the flat side down (anterior half shown here). A long blade is used to make 1 cm slices through the brain. If possible, avoid jagged sawing motions.* ***(Right)*** *One method for sectioning the cerebellum is to first separate brain stem from cerebellum. A scalpel is used to severe vascular and meningeal attachments and then cut through the middle cerebellar peduncle ➡ on each side.*

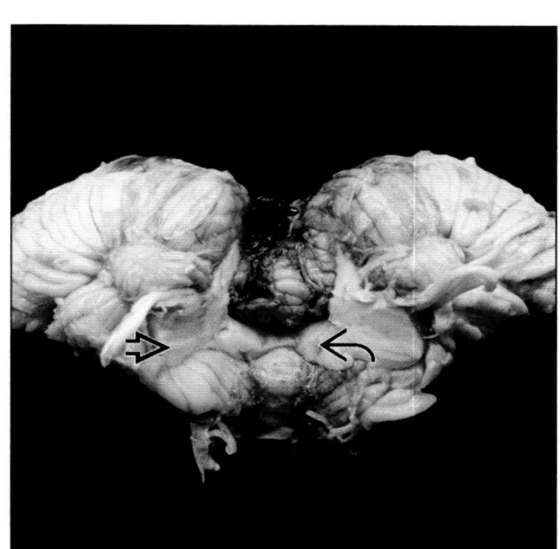

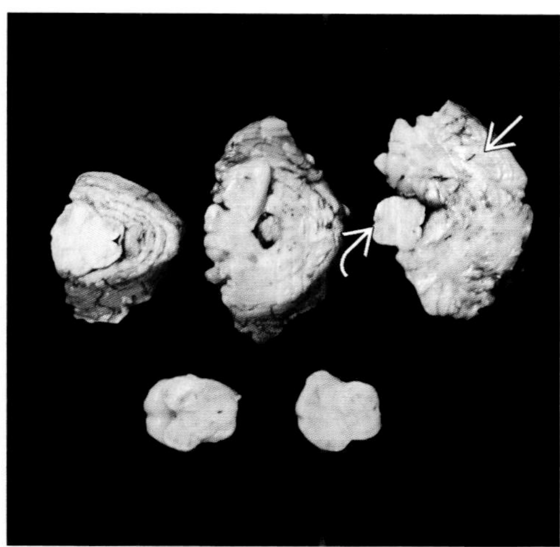

(Left) *Photograph shows the cerebellum after removal of the brainstem. Note the roof of 4th ventricle ➡ is cleanly separated from the cerebellar vermis and the middle peduncle ➡ is viewed en face.* ***(Right)*** *In this pediatric brain, the brainstem ➡ and cerebellum ➡ are kept intact and sectioned horizontally together. This may allow for better evaluation of suspected brainstem or cerebellar congenital malformations, such as a Dandy-Walker cyst.*

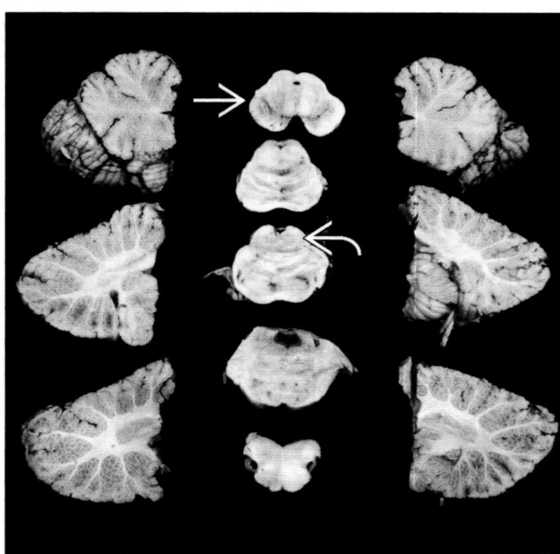

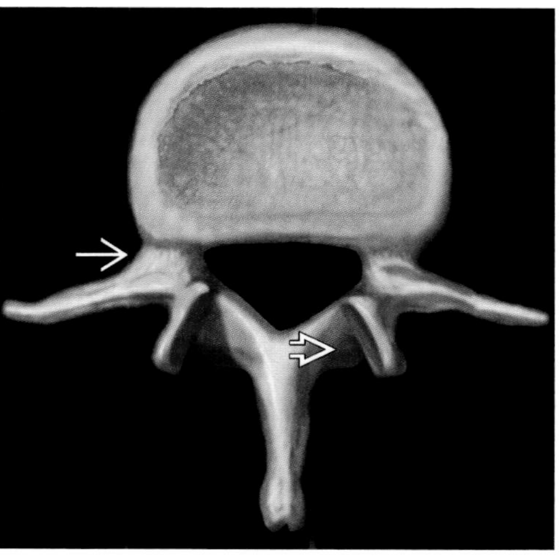

(Left) *Photograph shows axial sections through the brainstem and cerebellum in ~ 5 mm sections from rostral to caudal. Note the pigmentation of the substantia nigra ➡ and locus ceruleus ➡.* ***(Right)*** *In the anterior approach to cord removal, saw cuts are made at pedicles ➡. In the posterior approach, the cut is made through the lamina ➡. The angle of the saw cuts needs to be adjusted, as cervical, thoracic, and lumbar vertebrae have different shapes.*

PERIPHERAL NERVOUS SYSTEM

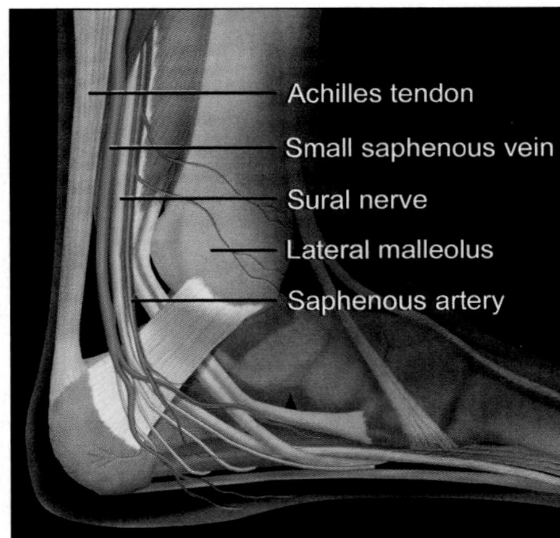

To remove a sural nerve sample, draw an arcuate line over the ankle posterior to the lateral malleolus, incise the skin, isolate the subcutaneous sural nerve, and remove a segment of at least 5 cm.

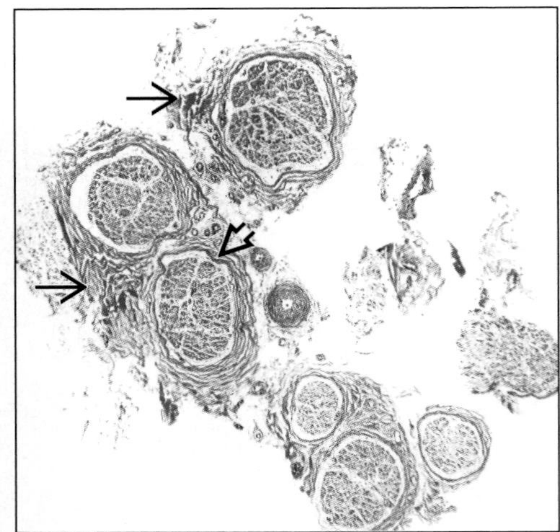

H&E stain of a sural nerve biopsy in cross section shows 6 fascicles with marked axonal loss. The small fascicles are surrounded by moderate epineurial ⇒ and mild perineurial ⇨ fibrosis.

CLINICAL IMPLICATIONS

Pertinent Antemortem Information

- Disease or syndrome with neuropathy
  - Biopsy report of peripheral neuropathy
  - Muscle biopsy report of neurogenic atrophy
- Electrophysiology
  - Nerve conduction studies
  - Electromyography (muscle innervation status)
- Magnetic resonance imaging
  - Compartment syndrome involving nerve

Anatomic Correlations

- Peripheral neuropathy distribution, e.g., dermatomes
- Focal: Compression/trauma, diabetes, vasculitis, herpes zoster virus, radiation, leprosy, sarcoidosis
- Multifocal: Demyelination, axonal degeneration
- Mononeuropathy: Single nerve involvement
- Mononeuropathy multiplex: Several nerve trunks
- Polyneuropathy: Acute, subacute/chronic, genetic

Cause of Death

- Associated disease: Amyloidosis, vasculitis, systemic lupus erythematosus, diabetes mellitus, liver disease, uremia, tumor
- Severe peripheral nerve damage
  - Amyotrophic lateral sclerosis, Guillain-Barré syndrome, toxin
- Nerve or familial syndrome-associated tumor
  - Malignant peripheral nerve sheath tumor (MPNST)
    - Up to 13% lifetime risk in neurofibromatosis type 1 (NF1)
  - Other NF1-associated malignancy

MACROSCOPIC FINDINGS

Anatomic Features

- Peripheral nerve-associated thickening or mass
- Schwannomatosis: Late-onset painful schwannomas
  - No classic stigmata of NF1 or NF2

Dissection Techniques

- Sural nerve (pure sensory; limited value)
  - Mark arcuate line over ankle starting 1.5 cm posterior to fibular tip, posterior to lateral malleolus
    - Incise into subcutaneous tissue, gently resect 5 cm
    - Divide for light and electron microscopy
  - Alternatively, remove nerve over gastrocnemius muscle belly
- Cervical plexus: Spinal nerves C1 (variable), C2-C4
  - Emerges deep to mid sternocleidomastoid muscle
    - Back of head, part of neck, diaphragm (with C5)
- Brachial plexus: Spinal nerves C4 (variable), C5-C8, T1
  - Passes through neck under mid clavicle to axilla
    - Chest, diaphragm, upper limb except trapezius
- Lumbar plexus: Spinal nerves T12 (variable), L1-L4; upper part of lumbosacral plexus
  - Forms lateral to intervertebral foramina, proceeds through psoas major muscle
  - Leaves pelvis posterior to inguinal ligament, partly as obturator nerve
    - Lower abdomen, buttocks, thigh, knee, genitalia
- Sacral plexus: Spinal nerves L4, L5, S1-S4 converge with lumbosacral trunk
  - Traverses pelvic bone's greater sciatic foramen, lies over retrorectal space
    - Pelvis, buttocks, genitalia, lower limb
- Coccygeal plexus: Spinal nerves S4, S5 and coccygeal nerve
  - Form anococcygeal nerves over levator ani muscle
- Posterior or anterior removal of spinal cord/dura
  - Include spinal nerve roots, cauda equina, some dorsal root ganglia (DRG)

Gross Evaluation/Sectioning

- Spinal nerve roots, DRG: Note spinal level
- Peripheral nerve/nerve lesion: Note nerve plexus, trunk, or branch

Distinguishing Features of NF1 vs. NF2

	NF1	NF2
Frequency	1/2,500	1/25,000
External clinical signs	> 6 café au lait macules, skin fold freckling, Lisch nodules (iris), skin neurofibromas	< 6 café au lait macules, cataracts, rarely skin neurofibromas
Internal exam findings	Plexiform neurofibromas (arising from underlying nerves), glial heterotopias (rare)	Schwannomas (especially vestibular division of CN8), supratentorial meningiomas, peripheral nerve schwannosis, ependymal/neural ectopia, syringomyelia, atypical glial nests
Associated tumors	MPNST, astrocytoma (2-3% lifetime risk), rhabdomyosarcoma, juvenile xanthogranuloma, GIST, carcinoid, pheochromocytoma, medullary thyroid carcinoma	Diffuse astrocytomas (rare)

NF1 = neurofibromatosis type 1; NF2 = neurofibromatosis type 2; MPNST = malignant peripheral nerve sheath tumor; GIST = gastrointestinal stromal tumor; CN8 = vestibulocochlear (acoustic) cranial nerve

Indications for Sampling Peripheral Nerve at Autopsy

- Guillain-Barré syndrome/chronic inflammatory demyelinating polyneuropathy (CIDP)
- History of
  - Systemic or peripheral nerve vasculitis
  - Amyloidosis
  - Hereditary neuropathy
  - Lipid storage disease
- Suspicion of
  - Inflammatory neuropathy
  - Paraneoplastic neuropathy

MICROSCOPIC FINDINGS

Normal Histology

- Peripheral nerve and spinal nerve roots
  - Connective tissue: Epi-, peri-, endoneurium
  - Axons, Schwann cells, myelin sheaths
    - Neurofilament stain: Unmyelinated axon density
  - Blood vessels
- Resin semithin sections: Nerve fascicle cross section
  - Large and small myelinated axon density, myelin sheath thickness
- Teased nerve preparation
  - Myelin sheath thickness, segmental demyelination, myelin ovoids (early wallerian degeneration following axonal lesion)
- DRG: Epineurium, sensory neurons, satellite glial cells, axons, Schwann cells, myelin, blood vessels

Disease/Histologic Findings of Neuropathy

- Inflammatory demyelinating neuropathy: Guillain-Barré syndrome, CIDP
- Other inflammatory: Sarcoidosis, perineuritis, insect bites
- Infectious: Leprosy, Lyme disease, human immunodeficiency virus, cytomegalovirus
- Vasculitis: Multisystem vasculitides, isolated peripheral nerve vasculitis
- Dysproteinemia: Immunoglobulin paraprotein, cryoglobulinemia, multiple myeloma
- Amyloidosis: Primary, familial
- Neoplasia associated: Paraneoplastic, infiltrative
- Endocrine: Diabetes, hypothyroidism, acromegaly
- Organ disease: Uremia, liver disease, chronic hypoxia
- Nutritional: Vitamins B12, B1, B5, and E deficiency
- Toxic: Alcohol, chloroquine, lead, mercury, vincristine
- Genetic
  - Hereditary motor sensory neuropathies (HMSN)
  - Hereditary sensory and autonomic neuropathies (HSAN)
  - Porphyric neuropathy
  - Dejerine-Sottas disease
  - Spinocerebellar degenerations (e.g., Friedreich ataxia)
  - Ataxia telangiectasia
- Storage: Sphingolipidoses, adrenoleukodystrophy
- Tumors
  - Neurofibromas (NFs), plexiform NFs
  - Schwannoma, plexiform schwannoma
  - Perineurioma
  - MPNST
- Others: Critical illness polyneuropathy, mitochondrial cytopathy, inflammatory sensory polyganglionopathy

SELECTED REFERENCES

1. Farid M et al: Malignant peripheral nerve sheath tumors. Oncologist. 19 (2):193-201, 2014
2. Hirbe AC et al: Neurofibromatosis type 1: a multidisciplinary approach to care. Lancet Neurol. 13(8):834-43, 2014
3. Lim SH et al: Systemic therapy inneurofibromatosis type 2. Cancer Treat Rev. 40(7):857-61, 2014
4. Ferner RE et al: Neurofibromatosis type 1 (NF1): diagnosis and management. Handb Clin Neurol. 115:939-55, 2013
5. Lloyd SK et al: Neurofibromatosis type 2 (NF2): diagnosis and management. Handb Clin Neurol. 115:957-67, 2013
6. Vranceanu AM et al: Quality of life among adult patients with neurofibromatosis 1, neurofibromatosis 2 and schwannomatosis: a systematic review of the literature. J Neurooncol. 114(3):257-62, 2013
7. King RHM: Atlas of Peripheral Nerve Pathology. London: Arnold, 1999
8. Midroni G et al: Biopsy Diagnosis of Peripheral Neuropathy. Boston: Butterworth-Heinemann, 1995

Microscopic Features

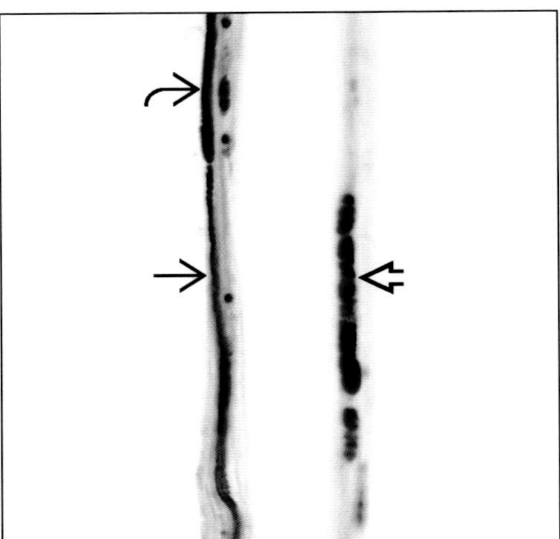

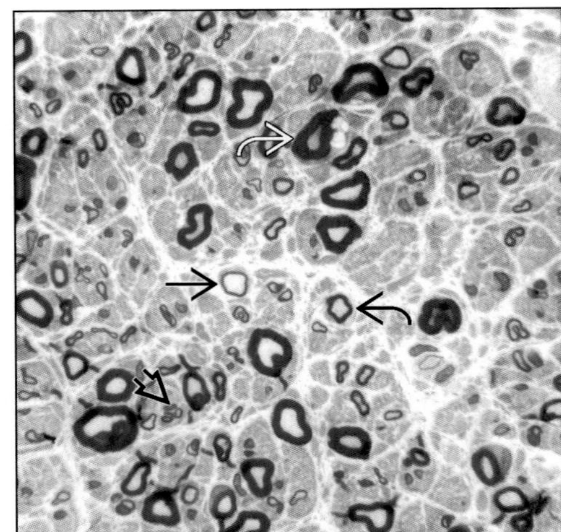

(Left) OsO_4 stain of 2 teased (separated) sural nerve axons shows remyelination of 1 with a thin myelin sheath → compared to the thick normal segment above →. The other has myelin ovoids → of wallerian degeneration secondary to axonal degeneration. **(Right)** Toluidine blue stain of a plastic section has axonal loss, large axons with normal myelin sheath thickness →, thin sheaths of remyelination → including an almost naked axon with little myelin →, and regenerative sprouts →.

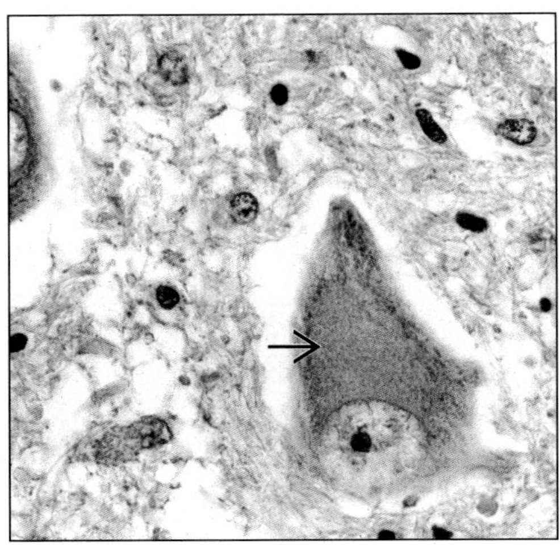

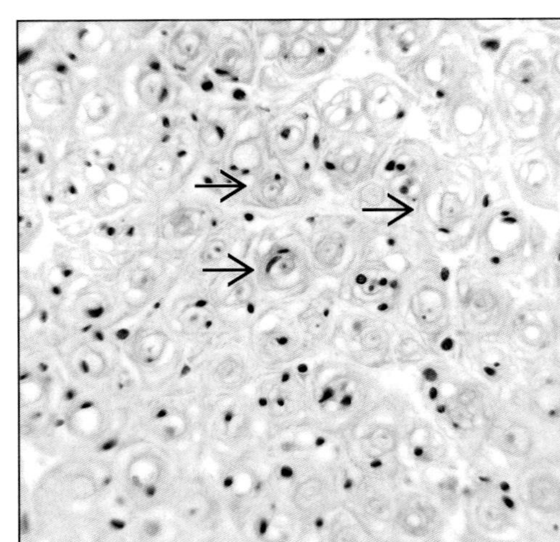

(Left) Lower extremity amputation removed the distal axon of this lumbar spinal cord anterior horn neuron causing reactive central chromatolysis →, as seen with an H&E stain. **(Right)** H&E stain shows "onion bulbs" → formed by Schwann cells in Charcot-Marie-Tooth disease in a cross section of the cauda equina. These accumulated Schwann cells encircle axons from the lower spinal cord in waves of unsuccessful attempted remyelination following primary or secondary wallerian degeneration.

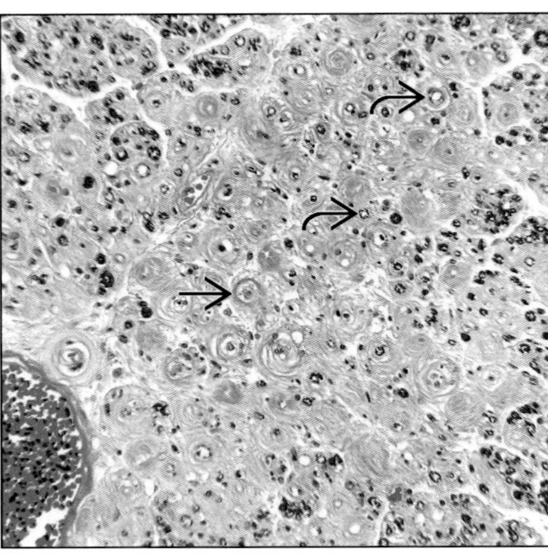

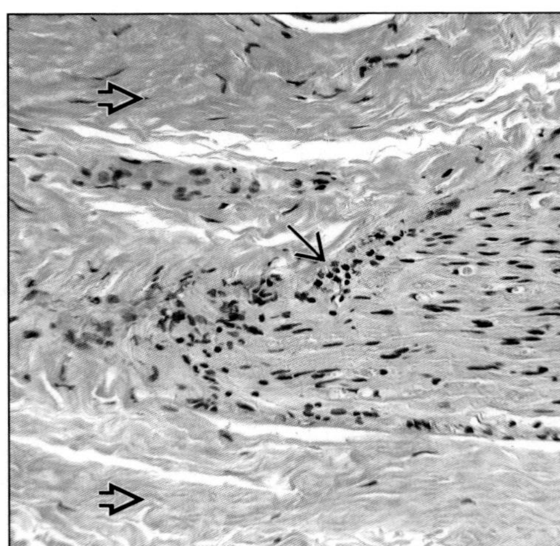

(Left) Luxol fast blue stain of the cauda equina in hereditary motor sensory neuropathies type 1 shows thinly myelinated axons →, indicating remyelination and "onion bulbs" with demyelinated axons →. **(Right)** A sural nerve from a patient with Lyme disease caused by Borrelia burgdorferi has chronic inflammatory neuritis, as seen with an H&E stain. Lymphocytes, scattered and in small aggregates →, are mostly in the perineurial covering of this fascicle. Epineurial fibrosis → shows the chronicity of the lesion.

Gross and Microscopic Features

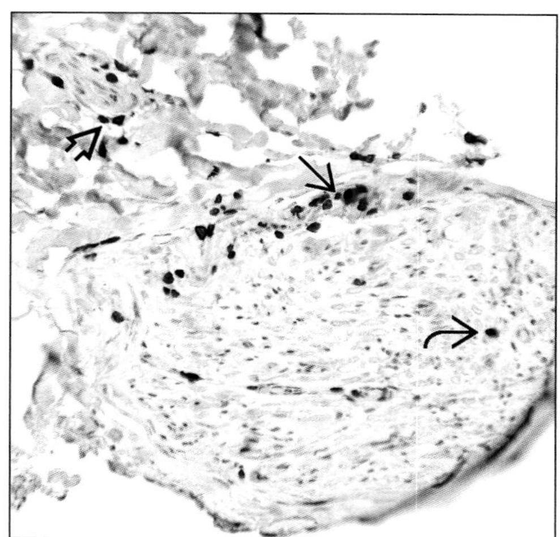

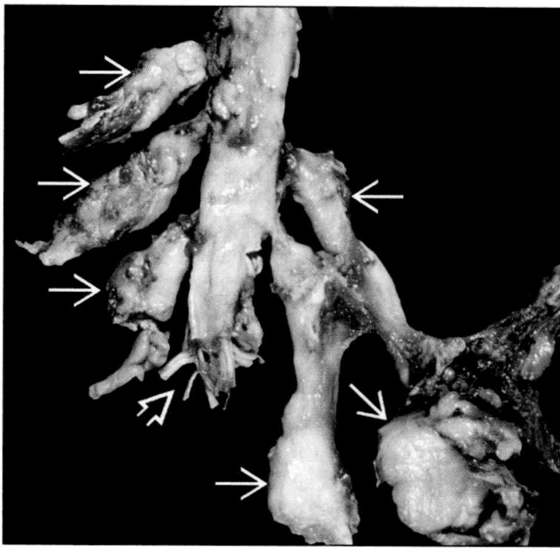

(Left) *Immunostain for CD3 shows T lymphocytes in Lyme neuritis along a fascicular blood vessel →, scattered in the endoneurium ↪, and in epineurial connective tissue, including in a perivascular space ⇨. This chronic inflammation affects axons and their vascular supply.* ***(Right)*** *Large neurofibromas ➡ expand multiple nerve roots of the lumbosacral spinal cord in NF1. The lumbosacral spinal cord is still enclosed in the dura with the upper cauda equina visible ➡.*

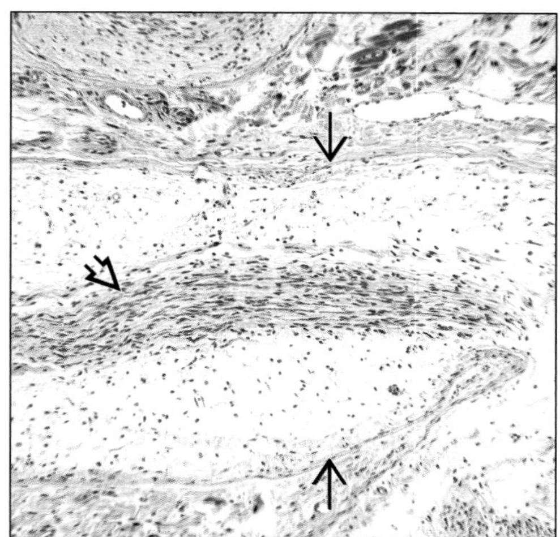

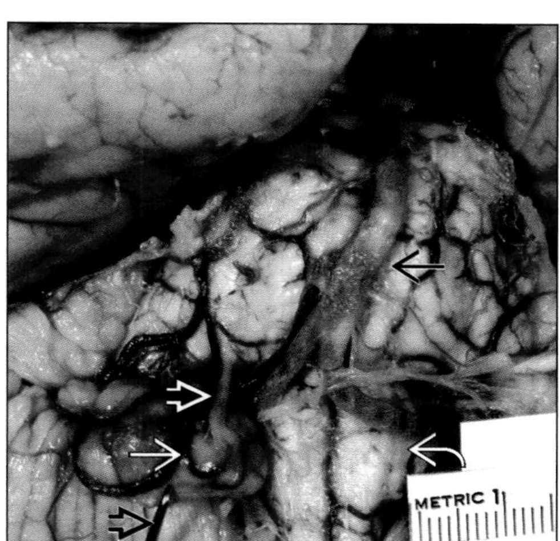

(Left) *Trichrome stain of this plexiform neurofibroma in the eyelid of a 5-year-old girl shows typical sparse cellularity. It surrounds the nerve radicle ⇨ and expands the perineurium →.* ***(Right)*** *This schwannoma ➡ of the vestibular division of CN8 ➡ is reflected by a probe ⇨ to lie by the medulla ↪. Vestibular division schwannomas may occur spontaneously and they are very common in NF2. The basilar artery → is seen over the belly of the pons.*

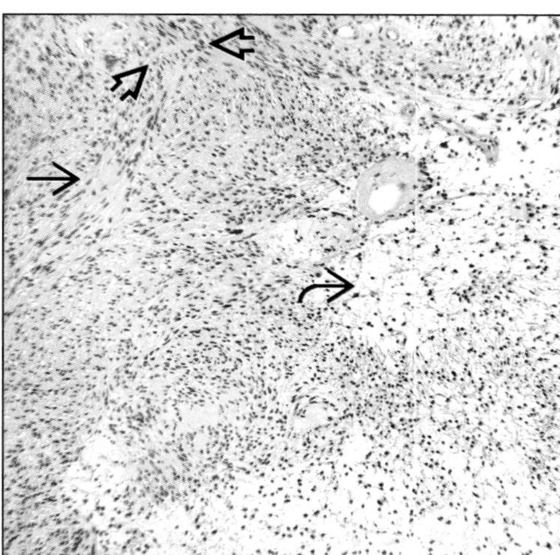

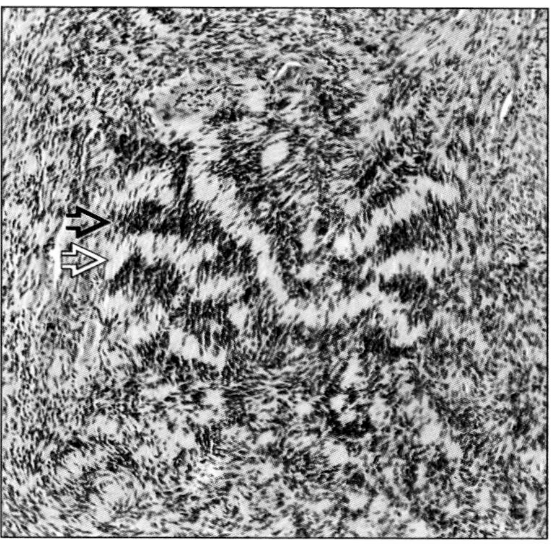

(Left) *This schwannoma of the median nerve in the arm displays the compact fascicular Antoni type A → and loose Antoni type B ↪ areas typical of this benign nerve sheath tumor, as seen with H&E stain. Focal palisading of nuclei ⇨ is typically found.* ***(Right)*** *A Verocay body, pathognomonic of schwannoma, has repeated picket fence-like cell palisades forming alternating nuclear ⇨ and cytoplasmic bands ➡ aligned in a prominent manner in this H&E stain.*

INTEGUMENTARY SYSTEM

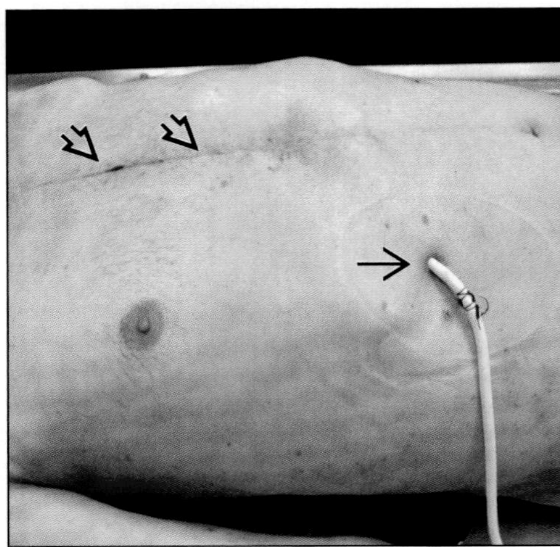

External examination findings at autopsy of a patient with a left ventricular assist device are shown. A recent medial sternotomy scar ⇨ is present. The driveline exit site ⇨ is well healed and noninflamed.

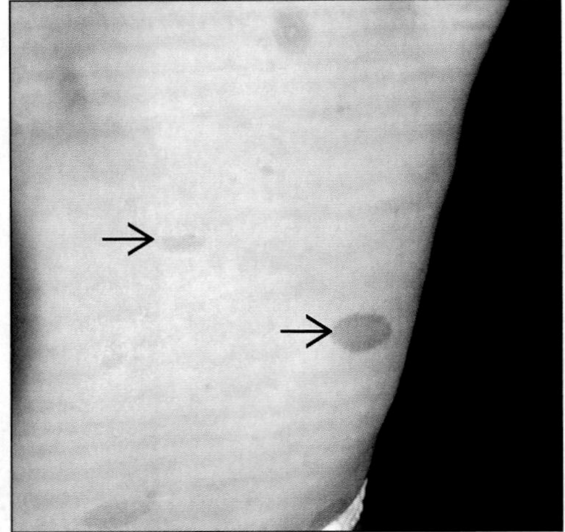

Multiple café au lait spots ⇨ represent an important cutaneous manifestation of neurofibromatosis syndromes. (From DP: Familial Cancer.)

MACROSCOPIC FINDINGS

External Examination

- Tattoos
  - May be present on any skin surface
  - Accessible mucosal membranes (e.g., inner lip) may also be tattooed
  - Professional
    - Colorful, intricate fine details; sharp lines, larger areas
  - Homemade
    - Coarse lines, irregular, crude; usually letters or digits
  - Fading may occur with age
  - Expansion and distortion may occur with skin stretching (e.g., weight gain)
- Piercings
  - Virtually anywhere on body
    - Ear, nose, lip, tongue, navel most common
  - Rings, studs, posts, chains, "gauges"
- Trauma and injuries
  - Bruises
    - Extravascular blood from damaged small arteries &/or venules/veins (not capillaries)
    - Exacerbated by &/or clotting disorders (platelet or clotting factor related)
    - Petechiae: Small (1-2 mm) round flat lesions
    - Purpura: Larger (> 3 mm) lesions that do not blanche under pressure; may be raised or firm
    - Ecchymoses: Largest (> 1 cm), flat; usually geographic or irregular shape
  - Abrasions
    - Superficial injury confined to epidermis/ superficial dermis
    - Pressure/crush type
    - Tangential/brush type
    - May bleed or crust depending on depth
    - May occur after death from moving the body
  - Lacerations
    - Tearing injury through full skin thickness
    - Jagged, irregular edges; often accompanied by bruising
    - May be caused by tangential force or crushing/ blunt force
    - More common on skin overlying rigid bony structures
  - Incised wounds
    - Cuts, punctures, stabbing
    - Traumatic vs. iatrogenic
    - May be stapled, sutured, dressed
  - Burns
    - 1st degree: Scald type, redness, and swelling
    - 2nd degree: Blistering
    - 3rd degree: Charring, full thickness
    - "Rule of 9's": Surface area of each side of each leg, each arm, abdomen, chest, lower back, upper back, head
  - Scars
    - Well healed: No remaining eschar; fade from red-pink to white over time (months to years)
    - Contracture (especially over flexor surfaces of joints)
    - Hypertrophic (keloid): Taut, protuberant, markedly exaggerated fibrotic response
- Lesions
  - Seborrheic keratosis
    - Raised, hyperpigmented lesions with pasted-on warty appearance
    - "Barnacles of old age": Benign behavior
  - Actinic keratosis
    - Scaly, plaque-like lesion on sun-exposed skin areas
    - Rough, sandpaper-like appearance with discoloration (red or brown)
    - Precancerous squamous lesion
  - Basal cell carcinoma
    - Shiny, pearly skin nodules
    - Sun-exposed or protected skin
    - May be destructive, erosive of adjacent structures

- Melanoma
  - Asymmetry
  - Borders (irregular)
  - Color (variegated)
  - Diameter (> 6 mm)
  - Evolving over time (growing, changing)
- Dermatitis (rash)
  - Intertrigo (intertriginous dermatitis): Inflammatory condition of skin folds; induced by heat, moisture, friction, lack of air circulation
  - Atopic: Eczema, allergy
  - Contact: Poisonous plants and insects, nickel, skin irritants
  - Stasis: Chronic edema
- Abscess
  - Subcutaneous fluctuant lesions
  - Red, indurated surrounding tissue

Specimen Handling

- Sampling skin at autopsy
  - Take care to keep skin integrity intact prior to embalming
  - Sampling along "Y" incision lines encouraged when necessary
  - Consider frozen samples for immunofluorescence studies (immunobullous disease, etc.)

COMMON DERMATOLOGIC DISEASES AT AUTOPSY

Genetic Syndromes

- Café au lait spots: Neurofibromatosis
- Ash leaf spots (under Wood's lamp), sebaceous adenoma: Tuberous sclerosis
- Prominent nevi: Dysplastic nevus syndrome
- Port-wine stain: Sturge–Weber syndrome

Disseminated Intravascular Coagulation

- Petechiae, purpura, haemorrhagica bullae
- Purpura fulminans: Diffuse microvascular clotting in superficial subcutaneous vessels
- Diffuse ecchymoses
- Bleeding from wounds or venipuncture sites

Pyoderma Gangrenosum

- Pustules or nodules that ulcerate and extend centrifugally
- Lower extremities most common
- Associated with
  - Rheumatoid arthritis
  - Inflammatory bowel disease
  - Paraproteinemia (multiple myeloma)

Erythema Multiforme/Stevens-Johnson Syndrome

- Cutaneous hypersensitivity reaction
  - Macules, papules, plaques, vesicles, or bullae
  - Often with targetoid or iris appearance
  - Acral distribution (extremities)
- Associated with
  - Infection (herpes simplex virus or *Mycoplasma)*
  - Drug sensitivity (sulfonamides, barbiturates, antibiotics)
- Erythema multiforme minor: Mild manifestation
- Erythema multiforme major or Stevens-Johnson syndrome: Severe manifestation with blistering

Scleroderma

- Autoimmune fibrosing skin disease
  - Localized (morphea)
  - Generalized (systemic sclerosis)
- Cutaneous findings
  - Localized lesions: Red patches evolve to hypopigmented plaques with dark borders, usually on trunk
  - Sclerodactyly ("sausage" fingers)
  - Taut, thickened facial skin
  - Telangiectasias, hypopigmentation
- Anti-centromere, Scl-70 antibodies positive

Connective Tissue Disorders (Ehlers-Danlos and Pseudoxanthoma Elasticum)

- Skin laxity
  - Especially on extensor surfaces on joints
- Pseudoxanthoma elasticum
  - Yellow papules over redundant skin folds on the neck, abdomen, and groin
  - Histologically, elastic fibers become brittle and calcified
  - Associated clinically with hypertension, peripheral vascular and coronary artery disease, retinal and gastrointestinal hemorrhage, and stroke
- Ehlers-Danlos
  - Multiple (at least 11) types
  - Clinical associations
    - Mitral valve prolapse
    - Blue sclerae
    - Vascular aneurysms, dissections
    - Peripheral vascular disease

REPORTING CRITERIA

Tattoos, Piercings

- Location, size, nature (photographs helpful)

Scars

- Location, orientation, length, color
- Contracture, keloid formation

Lesions

- Character, location, size

SELECTED REFERENCES

1. Kovarik CL et al: Forensic dermatopathology and internal disease. J Forensic Sci. 50(1):154-8, 2005
2. Rutty GN et al: The external examination. In: Hospital Autopsy. 2nd ed. London: Hodder Arnold. 42-51, 2001
3. Knight B et al: The autopsy: external examination. In: Forensic Pathology. London: Hodder Arnold. 12-17, 1996
4. Knight B et al: The pathology of wounds. In: Forensic Pathology. Arnold. London: Hodder Arnold. 133-70, 1996

Clinical Features

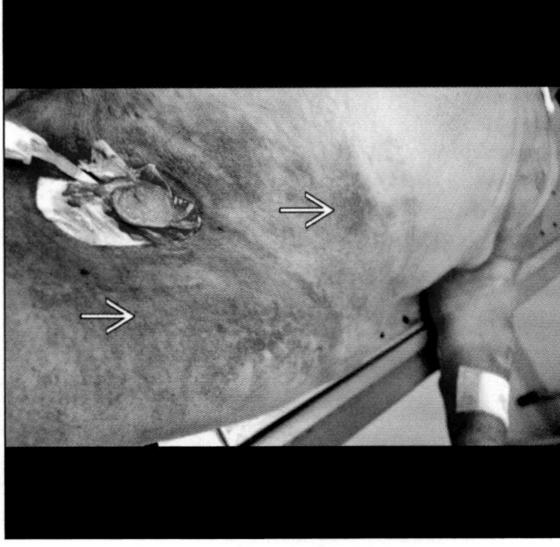

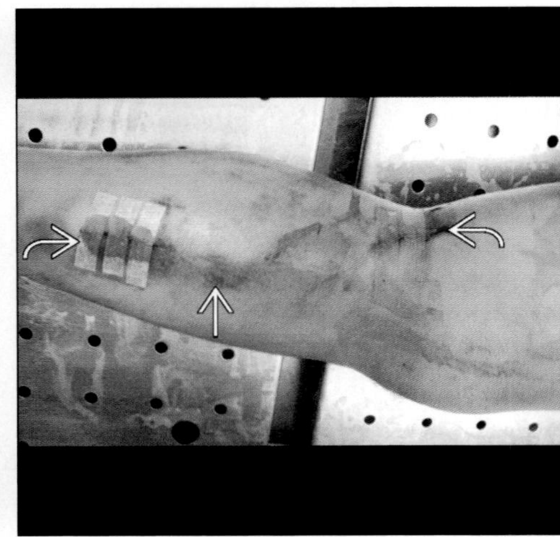

(Left) *This image shows massive ecchymoses ➔ surrounding a femoral cannulation site used for a temporary extracorporeal circulatory circuit prior to the death of this patient. She had developed a significant coagulopathy.* ***(Right)*** *This image shows dressed recent incisions ↪ from an endoscopic vein harvesting procedure. The veins were used in coronary artery bypass grafting. There is significant bruising along the harvesting tract ➔.*

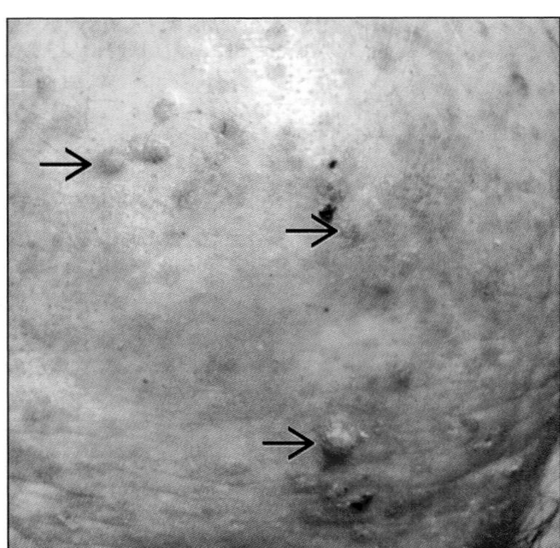

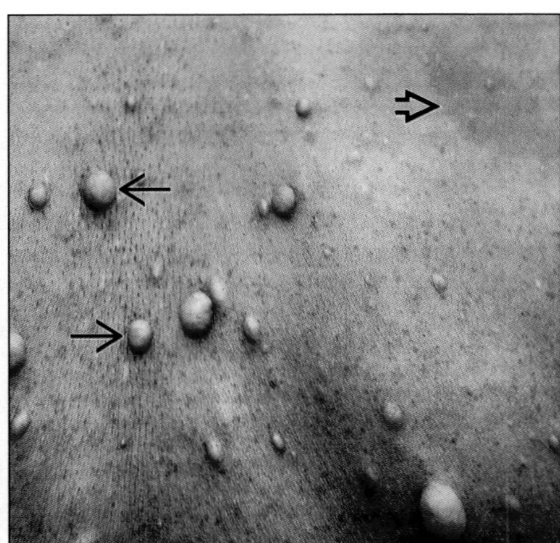

(Left) *Multiple actinic keratoses → are seen on the scalp of this patient. There is discoloration and prominent crusting. The texture is described as rough, like sandpaper. (DP: Neoplastic Derm.)* ***(Right)*** *Numerous cutaneous neurofibromas → may be seen in a diffuse distribution in patients with neurofibromatosis. They are characterized by sessile or pedunculated fibrous growths. A single café au lait spot is also present ⇨. (From DP: Familial Cancer.)*

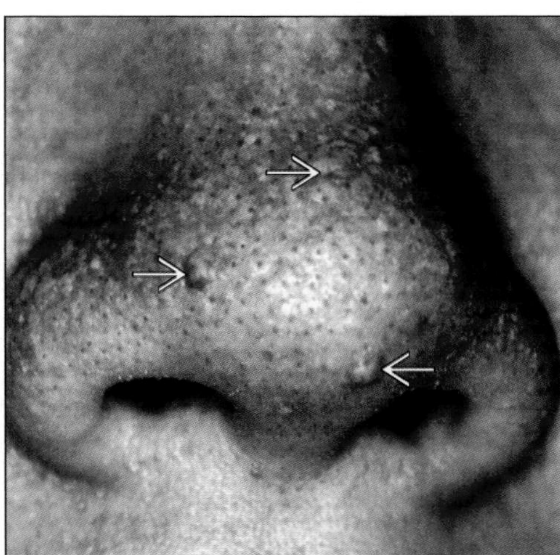

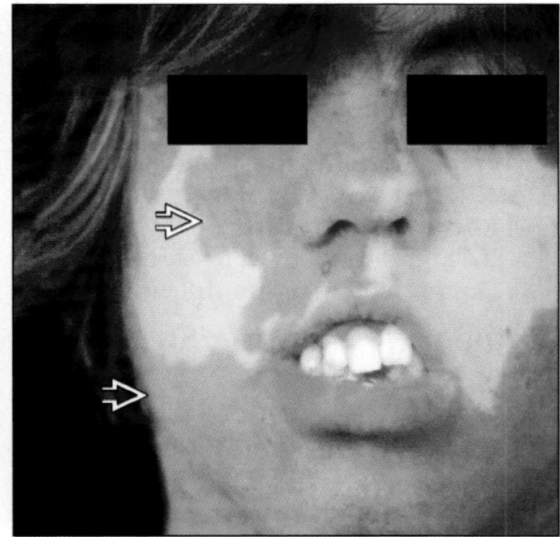

(Left) *This image shows the typical appearance of facial angiofibromas ➔ seen in tuberous sclerosis. These often appear before puberty and start in the nasolabial fold. They can be numerous and extensive on the face and scalp. (From DI: Obstetrics, 2e.)* ***(Right)*** *These port-wine stains ⇨ involving the distribution of the trigeminal nerve may be an external sign of Sturge-Weber syndrome. (From DP: Neoplastic Derm.)*

Microscopic Features

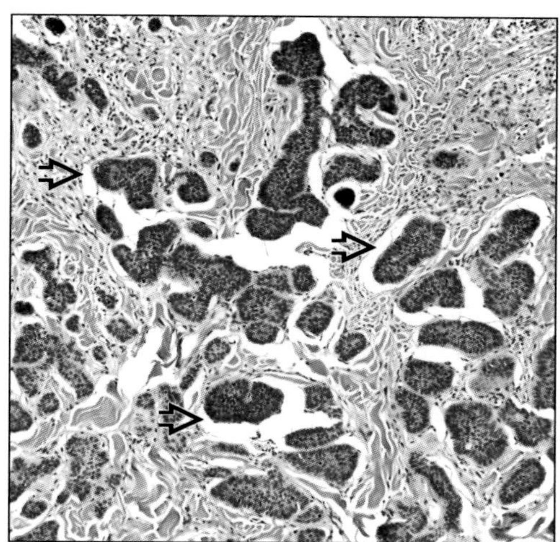

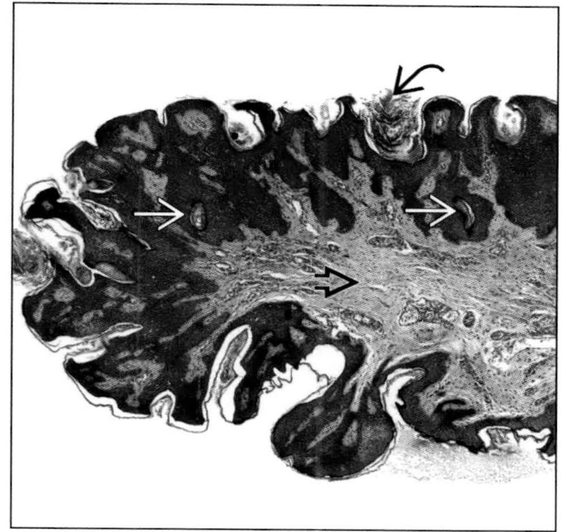

(Left) *This histologic section of a basal cell carcinoma shows a proliferation of small, infiltrative nests of basaloid cells with prominent retraction artifact ⇨ in a somewhat sclerotic-appearing stroma. (From DP: Neoplastic Derm.)* ***(Right)*** *This seborrheic keratosis with a papillary appearance shows hyperkeratosis ⇨, papillomatosis, acanthosis, and horn cysts/pseudocysts ➡. A fibrovascular stalk ⇨ may be present in some cases. (From DP: Neoplastic Derm.)*

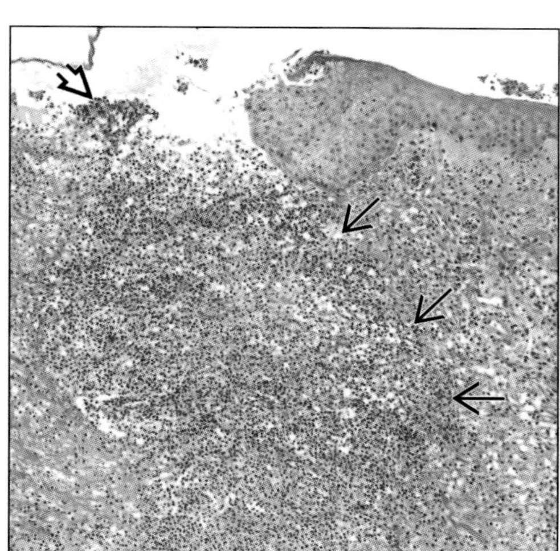

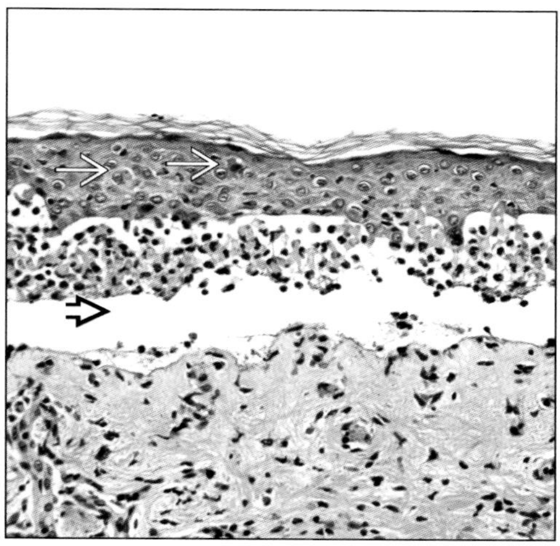

(Left) *Features of pyoderma gangrenosum are present in this skin section, with undermining of the epidermis by numerous neutrophils ⇨ and epidermal ulceration ⇨. (From DP: Nonneoplastic Derm.)* ***(Right)*** *This skin sample from a patient with erythema multiforme shows scattered necrotic (apoptotic) keratinocytes ➡ and subepidermal bulla formation ⇨. (From DP: Nonneoplastic Pediatrics.)*

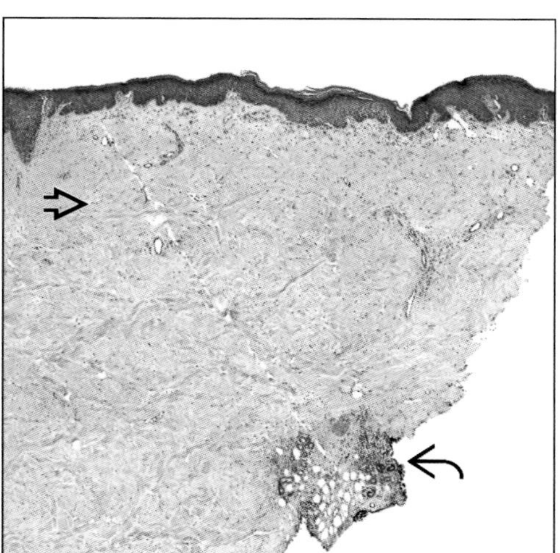

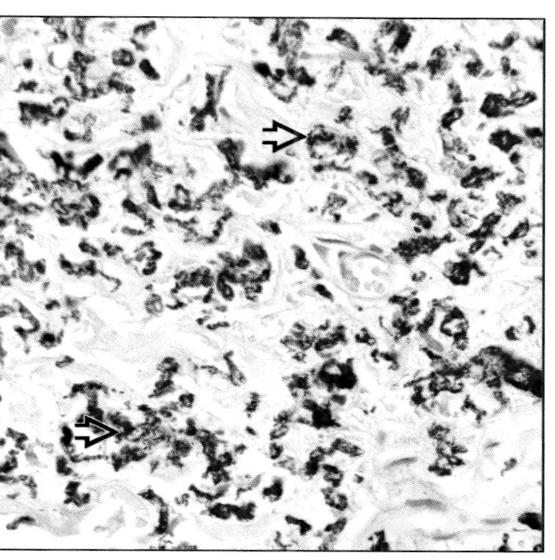

(Left) *This skin sample from a patient with systemic sclerosis (scleroderma) shows abundant dermal fibrosis ⇨, extending to involve adnexal structures ⇨ at the junction between the cutis and subcutis. (From DP: Nonneoplastic Derm.)* ***(Right)*** *This high-magnification photomicrograph from a skin section from a patient with pseudoxanthoma elasticum shows calcified elastic fibers ⇨ (von Kossa stain). (From DP: Nonneoplastic Derm.)*

ORAL CAVITY

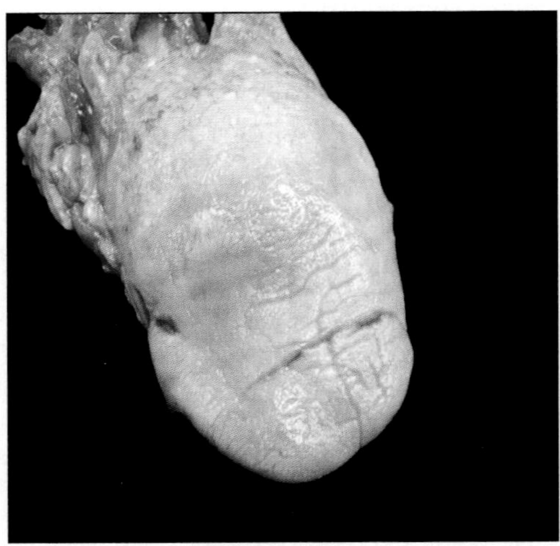

This tongue demonstrates extensive loss of papillae. This is atrophic glossitis that may be associated with nutritional deficiencies such as B12 deficiency. (Courtesy R. Irvine, MD.)

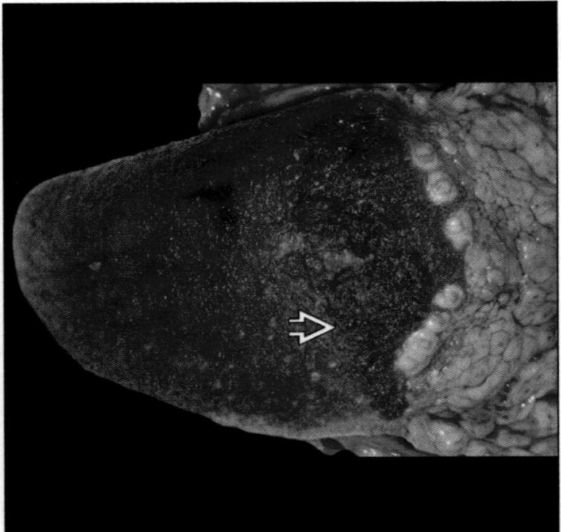

This strawberry tongue has hypertrophy of the tongue papillae ➡. This may be seen in scarlet fever, Kawasaki disease, and toxic shock syndrome. (Courtesy R. Irvine, MD.)

PRIMARY ORAL CAVITY DISEASE

Caries (Tooth Decay, Cavities)

- Bacterial infection of the mouth that causes breakdown of hard substances of tooth (enamel, dentin, and cementin)
  - May be a source for systemic infection, including infective endocarditis

Periodontitis

- Chronic, inflammatory process in the mouth affecting gingiva and other periodontal tissues (alveolar bone, periodontal ligament, and cementum) that causes loosening of the teeth and tooth loss
  - Related to excess of plaque: Biofilm normally found in the mouth
    - May also be a source for systemic infection, including infective endocarditis
    - May ↑ risk for coronary artery disease and ischemic heart disease
  - Gingival enlargement with periodontitis may be manifestation of monocytic leukemia, consider sampling tissue

Leukoplakia

- White plaque in the mouth that cannot be attributed to another entity (e.g., candidiasis, etc.)
  - Most often on buccal mucosa, floor of mouth, palate, gingiva, ventral tongue
  - White, often well-demarcated plaques that may be smooth or thick and even corrugated
  - Histology: Hyperkeratotic mucosa with acanthosis (thickening)
  - Premalignant lesion more commonly seen in the mouths of smokers and chewing tobacco users
    - May see a range of atypia → dysplasia → carcinoma in situ

Erythroplakia

- Red area in the mouth that cannot be attributed to another disease entity
  - Flat or depressed, occasionally with erosion
  - Commonly with dysplasia → carcinoma in situ → invasive carcinoma
  - Submucosal inflammatory infiltrate with dilated vessels → erythematous appearance
  - Smoking and alcohol are risk factors; 2:1 male predominance

Oral Squamous Cell Carcinoma

- Examination of oral cavity to exclude malignancy, particularly in decedents with history of tobacco use is mandatory
- Squamous cell carcinoma is most common oral cavity malignancy
  - Ventral tongue, floor of mouth, lower lip, soft palate, and gingiva are common locations
  - Early plague-like or verrucous lesions progress to ulcerated masses with indurated and rolled edges
  - Carcinoma in situ → invasion
    - Varying degrees of differentiation from well-differentiated keratinizing lesions to sarcomatoid tumors
    - If invasion is suspected, cervical node sampling should be considered on ipsilateral side of neck (with family permission)

ORAL CAVITY MANIFESTATIONS OF SYSTEMIC DISEASE

Angular Cheilitis

- Inflammation at 1 or more commonly both lip commissures (nutritional deficiency)

Glossitis

- Different patterns exist, some with systemic disease manifestations
  - Atrophic: Red smooth-appearing tongue due to inflammation with atrophy of papillae; may be associated with B12 deficiency
  - Strawberry tongue: Glossitis associated with hypertrophy of tongue papillae; associated with scarlet fever, Kawasaki disease, and toxic shock syndrome

Xerostomia

- "Dry mouth": Mucosal changes include redness and wrinkling
  - May be associated with many factors (medication, etc.) but characteristic of Sjögren syndrome
- If changes of xerostomia present, consider biopsy of salivary glands to examine for changes of Sjögren syndrome
  - Lymphoplasmacytic inflammation with occasional germinal center formation, gland fibrosis, and atrophy

Oral Thrush (Oral Candidiasis)

- May be manifestation of underlying immune deficiency

Pharyngitis/Tonsillitis

- Gingivitis, pharyngitis, and tonsillitis may be manifestation of immunodeficiency (pancytopenia and leukemia)

Bullae

- Autoimmune bullous diseases (pemphigus [most common], pemphigoid, linear IgA dermatosis)
- Erythema multiforme: Maculopapular vesiculobullous eruption
  - With involvement of lips and tongue is Stevens-Johnson syndrome
    - Symptomatic febrile form of erythema multiforme with extensive hemorrhagic crusting of lips and oral mucosa, often with secondary bacterial infection
  - EM associations
    - Infections, medications (sulfonamides, penicillin, barbiturates, salicylates, hydantoin, antimalarials), underlying malignancy, collagen vascular disease

Aphthous Ulcer

- Small round ulcers of the mouth with circumscribed borders, red margin, and gray/yellow base
  - May be manifestation of Crohn disease, ulcerative colitis, B12 or iron deficiency, folate deficiency, celiac disease, immunodeficiency (HIV, neutropenia), underlying malignancy, Sweet syndrome, medications (nonsteroidal anti-inflammatory drugs)
    - ~ 20-30% of Crohn disease and 10% of ulcerative colitis patients may have oral aphthous ulcers
    - Ulceration of mucosa with early chronic inflammatory infiltrate and late acute suppurative infiltrate due to superimposed bacterial infection

Tongue Laceration

- At autopsy, may be indication of seizure prior to and perhaps causing death

Gingival Hyperplasia

- Gingival fibrosis and enlargement may be seen with Dilantin (phenytoin) ingestion
  - When associated with tongue, laceration is good evidence for underlying epilepsy and possible death from seizure

Vascular Ectasias

- Telangiectatic vessels along oral mucosa and lips may indicate underlying Osler-Weber-Rendu syndrome
  - Autosomal dominant disorder with systemic vascular malformations (dilated veins and capillaries) that can involve respiratory, gastrointestinal, and genitourinary tract as well as oral cavity and may rupture and cause death

EXAMINATION OF ORAL CAVITY AND SPECIMEN HANDLING

Issues and Recommendations

- Oral cavity is difficult to examine due to presence of rigor at autopsy
  - Mouth wedge may be used to open cavity for examination
- If necessary, consider radiographic examination of teeth and jaw (rarely necessary)
- Examination should include entire oral cavity including dorsal and ventral aspect of tongue, buccal mucosa, and palate

Tissue Sampling

- Cosmetically considerate sampling mandatory to avoid disfiguring face/mouth
- Tissue sampling for immunofluorescence in blistering disease

SELECTED REFERENCES

1. Lankarani KB et al: Oral manifestation in inflammatory bowel disease: a review. World J Gastroenterol. 19(46):8571-9, 2013
2. Mays JW et al: Oral manifestations of systemic autoimmune and inflammatory diseases: diagnosis and clinical management. J Evid Based Dent Pract. 12(3 Suppl):265-82, 2012
3. Babu NC et al: Systemic manifestations of oral diseases. J Oral Maxillofac Pathol. 15(2):144-7, 2011
4. Islam NM et al: Common oral manifestations of systemic disease. Otolaryngol Clin North Am. 44(1):161-82, vi, 2011
5. Chi AC et al: Oral manifestations of systemic disease. Am Fam Physician. 82(11):1381-8, 2010

Clinical and Microscopic Features

*(**Left**) This oral ulcer has been complicated by candidal infection (thrush) identified by the pseudomembranes that are along the edge of the ulcer. (Courtesy R. Irvine, MD.) (**Right**) This area of superficial erosion of the buccal mucosa was from a ruptured bulla due to pemphigus. (From DP: H&N.)*

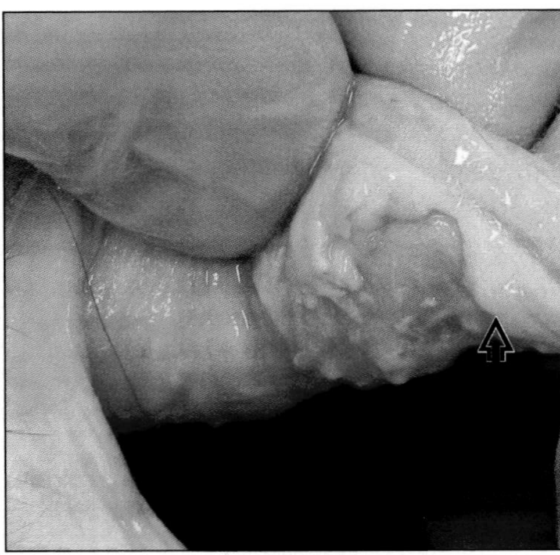

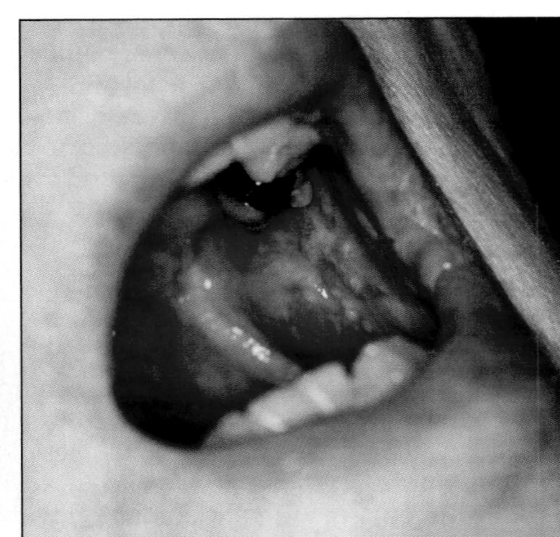

*(**Left**) The bulla in pemphigus is suprabasal, above the basal epithelial layer, with acanthosis of the cells within the bulla. (From DP: Nonneoplastic Derm.) (**Right**) Immunofluorescence with anti-IgG antibody reveals a lace-like pattern of staining around the epithelial cell membranes in pemphigus. (From DP: H&N.)*

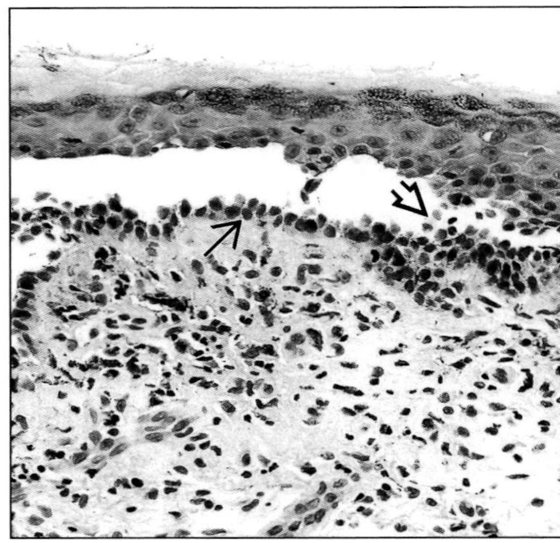

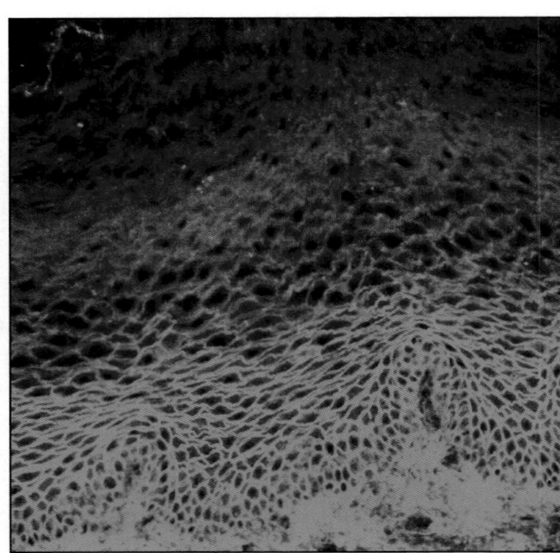

*(**Left**) This image of a rare cause of gingival enlargement, gingival fibromatosis, is virtually identical to the gingival enlargement related to phenytoin use. The enlarged gingiva extend onto the teeth and may cause gingivitis and periodontal disease. (From DP: Soft Tissue.) (**Right**) Erythroplakia of the palate shows white thick mucosa with scattered erythematous areas. Sample the erythematous areas as they are more likely to demonstrate dysplasia. (From DP: H&N.)*

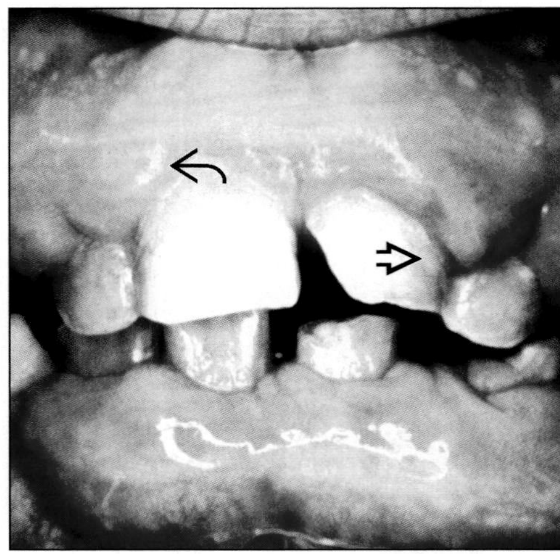

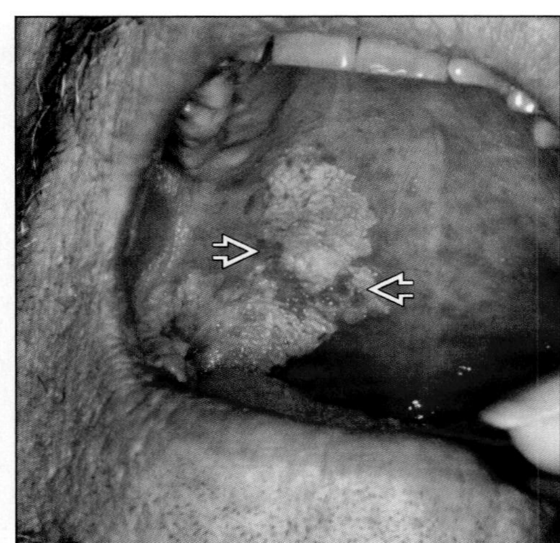

ORAL CAVITY

Gross, Radiographic, and Microscopic Features

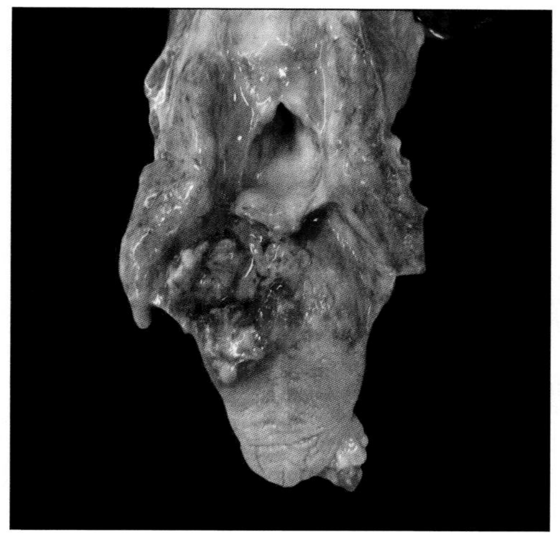

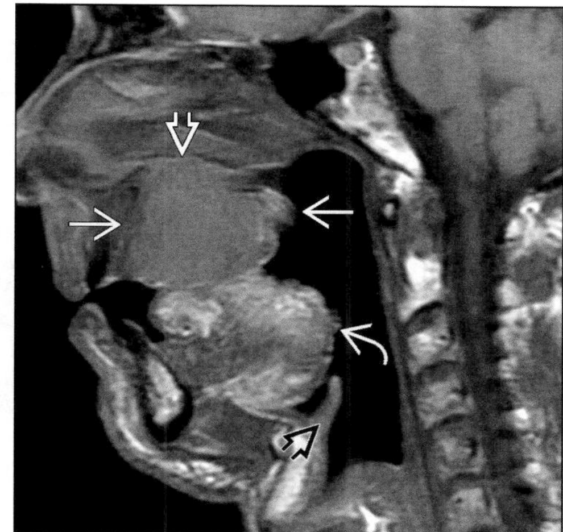

(Left) *This large fungating, ulcerated lesion at the posterior dorsum of the tongue extends into the pyriform sinuses. Sampling of the tumor and cervical nodes should be performed when these tumors are identified. (Courtesy R. Irvine, MD.)* ***(Right)*** *Sagittal MR shows a large oral cavity squamous cell carcinoma that destroys the hard palate and extends into the nasal cavity. The tongue and epiglottis are normal in appearance. (From DI: Oral & Maxillofacial.)*

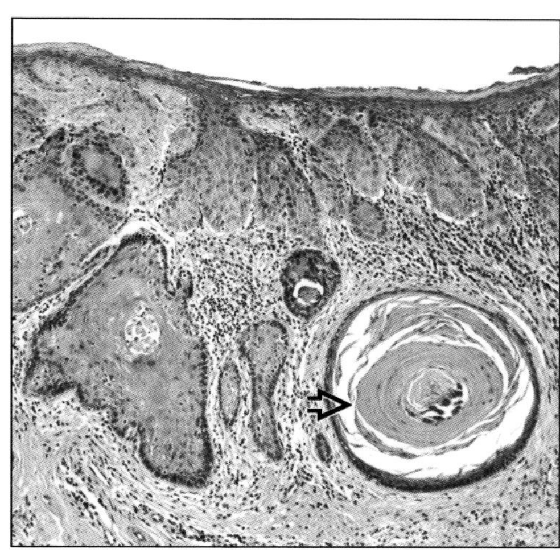

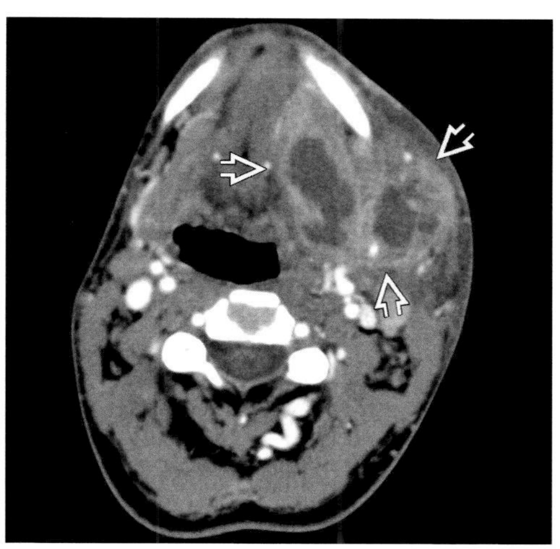

(Left) *This is a well-differentiated squamous cell carcinoma of the oral cavity. There are keratin pearls. The invasive tumor is arising from in situ carcinoma of the mucosa. (From DP: H&N.)* ***(Right)*** *Axial CT through the oral cavity shows an extensive thick-walled, multiloculated abscess cavity, which was a complication of a tooth abscess.*

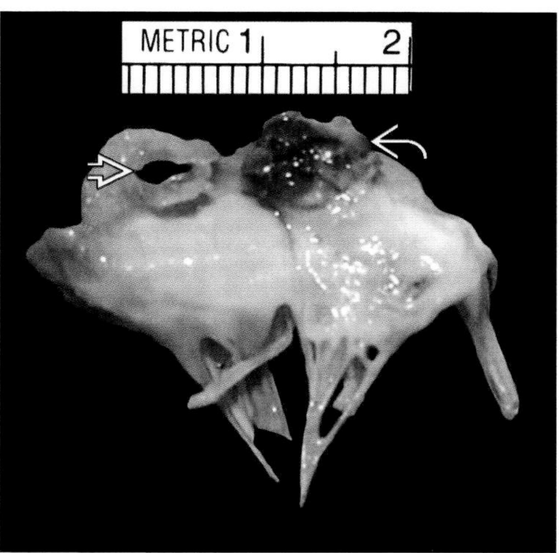

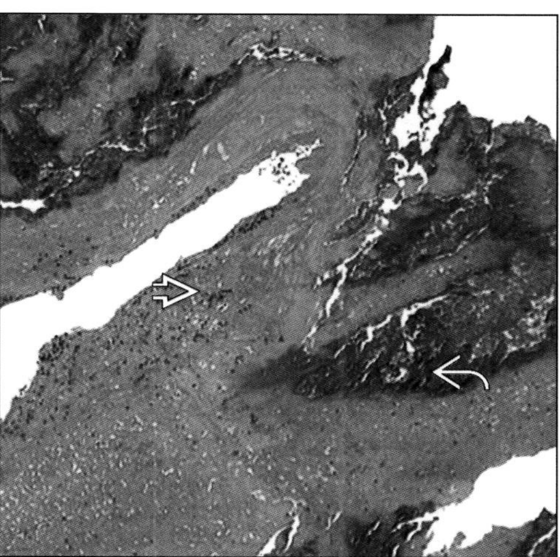

(Left) *This atrioventricular valve has an infective vegetation present with a focal perforation at the base of the valve. Oral cavity periodontitis and abscesses may be a source for infective endocarditis. (From DP: Cardiovascular.)* ***(Right)*** *Sections through the vegetation will reveal thrombus with acute inflammation and bacterial colonies. (From DP: Cardiovascular.)*

MEDICAL DEVICES

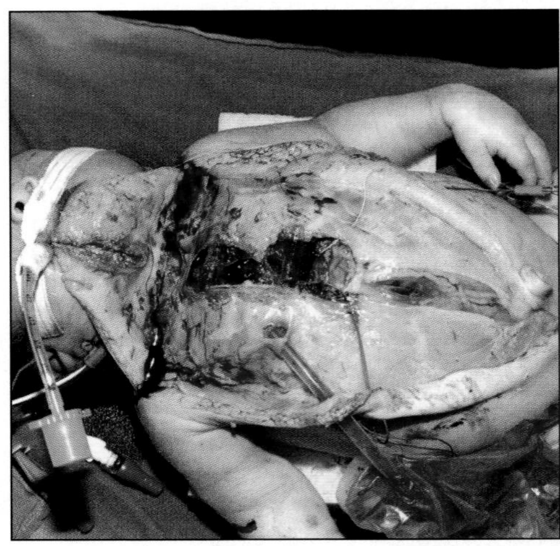

Multiple medical devices are often encountered at autopsy. Evaluation must include systematic examination of each device for location, evidence of failure, and complications related to failure.

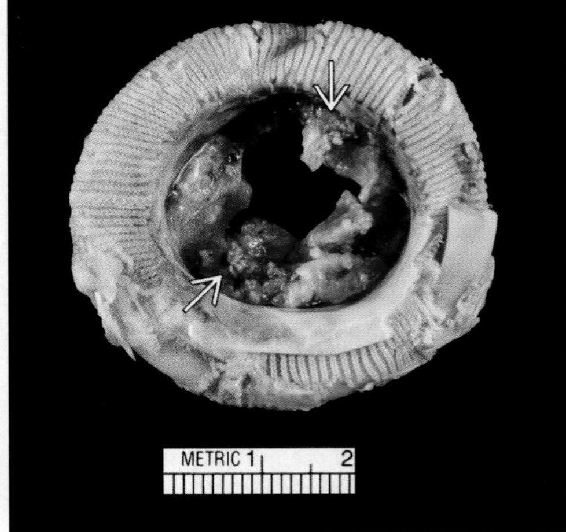

Structural deterioration is a common cause of failure of bioprosthetic devices. Here, a bioprosthetic tricuspid valve shows severe cusp calcification ➡ and retraction, causing severe regurgitation.

TERMINOLOGY

Definitions

- Medical devices relevant to hospital autopsy internal examination include all types of devices, regardless of
  - Time of implantation
  - Purpose of device
  - Location of device
  - Nature of device (mechanical vs. electronic)
  - Complexity of device

CLINICAL IMPLICATIONS

Preparation Before Autopsy

- Review decedent's medical records in detail
  - Past medical history
  - Past surgical history
  - Placement of medical devices
  - Nonsurgical interventions
  - Imaging findings
  - Laboratory findings
  - Events leading up to death
- Communicate with treating clinicians and surgeons
  - Clarify intraoperative findings or complications
  - Clarify devices that may be present and where devices are located
  - If automated implantable cardioverter-defibrillator (AICD) is present, ensure device is deactivated prior to beginning autopsy
  - Clarify specific questions to be answered

MACROSCOPIC FINDINGS

General Approach to Device Examination

- Examine anatomic location (external and internal)
  - Device in expected vs. unexpected location
- Examine for signs of infection
  - Purulence, vegetations, necrosis of tissues surrounding device
  - If suspicious for infection, obtain material for microbiologic cultures
- Examine for evidence of mechanical failure
  - Dehiscence from surrounding tissues/failed sutures
  - Separation or disconnection of components
  - Damage to device components
    - Fracture of leads
    - Structural deterioration of bioprosthetic devices (e.g., heart valves)
  - Obstruction of tubular device component
    - Thrombosis
    - Vegetations
    - Kinking (due to fixed or dynamic twisting of tubular component)
- Examine for evidence of electronic failure (if applicable, via interrogation of recorded data)
  - Discharged battery
  - Failed data recording
  - Other evidence of electronic malfunction
- Examine for immediate complications related to device insertion/implantation
  - Perforation of vascular structure
  - Accidental obstruction of vascular structure (e.g., suture through coronary artery during valve replacement)
  - Hemorrhage
  - Damage to nearby structure or surrounding tissues
  - Pneumothorax
  - Emboli and infarcts
- Examine for secondary systemic complications related to device failure
  - Sepsis
    - Obtain blood for microbiologic cultures if possible
  - Emboli and infarcts
    - Infarcts in brain, spleen, kidneys, etc. (due to thrombosis or infection of device)

- Global myocardial infarct (precipitated by massive hemorrhage and hypotension)
  - Organ failure
    - Pulmonary edema, effusions, edema (failed cardiac device)
    - Hepatic congestion or necrosis (failed cardiac device)

Common Medical Devices Encountered

- General surgical devices
  - Sutures/clips/staples
  - Surgical drains/chest tubes
  - Sponges/lap pads
- Neurologic devices
  - Intracranial pressure monitoring catheter
  - Ventriculoperitoneal shunt
  - Neurostimulator
  - Intrathecal drug pump
- Cardiovascular devices
  - Central venous catheters and other vascular access devices
  - Pacemaker
  - AICD (ensure deactivation prior to autopsy)
  - Ventricular assist device/total artificial heart
  - Coronary artery stents
  - Prosthetic valves
  - Vascular grafts/stents
  - Inferior vena cava filter
- Respiratory devices
  - Endotracheal/tracheostomy tube
- Gastrointestinal/hepatobiliary devices
  - Nasogastric/orogastric tube
  - Percutaneous endoscopic gastrostomy (PEG) tube
  - Laparoscopic adjustable gastric band device
  - Transjugular intrahepatic portosystemic shunt
  - Cholecystostomy tube
- Genitourinary devices
  - Suprapubic catheter
  - Foley catheter
  - Ureteral stents
  - Intrauterine contraceptive device
- Musculoskeletal devices
  - Prosthetic joints/orthopedic devices

Photography of Devices

- Essential for medical, legal, and educational purposes
- Include identifiers of decedent/case number in photograph
- Photographs of devices in situ usually best achieved with handheld, high-quality digital camera
- Photography of device in dissected organ usually best achieved using gross photography station
  - For complex devices (e.g., ventricular assist devices), also photograph components after disassembly to document pathology
- Ensure adequate lighting; use flash on handheld cameras, use proper light stands and shield ambient room lighting when using gross photography station
- Avoid distractions
  - Obscure nonessential elements with drapes
  - Clean away blood and body fluids
  - Keep retracting hands, instruments out of photograph
  - Frame shot close enough to visualize device well and avoid distracting elements, but far enough away that anatomic location and relationships are clearly discernible
- Have a low threshold for photographing medical devices: When in doubt, photograph!

Radiography of Devices

- Useful to document anatomic position
  - Location of coronary artery stents
  - Location of orthopedic devices
  - Position of tubes, drains, catheters
- Useful to document mechanical failure of device
  - Fracture of thin metallic components (e.g., wire leads, stent struts)
  - Inappropriate expansion of metallic stents
  - Obstruction of coronary artery stents (using contrast injection and postmortem angiography)
  - Structural failure of orthopedic devices

Reporting Considerations

- Elements to document (for each device present, if applicable)
  - Type of device
  - Name of manufacturer, model, serial number, lot number, and any other identifying data on device
  - Anatomic location of device (appropriate or expected vs. inappropriate)
  - Condition of device, leads, etc. (intact vs. damaged)
  - Evidence of secondary complications
- For electronic devices, also document
  - Results of device memory interrogation (if data recorded by device)
    - Time of most recent device memory interrogation
    - Recorded evidence of device malfunction
    - Battery charge status
    - Pacemaker: Arrhythmic events
    - AICD: Discharges (shocks delivered)

MICROSCOPIC FINDINGS

Histologic Features

- Thrombus
  - Alternating layers of RBCs/WBCs and platelets/fibrin; may be organizing
- Infection
  - Dense neutrophilic inflammation and abscess formation in surrounding soft tissues
  - Special stains (e.g. GMS, Gram) aid in identifying and characterizing microorganisms

SELECTED REFERENCES

1. Finkbeiner WE et al: Special dissection procedures. In: Finkbeiner WE et al: Autopsy Pathology: A Manual and Atlas, 2nd ed. Philadelphia: Saunders Elsevier. 67-79, 2009
2. Prahlow JA et al: Deaths due to medical therapy. In: Froede RC: Handbook of Forensic Pathology, 2nd ed. Northfield, Ill: College of American Pathologists. 381-92, 2003
3. Weitzman JB: Electronic medical devices: a primer for pathologists. Arch Pathol Lab Med. 127(7):814-25, 2003

Devices and Associated Infections

(Left) *For devices with extracorporeal components, autopsy examination should include external evaluation for infection. Here, pneumatic drivelines for a total artificial heart are sutured in place, without purulence, erythema of surrounding skin, or other evidence of infection.* ***(Right)*** *The external and internal anatomic locations of a device must be examined for correct placement. Here, a PEG tube traverses the abdominal wall and terminates appropriately in the stomach.*

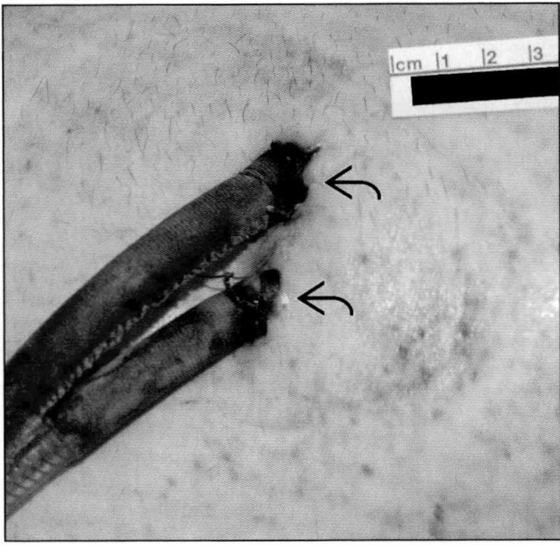

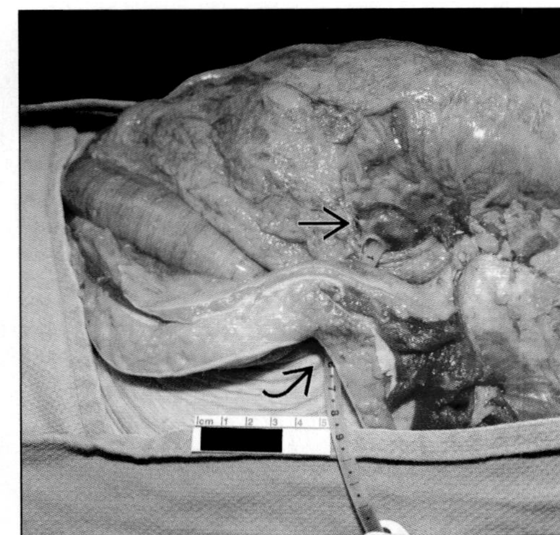

(Left) *Infection is an important complication of medical devices that may be fatal. In this case, intraabdominal misplacement of a PEG tube with subsequent introduction of food into the abdomen resulted in acute peritonitis, sepsis, multiorgan failure, and death. Note purulent serositis diffusely involving loops of small bowel.* ***(Right)*** *Infective endocarditis may cause failure of prosthetic cardiac valves. In this case, note multiple infective vegetations on prosthetic cusps.*

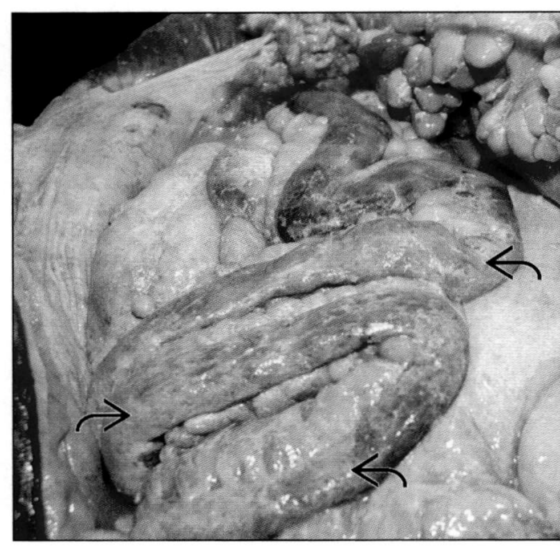

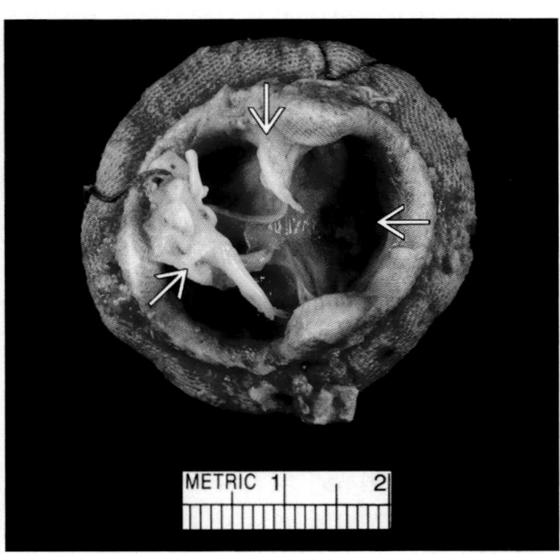

(Left) *This CardioWest total artificial heart has been appropriately connected to the main pulmonary artery and ascending aorta. Drivelines are also visible. Although clotted blood is present due to recent surgery, no signs of infection are seen.* ***(Right)*** *In contrast, this HeartMate II LVAD became infected, with purulent material coating the inflow cannula, pump, outflow conduit, and driveline. This material should be submitted for cultures.*

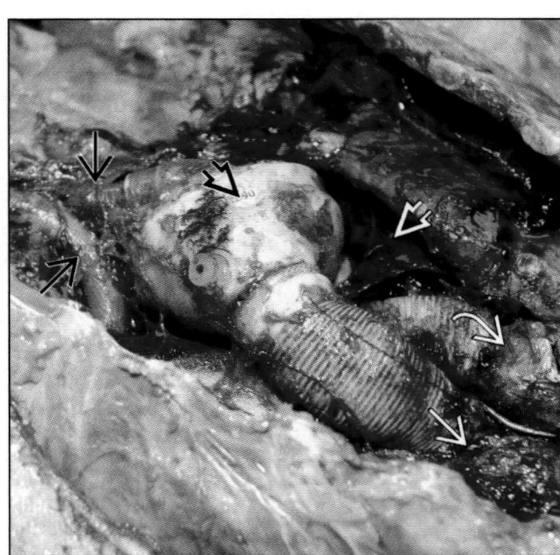

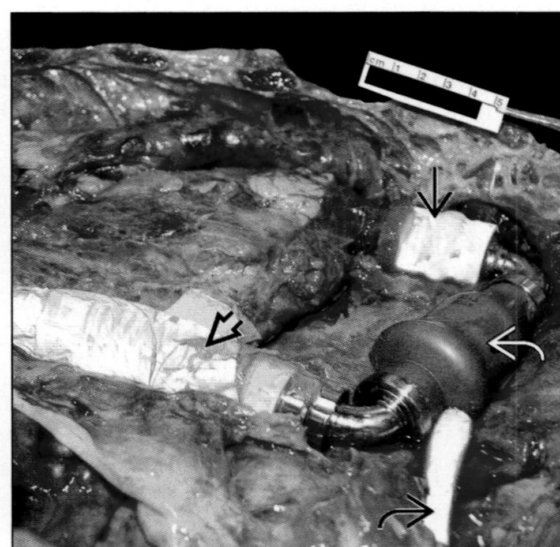

Devices and Associated Complications

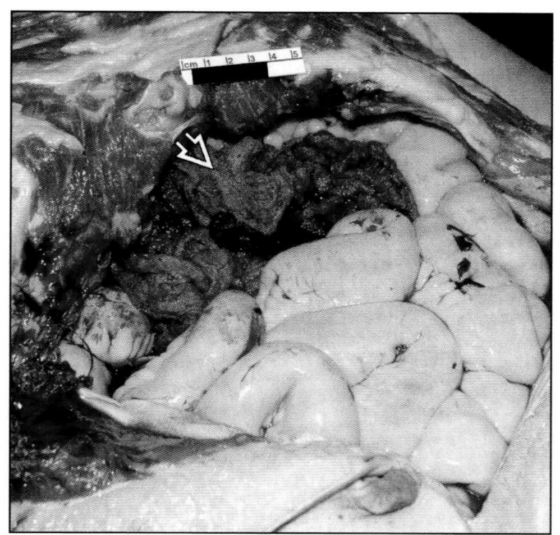

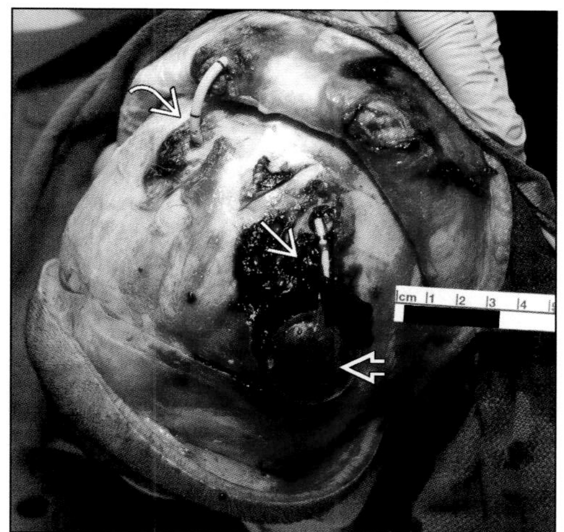

(Left) *Surgical sponges are occasionally seen at autopsy. Here, a lap pad soaked with fresh blood is present in the abdomen after intraoperative death. Unlike old retained sponges left behind accidentally by a surgeon, no fibrous adhesions, serositis, or evidence of infection is seen.* ***(Right)*** *This patient died of intracranial hemorrhage complicating placement of an Ommaya reservoir for intraventricular delivery of chemotherapy. Note separate ventriculostomy shunt.*

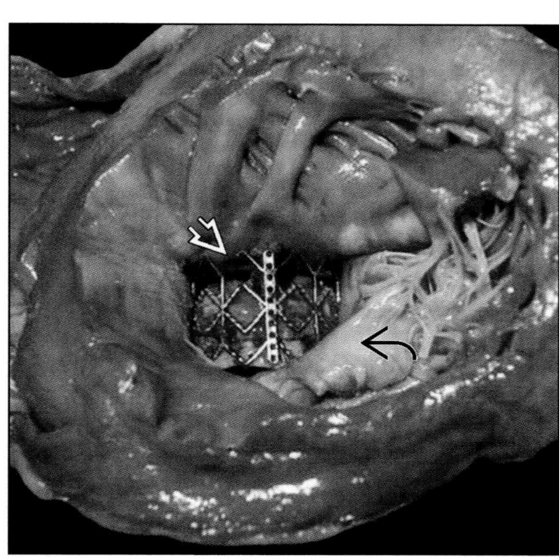

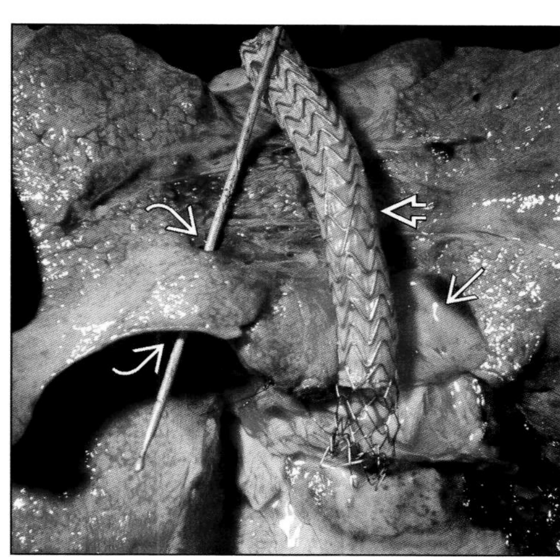

(Left) *Here, an improperly seated catheter-deployed bioprosthetic valve became loose and rotated within the LV outflow tract. Malorientation of the device caused obstruction and sudden death. Note anterior leaflet of mitral valve.* ***(Right)*** *In this case, placement of a transjugular intrahepatic portosystemic shunt into the portal vein was complicated by liver perforation by the initial guidewire (probe in perforation tract), resulting in fatal exsanguination.*

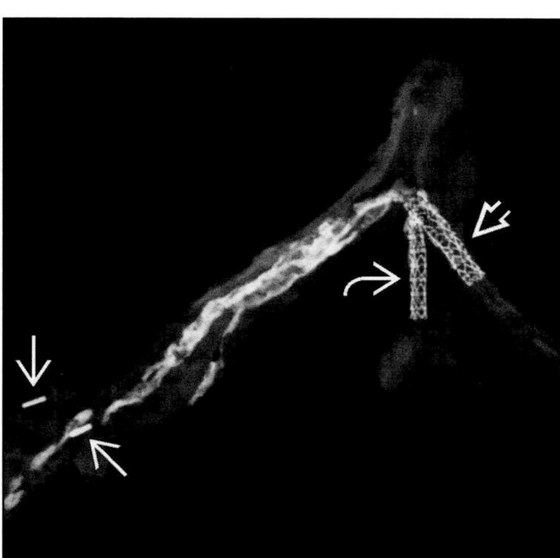

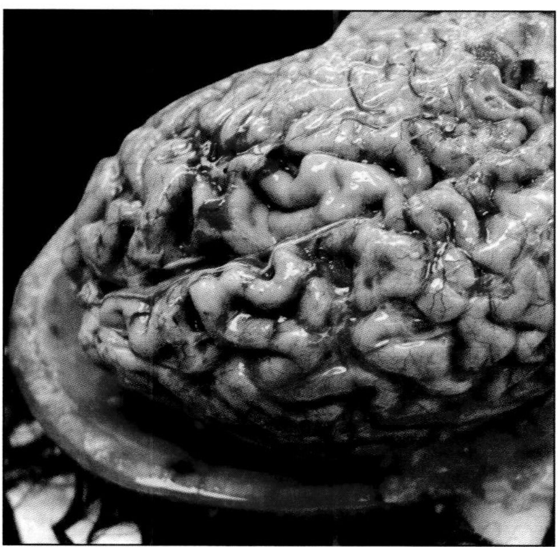

(Left) *Radiography aids evaluation of devices. Here, coronary stents are seen in the LCX and 1st OM branch. Note calcific atherosclerosis and clips on mid LAD due to LIMA graft.* ***(Right)*** *Remember that drugs are also medical devices. Although not visible themselves, evidence thereof may be readily visible at autopsy, as seen here after methylene blue infusion for treatment of vasoplegia syndrome associated with cardiac surgery. Note diffuse green discoloration of brain.*

CHEMISTRY

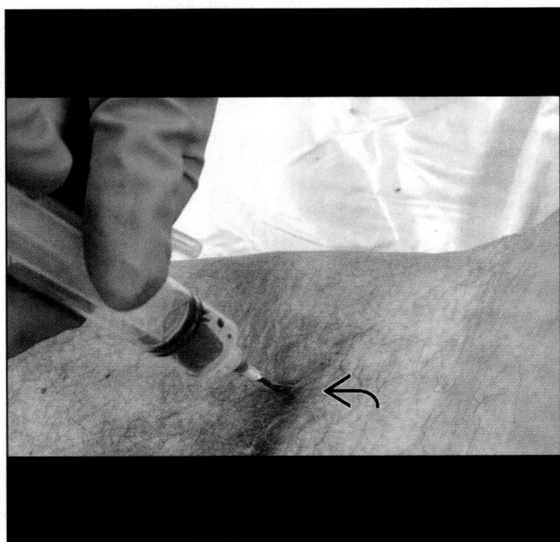

Blood can be obtained by performing a femoral artery/vein ⇗ puncture with a needle and applying gentle suction with a syringe. The sample can then be transferred to the appropriate test tube. (Courtesy B. Chung, MD.)

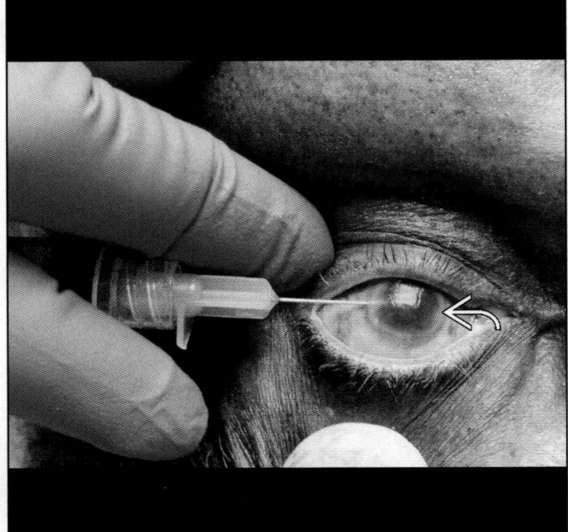

Best approached from the lateral canthus, a needle is inserted into the center of the globe to collect vitreous humor. Note the corneal clouding ⇗, which is an early postmortem ocular change.

TERMINOLOGY

Definitions

- This chapter covers utility and limitations of postmortem chemical analysis of blood, vitreous humor, and urine

ETIOLOGY/PATHOGENESIS

Postmortem Changes in Blood Components

- Clotting, hemolysis, and decomposition may interfere with results; most analytes only of value in early postmortem period (before putrefaction)
- Electrolytes
  - Sodium (Na), chloride (Cl), potassium (K), calcium (Ca), and magnesium (Mg): Unstable
    - Serum Na and Cl ↓, while K, Ca, and Mg ↑
  - Carbon dioxide: Stable
- Carbohydrates
  - Glucose: Unstable, ↓ rapidly due to glycolysis, may be ↑ after resuscitation or terminal stress
  - Glycated hemoglobin (A1c) and ketone bodies: Stable
- Proteins and nitrogen compounds
  - Blood urea nitrogen (BUN) and creatinine: Stable for days despite decomposition
  - Total protein and albumin/globulin ratio: Stable
  - Brain-natriuretic peptide (BNP): Aminoterminal portion of pro-BNP (NT-proBNP) more stable than BNP as a marker of cardiac function
  - Serum protein electrophoresis
    - Retains profile if hemolysis is minimal, except for slightly ↓ albumin and ↑ beta globulin
    - Otherwise useful for diagnosis of monoclonal gammopathy and agammaglobulinemia
  - Hemoglobin electrophoresis: Useful for hemoglobinopathies
  - Ammonia, oxypurines, and other amino acids: Unstable
- Enzymes
  - Generally unstable and rise unpredictably (e.g., transaminases, amylase, alkaline phosphatase)
  - Gamma glutamyl transferase (GGT) and carbohydrate-deficient transferrin: May be used to document chronic alcoholism when ↑
  - True cholinesterase: Stable
- Lipids
  - Total cholesterol: Relatively stable
  - Triglycerides and lipoproteins: May be stable within 24 hours postmortem but must consider premortem prandial state
- Hormones
  - Thyroid stimulating hormone, cortisol, parathormone, human chorionic gonadotropin, and luteinizing hormone: Stable
  - Free thyroxine (T4) and free triiodothyronine (T3): Relatively stable
  - Procalcitonin: Stable, ↑ in bacterial, fungal, or parasitic sepsis
  - Catecholamines: May not be reliable; levels vary and ↑ depending on premortem/perimortem factors
- Other
  - Bilirubin: Slightly ↑ postmortem, accurate only when significantly ↑ in icteric patients
  - Assays for specific antibodies (e.g., autoimmune diseases, infections) and PCR/other DNA tests generally accurate

Postmortem Changes in Urine Components

- Useful for certain organ-specific analytes
- Dipstick tests may be performed in autopsy suite
- Carbohydrates
  - Presence of glucose and ketone bodies for diabetes
- Bile pigments
  - Presence of bile or urobilinogen for hepatic disease
- Proteins

Patterns of Vitreous Humor Electrolyte Abnormalities

Pattern	Sodium	Chloride	Urea Nitrogen	Creatinine	Potassium
Dehydration/ hypertonic	↑ (> 155 mEq/L)	↑ (> 135 mEq/L)	↑	N/A	N/A
Uremic	No significant ↑	No significant ↑	↑	↑	N/A
Low salt/hypotonic	↓ (< 130 mEq/L)	↓ (< 105 mEq/L)	N/A	N/A	↓ (< 15 mEq/L)
Decomposition	↓	↓	N/A	N/A	↑ (> 20 mEq/L)

- No published data on stability of protein or utility of electrophoresis or immunofixation for detection of light chains
  - Interpret results with caution and compare to premortem data if available

Postmortem Changes in Vitreous Components

- Protected by blood-brain barrier, therefore some analytes not normally present (e.g., bile, most hormones, and enzymes)
- Embalming will usually not affect vitreous chemistries
- Electrolytes
  - Na and Cl: Stable
  - K: ↑ linearly, not helpful for premortem K status
  - Ca and Mg: Unstable
- Carbohydrates
  - Glucose: Relatively stable but undergoes some degree of glycolysis, may be useful when significantly ↑
  - Ketone bodies: Stable
- Proteins and nitrogen compounds
  - BUN and creatinine: Stable
- Other
  - May be more accurate for certain toxicology tests (e.g., alcohol, digoxin) than blood

Other Fluids

- Bile and gastric contents not usually relevant in hospital autopsy; used mainly in the forensic setting
- Cerebrospinal fluid, pericardial fluid, and synovial fluid rarely used in hospital autopsy; may occasionally be used for organ-specific disease

CLINICAL IMPLICATIONS

Methods of Collection of Body Fluids For Analysis

- Blood
  - Differences in levels of certain analytes (e.g., drugs) between right and left side of heart
  - Peripheral arteries or veins (e.g., femoral, subclavian) are preferred; best approximate antemortem values
  - May collect from inferior vena cava before removal of heart when large volume is required
  - Place sample in red top glass tube (without additives) or "tiger top/marbled" serum separator tube to obtain serum
  - Place sample in purple top tube containing EDTA to obtain plasma
- Urine
  - Can collect from Foley catheter
  - Can aspirate with large-bore needle and syringe directly from bladder before removal
  - May need to open bladder to obtain residual urine
- Vitreous humor
  - Insert 18-20 gauge needle with attached syringe into center of globe and apply gentle suction
  - Remove all fluid; should obtain 2-5 mL of clear, colorless fluid from each eye (will become cloudy and brown with decomposition)
  - Vitreous is very viscid; centrifugation with use of supernatant usually required
  - Sodium fluoride typically used as preservative
  - Can replace with same amount of saline to restore contour of eye

Diagnostic Examples

- Diabetes mellitus
  - Peripheral blood glucose > 600 mg/dL without other reasons for hyperglycemia (i.e., resuscitation, fatal hypothermia, asphyxia)
  - Vitreous glucose > 200 mg/dL, presence of ketone bodies
  - ↑ blood ketone bodies and hemoglobin A1c
  - Presence of glucose and ketone bodies in urine
- Liver failure
  - ↑ serum bilirubin with icterus/jaundice
  - ↓ serum total protein with inversion of albumin:globulin ratio
  - Presence of bile and urobilinogen in urine
- Renal failure
  - ↑ serum BUN and creatinine
  - ↑ vitreous BUN and creatinine without significant ↑ in Na and Cl
  - (+) proteins on urine dipstick

SELECTED REFERENCES

1. Palmiere C et al: Postmortem chemistry update part I. Int J Legal Med. 126(2):187-98, 2012
2. Coe JI: Postmortem chemistry update. Emphasis on forensic application. Am J Forensic Med Pathol. 14(2):91-117, 1993

MICROBIOLOGY

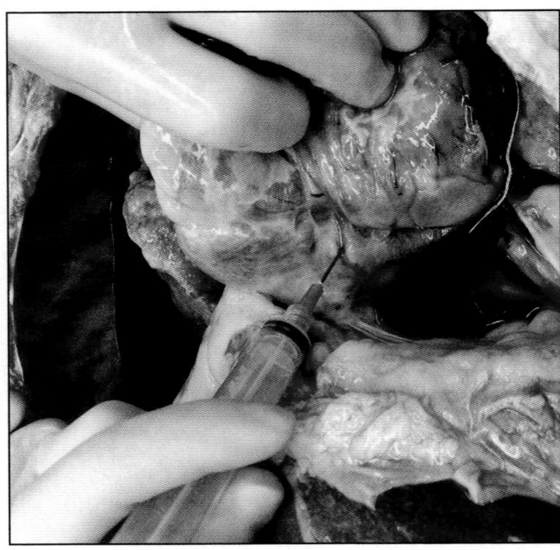

Shown here is the method for collecting heart blood for culture. In carefully selected cases and with attention to proper collection, autopsy cultures can yield important information.

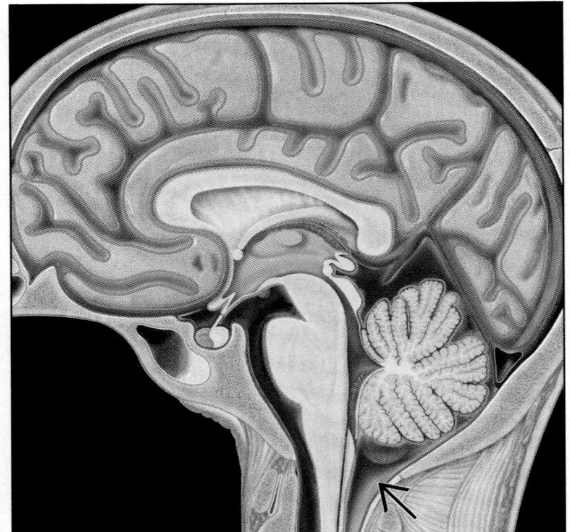

Postmortem collection of cerebrospinal fluid can be performed using a cisternal puncture technique In which a needle is introduced through the skin and soft tissue and into the cisterna magna ➔.

GENERAL PRINCIPLES

Utility of Postmortem Cultures

- Opinion in literature varies
  - Some authors oppose
    - Postmortem microbiologic testing not necessary for hospitalized patients
    - Unlikely to add important clinical information in a patient who has already undergone premortem infectious work-up
    - May yield confusing results: Multiple organisms, organisms that make no clinical sense (contaminant vs. invasive infection)
    - Adds additional cost for little return
  - Some authors encourage
    - Postmortem microbiologic testing at least in selected cases
    - Contamination avoided by careful collection techniques
    - Confusing results can be clarified by careful interpretation in clinical context, clinical judgment
    - Certain isolates from certain sites are unlikely to represent contaminants (e.g., TB from lung tissue)
- Practices that improve the chances for significant results
  - Attention to specimen collection technique
    - Sterile field
    - Aseptic technique
    - Anaerobic aspirate
  - Understanding of clinical context and microbiologic differential diagnosis
  - Appropriate culture/transport media
  - Appropriate test ordering
- Practices that may decrease chances for significant results
  - Poor preservation of remains/long postmortem interval
  - History of recent antimicrobial therapy
  - Poor sterile technique
  - Delayed submission of specimens to microbiology laboratory

Indications for Postmortem Microbiologic Testing

- Clinical history strongly suggests infectious etiology
  - Fever of unknown origin
  - Sepsis without known focus
- Uncertain cause of death in severely immunocompromised patient
  - HIV/AIDS
  - Patients on immunosuppressive medications
- Unexplained sudden death
  - Particularly true in unexpected infant death

Sample Collection Guidelines

- In adult patients who are not immunosuppressed by disease or therapy
  - Sample any organ with gross evidence of infection
  - Sample blood and spleen in cases of suspected bacterial sepsis
  - Sample abnormal collections of fluid, especially if they appear turbid or purulent
  - Sample any tissue or fluid implicated by clinical history/radiographic findings
- In immunosuppressed patients and infants who die suddenly and unexpectedly, immune response to infectious organisms may be blunted or absent
  - In addition to any grossly abnormal tissue or fluid, consider collecting
    - Blood
    - Cerebrospinal fluid
    - Urine
    - Lung tissue
    - Spleen

TECHNIQUES FOR BACTERIAL, FUNGAL, AND VIRAL CULTURES

General Principles

- Keep body refrigerated
- Begin autopsy as soon as possible
- Minimize number of people in room
- Take cultures before manipulation of organs or evisceration
- Use sterile gloves and instruments during specimen collection
- Carefully decontaminate surface of tissue to be sampled
- Deliver specimen to microbiology laboratory as soon as possible
- **Be familiar with and respect limitations of autopsy permit**
- **Use appropriate personal protective equipment**
  - Certain cases may call for additional precautions (e.g., HEPA masks/PAPRs in cases of suspected respiratory pathogens)
- Tissue samples and swabs for viral culture should be placed in appropriate viral transport liquid medium
- Fill out microbiology requisition form clearly and carefully
  - Indicate type of culture (bacterial, fungal, acid fast, viral)
  - Clearly identify source of specimen

Blood for Culture: Femoral Venipuncture

- Advantage: If properly done, minimizes contamination
- Disinfect inguinal skin
- Locate femoral vein
  - Place tip of index finger of nondominant hand on anterior superior iliac crest and tip of thumb on inguinal tubercle
    - Line between tips of thumb and index finger indicates course of inguinal ligament
  - Envision imaginary line perpendicular to inguinal crease drawn to crook of thumb and index finger
    - Perform venipuncture at intersection of imaginary line and inguinal crease
- Collect 20 mL of blood if possible
- Immediately inoculate labeled aerobic and anaerobic blood culture bottles
- Transport blood culture bottles to microbiology laboratory promptly

Blood for Culture: Heart Blood

- Open pericardium to expose heart
- Have an assistant lift apex of heart to expose entrance of inferior vena cava into right atrium
- Disinfect area
  - 1st alternative: Wipe away blood with alcohol swab, then cleanse area with antimicrobial swab
  - 2nd alternative: Heat a spatula blade and sear area
- Insert needle into inferior vena cava toward right ventricle
  - Be mindful of assistant's hands
- Collect 20 mL if possible
- Immediately inoculate labeled aerobic and anaerobic culture bottles
- Transport blood culture bottles to microbiology laboratory promptly

Cerebrospinal Fluid: Cisternal Puncture

- Disinfect skin in midline at base of occipital bone
- Insert needle with attached syringe in midline, just beneath occipital bone
- Collect several mL of CSF
- Eject CSF into labeled, sterile container
- Transport promptly to microbiology laboratory

Cerebrospinal Fluid: Ventricular Puncture

- Remove calvaria and dura to expose surface of cerebral hemispheres
- Disinfect portion of surface of cerebral hemisphere with antimicrobial swab
- Insert needle through cerebral cortex and into lateral ventricle
- Collect several mL of CSF
- Eject CSF into sterile labeled container
- Transport promptly to microbiology laboratory

Effusions: Pleural, Ascites, Joint

- Use needle and syringe to collect fluid percutaneously after appropriate skin disinfection
- Alternatively, collect ascites fluid/pleural effusion after opening body
  - Disadvantage: Increases likelihood of contamination

Abscesses

- Use needle and syringe to aspirate abscess contents after disinfection of surface
- Usually not necessary to culture abdominal abscesses
  - Typically polymicrobial and composed of enteric organisms

Tissue Biopsy for Culture

- When possible, sample organ in situ
- Use sterile scalpel and sterilized forceps
- Have assistant elevate organ to be sampled
- Disinfect surface of organ to be sampled
- Incise disinfected area with sterile scalpel blade
  - Be mindful of assistant's hands
- Use sterile scalpel and forceps to remove ~ 1 cm^3 of tissue
- Place tissue into labeled screw top sterile container
- Transport specimen promptly to microbiology laboratory

Tissue Swabs for Culture

- Prepare area to be sampled as for tissue biopsy culture
- Incise disinfected area
- Insert tip of swab into incision and swab incised surfaces
- Place swab into a labeled vial of appropriate transport medium
- Culture of biopsied tissue is preferred to swabs whenever possible

Urine for Culture

- Retract bowels to expose floor of peritoneal cavity
- Disinfect area in midline behind pubic bone

- Insert needle attached to syringe into disinfected area and through dome of bladder
- Collect urine, 20 mL if possible
- Expel contents of syringe into labeled screw top sterile container
- Transport promptly to microbiology laboratory

NONCULTURE METHODS

Histology

- Routine H&E and histochemical stains
  - Viral inclusions and viral cytopathic changes
    - May suggest specific etiology (e.g., herpes or CMV)
    - Useful to confirm histologic findings with immunoperoxidase if available
  - Bacteria may be visible
    - If tissue is inflamed (and bacteria potentially obscured), consider bacterial stain (e.g., Lisa stain)
  - Granulomas
    - Do acid-fast stain for mycobacteria and silver stain for fungi
    - Bear in mind that some bacteria (e.g., *Brucella* and *Yersinia*) may also cause granulomatous inflammation
  - Helminths and their ova may be visible on routine sections
- Immunoperoxidase
  - If index of suspicion is high for a particular pathogen, immunoperoxidase may be useful, even in absence of suggestive histology

Nucleic Acid Testing

- Advantages
  - Unlike cultures, do not depend on living organisms
  - May provide rapid identification
- Disadvantages
  - Require equipment and expertise that may not be available in all labs
  - Expense may be an obstacle
- Polymerase chain reaction (PCR) for specific organisms
  - Extremely sensitive and specific
  - Amplification inherent in technique means that very few organisms are needed for identification
  - May be done even on formalin-fixed, paraffin-embedded tissue
  - Drawback: Must have high index of suspicion for a particular organism and must have a specific probe for that organism
- PCR for bacterial DNA
  - Gene for 16S ribosomal RNA can be amplified using PCR probe
  - Sequence of amplified gene can be compared to database for identification
  - Technique is effective even in formalin-fixed, paraffin-embedded tissue
  - Not affected by antibiotic therapy
  - Drawbacks: Available only in limited number of labs

Enzyme-Linked Immunoassays

- May be collected with swabs of affected tissue
- Inferior sensitivity and specificity when compared to PCR
- Advantages: Comparatively rapid and inexpensive

INTERPRETATION OF TESTING RESULTS

Features of Clinically Relevant Result

- Identification of a single pathogenic organism
- Isolated organism was collected from normally sterile site
- Isolated organism is recognized pathogen at that site
- Isolated organism is never part of normal flora (e.g., *Mycobacterium tuberculosis* or *Salmonella typhi)*

Features of Isolation of Contaminants

- Multiple organisms recovered from usually sterile site
- Isolated organism is not a usual pathogen at site collected or does not make sense in clinical context
- Isolated organism is part of normal flora at site

SELECTED REFERENCES

1. Hart JD et al: Infectious diseases and tropical disease pathology: SC16-1 rRNA sequencing in molecular microbiological diagnosis of bacterial infections in the autopsy setting. Pathology. 46 Suppl 2:S26, 2014
2. Weber MA et al: Post-mortem interval and bacteriological culture yield in sudden unexpected death in infancy (SUDI). Forensic Sci Int. 198(1-3):121-5, 2010
3. Morris JA et al: Postmortem bacteriology: a re-evaluation. J Clin Pathol. 59(1):1-9, 2006

Gross and Microscopic Features

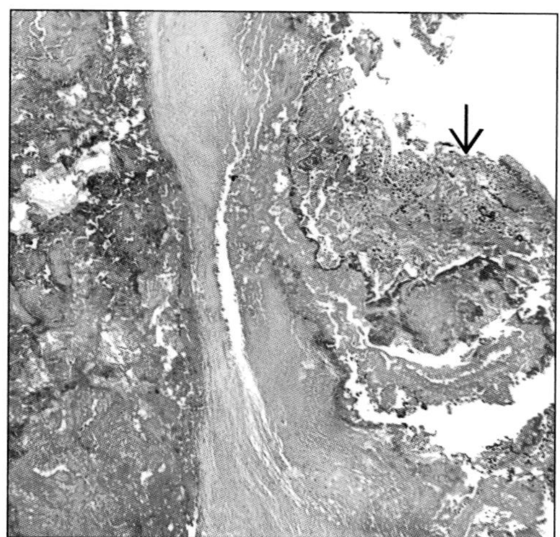

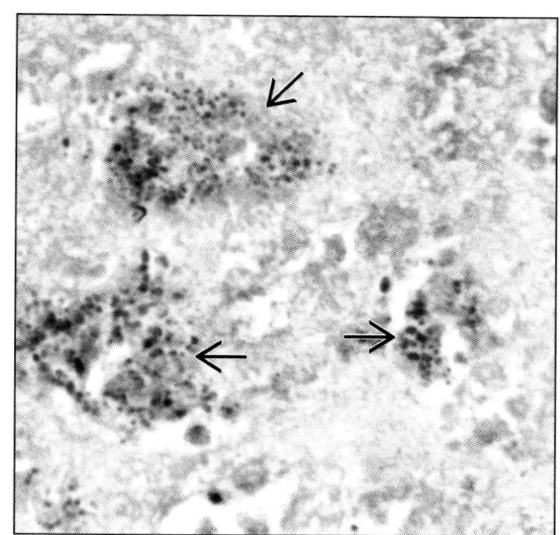

(Left) This section of aortic valve shows a fibrinous valvular vegetation ⇒. Bacterial endocarditis can be caused by a wide variety of organisms. Septic emboli may break off the vegetation, lodge in distant organs, and cause a bewildering constellation of symptoms. **(Right)** A higher power view of the same valve vegetation shows clusters of cocci ⇒, protected from host defenses and antibiotics deep within the fibrinous matrix.

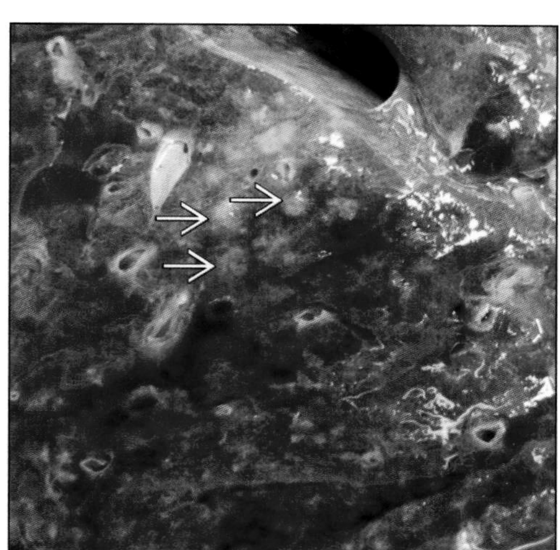

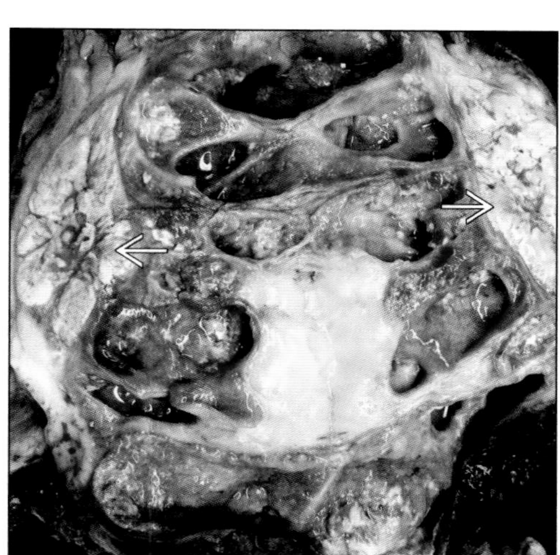

(Left) The cut surface of this lung shows many tan-yellow nodules ➡, which proved histologically to be caseating granulomas. Cultures were positive for Mycobacterium tuberculosis, an organism that is an obligate human pathogen and is never part of normal flora. **(Right)** This hydronephrotic kidney, from which staghorn calculi were removed, showed a mass ➡ on CT scan suspicious for renal cell carcinoma. It proved to be xanthogranulomatous pyelonephritis.

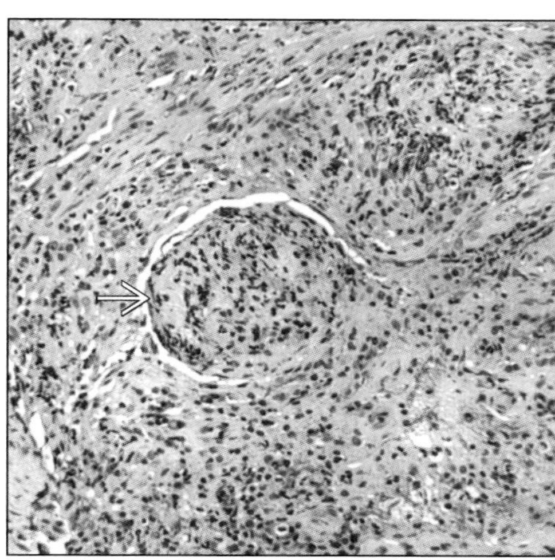

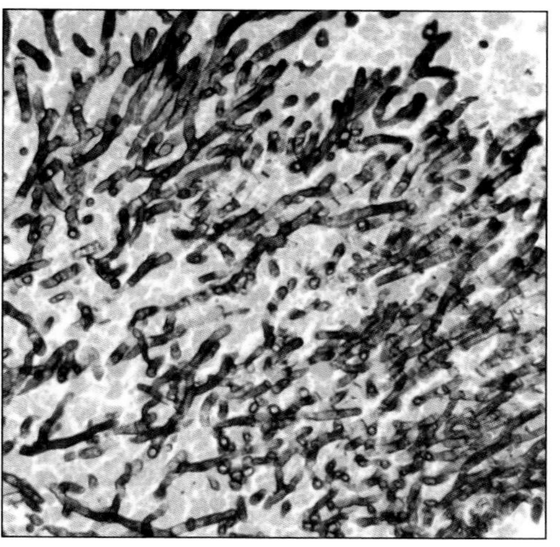

(Left) Granulomas, often thought of in association with mycobacterial or fungal infections, may be seen with other infectious and noninfectious etiologies. The granulomas ➡ found in this section from lumbar vertebra were thought suggestive of mycobacteria, but cultures grew Brucella melitensis. **(Right)** This silver-stained section taken from the lung of a patient who died with an unexplained infiltrate unresponsive to antibiotics shows fungal hyphae consistent with Aspergillus.

CYTOLOGY

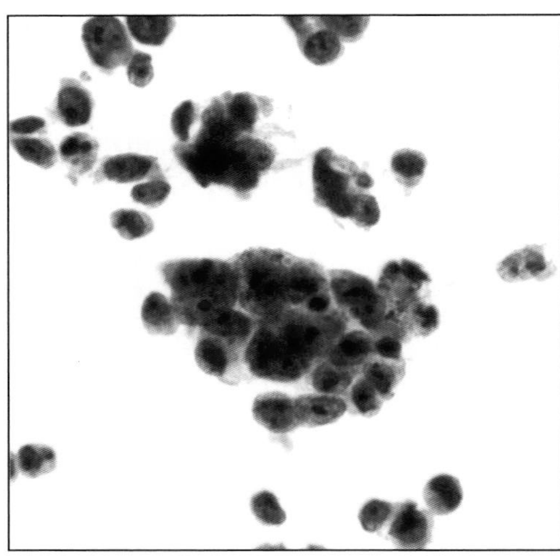

This FNA of an inguinal node (part of a limited autopsy) in a patient without a known primary tumor shows malignant cells with prominent nucleoli. A preliminary diagnosis of metastatic tumor was made.

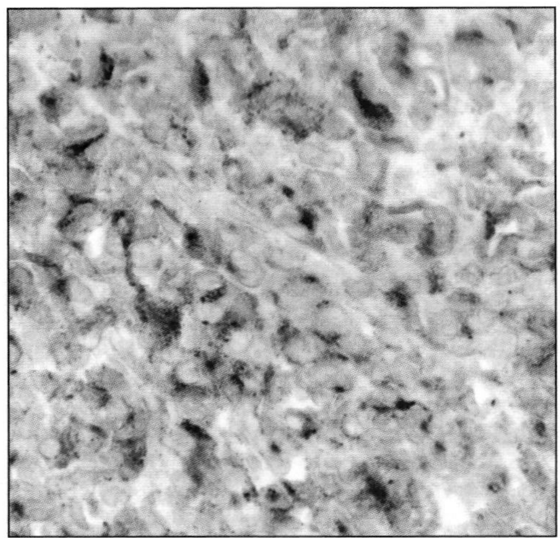

The cell block on the same case was positive for HMB-45 and MART1 consistent with malignant melanoma. No cutaneous lesion was found.

TECHNIQUES

Collection Methods

- Scrapings
  - Focal lesions, nodules
    - Cut into lesion
    - Scrape cut surface with fresh scalpel blade
    - Scraped material applied near frosted end of labeled glass slide
    - 2nd ("spreader") labeled slide lightly applied over scraped material
    - Spreader slide drawn down length of original slide
    - 1 slide **immediately** into alcohol
    - 1 slide air dried
- Impression/touch preparation (TP): For nodules or lymph nodes
  - Cut into lesion with fresh scalpel blade
  - Dab 1 cut surface onto absorbent paper towel
  - Touch dried cut surface of specimen to labeled glass slide
  - Using light pressure, draw cut surface down length of slide
  - 1 slide **immediately** into alcohol
  - 1 slide air dried
- Fine needle aspiration (FNA)
  - Palpable nodules; diffusely consolidated lung tissue
    - 16-21 gauge needle attached to 10 ml syringe
    - Insert needle into lesional tissue
    - Without withdrawing needle, move needle up and down within lesion while slightly changing angle (6-12 times)
    - Stop after 12 needle oscillations or if material appears in syringe
    - Remove needle from lesion
    - Detach needle from syringe
    - Pull back syringe plunger, reattach needle
    - Bring needle tip into light contact with labeled glass slide
    - Expel needle contents onto slide; avoid spraying through the air
    - Immediately spread expressed fluid with 2nd labeled glass slide
    - 1 slide **immediately** into alcohol
    - 1 slide air dried
    - Alternatively, expel needle contents into cytolyte solution and submit to cytology laboratory for thin prep
- Exfoliative cytology: Examination of cells spontaneously shed, e.g., into urine
  - Pericardial effusion, pleural effusion, ascites fluid, joint fluid, other fluid collections
    - Draw fluid into 20 ml syringe
    - Expel contents into labeled screw top specimen container
    - Submit to cytology laboratory

Cytologic Stains

- Papanicolaou stain
  - Used on rapidly alcohol-fixed smears
  - Advantages
    - Good preservation of nuclear features
  - Disadvantages
    - Procedure is comparatively long and complicated
    - Best done by cytology laboratory
- Romanowsky-type stains
  - Examples: Wright, Wright Giemsa, Diff-Quik
  - Used on air dried smears
  - Advantages
    - Fast and comparatively simple
    - Better preservation of cytoplasmic features
    - Certain features (colloid, mucin, endocrine granules) are seen better
    - Particularly useful for blood smears and lymph nodes
  - Disadvantages
    - Inferior preservation of nuclear features compared to Pap stain

- Rapid hematoxylin and eosin
  - Advantages
    - Usually readily available (same stain as frozen sections)
    - Fast and comparatively simple

CLINICAL IMPLICATIONS

Advantages of Autopsy Cytology

- Rapid, reliable preliminary microscopic results on suspicious lesions
  - More complete preliminary anatomic diagnosis (PAD)
  - Rapid feedback for clinicians and family members
    - Delay in microscopic results a frequent complaint by clinicians
    - Autopsy cytology provides limited histologic diagnosis within 24 hours of autopsy
  - Rapid information for hospital infection control
    - Useful for decisions regarding exposure prophylaxis and patient isolation
  - Useful for making decisions regarding transplant harvest
- Inexpensive and relatively simple
- Minimally invasive
  - May allow for microscopic evaluation in some limited autopsies
    - Note: Always assure that permit addresses autopsy limitations and honor limitations imposed
  - Allows for microscopic sampling without cosmetically unacceptable incisions
    - e.g., lesions of face and hands
  - Allows for evaluation of hard-to-sample areas
    - e.g., joint spaces for synovitis and crystal arthropathy
- Can direct decisions about ancillary special procedures
  - Flow cytometry, cytogenetics, culture
- Unlike frozen section, no potential for contamination of cryostat
- Aid for cytology training
  - Allows for correlation of autopsy cytology with histology

Disadvantages of Autopsy Cytology

- Not useful for diagnosis in many types of cases
  - e.g., myocardial infarction, pulmonary embolus
- Requires experience and training in specimen preparation and interpretation
- Will occasionally yield nondiagnostic specimen
- Still advisable to back up with 2nd method
  - Histology, culture

MACROSCOPIC FINDINGS

Lesions Amenable to Cytologic Evaluation at Autopsy

- Consolidated lungs
  - Often difficult to diagnose pneumonia grossly
  - FNA can demonstrate inflammation and provide material for culture
  - Suspicion of TB: Appropriate cultures and consultation with hospital infection control
- Enlarged lymph nodes
  - Benign vs. malignant
    - Reactive nodes can be cultured
  - Lymphoma vs. metastasis
    - Lymphoma: Tissue can be submitted for flow cytometry and other special studies
    - Metastasis: Prompts search for primary lesion
- Undiagnosed mass lesions
- Fluid collections
  - Pleural effusions
  - Ascites
  - Abscesses

MICROSCOPIC FINDINGS

Infectious Agents

- Bacteria: Typically difficult to see without special stains
- Acid fast bacteria
  - Granulomas &/or macrophages in appropriate setting are suggestive
  - Should be followed by acid fast stain
- Fungi
  - Granulomas &/or macrophages in appropriate setting are suggestive
  - Should be followed by silver stain or PAS stain
- Viruses
  - Viral cytopathic changes suggest DNA virus infection
    - HSV: Multiple nuclei with nuclear molding and ground-glass appearance
    - CMV: Giant cells with large nuclear inclusion and cytoplasmic inclusions

Tumors (Very Crude Guide)

- Carcinoma: Cohesive clusters of cells
  - Adenocarcinoma: 3-dimensional clusters ± mucin
  - Squamous cell carcinoma: Clusters of cells; orangeophilia on Pap stain; ± keratin pearls
- Melanoma: Clusters or dispersed large atypical cells with prominent nucleoli, ± pigment
- Lymphoma: Dyscohesive lymphocytes ± other inflammatory cells
  - Non-Hodgkin lymphoma: Monomorphous populations of lymphocytes
  - Hodgkin disease: Reed Sternberg cells or variants on background of mixed inflammatory cells

SELECTED REFERENCES

1. Uram-Tuculescu CG et al: Postmortem cytology: Alive and well in the practice of autopsy and forensic pathology. Cancer Cytopathol. Epub ahead of print, 2015
2. Sens MA et al: Unexpected neoplasia in autopsies: potential implications for tissue and organ safety. Arch Pathol Lab Med. 133(12):1923-31, 2009
3. Benbow EW et al: The autopsy: complete or not complete? Histopathology. 42(5):417-23, 2003
4. Atkins KA et al: The cytopathology of infectious diseases. Adv Anat Pathol. 9(1):52-64, 2002

CYTOLOGY

Fine-Needle Aspiration

*(**Left**) A 20-gauge needle attached to a 10 cc syringe is inserted into the mass. Without withdrawing the needle, it is moved up and down within the mass. The angle of the needle is changed slightly with each withdrawal. (**Right**) After 6 to 12 needle oscillations, or once fluid becomes visible in the syringe, withdraw the needle. Apply the tip of the needle lightly to the surface of a clean, labeled slide. Express a small drop of fluid near the middle of the slide.*

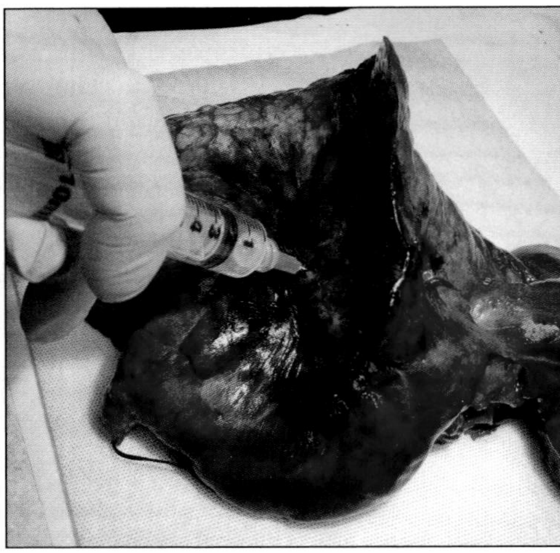

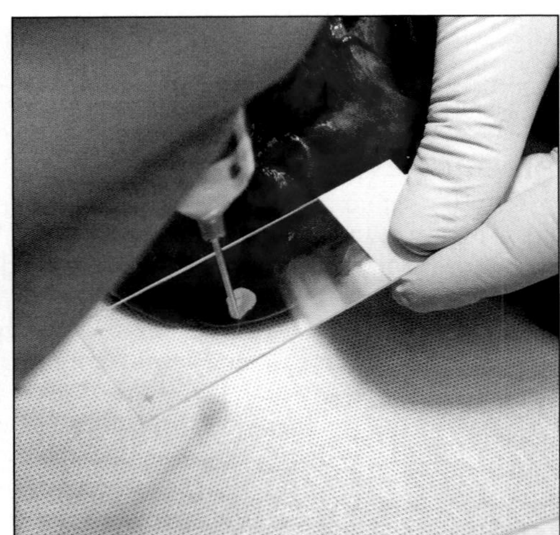

*(**Left**) Ideally the fluid on the slide will be cellular with a creamy appearance, but not bloody. No more than a small drop is needed. If more fluid is available, make more slides or squirt the fluid into fixative for Pap staining. (**Right**) Immediately apply a second clean labeled slide lightly to the first slide to slightly spread the drop of aspirate fluid. Maintain the light contact between the slides and draw them apart. The result is a thin smear of aspirate fluid on both slides.*

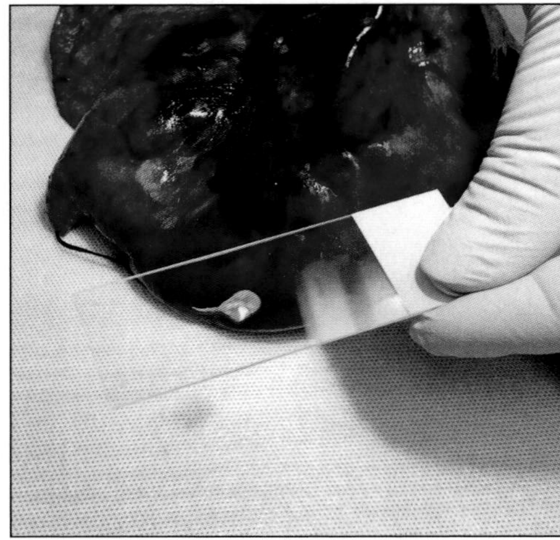

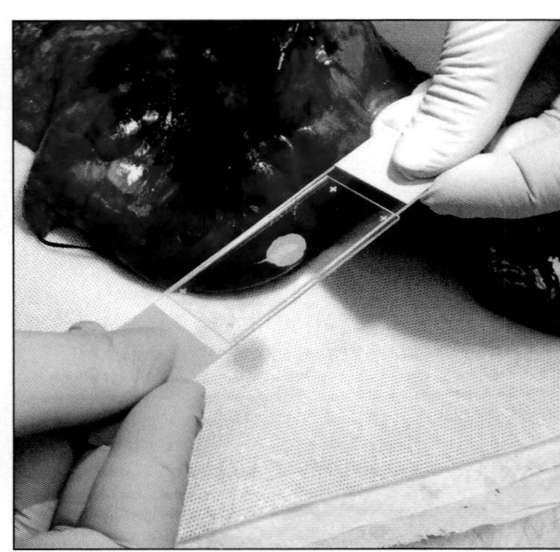

*(**Left**) At least 1 smeared slide (if not both) should be immediately immersed into fixative to avoid air drying artifact. The fixed slide can then be stained as you would a frozen section. Some pathologists like to air dry the 2nd smear and make a Wright stained slide. (**Right**) This FNA of an undiagnosed lung mass showed cohesive clusters of cells with abundant cytoplasm, some with the suggestion of keratinization ⇨. Histology showed a squamous cell carcinoma.*

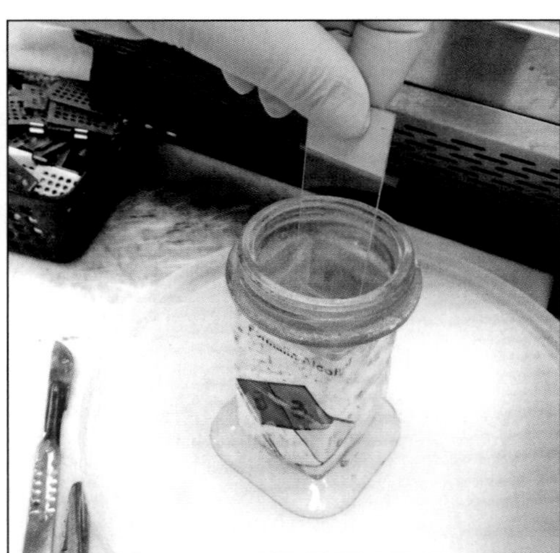

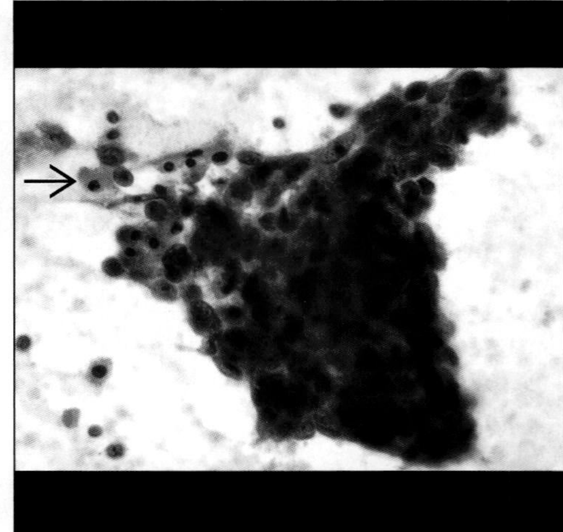

Scrape & Touch Preparations

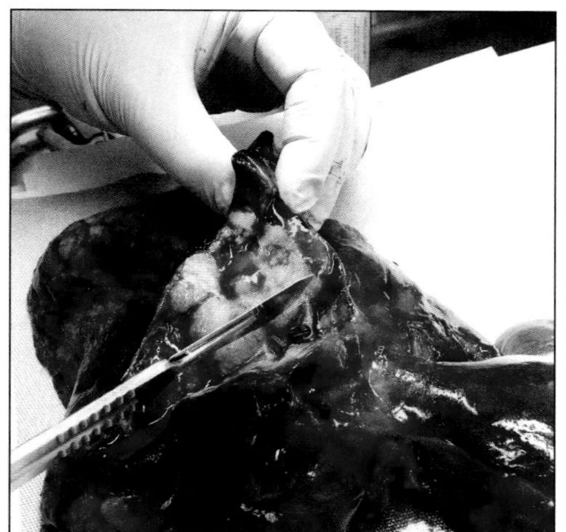

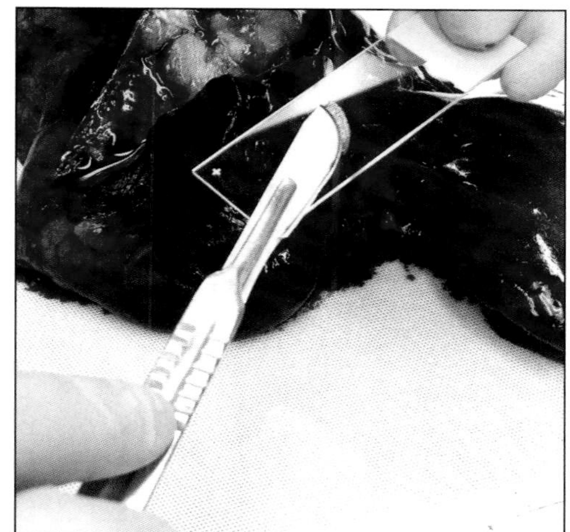

(Left) *To make a scrape preparation of a mass lesion, first incise the slide to expose a cut surface. The surface can be lightly scraped to clean any adherent blood or mucus. Change the scalpel blade and use the clean blade to gently but firmly scrape the cut surface of the mass.* ***(Right)*** *The blade should have an adherent small quantity of cellular fluid. Immediately apply the wet side of the blade lightly to a slide. Use a 2nd clean, labeled slide to smear the scraped fluid.*

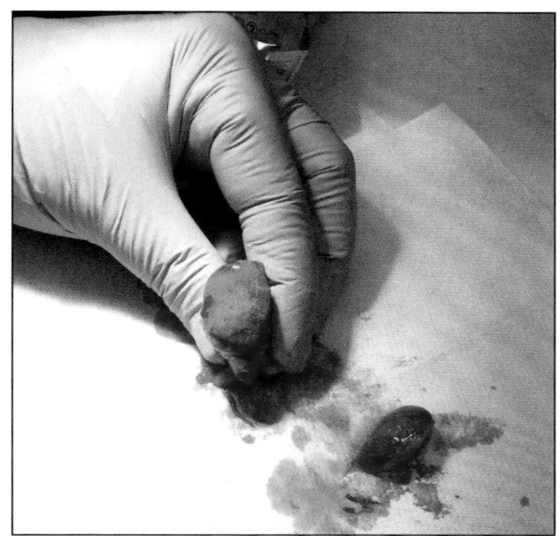

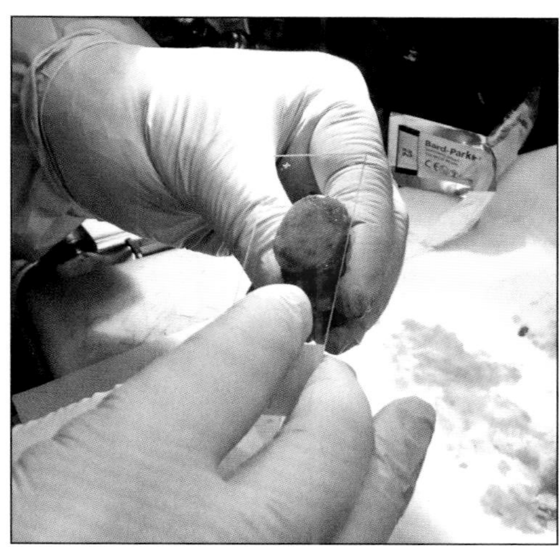

(Left) *To prepare a touch preparation of a lymph node, first section the node to expose a cut surface of a centimeter or 2. Touch the cut surface of the node lightly to a paper towel to remove excess fluid.* ***(Right)*** *Lightly touch the cleaned cut surface of the lymph node to a clean, labeled slide. While maintaining light contact between the node and the slide, draw the node downwards toward the end of the slide to make a thin smear. Place the slide immediately into fixative and stain.*

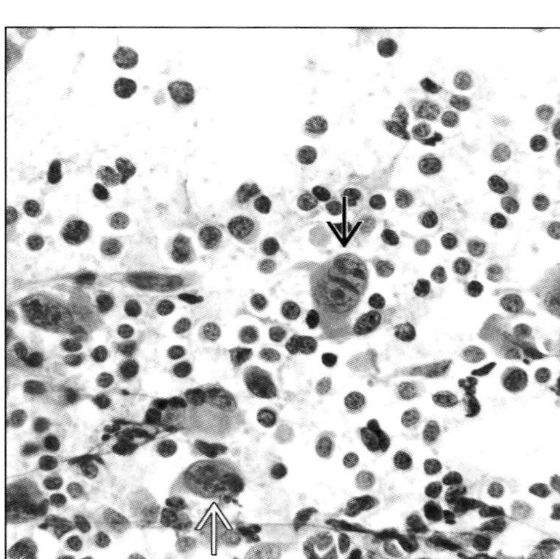

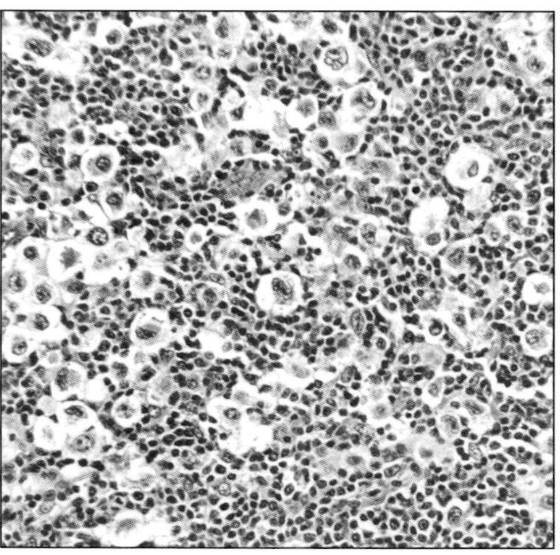

(Left) *This touch preparation of an enlarged mediastinal lymph nodes shows large atypical cells ➡, some of which were binucleated with prominent nucleoli ⇨ consistent with Reed Sternberg cells. The background is composed of small lymphocytes and occasional eosinophils. A preliminary diagnosis of Hodgkin lymphoma was made.* ***(Right)*** *A permanent section of the lymph node shows histologic features of Hodgkin disease. The diagnosis was confirmed with immunoperoxidase.*

CYTOLOGY

Microscopic Features

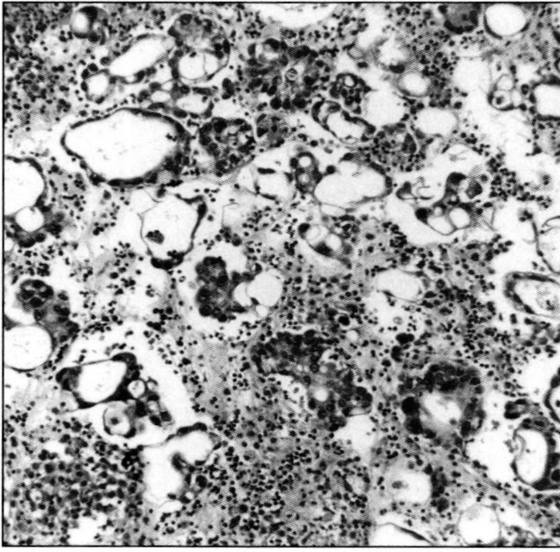
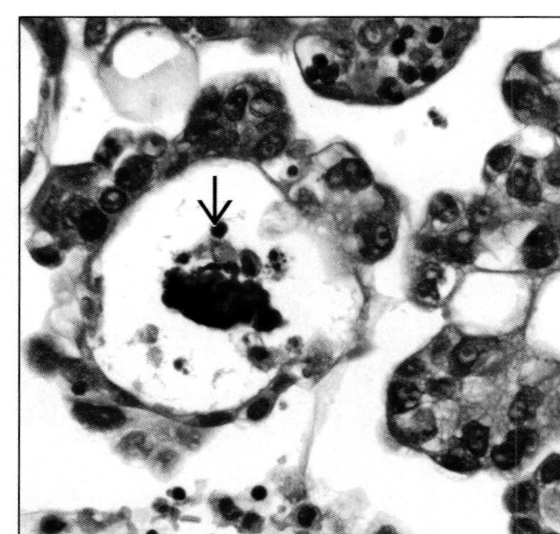

(Left) *Ascites fluid was taken from a patient with ascites, ovarian masses, and peritoneal nodules. The fluid is very cellular and composed of papillary collections of tumor cells.* ***(Right)*** *At higher power, the papillae are lined by cytologically atypical cells with prominent nucleoli. Some of the papillae had associated concentric calcifications ⇨ consistent with psammoma bodies. A preliminary diagnosis of papillary serous carcinoma was made and later confirmed.*

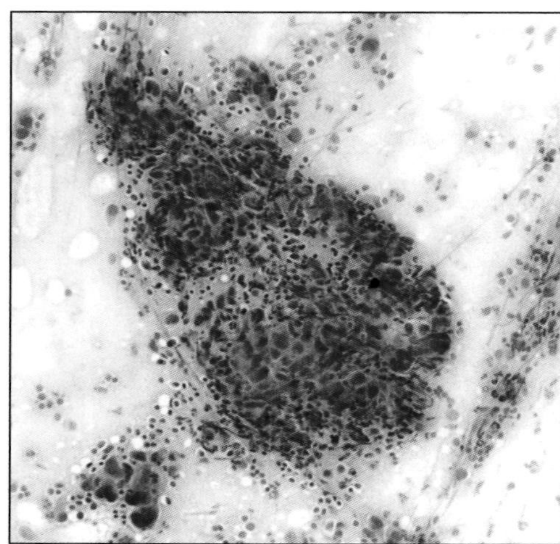
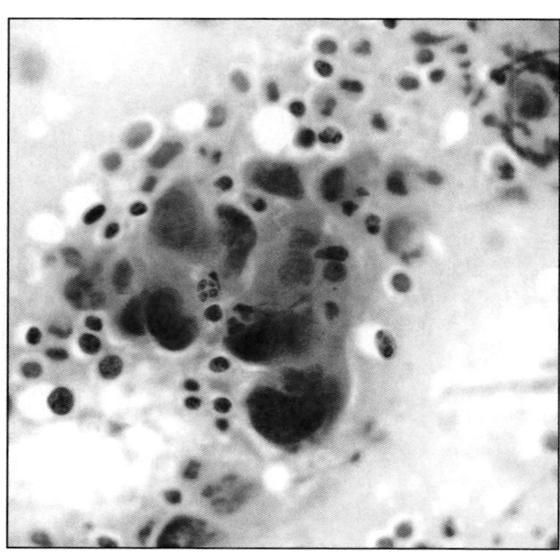

(Left) *This H&E-stained fine needle aspirate of an undiagnosed lung tumor showed cohesive clusters of cytologically atypical cells with eosinophilic cytoplasm. There was a single lung lesion as well as mediastinal lymphadenopathy and adrenal nodules.* ***(Right)*** *At higher power, the cells show nuclei with dark chromatin and relatively abundant eosinophilic cytoplasm. A preliminary diagnosis of non-small cell carcinoma was made. Histologic sections showed squamous cell carcinoma.*

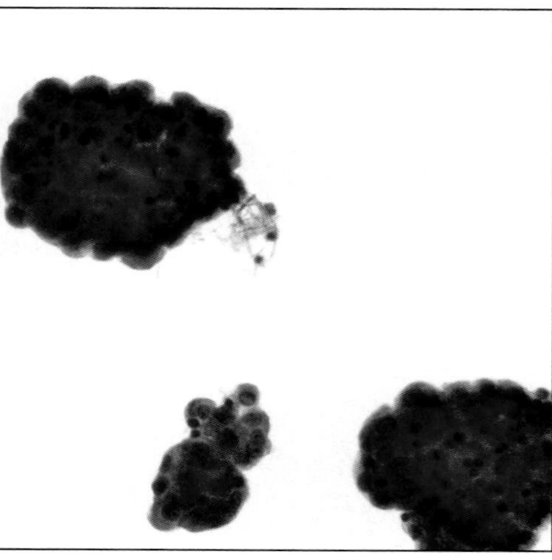
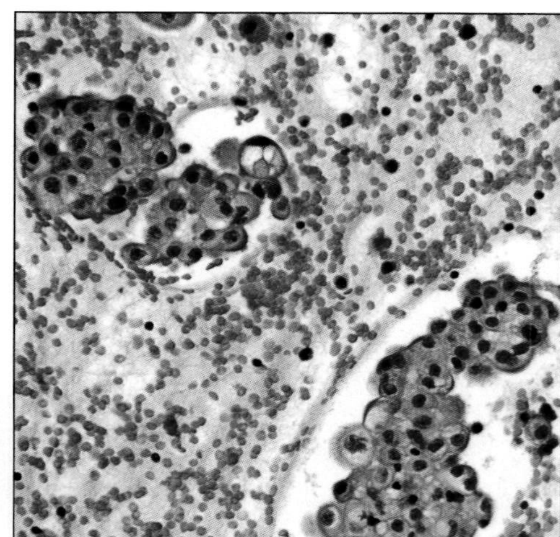

(Left) *This Papanicolaou-stained pleural effusion fluid was taken from a patient who had diffuse pleural thickening and a history of cigarette smoking and asbestos exposure. The clusters of cells are 3 dimensional and cytologically atypical. A distinction between carcinoma and mesothelioma could not be made.* ***(Right)*** *The cell block from the same pleural effusion is shown here. Immunoperoxidase stains on this material were consistent with mesothelioma.*

Cytology in Limited Cases

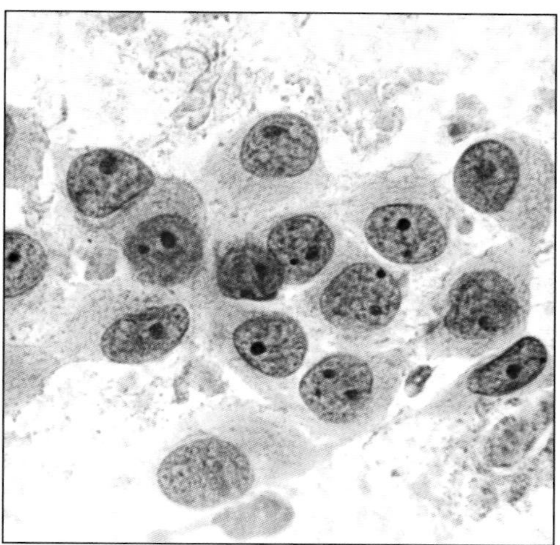

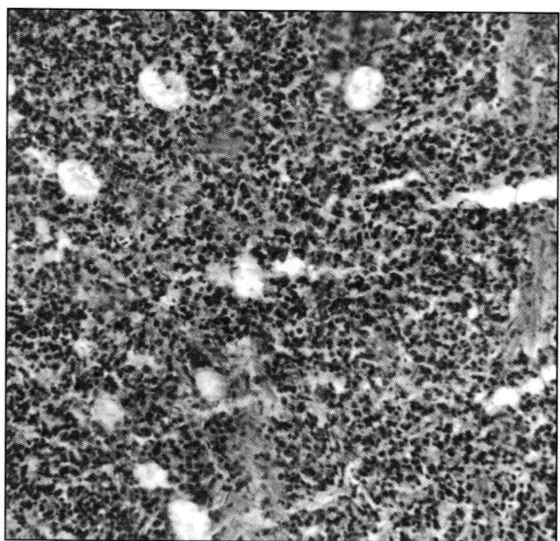

(Left) *These images were taken from an autopsy of a man who died with bony masses, possibly metastases, of unknown origin. The autopsy was limited to evaluation of rib lesions. This image is an H&E-stained touch preparation of a rib lesion. The cells have eccentric nuclei with fine chromatin and nucleoli.* ***(Right)*** *A frozen section of a rib lesion showed a hypercellular marrow space with with a monotonous infiltrate of cells that replaced the normal marrow elements.*

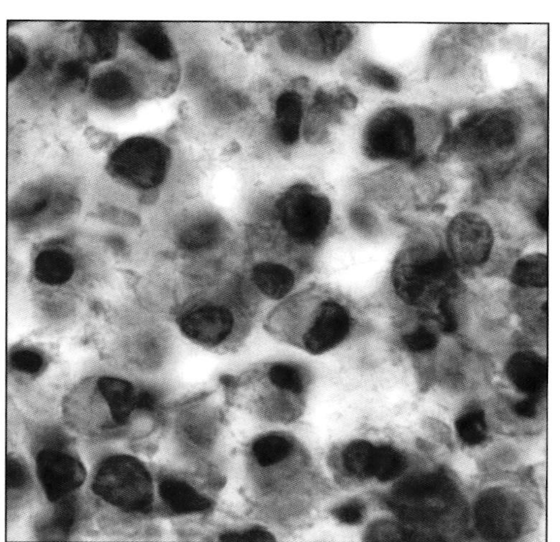

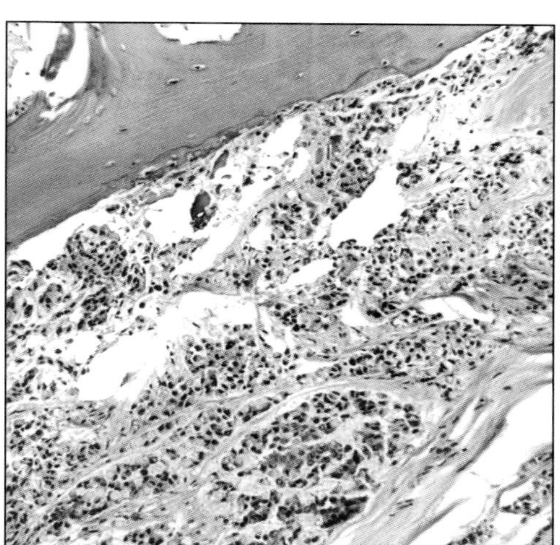

(Left) *At higher power, the infiltrate is composed of cells with eccentric nuclei. The cytoplasm is eosinophilic and uniform. The nuclei lack the clumped chromatin of plasma cells and the cytoplasm lacks the perinuclear hof zone of plasma cells. The cells were thought compatible with signet ring cells and a preliminary diagnosis of metastatic adenocarcinoma was made.* ***(Right)*** *This is the formalin fixed, paraffin embedded permanent section of the marrow.*

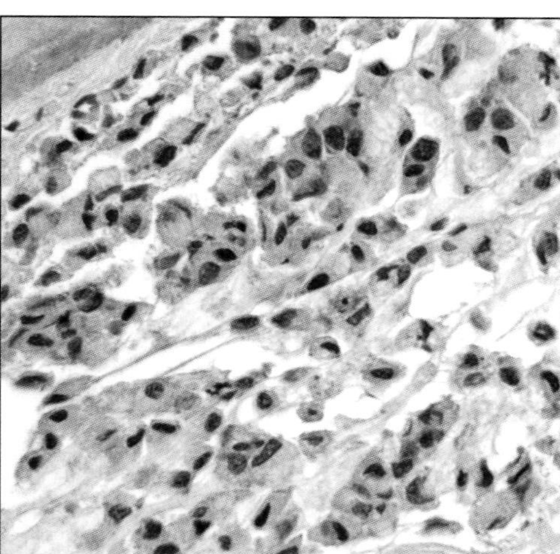

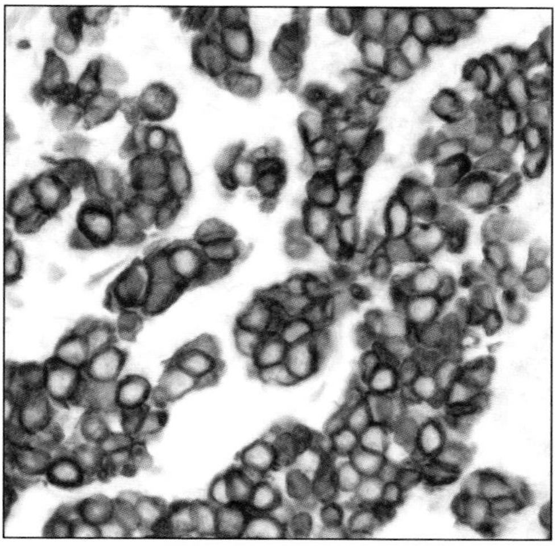

(Left) *At higher power, the infiltrating cells show intracellular mucin consistent with signet ring cell carcinoma.* ***(Right)*** *Immunoperoxidase studies were positive for CK20 and CDX2 and negative for CK7. A final diagnosis of disseminated signet ring cell carcinoma of probable gastrointestinal origin was made.*

POSTMORTEM RADIOGRAPHY AND VIRTUAL AUTOPSY

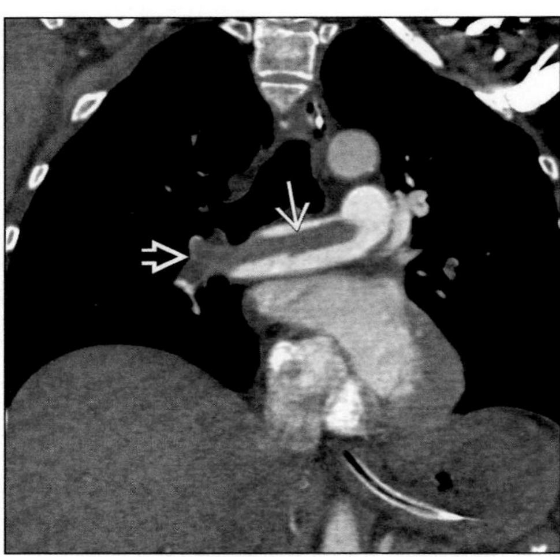

Coronal chest CT shows a large embolism ➡ in the main pulmonary artery, extending into the right branches ➡. This analysis is usually not necessary for routine autopsy for PE detection but does help with virtual autopsy.

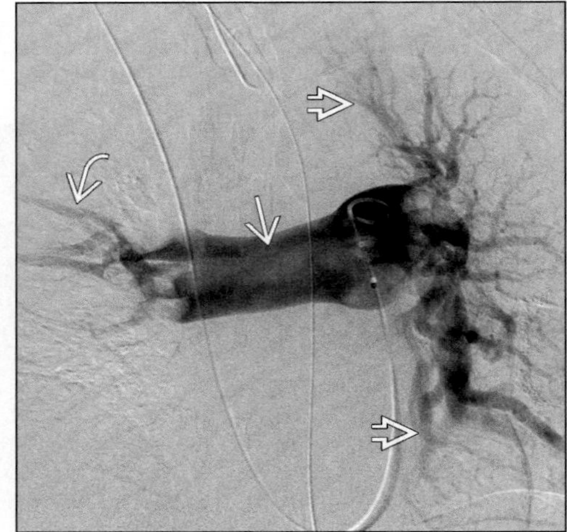

Angiogram of the pulmonary artery in the same case shows a large filling defect ➡ secondary to the embolism. There is normal arborization of pulmonary vessels on the left ➡ and a paucity of vessels on the right ➡.

TERMINOLOGY

Definitions

- Postmortem radiography (and other imaging modalities) are used to facilitate postmortem diagnoses in hospital autopsies
- Virtual autopsy: A minimally invasive autopsy that uses multislice CT and MR scans with 3D reformations to view exterior and interior of body
  - More frequently used in forensic, rather than hospital, autopsy setting

COMMON USES

Cardiovascular System

- Coronary arteries and grafts
  - Identification of coronary artery stents
    - Imaging of excised heart before dissection of coronary vasculature demonstrates placement of stents, gross pathology of stents (strut fractures, collapse)
    - Useful in patients with no available medical records to identify unsuspected stents
  - Postmortem angiographic analysis of coronary artery bypass grafts (1 method discussed; other more sophisticated methods exist)
    - Identify proximal graft insertion site and loosely place twine/string around proximal graft, do not secure
    - Draw contrast media (may use discarded contrast material from radiology department) into syringe and then insert intravenous catheter onto syringe
    - Inject media into graft and tie off proximal graft while removing catheter
    - Radiograph excised heart to visualize graft lumens
  - Bioprosthetic valve placement/struts/calcification
    - All bioprosthetic valves should be removed from heart after in-situ evaluation and radiographed separately for assessment of strut integrity and degenerative calcification of cusp material
    - Punctate calcification on bioprosthetic or native valves can indicate chronic infective endocarditis
  - Other findings on postmortem radiography of heart
    - Calcific coronary atherosclerosis
    - Mitral annular calcification
    - Aortic valve calcification
    - Artificial valve placement, structural integrity
- Aorta
  - Chest and abdominal x-ray at postmortem will reveal aortic aneurysm endografts or interposition grafts if present, can also be done on excised aorta
  - Ascending aortic, arch, and descending aortic atherosclerosis identified on chest radiograph
- Venous system
  - Abdominal x-ray at postmortem will reveal inferior vena cava filters (not a usual primary indication for postmortem radiography)
  - In cases of suspect placement, postmortem chest x-ray can identify placement of central lines
  - Radiographic evaluation of pacer and AICD generators and leads can show placement and abnormalities of lead wires

Respiratory System

- Chest x-ray before manipulation of chest can reveal pneumothorax, placement of endotracheal tube, chest tube placement
- Postmortem pulmonary angiography may reveal segmental pulmonary thromboemboli (localized lack of perfusion) or severe pulmonary hypertensive vasculopathy (diffuse pruning of distal pulmonary arterial tree)
  - Contrast media injected into right/left pulmonary artery (large syringe without needle), and proximal vessel clamped, tied, or sutured (leave long cuff of pulmonary artery if planning to do this analysis)

Virtual vs. Traditional Autopsy

Virtual Autopsy	Traditional Autopsy
Non- or minimally invasive; may appeal to families with religious objections	Invasive
In-situ viewing of wounds and ability to reconstruct complex trauma	More difficult
Pneumothorax and air embolism easily visualized	May be easily missed
Easy to visualize foreign bodies and medical devices in situ	Limited ability to document those findings without radiography
Bone fractures and lesions easy to identify	Difficult to impossible
Pulmonary thromboemboli, coronary artery disease and myocardial infarcts may be missed	Easily identified
Limited histologic sampling	Extensive histologic sampling
Limited color spectrum with radiographic examination of organs	Full color spectrum
Needs expensive equipment and trained personnel	No need for expensive equipment, do need trained personnel

  - X-ray excised lungs to evaluate pulmonary vasculature

Hepatobiliary System

- Radiograph can determine placement of biliary tube
- CT scan can reveal cirrhosis, metastatic or primary hepatic malignancy, cysts; but is not generally used for this indication in routine practice

Genitourinary System

- Abdominal x-ray may show presence and location of ureteral stent, renal stones

Skeletal System

- Hand/spine x-ray in suspected arthritis
- If extremity bruising or positioning is suspicious for trauma, x-ray can be performed to exclude fracture

Central Nervous System

- CT scan can reveal cysts, hemorrhage, metastatic disease, atrophy
- Must differentiate premortem disease from postmortem artifacts
  - Ventricles and sulci effaced, loss of gray-white distinction (autolysis)
  - Increased attenuation of vessels and dependent tissues (livor mortis)

Full-Body Imaging for Metastatic Disease

- Overall tumor burden easier to determine
- Skeletal metastases easier to document than at routine autopsy
- Extent of necrosis and growth of lesions can be documented (requires correlation with premortem imaging)

VIRTUAL AUTOPSY

Methodology

- Multidisciplinary approach (radiology and pathology) to postmortem investigation, developed at the University of Bern's Institute of Forensic Medicine
- Uses multislice CT and MR
  - Data can be shown in any plane including 3D reconstructions
- Newer methods combine a robotic biopsy device to perform image-guided tissue biopsy and fluid analysis
- Most widely used application is in forensic medicine
- Good for documenting trauma, fractures, bullet tracts, choking, drowning
- In hospital autopsy setting better than traditional autopsy for bone fractures and lesions, small effusions, foreign bodies, device placement
  - Pulmonary thromboembolism, coronary artery atherosclerosis, and myocardial infarction are less easily identified than with traditional autopsy
    - Newer angiographic techniques are being added to virtual autopsy to address this issue
- Barriers to clinical use include cost and training of personnel

SAFETY PRECAUTIONS

Routine

- Personnel should leave autopsy suite area when x-ray is being performed to avoid exposure
- When performing postmortem angiography maintain strict sharps safety after drawing up contrast media

REPORTING CRITERIA

Minimum Requirements

- Review of premortem imaging studies is a mandatory part of autopsy practice
  - Correlation of premortem imaging findings to postmortem findings (imaging, gross and microscopic pathology) is imperative for quality assurance and discrepancies should be discussed with radiologist/clinician
  - Consultation with radiologist to interpret postmortem imaging and correlate with premortem imaging

SELECTED REFERENCES

1. Wichmann D et al: Virtual autopsy with multiphase postmortem computed tomographic angiography versus traditional medical autopsy to investigate unexpected deaths of hospitalized patients: a cohort study. Ann Intern Med. 160(8):534-41, 2014

Radiographic Analysis of Cardiovascular System

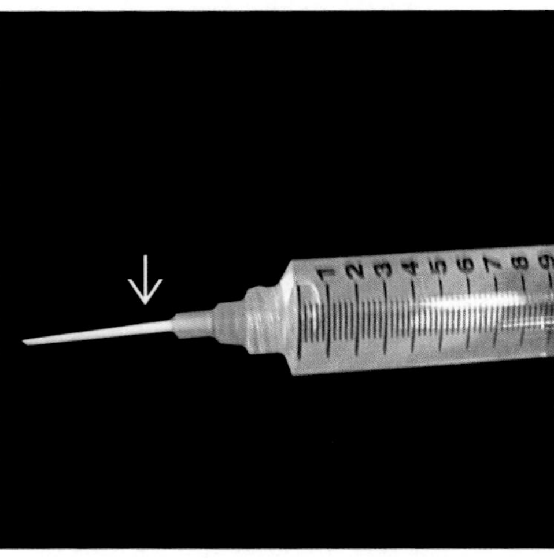

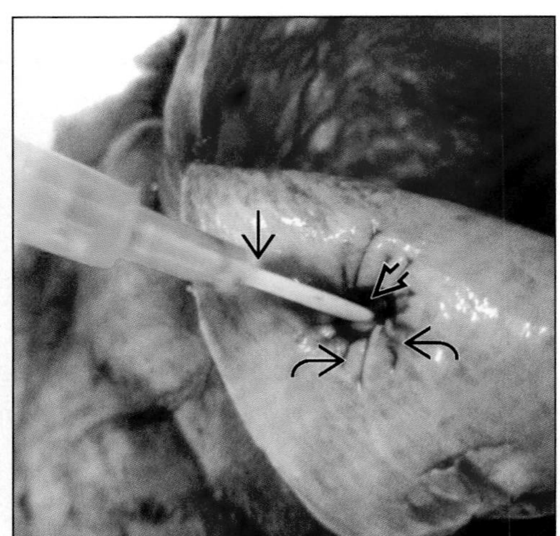

(Left) *This syringe has been filled with contrast media. An intravenous catheter attached to a syringe is a convenient way to inject contrast media into venous and arterial coronary artery bypass grafts.* ***(Right)*** *Here the intravenous catheter is inserted into the saphenous vein graft ostium. Sutures are radially oriented around the saphenous vein graft ostium.*

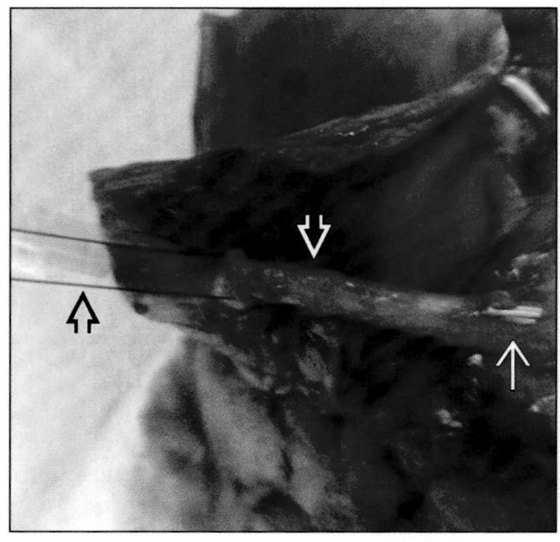

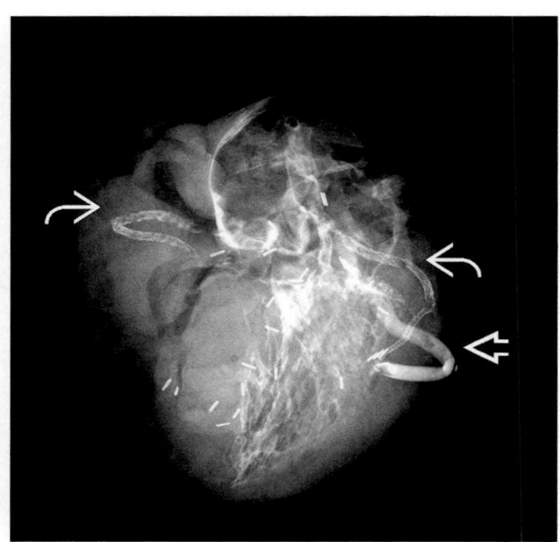

(Left) *A suture (if available) or string tied around the proximal graft and secured after injection of approximately 10 cc of contrast media prevents backflow of fluid. Metal clips along the saphenous vein graft are used intraoperatively to tie off tributary vessels.* ***(Right)*** *This postmortem heart x-ray with contrast reveals the saphenous vein graft to the left anterior descending coronary artery and multiple stents in the the left anterior descending and the right coronary artery.*

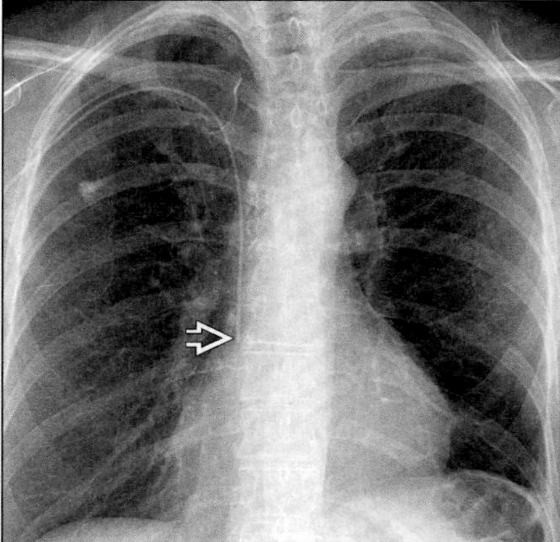

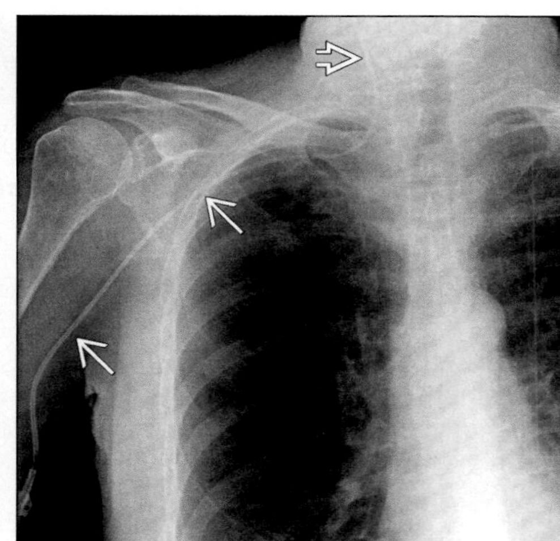

(Left) *This radiograph shows a normal peripherally inserted central catheter (PICC) line ending at cavoatrial junction. Radiography is the best way to document PICC position at autopsy especially if there is concern regarding placement.(From DI: Chest.)* ***(Right)*** *This radiograph demonstrates a malpositioned PICC line going into internal jugular vein instead of SVC. (From DI: Procedures.)*

Radiographic Examination of Iatrogenically Inserted Devices

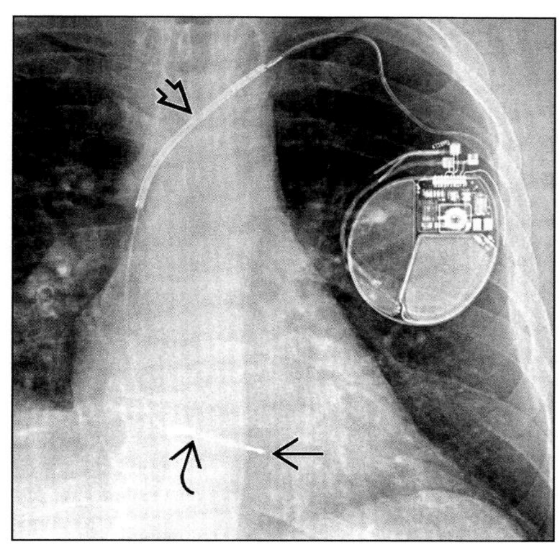

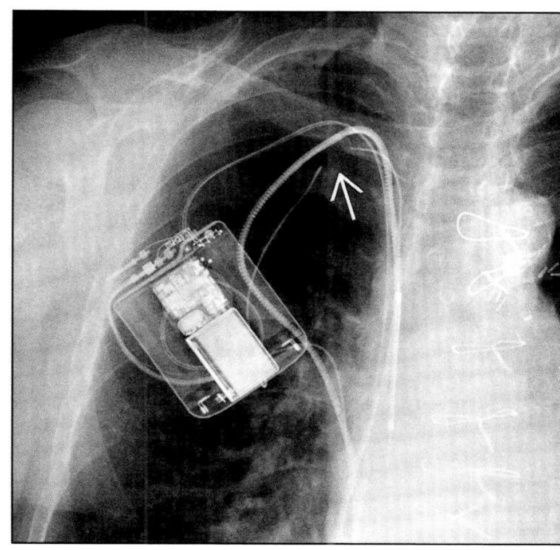

(Left) *Radiograph of the chest shows the typical location of a defibrillator lead terminating in the right ventricle. The defibrillator electrodes are typically in the superior vena cava ⇨ and the right ventricle ↗, with the sensing electrode at the tip →. (From DI: Cardiac.)* ***(Right)*** *This radiograph demonstrates a fractured pacer wire ➡. This diagnosis would be difficult to make at postmortem without x-ray analysis. (From DI: Cardiac.)*

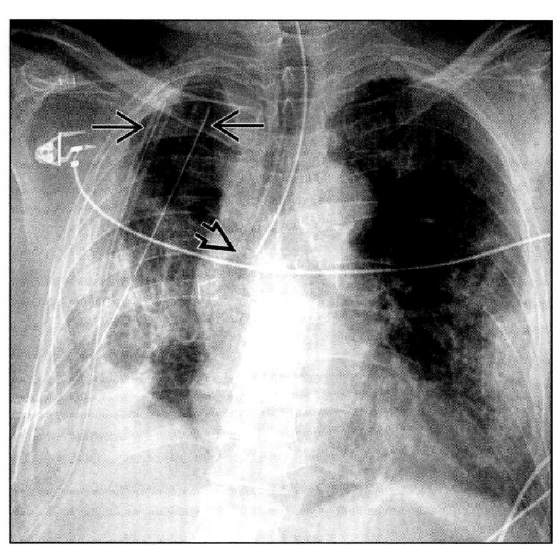

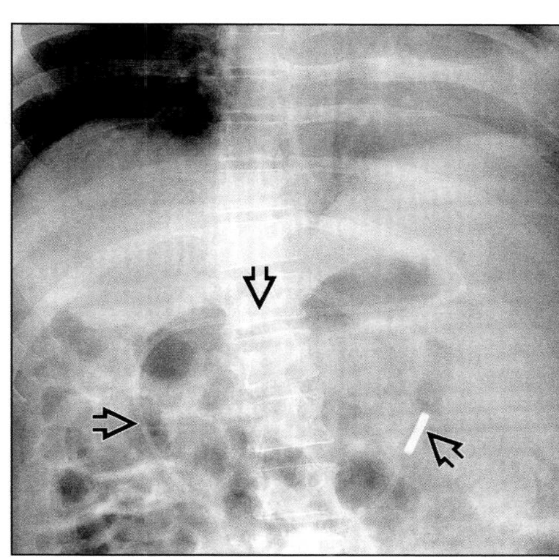

(Left) *When there is a question about placement of the endotracheal tube (ETT), postmortem x-ray can be very helpful. This radiograph shows an abnormally positioned ETT with the tip in the right mainstem bronchus ⇨. Two chest tubes are also in place → (From DI: Chest.)* ***(Right)*** *Radiograph of the upper abdomen shows a normally positioned feeding tube ⇨. (From DI: Chest.)*

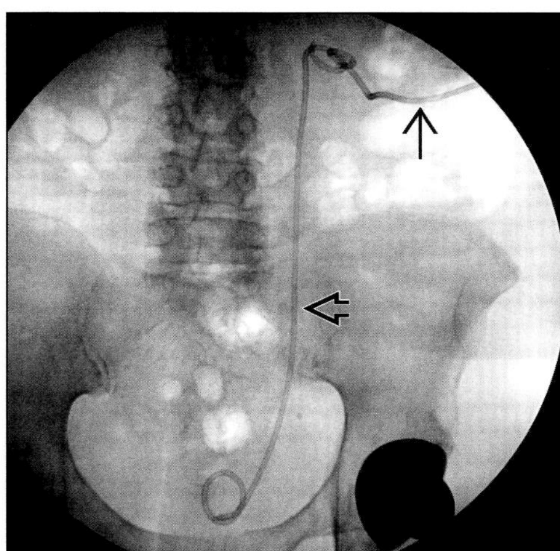

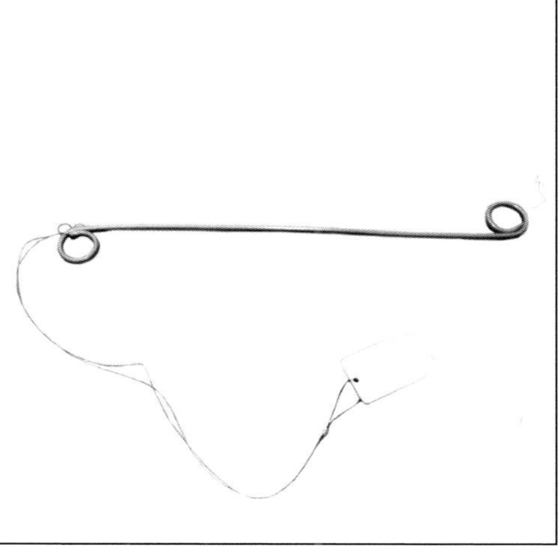

(Left) *This abdominal radiograph demonstrates a double J ureteral stent ⇨ and a percutaneous nephrostomy tube →. Postmortem radiographic imaging of these devices is usually not necessary unless there is a concern regarding placement. (From DI: Procedures.)* ***(Right)*** *Photograph of a double J ureteral stent. One end of the J should be in the renal pelvis and the other within the bladder.*

Radiographic Analysis of Stents and Foreign Material

(Left) This abdominal radiograph demonstrates a stent ➡ in the sigmoid colon. Stenting may be done for obstruction related to malignancy or radiation therapy. (From DI: Procedures.) ***(Right)*** Radiograph of the upper abdomen shows 2 overlapping stents ➡ in the 2nd and 3rd portions of the duodenum. (From DI: Procedures.)

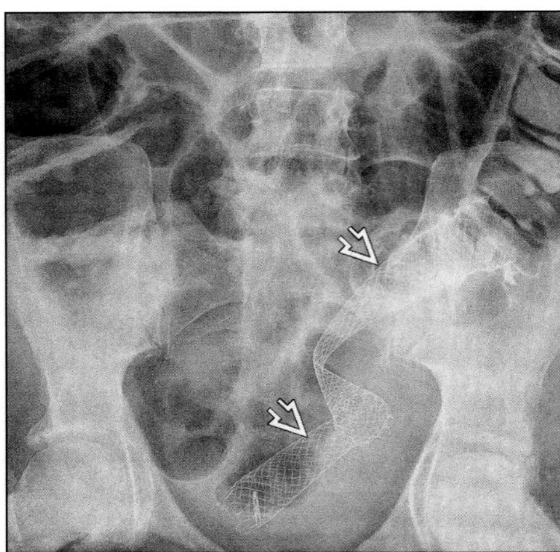

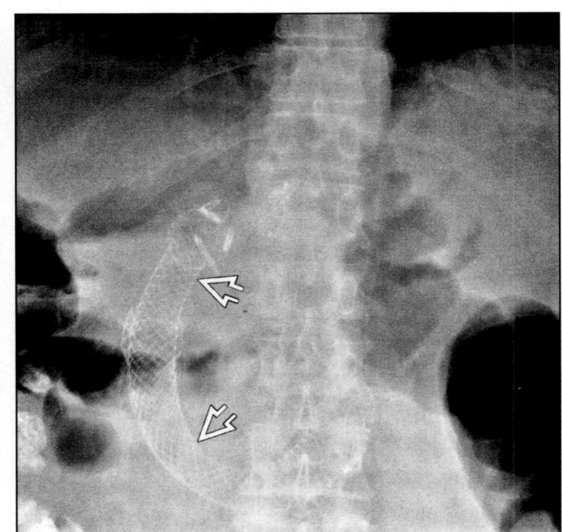

(Left) A 64-year-old man with metastatic gallbladder cancer shows multiple findings including 2 biliary stents ➡, a stent across ileocolic anastomosis ➡, and a feeding tube ➡. (From DI: Procedures.) ***(Right)*** Abdominal radiograph in a 47-year-old woman with metastatic gastric cancer producing extrinsic compression and obstruction of the colon is shown. Two overlapping colorectal stents ➡ are seen. (From DI: Procedures.)

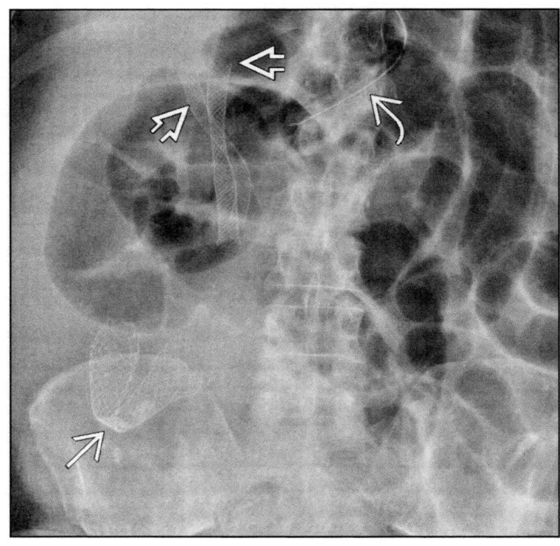

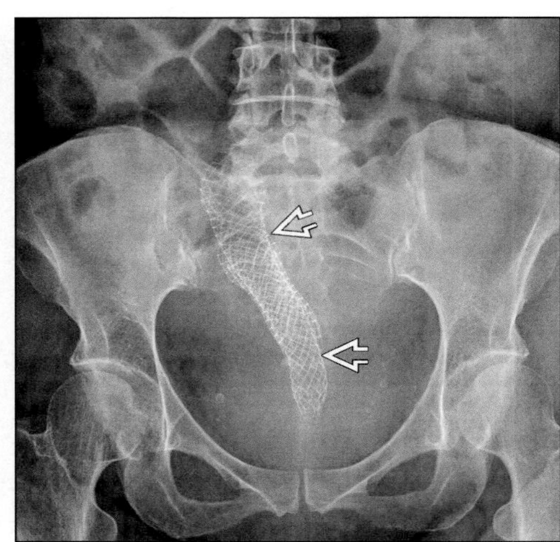

(Left) This is an example of a metallic stent. These are radiographically visible and the periodicity of the struts ➡ identifies stents from different manufacturers. ***(Right)*** CT shows a pencil pushed through the orbit into the brain. The inner lead ➡ is dense while the outer wood casing ➡ is lucent. Radiography, especially CT, is very helpful for locating lines, medical devices, and foreign bodies. (From DI: H&N.)

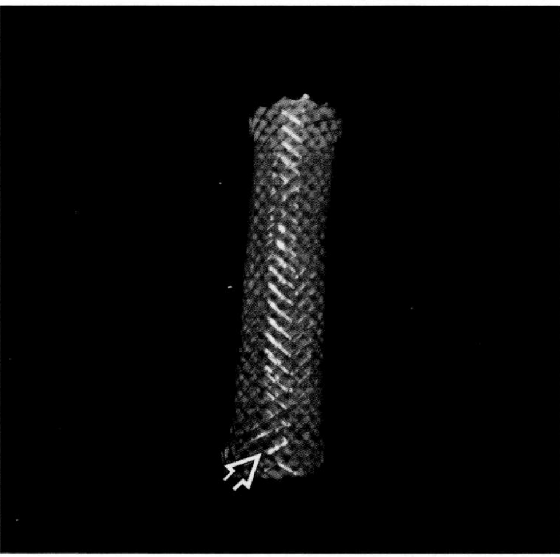

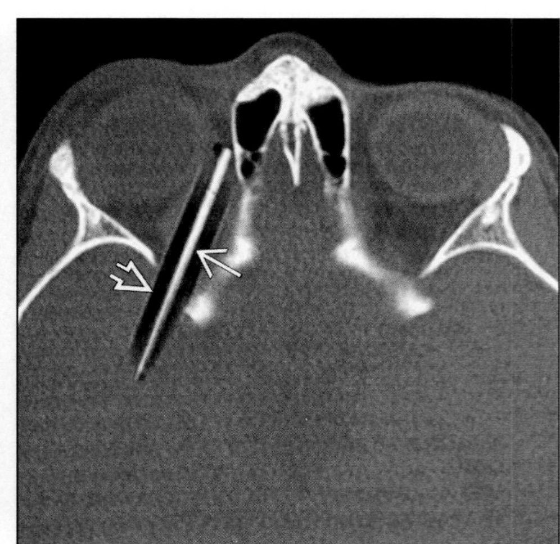

Virtual Autopsy-Type Imaging

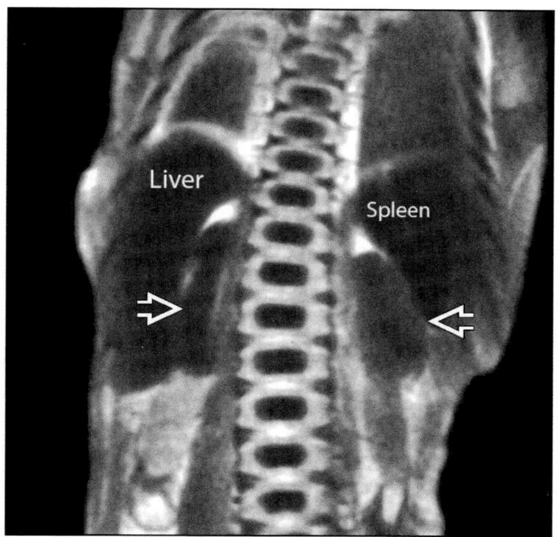

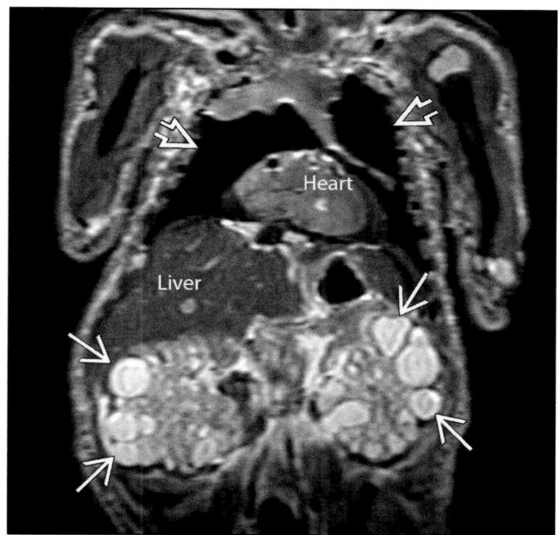

(Left) *This newborn died of respiratory distress. The parents declined autopsy but consented to MR examination (virtual autopsy). There is bilateral renal agenesis with flattened adrenal glands ➨ but no kidneys.* ***(Right)*** *Another MR virtual autopsy shows enlarged kidneys filled with cysts of varying sizes ➨ (multicystic dysplastic kidneys) and bilateral pneumothoraces ➨. MR or CT virtual autopsy can provide a reasonable alternative for internal exam when autopsy is refused.*

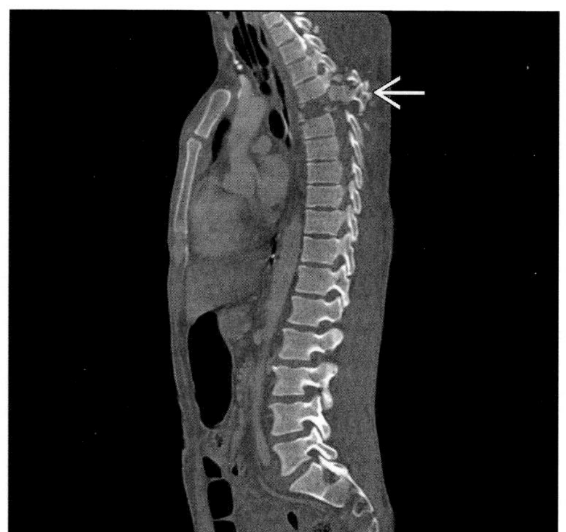

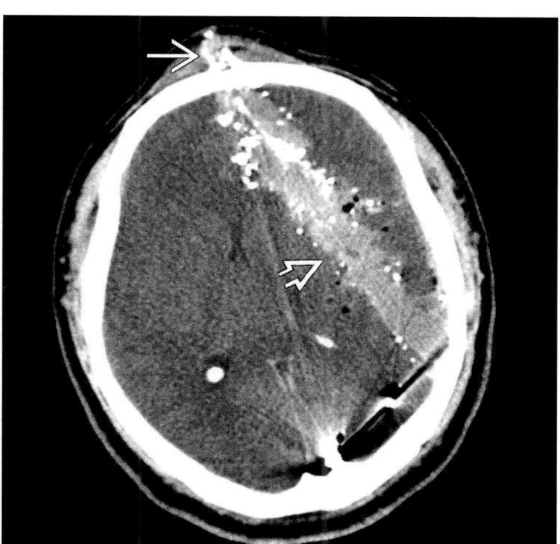

(Left) *CT images can be reconstructed in any plane to display the area of interest. This sagittal reconstruction of the spine shows a severely comminuted burst fracture of T5 ➨, which severed the cord. This type of imaging used in virtual autopsy is much better than traditional autopsy for documenting injury.* ***(Right)*** *CT of a gunshot wound shows the frontal entry site ➨ and the wide oblique hemorrhagic tract ➨ that extends to the left temporoparietal region. (From DI: Brain, 2e.)*

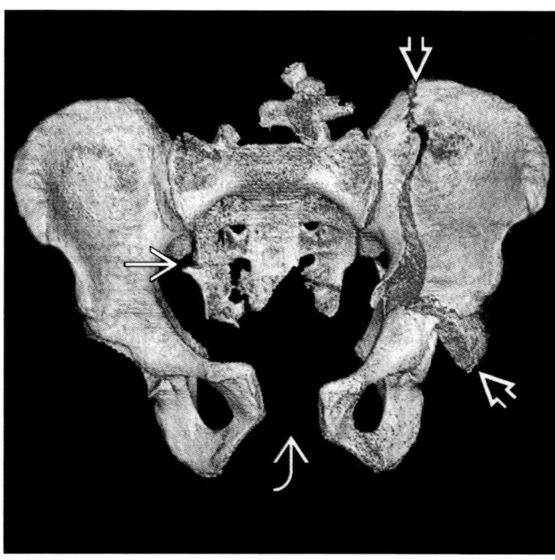

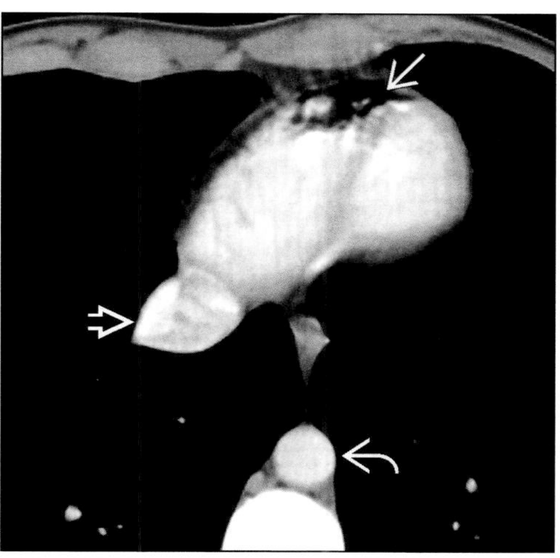

(Left) *CT data can also be used to reconstruct a 3D image as seen in this complex pelvic fracture. There are displaced fractures of the left iliac wing ➨ and sacrum ➨, with wide separation of the pubic symphysis ➨. (From DI: MSK Trauma.)* ***(Right)*** *Axial CT through the heart shows air ➨ in the right ventricle. Air is often better seen on CT than at autopsy (inferior vena cave ➨, aorta ➨). (From DI: Chest.)*

SECTION 3

Autopsy Consent and Reporting

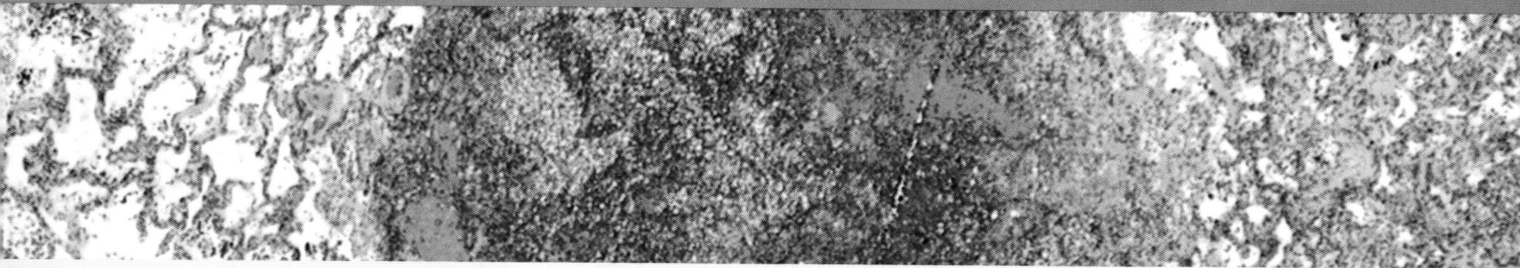

Autopsy Consent

Autopsy Reporting

CONSENT PROCESS AND LEGAL CONSIDERATIONS

AUTHORIZATION

Requesting Autopsy

- Attending physicians &/or housestaff caring for patient prior to death
  - Advantages
    - Established rapport with family members
    - 1st-hand knowledge of hospital course
  - Disadvantages
    - Implied admission of failure/fault
    - Rapport with family may also make approaching more difficult
- Decedent affairs or after-death services team
  - Advantages
    - Depth of knowledge
      - Logistics of hospital procedures
      - Legal issues
      - Commonly asked questions about autopsy
      - Funeral arrangements
      - Grief/bereavement counseling, pastoral care
    - Communication/liaison between family and hospital/pathology department
    - Coordination of multiple departments, agencies
  - Disadvantages
    - No prior relationship with family
    - Lacking medical fund of knowledge
- Pathologists, autopsy personnel
  - Advantages
    - Close communication regarding family concerns
    - Accurate expectations about potential autopsy benefits and limits
  - Disadvantages
    - Appearance of self-interest, promotion of department services
    - Affiliation with hospital (obligation to cover-up errors)
- Family members may be 1st to request autopsy

Authorizing Autopsy

- Legal next of kin
  - Definitions vary slightly by state and local statute
  - Typically in following order
    - Spouse
    - Adult daughter or son
    - Parent
    - Adult brother or sister
    - Grandparent
    - Other relative (cousin, aunt, nephew, etc.)
    - Friend or person responsible for burial, other affairs
- Decedent permission
  - Provisions vary by state and local statute
  - Patient may elect in advance to autopsy after their natural death
    - Such as part of a registry for rare diseases or donating to science
  - Spouse copermission often also required, reaffirmed at time of death
  - Objections from other next of kin should be taken seriously
    - Consider consultation with hospital ethics board or risk management

LIMITATIONS

Restricting Autopsy Extent

- Other than complete/full (chest, abdomen, brain, and spinal cord)
- Exclusion of brain (chest and abdomen only)
- Limited to 1 organ (liver only, heart only, etc.)
- Limited to 1 body cavity (chest only, brain only, etc.)

Special Requests

- Return all organs after microscopy samples taken
  - This significantly limits quality of brain examination especially
- Reflex clauses: Brain examined only if no cause of death found in chest and abdomen

Permission for Special Procedures

- Any potentially disfiguring procedures (that would preclude usual open casket viewing) should be specifically consented
  - Incisions on face, neck, or hands
  - Removal of bones, including spinal column
  - Removal of eyes
    - Permission may be obtained separately by eye bank or donation services
- May obtain special permission for DNA extraction and genetic testing

ORGAN AND TISSUE RETENTION

Communication and Documentation

- Family members may not be aware of long-term retention of entire organs (brain, heart, etc.)
- Permission should be expressly documented and discussed as part of consent process
- Nature of different tissue specimens may be delineated
  - Entire organs
  - Small "wet" samples (e.g., "stock jar")
  - Paraffin blocks, slides

DISPOSITION OF REMAINS

Suggestions

- Disposal after sufficient time has passed (to be determined at pathologists discretion)
- Documented provisions in consent for manner of disposal
  - Incineration/cremation
  - Tissue digester
  - Medical waste
- Exceptionally, families may request
  - Burial of tissues with body
  - Separate cremation of organs and return of ashes to family

COORDINATION WITH FUNERAL HOMES

Embalming

- Autopsy pathologists/technicians facilitate identification of major arteries after autopsy
- Autopsy examination of carotid arteries, leg vessels delayed until after embalming
- Autopsy after embalming
  - Awareness of trocar insertion sites

Cosmetic Considerations

- Ideally avoid incisions in face and neck, but for mishaps, communicate with funeral home so they can give attention to these
- Posterior placement of cranial incision for brain removal, notching skull cap to prevent rotation
  - Aids funeral directors in reconstructing for viewing
- Sewing Y incision
  - Often removed and resewn by funeral directors for embalming, "grain" placement, etc.

HUMAN TISSUE ACT OF 1961 (UNITED KINGDOM)

Purpose

- "With respect to the use of body parts of deceased persons for the therapeutic purposes and purposes of medical education and research"
- Federal statute governing postmortem examinations

Section 2(2)

- Hospital autopsy section
  - Necessity of consent (since not ordered by medical examiner/coroner)
  - Autopsies performed by "fully registered medical practitioner"
- Subsection 1
  - Relates to removal of organs at autopsy
  - Allows for decedents objections to be in force

Section 1(6)

- Limits authority of funeral directors
  - i.e., they may only do what next of kin indicates

Section 1(7)

- Relates to hospitals, nursing homes, care facilities

AUTOPSY CONSENT DOCUMENTS

Development/Revision

- Must reflect state and local statutes
- Recommendations
  - Clear choices for complete/full autopsy and autopsy with limitations (explicitly delineated)
  - Permission for autopsy pathologist to allow others to attend autopsy as appropriate
  - Permission for retention and eventual disposal of organs and tissues at discretion of autopsy pathologists
    - When necessary for diagnosis
    - For teaching, authoring, and other educational activities
    - For research activities
  - Documentation that person authorizing was given opportunity to have questions and concerns addressed adequately
  - Name, relationship to deceased, and contact information of person authorizing autopsy
  - Signature of person authorizing, witness, and person obtaining consent for autopsy

RISK MITIGATION

Suggestions

- Ensure appropriate notification of medical examiner/coroner in cases of potential medicolegal interest
- Practices in place and adopted for confirming patient identify prior to autopsy
- Review authorization documentation for completeness, any restrictions, and appropriate signatures (by legally authorized next of kin)
- Provide contact information to family and request it from them
  - Provide periodic updates until final report issued

SELECTED REFERENCES

1. van Diest PJ: No consent should be needed for using leftover body material for scientific purposes. For. BMJ. 325(7365):648-51, 2002
2. Bierig JR: Informed consent in the practice of pathology. Arch Pathol Lab Med. 125(11):1425-9, 2001
3. Nelkin D et al: Do the dead have interests? Policy issues for research after life. Am J Law Med. 24(2-3):261-91, 1998
4. Svendsen E et al: Autopsy legislation and practice in various countries. Arch Pathol Lab Med. 111(9):846-50, 1987
5. Human Tissues Act 1961. HMSO, London. 1961

DEATH CERTIFICATE

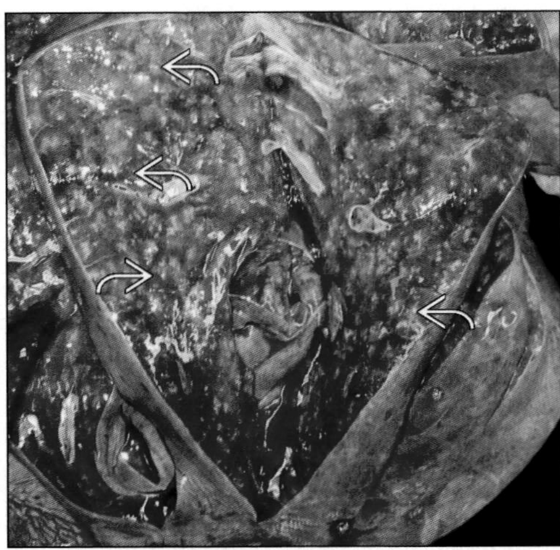

This patient had pneumonia evidenced by small yellow nodules ➡ diffusely throughout the lung. The immediate cause of death was cerebral hemorrhage; pneumonia was only a contributory cause. (Courtesy J. Hon, MD.)

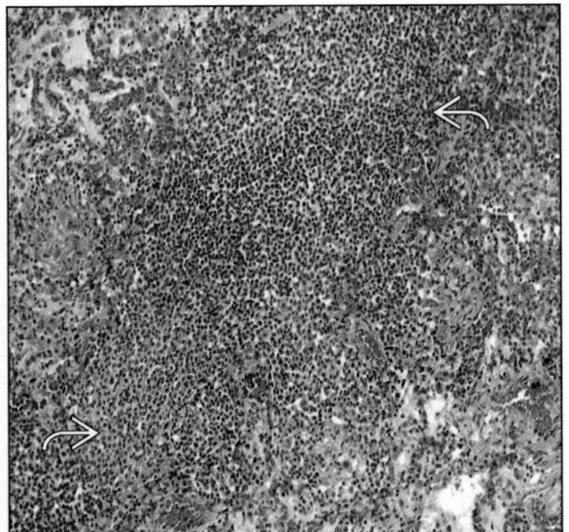

Histologically, pneumonia shows collections of leukocytes and fibrin within the alveoli ➡. This case was due to aspiration, which is common in the altered neurologic status seen in cerebral hemorrhage.

TERMINOLOGY

Definitions

- Death certificate (DC): Legal document recording fact of death, signed by physician who certifies manner and immediate and underlying cause of death and factors contributing to death
- States are responsible for registration of death and have their own DC; most follow outline proposed by federal government
- Physicians are responsible for medical portion of DC

PHYSICIAN RESPONSIBILITY

Pronouncement

- Date and time pronounced dead; actual or presumed date and time of death
  - Pronouncing physician pronounces death and completes pronouncement portion of DC
  - Medical examiner referral: Was medical examiner or coroner contacted? Y/N

Cause of Death

- Completed by certifying physician (usually same as pronouncing physician) but possibly pathologist or medical examiner who performed autopsy
  - Part I: Describes chain of events leading to death stating immediate and underlying cause of death as well as approximate duration in relation to death
  - Part II: Other significant conditions that contributed to death but did not result in underlying cause of death
  - Autopsy: Was autopsy performed? Y/N
  - Were autopsy findings available to complete cause of death? Y/N
- Immediate cause of death
  - Proximate (most recent) disease causing death
    - Should be specific with stated etiology: Cardiac arrest is unacceptable; acute myocardial infarction is acceptable
    - If organ system failure is reported as immediate cause of death, etiology must be reported on underlying cause of death
    - If neoplasm is reported as immediate cause of death, primary site (or unknown), tumor type, and metastatic disease should be reported
  - Timing of onset of cause of death
    - Approximate duration of immediate and underlying cause of death, usually based on clinical data
    - e.g., immediate cause acute myocardial infarction (3 days) due to coronary artery thrombosis (3-4 days), due to coronary artery atherosclerosis, years
- Underlying cause of death
  - Disease or pathophysiologic alteration that started chain of events that lead to death
    - If acute myocardial infarction immediate cause, underlying cause most commonly coronary artery atherosclerosis
    - May have more than one underlying cause of death: Acute myocardial infarction due to coronary artery atherosclerosis due to hypertension due to diabetes mellitus
- Other significant factors: Important factors that contributed to death but did not directly lead to underlying cause of death
  - e.g., bronchopneumonia in patient who died due to acute myocardial infarction

Manner of Death

- How death occurred: Natural or external (non-natural) causes (e.g., natural, homicide, accident, suicide, pending further investigation, and could not be determined)

- Physicians and non-forensic pathologists limited to certifying natural deaths; if manner questionable, consult medical examiner or coroner
- Medical examiner will either accept case and certify death ± autopsy or release case
- If medical examiner releases case but autopsy pathologist questions manner, refer again to medical examiner or coroner
- If injury (however remote) started chain of events leading to death, manner is external (nonnatural) (e.g., pneumonia in patient made paraplegic from homicide attempt months prior)

Other Questions

- Tobacco: Did tobacco contribute to death? Y/N, probably, or unknown
- If female: Was decedent pregnant within past year? Y/N

Amending Death Certificate to Revise Cause of Death

- If autopsy findings significantly change cause of death as listed on DC, certifying physician must report revised cause of death to appropriate state agency (usually vital records or local registrar)

DEATH CERTIFICATE DATA

State

- States are responsible for registering deaths and recording data
  - Under agreement with federal government, states share data to produce national vital statistics (National Vital Statistics System)

National

- Average life expectancy for USA population: 78.8 years (Center for Disease Control [CDC] 2013 Statistics)
- Age-adjusted death rate is 731.9/100,000 standard population (CDC 2013 Statistics)
- Mortality statistics are used to direct research funding

Leading Causes of Death (CDC 2013 Statistics)

- Heart disease, cancer, chronic lower respiratory tract disease, unintentional injury, stroke, Alzheimer disease, diabetes mellitus, influenza, pneumonia, kidney disease, suicide
  - Death rates decreased for heart disease, cancer, stroke, and Alzheimer disease and increased for influenza and pneumonia

UNCLEAR DEATH CERTIFICATION

Commonly Encountered Unclear Death Certifications

- Multisystem organ failure: No etiology specified
  - Better to state underlying etiology of multiorgan system failure, e.g., septic shock secondary to disseminated aspergillosis due to immunosuppression due to renal transplantation
- Cardiac arrest: Unacceptably vague
  - Better to state etiology of cardiac arrest, e.g., congestive heart failure secondary to chronic ischemic heart disease secondary to coronary artery atherosclerosis
- Respiratory arrest: Unacceptably vague
  - Better to state etiology of respiratory arrest, e.g., severe acute necrotizing bronchopneumonia due to *Streptococcus pneumonia* infection

REPORTING CRITERIA

Minimum Requirements

- Autopsy final reports must contain either direct statement as to immediate and underlying cause of death or enough information so that primary clinician can determine immediate and underlying cause of death
- If autopsy findings as to immediate and underlying cause of death are significantly different from what is listed on death certificate, this needs to be reported to certifying physician so that death certificate can be amended
  - This situation also likely indicates clinically unsuspected diagnosis, which alerts pathologist to report this according to institutional quality assurance procedure
  - Autopsy pathologist should be aware of how death was certified if certification was performed prior to autopsy or without use of available autopsy data
  - Even with modern imaging and diagnostic techniques, major discrepancies are still noted between certified causes of death and cause of death determined by autopsy

SELECTED REFERENCES

1. Hinchliffe SR et al: The impact of under and over-recording of cancer on death certificates in a competing risks analysis: a simulation study. Cancer Epidemiol. 37(1):11-9, 2013
2. Porter S et al: Death certification: a practical guide. Br J Hosp Med (Lond). 74(6):C82-5, 2013
3. Roulson J et al: Discrepancies between clinical and autopsy diagnosis and the value of post mortem histology; a meta-analysis and review. Histopathology. 47(6):551-9, 2005
4. Hanzlick R et al: Cause-of-death statements and certification of natural and unnatural deaths. Northfield: College of American Pathologists, 1997
5. Hetzel AM et al: History and organization of the vital statistics system. National Center for Health Statistics. Hyattsville, Maryland, 1997

Cause of Death Statements

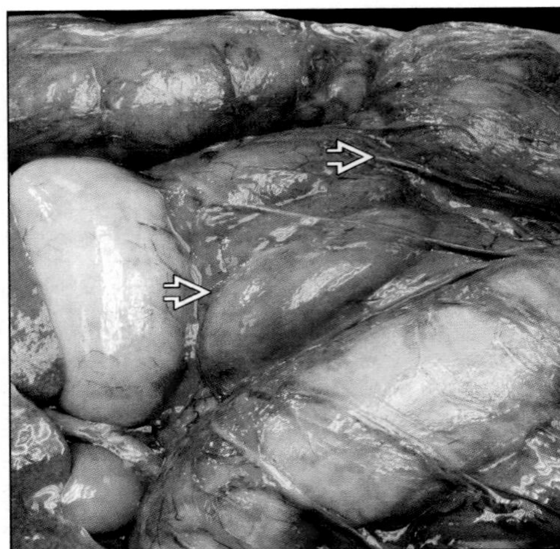

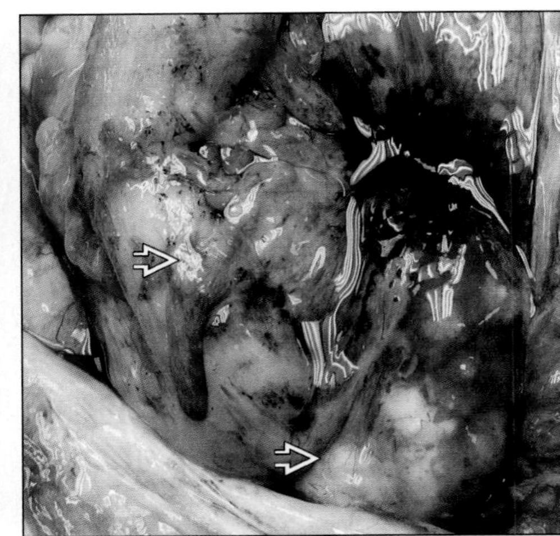

(Left) *This patient expired due to sepsis due to peritonitis ➡ that was due to bowel perforation.* ***(Right)*** *The underlying cause of bowel perforation in this patient was metastatic ovarian cancer ➡. The death certificate could read: Immediate cause of death sepsis (duration hours) due to peritonitis (duration hours) due to colon perforation (duration hours) due to metastatic ovarian carcinoma (duration months).*

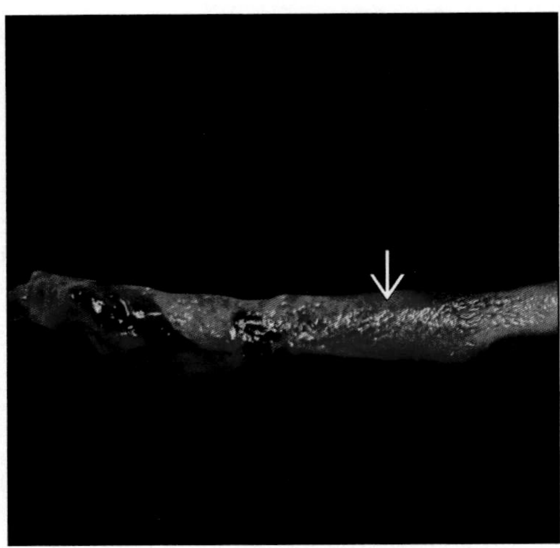

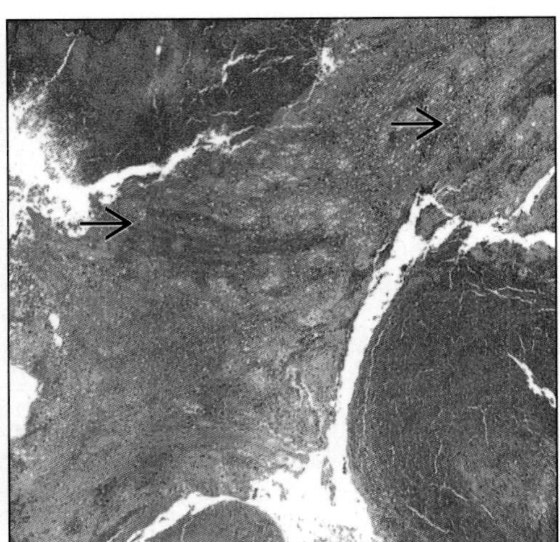

(Left) *This pulmonary thromboembolus was found in a patient who died suddenly. The granular appearance ➡ is due to fibrin. The immediate cause of death is pulmonary thromboembolism.* ***(Right)*** *The microscopic appearance of the thromboembolus highlights fibrin layering ➡. Without known risk factors, the cause of death is pulmonary thromboembolism. Otherwise, pulmonary thromboembolism is due to factors such as factor V Leiden mutation, pancreatic adenocarcinoma, etc.*

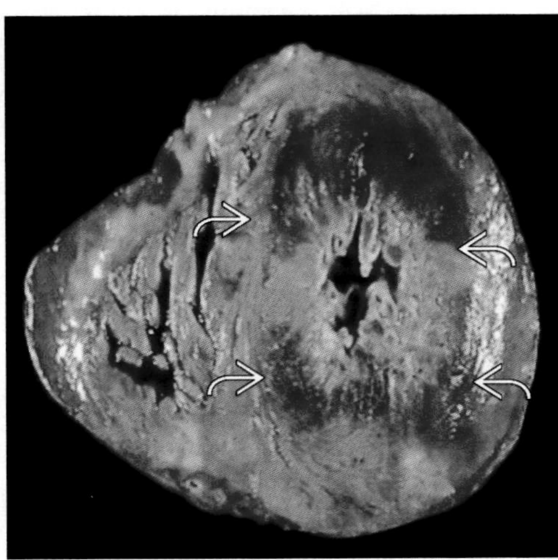

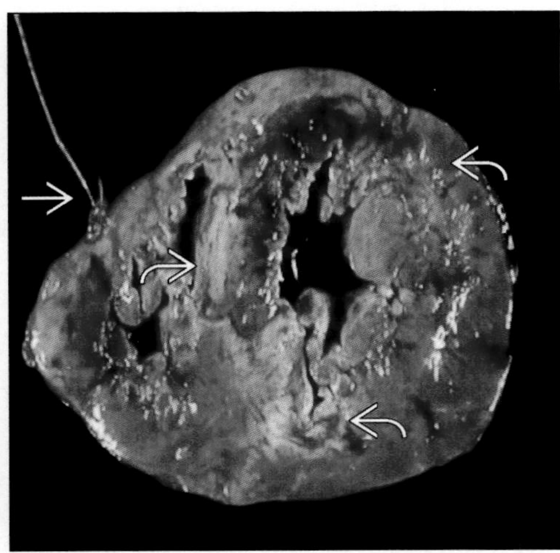

(Left) *This heart is extensively infarcted ➡. The immediate cause of death was cardiogenic shock due to acute myocardial infarction.* ***(Right)*** *This heart also shows extensive infarction ➡. Death was due to ventricular fibrillation. Immediate cause of death was ventricular fibrillation due to acute myocardial infarction. There is an epicardial pacer lead attached to the right ventricle ➡.*

Cause of Death Statements

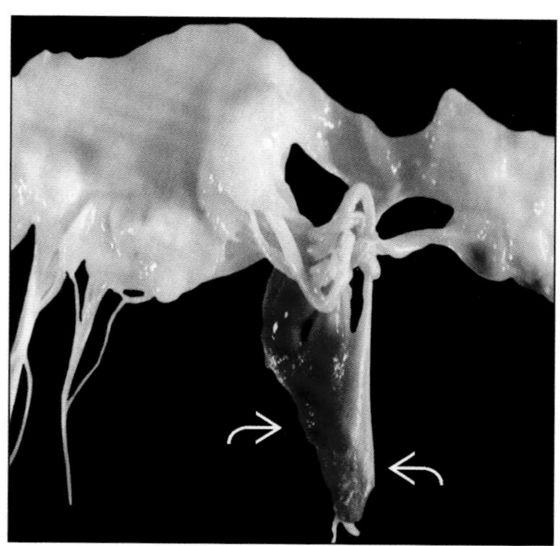

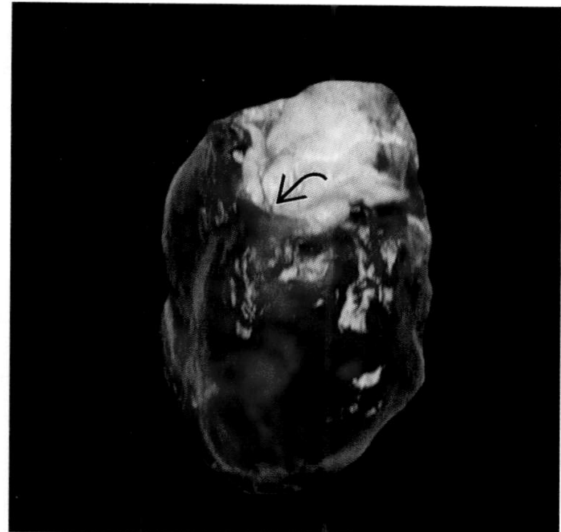

(Left) *Other mechanisms of death with acute myocardial infarction include rupture syndromes. This death was due to acute congestive heart failure due to ruptured papillary muscle ➨ due to acute myocardial infarction.* **(Right)** *This ruptured acute myocardial infarction caused hemopericardium ➨. The immediate cause of death was cardiac tamponade due to hemopericardium due to ruptured acute myocardial infarction.*

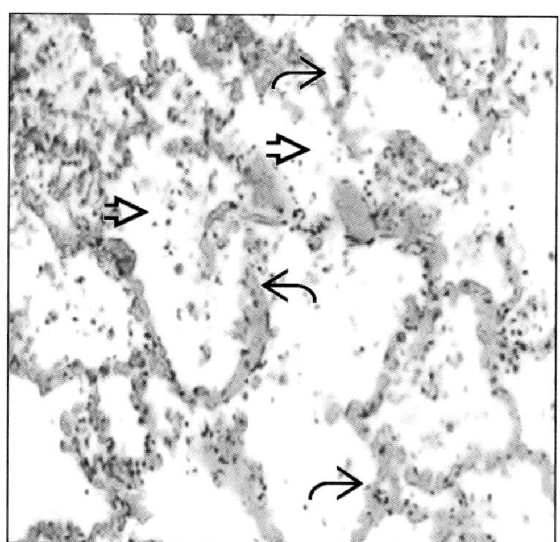

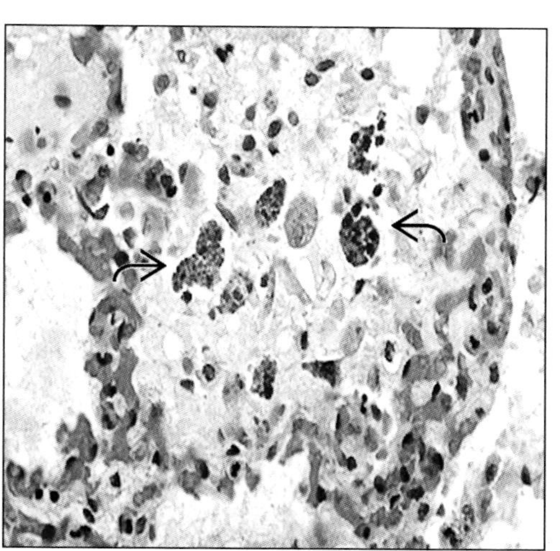

(Left) *This patient had pulmonary edema (pink material in the alveoli ➨), usually associated with congestion of the capillaries ➨. The most common cause of pulmonary edema is congestive heart failure.* **(Right)** *In CHF, hemosiderin-laden macrophages are seen in alveoli ➨ from prior intraalveolar hemorrhage. With lung histology like this, the immediate cause of death is commonly CHF and the underlying cause is the specific cardiac disease identified at autopsy.*

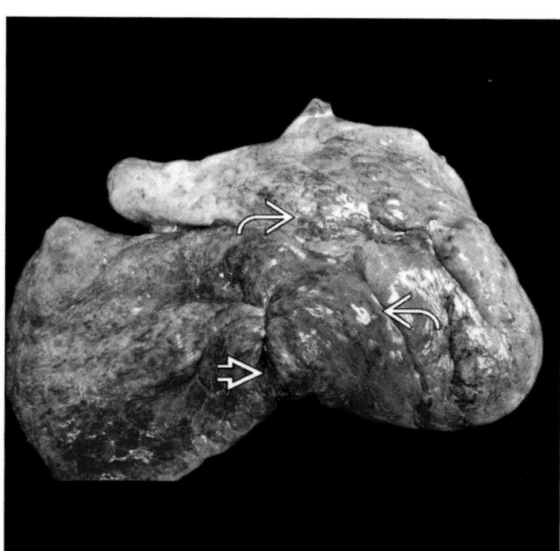

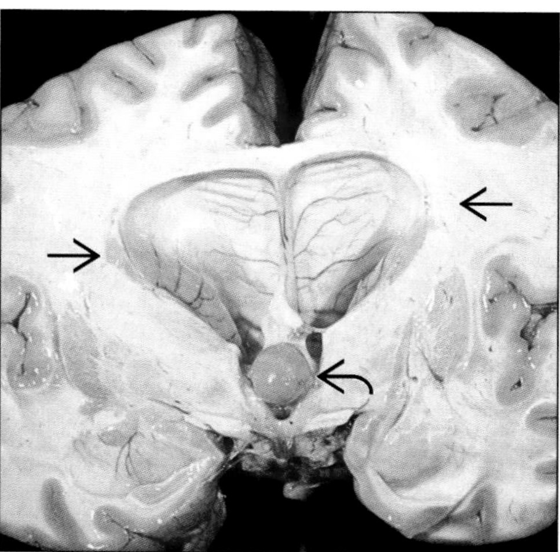

(Left) *This patient died from acute myocardial infarction. Emphysema (blebs ➨) with a small squamous cell cancer (SCC) ➨ were also noted. The lung findings are contributory causes of death. Tobacco was stated to have contributed to death.* **(Right)** *The immediate cause of death in this patient was acute hydrocephalus (dilated ventricles ➨) (days duration) due to colloid cyst ➨ (years duration) obstructing 3rd ventricle (underlying cause). (Courtesy R. Rhodes, PhD, MD.)*

AUTOPSY REPORT

OVERVIEW

Definitions

- Principal record of autopsy procedure, findings, and pathologic interpretations
- Report may be supplemented by photographs and diagrams, but clear and detailed written documentation is still required
- Intended audience
  - Clinical care team (becomes part of patient medical record)
  - Family members, who should be provided a copy
  - Administrators, evaluating quality of practice &/or patient care
  - Attorneys and their expert consultant pathologists (medical-legal document; part of patient medical record)
- Contains both objective findings and subjective interpretations of those findings
  - **Objective**
    - Case history (abstracted from medical records and 1st-hand reports)
    - "Protocol": Narrative of routine procedure and incident observations
    - External exam
    - Gross findings
    - Microscopic findings
    - Ancillary testing results
  - **Subjective**
    - Diagnostic summary
    - Additional comments
    - Clinical pathologic correlation
- Suggested structure and components below serve as a guideline
  - Institutions and pathologists can adapt report format as needed and appropriate

Turnaround Time Benchmarks

- Benchmarks from College of Americal Pathologists Laboratory Accreditation Program standards
- Provisional autopsy report: Within 2 working days of autopsy date
- Final report: 60 working days from autopsy date
  - 90% of reports should meet this benchmark
  - More complex cases may take longer (neuropathology and toxicology studies, etc.), but reason for delay should be documented

FINAL AUTOPSY REPORT

Components

- **Demographic information**
  - Name, birth date, medical record number
  - Date of death, place of death, date of autopsy
  - Pathology accession number, pathologist name, list of those present during autopsy
  - Ordering or requesting clinician contact information
  - Nature, location of identifying information on body
  - Name and relationship of person providing autopsy consent
  - Any limitations to extent of autopsy or other special considerations
  - Specific questions, concerns to be addressed (optional)
- **Clinical summary**
  - Written in past tense
  - Past medical history (brief)
    - Prior surgeries
    - Social history (substance use, occupational exposures, etc.)
    - Pertinent family history
  - Recent clinical course
    - Presentation
    - Imaging, laboratory studies
    - Description of procedures, complications
    - Events preceding death
  - Referencing sources of clinical data is recommended (especially if outside or handwritten records)
  - Summarizing prior pathology specimens (biopsies, surgical) in separate section helpful (optional)
    - Include information on specimens obtained and reviewed at outside institutions, if possible
  - Gross findings: External examination
    - Body length and weight
    - Livor, rigor, preservation, embalming
    - General description: Edema, jaundice, etc.
    - Identifying features: Scars, tattoos, etc.
    - Otherwise similar to physical exam
  - Gross findings: Internal examination
    - Templates often used as a guide and for documentation
    - Descriptions should provide objective information, not diagnoses
    - Medical interventions carefully documented (tube placements, anastomotic sites, etc.)
    - Group by organ system or anatomic compartment
    - Include organ weights and measurements
    - Organ system example
      - Central nervous system
      - Head and neck
      - Body cavities, including serosal surfaces and fluid collections
      - Cardiovascular system
      - Respiratory system
      - Hepatobiliary system
      - Gastrointestinal system
      - Lymphoreticular system
      - Urinary system
      - Internal genitalia
      - Endocrine system
      - Musculoskeletal system
    - Anatomic compartment example
      - Cranium
      - Ear, nose, and throat
      - Neck
      - Thoracic
      - Abdominal
      - Retroperitoneal
      - Pelvic
  - Microscopic findings
    - List of all histologic slides obtained, block designations

  - Common formats
    - Slide by slide, in order (A1, A2, etc.)
    - Narrative by organ system (with list of slides in each group)
  - Descriptions should include immunohistochemistry, special stains
- Additional studies
  - Cultures
  - PCR/molecular studies
  - Radiology
  - Chemistry
  - Toxicology
  - If "send-out" test, could include performing institution with contact information and case number
- Tissues preserved for additional studies or sent for approved research studies
  - Type of tissue and details of handling
  - Contact at agency receiving tissue
  - Recommend including this in final report outline for greater accessibility
- Consultants
  - Intra- and extradepartmental pathologic consultation
  - Include nature of review (gross review, specific slides, etc.)
- Final diagnosis (in outline form)
  - Often 1st page of report
  - Subjective interpretation synthesizing gross, microscopic, and ancillary tests
  - May include pertinent antemortem studies, findings supporting the diagnoses
  - Summarize findings in orderly fashion
    - By disease process (mirroring cause of death statement), preferred
    - By organ system, alternative
  - Incidental or miscellaneous findings may be included in separate heading
- Summary comments &/or clinical-pathologic correlation
  - Including a formal cause of death statement or sufficient information to accurately complete official cause of death statement on death certificate
  - At minimum, short comment including the following information
    - Brief statement of clinical situation
    - Brief statement of autopsy findings relevant to clinical questions
    - Explanation of any unanswered questions, limitations of autopsy diagnosis
    - Any recommendations of family screening, follow-up
  - Detailed clinical-pathologic correlations tend to be reserved for academic institutions
  - Complex cases may warrant a literature search with references provided

PROVISIONAL AUTOPSY REPORT

Primary Goal

- Communicate initial findings
- Alert to any concerns for communicable disease, etc.
- Indicate what further studies are pending

Components

- Diagnostic summary
  - Similar to FAR in structure and content
- Comment section
  - Narrative summary of initial findings and remaining questions
- Statement of preliminary nature of report
  - Include contact information for follow-up questions, obtaining final report
  - May include expected timeline for FAR release

SELECTED REFERENCES

1. Finkbeiner WF et al: The autopsy report. Autopsy Pathology: A Manual and Atlas. 2nd ed. Philadelphia: Saunders-Elsevier. 123-9, 2009
2. Adams VI: Guidelines for Reports by Autopsy Pathologists. New York City: Humana Press, 2008
3. Sheaff MT et al: Post Mortem Technique Handbook. 2nd ed. New York City: Springer. 338-49, 2005
4. Hanzlik RL et al: The autopsy lexicon: suggested headings for the autopsy report. In Collins KA et al: Autopsy Performance and Reporting. 2nd ed. Northfield, IL: College of American Pathologists. 275-85, 2003
5. Hutchins GM et al: autopsy reporting. In Collins KA et al: Autopsy Performance and Reporting. 2nd ed. Northfield, IL: College of American Pathologists. 265-74, 2003

PRESENTING AUTOPSY FINDINGS

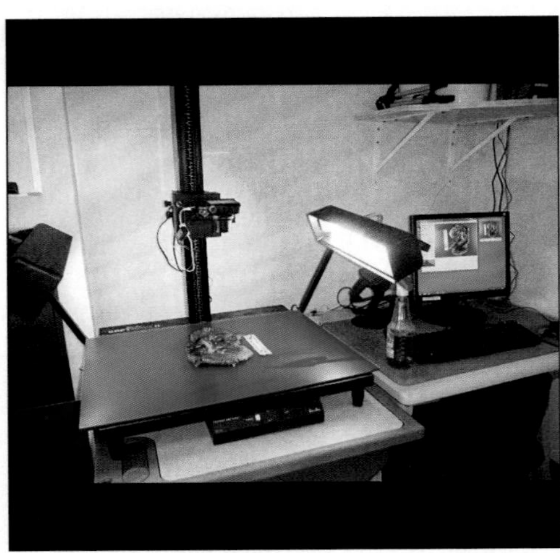

A dedicated photographic stand in the morgue facilitates the acquisition of high-quality images and encourages photographic documentation.

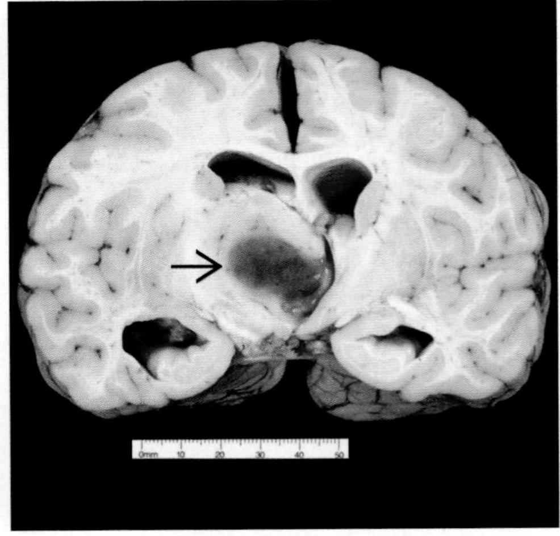

A well-composed autopsy photograph will show the organ and finding of interest ➔ on a clean background that is free of instruments and blood. It is very helpful to include the scale.

DAY OF AUTOPSY

General Comments

- Despite the availability of printed and digital teaching resources, there is no more effective way to correlate clinical findings and demonstrate pathologic changes than a properly performed complete autopsy

Involving Clinical Care Team

- Contact clinician(s) prior to performance of autopsy
  - Can provide valuable clinical information to supplement your chart review
  - Can clarify specific questions that clinicians or family may have
  - Provides opportunity to invite interested clinicians to autopsy
    - Scheduling may be difficult and autopsy and release of body should not be unduly delayed
- Invite interested medical students to view autopsy
- If clinicians cannot attend autopsy, consider contacting them directly afterwards
  - Especially important if autopsy reveals significant unexpected findings

DAY FOLLOWING AUTOPSY

General Comments

- Interest of clinical team is often at its peak immediately following death of patient
  - Use the opportunity to interact with clinical team
- Delays in communicating results or careless presentation of results may discourage future requests for autopsy

Preliminary Anatomic Diagnosis (PAD)

- Complete PAD within 24 hours whenever possible
  - 48 hours if selected sections have been submitted for histology
- **Clinicians often cite delay in autopsy diagnosis as shortcoming of hospital autopsies**
  - Clinical team may have rotated off of service by the time final diagnosis is complete
  - Prompt PAD helps maintain interest
- More complete and comprehensive PADs will have greater impact
  - Consider including frozen sections, cytology, or selected sections for rush histology as part of autopsy

Presentation of Fixed Dissected Organs

- **Be aware of limitations of autopsy permit and of local policy regarding retention of tissue**
  - Family wishes or local regulations may prohibit retention of tissue for teaching purposes
  - **Present organs only if it does not violate family wishes or local regulations**
- Organs can be presented to clinicians or pathologists/pathology residents
  - Consider inviting clinical care team to review organs
    - May be easier to schedule than attendance at actual autopsy
  - Consider using organ presentation as way to teach gross pathology to residents
- Carefully dissected organs should be thoroughly rinsed in cold water
  - If time permits, trim excess fat and extraneous tissues left from day of autopsy
  - Organs should be reasonably free of formalin odor
- Several shallow metal pans should be lined with moistened white paper towels
- Organs should be arranged in way that makes anatomic/clinical sense
  - e.g., thoracic organs on one pan, abdominal organs on a second, genitourinary tract on a third
  - Only a representative section or two of grossly normal liver, spleen should be included

- Only representative segments of grossly normal small and large intestine should be included
- Include demonstrations of all gross abnormalities mentioned in PAD
- Cover organs with moistened paper towels
- Encourage member of clinical team to present brief history
- Uncover organs and present findings
- Presentation of gross organs increasingly rare
  - Largely supplanted by presentation of photographs

AUTOPSY PHOTOGRAPHY

General Comments

- Recording images is important part of documenting significant findings
  - Images will be indispensable if findings are to be presented in conference
- In some cases, images may prove useful as part of future lectures or publications

Equipment

- Ideal: Dedicated photographic stand in morgue with adjustable dual lighting sources and dedicated camera
  - In practice, this may not be practical
- If photographic stand unavailable, any good quality digital camera will suffice

Composing Images

- Rinse away blood and mucus
- Background should be clean and free of extraneous fluids, tools, etc.
- Orient tissue in a way that makes anatomical sense
- Include scale to indicate size when possible
- Take several images
  - Overall (panoramic) image of organ
  - Close up of area of interest
  - Intact organ
  - Cut surface

INTERDEPARTMENTAL CASE CONFERENCE PRESENTATIONS

General Comments

- Presentations at interdepartmental meetings provide opportunity to represent your department and your specialty
- Thank organizers for opportunity to participate
- Show enthusiasm for case
  - Even cases that seem routine can be instructive

Preparation

- Know your role
  - Main presenter or adjunct to main presentation
  - If adjunct, consider submitting your presentation to presenting clinician beforehand
    - Will allow for incorporation of your presentation into larger presentation
    - Obviates time-consuming transitions
- Consult with clinicians beforehand
  - Clarify the history
  - Discuss your findings
  - Get sense of time allotted for your presentation
- Prepare your images
  - Add labels, arrows, or other indicators to highlight key findings

Presentation

- Present gross and then microscopic images
- Know your audience: Often most are not pathologists
  - Adapt your comments
    - Do not simply give diagnosis, explain features that allow for diagnosis
    - e.g., "acute inflammatory infiltrate in airspaces consistent with pneumonia" rather than "shows pneumonia"
  - Be sensitive to relationship care team had with deceased
    - Keep comments professional
    - Avoid accusations, assignments of blame
- Invite discussion and questions

After Presentation

- Remember to document case presentation in autopsy case file

SELECTED REFERENCES

1. Zampieri F et al: The clinico-pathological conference, based upon Giovanni Battista Morgagni's legacy, remains of fundamental importance even in the era of the vanishing autopsy. Virchows Arch. Epub ahead of print, 2015
2. Riley RS et al: Digital photography: a primer for pathologists. J Clin Lab Anal. 18(2):91-128, 2004
3. Belanger AJ et al: Implementation of a practical digital imaging system for routine gross photography in an autopsy environment. Arch Pathol Lab Med. 124(1):160-5, 2000
4. Edwards WD: Photography of medical specimens: experiences from teaching cardiovascular pathology. Mayo Clin Proc. 63(1):42-57, 1988

SECTION 1

Sudden and Unexpected Death

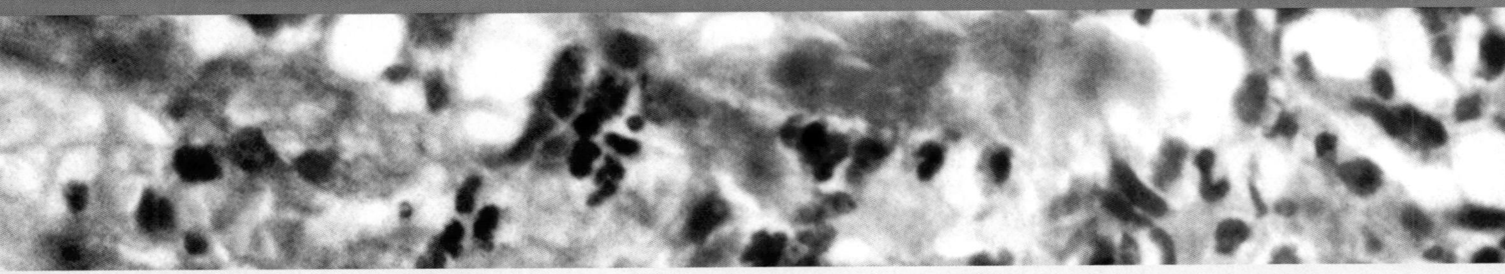

Cardiovascular

Respiratory

Gastrointestinal

Hepatobiliary

Genitourinary

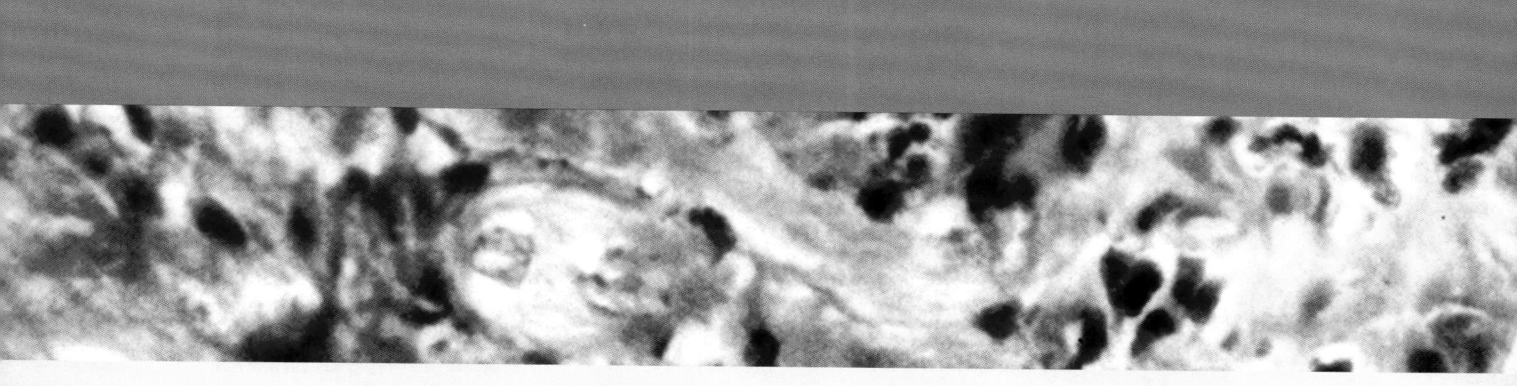

Endocrine

CNS

PULMONARY THROMBOEMBOLISM

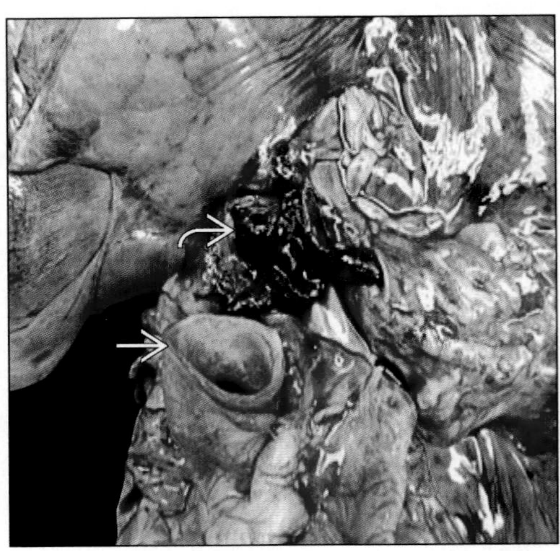

A large, serpiginous, dark red thromboembolus ➔ is present at the bifurcation of the main pulmonary artery (saddle embolus) of this thoracic organ block. Note the cut end of the aorta ➔.

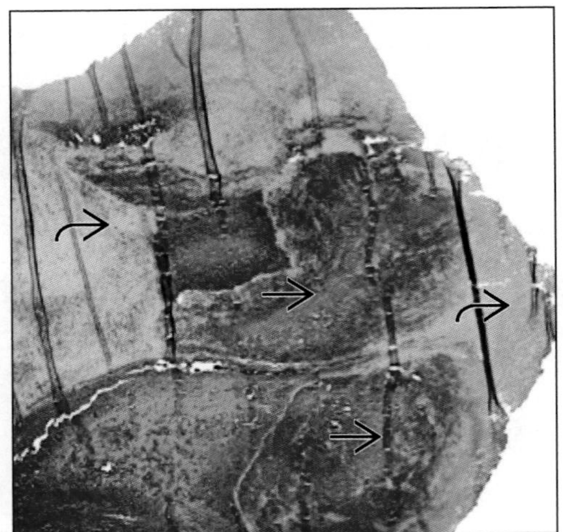

Alternating areas rich in fibrin and platelets ➔ and red blood cells ➔ (lines of Zahn) in a thromboembolus indicate that it arose from a thrombus that formed in flowing blood (i.e., antemortem).

TERMINOLOGY

Abbreviations

- Pulmonary thromboembolism (PTE)

Synonyms

- Venous thromboembolism (VTE)

Definitions

- Embolus: Solid, gaseous, or liquid mass that travels in circulation from its point of origin to distant location (usually an end artery)
  - Thromboembolus: Composed of thrombus material
  - PTE: Thromboemboli in pulmonary arterial circulation, virtually all arising from deep veins of lower extremity

CLINICAL ISSUES

Presentation

- Wells criteria: Clinical risk score for PTE (0-1 = low, 2-6 = intermediate, > 6 = high)
  - Clinical signs/symptoms of PTE (3)
  - PTE/VTE favored clinical diagnosis (3)
  - Heart rate > 100 (1.5)
  - Surgery/immobilization in last 30 days (1.5)
  - Prior VTE (1)
  - Hemoptysis (1)
  - Active or treated malignancy in last 6 months (1)

Laboratory Tests

- D dimer elevation
  - High negative predictive value
  - Nonspecific
  - Postmortem utility not proven

MACROSCOPIC FEATURES

External Examination

- Deep venous thrombosis
  - Swollen red lower extremity
    - Bilateral calf and thigh circumference

Internal Examination

- Often unremarkable or findings related to trauma, recent surgery, underlying malignancy
- After incising iliac veins, lower extremities elevated and "milked"
  - Free-flowing blood from iliacs = no obstruction

Organ Examination

- Cardiovascular system
  - Remove heart and lung block together to avoid disruption of pulmonary thromboembolus
    - Open pulmonary artery along anterior aspect of bifurcation
    - Check for PTE proximally ("saddle") or distally
    - Thromboembolus has shape of vessel of origin, has venous valve markings
  - Right ventricular dilatation, thromboembolus in transit
  - Patent foramen ovale (potential for paradoxical embolization)
  - IVC filter (postmortem radiograph helpful)
- Respiratory system
  - Pulmonary vasculature opened completely to identify PTE (may be multiple)
    - Webs within pulmonary artery indicate organized and recanalized thromboemboli
  - Pulmonary edema may indicate preexistent congestive heart failure, a contributory cause of PTE
- Hepatobiliary system
  - Liver congestion from acute cor pulmonale
- Malignancy: Occult tumor

PULMONARY THROMBOEMBOLISM

Key Facts

Terminology

- Thromboemboli in pulmonary arterial circulation, virtually all arising from deep veins of lower extremity

Macroscopic Pathology

- Signs of deep venous thrombosis include swollen red lower extremity; measure bilateral calf circumference to reveal subtle swelling
- Risk factors: Recent surgery, hip fracture, atrophy of lower extremities suggesting paralysis, trauma
- Remove heart and lung block together to avoid disruption of pulmonary thromboembolus, open pulmonary artery anteriorly
- Check for presence of thromboembolus either proximal within bifurcation (saddle embolus) or distal vasculature
- True thromboembolus has shape of vessel of origin, has venous valve markings on exterior

MICROSCOPIC PATHOLOGY

Histologic Features

- Thromboembolus
  - Recent
    - Red blood cells layered with fibrin and platelets (lines of Zahn)
    - May be subtle, thin, peripheral
  - Organizing
    - Cellular infiltration (macrophages and neovessels)
    - Starting at edges and progressing inward
- Lung
  - Congestion ± edema
  - Infarction: Coagulative necrosis with hemorrhage (red infarct)
- Hepatobiliary
  - Centrilobular congestion ± necrosis
- Malignancy
  - Tumor emboli

DIFFERENTIAL DIAGNOSIS

Postmortem Blood Clot

- "Chicken fat" (yellow gelatinous)
- "Currant jelly" (dark red)
- Random arrangement of coagulated serum and red blood cells
- Not adherent to wall

REPORTING CRITERIA

Presence and Location of Thromboembolus

- Cause of death or contributor?
- Underlying risk factors identified from chart review or postmortem

SELECTED REFERENCES

1. Tadlock MD et al: The origin of fatal pulmonary emboli: a postmortem analysis of 500 deaths from pulmonary embolism in trauma, surgical, and medical patients. Am J Surg. Epub ahead of print, 2014
2. Anderson FA Jr et al: Risk factors for venous thromboembolism. Circulation. 107(23 Suppl 1):I9-16, 2003
3. Wells PS et al: Use of a clinical model for safe management of patients with suspected pulmonary embolism. Ann Intern Med. 129(12):997-1005, 1998
4. Lindblad B et al: Autopsy-verified pulmonary embolism in a surgical department: analysis of the period from 1951 to 1988. Br J Surg. 78(7):849-52, 1991

IMAGE GALLERY

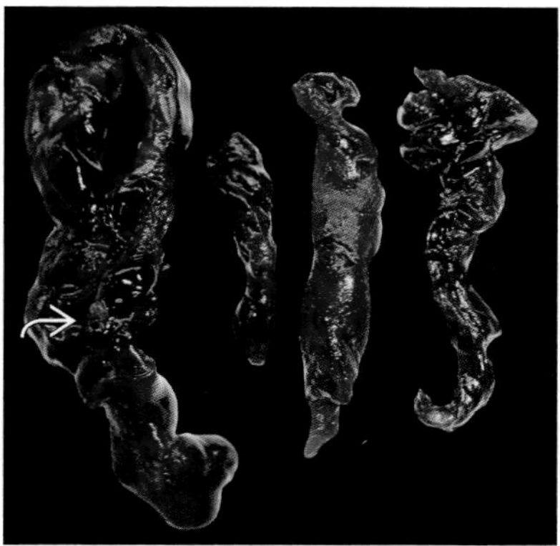

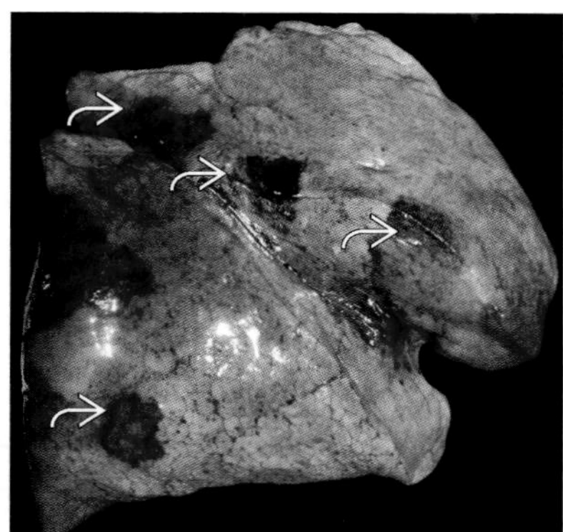

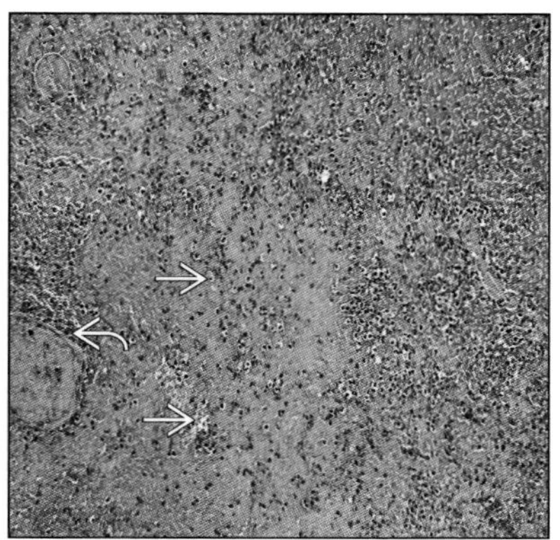

(Left) *These venous thromboemboli were removed from a pulmonary artery at autopsy. Their shape is a cast of the vein in which they formed. They are often coiled* ➢. ***(Center)*** *This lung contains multiple wedge-shaped hemorrhagic pulmonary infarcts* ➢. *The wedge base is located at the pleura. Lower lobe infarcts are most common.* ***(Right)*** *Pulmonary infarcts are hemorrhagic and show coagulative necrosis of the alveolar septa* ➡ *and vessels* ➢.

ACUTE MYOCARDIAL INFARCTION

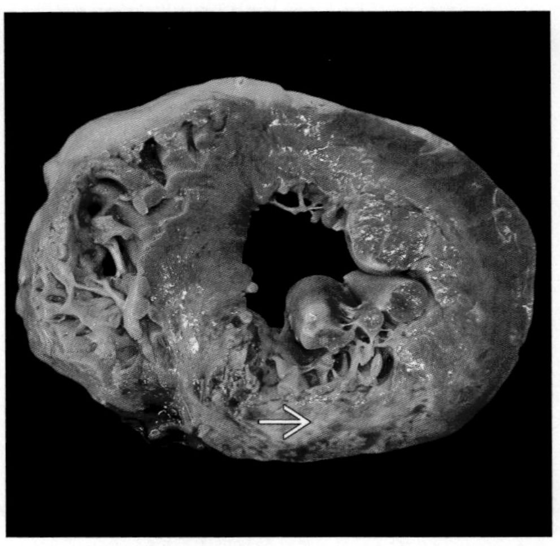

Recent transmural posterior/inferior wall myocardial infarction → is seen in this gross photograph with a marbled tan-red appearance and gross softening.

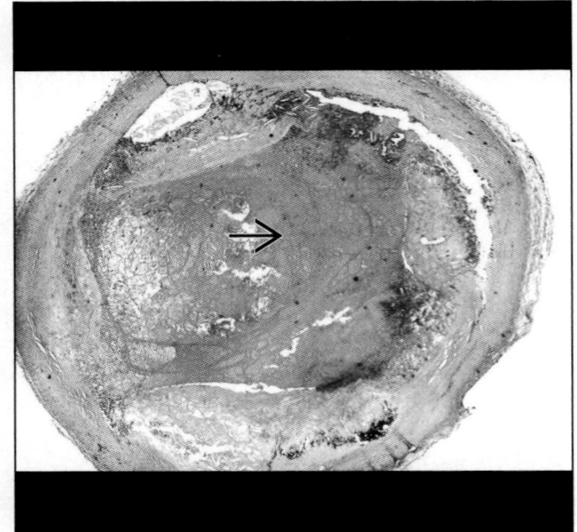

Photomicrograph shows a coronary artery with recent thrombus → occluding the lumen.

TERMINOLOGY

Synonyms

- Myocardial ischemia, heart attack, acute coronary syndrome

Definitions

- Myocardial infarction can be defined as irreversible myocardial muscle damage caused by prolonged ischemia, resulting from sustained imbalance of perfusion, supply, and demand

ETIOLOGY/PATHOGENESIS

Coronary Artery Atherosclerosis Risk Factors

- Smoking
- Hypertension
- Elevated low-density lipoprotein cholesterol
- Diabetes
- Increasing age

Nonatherosclerotic Coronary Disease

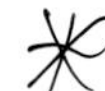

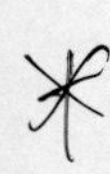

- Coronary artery vasculitis
- Coronary artery amyloidosis
- Coronary artery dissection
- Coronary artery spasm
- Coronary artery embolus (such as from endocarditis)

Other Causes of Mismatched Perfusion and Myocardial Demand

- Left ventricular hypertrophy (cardiomyopathy, hypertensive heart disease)
- Congenital heart disease
- Cardiac arrest (from nonischemic causes)
  - Metabolic, neurogenic, arrhythmia
- Impaired oxygen delivery (respiratory failure, severe anemia)

CLINICAL ISSUES

Epidemiology

- Incidence
  - Annual incidence of new myocardial infarction in USA has been estimated at 610,000 cases
  - Recurrent myocardial infarction accounts for 325,000 additional episodes
- Age
  - Average: 64.5 years for men and 70.3 years for women
- Gender
  - M > F
  - Women thought to be "protected" from coronary atherosclerosis in their reproductive years
- Ethnicity
  - Prevalence is highest in developed nations, presumably due to comparatively high-calorie diet, more sedentary lifestyle, and longer life expectancy
  - Significant variation in incidence across developed nations, with rates (per 100,000) such as
    - 30 in Japan
    - 39.8 in France
    - 65.2 in Italy
    - 94.9 in Canada
    - 106.5 in United States
    - 216 in Slovakia

Presentation

- Cardiac arrest without recognized antecedent symptoms
- Typical symptoms
  - Chest pain (angina) on exertion or rest
  - Mandibular, upper arm, or epigastric discomfort; usually lasts > 20 minutes
  - Associated nausea, diaphoresis, syncope
- No symptoms
  - In elderly, women, diabetic, postoperative, and critically ill

ACUTE MYOCARDIAL INFARCTION

Key Facts

Terminology
- Irreversible myocardial damage caused by prolonged ischemia, resulting from sustained imbalance of perfusion, supply, and demand

Clinical Issues
- Complications: Acute
  - Rupture of myocardium (tamponade, acquired ventricular septal defect, ruptured papillary muscle)
- Complications: Long term
  - Ischemic dilated cardiomyopathy
  - Ventricular true aneurysms (often with mural thrombus)

Macroscopic Pathology
- 12-24 hours: No changes or subtle mottling
- 7-10 days: Grossly softened and depressed with more prominent hyperemic edges
- 3-8 weeks: Grayish-white scar begins to form at edges and progresses to center

Microscopic Pathology
- 1-3 days: Coagulative necrosis with loss of nuclei, contraction bands, and heavy neutrophilic infiltration
- 3-7 days: Myocyte loss, karyorrhexis of neutrophils ("nuclear dust"), early phagocytosis by macrophages at infarct border
- 10-14 days: Well-established granulation tissue with new blood vessels and fibroblast infiltration
- 2-8 weeks: Increased collagen deposition with decreased cellularity

Treatment
- Surgical approaches
  - Coronary artery bypass grafting
  - Percutaneous coronary intervention (PCI)
    - Usually reserved for acute ST elevation myocardial infarction (salvageable myocardium)
    - Balloon angioplasty with coronary artery stenting
- Drugs
  - Sublingual nitroglycerin
  - Antiplatelet therapy (aspirin, clopidogrel)
  - Morphine for pain relief
  - Thrombolytic agents (effective only in 1st hours after acute coronary thrombosis)
    - 1st generation: Streptokinase, urokinase, acetylated plasminogen streptokinase activator complex (APSAC)
    - 2nd generation: t-PA, tenecteplase

Prognosis
- Median 30-day mortality: 16.6%
- Median 30-day readmission: 19.9%
- Complications
  - Acute
    - Cardiogenic shock
    - Rupture of myocardium (tamponade, acquired ventricular septal defect, ruptured papillary muscle)
    - Ventricular pseudoaneurysm (contained rupture)
    - Pericarditis (Dressler syndrome)
    - Arrhythmias
    - Sudden death
  - Longer term
    - Congestive heart failure
    - Ischemic dilated cardiomyopathy
    - Ventricular true aneurysms (often with mural thrombus)
    - Mitral regurgitation (scar retraction of papillary muscle)
    - Recurrent ventricular arrhythmias
- Risk of 2nd myocardial infarction

IMAGE FINDINGS

MR Findings
- Accurate assessment of myocardial function and motion and perfusion (with contrast)

Echocardiography
- Assesses myocardial thickness and motion
- Assesses myocardial perfusion and microvascular obstruction (coronary flow reserve)

Radionucleotide Imaging
- Commonly used to assess perfusion and viability

MACROSCOPIC FEATURES

General Features
- In initial few minutes to hours (up to 8-12 hours), there is no grossly apparent abnormality
- Thereafter
  - 12-24 hours: No change or subtle mottling and regional stiffness
  - 1-3 days: Mottling with yellow-tan center
  - 3-7 days: Yellow-tan center with hyperemic edges
  - 7-10 days: Grossly softened and depressed with more prominent hyperemic edges
  - 10-14 days: Edges become more gray in color
  - 3-8 weeks: Grayish-white scar begins to form at edges and progresses to center
  - 8-12 weeks: Grayish-white scar with early remodeling (wall thinning and chamber dilatation)

Hemorrhagic Infarct
- After revascularization (durable or failed), restoration of blood flow to damaged tissue may result in hemorrhagic infarction
  - Dark red-brown in color due to hemorrhage into ischemic tissues

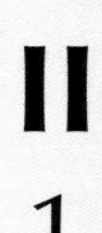

ACUTE MYOCARDIAL INFARCTION

Vital Staining of Fresh Heart Tissue (Autopsy)

- Triphenyltetrazolium chloride (TTC) or nitro blue tetrazolium (NBT) dye test
  - Redox indicator catalyzed by dehydrogenase enzymes in viable myocardium (but not infarcted myocardium)
  - TTC will stain viable myocardium brick red (infarcted myocardium will remain unchanged)
  - NBT will stain viable myocardium dark blue-purple (infarcted myocardium will remain unchanged)

MICROSCOPIC PATHOLOGY

Histologic Features

- After 4 hours (variable), myocytes may appear wavy and elongated, interstitial edema
- Within 24 hours, interstitial edema, focal hemorrhage, myocyte contraction bands, and infiltration of neutrophils (margination)
  - Staining for C4d may be positive in acutely ischemic myocytes due to complement activation
- 1-3 days: Coagulative necrosis with loss of nuclei, contraction bands, and heavy neutrophilic infiltration
- 3-7 days: Myocyte loss, karyorrhexis of neutrophils ("nuclear dust"), early phagocytosis by macrophages at infarct border
- 7-10 days: Well-developed phagocytosis with distended macrophages, granulation tissue at infarct border
- 10-14 days: Well-established granulation tissue with new blood vessels and fibroblast infiltration
- 2-8 weeks: Increased collagen deposition with decreased cellularity
- > 2 months: Dense collagenous scar
- Caveat: This sequence of changes assumes no revascularization (no reversal of ischemia)
  - Spontaneous or interventional reperfusion must be taken into account
- Reperfusion injury (after revascularization)
  - Prominent coagulative necrosis
  - Marked erythrocyte extravasation/hemorrhage
  - Small vessels may show small thrombi or atheroemboli

ANCILLARY TESTS

Immunohistochemistry

- C4d, C9: Positive staining in necrotic myocardium
- cTnT: Negative staining in necrotic myocardium

Electron Microscopy

- Transmission
  - Sarcolemmal disruption
  - Mitochondrial swelling, mitochondrial amorphous densities
  - Relaxation of myofibrils
  - Glycogen loss

DIFFERENTIAL DIAGNOSIS

Chest Pain

- Clinically, can be due to
  - Acute aortic dissection
  - Pericarditis
  - Gastrointestinal disorders (reflux, cholecystitis, gastritis)
  - Pneumonia
  - Pulmonary embolism
  - Pneumothorax

SELECTED REFERENCES

1. Chang J et al: Pathology of myocardial infarction. Diagnostic Histopathology. 19(1):7-12, 2013
2. Hoyert DL et al: Deaths: preliminary data for 2011. Natl Vital Stat Rep. 61(6):1-51, 2012
3. Hamm CW et al: ESC Guidelines for the management of acute coronary syndromes in patients presenting without persistent ST-segment elevation: The Task Force for the management of acute coronary syndromes (ACS) in patients presenting without persistent ST-segment elevation of the European Society of Cardiology (ESC). Eur Heart J. 32(23):2999-3054, 2011
4. Jenkins CP et al: The utility of C4d, C9, and troponin T immunohistochemistry in acute myocardial infarction. Arch Pathol Lab Med. 134(2):256-63, 2010
5. Krumholz HM et al: Patterns of hospital performance in acute myocardial infarction and heart failure 30-day mortality and readmission. Circ Cardiovasc Qual Outcomes. 2(5):407-13, 2009
6. Antman EM et al: ST-elevation myocardial infarction: Pathology, pathophysiology, and clinical features. In Libby P et al: Braunwald's Heart Disease: A Textbook of Cardiovascular Medicine. Philadelphia: Saunders Elsevier. 1207-32, 2008
7. Kung HC et al: Deaths: final data for 2005. Natl Vital Stat Rep. 56(10):1-120, 2008
8. Thygesen K et al: Universal definition of myocardial infarction. Eur Heart J. 28(20):2525-38, 2007
9. Pasotti M et al: The pathology of myocardial infarction in the pre- and post-interventional era. Heart. 92(11):1552-6, 2006
10. Olsen EGJ: Myocardial infarction. In The Pathology of the Heart. 2nd ed. Basingstoke and London: Macmillan Press. 99-132, 1980

ACUTE MYOCARDIAL INFARCTION

Gross and Microscopic Features

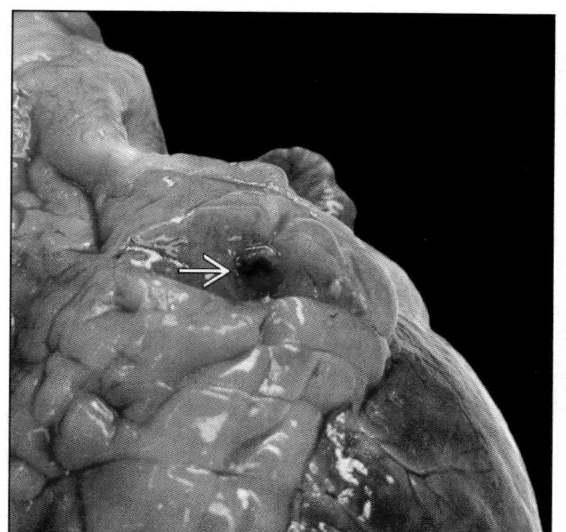

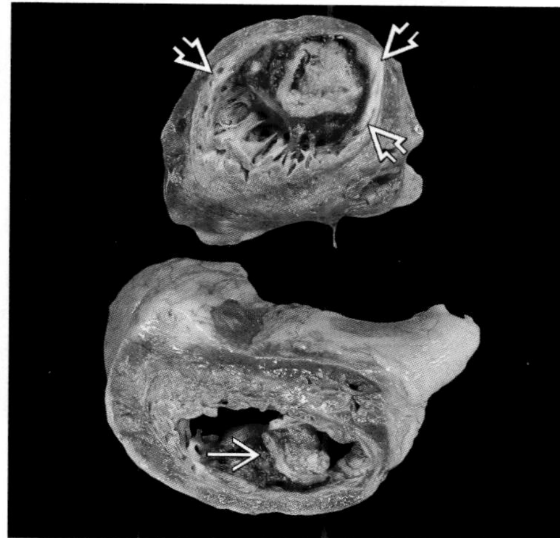

(Left) *This left anterior descending artery shows recent thrombus* → *occluding the lumen. This artery supplies the anterolateral wall of the left ventricle.* ***(Right)*** *This gross photograph shows an aneurysm* → *involving the apex of the left ventricle. The aneurysms are seen more frequently in healed transmural infarct than subendocardial infarct. A thrombus* → *is seen in the cavity of the aneurysm. (Courtesy J. Fernandes, MD.)*

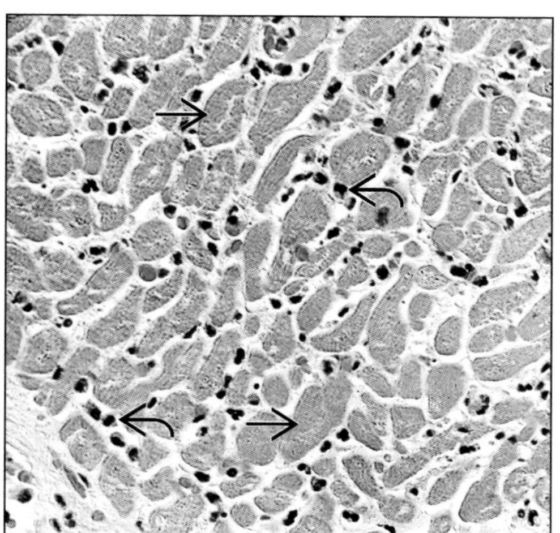

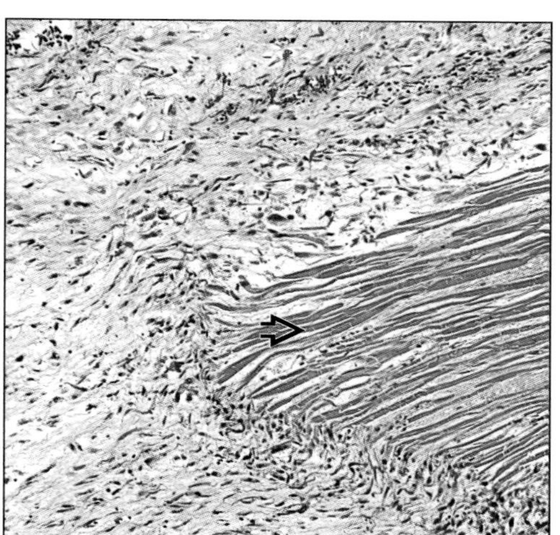

(Left) *Acute myocardial infarction that is 24-48 hours old shows anuclear hypereosinophilic myocytes* → *and acute inflammatory infiltrate* →*.* ***(Right)*** *Healing infarct that is 2 weeks old shows necrotic myocytes* → *in the center, surrounded by granulation tissue composed of fibroblasts, chronic inflammation, and neocapillaries.*

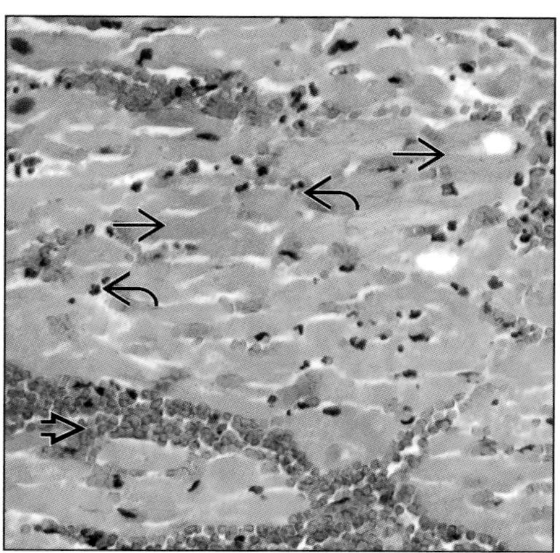

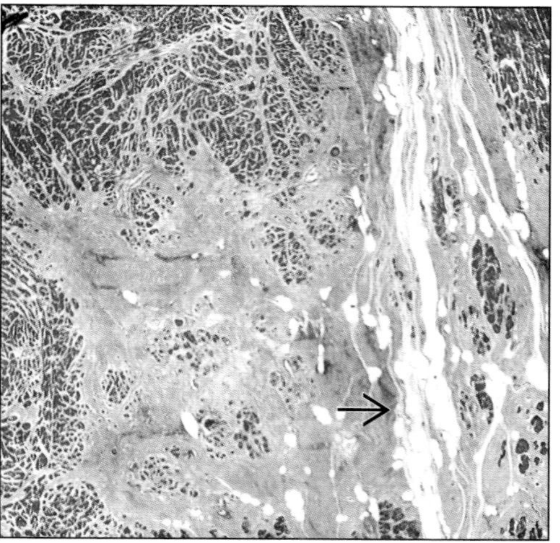

(Left) *Acute reperfusion infarct shows anuclear hypereosinophilic myocytes* →*, hemorrhage* →*, and neutrophils* →*. Reperfusion infarcts are usually hemorrhagic and can be extensive.* ***(Right)*** *Photomicrograph shows a well-healed transmural infarct. There is dense fibrosis* → *with focal fatty infiltration.*

CARDIOMYOPATHY

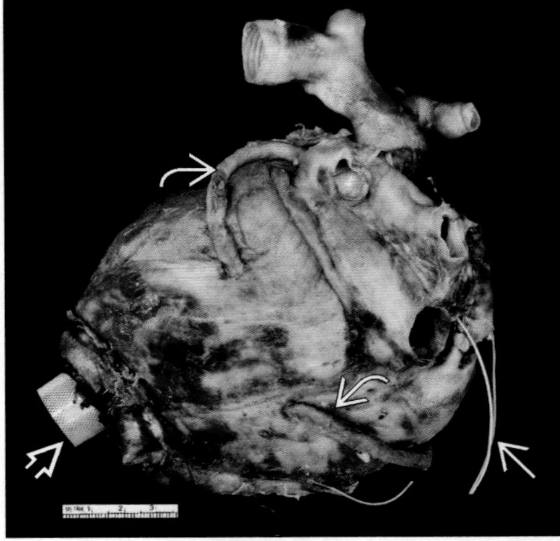

This autopsy heart specimen from a patient with multiple interventions (bypass grafts ➔, epicardial leads ➔, and left ventricular assist device conduits ➔) poses a challenge for cardiomyopathy evaluation.

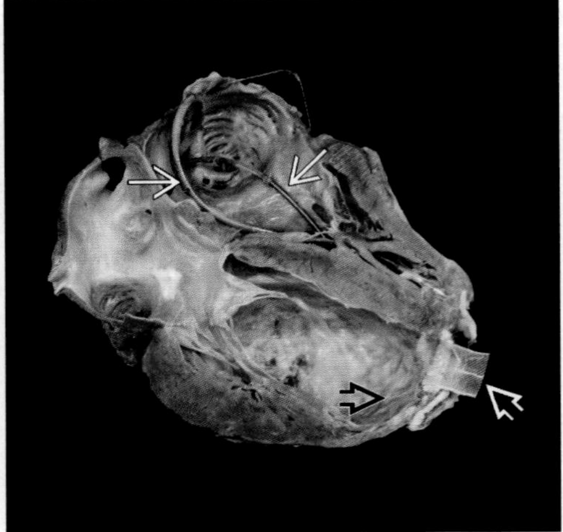

This 4 chamber long axis view of a heart at autopsy shows ischemic cardiomyopathy features with ventricular aneurysm ➔. Pacemaker leads ➔, and an LVAD inflow cannula ➔ is also seen.

TERMINOLOGY

Definitions

- Cardiomyopathies are a complex set of disorders often posing diagnostic challenges
- This chapter outlines a systematic approach to cardiomyopathies, primarily on basis of gross pathologic features

BASES FOR CLASSIFICATION

Etiology

- Primary
- Secondary
- Alcoholic
- Peripartum

Morphology

- Dilated
- Hypertrophic
- Restrictive

Physiology

- Systolic heart failure
- Diastolic: Preserved ejection fraction heart failure

AMERICAN HEART ASSOCIATION CLASSIFICATION (2006)

Primary

- Genetic
  - Hypertrophic cardiomyopathy
  - Arrhythmogenic cardiomyopathy
  - Left ventricular noncompaction/hypertrabeculation
  - Mitochondrial myopathies
  - Ion channel disorders
- Acquired
  - Inflammatory (myocarditis)
  - Stress provoked (Takotsubo/apical ballooning)
  - Tachycardia induced
  - Peripartum
- Mixed
  - Dilated cardiomyopathy
  - Primary restrictive cardiomyopathy

Secondary

- Amyloidosis
  - Primary (AL, AH)
  - Senile (ATTR)
  - Familial (numerous)
- Other infiltrative disease
  - Gaucher
  - Hurler
  - Hunter
- Storage disease
  - Fabry
  - Hemochromatosis
- Eosinophilic endomyocardial disease
- Sarcoidosis
- Endocrine
  - Diabetic cardiomyopathy
  - Thyroid dysfunction (hyper or hypo)
- Cardiofacial
  - Noonan syndrome
  - Lentiginosis
- Neuromuscular
  - Friedrich ataxia
  - Muscular dystrophy
- Nutritional
  - Beriberi
  - Pellagra
- Autoimmune/collagen vascular
  - Lupus
  - Rheumatoid
- Electrolyte imbalance
- Consequence of cancer therapy
  - Radiation induced

- Anthracycline toxicity

MACROSCOPIC FINDINGS

External Examination

- Lower extremity edema
- Ascites (abdominal distension)
- Pacemaker, implanted defibrillator
- Ventricular assist device

Internal Examination

- Cardiothoracic ratio
  - Heart:chest diameter in situ
- Pulmonary edema and congestion
  - Pleural effusions
- Liver enlargement (early) or "cardiac cirrhosis" (late)
- Nephrosclerosis
  - Possible indicator of hypertensive heart disease

Organ Examination

- Left ventricular hypertrophy
  - Heart weight > 150-175% of expected weight = moderate to severe hypertrophy
  - Ratio of septal:free wall thickness > 1.3 = asymmetric septal hypertrophy
    - Exclude papillary muscles when measuring free wall
- Left ventricle dilatation
  - Short axis left ventricle internal diameter
    - > 5 cm = severely dilated
    - Other chambers usually enlarged due to congestion from systolic failure
  - Dilated cardiomyopathy shows both dilatation and hypertrophy (by heart weight criteria)
- Right-sided effects
  - Pulmonary venous hypertension
    - Secondary to elevated left atrial pressure/ congestion
    - Dilated and tortuous vein branches in lobular septa
    - Septal edema and widening, prominent septal lymphatics
    - Intraalveolar hemosiderophages (heart failure cells)
  - Right ventricle enlargement
    - Complex chamber geometry precludes criteria for dilatation using width
    - "Gestalt" sense more useful
    - Right ventricle thickness (excluding trabeculation) > 0.6 = hypertrophy

Ventricular Assist Devices and Other Hardware

- Evaluate for pump thrombus, position and patency of cannulas
- Evaluate anastomotic connections for kinking, bending, extrinsic compression
- Deactivate implantable defibrillators
  - Coordinate with pacemaker nurse for institution, manufacturer
  - Potential for electric shock to autopsy personnel

MICROSCOPIC FINDINGS

Histologic Features

- Interstitial fibrosis
- Myocyte hypertrophy
  - Binucleation of myocytes (mild, early)
  - Enlarged, hyperchromatic "boxcar" nuclei (moderate, severe)
- Primary cardiomyopathy is a diagnosis of exclusion; must rule out the following
  - Chronic valvular disease
  - Hypertensive heart disease
  - Ischemic heart disease
- Etiology specific findings
  - Myocyte disarray: Hypertrophic cardiomyopathy
  - Hemosiderin: Hemochromatosis
  - Amyloid: Amyloidosis
  - Marked transmural myocyte vacuolization: Storage disease
  - Foamy macrophages: Gaucher

COMMON CARDIOMYOPATHIES

Idiopathic Dilated Cardiomyopathy

- Features
  - Moderate-severe LV dilatation (LVISD > 4 cm)
  - Moderate-severe LV hypertrophy (heart weight > 150% of expected weight)
  - Myocyte hypertrophy and interstitial fibrosis
- Etiology
  - Presumed to be late post myocarditis (viral or post viral) in most cases
  - Termed "idiopathic" due to lack of definitive causation
  - Wide age range (congenital to elderly)
  - Rare forms: Familial, alcoholic, peripartum, hemochromatosis, tachycardia induced
- Differential diagnosis
  - Mainly valvular disease, regurgitant valves (volume hypertrophy)

Hypertrophic Cardiomyopathy

- Features
  - Thick left ventricle walls, especially septum (septum to free wall ratio > 1.3)
  - Small left ventricle chamber volume
  - Moderate to severe LVH (heart weight > 150% of expected)
  - Myocyte hypertrophy, interstitial fibrosis, myocyte disarray
  - Left atrium and right chambers also enlarged
- Etiology
  - Mutations in sarcomeric or sarcomere-associated genes
  - Genetic testing for *MYH7*, *MBPC*, others
  - May manifest at any age
  - Common cause of sudden death in young people
- Differential diagnosis
  - Hypertensive heart disease
  - Aortic stenosis (pressure hypertrophy)
  - Storage disease (*LAMP2*-Danon)

- Athlete's heart

Restrictive Cardiomyopathy

- Features
  - Normal heart weight or mild hypertrophy (< 150% of expected heart weight)
  - Left atrial enlargement with normal-sized left ventricle and normal valves
  - Right chambers may be enlarged chronically
- Etiology
  - Primary: Mid to late adulthood, possible association with troponin I mutations
  - Secondary: Infiltrative, storage disease
- Differential diagnosis
  - Mitral stenosis
  - Constrictive pericarditis
  - Eosinophilic endomyocardial disease

Arrhythmogenic Cardiomyopathy

- Features
  - Often normal heart weight, only mild dilatation (right or left ventricle)
  - Fibrofatty transmural replacement of ventricular wall
  - Diverticular outpouchings from ventricles in areas of wall thinning
  - Right > left ventricle involvement
  - F > M, young adults
- Etiology
  - Viral and genetic factors are implicated in pathogenesis (possibly complex interaction of environment and genetic predisposition)
  - Screening for cell junction protein defects (desmoplakin, plakoglobin, plakophilin) by immunofluorescence
  - Monomorphic ventricular tachycardia on EKG
  - Sudden cardiac death in young patients
- Differential diagnosis
  - Normal mural fat, especially in right ventricle wall
  - Fatty degeneration/replacement of myocardium in dilated cardiomyopathy

DIAGNOSTIC CHECKLIST

Clinically Relevant Pathologic Features

- Exclude valvular, ischemic, and hypertensive heart disease
- Correlate with antemortem imaging (echocardiogram), EKG
  - Systolic or diastolic (preserved ejection fraction) failure
  - Chamber dilatation, enlargement
  - Wall thickness
  - High or low voltage EKG

Pathologic Interpretation Pearls

- Special stains for fibrosis, glycogen, iron, and amyloid
  - Selection can be guided by H&E appearance
- Autopsy examination approximates end systolic dimensions in clinical imaging
  - Rigor causes near maximal ventricular contraction
  - Subject to decomposition changes

Autopsy Considerations

- In cases of cardiomyopathy with potential heritability, consider storing frozen samples
  - Blood, myocardium, spleen

REPORTING CRITERIA

Gross Examination

- Accurate heart weight (great vessels, pericardium, blood removed)
- Accurate wall thickness (mid ventricle, exclude papillary muscles)
- Left ventricle internal short axis diameter

Microscopic Examination

- Degree and extent of fibrosis, hypertrophy
- Special stains to exclude iron, amyloid, glycogen storage disease, etc.
- Disarray in hypertrophic cardiomyopathy
- Severe myocyte vacuolization in storage disease

SELECTED REFERENCES

1. Rapezzi C et al: Diagnostic work-up in cardiomyopathies: bridging the gap between clinical phenotypes and final diagnosis. A position statement from the ESC Working Group on Myocardial and Pericardial Diseases. Eur Heart J. 34(19):1448-58, 2013
2. Asimaki A et al: The role of endomyocardial biopsy in ARVC: looking beyond histology in search of new diagnostic markers. J Cardiovasc Electrophysiol. 22(1):111-7, 2011
3. Basso C et al: Pathophysiology of arrhythmogenic cardiomyopathy. Nat Rev Cardiol. 9(4):223-33, 2011
4. Maron BJ et al: How should hypertrophic cardiomyopathy be classified?: What's in a name? Dilemmas in nomenclature characterizing hypertrophic cardiomyopathy and left ventricular hypertrophy. Circ Cardiovasc Genet. 2(1):81-5; discussion 86, 2009
5. McLeod CJ et al: Histologic characterization of hypertrophic cardiomyopathy with and without myofilament mutations. Am Heart J. 158(5):799-805, 2009
6. Maron BJ et al: Contemporary definitions and classification of the cardiomyopathies: an American Heart Association Scientific Statement from the Council on Clinical Cardiology, Heart Failure and Transplantation Committee; Quality of Care and Outcomes Research and Functional Genomics and Translational Biology Interdisciplinary Working Groups; and Council on Epidemiology and Prevention. Circulation. 113(14):1807-16, 2006
7. Lamke GT et al: Surgical pathology of subaortic septal myectomy associated with hypertrophic cardiomyopathy. A study of 204 cases (1996-2000). Cardiovasc Pathol. 12(3):149-58, 2003

Gross and Microscopic Features

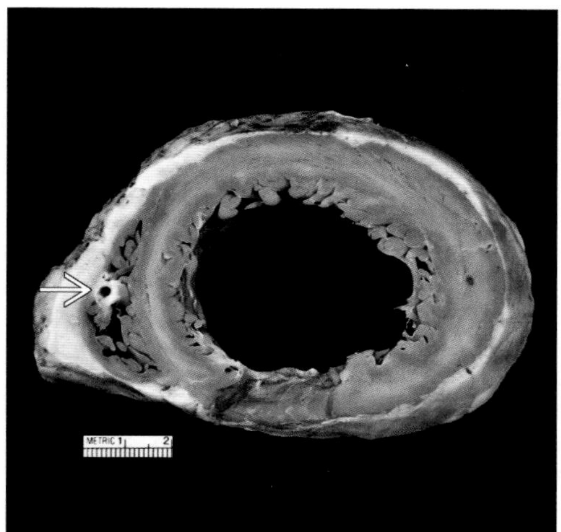

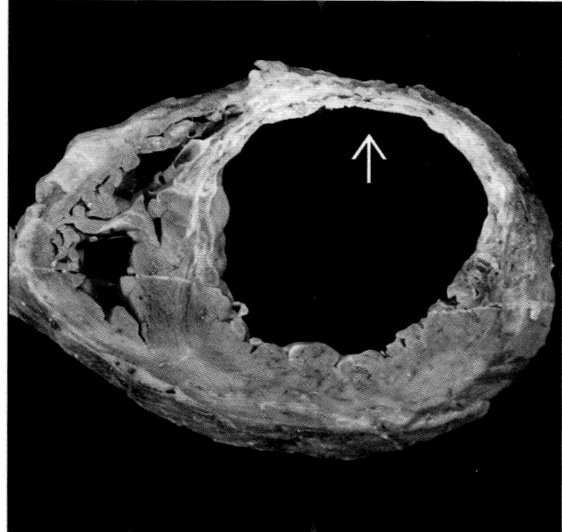

*(**Left**) This short-axis view of the ventricles demonstrates features of dilated cardiomyopathy. The internal short-axis diameter is ~ 5 cm. No regional ischemic changes are noted. The right ventricle is normal in size and shows fibrosis surrounding a pacemaker lead tract ➡. (**Right**) This short-axis section of the ventricles shows ischemic cardiomyopathy with massive transmural infarction of the anteroseptal wall ➡ with global left ventricle remodeling (dilatation and wall thinning).*

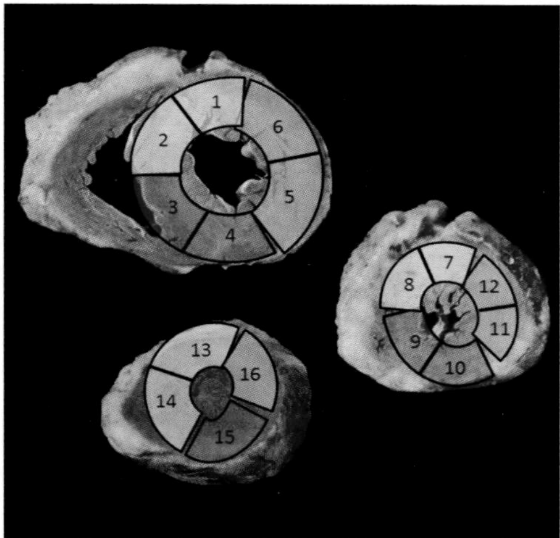

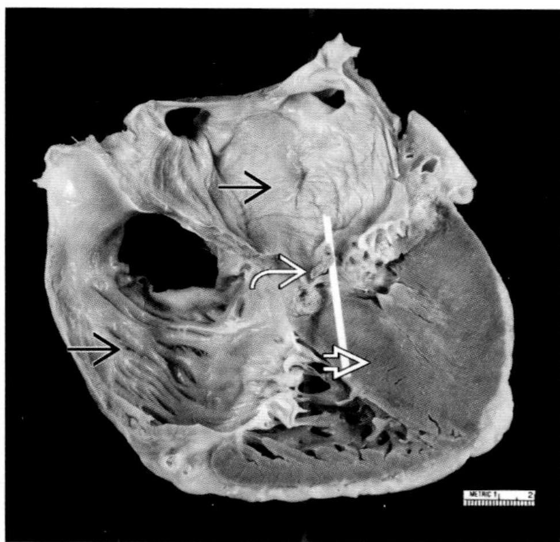

*(**Left**) The conventional regions or "segments" assessed by echocardiography have been superimposed on these short-axis views of the ventricles. Yellow = LAD territory, blue = LCX, and red = RCA (assuming right dominance). (**Right**) This autopsy heart shows hypertrophic cardiomyopathy. The left ventricle walls ➡ are thickened, and both atria are markedly dilated ➡ (diastolic failure). An incidental thrombotic-type vegetation is also seen ➡.*

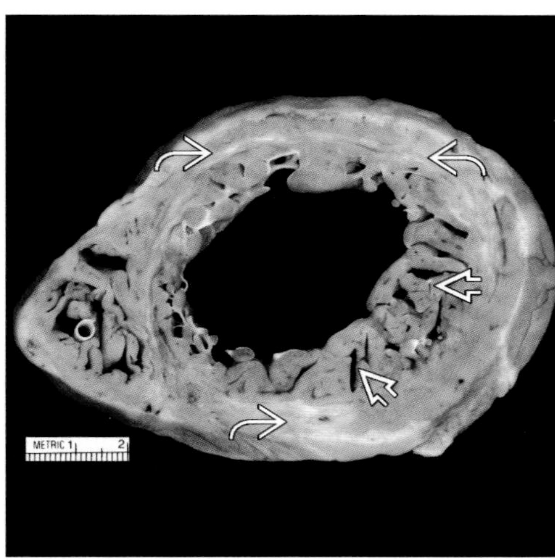

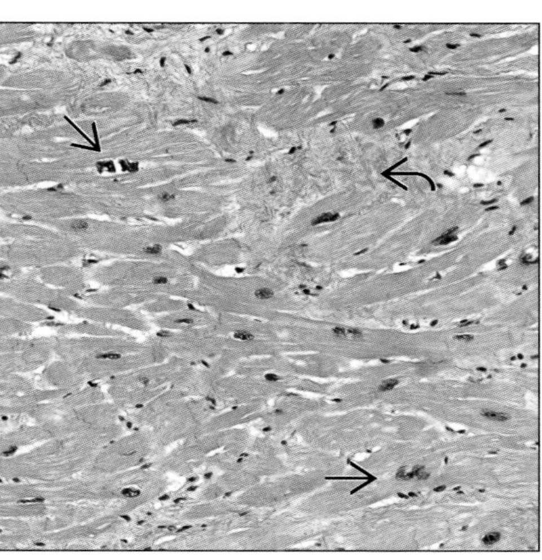

*(**Left**) This short-axis view of the left ventricle shows an unusual pattern. Besides left ventricular dilatation, there are features of hypertrabeculation/ noncompaction ➡ and fibrofatty infiltration of the left ventricle myocardium ➡. Not all cardiomyopathies are readily classified by morphology. (**Right**) This photomicrograph shows the typical features common to nearly all cardiomyopathies. The nuclei show features of myocyte hypertrophy ➡, and interstitial fibrosis ➡ is also seen.*

MYOCARDITIS

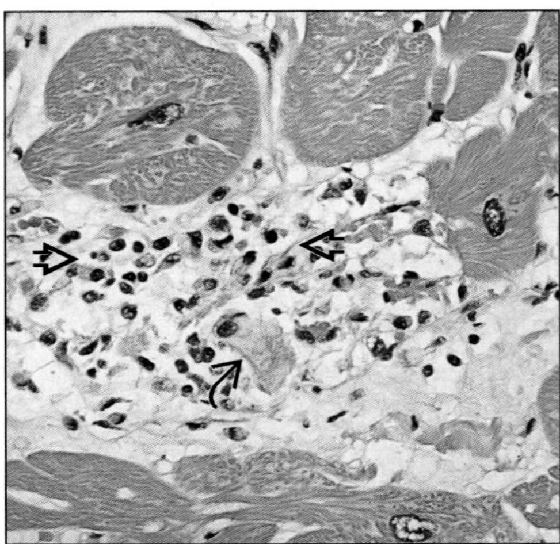

The definitive features of myocarditis are seen in this high-power image of myocardium, with interstitial inflammation ⊳ and myocyte damage ↗.

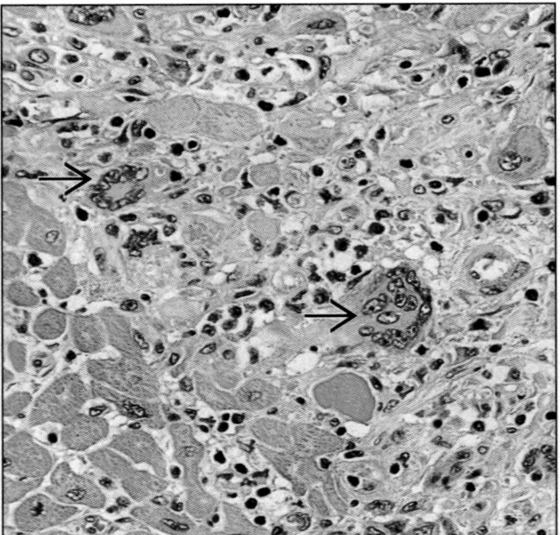

This image shows giant cell myocarditis with extensive inflammation, widespread myocyte destruction, and multinucleated giant cells →.

TERMINOLOGY

Definitions

- Inflammatory process involving myocardium with degeneration &/or necrosis of myocytes secondary to infection or autoimmune response

ETIOLOGY/PATHOGENESIS

Infectious Agents

- RNA virus
    - Coxsackie A and B
    - Influenza A and B
- DNA virus
    - Adenovirus
    - Herpesviridae (herpes simplex 1 & 2, varicella-zoster, cytomegalovirus [CMV], Epstein-Barr)
    - Poxvirus (variola, vaccinia)
- Bacteria
    - Gram-positive cocci
    - *Rickettsia*, *Borrelia*
- Fungus
    - *Candida*
    - *Aspergillus*
    - Zygomycosis (e.g., *Mucor*)
- Parasites
    - *Toxoplasma gondii*
    - *Trypanosoma cruzii* (Chagas)

Autoimmune

- Postviral/postinfectious sequela
- Rheumatic (pancarditis)
- Giant cell myocarditis
- Eosinophilic myocarditis
- Granulomatous myocarditis

Hypersensitivity

- Hypersensitivity myocarditis

CLINICAL ISSUES

Epidemiology

- Incidence
    - True incidence is unknown
    - Estimated that 10% of acute-onset heart failure is due to acute myocarditis
- Age
    - Any age, though incidence mirrors viral susceptibility (extremes of age)
- Gender
    - Slight male predominance

Presentation

- New onset of congestive heart failure
- Atrial/ventricular arrhythmias
- Embolic events
- Fatigue
- Chest pain
- Palpitations
- Sinus tachycardia
- Gallops, murmurs
- Pericardial friction rub
- Fever
- Eosinophilic myocarditis
    - Absolute eosinophil count > 1.5×10^9/L
    - ANCA to exclude Churg-Strauss

Laboratory Tests

- White blood cell count usually elevated
- Elevated cardiac-specific troponin in 1/3 of cases
- Elevated creatine kinase isoform MB in 10% of cases
- Autoantibodies to sarcolemma, alpha myosin, mitochondria, endothelial antigens
- Rising IgM/IgG titers to specific virus

Prognosis

- Mild cases of myocarditis may be asymptomatic, and patients can recover without sequelae

MYOCARDITIS

Key Facts

Etiology
- Viral
- Bacterial
- Fungal
- Parasitic
- Postviral/postinfectious sequela
- Giant cell myocarditis
- Eosinophilic myocarditis

Macroscopic Pathology
- Pericarditis may also be present (myopericarditis)
- No gross abnormalities (most common)

Microscopic Pathology
- Dallas criteria
  - No myocarditis: No inflammation or myocardial abnormalities
  - Borderline myocarditis: Inflammatory without myocyte damage
  - Myocarditis: Significant inflammation with myocyte damage
- Lymphocytic
  - T cells predominate
  - Neutrophils and rare eosinophils may also be seen (mixed)
- Eosinophilic
  - Prominent interstitial/perivascular eosinophils
  - Eosinophilic granulomas
- Giant cell
  - Diffuse myocardial infiltration and infarct-like damage
  - No recognizable granulomas
  - Prominent eosinophils in background

- Fulminant myocarditis more likely to have sequelae, but complete recovery is possible after support
- Progress to dilated cardiomyopathy in ~ 1/3 of cases
- Sudden death from circulatory failure in acute phase in some cases

IMAGE FINDINGS

Radiographic Findings
- Cardiomegaly on PA chest radiograph

Ultrasonographic Findings
- Global wall motion decreased
- Normal diastolic volumes
- Increased left ventricle wall thickness
- Right/left ventricular dysfunction

MR Findings
- Global relative gadolinium enhancement in myocardium compared to skeletal muscle
- Increased T2 signal in areas of myocardial inflammation
- Delayed enhancement in subepicardial region

EKG
- Elevation/depression of ST segment
- T wave changes
- Pathologic Q waves
- Atrial/ventricular arrhythmias
  - Premature beats
  - Tachycardia
  - Fibrillation
  - Conduction delays

MACROSCOPIC FEATURES

General Features
- Dilatation of left ventricle
- Cut myocardial surface with markedly variegated mottled appearance with pale foci alternating with minute hemorrhagic lesions
- Myocardium with flabby consistency
- Mural thrombi in any chamber
- Pericarditis may also be present (myopericarditis)
- No gross abnormalities (most common)
  - Thorough sampling is key
    - 10 full thickness sections from different parts of the ventricles (right, left, apical, mid, basal)
  - Single or rare microscopic foci may incite electrical instability
    - Substrate for sudden cardiac death

MICROSCOPIC PATHOLOGY

Histologic Features
- Dallas criteria
  - 1st diagnostic biopsy
    - No myocarditis: No inflammation or myocardial abnormalities
    - Borderline myocarditis: Sparse inflammatory infiltrate, but damage of myocytes is not demonstrated
    - Myocarditis: Significant inflammation with myocyte damage (necrosis, myocyte vacuolization)
  - 2nd/follow-up biopsy ± fibrosis
    - Ongoing (persistent) myocarditis: Morphology similar to that in prior biopsy
    - Resolving (healing) myocarditis: Fewer abnormalities than in prior biopsy
    - Resolved (healed) myocarditis: Fibrosis, no inflammation

Lymphocytic/Mixed Myocarditis
- T cells predominate
- Other mononuclear cells present (histiocytes, natural killer cells, etc.)
- Neutrophils and rare eosinophils may also be seen (mixed)
- Immunophenotyping not necessary for diagnosis
- Usually viral/postviral etiology but not specific

MYOCARDITIS

Eosinophilic Myocarditis
- Mixed inflammatory cell infiltrate with eosinophils in interstitial or perivascular distribution
- Eosinophilic granulomas
- Eosinophil degranulation and breakdown products (Charcot-Leyden crystals)
- Eosinophil-rich mural thrombus (eosinophilic endomyocardial disease)
- Careful exclusion of parasitic, fungal infection

Giant Cell Myocarditis
- Diffuse myocardial infiltration and infarct-like damage
- CD8 T cells and histiocytes with singly distributed multinucleated giant cells
- No recognizable granulomas
- Prominent eosinophils in background
- Individual entrapped cardiomyocytes common

ANCILLARY TESTS

Immunohistochemistry
- CD3 staining for T lymphocytes
- C4d or C9 staining to confirm microscopic foci of myocyte damage

In Situ Hybridization
- Viral genomic material demonstrated within myocytes

PCR
- Viral genomic material detected in nucleic acid extract from myocardial tissue

Special Stains
- Gram
- GMS/PAS
- AFB

DIFFERENTIAL DIAGNOSIS

Hypersensitivity Myocarditis
- History of recent medication use
- Skin rash, peripheral eosinophilia
- Eosinophilic myocardial infiltrates

Giant Cell Myocarditis
- Mixed myocardial inflammatory infiltrate with presence of giant cells
- Extensive areas of myocardial necrosis
- History of thymoma or autoimmune disorders

Sarcoidosis
- Noncaseating granulomas in myocardium, endocardium, or pericardium
- Hypercalcemia
- Lung or other organ involvement

CMV Myocarditis
- Viral inclusions identified in endothelial cells
- CMV DNA detection in myocardial tissue

Bacterial Myocarditis
- Interstitial infiltrate predominantly composed of neutrophils
- Microabscesses may be identified

DIAGNOSTIC CHECKLIST

Clinically Relevant Pathologic Features
- Sudden unexpected death
- New arrhythmias
- Recent flu-like illness
- Unexplained leukocytosis
- Hypereosinophilia (eosinophilic myocarditis)

Pathologic Interpretation Pearls
- Should be considered in absence of other anatomic causes of death
- Thorough myocardial sampling when no gross abnormalities seen
  - 10 sections, full thickness, multiple regions of both ventricles
- Diagnosis requires definite interstitial inflammation **and** myocyte necrosis or injury
- Ancillary tests (immunostains, ISH, PCR) not required for diagnosis

SELECTED REFERENCES

1. Kindermann I et al: Predictors of outcome in patients with suspected myocarditis. Circulation. 2008 Aug 5;118(6):639-48. Epub 2008 Jul 21. Erratum in: Circulation. 118(12): e493, 2008
2. Calabrese F et al: Myocarditis and inflammatory cardiomyopathy: microbiological and molecular biological aspects. Cardiovasc Res. 60(1):11-25, 2003
3. Mason JW: Myocarditis and dilated cardiomyopathy: an inflammatory link. Cardiovasc Res. 60(1):5-10, 2003
4. Calabrese F et al: Molecular diagnosis of myocarditis and dilated cardiomyopathy in children: clinicopathologic features and prognostic implications. Diagn Mol Pathol. 11(4):212-21, 2002
5. Kawai C: From myocarditis to cardiomyopathy: mechanisms of inflammation and cell death: learning from the past for the future. Circulation. 99(8):1091-100, 1999
6. Wojnicz R et al: Immunohistological diagnosis of myocarditis. Potential role of sarcolemmal induction of the MHC and ICAM-1 in the detection of autoimmune mediated myocyte injury. Eur Heart J. 19(10):1564-72, 1998
7. Aretz HT et al: Myocarditis. A histopathologic definition and classification. Am J Cardiovasc Pathol. 1(1):3-14, 1987
8. Aretz HT: Myocarditis: the Dallas criteria. Hum Pathol. 18(6):619-24, 1987

MR Findings and Microscopic Features

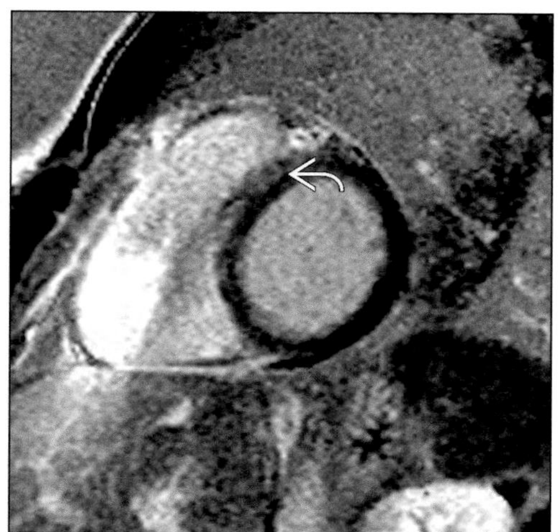

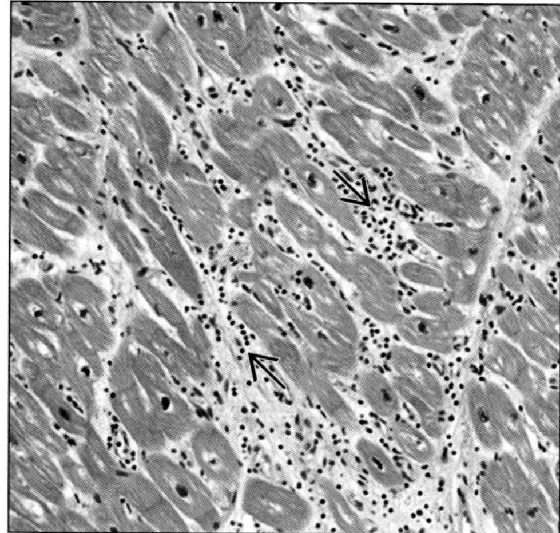

(Left) *Cardiac short axis MR shows septal delayed contrast enhancement* ➔ *suggestive of myocarditis. Antemortem findings like this can help guide tissue sampling at autopsy. (Courtesy C. McGann, MD.)* ***(Right)*** *This myocardial section from an autopsy demonstrates sparse mononuclear inflammation* ➔ *in the interstitium; however, no definite myocyte damage is seen. This is at most borderline myocarditis.*

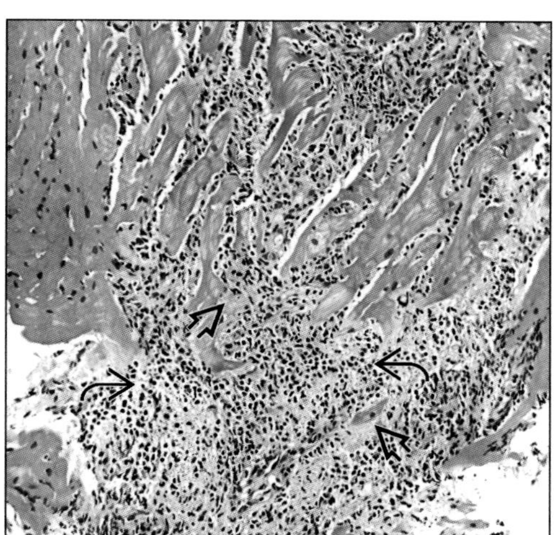

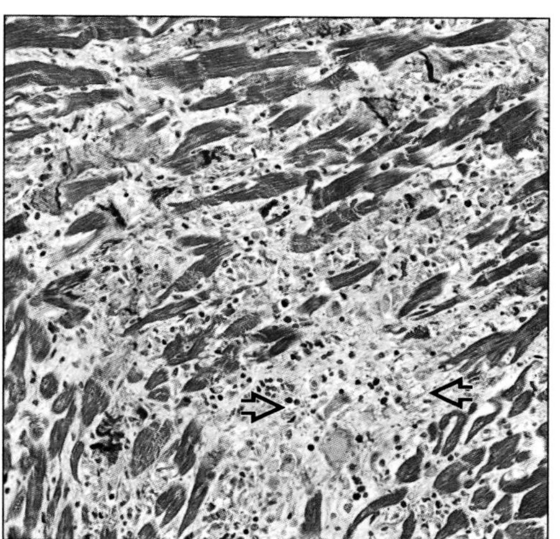

(Left) *This more fulminant example of lymphocytic myocarditis demonstrates a marked mononuclear inflammatory infiltrate* ➔ *and myocyte damage* ➔*.* ***(Right)*** *Subacutely, proliferating fibroblasts start to form areas of replacement-type fibrosis* ➔ *in place of the myocytes lost due to myocarditis.*

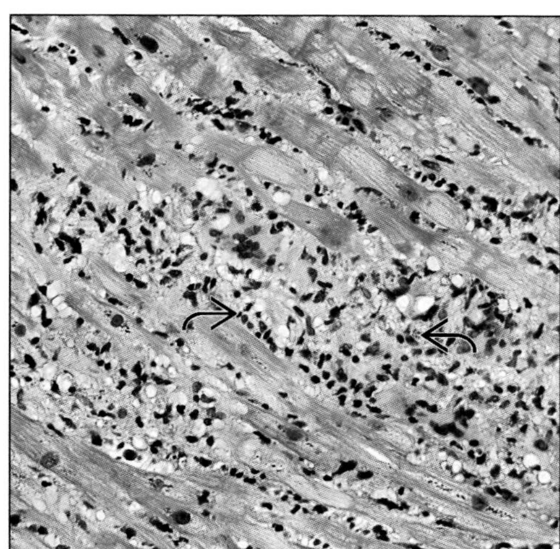

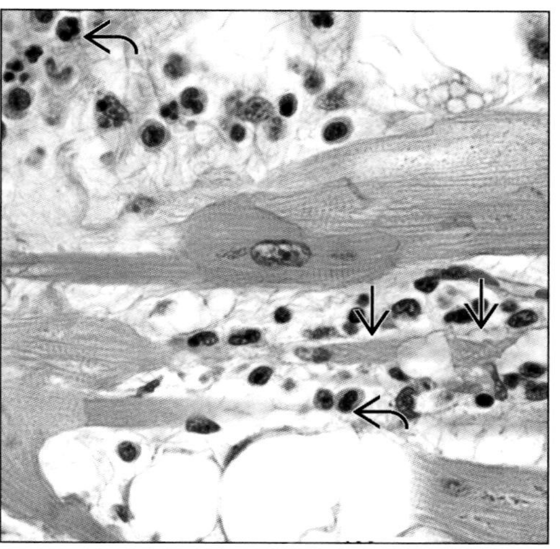

(Left) *This myocardial section demonstrates a predominantly mononuclear inflammatory infiltrate, though rare eosinophils* ➔ *are also present. Lymphocytic myocarditis can demonstrate occasional neutrophils and eosinophils.* ***(Right)*** *Myocyte damage* ➔ *can be subtle and difficult to recognize in some cases. Close inspection on high magnification is needed. This example of lymphocytic myocarditis also includes some eosinophils* ➔*.*

MYOCARDITIS

Microscopic Features

*(**Left**) This intermediate-magnification photomicrograph shows a focus of myocardial inflammation with myocyte destruction and a single multinucleated giant cell ⇾, diagnostic of giant cell myocarditis. (**Right**) This more typical view of giant cell myocarditis shows widespread destruction of myocardium with extensive mixed inflammation and singly distributed giant cells ⇾, without granuloma formation. Lymphocytic myocarditis is usually focal; giant cell myocarditis is usually diffuse.*

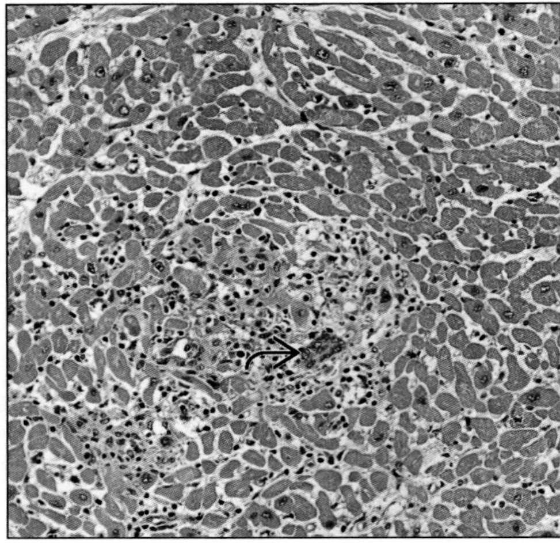

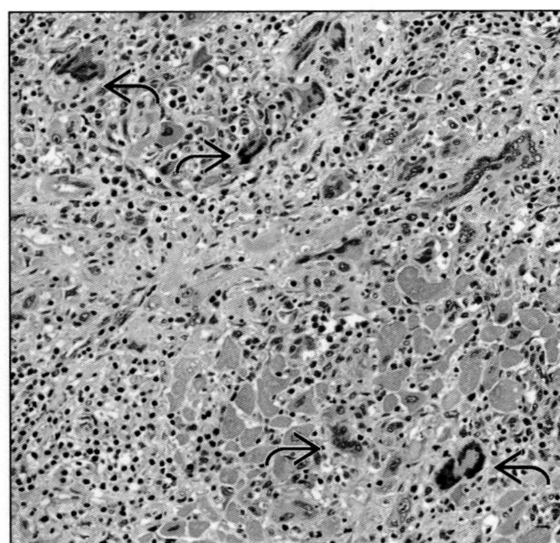

*(**Left**) This example of giant cell myocarditis shows some preserved myocardium ⇾ but otherwise extensive loss of cardiomyocytes with active myocyte damage ⇨. These myocytes are irreversibly injured, and replacement fibrosis will form in this area. (**Right**) Giant cells ⇾ may be small and inconspicuous, as seen in this high-magnification photomicrograph. Their presence is nonetheless diagnostic of giant cell myocarditis.*

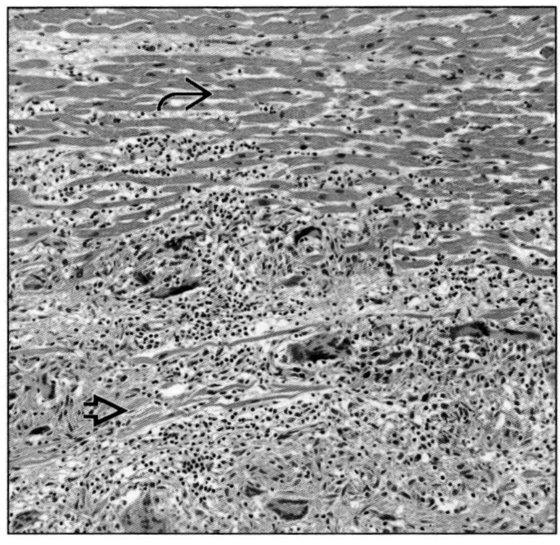

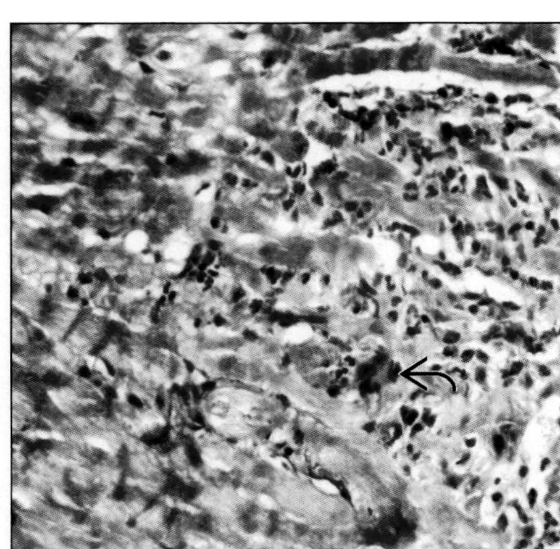

*(**Left**) In the later stages of giant cell myocarditis, extensive replacement fibrosis occurs with only rare islands of preserved (entrapped) myocytes ⇨. A single residual giant cell ⇾ indicates the type of myocarditis in this patient. Giant cell myocarditis is usually temporally uniform but may show more active areas of inflammation along with replacement fibrosis. (**Right**) This image shows healing/healed giant cell myocarditis ⇾ with entrapped preserved cardiomyocytes →.*

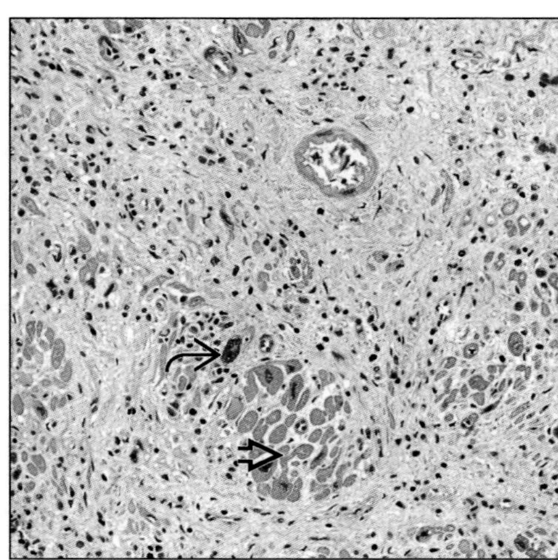

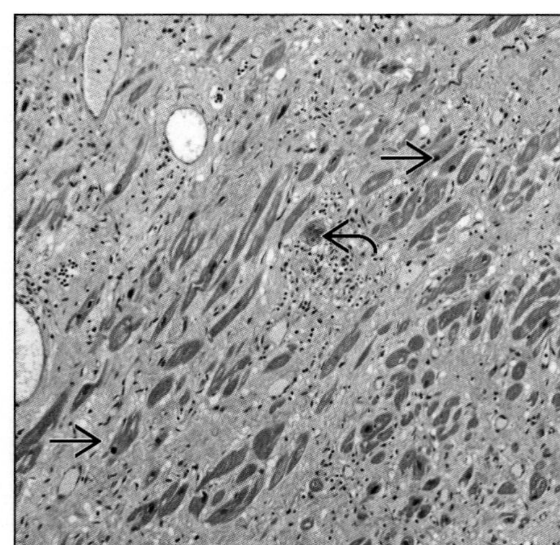

Microscopic Features

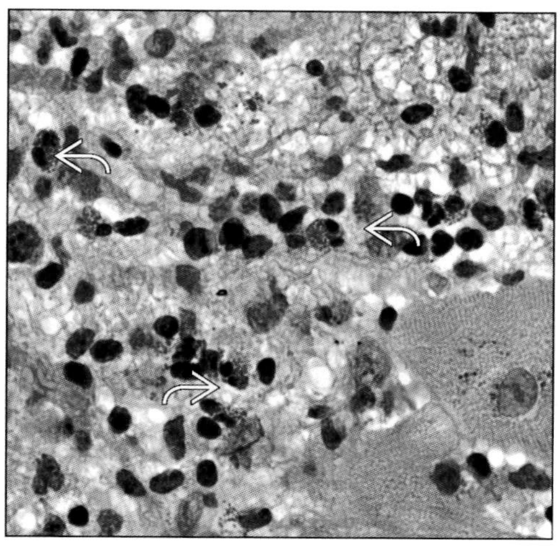

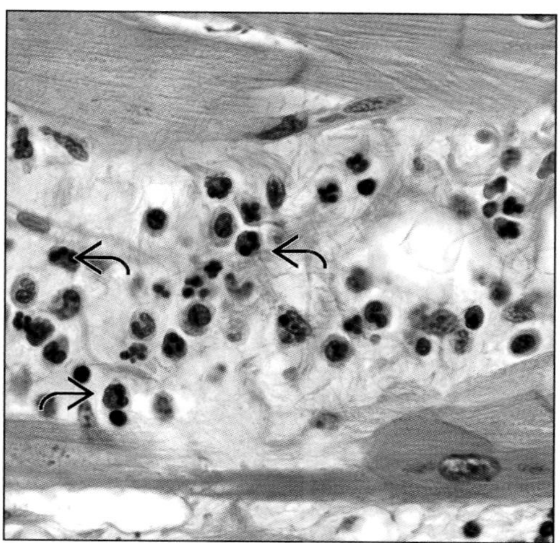

(Left) The abundance of eosinophils ➡ in this example of myocarditis is suggestive of eosinophilic myocarditis. Other inflammatory cells are present, but eosinophils at least equal the number of any other constituent inflammatory cell. (Right) While no definite myocyte damage is seen in this particular field, damage was present elsewhere. Again, eosinophils ➡ are a very prominent component of the inflammatory infiltrate.

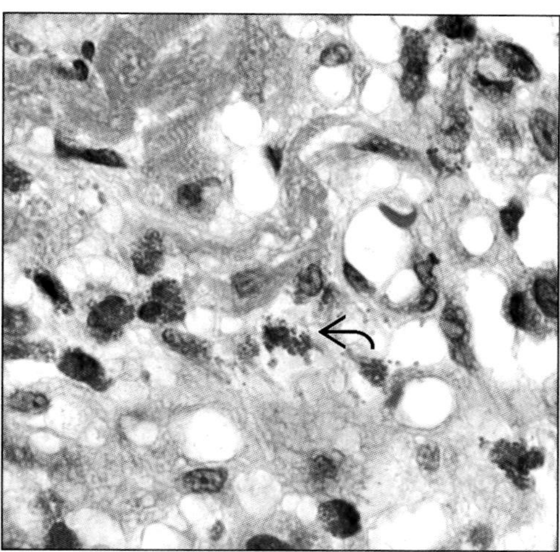

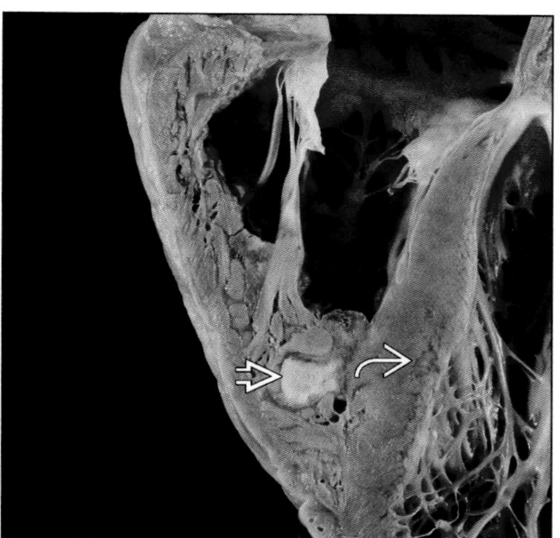

(Left) In this case of eosinophilic myocarditis, many of the eosinophils are releasing their cytoplasmic granules ➡ (degranulation). These granules contain the enzymes that damage the myocytes. (Right) This autopsy specimen from a patient with eosinophilic endomyocardial disease shows mottling of the myocardium ➡ (corresponding to eosinophilic myocarditis microscopically) and an eosinophil-rich mural thrombus in the right ventricle apex ➡.

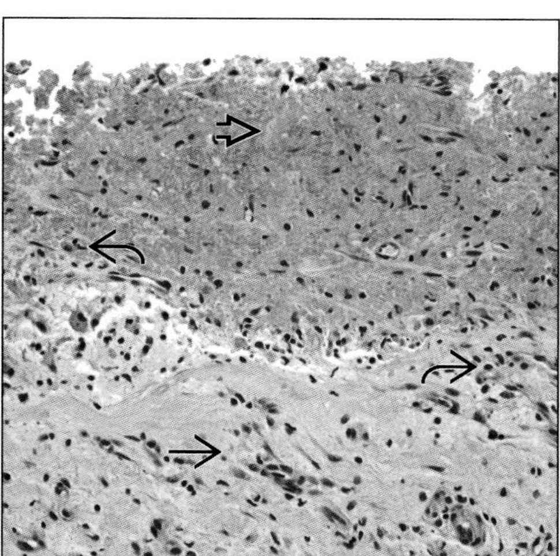

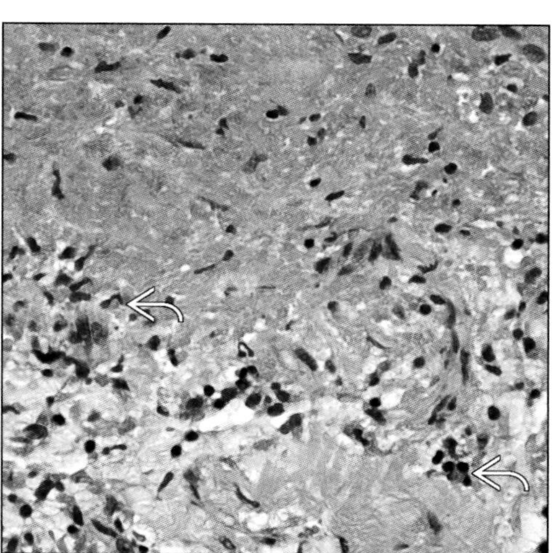

(Left) This photomicrograph shows mural thrombus with areas rich in eosinophils ➡ and progressive thrombus organization ➡ with fresh fibrin thrombus ➡ on top. (Right) The eosinophils in this clot ➡ are more difficult to recognize since many have degranulated. The characteristic bilobed nucleus can still be seen and is a helpful diagnostic clue to their identity.

CARDIAC CONDUCTION SYSTEM

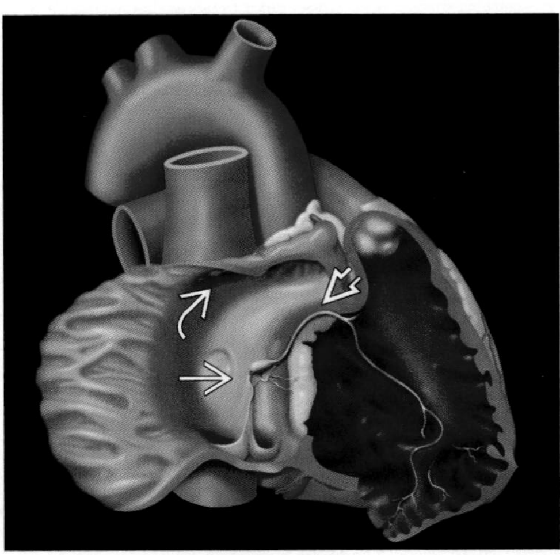

This illustration shows the approximate locations of the sinoatrial node ➔ (subepicardial), atrioventricular node ➔ (subendocardial), and His bundle ➔.

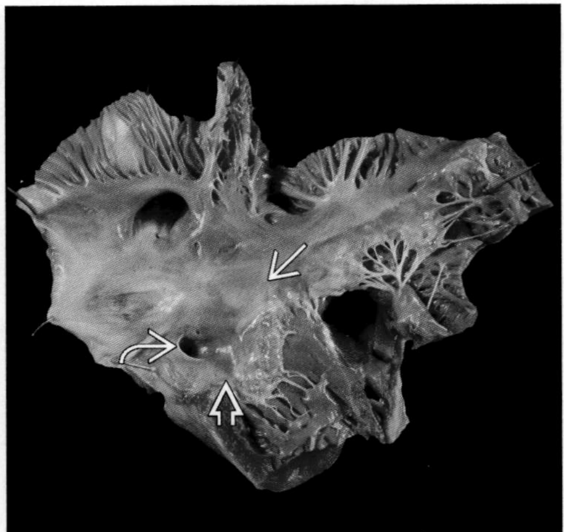

This view of the opened right heart shows the location of Koch triangle: Atrioventricular septum ➔, coronary sinus ostium ➔, and tricuspid annulus below the coronary sinus ostium ➔.

MACROSCOPIC FINDINGS

Sinoatrial (SA) Node

- Specialized "pacemaker" myocyte collection in right atrium
- Subepicardial structure near superior vena cava, overlying terminal crest (vertical crest on interior wall of right atrium that separates sinus of vena cava from rest of right atrium)
- Found at union of smooth-walled "sinus venosus" portion and trabecular portion of right atrium
- Supplied by sinus node artery (usually a branch from right coronary)

Atrioventricular (AV) Node

- Specialized conducting myocytes within tricuspid annulus near atrioventricular (membranous) septum
- Subendocardial structure found within Koch triangle, an anatomic area defined by these 3 vertices
  - Membranous septum
  - Roof of coronary sinus ostium
  - Tricuspid annulus at a point directly below coronary sinus ostium
- Supplied by AV nodal artery (usually from posterior descending artery)

MICROSCOPIC FINDINGS

SA Node

- Compact and polyhedral myocytes surrounded by dense collagenous tissue
- Sarcoplasm and cross-striations less prominent
- Sinus nodal artery courses through sinus node
- Autonomic nerve fibers and ganglia seen in vicinity
- Increased ratio of dense collagen to myocytes with increasing age reported

AV Node

- Compact "bulb" of smaller polyhedral myocytes merging with larger stellate to spindled myocytes with vacuolar sarcoplasm toward His bundle
- Mesothelial-like cells and cystic structures occasionally intermixed
- AV nodal artery courses through AV node
- Connective tissue surrounds node, "insulating" adjacent myocardium
- Autonomic nerves and lymphatics seen in vicinity
  - Rich supply of lymphatics may explain predilection for involvement in patients with sarcoidosis
  - Lymphatic drainage of endogenous toxins from distal infarcted myocardium causes "stunning" of AV node and transient heart block post myocardial infarction in some patients

His Bundle and Bundle Branches

- Constituent cells mostly smaller than myocardial myocytes and more vacuolated
- Right bundle branch is smaller and cord-like
- Left bundle branch is larger and splays out over leftward ventricular septum

Purkinje Cell

- Term applied to cells in left bundle branch and distal right bundle branch because they are larger than myocardial myocytes and have more vacuolar cytoplasm
- As with all conduction system cells, Purkinje cells are myocytes and contain myofibrils by electron microscopy
- Differ from normal cardiomyocytes by absence of T tubules and striking abundance of cell-cell junctions

Histochemical Stains

- Conduction system myocytes differ from contractile myocytes
  - Anaerobic oxidation predominates over aerobic

- Unique cholinesterases expressed in conduction system myocytes
- Abundant glycogen found in conduction system myocytes

Strategies for Processing and Examining Conduction System

- Given small size of these structures
  - It is difficult to grossly cut tissue blocks thinly enough to evaluate different segments in a single histologic section
  - Serial sectioning of paraffin blocks is necessary to identify structures and evaluate abnormalities
  - Some authors advocate exhaustive sectioning of paraffin blocks (1,200-1,600 total slides) to evaluate every conduction system cell

HISTOLOGIC PITFALLS

AV Node and Bundle Branches

- Normally occurring smooth muscle bundles in endocardium should not be mistaken for Purkinje cells or conduction system tracts

INDICATIONS FOR EXAMINATION OF CONDUCTION SYSTEM

SA Node

- Documented sinus node electrocardiographic abnormalities
  - Tachycardia-bradycardia syndrome
  - Sick sinus syndrome
  - Sinus arrest
  - **Not** atrial fibrillation or atrial flutter (in most cases, SA node is normal)
- Previous ablation procedure
- Sudden unexpected death without other cardiac cause(s) (pathologist's discretion)

AV Node

- Atrioventricular block
  - 1st degree
  - 2nd degree (Mobitz type 1 or Wenckebach type)
  - 2nd degree (Mobitz type 2)
  - 3rd degree
- Junctional arrhythmias
- Previous ablation procedure

His Bundle and Bundle Branches

- Variable, generally not indicated
- Very difficult to localize pathways of interest
- Previous ablation procedure

Preexcitation Electrocardiographic Changes

- Classic example is Wolff-Parkinson-White syndrome
- Anomalous connecting band of contractile myocardium between atria and ventricle
- Bypassing normal conduction delay coordinated in AV node
- Careful examination of entire coronary groove can be undertaken to identify a "myocardial bridge"

Transient Antemortem Conduction Disturbances

- Usually not associated with identifiable structural abnormality

MAJOR DISEASES AFFECTING CARDIAC CONDUCTION SYSTEM

Congenital Atrioventricular Block

- Usually "benign" clinically
  - Eventual pacemaker therapy
- Lack of connection to atrial myocytes
- Fatty replacement of AV nodal structures
- Fibrosis and septation (bands of fibrosis dividing nodal myocyte groups)
- Increased fibrosis of basal ventricular septal "summit"

Sarcoidosis

- Predilection for subendocardium and conduction pathways
- May relate to density of lymphatics in these areas
- Identical to sarcoidosis elsewhere
  - Nonnecrotizing granulomas
  - Fibrosis and chronic inflammation
  - Infectious causes should be excluded

Myocarditis

- Conduction disturbance may occur in acute or chronic phase
- Sinus node dysfunction usually reflect direct involvement of sinoatrial node myocytes
- AV node dysfunction
  - Direct involvement by inflammation
  - Stunning through lymphatic drainage of toxic substrates
- Can occur in all myocarditis etiologies
  - Infections (viral, bacterial, fungal)
  - Toxins (drug, chemotherapy)
  - Hypersensitivity
  - Autoimmune
- Ventricular arrhythmias also common in myocarditis
  - Foci of electrical excitability in damaged ventricular myocardium

Cystic Tumor of AV Node

- Biologically indolent
  - Slow growing
  - Never metastasizes
- May replace AV node entirely
- Wide age range at presentation
  - Diverse electrocardiogram manifestations
    - AV block (narrow QRS on EKG)
    - Ventricular arrhythmias (wide QRS on EKG)
  - Sudden death may be presenting sign
- Histopathology
  - Variably sized epithelial-lined cysts
  - Cyst lining ranging from squamoid (stratified) to simple cuboidal
  - Fibroblastic stroma and hemorrhage surrounding cysts
  - Often grossly inapparent

CARDIAC CONDUCTION SYSTEM

Lenègre Disease

- Idiopathic fibrosis of AV node
- Heritable component
- Several genes implicated
  - Cardiac morphogenesis
  - Cardiac structural proteins
  - Cardiac ion channels
- Histopathology
  - Fibrotic replacement, septation
  - Fatty infiltrate
  - Sparse inflammation in some cases

Others

- Amyloid
- Ischemic heart disease
  - SA nodal artery is typically a primary branch of the proximal right coronary artery
  - RCA territory infarction may be associated with direct AV node ischemic injury
  - Left bundle branches are most vulnerable in septal wall infarction
  - Chronic ischemia to nodal areas may result in increased fibrosis
- Metastasis
  - Any primary site possible
  - Disseminated lymphoma also reported

PATHOLOGY OF ENDOVASCULAR ABLATION PROCEDURES FOR ARRHYTHMIAS

Technical Aspects

- Increasingly common due to improved imaging guidance and catheter-based mapping and energy delivery
- Radiofrequency and high-frequency ultrasound energy
- Controlled "dose" delivery
- Catheter tip irrigation to limit scatter and improve precision

MR Mapping

- Used at some centers

3D Endovascular Electrophysiologic Mapping

- Used to identify target areas

Complications

- Possible injury to phrenic nerve, esophageal wall (in pulmonary vein isolation procedures)

Histopathologic Changes

- Acute
  - Cautery-like thermal injury
  - Infarct-like myocyte damage, edema, hemorrhage, with distinct borders
  - Influx of neutrophils
- Chronic
  - Discrete "punched out" areas of dense collagenous replacement fibrosis
  - Sharp interface with surrounding normal myocardium
  - Occasional mesenchymal heterotopia (chondroid, osseous)

SELECTED REFERENCES

1. Jongbloed MR et al: Normal and abnormal development of the cardiac conduction system; implications for conduction and rhythm disorders in the child and adult. Differentiation. 84(1):131-48, 2012
2. Arbustini E et al: Autosomal dominant dilated cardiomyopathy with atrioventricular block: a lamin A/C defect-related disease. J Am Coll Cardiol. 39(6):981-90, 2002
3. Wang JN et al: Complete atrioventricular block following myocarditis in children. Pediatr Cardiol. 23(5):518-21, 2002
4. Gollob MH et al: Identification of a gene responsible for familial Wolff-Parkinson-White syndrome. N Engl J Med. 344(24):1823-31, 2001
5. Tan HL et al: A sodium-channel mutation causes isolated cardiac conduction disease. Nature. 409(6823):1043-7, 2001
6. McGuire MA et al: Atrioventricular junctional tissue. Discrepancy between histological and electrophysiological characteristics. Circulation. 94(3):571-7, 1996
7. Bharati S et al: Cardiac conduction system involvement in sudden death of obese young people. Am Heart J. 129(2):273-81, 1995
8. Michaëlsson M et al: Isolated congenital complete atrioventricular block in adult life. A prospective study. Circulation. 92(3):442-9, 1995
9. Bharati S et al: The conduction system findings in sudden cardiac death. J Cardiovasc Electrophysiol. 5(4):356-66, 1994
10. Gamache MC et al: Histopathological study following catheter guided radiofrequency current ablation of the slow pathway in a patient with atrioventricular nodal reentrant tachycardia. Pacing Clin Electrophysiol. 17(2):247-51, 1994
11. James TN: Congenital disorders of cardiac rhythm and conduction. J Cardiovasc Electrophysiol. 4(6):702-18, 1993
12. Bharati S et al: The conduction system in transplanted hearts. Chest. 102(4):1182-8, 1992
13. Kurosawa H et al: The conduction bundle at the atrioventricular junction. An anatomical study. Eur J Cardiothorac Surg. 3(4):283-7, 1989
14. Carter JB et al: Congenital heart block. Anatomic correlations and review of the literature. Arch Pathol. 97(1):51-7, 1974
15. Lev M et al: The pathogenesis of atrioventricular block in coronary disease. Circulation. 42(3):409-25, 1970
16. Lev M: The pathology of complete atrioventricular block. Prog Cardiovasc Dis. 6:317-26, 1964

Gross and Microscopic Features

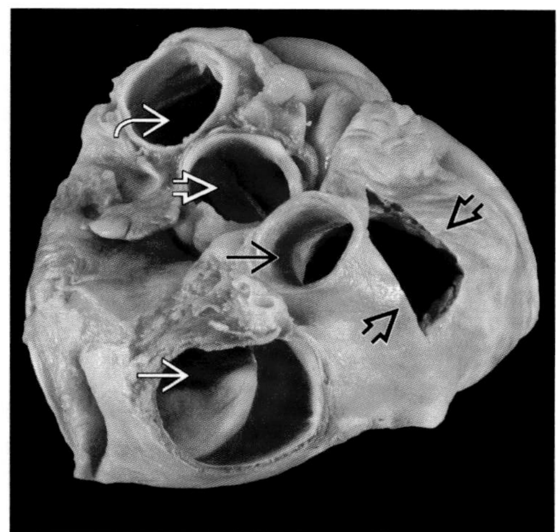

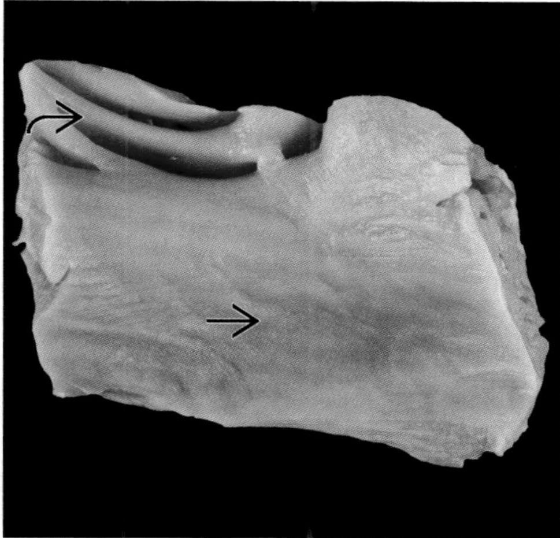

*(**Left**) This superior view of the heart shows the location of the tissue block removed for examination of the sinoatrial node ⇨. The pulmonary artery ➡, aorta ➡, superior vena cava →, and left atrium ➡ are labeled for orientation. (**Right**) Viewed from the endocardial aspect, this sinoatrial node tissue block consists of a portion of terminal crest → with a few pectinate muscles ↱ attached. The overlying epicardium (not seen, facing down) is intact.*

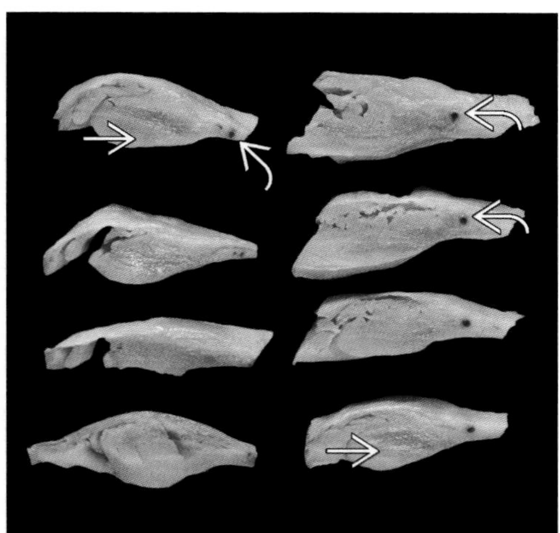

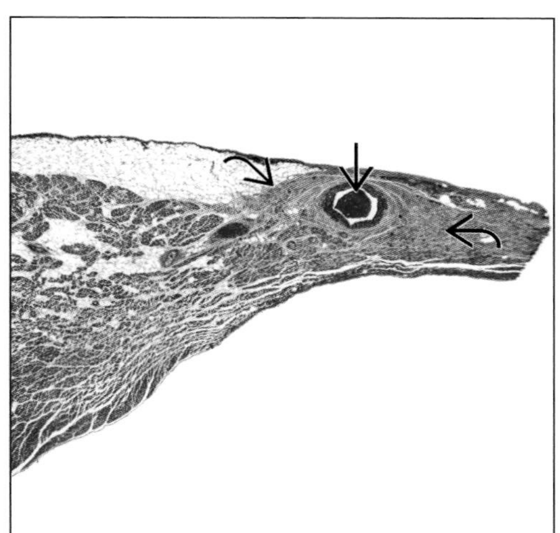

*(**Left**) After serial sectioning the tissue block, the belly of the terminal crest ➡ is now seen in cross section in each piece. The pinpoint sinus nodal artery ➡ can also be seen in many of the sections, identifying the location of the sinoatrial node. (**Right**) This cross section illustrates the dense connective tissue-rich sinoatrial node tissue ↱ surrounding the sinus node artery →.*

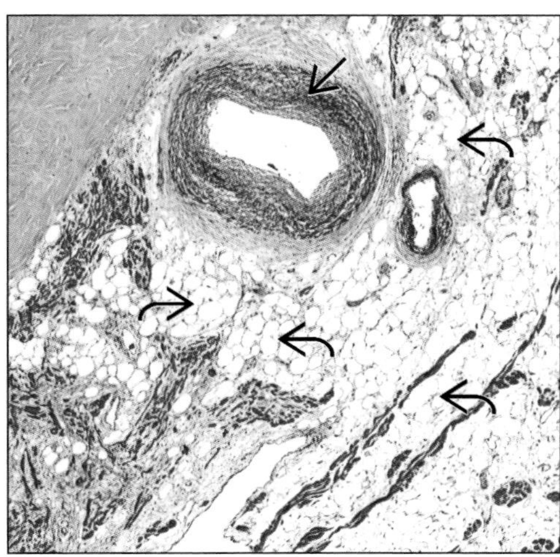

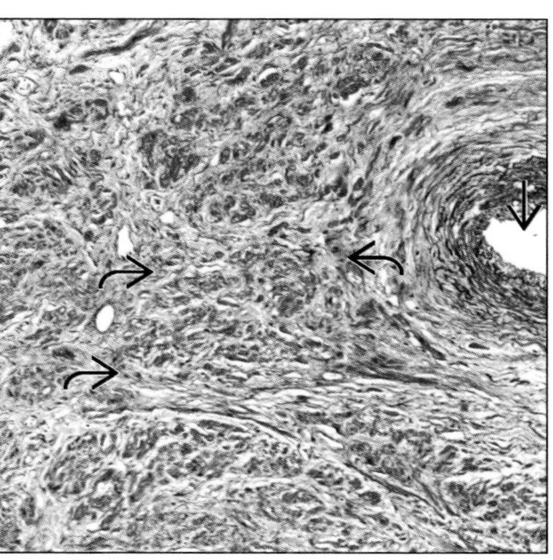

*(**Left**) This sinoatrial node from a 52-year-old man with sinus node dysfunction shows prominent fatty infiltration ↱ of the sinoatrial node. The sinus node artery is otherwise normal →. (**Right**) This sinoatrial node from a patient with sick sinus syndrome shows increased interstitial fibrosis (blue green) ↱ within the sinoatrial node. The sinus node artery is otherwise normal →. Clinical-pathologic correlation is essential in such cases.*

Gross and Microscopic Features

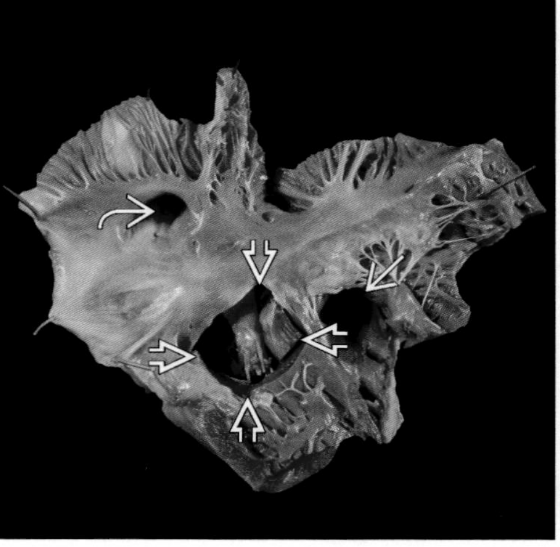

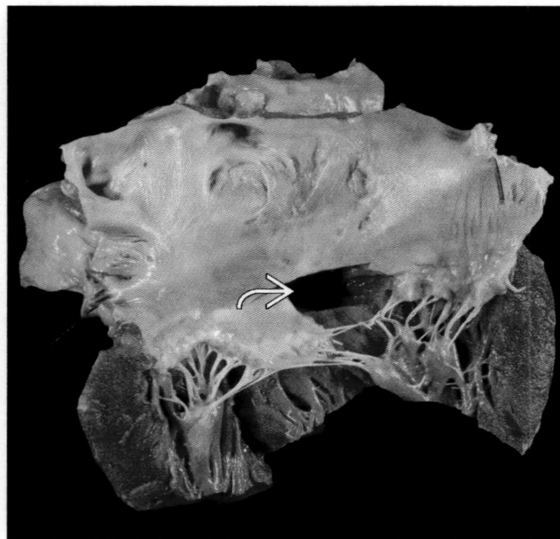

(Left) *This view of the opened right heart shows the defect ➡ after removing the tissue block containing the AV node (inside Koch triangle). The superior vena cava ➡ and pulmonary outflow tract ➡ are labeled for orientation.* ***(Right)*** *This view of the opened left heart demonstrates that the excised tissue block ➡ also includes a portion of anterior mitral valve leaflet (and aorto-mitral fibrous continuity).*

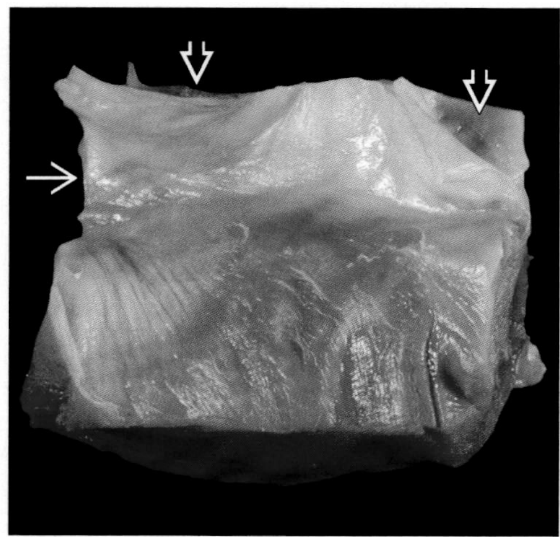

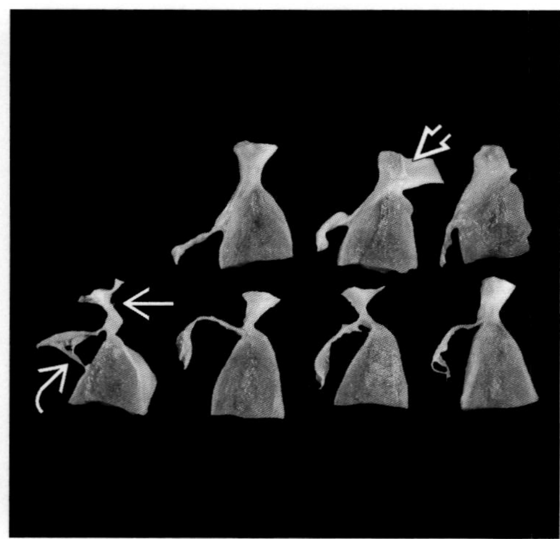

(Left) *The left-facing aspect of the AV node tissue block is shown here, with membranous septum ➡ and pockets of 2 aortic valve cusps ➡ labeled for orientation.* ***(Right)*** *Serial cross sections through the excised AV node tissue block illustrate portions of tricuspid valve leaflet ➡, membranous (atrioventricular) septum ➡, and aortic valve cusp ➡. Occasionally, the AV nodal artery may be seen grossly in the tricuspid annular fibrosa (not seen here).*

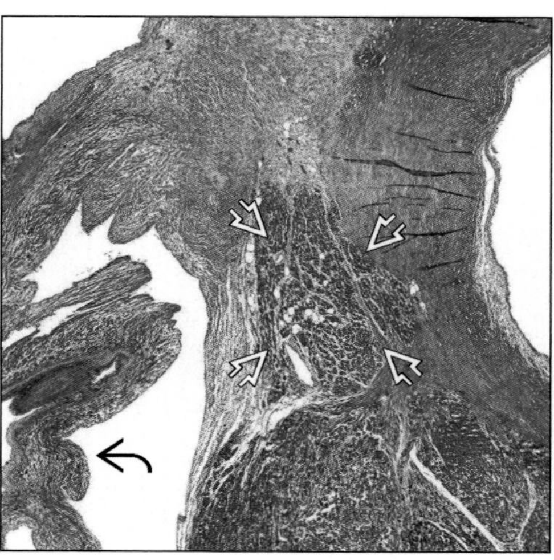

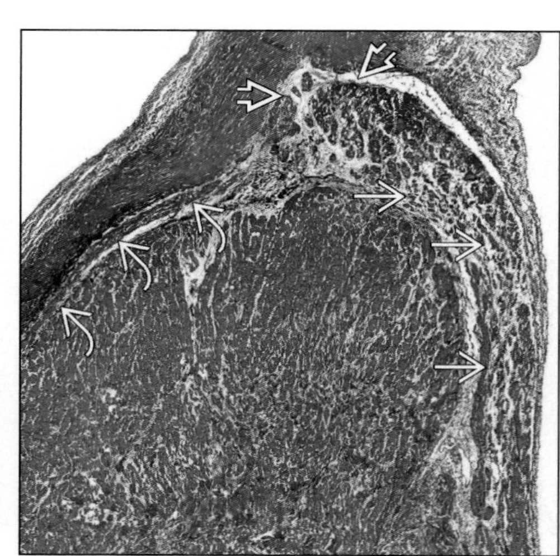

(Left) *The proximal bulbar portion of the atrioventricular node ➡ is shown here, seated within the annular fibrosa and insulated from the myocardium proper by dense collagen (blue). A portion of tricuspid valve leaflet ➡ is shown for orientation.* ***(Right)*** *This image shows the more distal bundle branches straddling the septal myocardium. The branches emanate from the His bundle ➡. The right bundle ➡ is thin and cord-like. The left bundle ➡ is typically thicker and splays widely across the septum.*

Gross and Microscopic Features

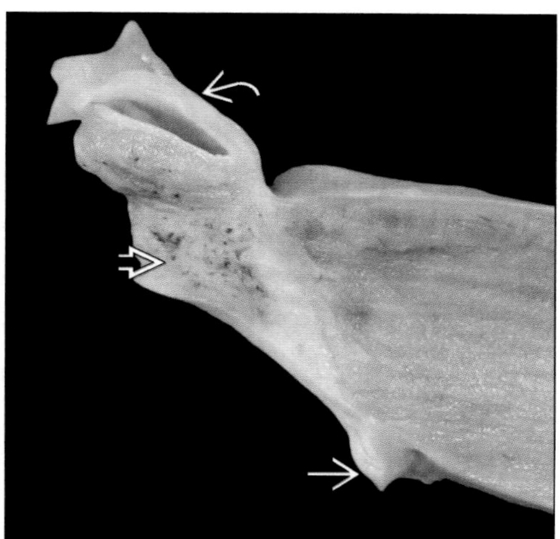

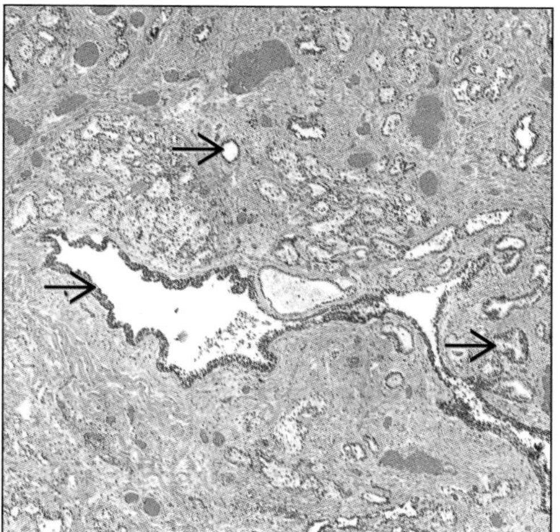

(Left) *This AV node tissue block section from a sudden cardiac death autopsy shows a grossly variegated, ill-defined mass lesion* ➲ *in the vicinity of the AV node. The aortic valve* ➲ *and tricuspid valve leaflets* ➲ *are labeled for orientation.* ***(Right)*** *Histologically, this mass shows multiple cystic structures* → *lined by squamoid to cuboidal epithelium, features diagnostic of cystic tumor of the atrioventricular node.*

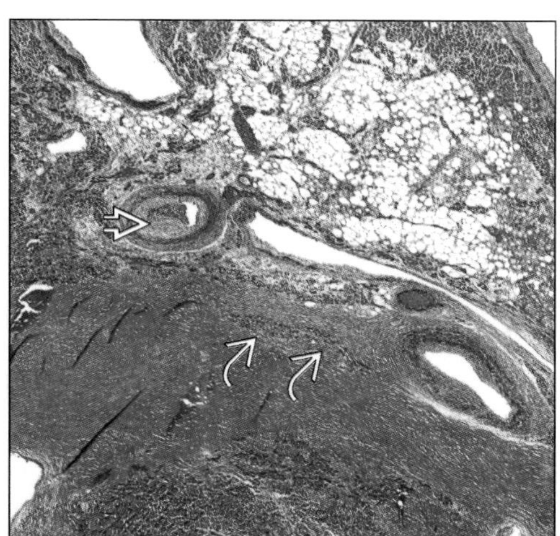

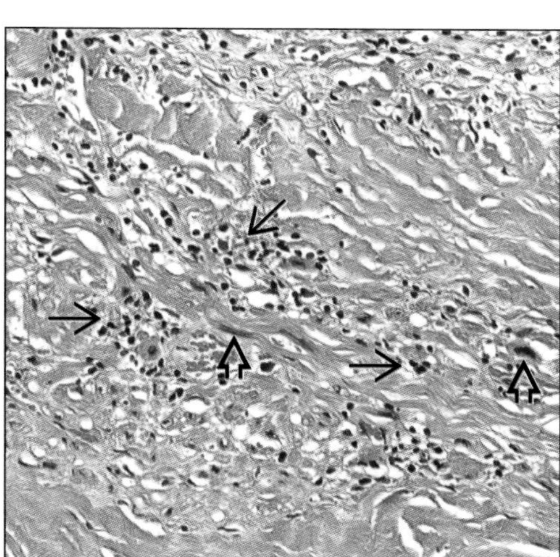

(Left) *This AV node section from cardiac allograft in a patient with Mobitz type 2 heart block shows cardiac allograft vasculopathy affecting the AV nodal artery* ➲ *and mononuclear inflammation associated with the AV node myocytes* ➲. ***(Right)*** *This higher magnification view from the heart shows a mix of mononuclear cells* → *with apparent injury to the AV nodal myocytes* ➲.

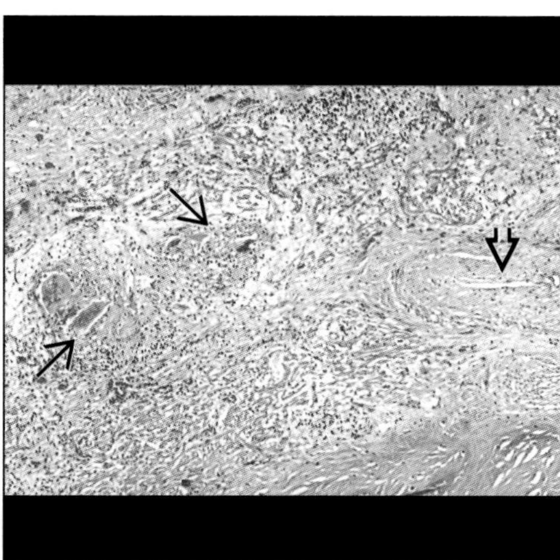

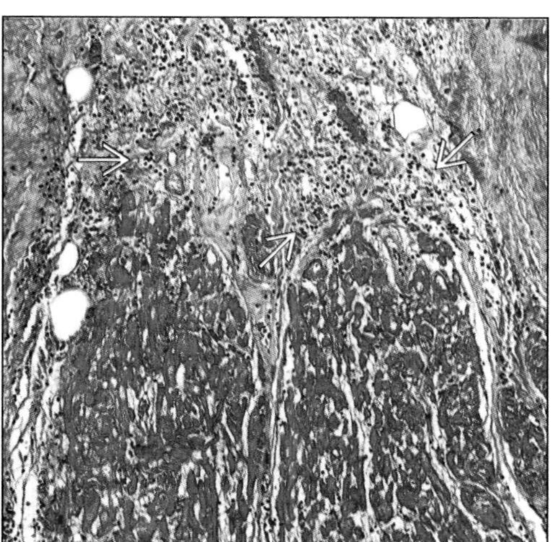

(Left) *This AV node section shows involvement by nonnecrotizing granulomatous inflammation* →*, consistent with sarcoidosis. The AV nodal artery* ➲ *is shown for orientation.* ***(Right)*** *This image shows acute lymphocytic myocarditis* ➲ *involving the superior portion of the bulbar atrioventricular node. In addition to systolic heart failure, the patient developed AV block.*

AORTIC DISSECTION

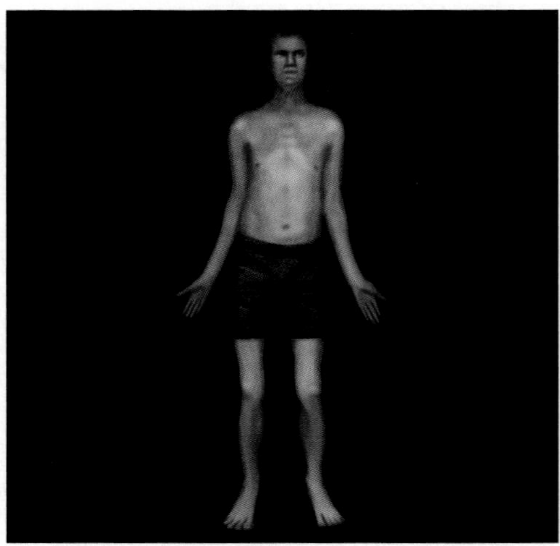

The Marfan syndrome phenotype includes a long thin body habitus with long limbs compared to trunk, long fingers (arachnodactyly), pectus excavatum, and scoliosis.

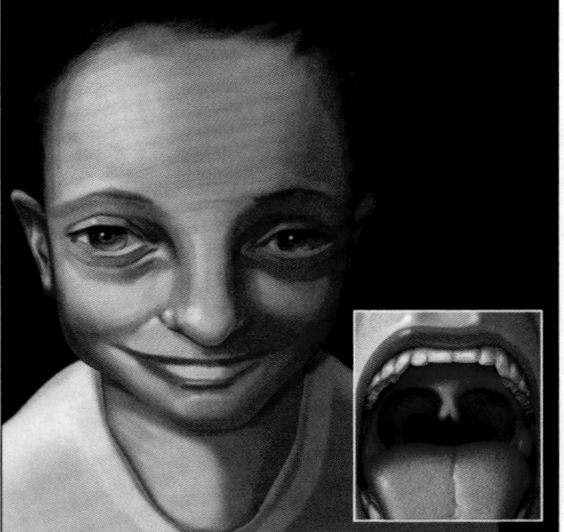

In Loeys-Dietz syndrome type 1, the phenotype includes hypertelorism (wide-set eyes) cleft palate/bifid uvula, and craniosynostosis. There is also overlap with Marfan phenotype.

TERMINOLOGY

Synonyms

- Dissecting aneurysm, dissecting hematoma

Definitions

- Presence of blood within media of aorta

ETIOLOGY/PATHOGENESIS

Hypertension

- Medial degenerative change (pressure and ischemia related)

Inherited or Acquired Connective Tissue Disorders

- Fibrillin 1 (*FBN1*) gene mutation: Marfan syndrome type 1
- *TGFB* receptor gene mutations: Marfan syndrome type 2 (classic Marfan phenotype with *TGFBR2* mutation), Loeys-Dietz (*TGFBR1* and *TGFBR2*)
- Various gene mutations (*FBN1*, *TGFBR1*, and *TGFBR2*) familial thoracic aortic aneurysm/dissection
  - Hereditary syndromes and nonsyndromic hereditary disorders of connective tissue
    - Marfan syndrome, Loeys-Dietz syndrome (types 1 and 2), vascular Ehlers-Danlos syndrome, familial thoracic aortic aneurysm syndrome, autosomal dominant polycystic kidney disease
    - Bicuspid aortic valve (2% of population, M > F); 5% develop dissection
  - Congenital diseases/syndromes
    - Turner syndrome, aortic coarctation, tetralogy of Fallot
  - Acquired disorders of connective tissue
    - Vitamin C deficiency, copper metabolism defects
  - Iatrogenic
    - Complication of cardiac surgery or cardiac catheterization and intraaortic balloon pump insertion
  - Trauma
    - Blunt trauma to thorax (vehicular accident) rarely causes dissection, most often full or partial rupture
  - Pregnancy (late) or puerperium (rare)

CLINICAL ISSUES

Epidemiology

- Incidence
  - ~ 2,000 cases per year in USA
- Age
  - Usually older (> 60 years)
  - If younger, ↑ suspicion for syndromic or nonsyndromic connective tissue disorder
- Gender
  - M > F (2-3:1)
- Risk factors
  - Hypertension, especially in older men

Presentation

- Clinical chart review
  - Presence of risk factors, family history
- Symptoms may be variable
  - Acute aortic syndrome (pain related to disruption of aortic media)
  - Obstruction of major branch vessels (MI, stroke, mesenteric angina)
  - Aortic valve insufficiency (acute aortic insufficiency, congestive heart failure,shock)
  - Rupture (cardiac tamponade, hypovolemic shock, hemothorax/peritoneum, retroperitoneal hematoma)

Laboratory Tests

- Hemoglobin and hematocrit
  - Expect decrease but may be normal in very acute blood loss without volume replacement

AORTIC DISSECTION

Key Facts

Clinical Issues

- If younger, ↑ suspicion for syndromic or nonsyndromic connective tissue disorder

Imaging Findings

- Widening of aortic silhouette or abnormal aortic contour on chest radiograph
- May be normal in 12-15% of patients with aortic dissection

Macroscopic Pathology

- Marfan syndrome: Thin habitus, long limbs (arm span > height), long digits (arachnodactyly)
- Loeys Dietz: Marfan features plus craniofacial abnormalities: Craniosynostosis, hypertelorism, bifid uvula &/or cleft palate
- Loeys-Dietz syndrome: Type 2 overlaps with vascular Ehlers-Danlos syndrome and Marfan syndrome
    - Fewer craniofacial abnormalities (only bifid uvula), pectus, joint laxity and arachnodactyly but no marfanoid body habitus, easy bruising (may see bruises), soft velvety translucent skin
- Vascular Ehlers-Danlos syndrome: Fewer overall physical findings; small joints with mild hypermobility, soft velvety translucent skin and easy bruising (may see bruises on body)
- Turner syndrome: Short stature, shield-like chest, webbed neck, short 4th metacarpal

IMAGE FINDINGS

Radiographic Findings

- Widening of aortic silhouette or abnormal aortic contour on chest radiograph
    - May be normal in 12-15% of patients with aortic dissection

CT Findings

- CT more sensitive for detection of dissection

MACROSCOPIC FEATURES

External Examination

- Pallor, body habitus suggesting underlying syndromic connective tissue disorder
    - Marfan syndrome: Thin habitus, long limbs (arm span > height), and long digits (arachnodactyly) are classic
        - Pectus excavatum (caved in or concave appearance of anterior chest wall), scoliosis, highly arched palate with crowding of teeth, and occasional skin striae and joint laxity may also be seen
    - Loeys-Dietz syndrome: Type 1 overlaps with Marfan syndrome with exceptions
        - Craniofacial abnormalities: Craniosynostosis, hypertelorism, bifid uvula &/or cleft palate
    - Loeys-Dietz syndrome: Type 2 overlaps with vascular Ehlers-Danlos syndrome and Marfan syndrome
        - Fewer craniofacial abnormalities (only bifid uvula), pectus, joint laxity and arachnodactyly but no Marfanoid body habitus, easy bruising (may see bruises), soft velvety translucent skin
    - Vascular Ehlers-Danlos syndrome: Fewer overall physical findings; small joints with mild hypermobility, soft velvety translucent skin and easy bruising (may see bruises on body)
    - Turner syndrome: Short stature, shield-like chest, webbed neck, short 4th metacarpal
- Medical/surgical intervention
    - Incision from operative or other invasive intervention that lead to or was in response to dissection
        - Sternotomy incisions, catheterization sites, abdominal incisions, etc.

Internal Examination

- Hemopericardium (blue appearance to unopened pericardium), hemothorax (usually left-sided), hemoperitoneum, retroperitoneal hematoma
    - Measure amount of blood in any individual cavity
    - Classic signs of hypovolemic shock occur with loss of 30-40% of blood volume (~ 1,500-2,000 cc)
        - Normal adult blood volume ~ 77mL/kg, with ↑ BMI and age it decreases

Organ Examination

- Aorta and aortic valve
    - Remove aorta and heart together, attached, and keep at least 0.5 cm of major branch vessels
    - Since most intimal tears are proximal, begin opening aorta distally and along posterior surface
    - Examine intima as aorta is opened to identify area of intimal tear
        - Most intimal tears within first 10 cm of aortic valve
        - Look for distal aortic intimal tear (double-barrel aorta)
    - Describe extent of dissection (proximal aorta, proximal and distal, distal aorta)
        - Type A: Ascending or ascending and descending aorta
        - Type B: Distal aorta without proximal involvement
    - Examine closed aortic valve from outflow (aortic) surface for absence of coaptation of leaflets (aortic insufficiency)
        - Assess for presence of bicuspid aortic valve: Fused cusp (usually right and left cusps fused, also called anterior fusion)
    - Measure ascending aorta and aortic valve circumference

AORTIC DISSECTION

- Check major branch vessels along route of dissection (coronary, carotid, subclavian, etc.) for involvement by dissection and presence of luminal obstruction
- Identify site of rupture if present
- Section through intimal tear, intramural hematoma, involved branch vessels, and noninvolved aorta
- Operative repair changes
  - Ascending aortic grafts ± aortic valve replacement/repair, coronary reimplantation or bypass
- Heart
  - Examine coronary arteries and interatrial septum closely for evidence of proximal extension of dissection
    - Right coronary artery involved more frequently than left coronary artery
  - Check for gross evidence of myocardial ischemia, myocardial hypertrophy (heart weight, LV wall thickness)
    - Subendocardial sampling (and papillary muscles): Area at highest risk for ischemia
  - Congenital heart disease (unusual in adult)
    - Tetralogy of Fallot (right ventricular hypertrophy, infundibular stenosis, ventricular septal defect, overriding aorta)
    - Aortic coarctation (narrowing of aortic lumen usually in region of ductus arteriosus [ligamentum arteriosum]) may be seen independently or in Turner syndrome
- Kidneys
  - Cortical pallor, infarct if dissection extends to renal artery
  - Granular pitting of cortical surface, ↓ size due to hypertension
- Gastrointestinal tract
  - Grossly examine for areas of ischemia especially "watershed areas" in transverse colon and splenic flexure
  - Infarct due to direct involvement of mesenteric artery by dissection
- CNS
  - Infarction related to obstruction of major vessels, lacunar infarcts from longstanding hypertension
    - Lacunar infarcts are small cystic areas in basal ganglia, subcortical white matter, and pons

MICROSCOPIC PATHOLOGY

Histologic Features

- Aorta
  - Intramural hematoma in media between inner 2/3 and outer 1/3; may show organization and neointima over time
  - Noninvolved aorta with varying degrees of medial degeneration, with cystic medial degeneration being most severe
    - Cystic medial degeneration: Fragmentation of elastic lamellae with formation of cystic spaces that are rich in mucopolysaccharides
- Aortic valve
  - May show myxoid changes
- Heart
  - Enlarged myocyte nuclei (hypertrophy) and perivascular fibrosis (hypertension changes)
  - Diffuse subendocardial coagulative myocyte necrosis (ischemia due to global hypoperfusion)
    - Due to hemorrhagic complication of dissection
  - Coagulative myocyte necrosis in territory of involved vessel
    - Due to involvement of coronary artery by dissection
- Kidneys
  - Hyaline arteriolosclerosis, small cortical scars, arterial sclerosis (hypertensive changes)
  - Coagulative necrosis (infarct)
- Gastrointestinal tract
  - Coagulative necrosis of epithelium, fibrin thrombi in submucosal vessels (ischemic injury)
- CNS
  - Hypertensive arteriolosclerosis, lacunar infarcts (small: < 15 mm) subcortical (basal ganglia, thalamus, pons, internal capsule) infarcts due to arterial sclerosis of single branch of a deep penetrating artery, cerebral hemorrhage
  - Due to dissection: Cerebral infarction in territory of an involved artery

ANCILLARY TESTS

Histochemistry

- Elastic Van Gieson: Highlights disruption of elastic lamellae and areas of cystic medial degeneration
- Alcian Blue pH 2.5 highlights acid mucopolysaccharides in areas of cystic medial degeneration

REPORTING CRITERIA

Final Report

- Document type of dissection (type A or B ± proximal aortic involvement), site of intimal tear, site of rupture and amount of hemorrhage, involvement of major branches and associated complications, any surgical interventions
- Underlying risk factors for aortic dissection
  - If considered to be possible hereditary syndrome, recommend follow-up evaluation for immediate family

SELECTED REFERENCES

1. Pyeritz RE: Heritable thoracic aortic disorders. Curr Opin Cardiol. 29(1):97-102, 2014
2. Van Laer L et al: Loeys-Dietz syndrome. Adv Exp Med Biol. 802:95-105, 2014

Gross Features

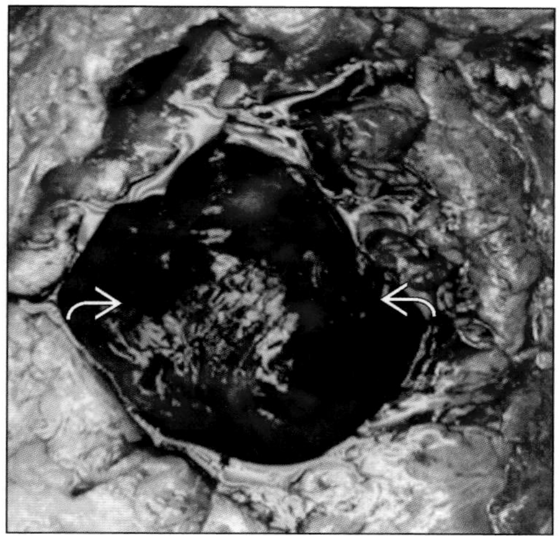

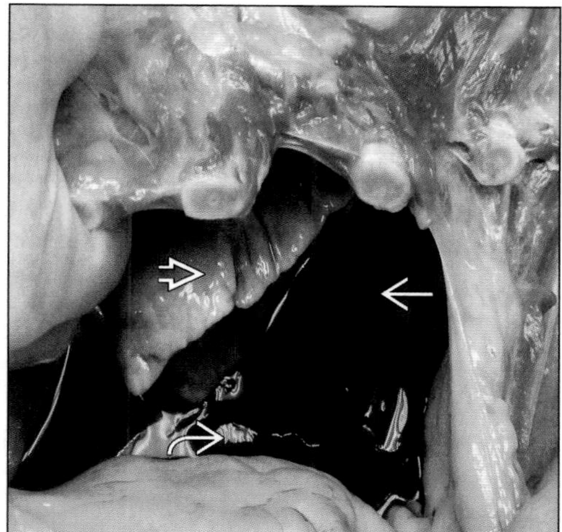

(Left) This hemopericardium with liquid and clotted blood ➔ surrounding the heart was noted in a case of aortic dissection with proximal rupture and clinical cardiac tamponade. (Right) There is liquid blood ➔ and blood clot ➔ in this left pleural cavity associated with compression of the left lung ➔, due to rupture of an aortic dissection. (From DP: Cardiovascular.)

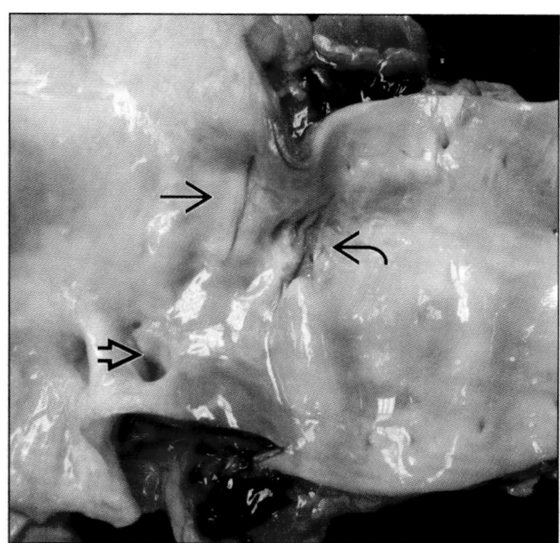

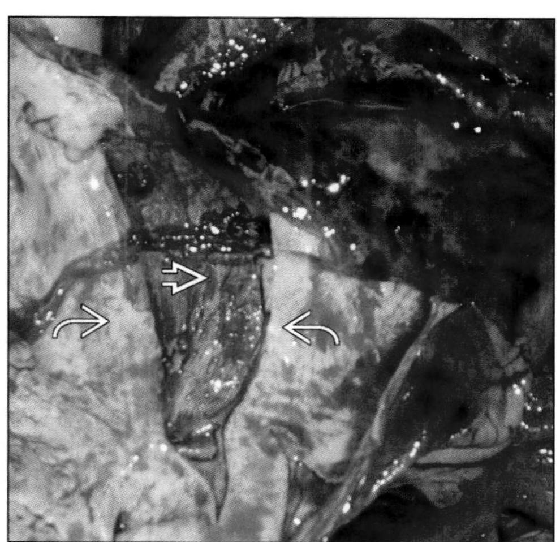

(Left) In this aorta, there were 2 intimal tears distal to the subclavian ostium ➔. One tear ➔ extended proximally into an aortic dissection. The other tear ➔ did not progress. (Right) In this aortic dissection there was a very large (almost circumferential) intimal tear in the proximal aorta ➔. The outer tissue present between the edges of the tear represents the outer aspect of the dissection ➔.

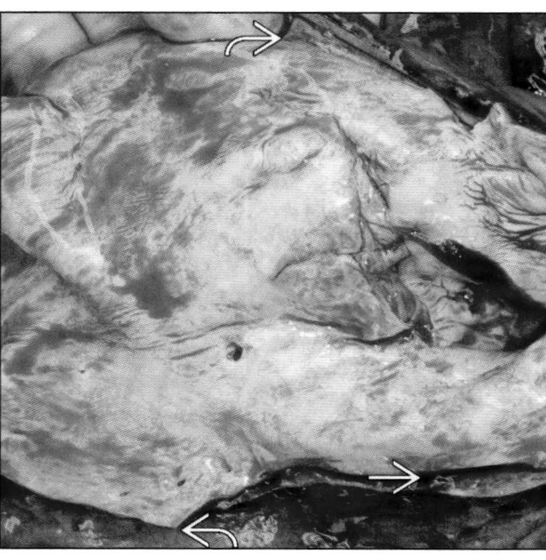

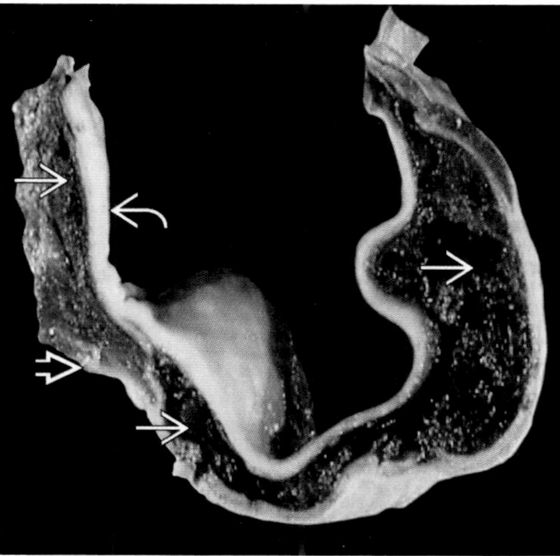

(Left) This ascending aorta with dissection ➔ is markedly dilatated ➔, a risk factor for dissection. (Right) This cross section through an aortic dissection shows medial blood clot ➔ located between the thicker inner ➔ and thinner outer ➔ portions of the media. (From DP: Cardiovascular.)

AORTIC DISSECTION

Aortic Dissection Extension and Risk Factors

*(**Left**) The probe ➔ in this aorta extends distally from an intimal tear within the false lumen of a dissection that involved the entire distal aorta to the iliac arteries. (**Right**) There was involvement of the left renal artery in this aortic dissection ➔ with an intimal flap ➔ from the left renal artery protruding into the lumen of the aorta.*

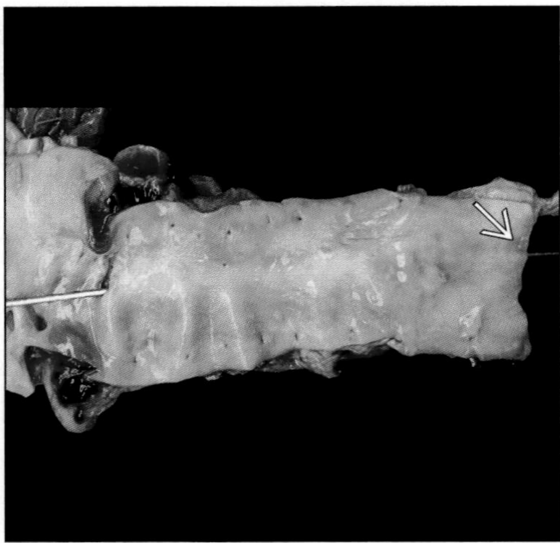

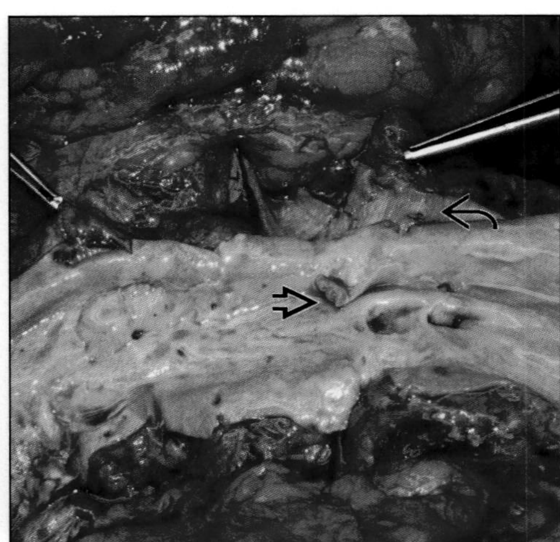

*(**Left**) This dissection highlights a bicuspid aortic valve that is viewed from the outflow (aortic) surface (abnormal cusp ➔) and cross sections through the associated aortic dissection (false lumen ➔). Of patients with bicuspid aortic valve, 5% will develop aortic dissection. (**Right**) A probe highlights the luminal narrowing in a resected segment of aorta with aortic coarctation. The intima is thickened and wrinkled ➔, and the wall is thick ➔.*

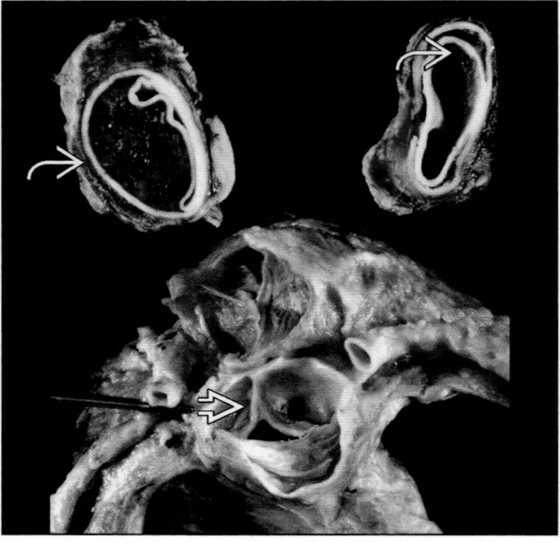

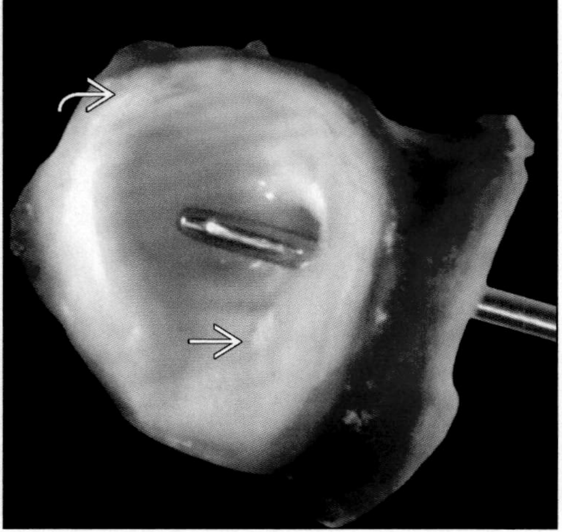

*(**Left**) This heart demonstrates concentric hypertrophy with left ventricular wall thickening ➔, as is often seen in hypertensive patients with aortic dissection. In addition, subendocardial infarction is present ➔, as may be seen in hypovolemic shock after rupture of an aortic dissection. (**Right**) Hypertensive renal changes such as nephrosclerosis are common in patients with aortic dissection. This kidney demonstrates the granular cortical surface seen in nephrosclerosis.*

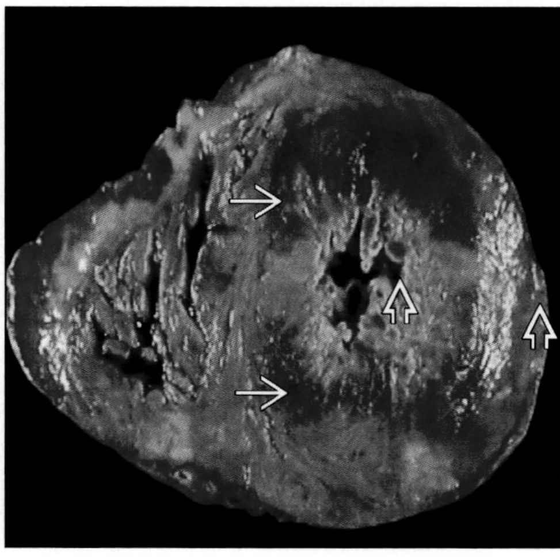

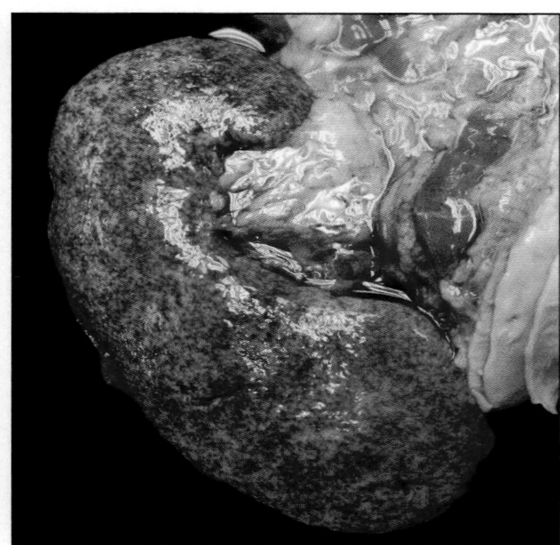

Operative Intervention and Microscopic Features

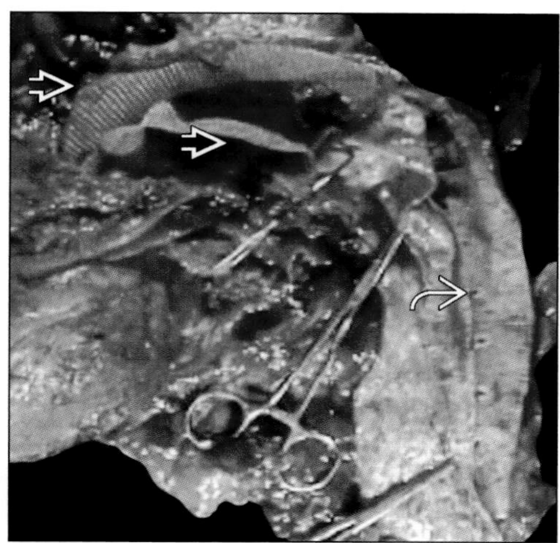

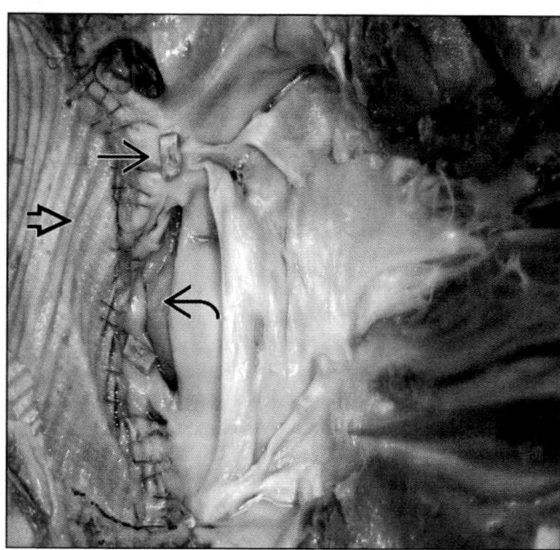

(Left) *This heart and thoracic aorta specimen shows surgical replacement of the ascending aorta with a Dacron graft ➨. There is also dissection of the descending thoracic aorta with a false lumen evident ➨. (From DP: Cardiovascular.)* ***(Right)*** *This is an example of an ascending aorta repair with a Dacron graft ➨; the intimal tear can be seen proximal to the graft ➨, and pledgeted sutures ➨ have been used to repair the aortic valve. (From DP: Cardiovascular.)*

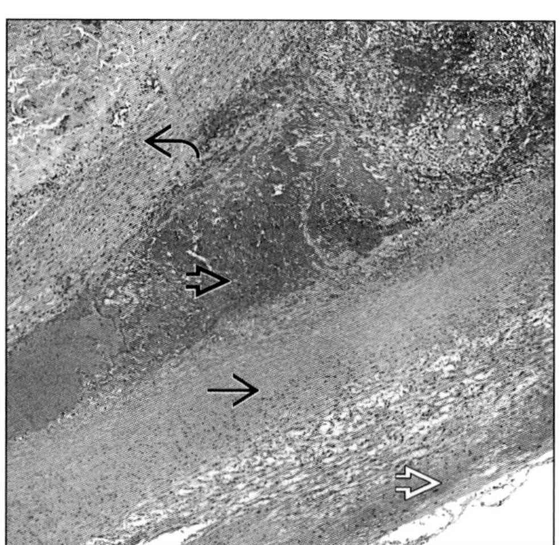

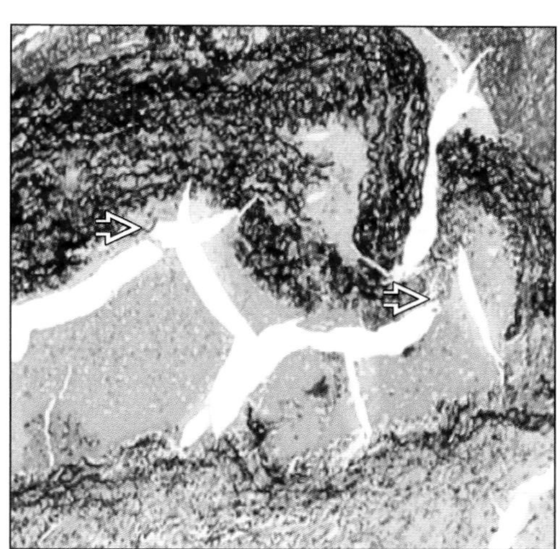

(Left) *Microscopic section through an aortic dissection shows the intramural hematoma ➨ located between the inner 2/3 ➨ and outer 1/3 ➨ of the aortic wall. The intima is on the bottom right ➨ and the adventitia is on the upper left. (From DP: Cardiovascular.)* ***(Right)*** *Elastic stain highlights the fragmentation of the elastic lamellae along the intramural hematoma ➨.*

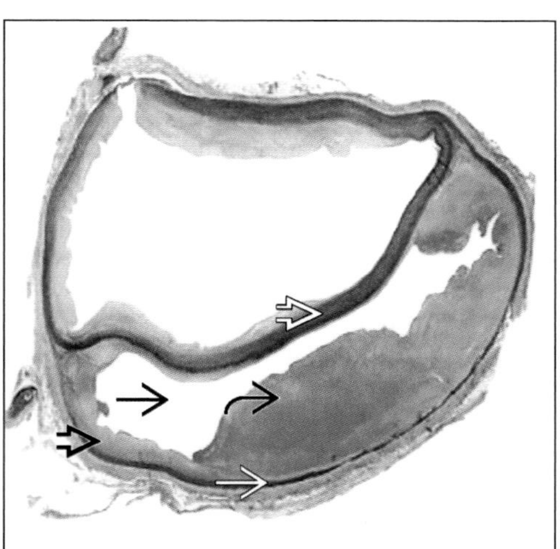

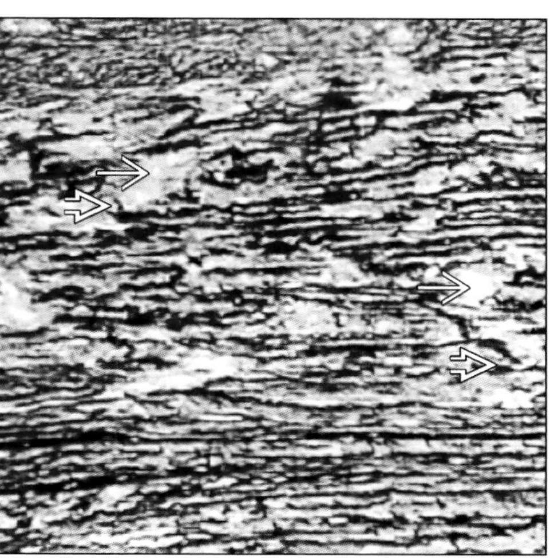

(Left) *Cross section through an aorta with a chronic dissection shows neointimal hyperplasia ➨ and unorganized hematoma ➨ along the false lumen ➨. The false lumen plane is in the outer aspect of the media between the inner 2/3 ➨ and outer 1/3 ➨.* ***(Right)*** *Elastic-stained aortic media demonstrates areas of elastic lamina fragmentation ➨ with cystic areas of accumulated mucopolysaccharides ➨ (cystic medial degeneration). (From DP: Cardiovascular.)*

ABDOMINAL AORTIC ANEURYSM

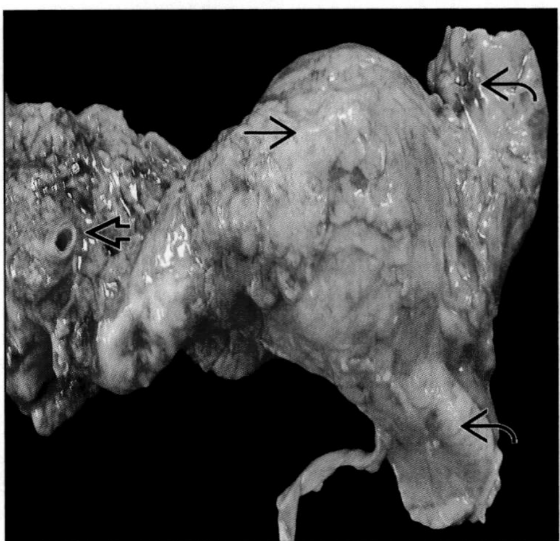

This infrarenal, saccular abdominal aortic aneurysm (AAA) ➞ is distal to the superior mesenteric artery ➞ and renal arteries (not well visualized) and ends at the iliac vessels ➞.

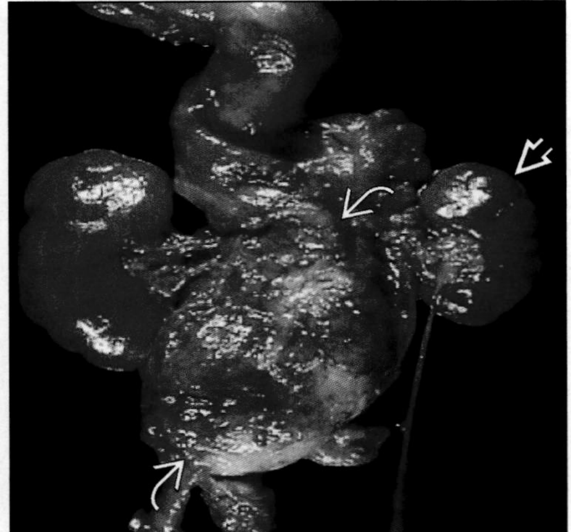

Obstructive complications of AAA include major branch obstruction. This juxtarenal AAA ➞ is associated with obstruction of the left renal artery as denoted by the atrophic left kidney ➞.

TERMINOLOGY

Abbreviations

- Abdominal aortic aneurysm (AAA)

Definitions

- Aneurysm: Localized permanent pathologic dilatation of vessel wall with diameter at least 50% > normal
  - Normal diameter ↑ with age, varies with aortic location and body habitus
  - Abdominal aortic diameter < 3 cm

CLINICAL ISSUES

Epidemiology

- Gender
  - M > F (4:1)
- Major risk factors
  - Nonmodifiable: ↑ age, male gender, family history
  - Modifiable: Hypertension, hyperlipidemia, smoking, diabetes

Presentation

- Usually due to complications of aneurysm/endografts
  - Rupture (abdominal pain/shock), emboli, compression (e.g., ureterazotemia), fistula (massive GI hemorrhage), infection (sepsis/shock), endoleaks

Laboratory Tests

- Hyperhomocysteinemia, hyperlipidemia, ↑ C-reactive protein (risk factor assessment)
- ↓ hemoglobin/hematocrit (normal if acute rupture, ↓ with slow leak), ↑ creatinine (acute tubular injury)
- Blood culture (infected aneurysm)

Clinical Chart Review

- Risk factors for atherosclerosis/aneurysm, family history, clinical presentation suggestive of rupture/other complication
- History of intervention: Endovascular aneurysm repair (EVAR) ± endoleak
- Other atherosclerotic complications (MI, stroke)

MACROSCOPIC FEATURES

External Examination

- Pallor &/or distended abdomen (rupture)
- Lower extremity changes related to aortic atherosclerotic disease/aneurysm
  - Loss of hair, thin skin, muscle atrophy, erythema, blue toe (embolic)
- Abdominal incision (aneurysm repair)
- Signs of risk factors for atherosclerosis
  - Xanthelasma (hypercholesterolemia)
  - Diagonal earlobe crease (Frank sign) (more sensitive in younger patients)

Internal Examination

- Hemoperitoneum or retroperitoneal hematoma

Organ Examination

- Aneurysm
  - Describe shape, length, position in relation to renal artery ostia (supra-/juxta-/infrarenal) and diameter
    - Rupture risk ↑ with ↑ diameter; 4-5 cm 1% per year, 5-6 cm 11% per year, 6 cm 25% per year: Repair usually at 5.5 cm
  - Abdominal or aorta x-ray highlights endografts
    - Review recent imaging; history of endoleaks
  - Look for rupture if hemoperitoneum or retroperitoneal hematoma present
    - Most common site: Left lateral infrarenal
  - Endoleaks: Continued growth of aneurysm due to continued perfusion after endograft
    - Type I at graft anastomosis, type II from branch vessels, type III between stents/ruptured graft, type IV through porous graft, type V unknown

ABDOMINAL AORTIC ANEURYSM

Key Facts

Macroscopic Pathology

- Describe shape, length, position in relation to renal artery ostia (supra-/juxta-/infrarenal) and diameter
- Rupture risk ↑ with ↑ diameter; 4-5 cm 1% per year, 5-6 cm 11% per year, 6 cm 25% per year: Repair usually at 5.5 cm
- Abdominal or aorta x-ray highlights endografts
- Look for rupture if hemoperitoneum or retroperitoneal hematoma present
- Most common site: Left lateral infrarenal

Microscopic Pathology

- Complications: Atheroemboli ± thrombosis/ vasculitis, infarcts (kidney, intestine, brain, spleen)

Top Differential Diagnoses

- IgG4-related disease/inflammatory aortic aneurysm
- Marked storiform adventitial fibrosis with extensive plasma cell infiltrate, composed of high percentage of IgG4 cells

        - Clinical diagnosis but recent thrombus around stent supports diagnosis, and radiograph of stent can identify rupture of graft
    - Aneurysm interior examination
        - Open aneurysm posteriorly examine contents, relationship to/obstruction of branch vessels, presence of rupture
        - Describe stent appearance, location, adherence to underlying aortic wall, obstruction of ostia
        - Graft can be kept intact with sampling of aneurysm around graft
- Systemic atherosclerosis ± complications
    - Acute/chronic MI, cerebral infarcts

MICROSCOPIC PATHOLOGY

Histologic Features

- Aneurysm: Atherosclerosis with marked degeneration of media, marked acute inflammation indicates possible infection (rare), malignancy related to stent (rare)
- Rest of cardiovascular system
    - Coronary/carotid atherosclerosis acute plaque events (rupture, thrombosis)
    - Acute/chronic myocardial infarction, acute subendocardial ischemia (terminal shock)
- Other: Emboli/shock
    - Atheroemboli ± thrombosis/vasculitis, infarcts (renal, intestine, spleen), acute tubular injury

ANCILLARY TESTS

Histochemistry

- Gram stain in cases of suspected infected aneurysms

Immunohistochemistry

- IgG4/IgG to exclude IgG4 disease (estimate % IgG4-positive cells)

DIFFERENTIAL DIAGNOSIS

IgG4-Related Disease/Inflammatory Aortic Aneurysm

- Marked storiform adventitial fibrosis with extensive plasma cell infiltrate, composed of high percentage of IgG4 cells

REPORTING CRITERIA

Aneurysm Incidental or Cause of Death

- Identify complications and risk factors for aneurysm

SELECTED REFERENCES

1. Kent KC: Clinical practice. Abdominal aortic aneurysms. N Engl J Med. 371(22):2101-8, 2014

IMAGE GALLERY

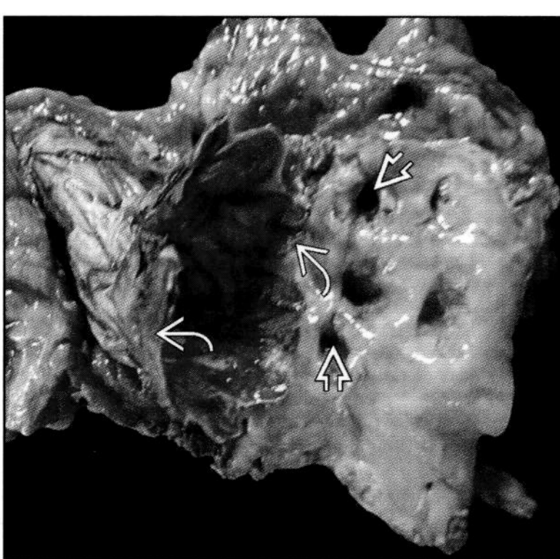

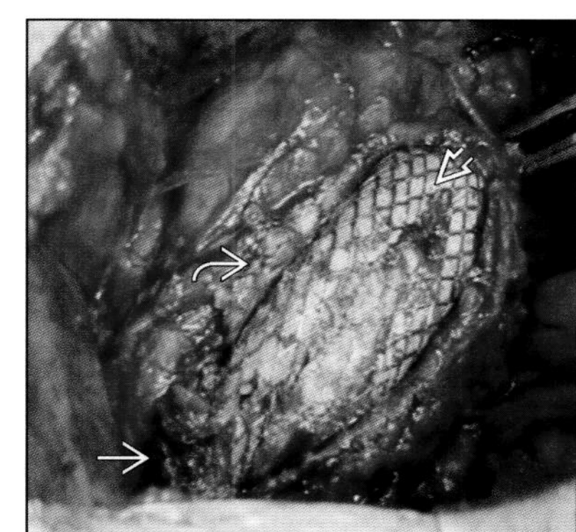

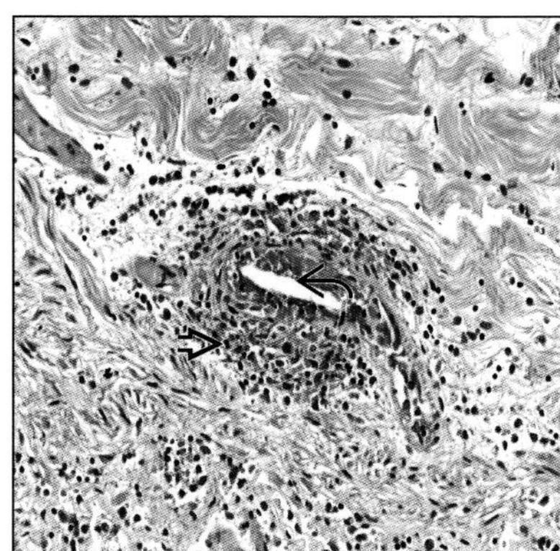

(Left) *This cloth-covered stent ➡ is attached proximally to the aorta beneath the renal artery ostia ➡. (Courtesy J. Chiaffarano, MD.)* ***(Center)*** *This ruptured infrarenal aneurysm has an endovascular stent ➡. The aneurysm wall ➡ is thin, and there is hematoma ➡ around the distal aneurysm due to rupture. (Courtesy S.A. Rahimi, MD.)* ***(Right)*** *Atheroemboli usually contain cholesterol crystals ➡ and may elicit a reactive vasculitis ➡.*

PULMONARY EDEMA

Pleural surface shows prominent interlobular septal markings as a consequence of excess fluid within the interstitial lymphatics that is present with severe pulmonary edema.

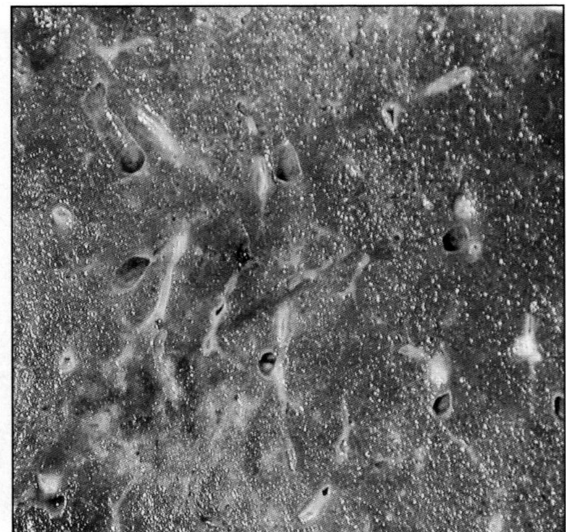

Gross appearance of pulmonary edema reflects the accumulation of fluid within the alveolar spaces.

TERMINOLOGY

Definitions

- Accumulation of fluid in alveolar spaces
  - 2 main etiologic categories
    - Cardiogenic pulmonary edema (CPE) (also referred to as hemodynamic edema)
    - Noncardiogenic pulmonary edema
  - Pathogenetic classification based on integrity of alveolar-capillary unit and intrinsic permeability of microvasculature
    - Nonpermeability edema of intact alveolar-capillary unit, usually seen with ↑ hydrostatic pressure; may also be due to ↓ oncotic pressure, lymphatic obstruction, and other less well understood factors
    - Permeability edema: Disruption of alveolar-capillary unit due to endothelial &/or epithelial damage
  - Diffuse alveolar damage (DAD) is classic noncardiogenic permeability edema and usual pathology seen in clinical acute respiratory distress syndrome (ARDS)
    - "Diffuse" refers to damage to all parts of alveolus, but not to widespread lung injury
    - DAD may be localized, but when clinically significant is usually widespread throughout lung

ETIOLOGY/PATHOGENESIS

Pathogenesis

- Lung fluid exchange based on Starling Law (balance of intra- and extravascular hydrostatic and oncotic pressures), normal permeability of microvasculature, and reserve capacity of lymphatics
  - Normal alveolar wall (alveolar/capillary unit) highly specialized to facilitate gas exchange
    - Normally, capillary endothelium is semipermeable to protein; allows escape of fluid and low molecular weight substances
    - Type I alveolar epithelial cells and endothelial cells are very thin and susceptible to damage
    - Direct injury to endothelium allows for escape of fibrin-rich exudates into interstitium and airspaces
    - Epithelial damage → epithelial necrosis, ↓ surfactant due to type II alveolar pneumocyte injury and alveolar collapse
  - CPE: Cardiac disease → accumulation of blood in pulmonary vasculature (passive congestion) → increased hydrostatic pressure → transudation of fluid from microvasculature into alveolar spaces
    - Acute passive congestion → small endothelial breaks → some release of red blood cells (alveolar microhemorrhage) in addition to fluid
    - Chronic passive congestion → repetitive alveolar microhemorrhage, ↑ hemosiderin-laden macrophages ("heart failure cells")
  - Noncardiogenic pulmonary edema: Mechanism of injury that → transudation/exudation of fluid varies according to etiology
  - In all cases, fluid in alveoli impairs gas exchange and can be fatal

Etiology

- Cardiogenic pulmonary edema
  - Ischemic and valvular heart disease, cardiomyopathy, myocarditis, cardiotoxic drugs and systemic toxins, hypertension and diabetes
- Noncardiogenic pulmonary edema including etiologies associated with diffuse alveolar damage
  - Infections
    - Pulmonary viral infections and sepsis (often with associated disseminated intravascular coagulation)
  - Trauma

PULMONARY EDEMA

Key Facts

Terminology

- Pulmonary edema is accumulation of fluid in alveolar spaces

Etiology

- Pulmonary edema divided into cardiogenic and noncardiogenic causes
- Diffuse alveolar damage is the prototypical example of noncardiogenic, permeability edema
  - Major histologic pattern associated with clinical syndrome of acute respiratory distress syndrome
- In hospitalized patients, etiology of pulmonary edema or diffuse alveolar damage is often multifactorial

Clinical Issues

- Significant cause of morbidity and mortality in hospitalized patients and is a common finding at autopsy

Macroscopic Pathology

- Heavy and fluid-filled lungs
- Diffuse alveolar damage results in airless and firm lungs

Microscopic Pathology

- Nonpermeability pulmonary edema
  - Fluid accumulation within alveolar spaces
- Diffuse alveolar damage
  - Hyaline membranes (early) and fibroblastic proliferation (late)

    - Major trauma and burns (burns often associated with smoke injury), fat embolism subsequent to trauma, near drowning
  - Chemical, toxin, drug, radiation exposure
    - Gastric acid (aspiration), smoke and other inhaled toxins (gases and chemicals), adverse drug reaction (including recreational drugs, oxygen toxicity, radiation injury, uremia)
  - Hypoalbuminemic states
    - Nephrotic syndrome, protein-losing enteropathies, chronic liver disease
  - Iatrogenic
    - Volume overload
  - Unknown exact mechanism of injury
    - Transfusion-related acute lung injury (TRALI), pancreatitis, high altitude pulmonary edema
  - Disseminated intravascular coagulation (DIC)
  - Cardiopulmonary bypass
    - Multifactorial, and in some cases may be associated with adverse reaction to protamine used to reverse heparin anticoagulation
  - Multifactorial/unknown
    - Pulmonary thromboembolism
    - Renal artery stenosis (often bilateral)
    - Eclampsia
    - Neurogenic
  - Lymphatic obstruction
  - Pulmonary vein obstruction

CLINICAL ISSUES

Presentation

- Depending on etiology, symptoms of pulmonary edema may appear suddenly or develop over time
  - Symptoms include shortness of breath, dyspnea, wheezing, cough, anxiety, chest pain, and rapid weight gain from build-up of fluid in body

MACROSCOPIC FEATURES

General Features

- Effect of formalin perfusion of lung on evaluation of pulmonary edema has long been debated
  - Cutting lungs in a fresh state enhances appreciation of pulmonary edema and might be appropriate in some circumstances and is favored by some pathologists
    - However, perfusion of lung allows for better overall appreciation of many other pathologic processes such as infection, parenchymal disease, and malignancy (many of which coexist in a hospital autopsy population), and perfusion is therefore recommended
    - Even with perfusion, it is still possible to satisfactorily document pulmonary edema by observation, pre-perfusion lung weights, and microscopic sections

External Examination

- Pulmonary edema often occurs in setting of congestive heart failure
  - Pitting edema and venous stasis changes may be present
  - Severe edema (anasarca) noted in hypoalbuminemic states
- Rapid infusion of fluids may result in iatrogenic volume overload and subsequent acute pulmonary edema
  - Note IV access and other central lines and correlate with clinical history of fluid administration as well as transfusions
- Sternal incision from recent coronary artery bypass graft surgery, valve surgery, ventricular assist device
- Burns (not encountered in hospital autopsy practice)
- Gastric contents in mouth (aspiration)
- Recent cesarean section scar (eclampsia-related pulmonary edema)

PULMONARY EDEMA

Internal Examination

- Absence or presence and character/quantitation of pleural effusions
  - Pleural effusion occurs when reserve capacity of lymphatic system to drain fluid from pulmonary extravascular spaces is exceeded and it is a good indicator of excess fluid in lungs
- Cardiac disease is the major cause of nonpermeability pulmonary edema
  - Special attention should be paid to examination of the 4 heart chambers, cardiac valves, coronary vessels, and major vessels for any abnormality
- Renal disease or renal artery stenosis can also cause noncardiogenic, nonpermeability pulmonary edema

Organ Examination

- Increased lung weights are a sensitive indicator of pulmonary disease and, in absence of another etiology such as infection or malignancy, reflect severity of fluid accumulation within lung
- Prominent interstitial markings are often present on pleural surface and reflect accumulation of fluid within lobular interstitium
- Sectioning of unfixed lung will result in exudation of fluid from cut surface
  - Assuming no other underlying pulmonary disease or longstanding cardiac disease resulting in chronic passive congestion, lungs in cardiogenic and noncardiogenic, nonpermeability pulmonary edema are fairly compliant
  - By contrast, lungs with evolving diffuse alveolar damage are airless and firm
- Presence of frothy fluid exuding into trachea and bronchi prior to fixation is another indication of pulmonary edema

MICROSCOPIC PATHOLOGY

Histologic Features

- Nonpermeability pulmonary edema
  - Fluid-filled alveolar spaces with pale granular eosinophilic precipitate, even with prior formalin perfusion
  - Most prominent changes are often in lower lobe sections where hydrostatic pressure is most increased
  - Alveolar capillaries are often distended reflecting antecedent capillary congestion
    - Additional finding of increased hemosiderin-laden macrophages supports a diagnosis of chronic passive congestion in appropriate clinical setting
- Permeability pulmonary edema (diffuse alveolar damage)
  - Early phase (also referred to as acute or exudative phase)
    - Hyaline membranes (formed by escape of fibrin-rich exudates and epithelial cell necrosis)
    - Interstitial edema
    - Alveolar collapse secondary to loss of surfactant
    - Fibrin thrombi reflecting endothelial damage
  - Late phase (also referred to as proliferative or organizing phase)
    - Fibroblastic proliferation and type II pneumocyte hyperplasia predominate
    - Squamous metaplasia

DIFFERENTIAL DIAGNOSIS

Acute Fibrinous and Organizing Pneumonia (AFOP)

- Alveolar spaces filled with organizing balls of fibrin rather than classic hyaline membranes found in diffuse alveolar damage

DIAGNOSTIC CHECKLIST

Pathologic Interpretation Pearls

- In cardiogenic pulmonary edema, etiology is often directly attributable to a specific injury such as acute myocardial infarction
- In hospitalized patients, particularly within an intensive care setting, etiology of pulmonary edema or diffuse alveolar damage is often multifactorial
  - Include major contributory causes when multifactorial

REPORTING CRITERIA

Pulmonary Edema as Primary or Contributory Cause of Death

- Example: Patient maintained on life support after major intracerebral hemorrhage eventually sustains cerebral herniation and expires, lungs with permeability pulmonary edema
  - Permeability edema is a contributory cause of death

SELECTED REFERENCES

1. Mac Sweeney R et al: Acute lung failure. Semin Respir Crit Care Med. 32(5):607-25, 2011
2. Matthay MA et al: The acute respiratory distress syndrome: pathogenesis and treatment. Annu Rev Pathol. 6:147-63, 2011
3. Beasley MB: The pathologist's approach to acute lung injury. Arch Pathol Lab Med. 134(5):719-27, 2010

Pulmonary Edema and Early Diffuse Alveolar Damage

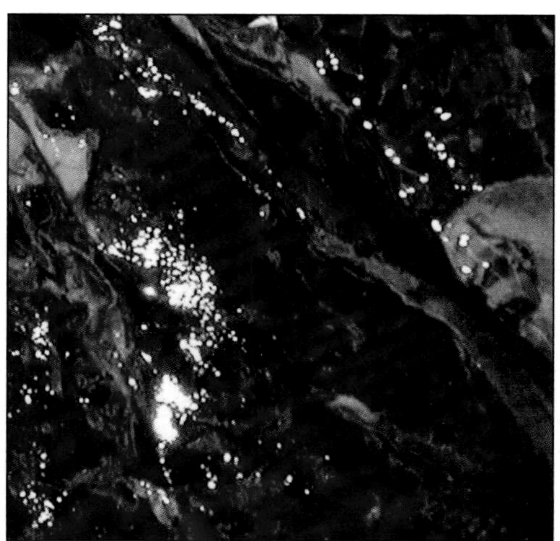

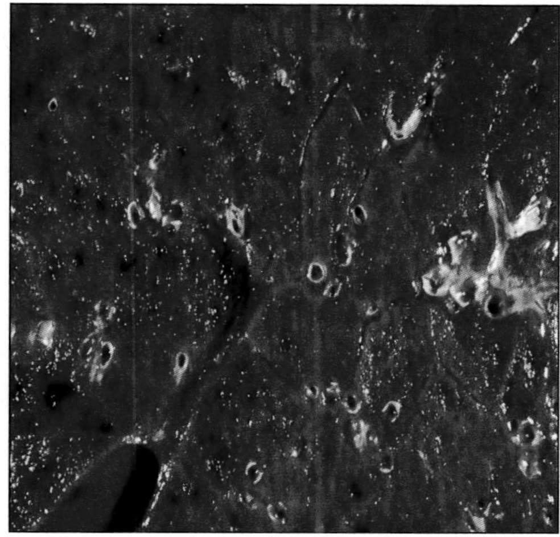

(Left) Gross photograph demonstrates pulmonary edema with fluid exuding from the fresh cut surface of the lung. ***(Right)*** Early diffuse alveolar damage with a beefy red cut surface is seen in this gross photo. The lung is palpably firm and airless.

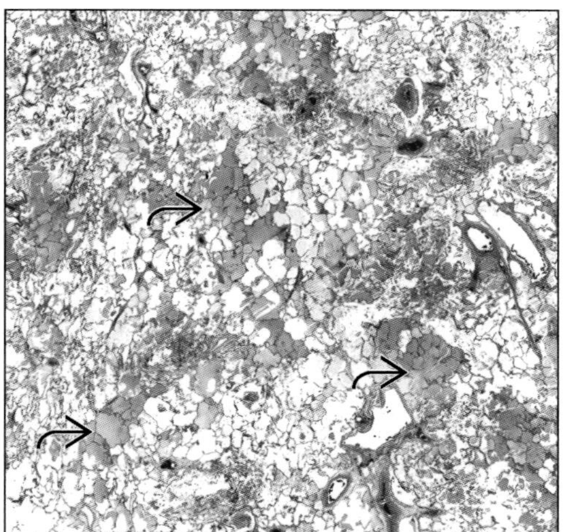

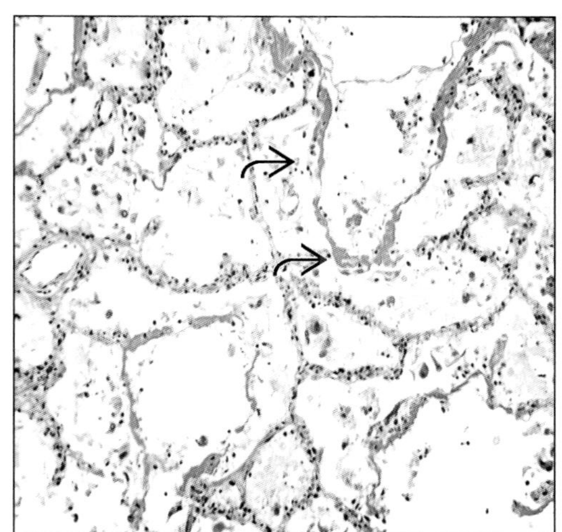

(Left) Low-power image of pulmonary edema shows fluid-filled alveolar spaces ⇗. ***(Right)*** Low-power view shows acute diffuse alveolar damage with hyaline membranes ⇗.

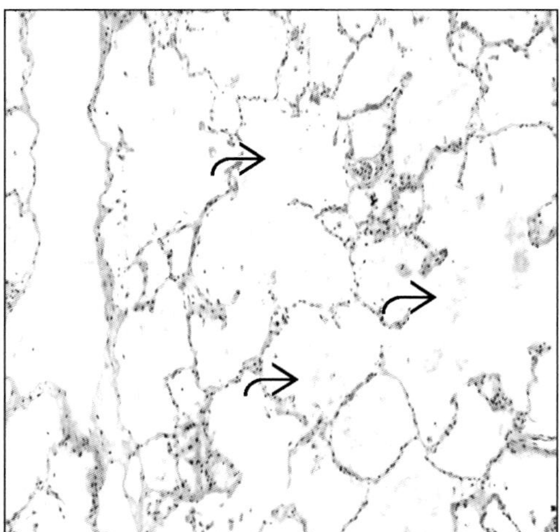

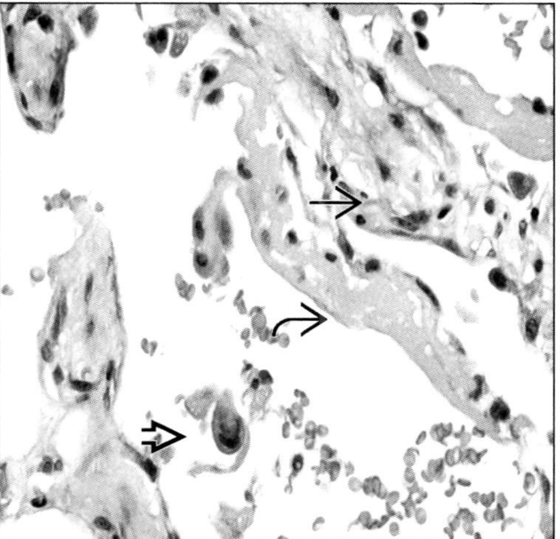

(Left) High-power photo shows pulmonary edema. Even with prior formalin fixation, there is a patchy pale granular eosinophilic precipitate ⇗. ***(Right)*** High-power view shows acute diffuse alveolar damage and hyaline membrane ⇗. The adjacent alveolar wall is edematous →, and there are desquamated epithelial cells ⇨.

PULMONARY HEMORRHAGE

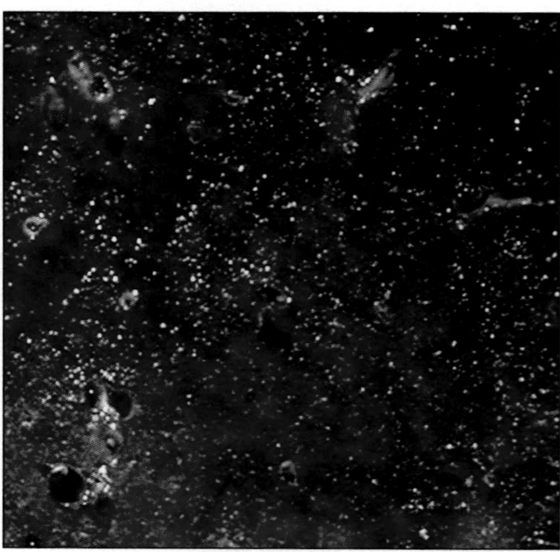

Diffuse pulmonary hemorrhage imparts a dark-red appearance to the lung parenchyma.

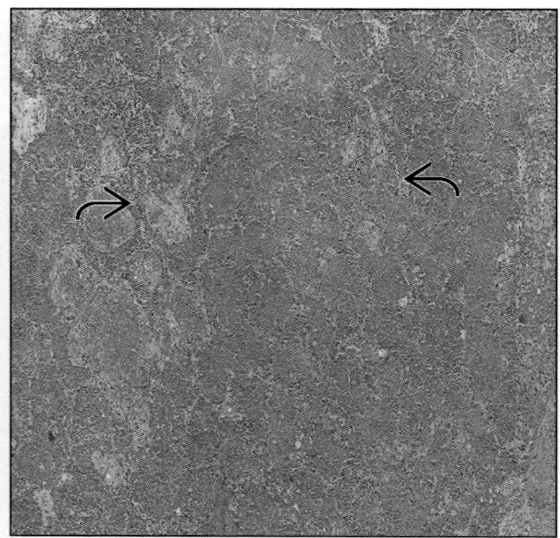

DAH in Goodpasture syndrome has a bland appearance without vasculitis or necrosis of alveolar septa (note intact septa ➔).

TERMINOLOGY

Definitions

- Diffuse alveolar hemorrhage (DAH) refers to accumulation of intraalveolar red blood cells that originate from pulmonary microcirculation
  - Excludes other intraparenchymal and extrapulmonary sources of blood

ETIOLOGY/PATHOGENESIS

Pathogenesis

- All DAH is result of injury to pulmonary microcirculation: Pathogenetic classification: Seropositive systemic vasculitides and autoimmune disorders, coagulation disorders, drug toxicity, and infections
  - ANCA-associated vasculitides
    - Granulomatosis with polyangiitis (Wegener granulomatosis)
    - Microscopic polyangiitis
    - Eosinophilic granulomatosis with polyangiitis (Churg-Strauss syndrome) (uncommon)
  - Goodpasture syndrome (antiglomerular basement membrane [GBM] disease)
  - Isolated pulmonary capillaritis (seronegative vasculitis limited to lung)
  - Autoimmune
    - Systemic lupus erythematosus (SLE): ~ 4% of patients with SLE have DAH, usually associated glomerulonephritis
    - Uncommonly associated with DAH: Rheumatoid arthritis, scleroderma, mixed connective tissue disorder, polymyositis, antiphospholipid antibody syndrome, cryoglobulinemia, Henoch-Schönlein purpura/IgA nephropathy, Behçet syndrome
    - Pre- and postmortem serologic studies, immunofluorescence and ultrastructural studies should help identify and distinguish among autoimmune disease
  - Drug (therapeutic and recreational) toxicity
    - Cytotoxic drugs: Cyclophosphamide, mitomycin, cytarabine
    - Anticoagulants
    - Chelator: Penicillamine
    - Antithyroid medication: Propylthiouracil (may be via drug-induced ANCA-mediated vasculitis)
    - Crack cocaine inhalation
  - Infection
    - H1N1 and other viral and bacterial infections and parasitic infestation
  - Bone marrow/stem cell transplantation
  - Radiation therapy
  - Idiopathic pulmonary hemosiderosis
    - Rare disease usually seen in children characterized by recurrent episodes of DAH with resultant fibrosis and hemosiderosis
    - Pathogenesis unknown
  - Malignancy
    - Kaposi sarcoma and metastatic malignancy

CLINICAL ISSUES

Presentation

- Most common presenting symptom is hemoptysis; however, hemoptysis absent in up to 1/3 of patients
  - Hemoptysis may be abrupt in onset or slowly evolve over period of days to weeks
  - Other symptoms and signs include fever, cough, chest pain, dyspnea, and anemia
- Radiographs demonstrate nonspecific diffuse pulmonary infiltrates
- Sequential bronchoalveolar lavage (BAL) can be confirmatory in patients without obvious hemoptysis

PULMONARY HEMORRHAGE

Key Facts

Terminology
- Diffuse alveolar hemorrhage is accumulation of intraalveolar red blood cells that originate from pulmonary microcirculation

Etiology
- Result of injury to pulmonary microcirculation
- Pathogenesis varies according to etiology
- Differential diagnosis includes seropositive systemic vasculitides and autoimmune disorders, coagulation disorders, drug toxicity, and infections

Clinical Issues
- Patients often (but not always) present with hemoptysis, diffuse radiographic pulmonary infiltrates, and hypoxemic respiratory failure

Macroscopic Pathology
- Diffusely heavy and blood-filled lungs with exclusion of localized sources of bleeding

Microscopic Pathology
- Intraalveolar red blood cells and fibrin with accumulation of hemosiderin-laden macrophages and organizing pneumonia in later phase
- 3 major histologic patterns
  - Pulmonary capillaritis
  - Bland hemorrhage
  - Diffuse alveolar damage

Diagnostic Checklist
- Clinical history and ancillary studies are essential for diagnostic interpretation

Prognosis
- Most patients develop hypoxemic respiratory failure that is often severe and fatal

MACROSCOPIC FEATURES

External Examination
- Examine skin and extremities for signs of generalized thrombocytopenia or coagulation disorder
  - Skin petechiae, mucosal petechiae, or oral blood
- Check for rash that may indicate drug reaction, vasculitis, or autoimmune disorder

Internal Examination
- Check for internal signs of generalized thrombocytopenia, coagulation disorder, vasculitis, or autoimmune disorder
- Evidence of active or remote episodes of pleuritis, pericarditis, and abdominal serositis may indicate underlying connective tissue disease
  - Look for shaggy serosal surfaces (acute), fibrosis/ adhesions (chronic)

Organ Examination
- Lungs
  - Obtain fresh tissue for immunofluorescence
  - Alveolar hemorrhage should involve lung diffusely
    - Consider alternative diagnosis for more localized patterns of blood
    - Alveolar hemorrhage can be distinguished from pulmonary edema by consolidation and exudation of blood from cut surface, even after formalin perfusion and fixation
- Kidneys
  - Renal involvement is a prominent feature of ANCA-associated granulomatosis with vasculitis (Wegener granulomatosis), SLE, and Goodpasture syndrome
    - Petechiae (flea-bitten appearance), edema of kidneys
  - Obtain fresh samples for immunofluorescence and electron microscopic studies
- Skin
  - May be involved in autoimmune diseases
  - Sample rashes, petechiae, purpura
  - Collect fresh tissue for immunofluorescence

MICROSCOPIC PATHOLOGY

Histologic Features
- Lung: Intraalveolar red blood cells and fibrin with accumulation of hemosiderin-laden macrophages and organizing pneumonia over time
- 3 major histologic patterns are associated with diffuse alveolar hemorrhage
  - Pulmonary capillaritis
    - Interstitial neutrophilic infiltrate, leukocytoclasia, and fibrinoid necrosis of alveolar walls
  - Bland alveolar hemorrhage (classic for Goodpasture syndrome but other potential etiologies)
  - Diffuse alveolar damage
- Although less common cause of DAH, consider infectious etiology
  - Secondary infection as a result of immunosuppressive therapy is common
  - Common infections associated with DAH in immunocompromised patients
    - Cytomegalovirus, adenovirus, invasive aspergillosis, *Mycoplasma*, *Legionella*, *Strongyloides*
  - Common infections associated with DAH in immunocompetent patients
    - Influenza (H1N1), dengue, leptospirosis, malaria, *Staphylococcus aureus*
  - Appropriate microbiologic/virologic studies should be performed, such as nasal swab for suspected H1N1
- Kidney: Glomerular inflammation/necrosis/crescent (glomerulitis), red blood cell casts in tubules associated with glomerulonephritis and also may indicate anticoagulant effect (warfarin nephropathy)

PULMONARY HEMORRHAGE

Cytologic Features

- Bronchoalveolar lavage with fresh and degenerated red blood cells, hemosiderin macrophages
  - May also reveal evidence of viral/bacterial infection, parasitic infestation, or malignancy

ANCILLARY TESTS

Immunofluorescence

- Procure fresh frozen lung, kidney, or skin (if rash present) for full immunofluorescence panel with immunoglobulin and complement staining
  - Diffuse, linear alveolar capillary and glomerular capillary basement membrane staining with IgG indicates Goodpasture syndrome
  - Granular deposits of immune complexes (immunoglobulin and complement)
    - SLE and other connective tissue disorders
    - Glomerulonephritis associated with infection (e.g., *Staphylococcus*)
    - Cryoglobulinemia
    - HSP (IgA dominant immune complex deposit in glomeruli)
  - Skin immunofluorescence may reveal immunoglobulin ± complement deposition in lesions of SLE, vascular IgA deposition in HSP, immunoglobulin and light chain deposition in cryoglobulinemia

Serologic Testing

- Premortem serum should be sequestered and postmortem serum obtained by cardiac puncture
  - Seropositivity may be rapidly diminished by initiation of immunosuppressive therapy or plasmapheresis
- ANCA, anti-GBM, ANA, and expanded panel of connective tissue disease serologies as indicated

Electron Microscopy

- Transmission
  - In DAH with renal involvement (pulmonary renal syndrome), may help in differential diagnosis
    - Disruption of GBM with fibrin and inflammatory cells indicate crescent formation (ANCA, anti-GBM, occasional lupus)
    - Electron-dense immune complex-type deposits (not seen in ANCA or anti-GBM disease) support SLE or other connective tissue disorder
    - Deposits with organized appearance (tubular or thumbprint [SLE, fibrillary], cryoglobulin)

DIFFERENTIAL DIAGNOSIS

Pulmonary Arterial Bleeding

- Small, medium, or large-sized pulmonary vessels involved by vasculitides such as ANCA-positive granulomatous vasculitis, microscopic polyangiitis, and Churg-Strauss syndrome
- Other causes of thromboembolism with adjacent infarction

Bronchial Arterial Bleeding

- Common source of blood with bronchiectasis or chronic cavitary lesions

Extrinsic Blood

- Aspirated blood from gastrointestinal source
- Aspirated blood from upper respiratory source

Malignancy

- Metastatic angiosarcoma as well as Kaposi sarcoma may present with extensive alveolar hemorrhage

Outflow Obstruction

- Postsurgical acute pulmonary venous outflow obstruction with lung transplantation
- Cardiac causes such as mitral stenosis and mitral regurgitation in addition to pulmonary venoocclusive disease

Traumatic Injury or Postsurgical Bleeding

- Also includes cardiopulmonary resuscitation (CPR)

DIAGNOSTIC CHECKLIST

Pathologic Interpretation Pearls

- Gross and histologic findings of diffuse alveolar hemorrhage are not specific as to etiology
- If possible, premortem serum samples should be sequestered and postmortem blood should be obtained for serologic studies
- Fresh frozen lung tissue should be procured for immunofluorescence, if indicated
- Clinical history and premortem laboratory data should be carefully reviewed for evidence of evolving coagulation disorder, thrombolytic therapy complications, infection, and drug toxicity
  - Common etiologies for alveolar hemorrhage in hospital setting, particularly if patient did not initially present with findings suggesting diffuse alveolar hemorrhage syndrome

REPORTING CRITERIA

Presence/Extent of DAH

- Was DAH cause of death
- Etiology of DAH if known

SELECTED REFERENCES

1. West S et al: Diffuse alveolar haemorrhage in ANCA-associated vasculitis. Intern Med. 52(1):5-13, 2013
2. Marchiori E et al: Diffuse alveolar hemorrhage in infectious diseases. Chest. 139(1):228, 2011
3. McCabe C et al: Pulmonary-renal syndromes: an update for respiratory physicians. Respir Med. 105(10):1413-21, 2011
4. Lara AR et al: Diffuse alveolar hemorrhage. Chest. 137(5):1164-71, 2010
5. Colby TV et al: Pathologic approach to pulmonary hemorrhage. Ann Diagn Pathol. 5(5):309-19, 2001

Gross and Microscopic Appearance of Diffuse Alveolar Hemorrhage

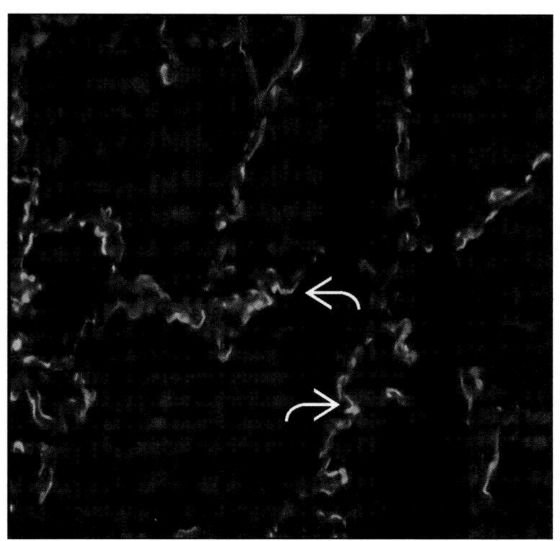

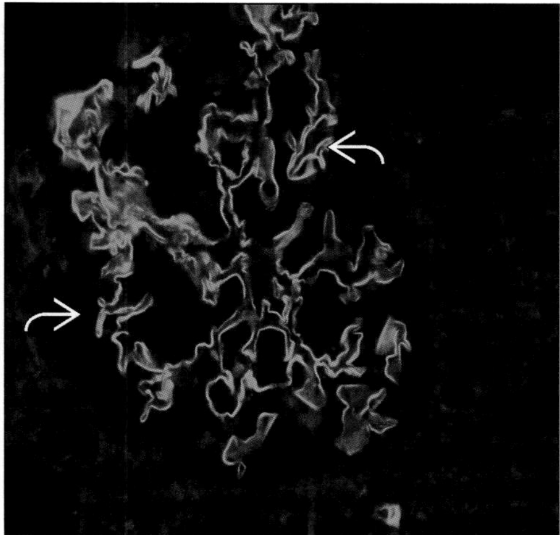

(Left) *Immunofluorescence study of lung from the same patient with DAH reveals linear IgG deposition* ➔ *in the alveolar walls, supporting the diagnosis of Goodpasture syndrome.* *(Right)* *In anti-GBM disease, there is strong linear staining with IgG along the glomerular capillary basement membrane* ➔. *Anti-GBM antibody is most often IgG subclass 1 or 3 and rarely IgA or M. The antigen is the NC1 domain of the alpha 3 chain of type IV collagen.*

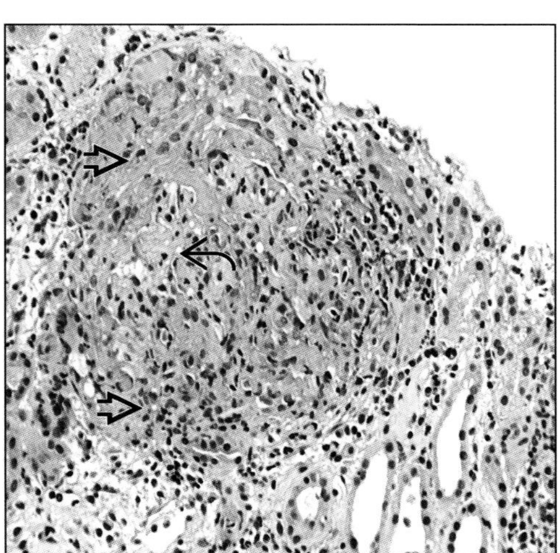

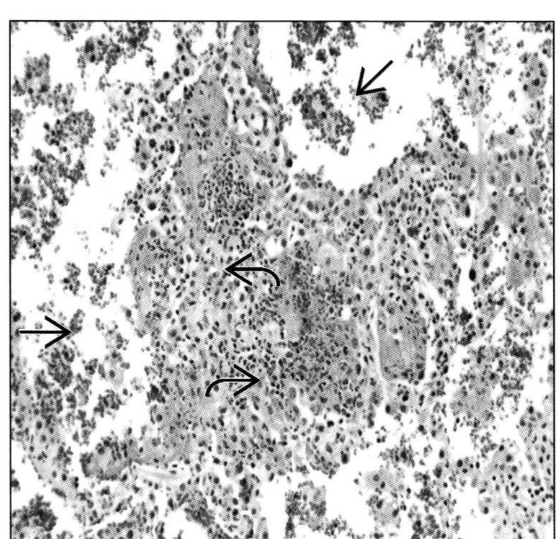

(Left) *The glomerular tuft* ➔ *in this glomerulus is difficult to see because of a circumferential crescent* ➔. *Crescents can be seen in many renal diseases but are most often associated with anti-GBM disease or ANCA vasculitis.* *(Right)* *In this example of DAH due to neutrophilic capillaritis, there is interstitial neutrophilia* ➔ *as well as a background of acute intraalveolar hemorrhage* ➔ *(intact, nondegenerated red blood cells without hemosiderin macrophages).*

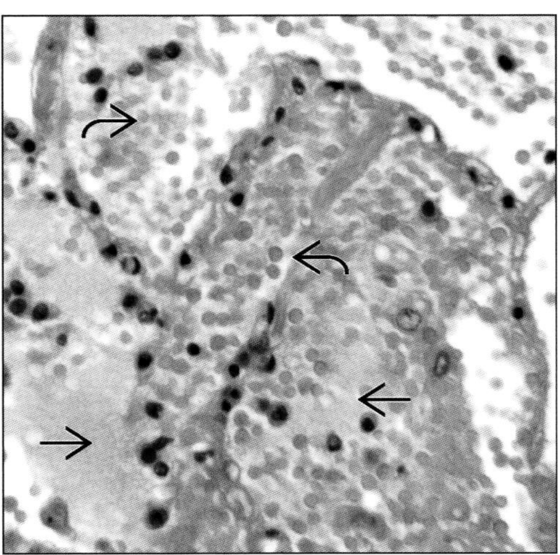

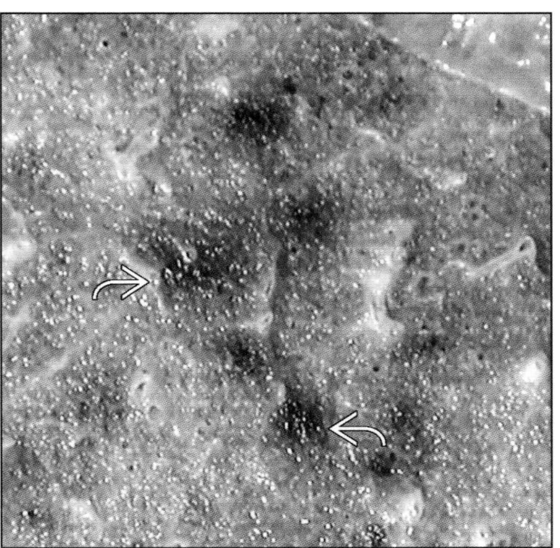

(Left) *This lung section from a patient with terminal thrombocytopenia demonstrates nonspecific acute intraalveolar hemorrhage* ➔ *and fibrin* ➔. *(Right)* *This is an example of nonspecific hemorrhagic foci* ➔ *in a coagulopathic patient. Microscopic sections should always be taken to exclude the possibility of infection.*

TENSION PNEUMOTHORAX

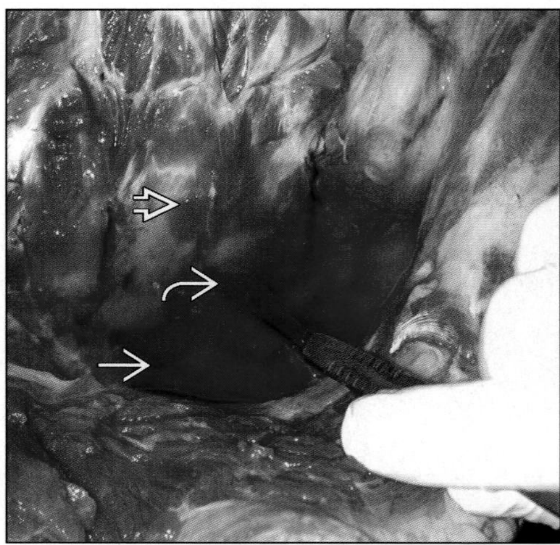

This photograph shows the technique for demonstrating pneumothorax using a pocket of water ➡ and scalpel incision ➡ under the water and into the chest wall ➡.

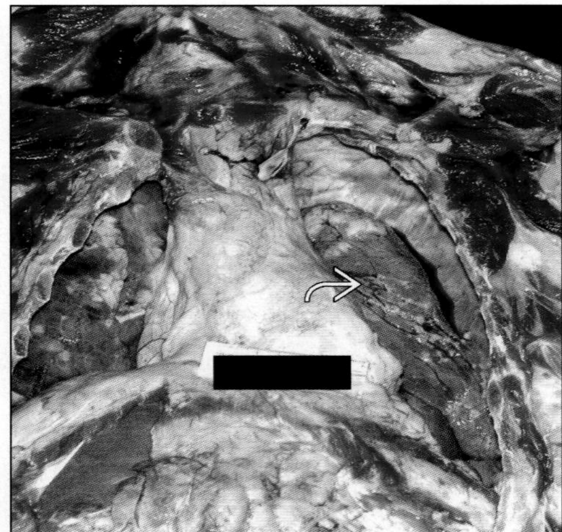

This opened chest cavity demonstrates collapse of the left lung ➡ with tension pneumothorax in a patient with widely metastatic carcinoma.

TERMINOLOGY

Definitions

- Air in pleural space
  - Classified as simple or tension pneumothorax
    - Tension pneumothorax: Progressive accumulation of entrapped air in pleural space that → pressure-induced displacement of mediastinum and heart; may result in potentially fatal hemodynamic compromise
- Primary (spontaneous) pneumothorax: Pneumothorax in patients with no known underlying lung disease
- Secondary pneumothorax: Pneumothorax associated with known underlying lung disease, trauma, or iatrogenic injury
- Pleural bleb: Airspace within pleura and separated from pleural space and alveoli by thin pleural membrane that may rupture and lead to pneumothorax
- Bullae: Airspaces that are characteristically subpleural and associated with destruction of lung tissue
- Pneumomediastinum, pneumopericardium, pneumoperitoneum, and subcutaneous emphysema: Air in mediastinum, pericardial space, peritoneal cavity, or subcutaneous tissue

ETIOLOGY/PATHOGENESIS

Pathogenesis

- Injury to lung or pleura → communication between airspace and pleural space with so-called valve effect
- When valve is created, air accumulates in pleural cavity during respiratory cycle
  - Valve is 1-way only, allowing for entry of air during inspiration but not for its escape during expiration
- Accumulation of air ↑ intrapleural pressure and interferes with lung expansion on pneumothorax side
- ↑ intrapleural pressure ↑ effect of ipsilateral lung collapse and pushes mediastinal structures and heart toward opposite side
- Compression of vena cava and right heart compromises venous return, diastolic filling, and cardiac output
- Significant shunting with ventilation-perfusion mismatch leads to hypoxemia, acidosis, and shock
- Decompression of pleural space must be prompt to avoid fatal hemodynamic compromise
- If air escapes into interstitial tissue planes, pneumomediastinum, pneumopericardium, pneumoperitoneum, and subcutaneous emphysema may result

Etiology of Pneumothorax

- Primary
  - Unknown; also termed spontaneous idiopathic pneumothorax
  - Entity occurring in relatively younger patients that appears related to rupture of small peripheral and usually apical blebs
- Secondary pneumothorax
  - Trauma including esophageal rupture and foreign body obstructing bronchus
  - Iatrogenic
    - Lung or pleural biopsy, thoracotomy, mechanical ventilation, subclavian vein catheterization, and cardiopulmonary resuscitation
  - Genetic
    - Cystic fibrosis, Ehlers-Danlos syndrome, Marfan syndrome, α-1-antitrypsin deficiency associated emphysema, Birt-Hogg-Dubé syndrome
  - Hemodynamic
    - Pulmonary Infarction
  - Infectious
    - Necrotizing cavitary lesions (TB, coccidiomycosis), *Pneumocystis jirovecii* pneumonia, and HIV
  - Inflammatory/immune

TENSION PNEUMOTHORAX

Key Facts

Terminology

- Pneumothorax is defined as presence of air in pleural space
- Tension pneumothorax is progressive accumulation of entrapped air within pleural space that results in pressure-induced displacement of mediastinum and heart, resulting in potentially fatal hemodynamic compromise

Etiology

- Extensive number of underlying lung diseases, as well as traumatic and iatrogenic injury

Clinical Issues

- Differences in presentation and outcome based on whether patient is spontaneously breathing or on mechanical ventilation, with the latter being more difficult to recognize and more likely to result in mortality

Macroscopic Pathology

- Tracheal deviation, mediastinal shift, and pneumomediastinum
- Unilateral lung collapse with positive test for air in pleural space
- Signs of prior intervention

Microscopic Pathology

- Findings consistent with specific underlying lung disease predisposing to pneumothorax or recent lung injury

Top Differential Diagnoses

- Terminal cardiopulmonary resuscitation
- Simple pneumothorax

        - Usual interstitial pneumonia, respiratory bronchiolitis, asthma, hypersensitivity pneumonitis, sarcoidosis, constrictive bronchiolitis following bone marrow transplantation
    - Neoplastic
        - Primary and metastatic pulmonary malignancy, especially when necrotic and cavitary
        - Pleural malignancy: Malignant mesothelioma and metastatic disease
    - Emphysema
        - Paraseptal emphysema with bullae (emphysematous cystic spaces > 1 cm)
    - Other
        - Endometriosis (catamenial pneumothorax), lymphangioleiomyomatosis, Langerhans cell histiocytosis

CLINICAL ISSUES

Presentation

- Tension pneumothorax can occur abruptly, but cardiovascular compromise may occur more gradually
    - Incidence of tension pneumothorax varies from ~ 3.5-30%
    - Tension pneumothorax is not uncommon in hospitalized patients, but fatal tension pneumothorax is relatively rare
        - Possibility is expectantly managed in certain patient populations and promptly treated
        - Estimates of missed diagnosis of patients dying in ICU setting range from 1% to almost 4%
        - Missed diagnosis is more likely with ventilation, if cardiopulmonary resuscitation has occurred, or if delay in diagnosis of simple pneumothorax
        - Majority of ventilated patients with pneumothorax will require emergent treatment with tube thoracostomy, given high risk of progression to tension pneumothorax
        - Tension pneumothorax should also be suspected in patients who already have chest tube placed for pneumothorax, because tube may have become kinked or obstructed
- Symptoms: Ipsilateral pleuritic chest pain, progressive tachycardia, respiratory distress, diaphoresis, hypotension and pallor from hypoxemia, mediastinal shift, and reduced venous return

Treatment

- Early recognition and prompt intervention before hemodynamic deterioration is essential
- Hemodynamic improvement is achieved through release of entrapped air, usually by tube thoracostomy
- Following decompression, patients are at risk for reexpansion pulmonary edema (REPE) that may further complicate recovery

Prognosis

- If untreated, fatal cardiovascular collapse can occur even in healthy, young individuals
- As would be expected, mortality is increased in patients with more severe comorbidities who are less able to tolerate hemodynamic compromise and particularly in ventilated patients in ICU setting

IMAGE FINDINGS

Radiographic Findings

- Tracheal deviation toward opposite side from pneumothorax, flattening of diaphragmatic contour, displaced cardiac silhouette, shifting of left cardiac border

MACROSCOPIC FEATURES

General Features

- Role of pneumothorax as immediate or contributory cause of death may be difficult to evaluate because of coexistence with other major potentially fatal conditions and because time of onset is often unknown

- Chart review for premortem signs of tension pneumothorax
  - May be more difficult to identify these signs in critically ill, ventilated patients
- Even if pneumothorax is detected and treated, intervention may not have been sufficient to restore hemodynamic function
- Forceful terminal CPR may cause tension pneumothorax and should be excluded as a contributing cause of death

External Examination

- Crepitant subcutaneous emphysema
- Craniofacial congestion secondary to central venous compression
- Tracheal deviation toward opposite side of suspected pneumothorax
- Signs of intervention such as puncture wound or chest tube
- Postmortem radiograph of chest is most sensitive method for distinguishing simple from tension pneumothorax

Internal Examination

- Methods to detect pneumothorax prior to opening body cavities
  - Once thoracic skin is reflected, create pocket of water between reflected skin and rib cage, open pleural cavity under water with scalpel inserted between 2 ribs
    - Air bubbles in the water indicate tension pneumothorax
  - Insert needle attached to syringe filled with water into pleural space (can be inserted through skin before making thoracic skin flap)
    - Air bubbles in water indicate tension pneumothorax
- Unilateral lung collapse
- Depression of diaphragm
  - If viewed from abdominal cavity, dome of diaphragm may be displaced downward
  - In severe cases, pneumoperitoneum may be present
- Pneumomediastinum and mediastinal displacement toward opposite side of suspected pneumothorax
- Pneumopericardium and cardiac displacement toward opposite side of suspected pneumothorax
- Look for mechanism of injury
  - Rib fracture with lung puncture wound
  - Bronchopleural fistula
  - If prior chest tube placed, determine that tube is appropriately placed without kinks or obstruction

Organ Examination

- Examine for pleural blebs, bullae, evidence of underlying lung disease or localized traumatic injury

MICROSCOPIC PATHOLOGY

Histologic Features

- With prolonged time interval between pneumothorax and death, characteristic histologic findings may be present
  - Eosinophilic pleuritis
  - Reactive mesothelial hyperplasia
  - Fibrinous exudate
  - Pleural and subpleural parenchymal fibrosis
  - Giant cells consistent with persistent interstitial air
  - Chronic inflammation and hemosiderin deposition
- Findings that suggest or are consistent with specific underlying lung disease predisposing to pneumothorax
  - Asthma, emphysema, and tuberculosis are some lung diseases that are most frequently associated with pneumothorax

DIFFERENTIAL DIAGNOSIS

Cardiopulmonary Resuscitation (CPR)

- A test for air bubbles should be performed bilaterally
  - Bilateral disease would indicate CPR injury
- Correlate clinical events immediately preceding terminal resuscitation efforts with autopsy findings
- Bilateral lung collapse more consistent with vigorous resuscitation than tension pneumothorax
  - Differential for bilateral collapse includes simple pneumothorax on one side and tension pneumothorax on other

Simple Pneumothorax

- Diagnosis of tension pneumothorax rests on documentation of unequivocal mediastinal shifting to opposite side
- If absent, diagnosis defaults to simple pneumothorax

SELECTED REFERENCES

1. Schneider F et al: Approach to lung biopsies from patients with pneumothorax. Arch Pathol Lab Med. 138(2):257-65, 2014
2. Yarmus L et al: Pneumothorax in the critically ill patient. Chest. 141(4):1098-105, 2012
3. Celik B et al: Iatrogenic pneumothorax: etiology, incidence and risk factors. Thorac Cardiovasc Surg. 57(5):286-90, 2009
4. Leigh-Smith S et al: Tension pneumothorax--time for a re-think? Emerg Med J. 22(1):8-16, 2005
5. Weissberg D et al: Pneumothorax: experience with 1,199 patients. Chest. 117(5):1279-85, 2000
6. Barton ED: Tension pneumothorax. Curr Opin Pulm Med. 5(4):269-74, 1999

Gross and Microscopic Features

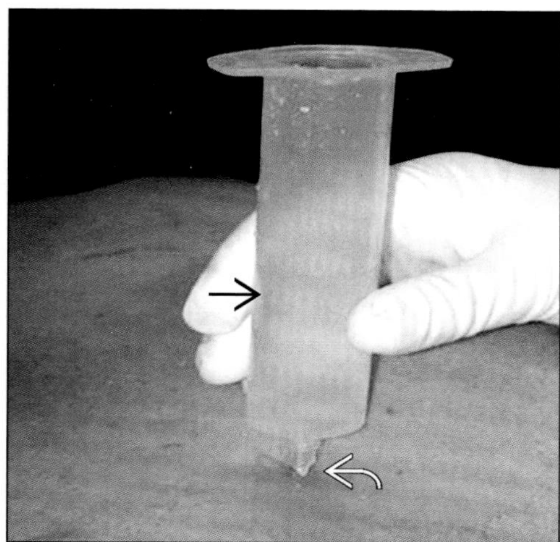

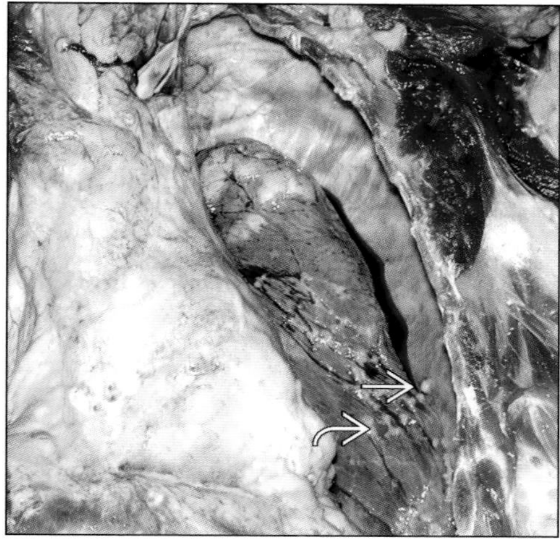

(Left) *This photograph demonstrates the water-filled syringe test for pneumothorax. A needle is attached to a syringe filled with water* ➔ *and is inserted through the thoracic skin* ➔ *into the pleural space. Air bubbles in the syringe indicate a tension pneumothorax.* ***(Right)*** *This view shows a collapsed left lung and chest wall of a patient with metastatic carcinoma and tension pneumothorax. Nodules of metastatic tumor are present on the lung* ➔ *and chest wall* ➔*.*

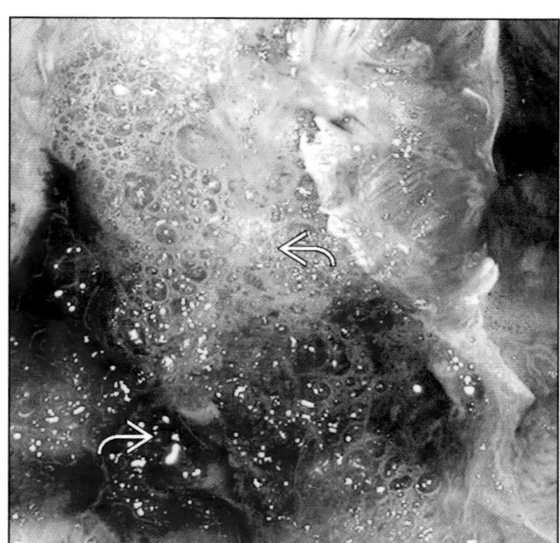

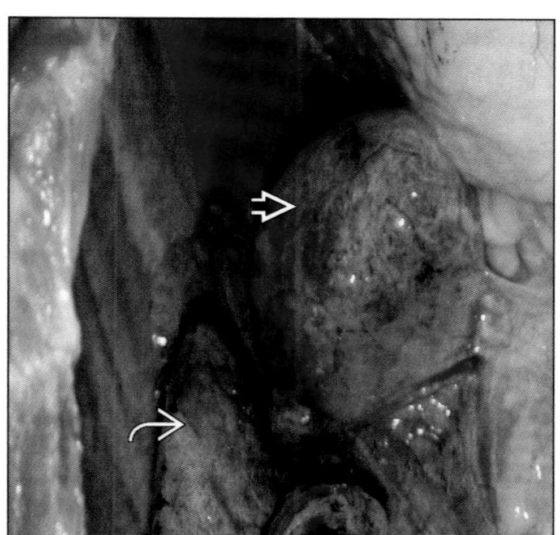

(Left) *Air bubbles* ➔ *in mediastinal soft tissue are consistent with pneumomediastinum in tension pneumothorax.* ***(Right)*** *This patient with severe chronic obstructive pulmonary disease (COPD) and ruptured bulla had tension pneumothorax. The lung* ➔ *is collapsed, and an additional intact bulla* ➔ *is present. Bullae are air-filled spaces beneath the pleura that are usually associated with destruction of lung tissue as seen in emphysema.*

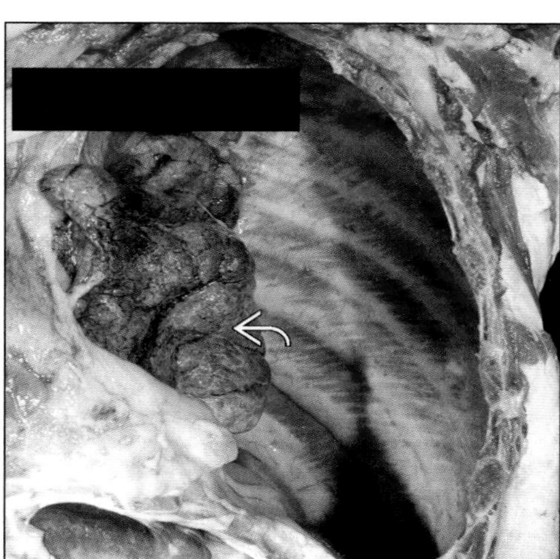

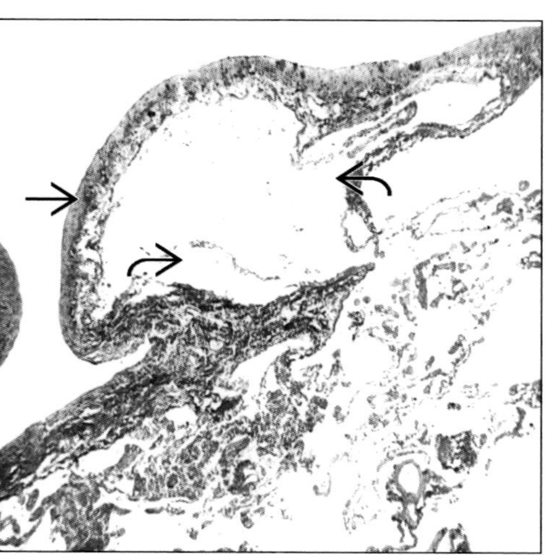

(Left) *This is an example of a collapsed left lung* ➔ *secondary to forceful and prolonged CPR. The contralateral lung was adhesed due to prior surgery. Terminal CPR may be associated with a tension pneumothorax that should not be considered a contributory cause of death.* ***(Right)*** *This is a histologic section of bullous paraseptal (distal acinar) emphysema. The bulla is the large airspace* ➔ *in the subpleural* ➔ *location.*

UPPER GASTROINTESTINAL HEMORRHAGE

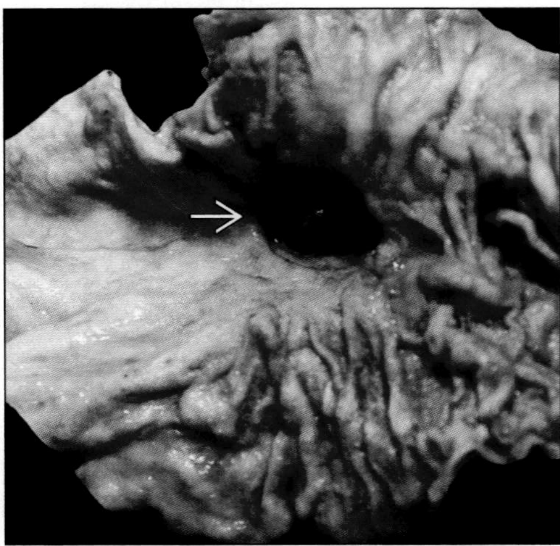

This peptic ulcer ➡ has a characteristic sharply punched out appearance with edges that are level with the surrounding mucosa. Intestinal type tumors tend to rise above surrounding mucosa.

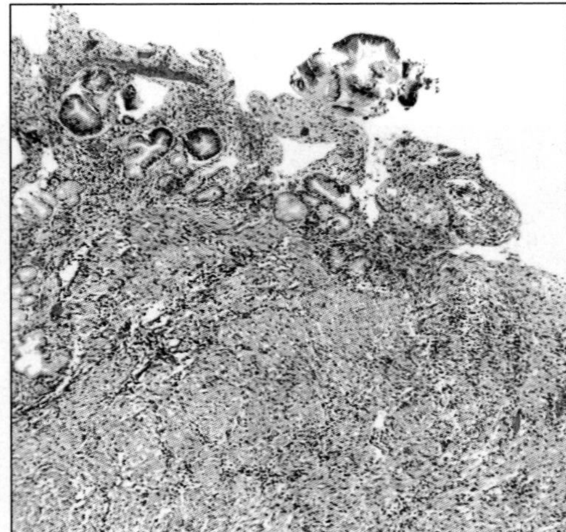

This H&E section from the stomach shows chronic gastritis and mucosal erosion. The patient had a history of NSAID use, and a special stain for Helicobacter was negative.

TERMINOLOGY

Synonyms

- Upper GI bleed

Definitions

- Upper gastrointestinal (UGI) hemorrhage: Gastrointestinal hemorrhage that originates proximal to ligament of Treitz
  - Severe; → shock, > 6% ↓ hematocrit, > 2% ↓ hemoglobin, or transfusion of ≥ 2 units RBC
- Hematemesis: Vomiting of blood; almost always associated with hemorrhage from esophagus, stomach, or duodenum
  - Bright red blood: Recent hemorrhage
  - "Coffee grounds": Result of gastric acid effect on blood
- Melena: Black, tarry stool usually due to UGI hemorrhage but may be seen with bleeding as far down as cecum
  - Result of digestive action by GI tract and bacteria on blood
- Hematochezia: Bright red blood in stool; typically result of lower GI hemorrhage but can be seen with large, rapid UGI bleed

ETIOLOGY/PATHOGENESIS

Peptic Ulcer Disease (PUD)

- **Most common cause of significant UGI bleeding**
- Acid-induced injury to damaged gastric or duodenal mucosa
- Mucosal injury
  - *Helicobacter pylori*: Colonizes mucous layer of stomach with resulting inflammation and mucosal injury
    - Most frequent cause of duodenal ulcers
  - Aspirin/NSAIDs: Used by 11% of adults; causes mucosal injury in part by inhibiting production of protective prostaglandins
  - Predictors of poor outcome: Age > 60, onset while inpatient, comorbid conditions, shock/orthostasis, coagulopathy, multiple transfusions, endoscopically visible vessel, or arterial bleeding
  - Complications of PUD: Potentially life threatening; unusual because of effective medical therapy
    - Perforation: Ulcer erodes through free wall of stomach or duodenum with bleeding and peritonitis
    - Penetration: Ulcer erodes into adjacent structures
    - Obstruction: Chronic gastroduodenitis leads to fibrosis and stenosis of gastric outlet
- Excess acid production
  - Gastrinoma (Zollinger-Ellison syndrome): Endocrine tumors, usually pancreatic; may cause multiple ulcers or ulcers in unusual locations
  - Mast cell tumors: Produce high levels of histamine (potent stimulator of gastric acid secretion)

Esophageal Varices

- **2nd most common cause of significant UGI bleeding**
- Result of portal hypertension, usually in setting of hepatic cirrhosis
- Clinical: 30% mortality with each episode of bleeding
  - Hematemesis with potentially massive blood loss
  - Prognosis depends in part on severity of underlying hepatic disease

Mallory-Weiss Tear

- Etiology: Sudden increases in intraabdominal pressure with transmural pressure gradient across distal esophagus; often associated with hiatal hernia
  - Severe vomiting, retching, coughing, straining; rarely reported with hiccups, CPR, trauma, convulsions

UPPER GASTROINTESTINAL HEMORRHAGE

Key Facts

Etiology

- Predictors of poor outcome: Age > 60, onset while inpatient, comorbid conditions, shock/orthostasis, coagulopathy, multiple transfusions, endoscopically visible vessel, or arterial bleedings

Top Differential Diagnoses

- Peptic ulcer disease: Most common cause of severe UGI hemorrhage
  - Typical gross appearance: Sharply punched-out gastric or duodenal ulcers with nonraised edges and clean ulcer base
  - Histology is crucial to exclude malignancy
- Esophageal varices: 2nd most common cause of severe UGI hemorrhage
  - Esophageal varices collapse after death and are notoriously difficult to demonstrate
  - Eversion of unopened esophagus is a simple means of demonstrating esophageal varices
- UGI tumors (primary and metastatic): 7% of UGI hemorrhage
  - Usually in late-stage disease
  - Poor prognosis

Diagnostic Checklist

- Gross findings may be subtle
  - Clinical presentation, age, and premortem diagnostic studies should guide dissection
  - Other significant history of (NSAID use, gastritis, cirrhosis, trauma, aortic surgery, etc.) may lead to index of suspicion
- Acuity **and** volume of blood influence the differential diagnosis

- Clinical: Typical presentation is retching and vomiting followed by hematemesis (often painless)
  - Blood loss is usually small, and episode is self-limited (90%)
  - Most of these lesions will resolve spontaneously within 48 hours
  - 10% will have severe UGI bleed

Tumors

- Primary (epithelial, stromal, lymphoid) and metastatic (melanoma, carcinoma, etc.) UGI tumors can cause significant UGI bleeding
  - Oncology patients can also have bleeding from PUD, varices, or other nonneoplastic causes
- **UGI bleeding is usually a complication of late-stage disease and carries poor prognosis**

Aortoduodenal Fistula

- Rare and easily missed cause of catastrophic UGI bleeding
- Typically between aneurysmal abdominal aorta and 3rd portion of duodenum
  - May be preceded by a small UGI bleed (herald bleed)
- Aortoenteric fistulas may rarely result from swallowed sharp objects (needles, pins, swizzle sticks) and arise elsewhere in GI tract (e.g., aortoesophageal fistula)

Hematobilia

- Rare cause of UGI hemorrhage
- Abnormal communication between biliary tree and blood vessels
- Can result from trauma, iatrogenic injury, cholecystitis, bile duct tumors, or arterial aneurysms
- Hemosuccus pancreaticus
  - Bleeding through pancreatic duct into ampulla of Vater

Other Vascular Lesions

- Gastric antral vascular ectasia
  - Uncommon cause of chronic UGI hemorrhage and anemia
  - Typically older patients; **striking female preponderance**
  - Associated with portal hypertension in 30% of cases but is also seen with systemic sclerosis and a number of other conditions
- Portal hypertensive gastropathy
  - Seen exclusively in patients with portal hypertension; can sometimes cause chronic hemorrhage and anemia
- Dieulafoy lesion (caliber-persistent artery): Thought to result from congenital vascular malformation
  - Bleeding is typically self-limited but may be severe; can cause recurrent hemorrhage
- Cameron lesion: Ulcers that arise in ~ 5% of hiatal hernias
  - Most will be asymptomatic but some will cause chronic hemorrhage; rare cases of acute UGI hemorrhage are reported

MACROSCOPIC FEATURES

Peptic Ulcer

- Sharply punched-out ulcers without raised edges in stomach/duodenum
  - Gross features can overlap, but carcinomas usually have raised edges
- Clean ulcer base
- "Coffee ground" gastric contents

Esophageal Varices

- External examination: Stigmata of portal hypertension
  - Jaundice, caput medusa, spider angiomata
- Internal examination: Changes of portal hypertension
  - Cirrhosis, splenomegaly, ascites
- Esophagus: **Varices collapse after death and are notoriously hard to demonstrate**
  - Technique: Open stomach along greater curvature, leave esophagus unopened, tie off proximal end of esophagus, use a clamp to reach up the esophageal lumen, grasp proximal end, and evert esophagus

UPPER GASTROINTESTINAL HEMORRHAGE

Causes of Upper Gastrointestinal Hemorrhage

Cause	Frequency
Peptic ulcer disease*	38%
Esophageal varices*	16%
Esophagitis	13%
Unknown	8%
Upper gastrointestinal tumors (primary and metastatic)	7%
Angioma	6%
Mallory-Weiss Tear	4%
Other	8%

*Percentages based on a clinical series. Other causes include mucosal erosion, Dieulafoy lesions, Cameron lesions, aortoduodenal fistula, hemobilia, hemosuccus pancreaticus, gastric antral vascular ectasia, and UGI involvement by amyloidosis. *Most common causes of fatal UGI hemorrhage*

Mallory-Weiss Tear

- Usually single (rarely multiple), linear, longitudinal defect in mucosa and submucosa
- Distal esophagus with occasional extension into proximal stomach

Tumors

- Primary intestinal-type gastric tumors
  - Polypoid or fungating tumors with central ulceration
  - Ulcerated: Gross features can overlap with peptic ulcers
    - Nodular, shaggy, necrotic ulcer base
- Diffuse-type gastric carcinoma (linitis plastica): Rarely presents with bleeding

Aortoduodenal Fistula

- Primary: Fistula between abdominal aortic aneurysm and duodenum
- Secondary: Fistula between surgically repaired aorta and duodenum; usually 3-5 years postoperatively

Hematobilia/Hemosuccus Pancreaticus

- Pancreatic tumor or pseudocyst erodes into vessel (difficult to demonstrate at autopsy)
- Affected vessel often aneurysmal

Other Vascular Lesions

- Gastric antral vascular ectasia: 2 patterns
  - "Watermelon" stomach: Submucosal vascular ectasia with erythematous mucosal crests in parallel linear pattern
  - Diffuse antral mucosal spots separated by grossly normal mucosa
    - Often seen with portal hypertension
- Portal hypertensive gastropathy
  - Mosaic or "snakeskin" appearance seen endoscopically
  - Beefy red mucosa with petechiae, erosions, and ulcers
- Dieulafoy lesion
  - Usually single lesion in distal esophagus/proximal stomach **within 5 cm of GEJ** (can be seen elsewhere)
  - Typically small (0.2-0.5 cm) mucosal defect
  - Easily missed; requires careful inspection of esophageal and gastric mucosa
- Cameron lesions
  - Most arise in distal neck of hiatal hernia
  - Small, linear, erythematous erosions

MICROSCOPIC PATHOLOGY

Peptic Ulcer Disease

- Ulceration and acute and chronic gastroduodenitis
- *Helicobacter* easier to see with histochemical stains or immunoperoxidase

Esophageal Varices

- Dilated submucosal vessels

Other Vascular Lesions

- Gastric antral vascular ectasia
  - Dilated submucosal vessels with fibrohyalinosis and thrombosis
- Portal hypertensive gastropathy
  - Dilated mucosal and submucosal veins and capillaries
- Dieulafoy lesion (caliber-persistent artery)
  - Single, dilated (0.1-0.5 cm) muscular artery under a small mucosal erosion
  - Muscular artery histologically unremarkable, but larger than surrounding mucosal vessels
- Cameron lesions
  - Histologic changes resemble those of ischemic gastritis
  - Clinical/endoscopic information is essential

SELECTED REFERENCES

1. Feinman M et al: Upper gastrointestinal bleeding. Surg Clin North Am. 94(1):43-53, 2014
2. Kapadia S et al: Cameron ulcers: an atypical source for a massive upper gastrointestinal bleed. World J Gastroenterol. 18(35):4959-61, 2012
3. Fenoglio-Preiser CM et al: Gastrointestinal Pathology: An Atlas and Text. 3rd ed. Philadelphia: Lippincott Williams & Wilkins, 2008
4. Merrell SW et al: Hemobilia--evolution of current diagnosis and treatment. West J Med. 155(6):621-5, 1991
5. Clay RP et al: Hemosuccus pancreaticus. An unusual cause of upper gastrointestinal bleeding. Ann Surg. 202(1):75-9, 1985
6. Zimmerman MR: Postmortem demonstration of esophageal varices. Am J Clin Pathol. 65(5):729, 1976

Gross and Microscopic Features

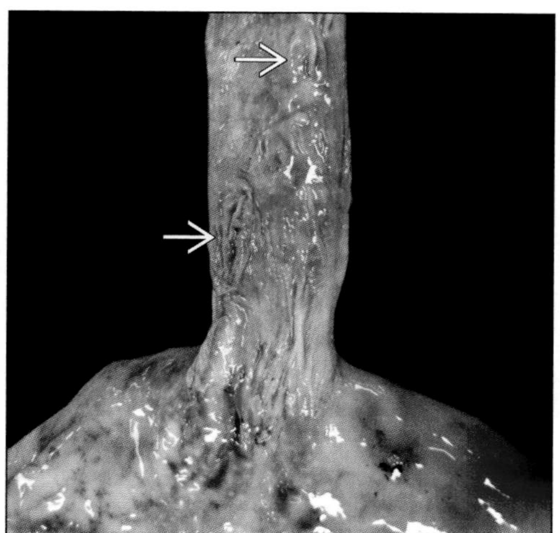

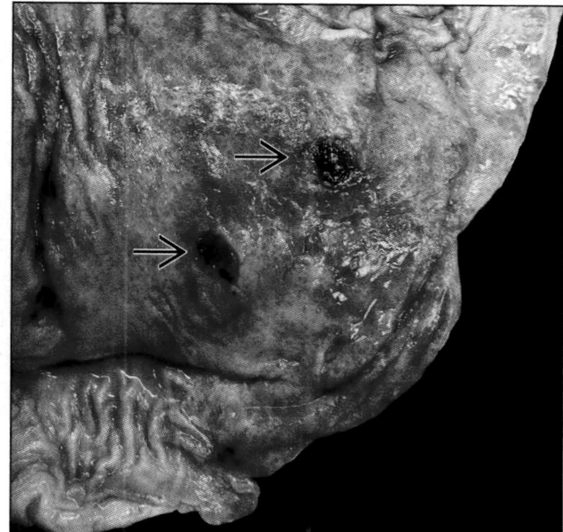

(Left) *This image shows the mucosal surface of an unopened, everted esophagus from a patient with cirrhosis and portal hypertension. Flaccid, dilated submucosal vessels* ➔ *can be seen. During life, these vessels would be visible endoscopically as distended esophageal varices.* ***(Right)*** *This stomach image shows the beefy red mucosa, punctate erythema, and focal ulceration* ➔ *characteristic of portal hypertensive gastropathy. The patient also had cirrhosis and splenomegaly.*

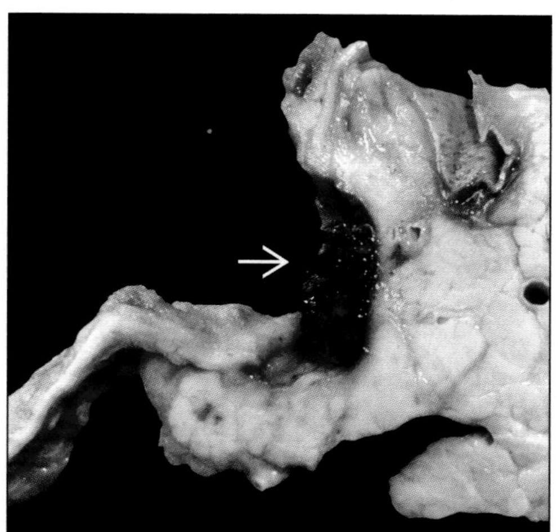

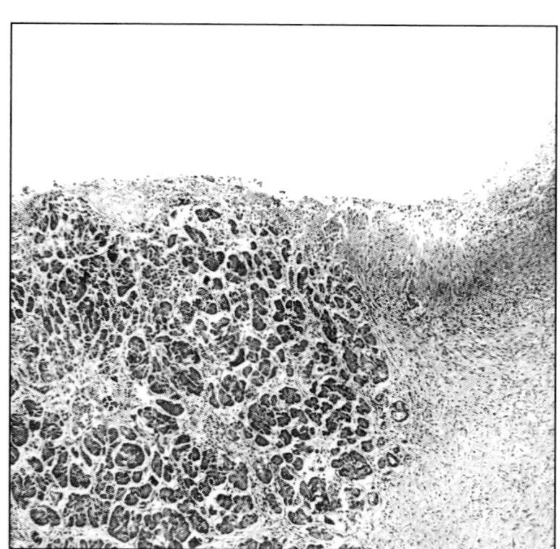

(Left) *This image shows a section through the duodenum and pancreas from a case of penetrating duodenal ulcer. The ulcer* ➔*, which extends through the full thickness of the duodenum and into the adjacent pancreas, resulted in fatal hemorrhage* ***(Right)*** *H&E section of a penetrating duodenal ulcer shows the pancreatic tissue in the ulcer bed. With effective medical therapy, complications of peptic ulcer disease (perforation, penetration, and obstruction) have become unusual.*

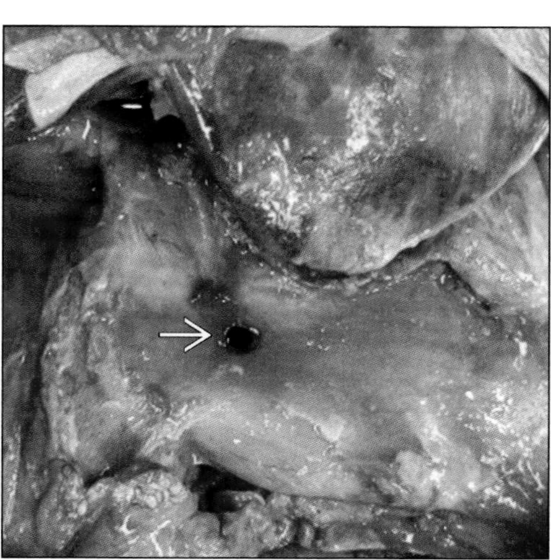

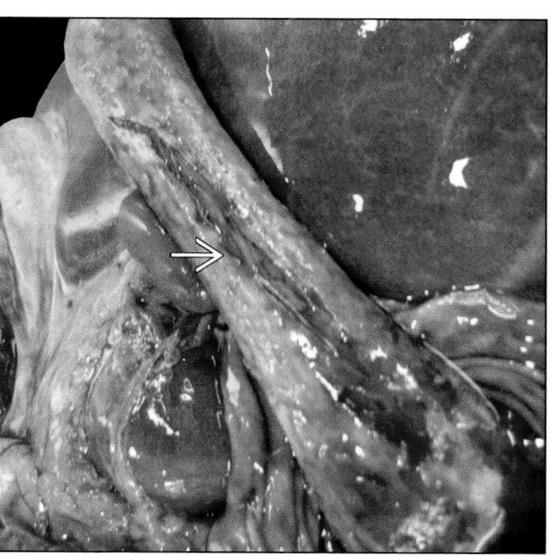

(Left) *In situ photograph of a perforated gastric ulcer shows a sharply punched out, full-thickness ulcer* ➔ *with surrounding serositis and evidence of fat necrosis.* ***(Right)*** *This image of an unopened, everted esophagus shows a single linear, longitudinal defect* ➔ *that involves the mucosa and submucosa of the distal esophagus, features characteristic of a Mallory-Weiss tear. This patient had prolonged severe vomiting followed by hematemesis.*

LOWER GASTROINTESTINAL HEMORRHAGE

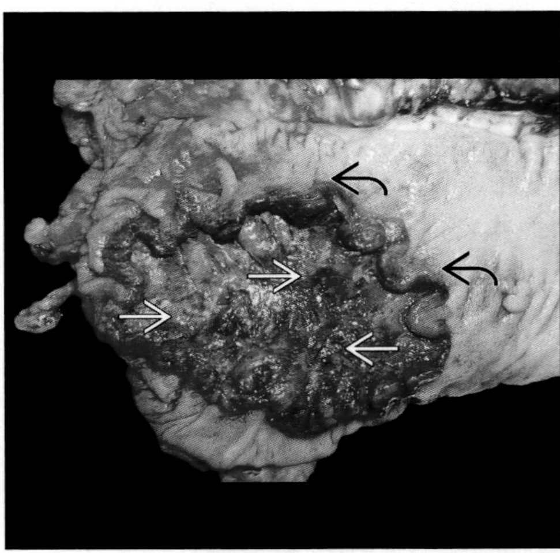

This large rectosigmoid adenocarcinoma with rolled, heaped-up edges ⇨ has a central ulcer ➡ and hemorrhagic foci.

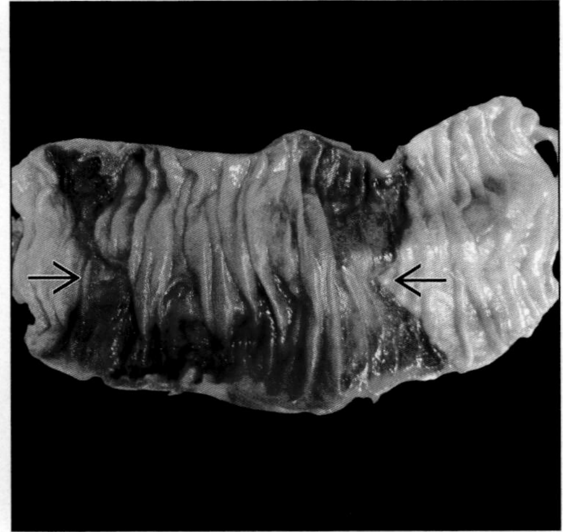

This portion of small bowel shows an area of ischemic enteritis with a discrete, well-demarcated segment of dark red-purple hemorrhagic mucosa ⇨.

TERMINOLOGY

Synonyms

- Lower gastrointestinal bleed (LGIB)

Definitions

- Lower GI hemorrhage
  - Traditional: Blood loss from GI tract distal to ligament of Treitz
  - Current: Blood loss from colon or anorectum
- Hematochezia: Bright red blood upon defecation
- Melena: Black tarry stool due to breakdown of hemoglobin
- Occult bleed: Slow, chronic bleeding not seen grossly

ETIOLOGY/PATHOGENESIS

Common Causes

- Diverticular disease
  - 30-40% of LGIB in adults, ↑ incidence in elderly
  - Most commonly in left colon
  - Acquired pseudodiverticula
    - Herniation through defect in muscularis
    - Contains mucosa and submucosa only
- Meckel diverticulum
  - Common cause of LGIB in children
  - Congenital true diverticulum (all layers of bowel wall) in ileum
- Ischemic enterocolitis
  - Nonocclusive: Low blood flow, vasospasm, medications/drugs
  - Occlusive: Atherosclerosis, thromboembolic, vasculitis
  - External: Volvulus, tumor, intussusception, obstruction
- Stercoral ulcer
  - Rectosigmoid ulcer due to stool impaction in elderly
- Angiodysplasia
  - Acquired vascular lesion in elderly, usually right colon
- Arteriovenous malformation
  - Developmental vascular defect in small/large bowel
- Neoplasia
  - Benign polyps > 1 cm may bleed from surface erosion
  - Postpolypectomy bleeding may occur up to 2 weeks after procedure
    - Incidence is 1-6%, results from inadequate hemostasis, risk ↑ with size of polyp
  - Carcinomas usually cause occult-type bleeding
    - Hematochezia may occur with distal tumors
- Anorectal disease
  - Hemorrhoids
    - Cushions of fibrovascular tissue (engorged veins) ± thrombosis
    - Bleeding may occur due to prolapse or ↑ sphincter or intraabdominal pressure
  - Radiation-induced proctitis/colitis
    - Consequence of irradiation for pelvic malignancies
  - Mucosal/rectal prolapse
    - Due to abnormal pelvic floor muscle function during defecation causing excessive straining
- Other inflammatory diseases
  - Inflammatory bowel disease (IBD) (e.g., ulcerative colitis, Crohn disease), usually bloody diarrhea (severe LGIB < 1%)
  - Medications (e.g., NSAIDs, sodium polystyrene)
  - Infections
    - Bloody diarrhea/dysentery (enterohemorrhagic *Escherichia coli*, *Salmonella*, *Shigella*)
    - Pseudomembranous (*Clostridium difficile*)
    - Ulcerative (viral, *Entamoeba histolytica*)
    - IBD-like (*Yersinia*)

LOWER GASTROINTESTINAL HEMORRHAGE

Key Facts

Terminology
- Lower GI hemorrhage
  - Traditional: Blood loss from GI tract distal to ligament of Treitz
  - Recent: Blood loss from colon or anorectum

Etiology
- Diverticular disease
- Infections
  - Bloody diarrhea/dysentery (enterohemorrhagic *E. coli*, *Salmonella*, *Shigella*)
  - Pseudomembranous (*C. difficile*)
  - Ulcerative (viral, *E. histolytica*)
  - IBD-like (*Yersinia*)
- IBD (ulcerative colitis, Crohn disease), usually bloody diarrhea (severe LGIB < 1%)

Clinical Issues
- LGIB accounts for 20% of all GI bleeding
- Exact location of bleed not identified clinically in 10% of cases
- Important elements of chart review
  - Type of bleeding, frequency, severity, duration
  - Factors affecting coagulation (cirrhosis, medications)
  - Medications (NSAIDs, sodium polystyrene)
  - Underlying GI disease
  - Prior therapy

Top Differential Diagnoses
- Postmortem autolysis occurs rapidly in luminal GI tract, may obscure diagnostic features of some diseases

CLINICAL ISSUES

Epidemiology
- Incidence
  - 20-30 cases/100,000 adults in US
  - 20% of all GI bleeds are LGIB
  - Exact location of bleed not identified clinically in 10% of cases

Presentation
- Hematochezia, melena, occult bleed, anemia, abdominal pain
- Important elements of chart review
  - Type of bleeding, frequency, severity, duration
  - Factors affecting coagulation (cirrhosis, medications)
  - Medications (NSAIDs, sodium polystyrene)
  - Underlying GI disease
    - Diverticular disease, neoplasm, IBD
  - Prior therapy
    - Radiation, endoscopic biopsy/clips/cautery/ injection, angiographic embolization/vasopressin infusion

Laboratory Tests
- ↓ hemoglobin/hematocrit, iron deficiency anemia
- Thrombocytopenia, ↑ prothrombin & partial thromboplastin times
- (+) fecal occult blood test, ± stool bacteria cultures, ova and parasite tests, *C. difficile* toxin assay, blood cultures

Prognosis
- Mortality ≤ 5% but ↑ if bleeding occurs after hospitalization
- ↑ morbidity in older patients
- Spontaneous cessation in 80% of cases
- May vary with etiology
  - Stercoral ulcer: High risk of perforation
  - Meckel diverticulum: Intussusception or volvulus
  - Angiodysplasia: May cause massive hemorrhage

IMAGE FINDINGS

CT Findings
- Thickened bowel wall, edema, pericolonic stranding, obstruction, mass, diverticula

Nuclear Medicine Findings
- CT angiography or nuclear scintigraphy/RBC scan may localize bleed

MACROSCOPIC FEATURES

External Examination
- Pallor of skin, mucous membranes, conjunctiva
- Koilonychia, oral ulcers, glossitis
- External hemorrhoids, perianal ulcers/fissures, hernias

Internal Examination
- Ascites, hemoperitoneum, perforations ± peritonitis, adhesions, strictures
- Surgical anastomoses: Ulcers, ischemia, perforation, dehiscence

Organ Examination
- Diverticular disease
  - Outpouchings of mucosa through muscularis propria (pseudodiverticula), strictures, subserosal abscess cavities, perforation
- Meckel diverticulum
  - Outpouching of bowel wall along antimesenteric border of ileum
- Ischemic enterocolitis
  - Segmental vs. diffuse, watershed areas (splenic flexure, rectosigmoid junction)
  - Mucosal congestion, edema, ulceration ± perforation, serosal fibrinous exudate, pseudomembranes, gross thrombi in mesenteric vessels
- Benign ulcers (stercoral, medication induced)
  - Hemorrhagic mucosa and ulcer with purulent exudate

LOWER GASTROINTESTINAL HEMORRHAGE

- Angiodysplasia
  - Gross appearance usually subtle, appears as foci of mucosal/submucosal erythema
- Arteriovenous malformation
  - Mass of tortuous dilated vessels usually in subserosa
- Neoplasia
  - Polyp or mass with surface erosion/ulcer
  - Following polypectomy or biopsy of mass: Hemorrhagic biopsy site ± mucosal defect
- Anorectal disease
  - Hemorrhoids
    - Dilated, engorged submucosal vessels ± ulceration, thrombosis
  - Radiation-induced proctitis/colitis
    - Acute: Friable mucosa with erosions and edema
    - Chronic: Result of vascular injury & ischemia (ulcers, mucosal telangiectasias, strictures, fistulas, serosal adhesions)
  - Mucosal/rectal prolapse
    - Well-demarcated ulcers, polypoid erythematous mass-like lesions
- Other inflammatory diseases
  - Ulcerative colitis: Diffuse continuous hemorrhagic granular mucosa from rectum proximally, ± ulcers
  - Crohn disease: Patchy involvement of small ± large bowel by deep ulcers, cobblestone mucosa, creeping fat, strictures, fistulas, usually rectal sparing
  - Infections: Variable, typically diffuse erythema

Sections to Be Submitted

- Gross mucosal abnormalities, ulcers, perforations
- Mesenteric vessels in cases of ischemia (emboli, thrombosis)
- Large polyps/masses + grossly positive lymph nodes

MICROSCOPIC PATHOLOGY

Histologic Features

- Diverticular disease
  - Peridiverticular abscess, foreign body giant cell reaction, cryptitis, congestion, erosion with hemorrhage
- Meckel diverticulum
  - All 3 layers of bowel wall, ileal-type epithelium ± various heterotopias
- Ischemic enterocolitis
  - Early: Submucosal edema, congestion, hemorrhage
  - Ulcers, mucopurulent exudate (pseudomembranes), loss of epithelium, mucosal/transmural necrosis
  - Remaining crypts have withered appearance with hyalinized lamina propria
  - Mesenteric vessels ± organizing thrombi, atherosclerosis, cholesterol emboli, vasculitis
- Benign ulcers (stercoral, medication induced)
  - Erosions, nonspecific inflammation, fibrinopurulent exudate, deep ulcers with hemorrhage
- Angiodysplasia
  - Submucosal cluster of dilated thin-walled veins, arterioles, capillaries
- Arteriovenous malformation
  - Subserosal clusters of dilated arteries and veins with arterialization of veins (thickened wall with myointimal hyperplasia)
- Radiation proctitis/colitis
  - Acute: Erosions, submucosal edema, regenerative epithelial changes
  - Chronic: Ulcers, dilated mucosal capillaries, hyalinized lamina propria and submucosal vessels, atypical fibroblasts
- Mucosal/rectal prolapse
  - Mucosal erosion, vascular congestion, distorted and dilated crypts, lamina propria fibrosis
  - Thickened muscularis mucosa with splayed muscle fibers extending up into mucosa
- Inflammatory bowel disease
  - Ulcerative colitis: Chronic active colitis ± ulcers affecting mucosa only
  - Crohn disease: Chronic active colitis/enteritis ± ulcers and granulomas, transmural inflammation

ANCILLARY TESTS

Microbiology

- Stool cultures and other tests (ova and parasites, PCR, etc.) can be performed on postmortem samples
- Blood cultures in suspected infection/sepsis

DIFFERENTIAL DIAGNOSIS

Autolysis

- Occurs rapidly post mortem
- Affects mucosa first with fading of histologic detail, loss of epithelial cells, ghosts of normal structures
  - May mimic ischemic colitis, but lack of vital reaction and vascular thrombosis helps to distinguish
  - May obscure diagnostic features of other diseases

REPORTING CONSIDERATIONS

Key Elements to Report

- Location and etiology of hemorrhage
  - Cause of death, contributing factor, or incidental
- Underlying GI disease and risk factors for hemorrhage
- Effects of hemorrhage/disease on other organs

SELECTED REFERENCES

1. Barnert J et al: Diagnosis and management of lower gastrointestinal bleeding. Nat Rev Gastroenterol Hepatol. 6(11):637-46, 2009
2. West A.B. et al: Vascular disorders of the GI tract. In R.D. Odz et al: Surgical Pathology of the GI Tract, Liver, Biliary Tract, and Pancreas. 2nd ed. Philadelphia: Saunders/ Elsevier. 185-230, 2009
3. Edelman DA et al: Lower gastrointestinal bleeding: a review. Surg Endosc. 21(4):514-20, 2007

Gross and Microscopic Features

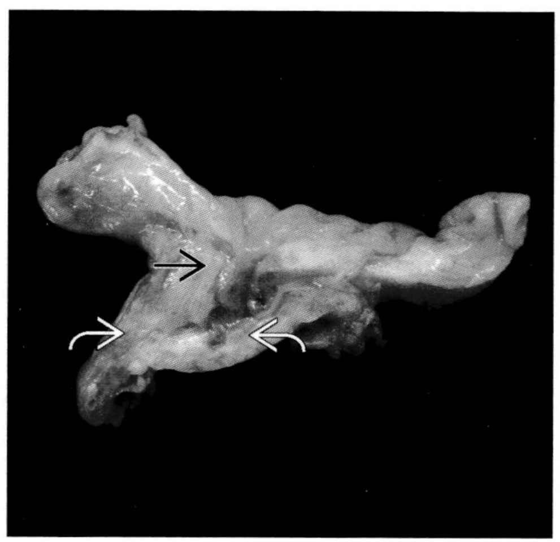

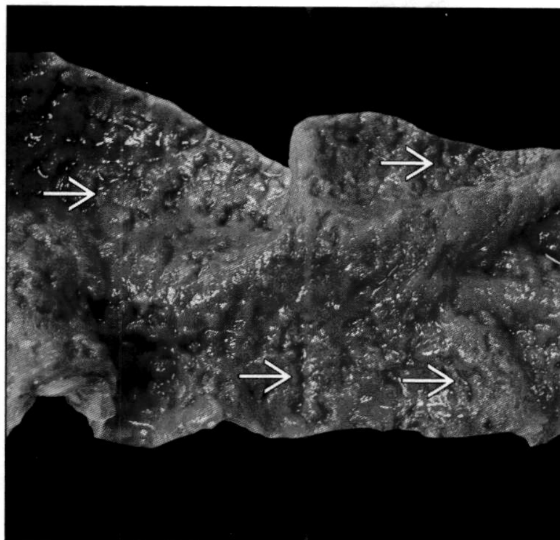

(Left) *This is a cross section of a diverticulum in the sigmoid colon showing outpouching of the mucosa through the muscularis propria ➔ with a peridiverticular abscess cavity and associated fibrosis ➔.* ***(Right)*** *The entire colonic mucosa is diffusely hemorrhagic and granular with numerous irregular ulcers ➔ in this patient with ulcerative colitis.*

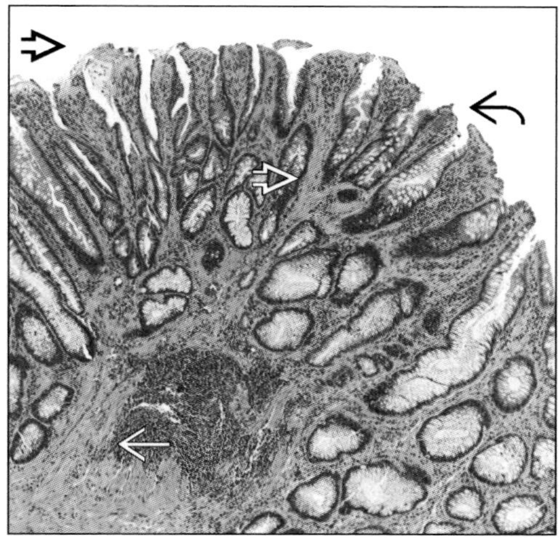

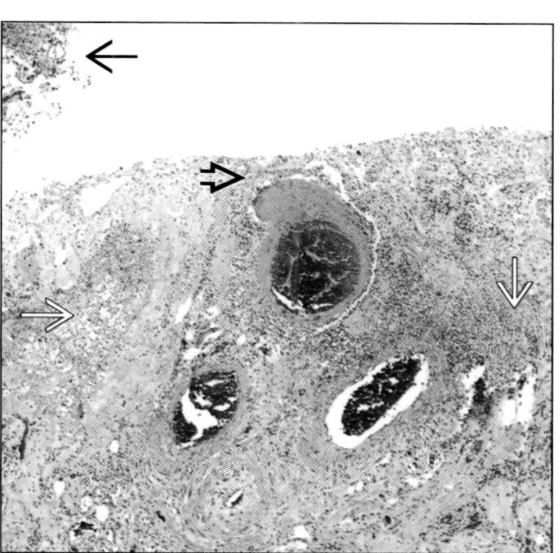

(Left) *This example of rectal prolapse shows polypoid mucosa with surface erosion and ischemic-type injury ➔, exposed mucosal capillaries ➔, and splayed muscularis mucosa ➔ with smooth muscle fibers extending vertically toward the lumen ➔.* ***(Right)*** *The mucosa in this NSAID-associated cecal ulcer is completely eroded, exposing a large submucosal vessel ➔. Submucosal acute inflammation and necrosis ➔ and purulent exudate within the lumen ➔ are also present.*

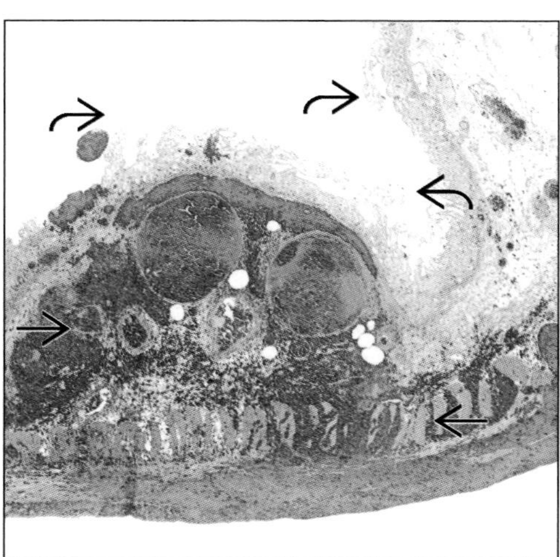

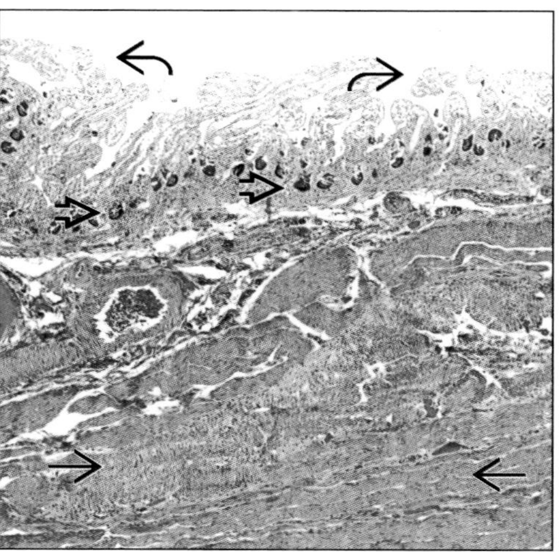

(Left) *This case of ischemic enteritis shows complete epithelial loss and "ghosts" of villi ➔. Full-thickness coagulative necrosis ➔, hemorrhage, and transmural acute inflammation are also present.* ***(Right)*** *Autolyzed small bowel with near total epithelial loss and "ghosts" of villi ➔ mimics ischemic enteritis. Basal crypt epithelial cells are preserved ➔. The muscularis propria ➔ is intact and viable without evidence of transmural hemorrhage, necrosis, or inflammation.*

INTESTINAL ISCHEMIA

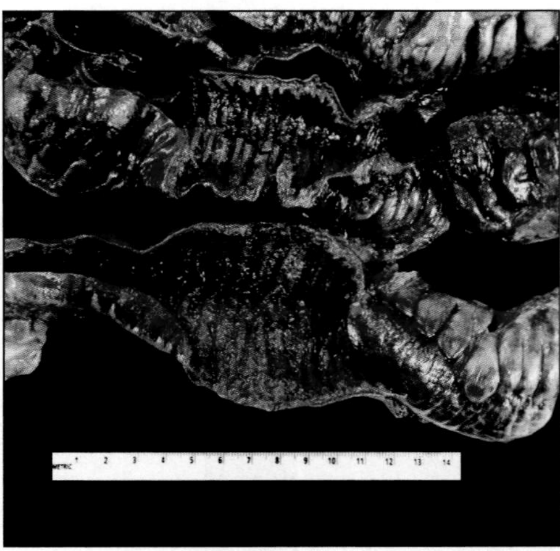

This segment of infarcted small bowel with a red-black hemorrhagic appearance was due to mesenteric vein thrombosis in a hypercoagulable patient with portal vein thrombosis and pulmonary embolism.

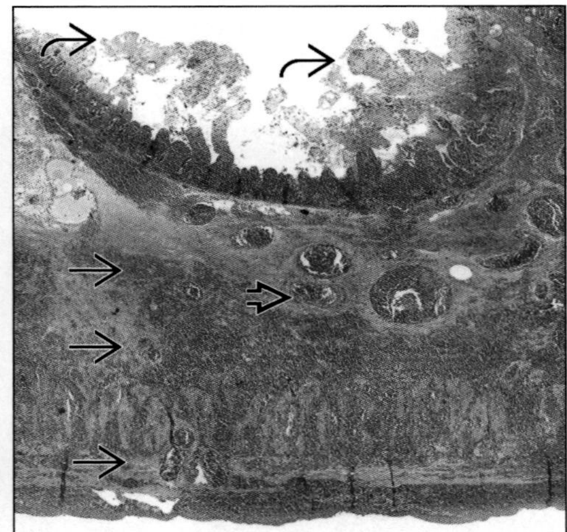

Histologic sections of the infarcted small bowel show transmural hemorrhage ➔, vascular congestion ➔, and mucosal necrosis ➔.

TERMINOLOGY

Definitions

- Reduction in intestinal blood flow resulting in bowel injury ± infarction, necrosis, and perforation

ETIOLOGY/PATHOGENESIS

Acute Mesenteric Ischemia (AMI)

- Mesenteric artery embolism
  - 50% of AMI cases
  - Usually involves superior mesenteric artery (SMA)
    - SMA anatomy → risk for obstruction: High basal flow rate and acute angle of take-off from aorta
  - Risk factors: Atrial fibrillation, other arrhythmia, myocardial infarction, valvular disease, endocarditis, cardiac catheterization
- Mesenteric artery thrombosis
  - 15-25% of AMI, usually at SMA origin or celiac axis
  - Usually thrombosis superimposed on a critical atherosclerotic lesion
  - Less common: Vasculitis, SMA aneurysm/dissection, thrombophilia, fibromuscular dysplasia, vascular amyloid
- Nonocclusive mesenteric ischemia (NOMI)
  - 20-30% of AMI, many etiologies all → vasoconstriction of intestinal vessels and ↓ flow
  - Risk factors: Cardiogenic, hypovolemic, or septic shock, congestive heart failure, cardiac/major abdominal surgery, vasoconstricting drugs (e.g., digoxin, α-adrenergic agonists, cocaine, ergot)
- Mesenteric venous thrombosis
  - 5% of AMI cases, impaired venous return, bowel wall edema, impaired microvascular perfusion, ↓ arterial flow, and hemorrhage
  - Risk factors: Inherited or acquired hypercoagulable states, abdominal infections/trauma, portal hypertension, periportal malignancy, pancreatitis, severe dehydration
- Secondary to mechanical obstruction
  - Strangulated hernia, intussusception, volvulus, tumors, adhesions

Chronic Mesenteric Ischemia (CMI)

- Rare due to rich collateral networks
  - Need to have ≥ 2 mesenteric arterial branches involved by atherosclerosis/stenosis to occur
- F > M, 50-60 years; associated with systemic atherosclerosis, coronary artery disease, tobacco use, and hypertension

Ischemic Colitis

- Specific occluding lesion rarely identified, may be transient and reversible or chronic
- Usually acutely ↓ blood flow
  - "Watershed" areas with limited collateral flow vulnerable (i.e., splenic flexure, right colon, rectosigmoid junction)
- Risk factors: Hypotension/shock, hypercoagulable states, mechanical obstruction (adhesions, diverticulitis, prolapse, tumors, volvulus), aortoiliac or cardiac bypass surgery
- Drugs/medications: Antihypertensives, cocaine, sodium polystyrene (Kayexalate), oral contraceptives, digoxin, nonsteroidals, diuretics, pseudoephedrine
- Infectious ischemic-type colitis (e.g., *Escherichia coli* 0157:H7, *Clostridium difficile* [C. diff], *Salmonella*, *Shigella*, *Entamoeba histolytica*)

CLINICAL ISSUES

Presentation

- Abdominal pain (out of proportion to physical exam findings in AMI), nausea, vomiting, diarrhea, hematochezia, melena

INTESTINAL ISCHEMIA

Key Facts

Terminology
- Reduction in intestinal blood flow resulting in bowel injury ± infarction, necrosis, and perforation

Etiology
- Mesenteric artery embolism
- Mesenteric artery thrombosis
- Nonocclusive mesenteric ischemia (NOMI)
- Mesenteric venous thrombosis
- Secondary to mechanical obstruction
- Ischemic colitis
- Drugs, infections

Macroscopic Pathology
- Evaluate small and large intestine in situ for perforations, adhesions, volvulus, strangulated hernias, intussusception, masses
- Examine aorta and branches for atherosclerosis, stenosis/occlusion, thrombi, status of stents
- Examine branches of inferior vena cava for thrombi

Microscopic Pathology
- Epithelial degenerative/reactive changes with loss of cytoplasmic mucin and hyperchromatic nuclei, sloughing, necrosis, ulcers
- Submucosal edema, congestion, lamina propria hemorrhage, transmural necrosis/hemorrhage, serositis
- Vascular findings: Thromboemboli, cholesterol emboli, atherosclerosis, vasculitis, amyloid deposition, tumor thrombi, pyelophlebitis

Top Differential Diagnoses
- Autolysis

- Weight loss, postprandial pain, early satiety, and food aversion (CMI)
- Tachycardia, tachypnea, arrhythmia, altered mental status, fever, anorexia, abdominal tenderness, peritoneal signs (late), shock
  - Indirect signs of atherosclerosis (↓ peripheral pulses, carotid/femoral bruits, stigmata of prior stroke)
- Important elements of chart review
  - General risk factors: Older age, tobacco use, hypertension, thrombophilia, obesity (↑ risk for venous thrombi), dyslipidemia
  - Cardiac risk factors: Myocardial infarction, arrhythmia, cardiac valve disease ± endocarditis (nonbacterial thrombotic or infectious), congestive heart failure, known aneurysm (heart, aorta)
  - Prior procedures: Cardiac catheterization, cardiac/abdominal surgery, arterial bypass surgery
  - Medications/drugs, history of malignancy or cirrhosis
  - Surgical/other interventions performed, postintervention course

Laboratory Tests
- Hemoconcentration, leukocytosis, metabolic acidosis with ↑ anion gap
- ↑ amylase, lactate dehydrogenase, alkaline phosphatase
- ↑ digoxin level, (+) cocaine metabolites
- (+) fecal occult blood, blood culture, stool culture/C. diff toxin assay/parasites

Prognosis
- Mortality varies depending on cause
  - Mesenteric artery embolus ~ 70%
  - Mesenteric artery thrombosis ~ 90%
  - NOMI ~ 70-90%
  - Mesenteric venous thrombosis ~ 20-50%
  - Ischemic colitis (if gangrenous) ~ 50%

Complications
- Ileus, perforation, peritonitis, gastrointestinal bleeding, sepsis, multiorgan failure

IMAGE FINDINGS

Ultrasonographic Findings
- Arterial occlusion/stenosis (with Doppler)

CT Findings
- Segmental circumferential bowel wall thickening, mesenteric stranding/edema, vascular occlusions, atherosclerosis, pneumatosis, portal venous gas
- Masses/obstructions, volvulus, intussusception
- Ascites, intraabdominal free air

Mesenteric Angiography
- Diagnostic and therapeutic (not typically used for ischemic colitis)

MACROSCOPIC FEATURES

External Examination
- Surgical interventions: Wound status, drains
- Abdominal/inguinal/incisional hernias
- Sepsis changes: Petechiae, jaundice, acrocyanosis

Internal Examination
- Ascites ± feculent debris
- Peritonitis (green fibrinous exudates on peritoneal/serosal surfaces), adhesions, masses
- Evaluate small and large intestine in situ for perforations, adhesions, volvulus, strangulated hernias, intussusception, masses

Organ Examination
- Examine aorta and major branches for atherosclerosis, aneurysms, dissection, stenosis/occlusion, thrombi, presence and status of stents
- Examine for evidence of thrombophilia and presence of venous thrombi/thromboemboli
  - Inferior vena cava thrombi, presence and status of previously inserted IVC filter
  - Portal vein thrombosis
  - Pulmonary artery venous thromboembolism

INTESTINAL ISCHEMIA

- Legs can be "milked" for evaluation of deep vein thrombosis once organs are removed
- Small and large intestine
  - Early/acute ischemia
    - Friable, erythematous mucosa ± ulcers, pseudomembranes
    - Thickened edematous or thin friable bowel wall, pneumatosis (submucosal/subserosal bubbles/ cystic nodules), perforation
    - Red/black hemorrhagic mucosa and boggy hemorrhagic wall (usually in venous insufficiency)
  - Chronic ischemia
    - Circumferential bowel wall thickening, strictures
  - Segmental, patchy, or diffuse involvement
  - Mesenteric/subserosal vessels: Thrombi, atherosclerotic lesions, stenosis
- Lungs: Edema, congestion, infection (pneumonia may be possible source of septic shock → ischemic bowel)
- Liver: Congestion/necrosis (shock), cholestasis (sepsis), portal vein thrombosis
- Kidneys: Cortical pallor, medullary congestion
- Heart and vasculature
  - Atherosclerotic coronary and aortic disease ± myocardial acute/chronic ischemia
    - Check for vascular thrombi, dissection, aneurysm
  - Thromboembolic foci
    - Atrial/ventricular thrombi (also check for patent foramen ovale → paradoxical embolization venous to arterial), vegetations on valves (thrombotic or endocarditis), neoplasms (rare: Atrial myxoma, papillary fibroelastoma of aortic valve)

MICROSCOPIC PATHOLOGY

Histologic Features

- Small and large intestine
  - Early/acute ischemia
    - Epithelial degenerative/reactive changes with loss of cytoplasmic mucin and hyperchromatic nuclei, sloughing, necrosis
    - Ulcers, fibrinopurulent exudate
    - Submucosal edema, congestion, lamina propria hemorrhage, transmural necrosis/hemorrhage, acute/organizing serositis
    - Remaining crypts are "withered"
    - Pneumatosis: Cystic spaces lined by macrophages and multinucleated giant cells
  - Chronic ischemia
    - Fibrosis of all layers of bowel wall ± ulcers
  - Vascular findings: Thromboemboli, cholesterol emboli, atherosclerotic changes, vasculitis, amyloid deposition (Congo red stain [+]), tumor thrombi, pyelophlebitis
  - Sodium polystyrene (Kayexalate) crystals: Nonpolarizable, basophilic crystals with fish scale or mosaic appearance present in ulcer exudate
- Liver
  - Sepsis changes: Hepatocellular, canalicular, and ductular cholestasis
  - Shock changes: Centrilobular/perivenular congestion ± hepatocellular necrosis
- Lungs: Bronchopneumonia, diffuse alveolar damage (alveolar hyaline membranes, neutrophils, fibrin deposition, edema), thromboemboli, intraalveolar hemorrhage
- Kidneys
  - Dilated tubules and tubal epithelial necrosis/ sloughing (acute tubular injury), coagulative necrosis of cortex (cortical necrosis)
  - Arteriolosclerosis, glomerular capillary thrombi (disseminated intravascular coagulation from sepsis)
- Heart
  - Subendocardial/myocardial contraction band injury, coagulative necrosis, edema, hemorrhage, scarred thinned aneurysm wall usually with mural thrombus
  - Nonbacterial thrombotic endocarditis (bland [noninfected] thrombi along closing edge of valve), infected vegetation with fibrin, scattered leukocytes, bacterial/fungal colonies

ANCILLARY TESTS

Microbiology

- Blood, fluid collection, stool cultures, and other stool studies (e.g., ova and parasites, toxin assays) can be performed postmortem
- Gram/fungal stains on possible infected vegetations, other areas of suppurative inflammation

DIFFERENTIAL DIAGNOSIS

Autolysis

- Occurs rapidly postmortem
- Affects mucosa first with fading of histologic detail, loss of epithelial cells, ghosts of normal structures
- Lack of vital reaction (hemorrhage, inflammation, necrosis) or vascular thrombosis

REPORTING CONSIDERATIONS

Key Elements to Report

- Immediate cause of death and how it relates to intestinal ischemia
- Etiology of intestinal ischemia and subsequent complications
- Underlying conditions association with development of intestinal ischemia

SELECTED REFERENCES

1. Bobadilla JL: Mesenteric ischemia. Surg Clin North Am. 93(4):925-40, ix, 2013
2. Byard RW: Acute mesenteric ischaemia and unexpected death. J Forensic Leg Med. 19(4):185-90, 2012
3. Florian A et al: Mesenteric ischemia--a complex disease requiring an interdisciplinary approach. A review of the current literature. Rom J Intern Med. 48(3):207-22, 2010
4. Harnik IG et al: Mesenteric venous thrombosis. Vasc Med. 15(5):407-18, 2010

Gross and Microscopic Features

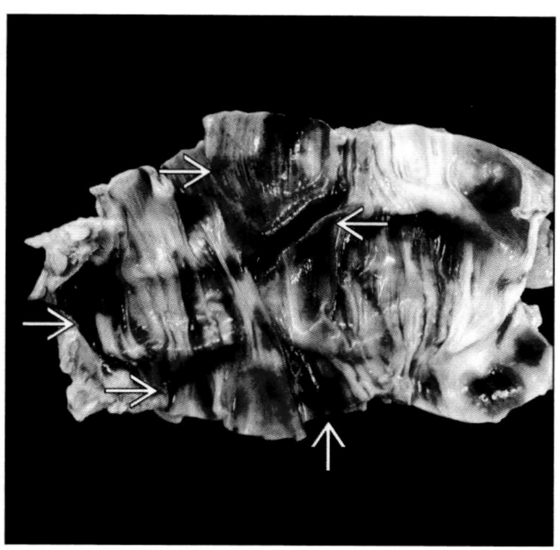

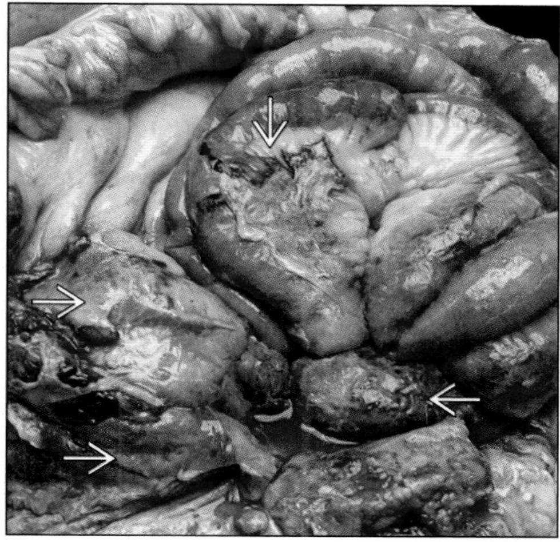

(Left) *This segment of small bowel from a patient with multiple abdominal adhesions shows patchy red-black mucosal discoloration ➡ in areas of ischemic injury.* ***(Right)*** *Acute peritonitis and serositis ➡ developed in a patient with ischemic colitis due to multiple hypotensive episodes that resulted in rectosigmoid perforation and sepsis.*

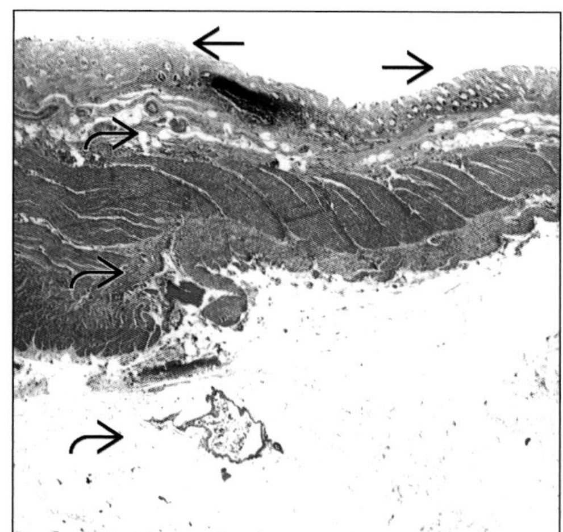

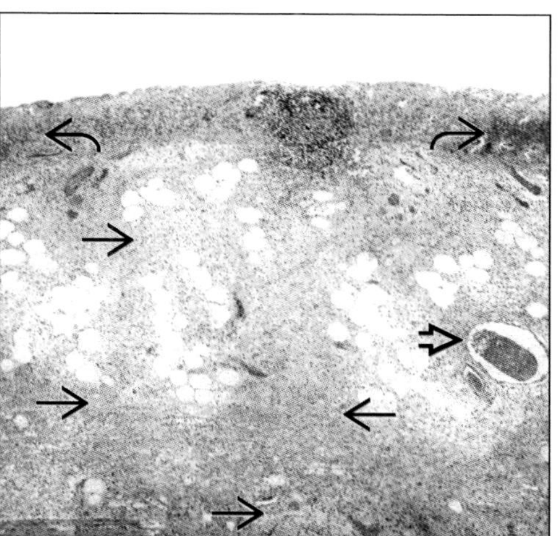

(Left) *This section of normal colon shows changes of autolysis without evidence of injury. The surface epithelium has faded with loss of epithelial cells in crypts ➡. The submucosa, muscularis propria, and subserosa are intact ➡.* ***(Right)*** *Although the mucosa is autolyzed, ischemic colitis can still be diagnosed by the presence of a "vital reaction" in the tissue (i.e., lamina propria hemorrhage ➡, transmural inflammation ➡, and vascular congestion ➡).*

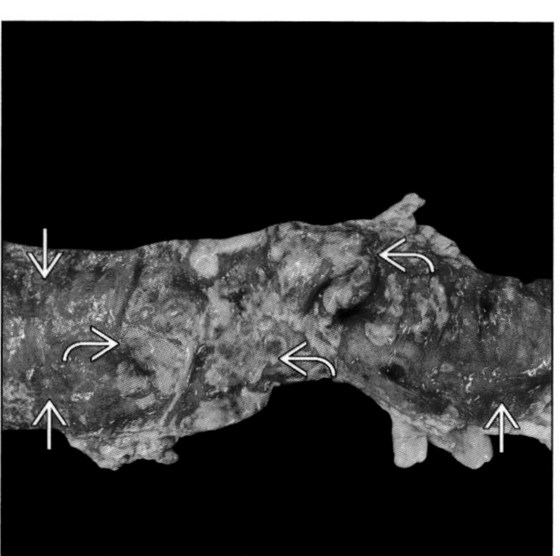

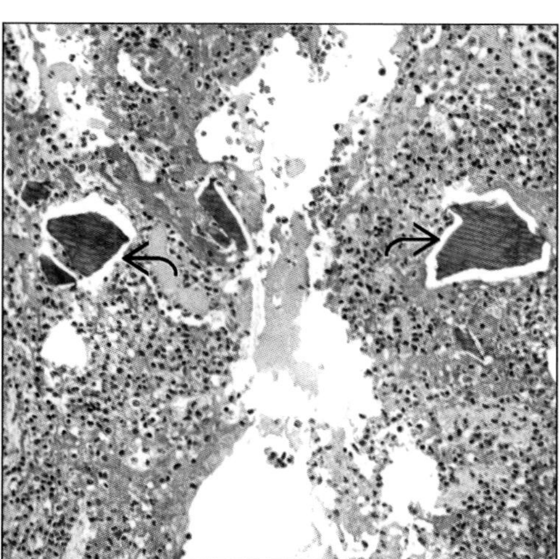

(Left) *This segment of colon has an erythematous, granular mucosa ➡ with multiple tan-brown ulcers ➡ in this case of ischemic colitis due to sodium polystyrene use in a patient with chronic kidney failure.* ***(Right)*** *Sodium polystyrene crystals ➡ (basophilic with a mosaic or fish scale appearance) are present in the fibrinopurulent ulcer exudate in this patient with ischemic colitis.*

HEPATIC HEMORRHAGE

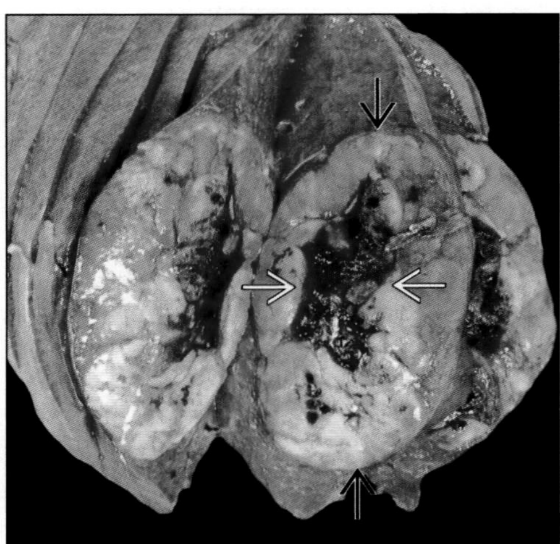

The cut surface of this hepatocellular carcinoma ⇒ shows intratumoral hemorrhage/hematoma ➡.

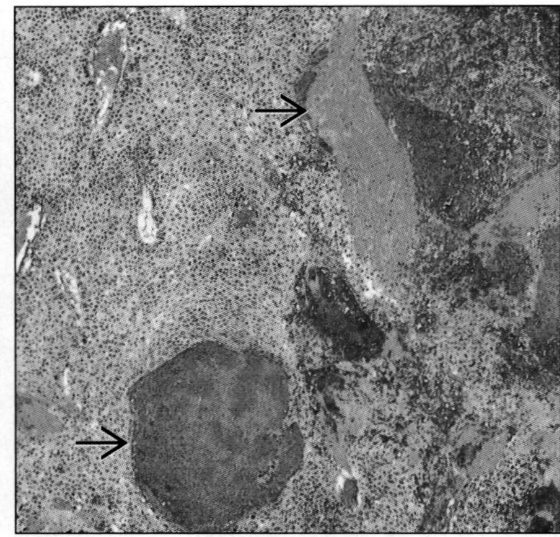

A histologic section of this hepatocellular carcinoma shows sheets of malignant hepatocytes with intratumoral hemorrhage/hematoma ⇒.

TERMINOLOGY

Definitions

- Intraparenchymal with hematoma ± hemobilia or hepatic rupture with hemoperitoneum

ETIOLOGY/PATHOGENESIS

Tumors

- Pathogenesis of rupture
  - ↑ intravascular/intratumoral pressure resulting from thrombi → venous outflow obstruction, vascular rupture and intratumoral/intraparenchymal hemorrhage
  - Direct pressure of tumor on capsule, extrahepatic invasion
- Hepatocellular carcinoma
  - Rupture in 3-26%
  - Risk factors for rupture: Cirrhosis, hypertension, size > 5 cm, protrusion from surface, vascular thrombi, extrahepatic invasion
- Hepatocellular adenoma
  - 4 major subtypes: *HNF1A* mutated type (steatotic), β-catenin mutated type, inflammatory (a.k.a. telangiectatic) type, unclassified type (no mutations or specific features)
  - Rupture in up to 25%
  - Risk factors for rupture: Size > 5 cm, recent hormone use or pregnancy, inflammatory type due to presence of sinusoidal dilatation/peliosis
- Hemangioma
  - Rupture in 1-4%
  - Risk factors for rupture: Large size, coagulopathy
- Metastatic neoplasms
  - Rupture is rare; exact incidence unknown
  - Risk factors for rupture: Large size, subcapsular location
- Other rare primary hepatic tumors
  - Benign cysts/polycystic liver disease, angiosarcoma, epithelioid hemangioendothelioma

Pregnancy Related

- Rupture in ~ 1-2% with severe preeclampsia/eclampsia ± hemolysis, elevated liver enzymes, and low platelet count (HELLP) syndrome
- Usually multiparous, 30-40 years old
- Exact cause unknown; hypotheses include hypertension, hemolysis, vasospasm → fibrin deposition, ischemia, infarction, sinusoidal obstruction, neovascularization → microhemorrhage, hematoma, rupture

Iatrogenic

- Status post percutaneous biliary drain placement
  - Incidence of significant hemorrhage is ~ 2-3%
  - Causes: Injury to hepatic artery, portal vein, or intercostal artery resulting in (peri)hepatic or gastrointestinal hemorrhage, bleeding into biliary drain, or hemothorax
- Status post core biopsy
  - Incidence of significant hemorrhage is ~ 0.3-0.5%
  - Risk factors for hemorrhage: ↑ age, cirrhosis, > 3 passes performed
  - Early/immediate hemorrhage due to capsular laceration or vascular injury
  - Delayed hemorrhage (days after biopsy) from pseudoaneurysm formation
- Status post cholecystectomy
  - Incidence of postoperative hemorrhage is ~ 0.1-0.2%
  - Causes: Parenchymal injury to gallbladder bed, puncture of liver with trocar, capsular tears from traction
- Status post transjugular intrahepatic portosystemic shunt (TIPS) procedure
  - Incidence of significant hemorrhage is < 1%
  - Causes: Capsular laceration during venogram for portal vein localization, portal vein perforation while obtaining portal vein access, inferior vena

HEPATIC HEMORRHAGE

Key Facts

Terminology
- Intraparenchymal with hematoma ± hemobilia or hepatic rupture with hemoperitoneum

Clinical Issues
- Incidence of hepatic hemorrhage is rare, differs depending on etiology
- Mortality of hepatic rupture is high (30-75%)
- Patient chart review
  - Cirrhosis/chronic liver disease, viral hepatitis, malignancy, pregnancy
  - Coagulopathy, medications, vasculitis/connective tissue disease
  - Recent hepatobiliary surgery, liver biopsy, or TIPS procedure

Macroscopic Pathology
- Examine Glisson capsule for disruption; check location and status of stents and drains
- Assess presence of underlying liver disease
- Common etiologies of hemorrhage
  - Tumors
  - Pregnancy related
  - Iatrogenic
  - Peliosis hepatis

Microscopic Pathology
- Submit representative sections of masses, hemorrhagic areas/hematomas, gross vascular lesions
- Evaluate uninvolved liver with iron and trichrome ± reticulin stains for intrinsic disease
- Very rarely, no underlying pathology identified

cava laceration during transcaval puncture, hepatic artery injury

Peliosis Hepatis
- Rare, incidence of significant hemorrhage/rupture unknown
- Exact etiology unknown, variety of associations
  - Drugs/toxins: Anabolic steroids, oral contraceptives, tamoxifen, azathioprine, 6-mercaptopurine, corticosteroids, vinyl chloride, arsenic acid
  - Infections: Tuberculosis, HIV, *Bartonella henselae*
  - Malignancies: Hematologic and nonhematologic
  - Other: Organ transplantation, hemodialysis, celiac disease, glycogenosis type I

Other Rare Causes
- Vasculitis/connective tissue diseases (e.g., polyarteritis nodosa, lupus erythematosus), hypereosinophilic syndrome, microaneurysms secondary to inflammatory processes, hepatic amyloidosis (variable data regarding ↑ risk)

CLINICAL ISSUES

Epidemiology
- Incidence
  - Rare; incidence differs depending on etiology

Presentation
- Sudden right upper quadrant pain ± radiation to shoulder, nausea, vomiting
- Tachycardia, hypotension, hypovolemic shock, hemobilia (melena, jaundice, biliary pain)
- Important elements of chart review
  - Cirrhosis/chronic liver disease, alcohol use, viral hepatitis, malignancy, pregnancy, coagulopathy, hypertensive disease, vasculitis/connective tissue diseases
  - Recent hepatobiliary surgery, liver biopsy, biliary drain placement, or TIPS procedure
  - Medications, e.g., anticoagulants, antiplatelet agents, oral contraceptives, anabolic steroids, other hormone therapy, immunosuppressive drugs

Laboratory Tests
- ↓ hemoglobin/hematocrit, thrombocytopenia, ↑ prothrombin and partial thromboplastin times
- ↑ transaminases, alkaline phosphatase, bilirubin, and ammonia, ↓ albumin
- (+) viral hepatitis serologies, ↑ α-fetoprotein/other tumor markers

Prognosis
- Mortality of hepatic rupture is high (30-75%)
- Pregnancy-related hemorrhage: Maternal mortality ~ 40%, fetal mortality ~ 30%

IMAGE FINDINGS

Radiographic Findings
- Ultrasound, CT scan, MR for evidence of bleeding/rupture ± underlying masses, cirrhosis, other diffuse liver disease

Angiography
- Diagnosis of vascular lesions (e.g., hemangiomas, pseudoaneurysms, peliosis hepatis) ± therapeutic interventions (e.g., embolization)

MACROSCOPIC FEATURES

Sections to Be Submitted
- Masses, hemorrhagic areas/hematomas, gross vascular lesions
- Uninvolved liver with iron and trichrome stains for evaluation of hemosiderosis and fibrosis, ± reticulin stain for evaluation of sinusoidal architecture

External Examination
- Pallor of skin, mucous membranes, conjunctiva

HEPATIC HEMORRHAGE

- Jaundice/scleral icterus, periumbilical caput medusae, skin spider angiomas
- Evidence of recent surgical procedures, drains

Internal Examination

- Hemoperitoneum, hemothorax, ascites, hepatosplenomegaly
- Disruption of Glisson capsule, location and status of stents and drains

Organ Examination

- Location of hemorrhage/hematoma: Intraparenchymal, subcapsular ± rupture, gallbladder bed, in bile ducts/gallbladder
- Underlying liver disease, cirrhosis/nodularity, gross thrombi in large vessels
- Tumors
  - Hepatocellular carcinoma
    - Single, multiple or diffusely nodular, color variable, ± capsule, ± tumor thrombi in veins/inferior vena cava; usually in background of cirrhosis
  - Hepatocellular adenoma
    - Single, rarely multiple, color variable, well circumscribed, usually not encapsulated, noncirrhotic background
  - Hemangioma
    - Usually single, subcapsular, well circumscribed, nonencapsulated, spongy, soft, red-purple, blood filled ± thrombosis, fibrosis, and calcification
  - Metastatic neoplasms
    - Usually multiple, variable in size, location, and gross appearance; noncirrhotic background
- Pregnancy related
  - Subcapsular hematoma ± rupture, right lobe > left lobe
  - Patchy necrosis
- Peliosis hepatis
  - Multiple blood-filled cystic spaces ranging from few mm to few cm in diameter, randomly distributed, ± necrosis
- Amyloidosis
  - Pale, friable parenchyma, ± capsular tears

MICROSCOPIC PATHOLOGY

Histologic Features

- Hepatocellular carcinoma
  - Many histologic patterns, all show abnormal or loss of reticulin framework
  - Endothelial cells/sinusoidal vessels surrounding tumor cells, i.e., "capillarization of sinusoids" ([+] immunostain for CD34)
  - Cells are polygonal with abundant eosinophilic or less often clear cytoplasm, high N:C ratio, nuclei with coarse chromatin ± nucleoli, ± steatosis, Mallory-Denk bodies, or bile production
  - Vascular invasion and mitotic figures common
- Hepatocellular adenoma
  - Normal-appearing hepatocytes present in cords/sheets 1-3 cells thick with normal reticulin framework
  - Absence of normal portal tracts within tumor, scattered isolated arteries/veins, no cytologic atypia, nucleoli, mitoses, or vascular invasion
  - Portal tract-like structures with inflammation, ductular reaction and vessels, but no bile ducts (inflammatory type)
- Hemangioma
  - Usually cavernous type
  - Vascular spaces lined by single layer of bland, flattened endothelial cells
  - ± fibrosis, thrombosis, calcification
- Preeclampsia/eclampsia ± HELLP syndrome
  - Periportal hemorrhage, fibrin deposition, and hepatocellular necrosis
  - Fibrin thrombi in portal vessels, infarction, nonspecific portal inflammation
- Peliosis hepatis
  - Parenchymal pattern: Irregular blood-filled spaces/blood lakes without endothelial lining ± hepatocellular necrosis
  - Phlebectatic pattern: Rounded centrilobular blood-filled spaces lined by endothelial cells or fibrous tissue, compresses adjacent parenchyma without significant necrosis, ± perisinusoidal fibrosis
  - *B. henselae* infection (bacillary peliosis hepatis): Gram-negative bacilli, (+) Warthin-Starry stain, bacteria in clumps within smudge-like, granular material in a myxoid stroma, dilated vascular spaces
- Amyloidosis
  - Deposition of hyaline material that is Congo red positive, usually in periportal space of Disse or sometimes central; may obstruct sinusoids or involve portal vessels, loss of normal reticulin framework
- Very rarely, no underlying pathology is identified

REPORTING CRITERIA

Key Elements to Report

- Location and type of hemorrhage
- Etiology and risk factors for hemorrhage
- Presence of underlying liver disease
- Effect of hemorrhage and underlying disease on other organs

SELECTED REFERENCES

1. Vigil-De Gracia P et al: Pre-eclampsia/eclampsia and hepatic rupture. Int J Gynaecol Obstet. 118(3):186-9, 2012
2. Zhu Q et al: Predictors and clinical outcomes for spontaneous rupture of hepatocellular carcinoma. World J Gastroenterol. 18(48):7302-7, 2012
3. Jr MA et al: Spontaneous rupture of hepatic hemangiomas: A review of the literature. World J Hepatol. 2(12):428-33, 2010
4. Ripamonti R et al: Transjugular intrahepatic portosystemic shunt-related complications and practical solutions. Semin Intervent Radiol. 23(2):165-76, 2006

Gross and Microscopic Features

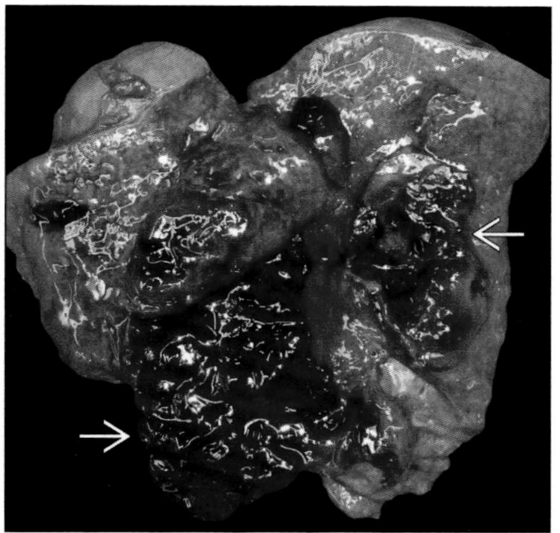

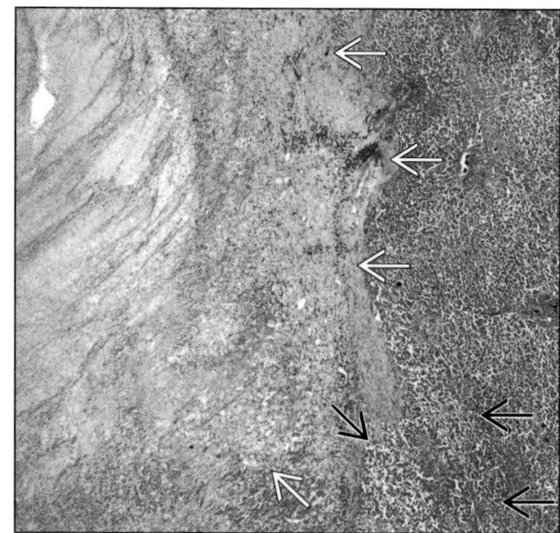

(Left) *This hepatic hematoma ➔ occurred after percutaneous biliary drain placement, which resulted in portal vein injury and arterial-portal venous fistula formation (confirmed on premortem hepatic angiogram).* ***(Right)*** *Section through the hematoma ➔ shows adjacent hepatic parenchyma with patchy coagulative necrosis ➔.*

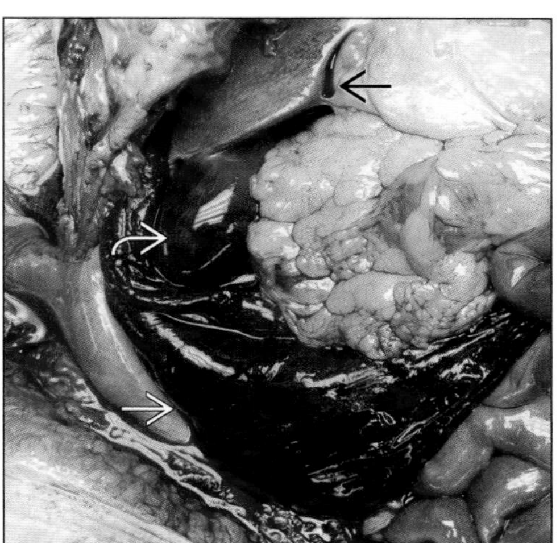

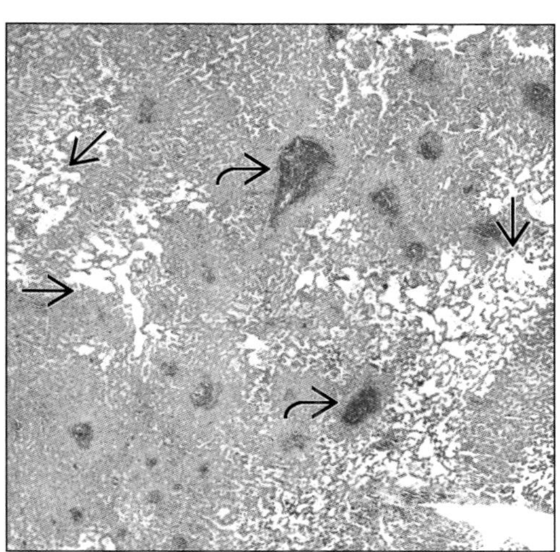

(Left) *Hemoperitoneum ➔ occurred after percutaneous liver biopsy in a patient on anticoagulant therapy. Note the liver ➔ and gallbladder ➔.* ***(Right)*** *The inflammatory (a.k.a. telangiectatic) type of hepatocellular adenoma is characterized by portal tract-like structures containing inflammatory infiltrates ➔ and marked sinusoidal dilatation ➔.*

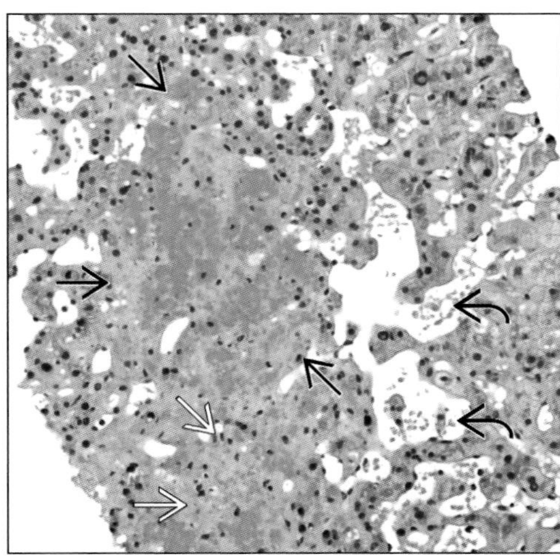

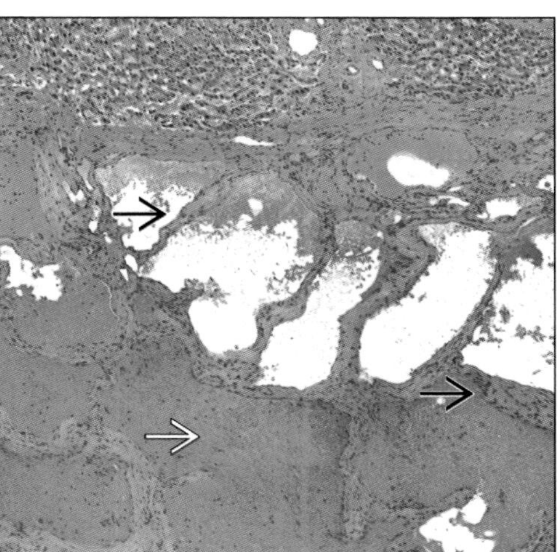

(Left) *A microscopic focus of the parenchymal pattern of peliosis hepatis in a patient with a history of anabolic steroid use shows sinusoidal dilatation ➔ and an irregular blood-filled space ➔ with associated hepatocellular necrosis ➔.* ***(Right)*** *A cavernous hemangioma is composed of blood-filled spaces ➔ lined by bland, flattened endothelial cells ➔.*

HEMORRHAGIC PANCREATITIS

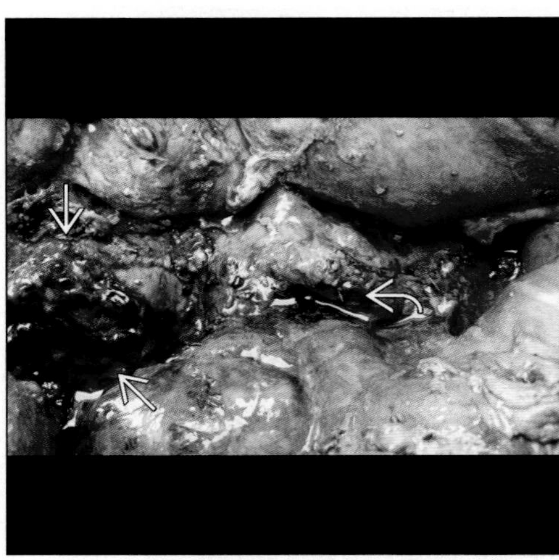

Hemorrhagic necrosis of the head ➡ and body ➡ of the pancreas developed following distal pancreatectomy/ splenectomy for tumor.

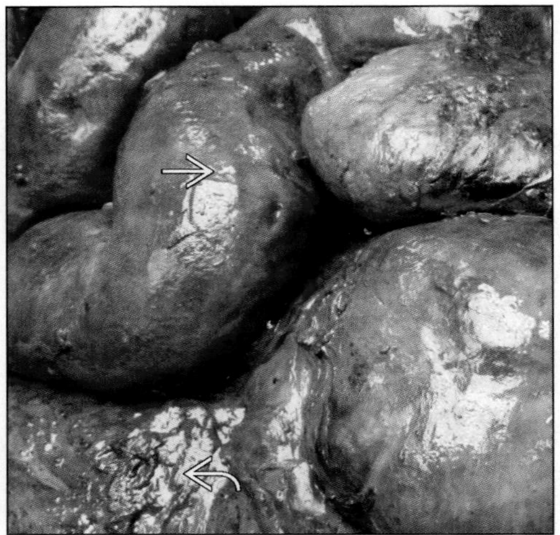

There is also peritonitis with dullness and green-brown-black discoloration of the serosal ➡ and peritoneal ➡ surfaces in the same patient.

TERMINOLOGY

Definitions

- Acute hemorrhagic pancreatitis: Necrotizing pancreatitis with disruption of microvasculature, leading to severe systemic complications
- Grey Turner sign: Bruising of flanks due to retroperitoneal hemorrhage
- Cullen sign: Periumbilical bruising due to subcutaneous hemorrhage

ETIOLOGY/PATHOGENESIS

Etiologies of Acute Pancreatitis

- Choledocholithiasis and alcohol-related: Most common
- Metabolic (hyperlipidemia, hypercalcemia)
- Infections (viral, bacterial, parasitic)
- Medications/toxins (antiretroviral drugs, valproic acid, diuretics, scorpion venom)
- Postoperative (pancreaticobiliary or other abdominal surgery), post endoscopic retrograde cholangiopancreatography (ERCP)
- Anatomic abnormalities/obstruction (pancreas divisum, tumors)
- Ischemia related (shock, vasculitis, thromboemboli)
- Trauma

Pathogenesis of Hemorrhage in Pancreatitis

- Necrosis and enzyme leakage causing pseudoaneurysm formation or vascular rupture with bleeding into peritoneal cavity, retroperitoneal space, and other organs
- Bleeding into pancreatic/peripancreatic collections (abscesses, pseudocysts) with rupture ± erosion of adjacent vessels
- Splenic vein thrombosis resulting in left-sided portal hypertension and bleeding from upper GI varices

Risk Factors for Hemorrhage

- Necrosis, organ failure, sepsis, pancreatic/ peripancreatic collections, status post surgery for debridement

CLINICAL ISSUES

Epidemiology

- Incidence
  - Occurs in 20-30% of all patients with acute pancreatitis
  - Fatal hemorrhagic complications ~ 2-15%

Presentation

- Symptoms: Epigastric pain ± radiation to back, nausea, vomiting, anorexia
- Signs: Fever, hypovolemic shock, disseminated intravascular coagulation (DIC), respiratory distress, sepsis, hematemesis, melena, Grey Turner or Cullen sign, peritoneal signs

Laboratory Tests

- ↑ serum amylase and lipase, ↓ hemoglobin and hematocrit
- Leukocytosis, hyperglycemia, hypocalcemia
- Multiorgan failure (↑ BUN and creatinine, abnormal LFTs, ↓ arterial pO_2)

Prognosis

- Overall mortality due to hemorrhage ~ 20-50%
- Usually diagnosed premortem, but can occasionally result in sudden death due to multiorgan failure

IMAGE FINDINGS

CT Findings

- Enlarged pancreas, edema, necrotic areas, hematomas, abscesses, pseudocysts

HEMORRHAGIC PANCREATITIS

Key Facts

Terminology
- Acute hemorrhagic pancreatitis: Necrotizing pancreatitis with disruption of microvasculature, leading to severe systemic complications

Etiology
- Choledocholithiasis and alcohol related are most common
- Metabolic disorders, infections, medications/toxins, obstruction, postoperative, ischemia, trauma

Clinical Issues
- Incidence of fatal hemorrhagic complications ~ 2-15%
- Overall mortality due to hemorrhage ~ 20-50%

Macroscopic Pathology
- Signs of sepsis, Grey Turner or Cullen sign
- Hemoperitoneum, ascites, peritonitis
- Pancreatic/peripancreatic abscesses or pseudocysts
- Indurated, edematous, red-black hemorrhagic parenchyma ± necrosis
- Peripancreatic/mesenteric fat necrosis
- Peripancreatic vascular lesions (thromboses, ruptures, pseudoaneurysms)
- Gastric/esophageal varices, stress ulcers, perforations, fistulas, strictures

Microscopic Pathology
- Interstitial edema and hemorrhage
- Acute inflammation ± necrosis involving acini, ducts, and islets of Langerhans
- Other organs: Diffuse alveolar damage, bronchopneumonia, acute tubular injury/necrosis, hepatic centrilobular congestion/necrosis

Angiography
- Diagnostic (thrombosed vessels, pseudoaneurysms, active bleeding) and therapeutic (embolization)

MACROSCOPIC FEATURES

External Examination
- Skin: Grey Turner or Cullen sign, jaundice, surgical incisions/drains, erythematous nodules (usually pretibial due to subcutaneous fat necrosis)
- Signs of sepsis: Petechiae, peripheral edema/anasarca

Internal Examination
- Hemoperitoneum, ascites, peritonitis (dull surfaces ± green/yellow fibrinopurulent exudate)
- Surgical anastomoses, vascular therapeutic interventions
- Pleural or pericardial effusions

Organ Examination
- Pancreas
  - Indurated, edematous, red-black hemorrhagic parenchyma ± necrosis
  - Peripancreatic/mesenteric fat necrosis: Yellow-white chalky nodules in adipose tissue
  - Peripancreatic vascular lesions (thromboses, ruptures, pseudoaneurysms)
  - Pseudocyst: Usually unilocular with thick fibrous wall, smooth or roughened inner lining with adherent debris and cloudy, brown, or hemorrhagic fluid contents, usually not connected to pancreatic ductal system
  - Abscess: Purulent debris/pus within a fibrous tissue wall around or within pancreas
  - Fistulas from pancreas to other organs
- Gastrointestinal tract
  - Gastric/esophageal varices, gastric stress ulcers
  - Perforations, fistulas, strictures
- Lungs: Edema/congestion, consolidation, abscesses
- Kidneys: Cortical pallor and medullary congestion (acute tubular injury/necrosis)
- Liver: Congestion and patchy necrosis (shock), portal vein thrombosis

MICROSCOPIC PATHOLOGY

Histologic Features
- Pancreas
  - Interstitial edema and hemorrhage
  - Acute inflammation ± necrosis involving acini, ducts, and islets of Langerhans
  - Vascular injury with necrosis of vessel wall
  - Fat necrosis ± calcification
  - Pseudocysts: Fibrous wall with granulation tissue, calcifications, cholesterol clefts, inflammation, and giant cells **without** epithelial lining, filled with necrotic/hemorrhagic debris
- Other organs: Diffuse alveolar damage, bronchopneumonia, acute tubular injury/necrosis, hepatic centrilobular congestion/necrosis

REPORTING CRITERIA

Key Elements to Report
- Risk factors for developing pancreatitis, risk factors for hemorrhagic complications, effects on other organs

SELECTED REFERENCES

1. Banks PA et al: Classification of acute pancreatitis--2012: revision of the Atlanta classification and definitions by international consensus. Gut. 62(1):102-11, 2013
2. Sharma PK et al: Hemorrhage in acute pancreatitis: should gastrointestinal bleeding be considered an organ failure? Pancreas. 36(2):141-5, 2008
3. Fu CY et al: Timing of mortality in severe acute pancreatitis: experience from 643 patients. World J Gastroenterol. 13(13):1966-9, 2007
4. Flati G et al: Potentially fatal bleeding in acute pancreatitis: pathophysiology, prevention, and treatment. Pancreas. 26(1):8-14, 2003

HEMORRHAGIC PANCREATITIS

Pancreatic and Peripancreatic Findings

*(**Left**) This case of acute pancreatitis with peripancreatic hemorrhage/ hematoma ➡ developed status post ERCP. (**Right**) Histologic section from the same patient shows intraparenchymal and peripancreatic hemorrhage/ hematoma ↷ and a residual islet ➡.*

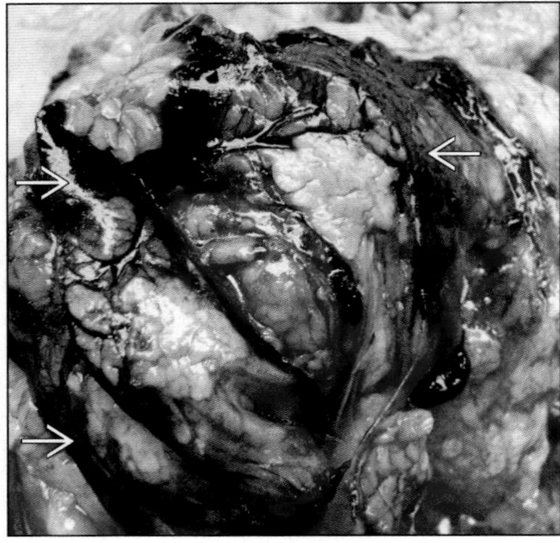

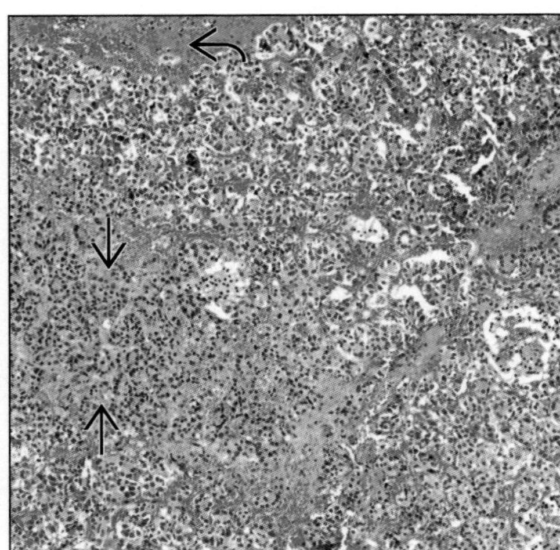

*(**Left**) Neutrophils ➡ are infiltrating the pancreatic parenchyma in this case of acute pancreatitis. (**Right**) Peripancreatic fat necrosis is composed of "ghosts" of adipocytes with blue-gray to pink cytoplasm and loss of nuclei ➡. Adjacent hemorrhage ⇨ is also present.*

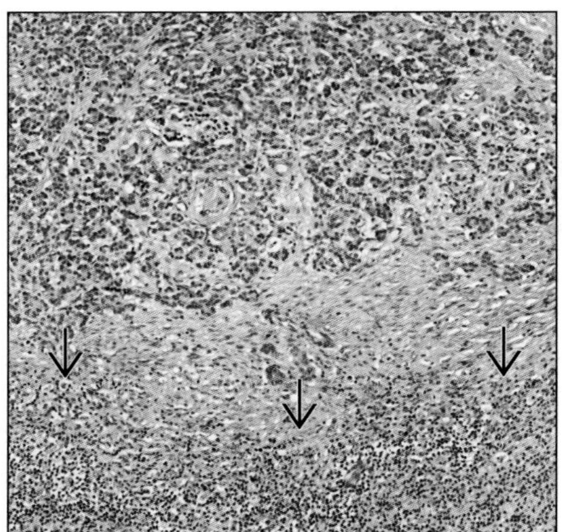

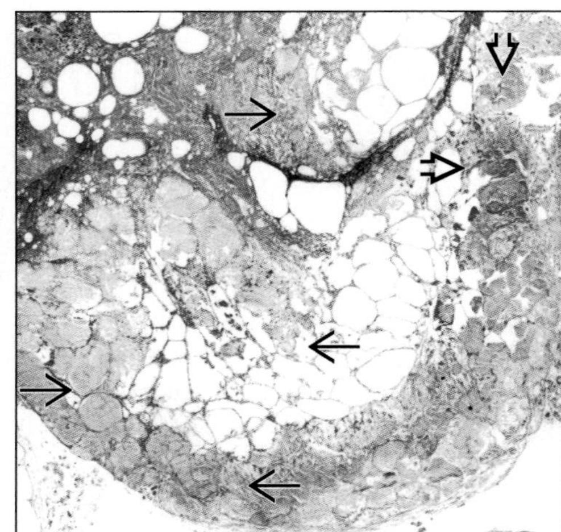

*(**Left**) This bivalved peripancreatic pseudocyst has a thin, partially calcified fibrous wall ➡ and necrotic hemorrhagic cyst contents ↷. (**Right**) Histologic sections of the peripancreatic pseudocyst show a fibrous wall ➡ containing scattered calcifications ↷. No epithelial lining is present. Hemorrhagic, fibrinous, and necrotic debris is present within the pseudocyst ➡.*

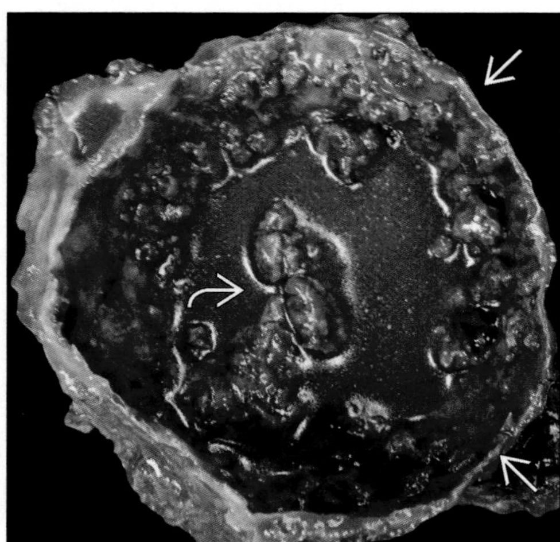

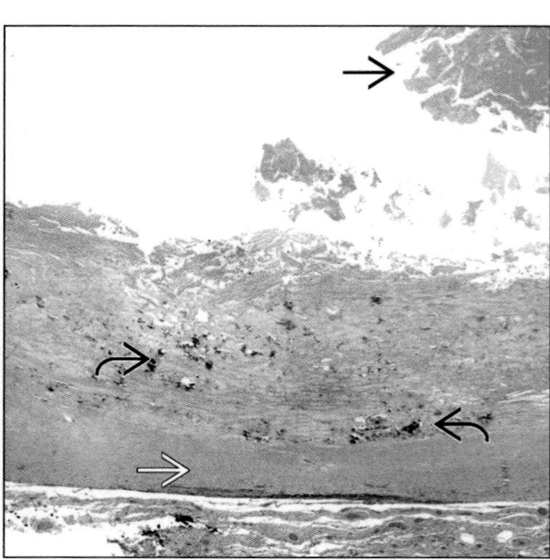

Other Organ Changes

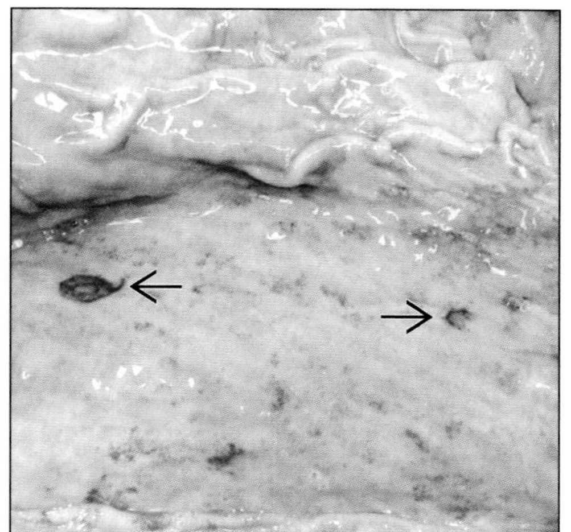

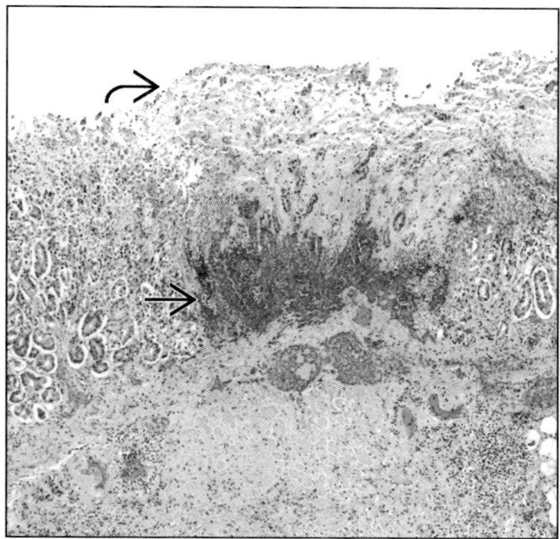

(Left) *Gastric stress ulcers with a round, punched-out appearance and smooth, flat, nonindurated borders ➔ can occur in patients with hemorrhagic pancreatitis.* ***(Right)*** *A section through a gastric stress ulcer shows mucosal erosion ➔ and hemorrhage ➔. The adjacent mucosa is normal and partially autolyzed.*

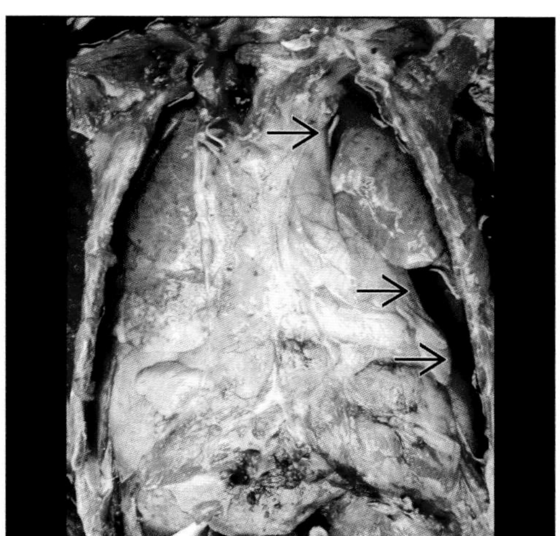

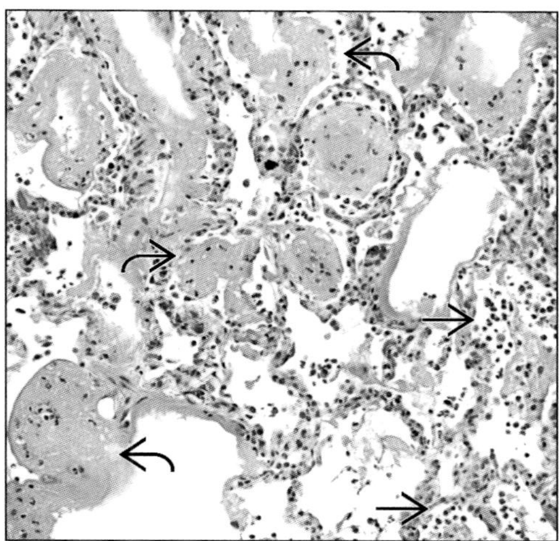

(Left) *A left-sided pleural effusion composed of clear, yellow serous fluid ➔ occurred in a patient with hemorrhagic pancreatitis.* ***(Right)*** *Diffuse alveolar damage, as seen in acute respiratory distress syndrome, with alveolar hyaline membranes ➔, fibrin deposition, and acute inflammation ➔ in alveolar spaces can be a complication of pancreatitis.*

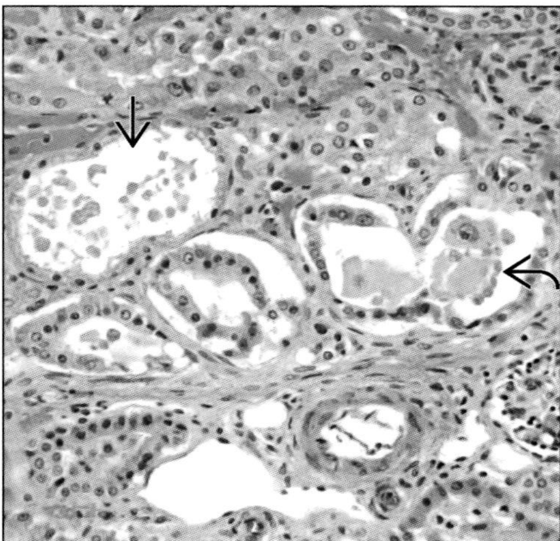

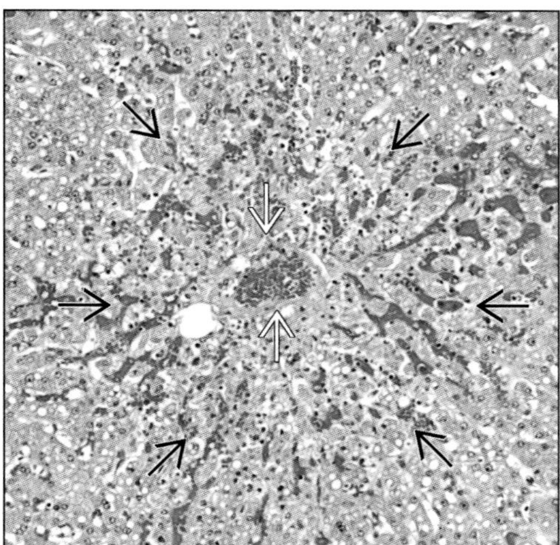

(Left) *This section from the kidney shows acute tubular injury with dilated tubules, epithelial necrosis and sloughing ➔, and pigmented tubular casts ➔.* ***(Right)*** *Centrilobular/perivenular congestion and hepatocellular necrosis ➔ are due to shock resulting from hemorrhagic pancreatitis. Note the central vein ➔.*

ACUTE LIVER FAILURE

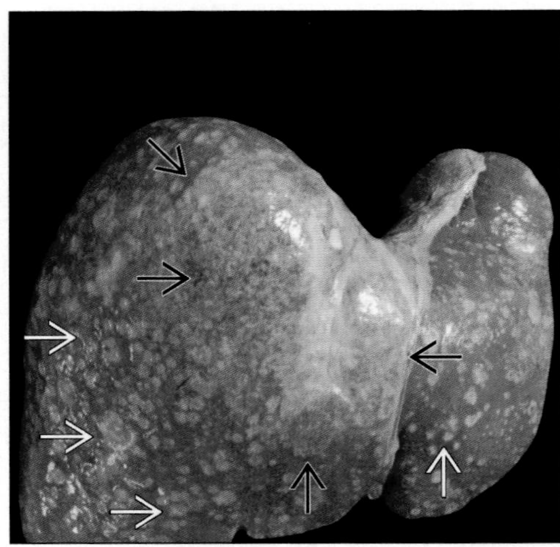

Liver with innumerable tan-yellow metastatic deposits ➡ and associated parenchymal necrosis ⇨ is from a patient with breast cancer who presented with acute liver failure.

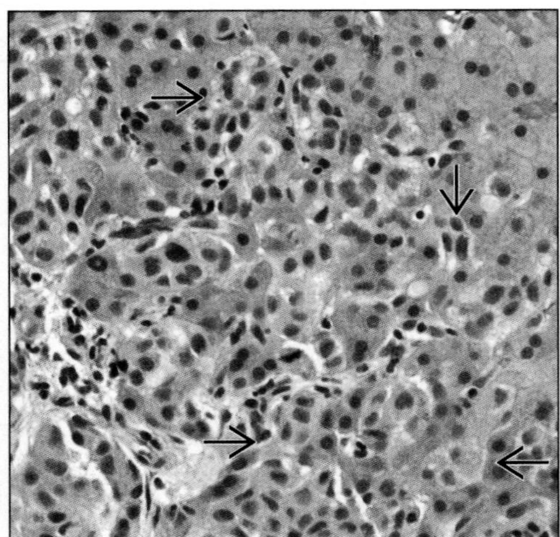

Histologic section of the liver shows metastatic breast carcinoma ⇨ infiltrating through the sinusoidal spaces.

TERMINOLOGY

Abbreviations

- Acute liver failure (ALF)

Definitions

- Coagulopathy (international normalized ratio [INR] ≥ 1.5) and encephalopathy (any degree of mental alteration) resulting from severe liver injury for < 26 weeks duration without preexisting liver disease/cirrhosis

ETIOLOGY/PATHOGENESIS

Drug/Toxin Induced

- Acetaminophen: Leading cause of liver failure in USA, dose-related toxicity
- Idiosyncratic drug reaction: Antibiotics, nonsteroidals, anticonvulsants, statins, herbals, supplements
- Mushroom poisoning: Toxin produced by fungal cells of toxic mushrooms, usually *Amanita phalloides*

Viral Hepatitis

- Leading cause of ALF worldwide
- Common: Hepatitis A, E, B (either new infection or reactivation), or D (coinfection with hepatitis B vs. superinfection)
- Uncommon: Herpes simplex virus (HSV), Epstein-Barr virus (EBV), cytomegalovirus (CMV), human herpesvirus 6 (HHV-6), or varicella-zoster virus (VZV), in setting of immunosuppression

Ischemic/Hemodynamic

- Shock liver after cardiac arrest, hypovolemia/hypotension, severe congestive heart failure, heat stroke
- Drug related (cocaine, methamphetamine)
- Budd-Chiari syndrome: Acute hepatic vein or inferior vena cava thrombosis → venous outflow obstruction
  - Contraceptive steroids, pregnancy, myeloproliferative disorders, thrombophilia, hepatocellular carcinoma

Autoimmune Hepatitis

- Usually causes chronic hepatitis but occasionally presents with ALF

Metabolic Disorders

- Wilson disease: Uncommon; usually seen in young patients
- Acute fatty liver of pregnancy: 3rd trimester, enzyme deficiency → defects in fatty acid oxidation
- Metabolic disorders and neonatal hemochromatosis in children < 1 year old are rare

Malignant Infiltration of Liver

- Lymphomas, melanoma, breast carcinoma, and small cell carcinoma are most likely to cause ALF

Indeterminate

- ~ 15% of cases

CLINICAL ISSUES

Epidemiology

- Incidence
  - Rare; ~ 2,000 cases/year in USA, usually young patients
  - ~ 5-10% of liver transplants annually

Presentation

- Jaundice, fatigue, fever, right upper quadrant pain, altered mental status, seizures
- **No** history or signs of chronic liver failure/cirrhosis

Laboratory Tests

- ↑ prothrombin and partial thromboplastin times, INR ≥ 1.5; ↑ transaminases, bilirubin, ammonia
- Hypoglycemia, hyponatremia, lactic acidosis

ACUTE LIVER FAILURE

Key Facts

Terminology
- ALF: Coagulopathy (INR ≥ 1.5) and encephalopathy (any degree of mental alteration) resulting from liver injury for < 26 weeks duration without preexisting liver disease/cirrhosis

Etiology
- Drug-/toxin-induced viral hepatitis: Most common
- Ischemic/hemodynamic causes (shock liver, severe congestive heart failure, heat stroke, drug related, Budd-Chiari syndrome)
- Autoimmune hepatitis
- Metabolic disorders (Wilson disease, acute fatty liver of pregnancy)
- Malignancy
- Indeterminate etiology (~ 15% of cases)

Clinical Issues
- ~ 2,000 cases/year in USA, usually young patients, mortality ~ 30%
- Common immediate causes of death: Cerebral edema/herniation, multiorgan failure, infection/sepsis

Macroscopic Pathology
- Wrinkled capsule, nodular surface, necrosis

Microscopic Pathology
- Findings may differ depending on cause of ALF
- Varying degrees of necrosis, ± parenchymal collapse, ductular reaction, regeneration

Top Differential Diagnoses
- Cirrhosis/chronic liver failure

- Thrombocytopenia, ↑ fibrin degradation products, ↓ fibrinogen (in disseminated intravascular coagulation [DIC])
- ↑ IgG and (+) autoantibodies (autoimmune hepatitis)
- Hemolytic anemia, ↓ serum ceruloplasmin, ↑ urine and hepatic copper levels (Wilson disease)
- Viral antibodies/antigens (+)
- ↑ acetaminophen levels (depending on time of ingestion), other drug levels

Prognosis
- Mortality ~ 30%, differs depending on etiology
- Common immediate causes of death
  - Cerebral edema/intracranial hypertension ± herniation, multiorgan failure, infection/sepsis

IMAGE FINDINGS

Radiographic Findings
- Hepatic atrophy or hepatomegaly ± heterogeneous, hypoattenuated foci (necrosis)
- Surface nodularity due to alternating necrosis and regeneration (may mimic cirrhosis)
- Evidence of portal hypertension (also present in cirrhosis), i.e., splenomegaly, ascites, collateral vessel formation, hepatofugal (reverse) flow in portal vein

MACROSCOPIC FEATURES

External Examination
- Jaundice/scleral icterus
- Petechiae/purpura, gangrene (sepsis, DIC)
- Mucocutaneous hemorrhage, bleeding from surgical/procedural sites (DIC)

Internal Examination
- Ascites, splenomegaly

Organ Examination
- Liver
  - Atrophic or enlarged
  - Wrinkled capsule, nodular surface
  - Soft cut surface, necrotic areas, regenerative nodules, congestion, green discoloration (cholestasis)
  - Yellow fatty liver (acute fatty liver of pregnancy, drug reaction)
  - Thrombi in hepatic veins/inferior vena cava (Budd-Chiari syndrome)
- GI tract: Ulcers, ischemic enterocolitis, rarely hemorrhagic/necrotizing pancreatitis
- Kidneys: Cortical pallor, medullary congestion
- Lungs: Edema/congestion, consolidation, abscesses
- Brain: Flattened gyri, narrowed sulci and ventricular compression (cerebral edema), herniation (subfalcine, transtentorial/uncinate, tonsillar), hemorrhagic foci in midbrain and pons with transtentorial herniation
- Heart: Subendocardial/myocardial mottling ± yellow-tan areas with hyperemic borders (infarction)

MICROSCOPIC PATHOLOGY

Histologic Features
- Hepatic findings
  - May differ depending on cause of ALF
  - Varying degrees of necrosis (zonal, confluent, multiacinar, bridging, panacinar), ± parenchymal collapse, ductular reaction, regeneration
  - Canalicular ± ductular cholestasis (sepsis)
- Other organs
  - Lungs: Aspiration pneumonitis, bronchopneumonia, abscesses, diffuse alveolar damage
  - GI tract: Mucosal ulcers, ischemic enterocolitis, acute pancreatitis
  - Kidneys: Acute tubular injury/necrosis
  - Heart: Subendocardial/myocardial contraction band/coagulative necrosis, edema, hemorrhage, inflammation (infarction)
  - Brain: Hemorrhage in areas of herniation
  - DIC: Widespread microthrombi ± ischemic necrosis of various organs/tissues, schistocytes on peripheral blood smear

ACUTE LIVER FAILURE

Histologic Features of Acute Liver Failure Etiologies

Etiology	Necrosis	Inflammation	Steatosis	Cholestasis	Bile Duct Injury	Other Findings
Acetaminophen toxicity	+ coagulative, perivenular → midzonal	-	+ in remaining hepatocytes	-	-	
Idiosyncratic drug reaction	+	+	+	+	+	Varies depending on drug
Mushroom poisoning	+ perivenular	-	+	-	-	
Hepatitis A	+ periportal	+ periportal	-	+ perivenular	-	± plasma cells
Hepatitis B ± D	+	+ active ± chronic hepatitis	-	-	-	Ground-glass hepatocytes, "sanded" nuclei (pale pink inclusions)
Hepatitis E	+	+	-	±	-	
HSV	+ irregular/ geographic coagulative	±	-	-	-	Intranuclear inclusions, chromatin margination, multinucleation
EBV	+ (rare)	+ diffuse sinusoidal lymphocytic infiltrate	-	-	-	-
CMV	+ (rare)	+ neutrophilic microabscesses	-	-	-	Intranuclear & intracytoplasmic inclusions
Acute ischemic injury	+ coagulative, perivenular → midzonal	- or scant	+ in remaining hepatocytes	-	-	± congestion
Budd-Chiari syndrome	±	-	-	-	-	Severe congestion, sinusoidal dilatation, preserved portal tracts, ± portal vein thrombi
Autoimmune hepatitis	+ perivenular, confluent ± bridging	+ lymphoplasmacytic interface	-	-	-	Hepatocyte rosettes
Wilson disease	±	+ chronic or active	+	+	-	Mallory-Denk bodies
Acute fatty liver of pregnancy	-	+ lobular	+ microvesicular	±	-	

HSV = herpes simplex virus; EBV = Epstein-Barr virus; CMV = cytomegalovirus

ANCILLARY TESTS

Immunohistochemistry

- Immunostains for hepatitis B surface/core antigens, HSV, CMV, VZV, HHV6

In Situ Hybridization

- EBER for EBV

Special Stains

- Hepatocellular copper/copper-binding protein stains (+) in Wilson disease
  - May be patchy or absent, not specific for Wilson disease, may be present in chronic cholestasis

DIFFERENTIAL DIAGNOSIS

Cirrhosis/Chronic Liver Failure

- Similar clinical presentation but ≥ 26 weeks duration and history/signs of underlying chronic liver disease
- Some similar etiologies (hepatitis B ± D, autoimmune hepatitis, Wilson disease, drug-induced hepatitis)
- Radiographic: Surface/parenchymal nodularity, atrophy or hepatomegaly, evidence of portal hypertension
- Macroscopic: Diffusely (micro- or macro-) nodular parenchyma composed of regenerative nodules separated by fibrous bands, ascites, splenomegaly
- Microscopic: Disruption of normal architecture by scarring/bridging fibrosis surrounding nodules of hepatocytes without central veins

DIAGNOSTIC CHECKLIST

Final Report Should Include

- Etiology and whether it was cause of death or contributing factor
- ALF risk factors, effects on other organs

SELECTED REFERENCES

1. Bernal W et al: Acute liver failure. N Engl J Med. 369(26):2525-34, 2013
2. Das P et al: A retrospective autopsy study of histopathologic spectrum and etiologic trend of fulminant hepatic failure from north India. Diagn Pathol. 2:27, 2007

Microscopic and Gross Features

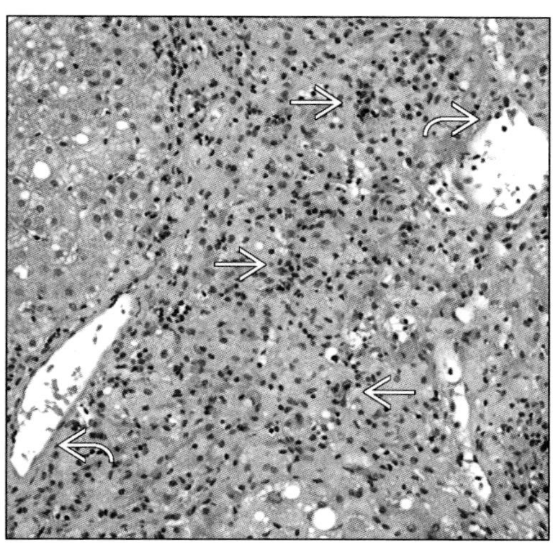

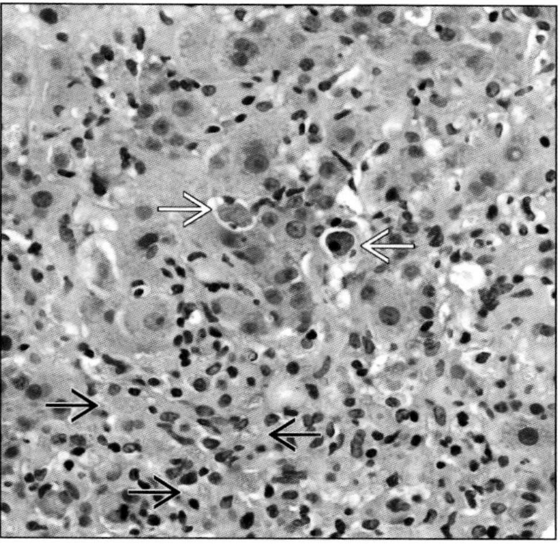

(Left) *Bridging necrosis extends from one central vein ➔ to another in this case of autoimmune hepatitis. Clusters of plasma cells ➔ are present in the inflammatory infiltrate.* ***(Right)*** *Acute imatinib (Gleevec)-induced liver injury is characterized by diffuse, predominantly lymphocytic lobular inflammation, scattered acidophil bodies ➔, and canalicular and hepatocellular cholestasis ➔.*

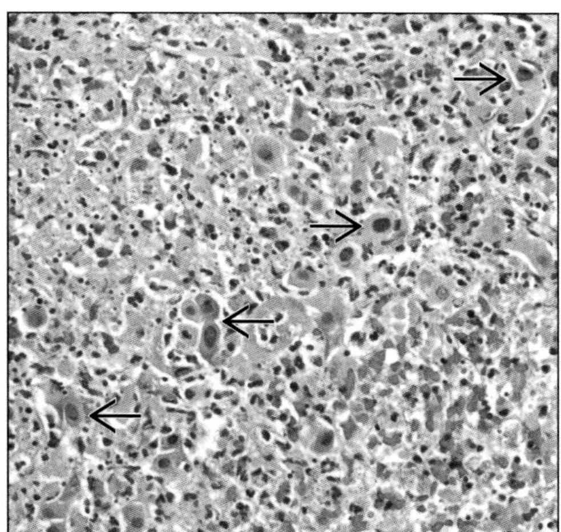

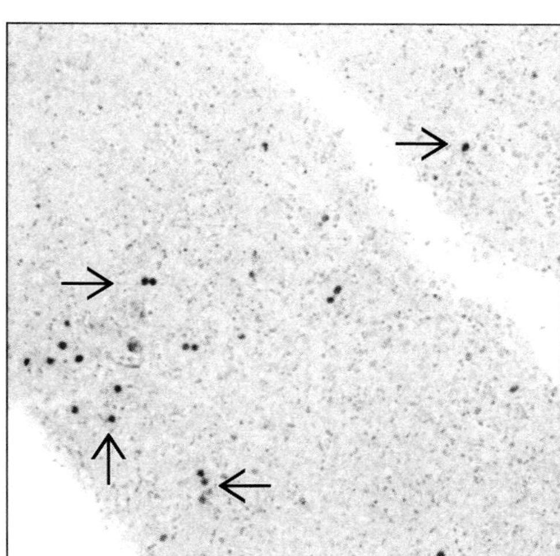

(Left) *This liver is from an immunosuppressed patient presented with acute liver failure due to herpes simplex virus (HSV) infection. The liver parenchyma is extensively necrotic. The nuclei in scattered residual hepatocytes show glassy intranuclear inclusions with chromatin margination ➔.* ***(Right)*** *Immunostain for HSV1/2 of the same case highlights numerous infected hepatocytes. Note nuclear staining ➔.*

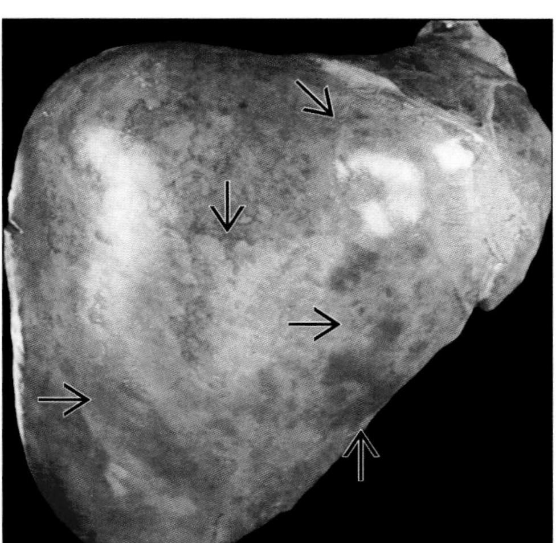

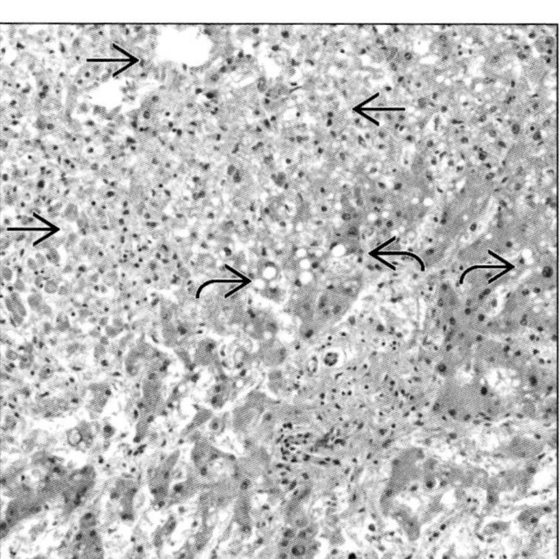

(Left) *Large irregular areas of hepatic parenchymal necrosis ➔ are the result of ischemia due to hypovolemic shock. (Courtesy D. Rubin, MD.)* ***(Right)*** *The hepatic parenchyma in this case of hypovolemic shock shows submassive necrosis involving centrilobular/perivenular and midzonal regions ➔. Viable periportal hepatocytes show fatty change ➔.*

PREGNANCY COMPLICATIONS

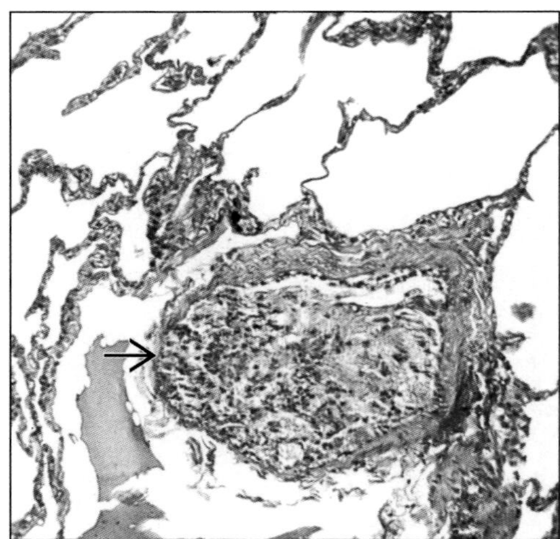

H&E stain of the lung in a case of a postpartum maternal death shows amorphous material within a vascular space ➔ consistent with an amniotic fluid embolism.

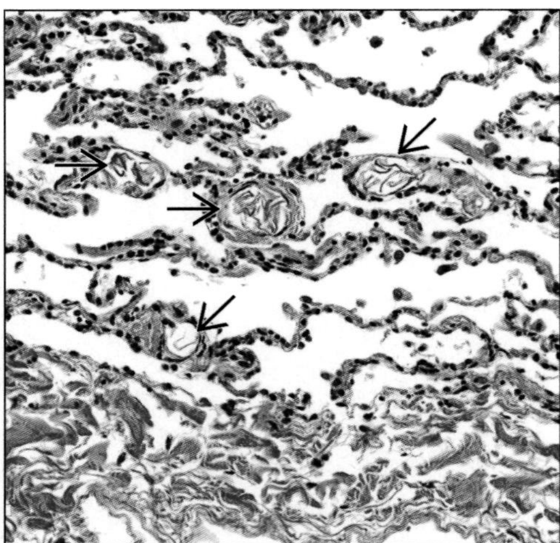

H&E photomicrograph from an autopsy lung in an amniotic fluid embolism death shows fetal "squames" ➔ or sloughed amniotic lining cells lodged in distal (subpleural) pulmonary arterioles.

TERMINOLOGY

Definitions

- Maternal mortality (WHO)
  - Death of a woman while pregnant or within 42 days of termination of pregnancy (delivery)
    - Irrespective of gestational duration or site (e.g., ectopic)
    - Any cause related to or aggravated by pregnancy or its management
    - Not from accidental or incidental causes
  - Late maternal mortality
    - From 42 days to 1 year after termination

EPIDEMIOLOGY

Incidence

- Maternal mortality rate
  - Developed nations: < 10/100,000 live births
  - Developing nations: 100-1,000/100,000 live births

Presentation

- Direct obstetric death
  - Result from obstetric complications (pregnancy, labor, and puerperium)
  - Examples
    - Amniotic fluid embolism
    - Uterine rupture
    - Peripartum cardiomyopathy
- Indirect obstetric death
  - Result from preexisting disease or disease that developed during pregnancy
    - Not directly due to obstetric cause, but aggravated by pregnancy
  - Examples
    - Congenital heart defect
    - Idiopathic pulmonary hypertension
    - Aortic dissection in Marfan syndrome
- Coincidental maternal death
  - Result from diseases or injuries not related to pregnancy
  - Examples
    - Homicide
    - Accidents
- Risk factors associated with maternal death
  - Inadequate maternal care
  - Substance abuse
  - Medical comorbidities
  - Previous pregnancy problems
  - Hypertensive disorders of pregnancy

CLINICAL SUMMARY

Clinical Information

- Current pregnancy history
- Gravida/para status
- Mode of delivery
  - Delivery procedures (cesarean section, vacuum assisted, forceps)
- APGAR scores
- Infection serologies
  - TORCH, group B Streptococcus

Past Medical History

- Heart or lung disease, anemia, hypertension, thrombophilia/coagulopathy
- Medications

MACROSCOPIC FINDINGS

Autopsy, Mother

- Per normal routine
- Extensive sampling of lungs
- Photograph liberally
- Consider fixing pelvic organs en bloc and examining with obstetrician present

Autopsy, Fetus

- Per normal routine
- Cultures (blood, CSF)

Surgical Specimens

- Obtain placenta, hysterectomy, or other organs removed in proximity to death
  - After surgical report is finalized

MICROSCOPIC FINDINGS

Amniotic Fluid Embolism

- Amniotic fluid, fetal cells, lanugo hair, and other debris enter maternal blood stream causing cardiorespiratory collapse and disseminated intravascular coagulation (DIC)
  - Can occur during active labor, delivery, or post delivery
  - Mortality rate: 11-44%
  - Risk factors include
    - Maternal age ≥ 35 years
    - Cesarean section
    - Placenta previa
    - Multiparity
- Pathophysiology poorly understood as fetal cells often found in asymptomatic women
  - Immunologic mechanisms, amniotic fluid-dependent anaphylactic reaction, and complement activation have been proposed as potential pathophysiologic mechanisms
- Amniotic "squames" within pulmonary arterioles and capillaries, parauterine vessels
  - Cytokeratin staining used to highlight
  - Other supplemental stains may be used
    - PAS or Alcian blue to visualize mucus
    - Sudan III to show fatty substances

Postpartum Hemorrhage

- Uterine atony
- Uterine rupture or genital tract trauma
  - Risk factors include prior cesarean section, connective tissue disorders, instrumentation
- Retained placenta

Prepartum Hemorrhage

- Ectopic pregnancy
  - Those occurring in intramural portion of tube (cornual ectopic) and cesarean section scar are covered by myometrium and grow to larger size than typical tubal ectopic before symptomatic
    - Rupture later than tubal ectopic
    - More likely to cause catastrophic bleeding and death
- Unskilled abortion
- Placenta previa
- Placental abruption

Placenta Accreta

- Placental invasion of myometrium
  - Villi in direct contact with superficial myometrial smooth muscle (no intervening decidua)
  - Associated with previous uterine surgical scar sites, especially cesarean section scars
    - Risk increases with number of prior cesarean sections
  - Most associated with placenta previa
- Increta
  - Invasion deep into myometrium
- Percreta
  - Invasion through myometrium into peritoneal space
  - Invasion into other organs, typically bladder
- Maternal death: 4-7%
  - Hemorrhage with cardiovascular collapse
    - Average blood loss 3,000-5,000 mL but can be much higher
  - Secondary causes of death include DIC, renal failure, acute respiratory distress

Puerperal Sepsis

- Genital tract nidus of infection
  - Occurring between rupture of membranes or labor and postpartum day 42
- 2 or more of following present
  - Pelvic pain
  - Fever
  - Abnormal vaginal discharge
  - Abnormal smell of discharge
  - Delay in reduction of size of uterus
- Possible sources
  - Chorioamnionitis
  - Laceration with necrotizing fasciitis
  - Nosocomial infection

Preeclampsia/Eclampsia

- Hypertension (> 140/> 90), proteinuria, hyperreflexia
- Maternal complications
  - Seizures
  - Stroke
  - Renal failure
    - Glomerular endotheliosis at autopsy
  - Liver failure
    - Hepatic necrosis in periportal zone 1
  - Adult respiratory distress syndrome, severe pulmonary edema
  - Cardiopulmonary arrest
- Fetal complications
  - Intrauterine growth restriction
  - Stillbirth
  - Complications associated with prematurity
- Placental changes
  - Decidual vasculopathy
  - Atherosis
  - Ischemic changes/pressure-related injury
    - Infarcts: Large, central, and of variable age
    - Hypermaturity of villi
- HELLP syndrome develops in 10-20% of preeclampsia cases
  - H = hemolysis (breakdown of red blood cells)
  - EL = elevated liver enzymes
  - LP = low platelet count
  - Overall maternal mortality: 3.5%
    - Approaches 50% in cases of liver rupture

PREGNANCY COMPLICATIONS

Pregnancy-Associated Hematologic Disorders

- Thrombophilia
  - Combined with extrinsic compression of iliac veins and vena cava increases risk of thromboembolism
- Microangiopathic thrombocytopenia in preeclampsia/eclampsia and HELLP syndrome
- Thrombocytopenic purpura (TTP)
- Atypical hemolytic uremic syndrome

Spontaneous Coronary Dissection

- Constitutional or acquired arterial wall weakness added to mechanical stress

Peripartum Cardiomyopathy

- Dilated cardiomyopathy that develops between last month of pregnancy and 1st 5 months after delivery
- Relationship between pregnancy and dilated cardiomyopathy is unclear but may involve hormonal, inflammatory, familial, or hemodynamic factors
- Death may occur form progressive heart failure, arrhythmia, or thromboembolism
  - USA death rate: 3.3-9.6%

ANCILLARY STUDIES

Postmortem Samples

- Blood cultures (aerobic and anaerobic)
- Genital tract, perineum cultures
- Toxicology

Antemortem Samples

- Retrieve and store
- Remain aware of sample stability issues

DIAGNOSTIC CHECKLIST

Clinically Relevant Pathologic Features

- In event of unexplained maternal death, autopsy must be performed
- Carefully sample lungs to look for amniotic fluid embolism
  - Leading cause of unexplained death

SELECTED REFERENCES

1. Jariwala MC Sr: [51-OR.] Pregnancy Hypertens. 5(1):26, 2015
2. Mehrabadi A et al: Contribution of placenta accreta to the incidence of postpartum hemorrhage and severe postpartum hemorrhage. Obstet Gynecol. 125(4):814-21, 2015
3. Nair M et al: Factors associated with maternal death from direct pregnancy complications: a UK national case-control study. BJOG. 122(5):653-62, 2015
4. Woo YS et al: Ischemic stroke related to an amniotic fluid embolism during labor. J Clin Neurosci. 22(4):767-768, 2015
5. Clark SL: Amniotic fluid embolism. Obstet Gynecol. 123(2 Pt 1):337-48, 2014
6. Fitzpatrick KE et al: The management and outcomes of placenta accreta, increta, and percreta in the UK: a population-based descriptive study. BJOG. 121(1):62-70; discussion 70-1, 2014
7. Ito F et al: Incidence, diagnosis and pathophysiology of amniotic fluid embolism. J Obstet Gynaecol. 34(7):580-4, 2014
8. Yoneyama K et al: Clinical characteristics of amniotic fluid embolism: an experience of 29 years. J Obstet Gynaecol Res. 40(7):1862-70, 2014
9. Zosmer N et al: The morbidly adherent placenta: early accurate diagnosis is essential for the meaningful interpretation of outcomes. BJOG. 121(10):1314-5, 2014
10. Abildgaard U et al: Pathogenesis of the syndrome of hemolysis, elevated liver enzymes, and low platelet count (HELLP): a review. Eur J Obstet Gynecol Reprod Biol. 166(2):117-23, 2013
11. Guillaume A et al: Amniotic fluid embolism: 10-year retrospective study in a level III maternity hospital. Eur J Obstet Gynecol Reprod Biol. 169(2):189-92, 2013
12. Hikiji W et al: Fatal amniotic fluid embolism with typical pathohistological, histochemical and clinical features. Forensic Sci Int. 226(1-3):e16-9, 2013
13. Saucedo M et al: Ten years of confidential inquiries into maternal deaths in France, 1998-2007. Obstet Gynecol. 122(4):752-60, 2013
14. Kanayama N et al: Maternal death analysis from the Japanese autopsy registry for recent 16 years: significance of amniotic fluid embolism. J Obstet Gynaecol Res. 37(1):58-63, 2011
15. Sinicina I et al: Forensic aspects of post-mortem histological detection of amniotic fluid embolism. Int J Legal Med. 124(1):55-62, 2010
16. Sliwa K et al: Current state of knowledge on aetiology, diagnosis, management, and therapy of peripartum cardiomyopathy: a position statement from the Heart Failure Association of the European Society of Cardiology Working Group on peripartum cardiomyopathy. Eur J Heart Fail. 12(8):767-78, 2010
17. Turillazzi E et al: Amniotic fluid embolism: still a diagnostic enigma for obstetrician and pathologist? Acta Obstet Gynecol Scand. 88(7):839-41, 2009
18. Silver RM et al: Maternal morbidity associated with multiple repeat cesarean deliveries. Obstet Gynecol. 107(6):1226-32, 2006

Microscopic and Gross Features

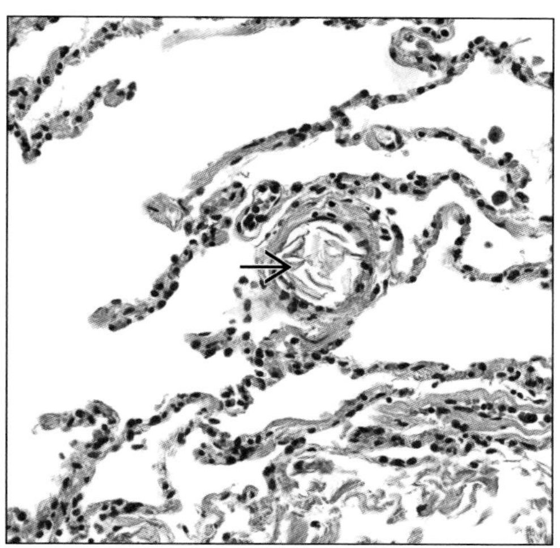

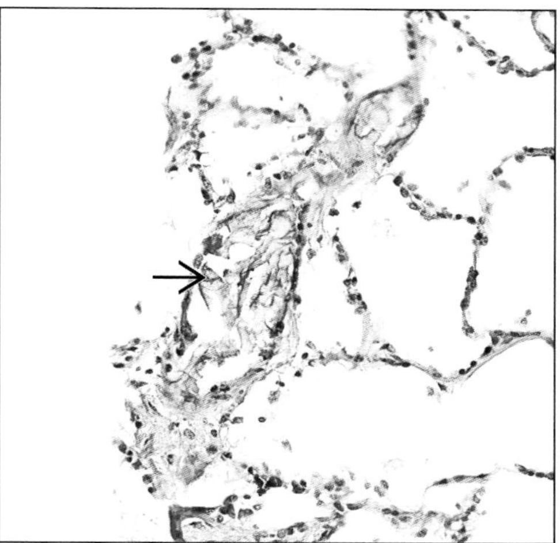

(Left) *The presence of fetal "squames" ⇒ within the pulmonary arterial circulation is pathognomonic for amniotic fluid embolism in a postpartum death. This is often associated with disseminated intravascular coagulation systemically.* ***(Right)*** *Mucicarmine staining can be used to help highlight fetal "squames" ⇒ in the pulmonary arterial branches. They stain positive for mucin (pink) due to their rich mucopolysaccharide content.*

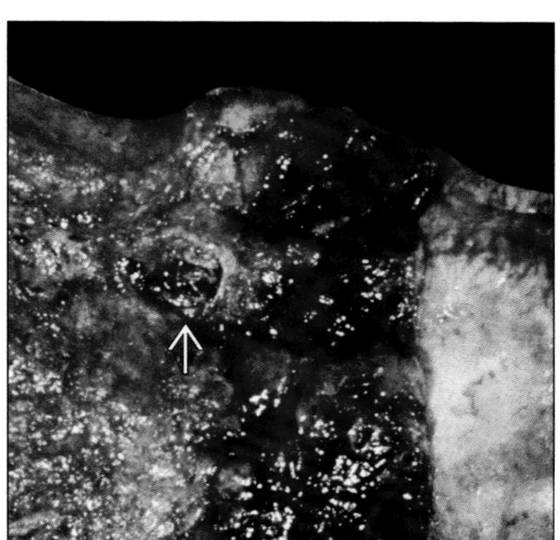

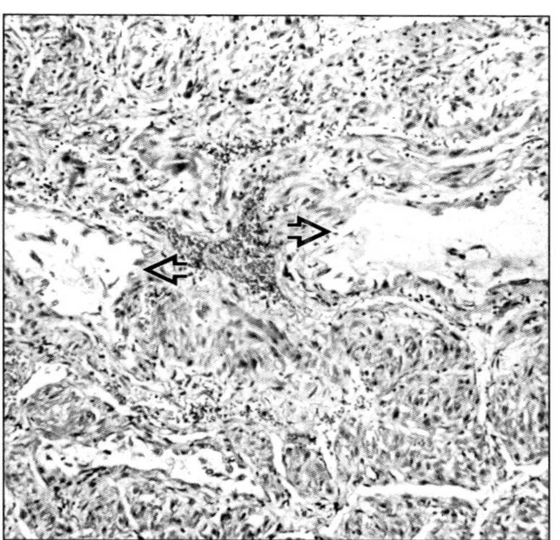

(Left) *Gross image of a term uterus shows a large amniotic fluid embolism located within a dilated vessel ➡ of the lower uterine segment.* ***(Right)*** *Section of myocardium shows 2 moderately dilated vascular spaces that contain amorphous material ⇨ consistent with amniotic fluid emboli.*

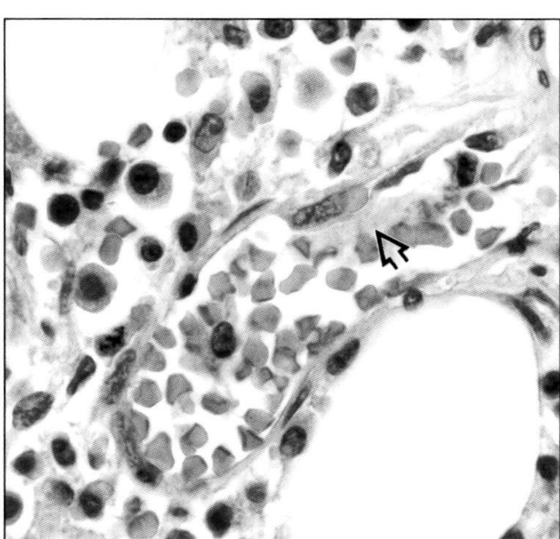

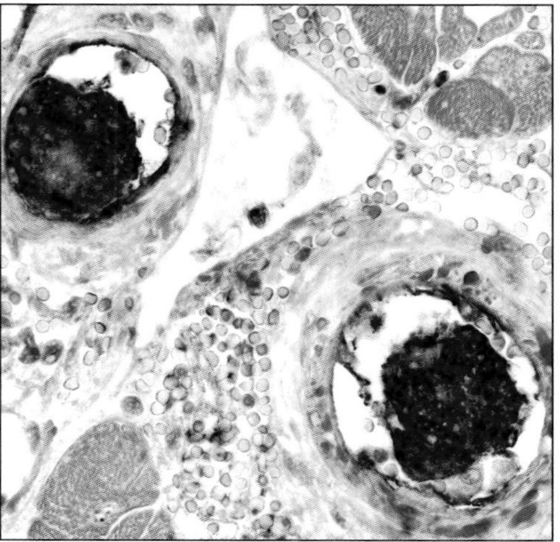

(Left) *Blood vessel from bone marrow taken at autopsy shows a small eosinophilic thrombus ⇨. Thrombi within the microvasculature are responsible for RBC fragmentation and thrombocytopenia in TTP as a complication of pregnancy. (From DP: Blood & Bone Marrow.)* ***(Right)*** *Intravascular thrombi are highlighted by immunoperoxidase staining for CD31 in this case of fatal TTP. Note the compromise of vascular lumina. (From DP: Blood & Bone Marrow.)*

PREGNANCY COMPLICATIONS

Gross and Microscopic Features

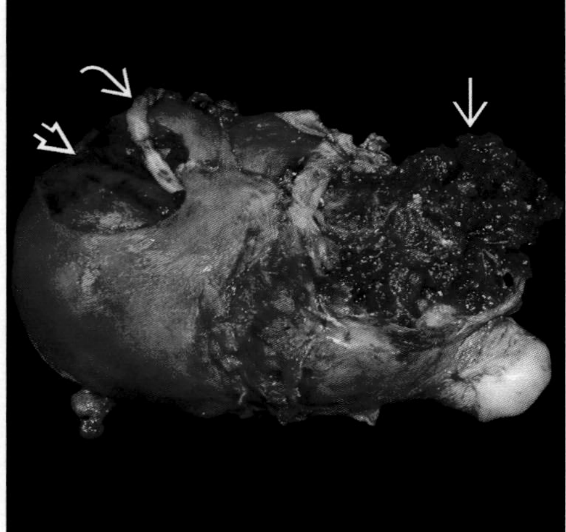

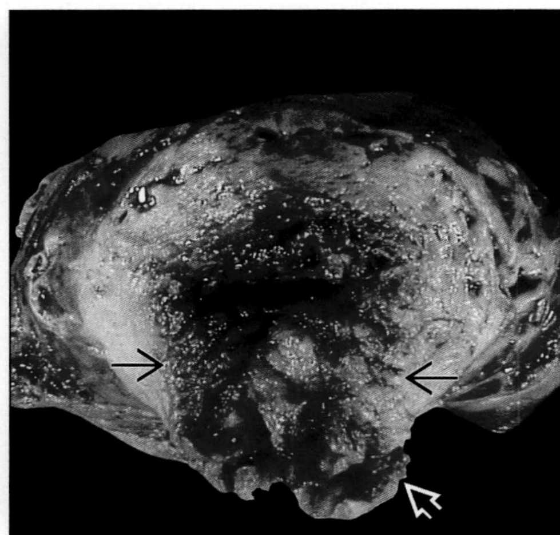

*(**Left**) Gross photograph of the uterus in a case of placenta percreta shows the umbilical cord ➔ going through the fundal hysterotomy ➔. There is a frank breech of the anterior uterine wall with the placenta appearing as a fungating mass ➔. (**Right**) Transverse section through the lower uterine segment in another case shows placental invasion into the myometrium ➔ and through the serosal surface ➔. Invasion into surrounding structures, typically bladder, can result in massive hemorrhage and death.*

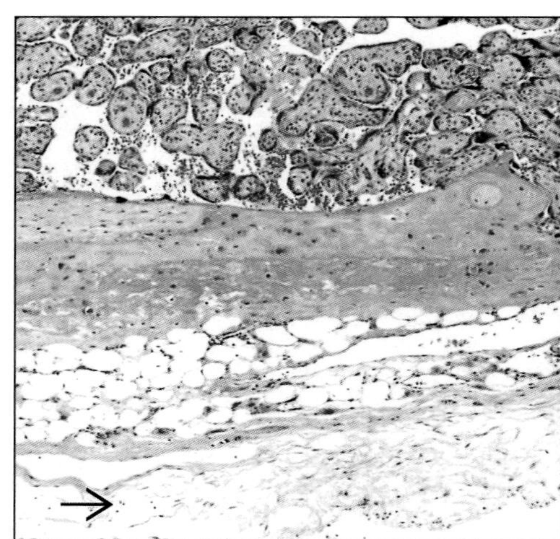

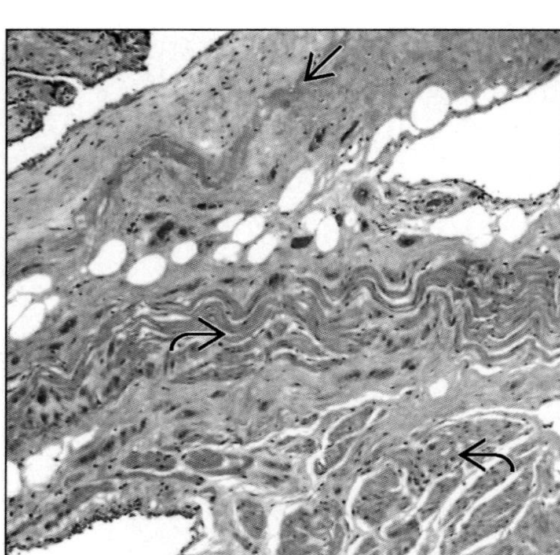

*(**Left**) A section taken from the lower uterine segment shows placenta percreta with absent decidua, absent myometrium, and omental adipose tissue ➔ adherent to the uterine serosa. (From DP: Placenta.) (**Right**) In this section taken from an area of placenta percreta, fibrinoid at the base of the placenta ➔ is adjacent to omental adipose tissue and bundles of smooth muscle ➔ from the bladder. (From DP: Placenta.)*

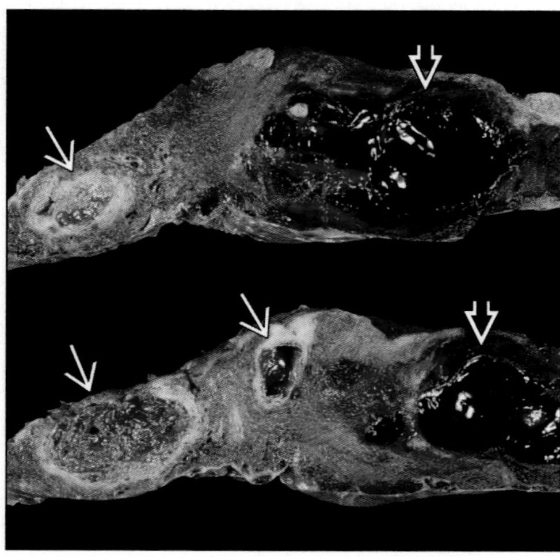

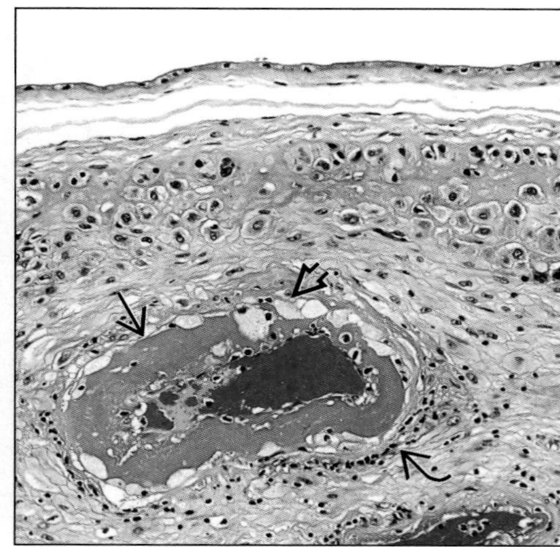

*(**Left**) This small placenta has multiple infarcts of variable age, including infarction hematomas, as most commonly seen in preterm preeclampsia. White infarcts ➔ are ≥ 7 days old, whereas red infarcts ➔ are more recent (2-3 days). (From DP: Placenta.) (**Right**) This section from the free membranes in a case of preeclampsia shows an acute atheroma within a maternal vessel of the decidua parietalis. There is fibrinoid necrosis ➔, foamy macrophages ➔, and a cuff of surrounding lymphocytes ➔. (From DP: Placenta.)*

Radiologic, Microscopic, and Gross Features

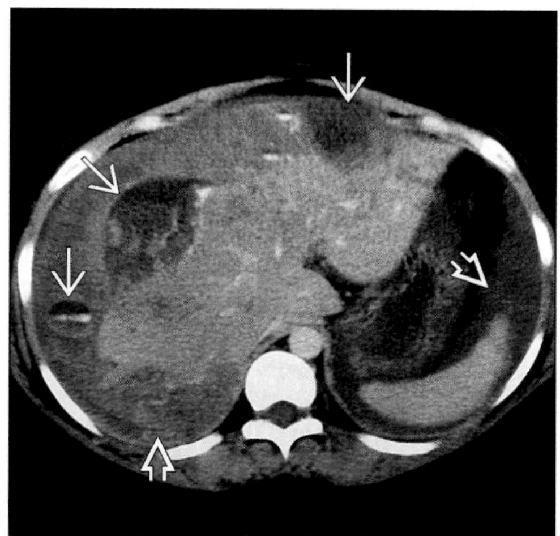

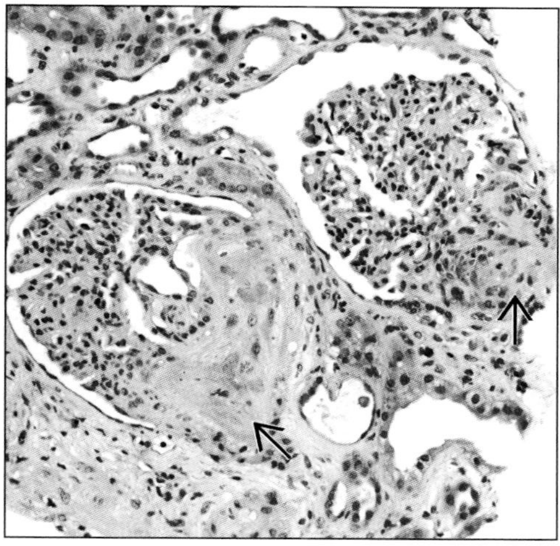

(Left) *CT scan of the liver shows a woman with severe preeclampsia and HELLP syndrome. There are intrahepatic hemorrhages ➡ and a hemoperitoneum ⇨. Maternal death approaches 50% in cases of liver rupture. (From DI: Abdomen.)* ***(Right)*** *H&E stain highlights large thrombi with entrapped red blood cells and red cell fragments in the hilar arterioles ➡ of 2 adjacent glomeruli from a pregnant woman with HELLP syndrome. (From DP: Kidney.)*

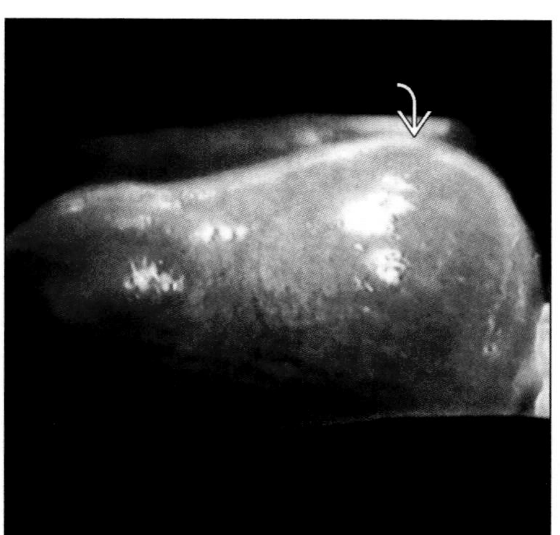

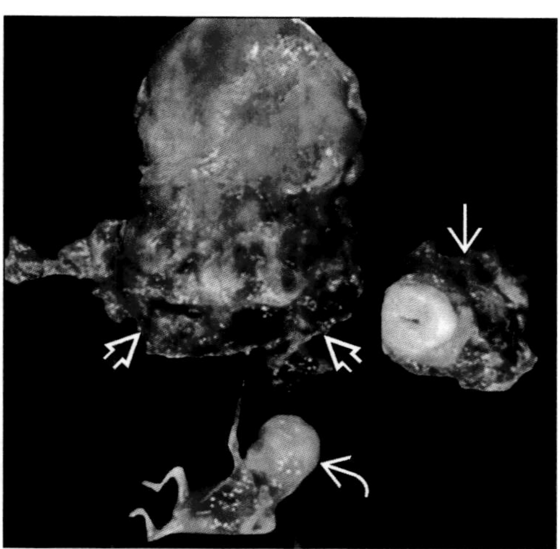

(Left) *Intraoperative photo of a cornual ectopic shows an obvious bulge and thinning of the overlying myometrium ↷. These often rupture later in pregnancy than a tubal ectopic and are, therefore, more likely to cause catastrophic bleeding and death. (From DI: Obstetrics.)* ***(Right)*** *Gross pathology shows a ruptured uterus secondary to a cesarean section ectopic pregnancy. A 13-week fetus ↷ is still attached to the hemorrhagic placenta ⇨. The cervix ➡ is detached. (From DI: Obstetrics.)*

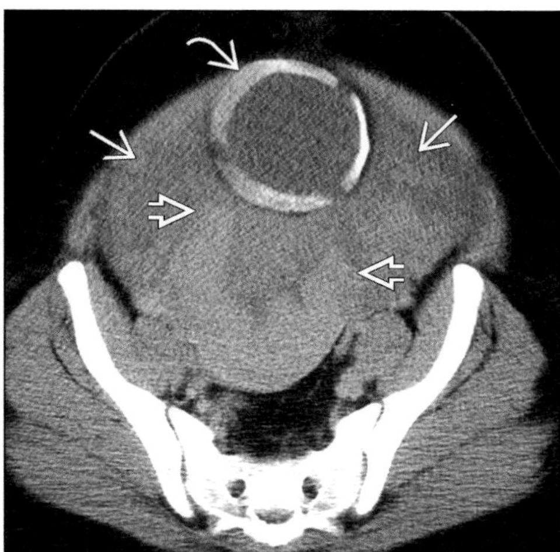

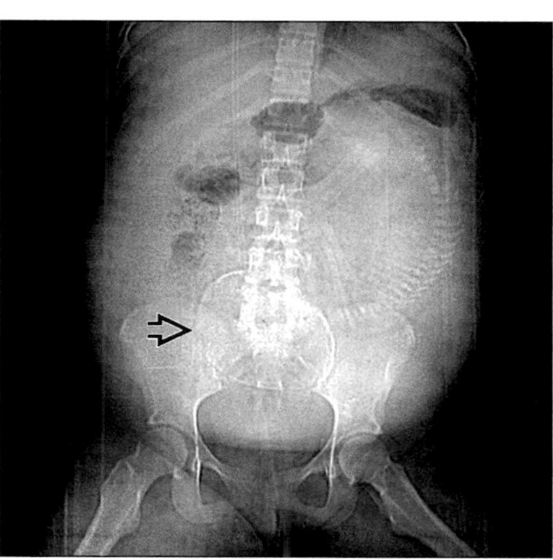

(Left) *CT scan in a patient with acute uterine rupture shows the open anterior margins of the uterus ⇨. The fetal head ↷ is within the maternal peritoneal cavity and is surrounded by a large hemoperitoneum ➡, which is making the borders of the uterus difficult to see.* ***(Right)*** *Radiograph of the abdomen in the same patient shows the the fetal head ⇨ high in the maternal abdomen. It is being displaced out the pelvis by the massive hemorrhage.*

ACUTE RENAL FAILURE

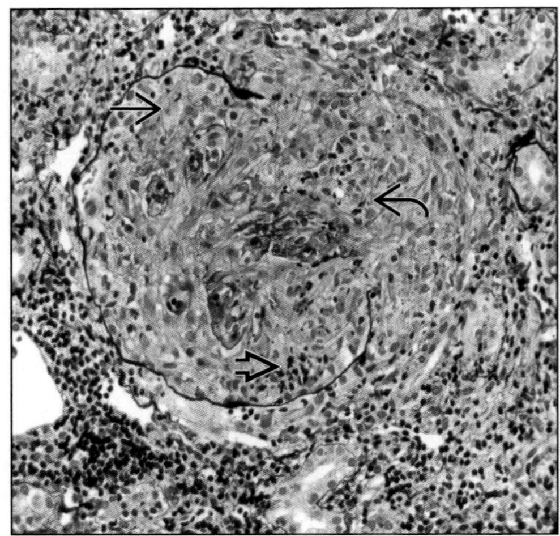

In this case of anti-GBM crescentic glomerulonephritis, the glomerulus shows marked parietal epithelial cell proliferation (crescent) ➡ with associated inflammatory cells ➡ and fibrinoid necrosis ➡.

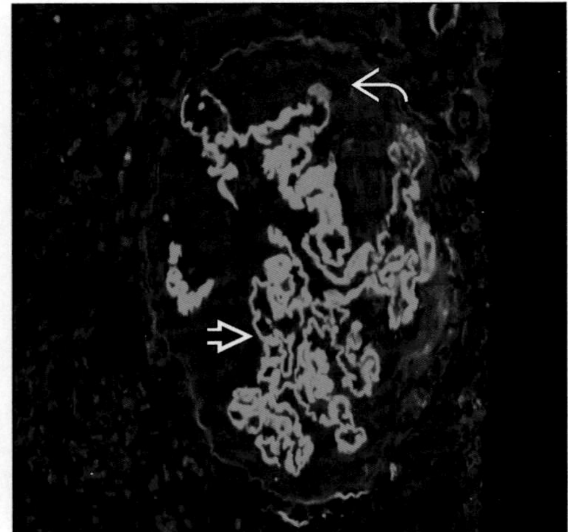

In anti-glomerular basement membrane-mediated glomerulonephritis, there is bright linear glomerular basement staining for IgG ➡. In Bowman space, a crescent can be identified ➡.

TERMINOLOGY

Abbreviations

- Acute renal failure (ARF)

Synonyms

- Acute kidney injury (AKI)

Definitions

- Sudden sustained decline of glomerular filtration rate (GFR) associated with uremia, fall in urine output, and serum creatinine (SCr) increase of
  - ≥ 0.5 mg/dL in patients with baseline SCr ≤ 1.9 mg/dL
  - ≥ 1 mg/dL in patients with baseline SCr between 2 and 4.9 mg/dL
  - ≥ 1.5 mg/dL in patients with baseline SCr ≥ 5 mg/dL

ETIOLOGY/PATHOGENESIS

Glomerular Diseases

- Crescentic glomerulonephritis: ANCA-related small vessel vasculitis, anti-GBM crescentic glomerulonephritis, immune complex-related glomerulonephritis
- Acute postinfectious glomerulonephritis
- Thrombotic microangiopathy (TMA)

Drug/Toxin Induced

- Hypersensitivity reaction: Antibiotics, nonsteroidals, protein supplements, proton pump inhibitors
- Cocaine

Systemic Disorders

- Hypotension
- Hypertension
- Hypovolemia
- Sepsis
- Rhabdomyolysis
- Post surgery

Urinary Obstruction

- Nephrolithiasis
- Malignancies in urinary tract and prostate

Vascular

- Renal vein thrombosis
- Renal artery thrombosis
- Atheroembolic disease

Infections

- Acute pyelonephritis

CLINICAL ISSUES

Epidemiology

- Incidence
  - Prerenal causes: 55-60%
  - Renal parenchymal diseases: 35-40%
  - Postrenal causes: < 5%
  - AKI in hospitalized patient: 3-7%
- Age
  - All ages are affected
  - Etiology varies according to age

Presentation

- Glomerular diseases
  - Nephritic/nephrotic syndrome
  - Increased creatinine
  - Oliguria/anuria
  - Microangiopathic hemolytic anemia
  - Thrombocytopenia
  - ± systemic manifestations: Fever, arthralgias, flu-like symptoms
  - Other organ involvement: Upper respiratory tract, central nervous system, lung, heart
- Tubular/interstitial
  - Oliguria/anuria

ACUTE RENAL FAILURE

Key Facts

Terminology
- Sudden sustained decline of glomerular filtration rate (GFR) associated with uremia, fall in urine output, and serum creatinine (SCr) increase

Etiology
- Crescentic glomerulonephritis: ANCA-related small vessel vasculitis, anti-GBM crescentic glomerulonephritis, immune complex-related glomerulonephritis
- Acute postinfectious glomerulonephritis
- Thrombotic microangiopathy (TMA)
- Hypersensitivity reaction: Antibiotics, nonsteroidals, protein supplements, proton pump inhibitors
- Systemic disorders: Hypotension, hypovolemia, sepsis, rhabdomyolysis, post surgery
- Vascular: Renal vein or artery thrombosis, atheroembolic disease
- Infections: Acute pyelonephritis

Clinical Issues
- Prerenal causes: 55-60%
- Renal parenchymal diseases: 35-40%
- Postrenal causes: < 5%
- AKI in hospitalized patient: 3-7%
- All ages are affected, and etiology varies according to age

Microscopic Pathology
- Microscopic findings vary according to processes causing renal failure

  - Hyaline, granular, pigmented casts in urine
  - Fever in case of infections
  - Creatinine increase
- Vascular
  - ARF
  - Eosinophilia
  - Hypertension
  - Skin petechial hemorrhages

Laboratory Tests
- Serum/blood
  - Serum creatinine
  - Blood urea nitrogen (BUN)
  - Antineutrophil cytoplasmic antibodies (ANCA/PR3, MPO)
  - Antiglomerular basement membrane antibodies (anti-GBM)
  - Antinuclear antibodies (ANA)
  - Cryoglobulins
  - Complement (C3, C4)
  - SPEP/immunofixation
  - Antistreptolysin antibody (ASO)
  - Complete blood count (CBC)
  - Electrolytes: Na, K, Ca, HCO_3, Cl, PO_4
- Urinalysis
  - Microscopic examination for crystals, casts, cells
  - Eosinophil count
  - Urine protein electrophoresis (UPEP)

Treatment
- Drugs
  - Hypertensive medication
  - Diuretics
  - Immunosuppressors in case of glomerulonephritis
- Renal replacement therapy
  - Hemodialysis, peritoneal dialysis
- Plasma exchange

Prognosis
- Mortality rate in hospitalized patients ~ 21.3%; varies depending on etiology
- Long-term prognosis varies depending on cause and clinical setting, as well as pre- and post-AKI kidney function
- Recovery can occur
- Progression to end-stage renal disease is a risk in older patients with comorbidities
- Risk factors for poor outcome
  - Male gender
  - Advanced age
  - Oliguria
  - Creatinine > 3 mg/dL at presentation
  - More severe renal injury
  - Failure involving other organs

IMAGE FINDINGS

Ultrasonographic Findings
- Enlarged or normal-sized kidneys
- Vascular obstruction of vein or artery can be detected
- Pyelocalyceal system dilatation in case of obstruction

CT Findings
- CT angiography useful to detect artery or vein occlusions

MACROSCOPIC FEATURES

External Examination
- Generalized edema, palpable purpura (vasculitis)
- Blood in mouth (pulmonary renal syndome: Anti-GBM or ANCA)
- Pallor, hemorrhagic shock (ATN)

Internal Examination
- Pleural effusions
- Ascites

Organ Examination
- Gross examination of kidney
  - Remove fat for accurate weight
  - Bisect kidneys in antero/posterior (coronal) plane

ACUTE RENAL FAILURE

    - Measurement of cortex and medulla
    - Assessment of cortex and medullary pyramids and pelvis
    - Opening of calyces major and minor
- Tissue allocation
    - Light microscopy
        - Sample from cortex and medulla should be submitted in formaldehyde from each kidney
        - H&E, PAS, trichrome, and Jones silver stains requested
    - Immunofluorescence
        - Sample from cortex (2-3 mm thickness) snap frozen or placed in Michel or Zeus transport media should be saved
        - In case of glomerular diseases stains with IgG, IgA, IgM, C3, C1q, fibrinogen, and light chains should be requested
    - Electron microscopy
        - Sample from cortex 2 x 3 mm cubes placed in glutaraldehyde should be saved and submitted for examination in cases of glomerular diseases
- Kidney gross appearance according to disease processes
    - Glomerular diseases
        - Enlarged kidney with petechial hemorrhage
        - Extensive cortical necrosis in TMA
    - Tubular diseases
        - Enlarged pale kidney
        - Swollen appearance and bulging from capsule
        - Widened cortex
        - Accentuation of cortico/medullary junction
        - Darker medulla
    - Interstitial diseases/pyelonephritis
        - Enlarged kidney
        - Yellow or white microabscesses on the surface
        - Pale streaks extending from medulla into cortex
        - Mucosa of pyelocaliceal system show edema and erythema; may be covered by purulent material
    - Vascular diseases
        - Malignant hypertension: Enlarged/normal size/ small kidney, chronic arterionephrosclerosis changes may be present; petechial hemorrhage flea-bitten appearance
        - Renal vein thrombosis: Enlarged kidney with vascular congestion; thrombus identified in vein and venules
        - Renal artery thrombosis: Thrombus in main renal artery and branches; renal artery stenosis and atheromatous plaque may be present; wedge peripheral infarcts
        - Atheroembolic disease: Cortical wedge infarcts when large artery involved

MICROSCOPIC PATHOLOGY

Histologic Features

- Glomerular diseases
    - Crescentic glomerulonephritis
        - ANCA related: Glomerular tuft fibrinoid necrosis; crescents; variable degree of interstitial inflammation; tubular injury
        - Anti-GBM crescentic glomerulonephritis: Glomerular tuft fibrinoid necrosis; crescents; variable degree of interstitial inflammation; tubular injury
        - Immune complex glomerulonephritis: Glomerular tuft fibrinoid necrosis; crescents; variable degree of interstitial inflammation; tubular injury
    - Acute postinfectious glomerulonephritis
        - Enlarged glomeruli with endocapillary proliferation and numerous intracapillary neutrophils
    - Thrombotic microangiopathy
        - Acute: Bloodless glomeruli, fibrin thrombi, glomerular capillary congestion and neutrophilic accumulation; mesangiolysis; arterioles and small arteries may contain fibrin thrombi
- Tubular diseases
    - Acute tubular necrosis
        - Ischemic: Tubular epithelial cell damage in multiple, patchy segments of proximal tubule; breaks in tubular basement membranes; luminal casts (hyaline, granular)
        - Toxic: Extensive tubular epithelial cell necrosis in proximal tubules
    - Cast nephropathy
        - Intratubular casts positive for κ light chain (75%) within distal tubules; with pale (on PAS) fractured appearance associated with inflammatory or giant cell reaction; mixed interstitial inflammation
    - Acute phosphate nephropathy
        - Calcium phosphate crystals within tubular lumens with basophilic/purple color on H&E stain; not polarizable; mild interstitial inflammation; fibrosis and tubular atrophy; glomeruli not involved
    - Bile (bilirubin) cast nephropathy
        - Bile casts in distal tubules; acellular and greenish-tinged brown on H&E; green in Hall stain; tubular injury
    - Oxalate nephropathy
        - Intratubular oxalate crystals with fan-like or irregular shapes and translucent on H&E stain; birefringent under polarized light; tubular injury; interstitial inflammation in fibrotic areas
    - Rhabdomyolysis
        - Tubular epithelial injury, hyaline, granular and pigmented (hemoglobin/myoglobin) casts; interstitial edema; glomeruli are spared
- Intersitial diseases
    - Acute interstitial nephritis: Mixed interstitial inflammation with frequent eosinophils; tubulitis; interstitial edema; multinucleated giant cells; nonnecrotizing granulomas
    - Acute pyelonephritis: Neutrophilic interstitial inflammation with neutrophilic casts; interstitial edema
- Vascular diseases
    - Malignant hypertension: Mucoid intima change; fibrinoid necrosis involving arterioles; corrugation/ reduplication of GBM; "onion skin" change in arterioles
    - Renal vein thrombosis: Organized thrombus within renal vein and venules; glomerular capillary and

peritubular capillary congestion; neutrophilic margination; interstitial edema and hemorrhage
  - Renal artery thrombosis: Cortical necrosis; interstitial hemorrhage
  - Atheroembolic disease: Elongated cholesterol clefts in small arteries (100-200 nm in diameter) &/or glomerular capillaries; clefts may be surrounded by debris and fibrin or englobed by macrophages or giant cells
- Cortical necrosis
  - Multifactorial etiology
  - Multifocal or diffuse coagulative necrosis of cortex with glomerular and tubular involvement
  - Thrombi may be identified in vasculature

ANCILLARY TESTS

Immunohistochemistry

- Myoglobin immunostain useful identifying casts in rhabdomyolysis
- von Kossa stain highlights phosphate crystals

Immunofluorescence

- Glomerular diseases
  - ANCA related: No or minimal deposits
  - Anti-GBM crescentic glomerulonephritis: Linear IgG deposits
  - Immune-complex glomerulonephritis: Deposits of IgG, IgA, IgM, C3, C1q, and light chains in subendothelial, mesangial, &/or subepithelial distribution
  - Acute postinfectious glomerulonephritis: Immune-complex type deposits positive for C3 and in lesser intensity for IgG or IgM
  - Thrombotic microangiopathy: Fibrinogen stain is seen in thrombi; nonspecific trapping of IgM and C3 in mesangium

Electron Microscopy

- Glomerular diseases
  - ANCA related: No or minimal deposits
  - Anti-GBM crescentic glomerulonephritis: No deposits
  - Immune-complex glomerulonephritis: Electron-dense deposits in subendothelial, mesangial, &/or subepithelial distribution
  - Acute postinfectious glomerulonephritis: Electron-dense deposits in subendothelial, mesangial, &/or subepithelial distribution (hump-like configuration)
  - Thrombotic microangiopathy: Fibrin tactoids, lamina rara interna expansion, mesangiolysis
- Tubular diseases
  - Rhabdomyolysis: Casts containing electron-dense granules
- Vascular diseases
  - Malignant hypertension: Expansion of lamina rara interna and mesangial interposition

DIFFERENTIAL DIAGNOSIS

Acute Tubular Necrosis

- Autolysis
  - Widespread tubular degenerative changes
  - Pyknosis of tubular epithelial cell nuclei
  - Detachment of tubular epithelial cells

REPORTING CRITERIA

Final Report Should Include

- Etiology of ARF and complications
- Effects in other organs
- Whether it was cause of death or contributing factor

SELECTED REFERENCES

1. Ford SL et al: Histopathologic and clinical predictors of kidney outcomes in ANCA-associated vasculitis. Am J Kidney Dis. 63(2):227-35, 2014
2. Hellmark T et al: Diagnosis and classification of Goodpasture's disease (anti-GBM). J Autoimmun. 48-49:108-12, 2014
3. Jennette JC et al: Pathogenesis of antineutrophil cytoplasmic autoantibody-mediated disease. Nat Rev Rheumatol. 10(8):463-73, 2014
4. Li Z et al: Clinical and pathological features of acute kidney injury in children. Ren Fail. 36(7):1023-8, 2014
5. Muriithi AK et al: Biopsy-proven acute interstitial nephritis, 1993-2011: a case series. Am J Kidney Dis. 64(4):558-66, 2014
6. Muriithi AK et al: Clinical characteristics, causes and outcomes of acute interstitial nephritis in the elderly. Kidney Int. Epub ahead of print, 2014
7. Tang X et al: Acute and chronic kidney injury in nephrolithiasis. Curr Opin Nephrol Hypertens. 23(4):385-90, 2014
8. Tanna A et al: Long-term outcome of anti-neutrophil cytoplasm antibody-associated glomerulonephritis: evaluation of the international histological classification and other prognostic factors. Nephrol Dial Transplant. Epub ahead of print, 2014
9. Valluri A et al: Acute tubulointerstitial nephritis in Scotland. QJM. Epub ahead of print, 2014
10. Nasr SH et al: Clinicopathologic correlations in multiple myeloma: a case series of 190 patients with kidney biopsies. Am J Kidney Dis. 59(6):786-94, 2012
11. Hutchison CA et al: The pathogenesis and diagnosis of acute kidney injury in multiple myeloma. Nat Rev Nephrol. 8(1):43-51, 2011
12. Williamson SR et al: A 25-year experience with pediatric anti-glomerular basement membrane disease. Pediatr Nephrol. 26(1):85-91, 2011
13. Kocovski L et al: Can renal acute tubular necrosis be differentiated from autolysis at autopsy? J Forensic Sci. 54(2):439-42, 2009
14. Markowitz GS et al: Acute phosphate nephropathy. Kidney Int. 76(10):1027-34, 2009
15. Iwasa S et al: Autopsy case of microscopic polyangiitis with crescentic glomerulonephritis and necrotizing pancreatitis. Pathol Int. 55(8):520-3, 2005
16. Herrera GA et al: Renal pathologic spectrum in an autopsy series of patients with plasma cell dyscrasia. Arch Pathol Lab Med. 128(8):875-9, 2004

Variant Microscopic Features

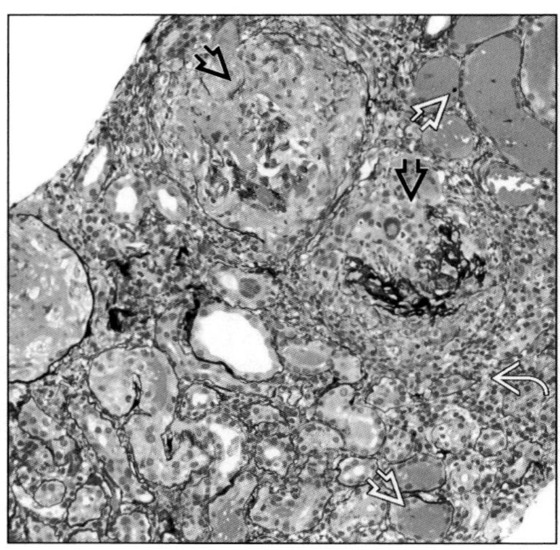

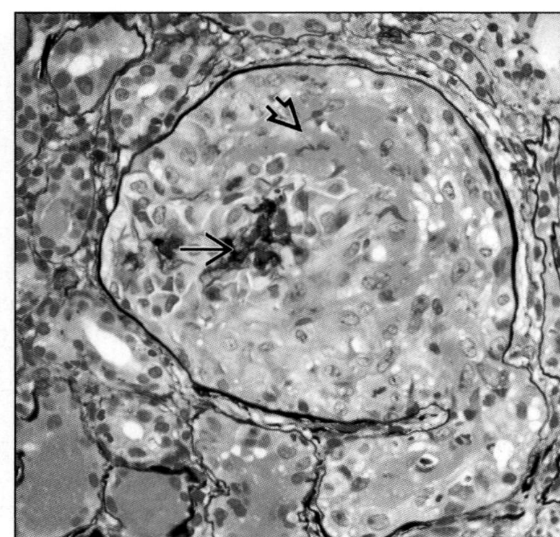

***(Left)** In this case of ANCA-related necrotizing crescentic glomerulonephritis, several glomeruli show cellular crescents, and there is inflammatory infiltrate in the interstitium, and numerous red blood cell casts are seen within tubules. **(Right)** In this case of ANCA-related necrotizing crescentic glomerulonephritis, a large circumferential cellular crescent admixed with fibrin is seen with collapse of the capillary loops.*

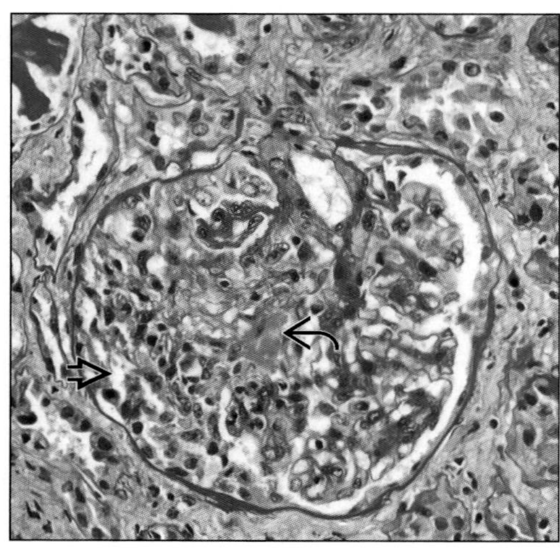

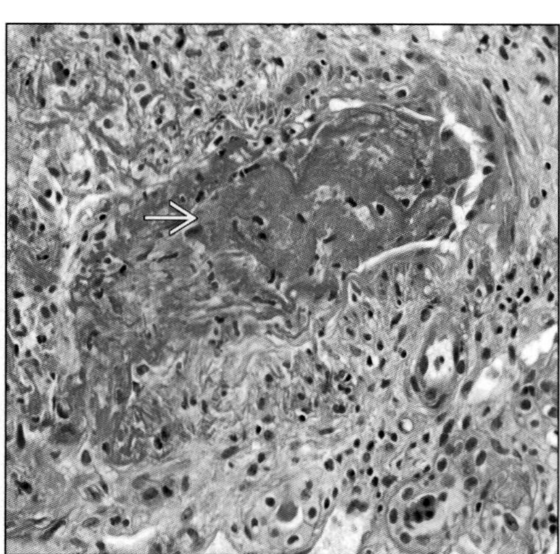

***(Left)** In ANCA-related necrotizing crescentic glomerulonephritis, areas of fibrinoid necrosis and crescents can be identified. There is no significant proliferation in the portion of uninvolved glomerulus, which is different from immune complex crescentic glomerulonephritis. **(Right)** In ANCA-associated necrotizing crescentic glomerulonephritis, arteritis is an occasional finding, as is shown in this case, where extensive fibrinoid necrosis of the interlobular artery is seen.*

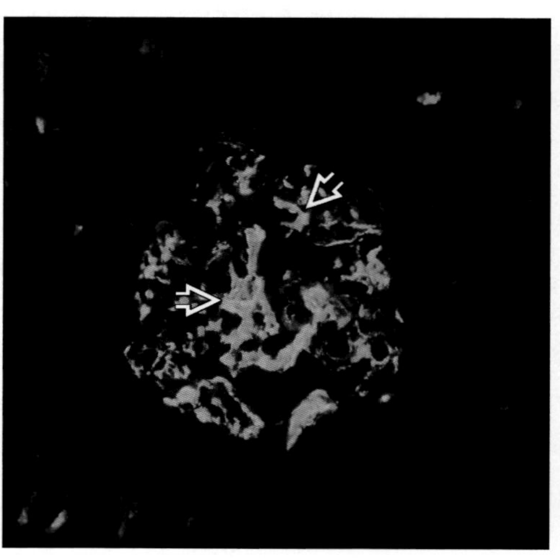

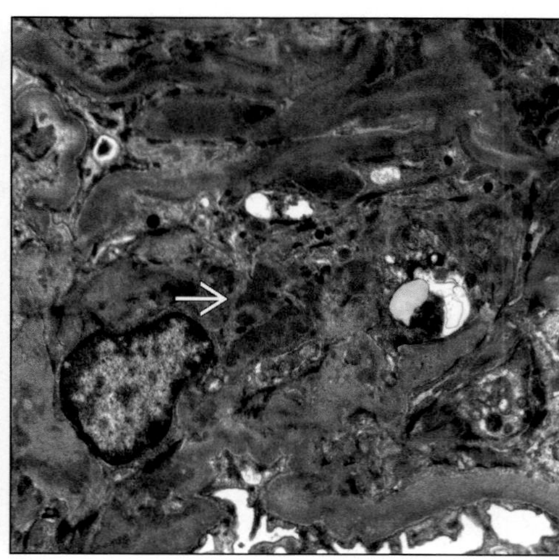

***(Left)** IgA nephropathy shows a bright granular staining in mesangium for IgA by immunofluorescence. The staining may be dominant, or codominant with other immunoglobulins (IgG or IgM). C3 and light chain staining are also present. **(Right)** Electron microscopy shows mesangial electron-dense deposits, usually attached to paramesangial basement membranes.*

Gross and Microscopic Features

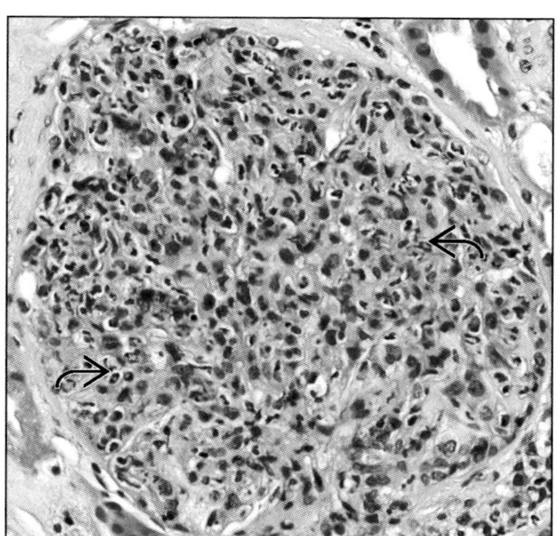

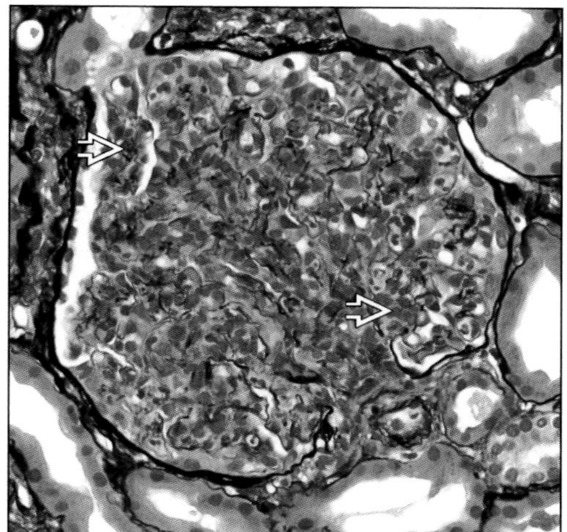

(Left) *In acute postinfectious glomerulonephritis, there is marked endocapillary hypercellularity with lobular accentuation and presence of numerous neutrophils* ➩ *within the capillary lumina, as well as swollen endothelial cells.* ***(Right)*** *On Jones silver stain, the endocapillary proliferation is evident, and no significant changes are seen in the glomerular basement membranes. Frequent neutrophils are present* ➩.

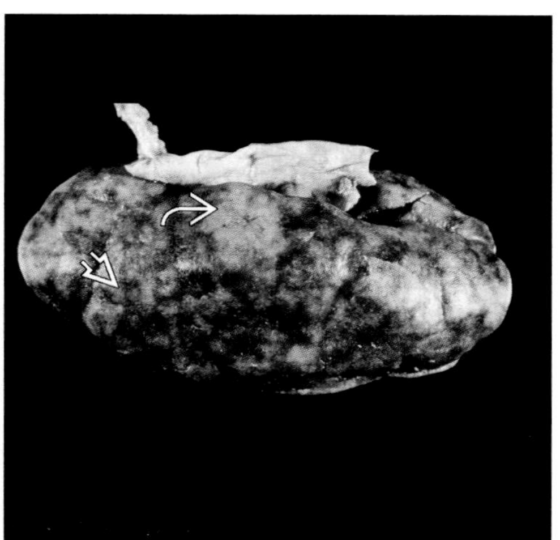

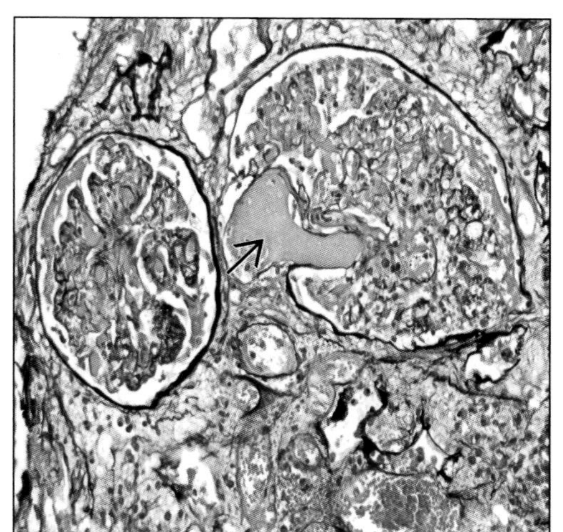

(Left) *Gross specimen from patient with hemolytic uremic syndrome show multiples areas of hemorrhage in the surface of the kidney* ➩ *as well as areas of white coloration corresponding to cortical infarcts* ➩. ***(Right)*** *Thrombotic microangiopathy in Hemolytic uremic syndrome shows extensive fibrin thrombi in glomerular capillaries* → *at the vascular pole. Thrombi may also involve small arteries.*

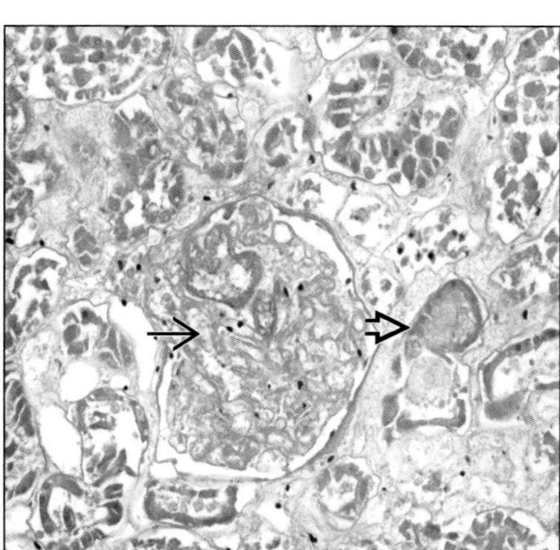

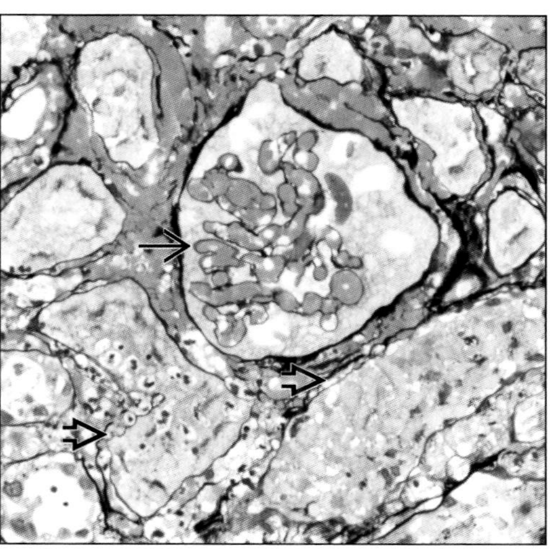

(Left) *Cortical necrosis is characterized by glomerular necrosis* → *and acute tubular necrosis* ➩. *This process may be secondary to obstetric complications such as abruptio placenta, placenta previa, septic abortion, etc. Other etiologies include transfusion reactions, thrombotic microangiopathy, shock, and antibody-mediated rejection.* ***(Right)*** *On silver stain in this case of cortical necrosis, the glomerulus appears congested and only the GBM* → *and TBM* ➩ *are preserved.*

ACUTE RENAL FAILURE

Variant Microscopic Features

(Left) Acute tubular injury is characterized by extensive flattening of tubular epithelial cell lining ➔, dilatation of the tubular lumina, and presence of proteinaceous material within tubular lumina. Interstitial inflammation is not seen, and only inflammatory cells within peritubular capillaries may be present. ***(Right)*** *In acute phosphate nephropathy, there is tubular epithelial injury ➔, and numerous calcium phosphate crystals are present in tubular lumina ➔.*

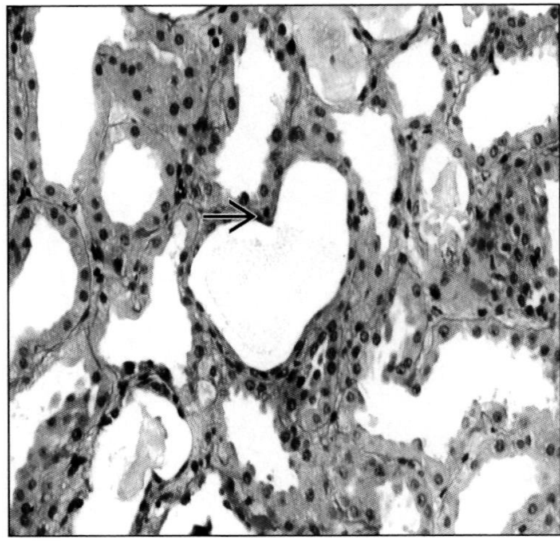

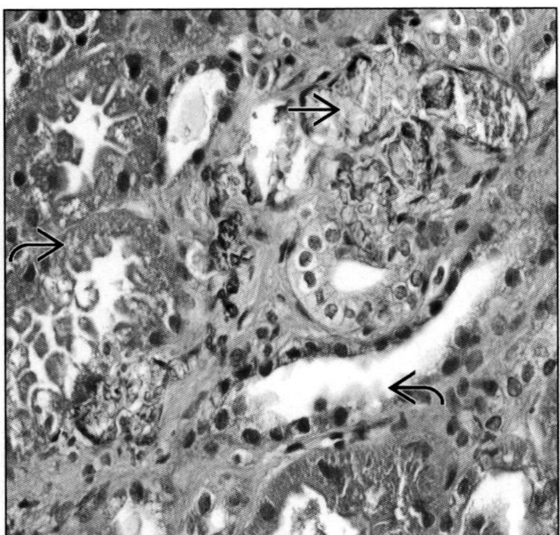

(Left) Bile (bilirubin) casts are seen as brownish casts ➔ with slight green tinge with associated acute tubular injury with flattened epithelial cell lining ➔. ***(Right)*** *Bile (bilirubin) casts are seen as distinctly green ➔ with special stain for bilirubin (Hall stain).*

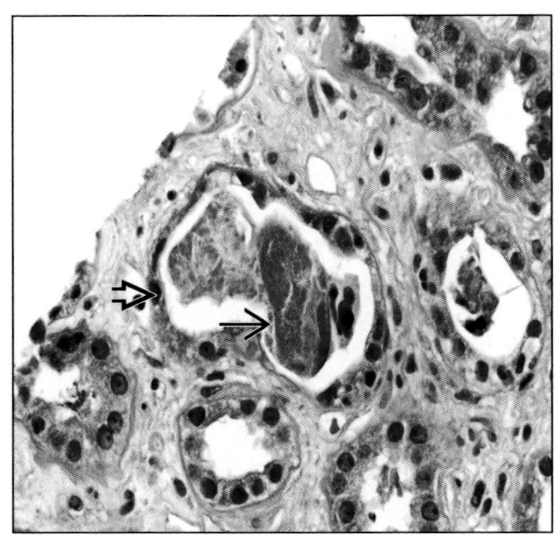

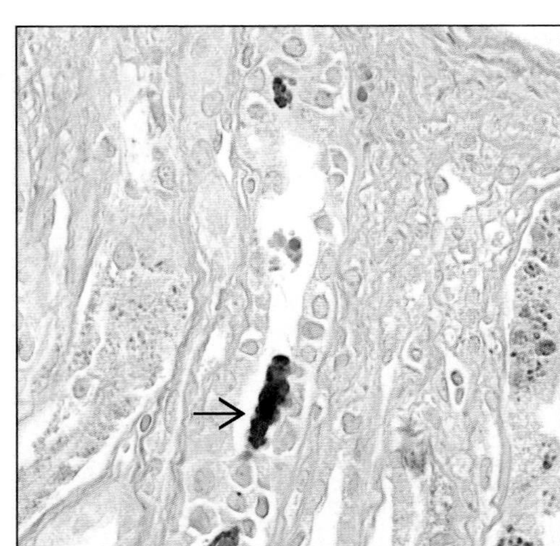

(Left) In acute renal failure caused by ethylene glycol, there is extensive acute tubular injury with associated calcium oxalate crystals which are clear and may not be discernible by light microscopy ➔. ***(Right)*** *Calcium oxalate crystals are seen under polarized light as birefringent polarizable fan-shaped crystals ➔.*

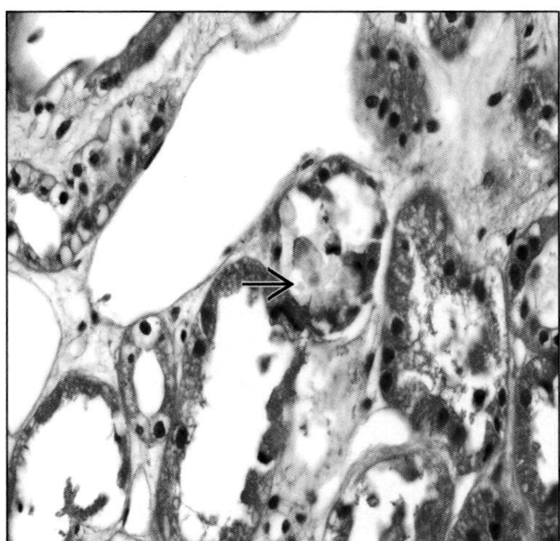

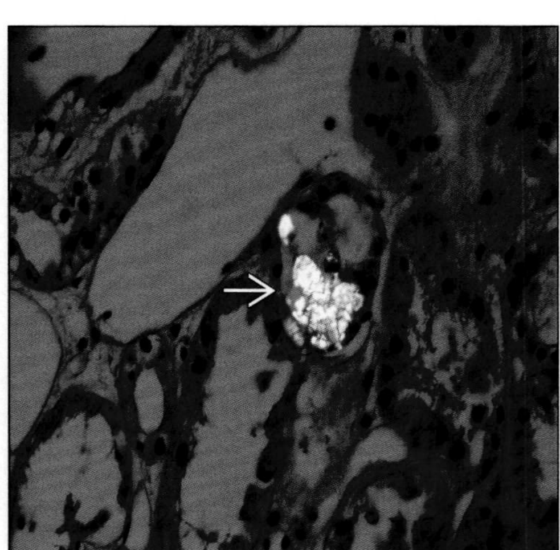

Variant Microscopic Features

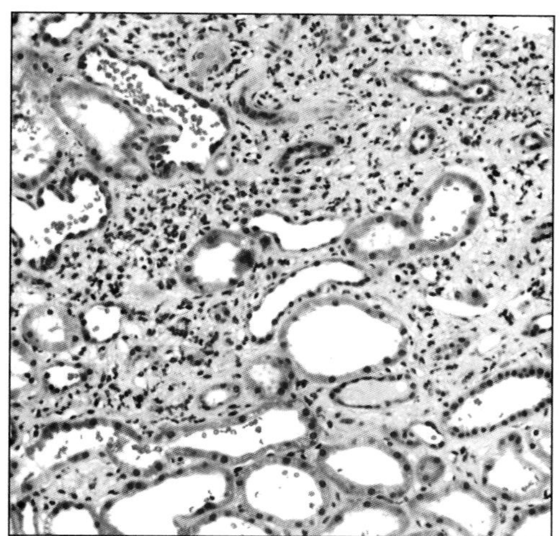

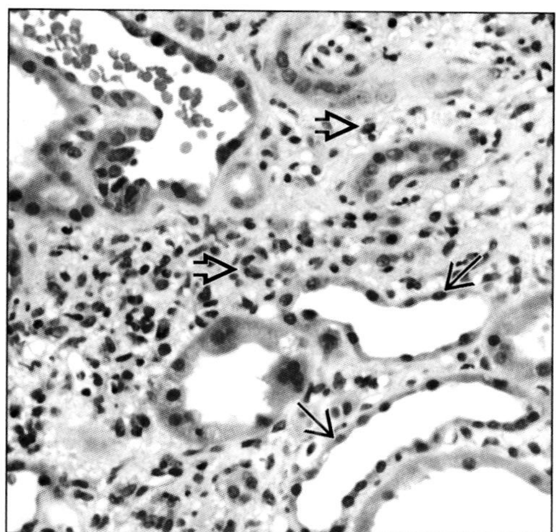

(Left) *A case of acute interstitial nephritis caused by drug-induced hypersensitivity reaction shows extensive interstitial edema with associated mixed interstitial infiltrate containing mononuclear cells (lymphocytes, plasma cells, macrophages) and eosinophils.* ***(Right)*** *High-power view shows acute interstitial nephritis with scattered interstitial eosinophils ➨ in a background of interstitial edema and tubular injury characterized by flattening of epithelial cells ➔.*

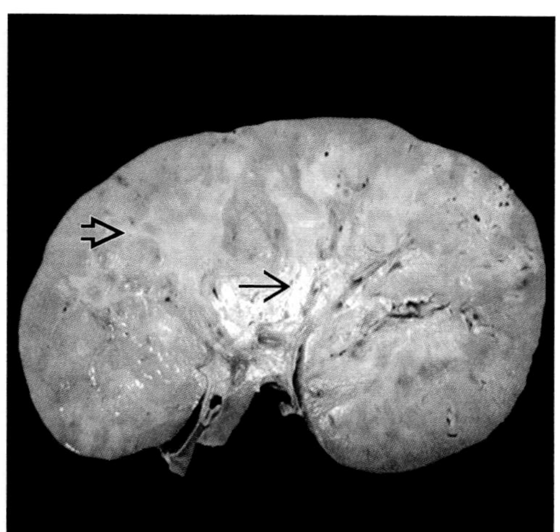

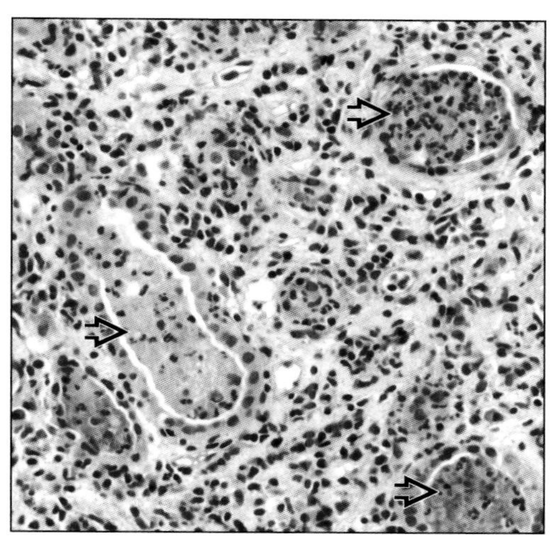

(Left) *In this case of acute pyelonephritis, the kidney is enlarged and swollen. There are diffuse white streaks ➔ along the major and minor calyces ➨ that correspond to collecting ducts filled with purulent material.* ***(Right)*** *Section shows marked inflammatory infiltrate composed of mononuclear cells with numerous neutrophils as well as presence of neutrophilic casts ➨, which are characteristic of acute pyelonephritis. Interstitial edema is also present.*

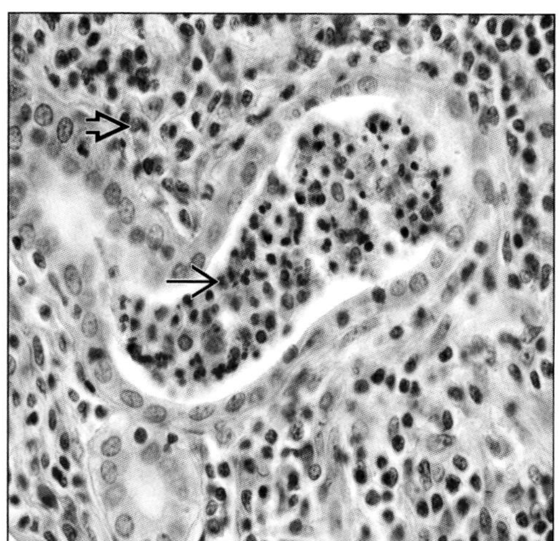

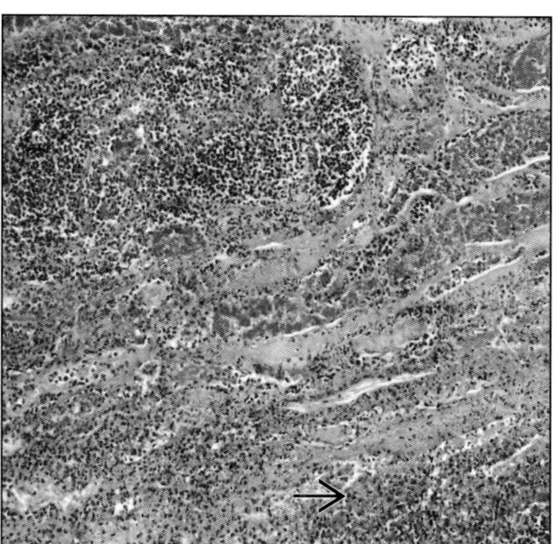

(Left) *The characteristic findings of acute pyelonephritis are neutrophils present in tubular lumina forming neutrophilic plugs ➔ as well as neutrophils invading tubular epithelium and interstitium ➨.* ***(Right)*** *Papillary necrosis can occur in severe cases of acute pyelonephritis. In this case, there is coagulative necrosis ➔ with retention of medulla outlines but little cellular detail.*

ACUTE RENAL FAILURE

Variant Microscopic Features

*(**Left**) In acute rhabdomyolysis, myoglobin casts are present within the tubules. They show a characteristic granular reddish-brown globular appearance ➔, and there is associated acute tubular injury. (**Right**) The composition of the casts in rhabdomyolysis can be determined by immunohistochemistry for myoglobin. In this case, the cast is strongly positive for myoglobin ➔.*

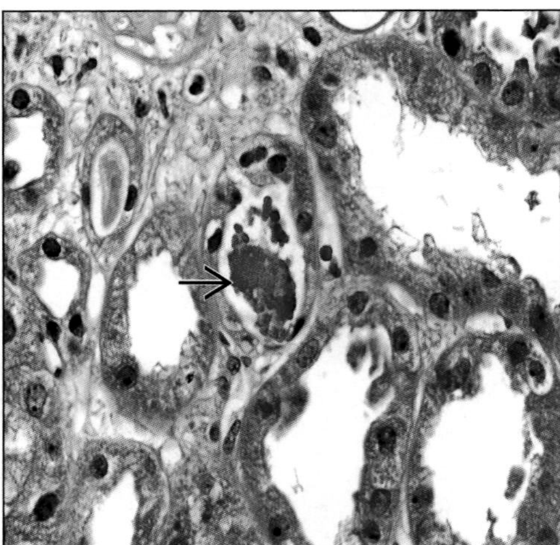

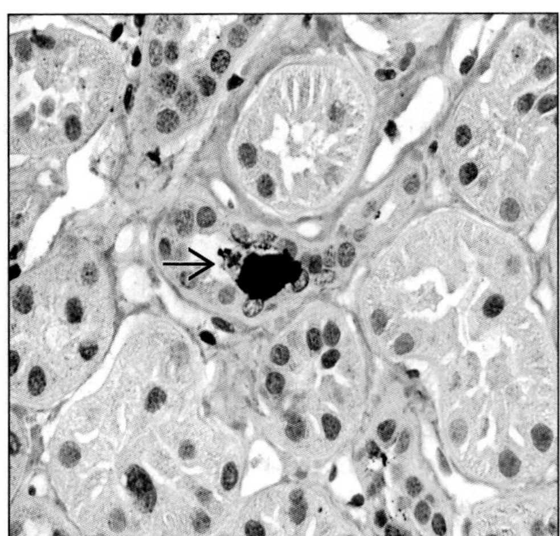

*(**Left**) In acute phase of malignant hypertension, there is marked mucoid degeneration ➔ characterized by basophilic change in the intima of arteries with reduction of the lumina. (**Right**) In malignant hypertension, the arterioles show intimal proliferation of myofibroblasts ➔ and lamination of internal elastic lamina with a characteristic onion skin appearance.*

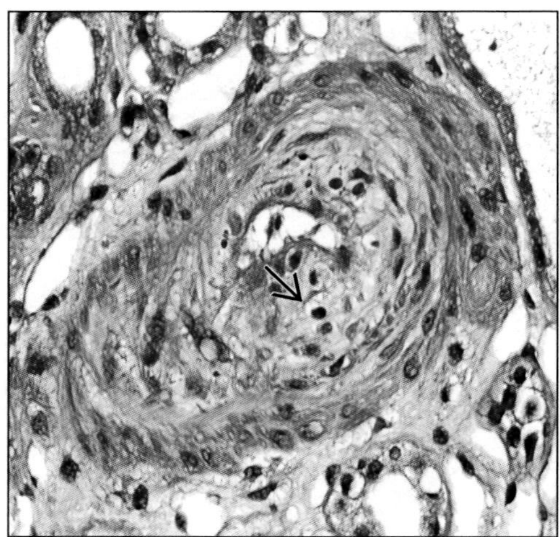

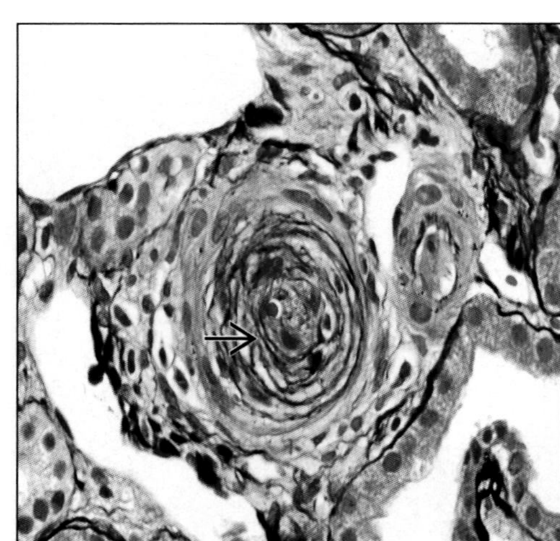

*(**Left**) The arterioles in malignant hypertension may show areas of fibrinoid necrosis in the wall, which appears as a pink-red material ⇨. (**Right**) In malignant hypertension, the glomeruli usually show ischemic appearance and may also show fibrin thrombi ➔; however, glomeruli are not the dominant site of injury.*

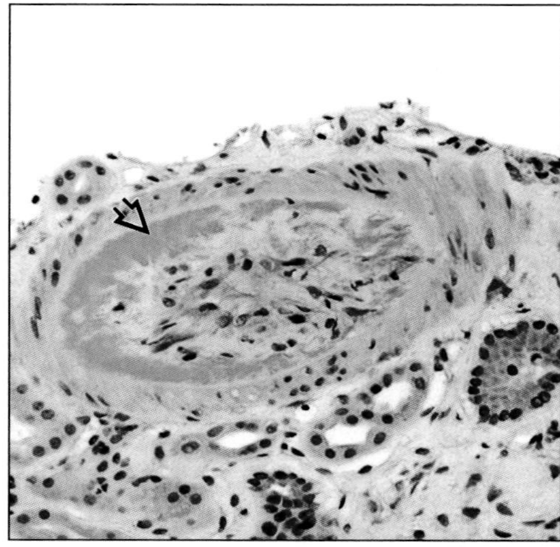

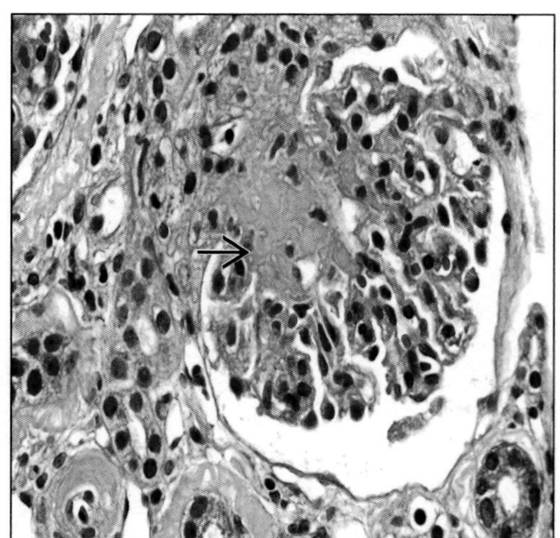

Gross and Microscopic Features

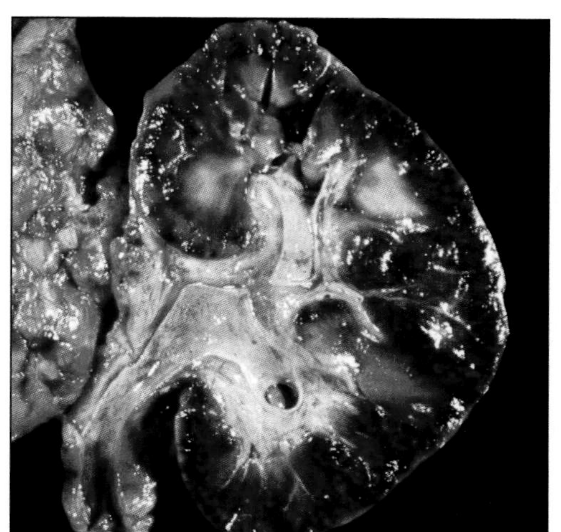

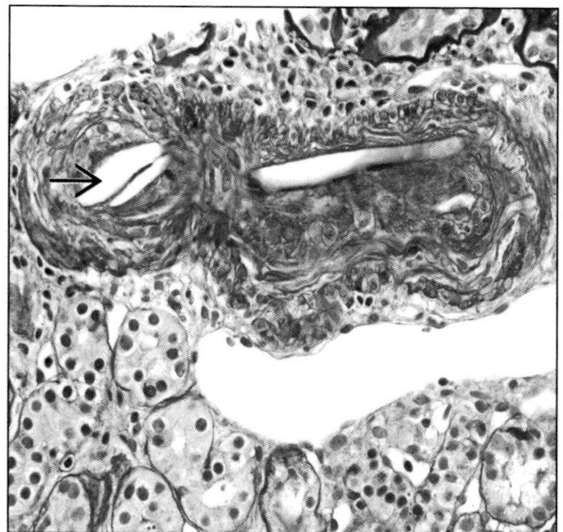

(Left) *Gross image in a case of thromboembolization in the kidney shows areas of cortical hemorrhage alternating with white areas that correspond to ischemic infarcts. Acute embolization may occur from atherosclerotic lesions.* ***(Right)*** *Atheroembolization is characterized by the presence of elongated clefts of cholesterol ⇒ in the lumina of small arteries (100-200 μm in diameter). There may be associated inflammatory reaction surrounding clefts.*

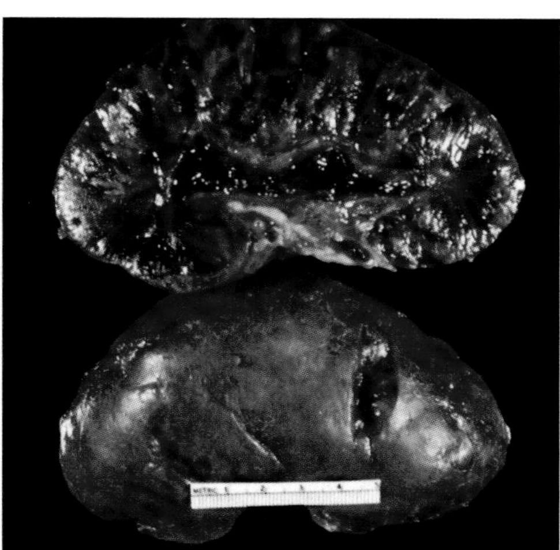

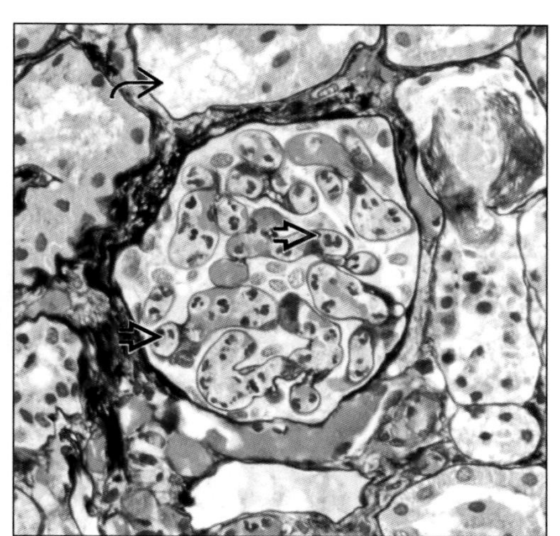

(Left) *In renal vein thrombosis, the kidney shows enlargement and swelling with extensive hemorrhage involving cortex and medulla. Thrombosis of renal vein may occur in nephrotic syndrome, anti-phospholipid antibody syndrome, malignancies, infections, trauma, etc.* ***(Right)*** *In this case of renal vein thrombosis, the glomerular capillaries are congested with marginating neutrophils ⇨ in the lumina. Tubular epithelial cell necrosis ↷ and interstitial hemorrhage are also present.*

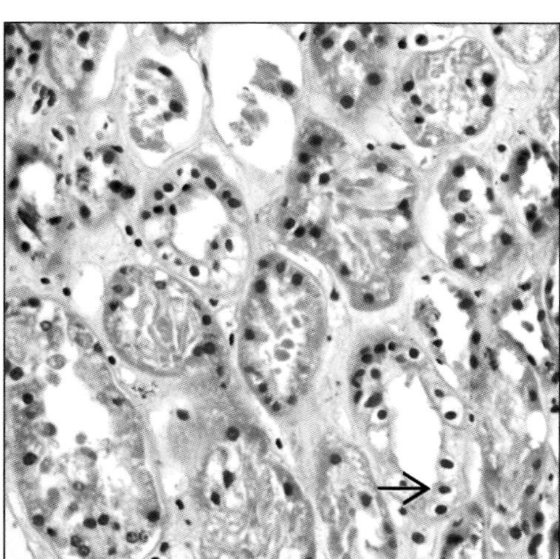

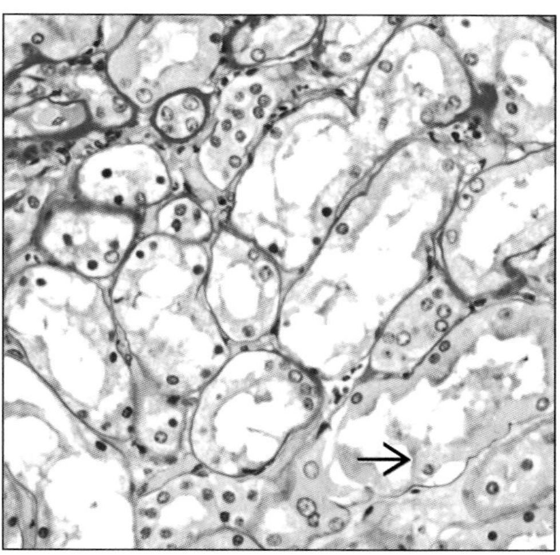

(Left) *Autolysis is a common finding in autopsy kidneys, and it is difficult to differentiate from acute tubular injury; however, it is a more diffuse process with detachment of epithelial cells from tubular basement membranes and nuclear pyknosis ⇒.* ***(Right)*** *On PAS stain, the separation of tubular epithelial cells ⇒ from the basement membranes is more evident. The degree of autolysis varies depending of post mortem interval, cooling time, and body mass.*

ADRENAL INSUFFICIENCY

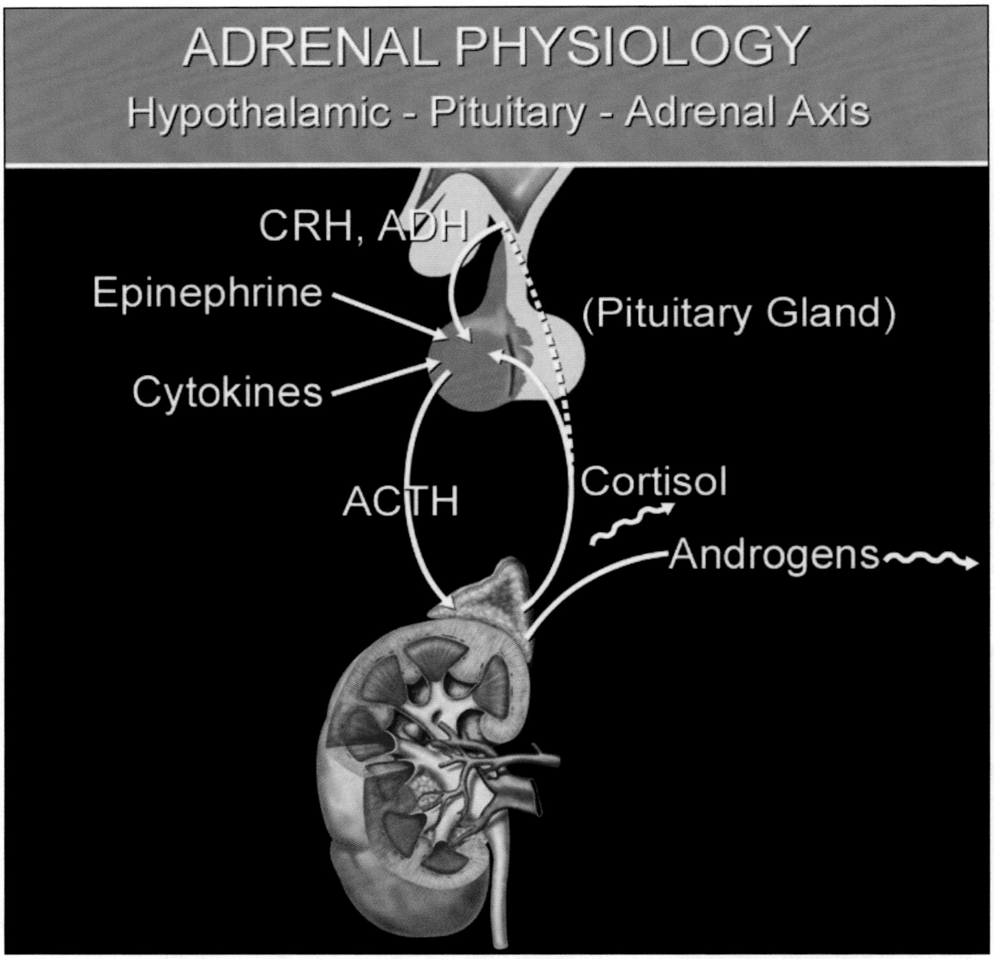

The relationship between hypothalamus, pituitary, and adrenal gland is shown. Various stimuli affect the anterior pituitary (including corticotropin-releasing hormone [CRH], antidiuretic hormone [ADH], and cytokines), leading to release of adrenocorticotrophic hormone (ACTH). Under the influence of ACTH, the adrenal glands increase secretion of various steroid-based hormones including cortisol and androgens. Negative feedback loops also inhibit the release of ACTH and the hormones produced by the adrenal glands. Abnormal or inappropriate inhibition of these adrenal hormones leads to adrenal insufficiency.

TERMINOLOGY

Synonyms

- Adrenal hypofunction
- Addison disease

ETIOLOGY/PATHOGENESIS

Primary Causes

- Primary chronic adrenocortical insufficiency (Addison disease)
  - Most often due to autoimmune adrenalitis
- Autoimmune adrenalitis
  - 50% of cases associated with other autoimmune endocrine disorder
    - Esp. thyroid, parathyroid disease
    - May be part of "autoimmune polyglandular syndromes"
  - Almost complete loss of adrenal cortical cells achieved before symptoms manifest
    - "Tipping point" may occur under stressful conditions (basal needs can be met, but stress levels cannot)
  - Presumed autoantibody to adrenal cortical cell epitopes
- Adrenal hemorrhage
  - Often associated with sepsis due to bacterial infection
  - Causative organisms
    - *Neisseria meningitidis*
    - Gram-positive cocci (*Staphylococcus* and *Streptococcus*)
    - *Haemophilus influenzae*
    - *Klebsiella* spp.
    - *Pseudomonas* spp.
    - Opportunistic fungi: *Candida* spp.
  - Waterhouse-Friderichsen syndrome
    - Bilateral adrenal hemorrhage (massive)

ADRENAL INSUFFICIENCY

Key Facts

Etiology
- Autoimmune adrenalitis (Addison disease)
- Adrenal hemorrhage (Waterhouse-Friderichsen syndrome)
  - Often associated with sepsis due to bacterial infection
- Tuberculosis
- Congenital defects
  - Adrenal agenesis
  - Congenital adrenal hypoplasia
  - Adrenoleukodystrophy
- Adrenal metastasis
- Iatrogenic (rapid steroid withdrawal)
- Postpartum pituitary infarction (Sheehan syndrome)

Clinical Issues
- Acute insufficiency (Addisonian crisis)
  - Back, abdominal &/or leg pain
  - Severe vomiting and diarrhea (volume depletion)
  - Hypotension, shock
  - Altered mental status (even coma)
  - Hyperkalemia

Macroscopic Pathology
- Adrenal glands
  - Glands initially normal size (4-7 g)
- Marked bilateral atrophy in end stages
  - Can weigh < 2 g

Microscopic Pathology
- Autoimmune adrenalitis
  - Lymphoplasmacytic inflammation
  - Medulla is relatively preserved and can extend to capsule

---

    - More common in children
    - Classically due to *Neisseria meningitidis* sepsis
  - Other noninfectious etiologies (rare)
    - Cardiogenic shock
    - Severe burns
    - Hypercoagulable states (including pregnancy)
    - Excessive anticoagulation or thrombolytic therapy
    - Hypothermia
- Tuberculosis
  - Most common cause of adrenalitis worldwide, but rare in developed countries
  - 6% of patients with active infection
- Congenital defects
  - Adrenal agenesis
    - 10% of unilateral renal agenesis also ipsilateral adrenal agenesis
  - Congenital adrenal hypoplasia
    - Association with anencephaly and congenital hypothalamus-pituitary axis anomalies
    - X-linked adrenal hypoplasia congenita (*DAX1* mutation)
    - Familial glucocorticoid deficiency (mutations of ACTH receptor)
  - Adrenoleukodystrophy
    - Fatty acid metabolism disorder (very long chain fatty acids [VLCFA])
    - Clinically and genetically heterogeneous
    - Signs and symptoms include myeloneuropathy (defect in myelination) and adrenal insufficiency
    - Rare "Addison only" form
- Adrenal metastasis
  - Primary (carcinomas): Lung, breast, upper GI, liver, renal, ovarian
  - Non-carcinomas: Lymphoma, sarcoma
  - Bilateral in 50%
  - 80-90% replacement of adrenal tissue before symptoms manifest
- Genetic
  - Autoimmune polyendocrinopathy syndrome 1 (*AIRE* gene on 21q22)
  - Autoimmune polyendocrinopathy syndrome 2 (polygenic)
- Iatrogenic
  - Rapid withdrawal of corticosteroids

Secondary Causes
- Secondary chronic adrenocortical insufficiency
  - Most commonly from hypothalamic suppression due to long-term corticosteroid use
  - No hyperpigmentation or electrolyte imbalances
- Postpartum pituitary infarction (Sheehan syndrome)
  - Complication of massive hemorrhage during delivery
    - Mechanism not completely understood (localized vasospasm?)
    - 10% of cases without clinically recognized peripartum volume loss
  - Acute: Liquefactive necrosis
  - Chronic: Fibrotic replacement
  - Pituitary "apoplexy": Similar to Sheehan syndrome, but infarction due to adenoma
  - Partial or complete (pan) hypopituitarism
    - Hypogonadism: 100% of cases
    - Prolactin and growth hormone: 100% of cases
    - Hypothyroidism: 90% of cases
    - Hypocortisolism: 50% of cases
  - Latency between event and symptoms varies widely (2 months to decades later)

CLINICAL ISSUES

Presentation
- Signs and symptoms
  - Chronic insufficiency
    - Muscle weakness and fatigue
    - Weight loss and decreased appetite
    - Hyperpigmentation of skin
    - Hypotension, lightheadedness
    - Salt craving
    - Electrolyte disturbances: ↑ K, ↓ Na
    - Hypoglycemia

ADRENAL INSUFFICIENCY

- Nausea, vomiting, diarrhea
- Myalgias, arthralgias
- Depression
- Body hair loss or sexual dysfunction (in women)
- Acute insufficiency (Addisonian crisis)
  - Back, abdominal, &/or leg pain
  - Severe vomiting and diarrhea (volume depletion)
  - Hypotension, shock
  - Altered mental status (even coma)
  - Hyperkalemia

Laboratory Tests

- Adrenocorticotrophic hormone (ACTH) (antemortem)
  - Can be used to distinguish between patients with
    - Primary adrenal insufficiency (↑ ACTH, ↓ cortisol)
    - Secondary causes (e.g., pituitary) (nl or ↓ ACTH, ↓ cortisol)

IMAGE FINDINGS

CT Findings

- Adrenal gland enlargement
  - Hemorrhage
  - Metastatic tumor
- Adrenal gland atrophy

MACROSCOPIC FEATURES

External Examination

- Hyperpigmentation: Addison disease
- Hair distribution: Addison disease
- Ecchymoses, petechiae: Adrenal hemorrhage

Internal Examination

- Pituitary necrosis, fibrosis
- Cardiomyopathy
- Metastatic malignancy
- Gonadal atrophy
- Renal pallor

Organ Examination

- Adrenal glands
  - Glands initially normal size
    - Normal weight range: 4-7 g each (with fat removed)
  - Marked bilateral atrophy in end stages
    - Can weigh < 2 g

MICROSCOPIC PATHOLOGY

Histologic Features

- Autoimmune adrenalitis
  - Lymphocytic and lymphoplasmacytic inflammatory infiltrate
  - Cortical cell necrosis and loss
  - Medulla is relatively preserved and can extend to capsule
- Adrenal hemorrhage
  - Recent hemorrhage
  - Loss of cortical parenchymal cells
  - Acute inflammation
  - Exclude renal vein branch thrombosis
- Tuberculosis
  - Chronic inflammation, giant cells, and caseation
  - Granulomas may be less developed than in other sites
  - Subcapsular granulation tissue and calcifications in older lesions

SELECTED REFERENCES

1. Marti JL et al: Spontaneous adrenal hemorrhage with associated masses: etiology and management in 6 cases and a review of 133 reported cases. World J Surg. 36(1):75-82, 2012
2. Sethuraman C et al: Bilateral absence of adrenal glands: a case series that expands the spectrum of associations and highlights the difficulties in prenatal diagnosis. Fetal Pediatr Pathol. 30(2):137-43, 2011
3. Guarner J et al: Adrenal gland hemorrhage in patients with fatal bacterial infections. Mod Pathol. 21(9):1113-20, 2008
4. Dökmetaş HS et al: Characteristic features of 20 patients with Sheehan's syndrome. Gynecol Endocrinol. 22(5):279-83, 2006
5. Lam KY et al: Metastatic tumours of the adrenal glands: a 30-year experience in a teaching hospital. Clin Endocrinol (Oxf). 56(1):95-101, 2002
6. Lack EE et al: Embryology, developmental anatomy, and selected aspects of non-neoplastic pathology. In Pathology of the Adrenal Glands. New York: Churchill Livingstone. 1-74, 1990
7. Petri M et al: Addison's adrenalitis. Studies on diffuse lymphocytic adrenalitis (idiopathic Addison's disease) and focal lymphocytic infiltration in a control material. Acta Pathol Microbiol Scand A. 79(4):381-8, 1971

ADRENAL INSUFFICIENCY

Gross, Radiologic, and Microscopic Features

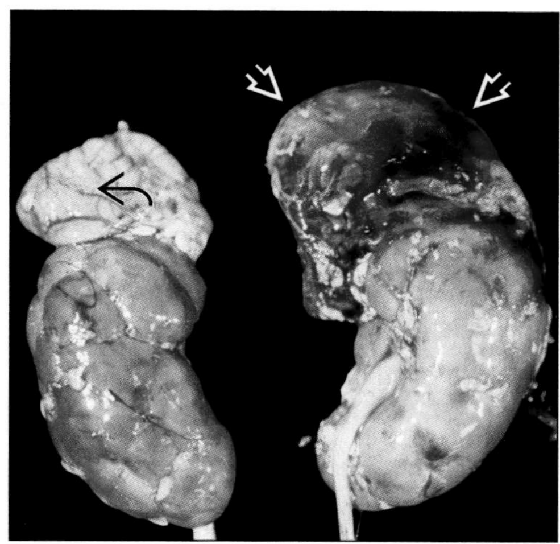
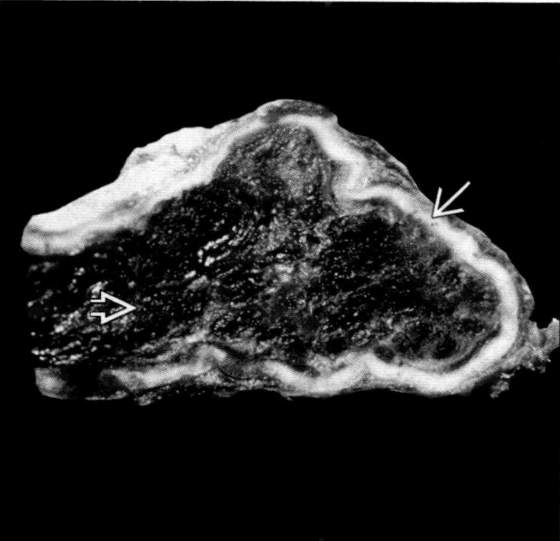

*(**Left**) Unilateral hemorrhage of adrenal gland is present on the right. Note the discrepancy in size between the 2 adrenals due to massive hemorrhage . The left adrenal gland is normal size for age in this neonate. (From DP: Nonneoplastic Pediatrics.) (**Right**) This gross photograph on an adrenal gland at autopsy shows hemorrhage into the interior of the gland. A thin rim of yellow adrenal cortex remains .*

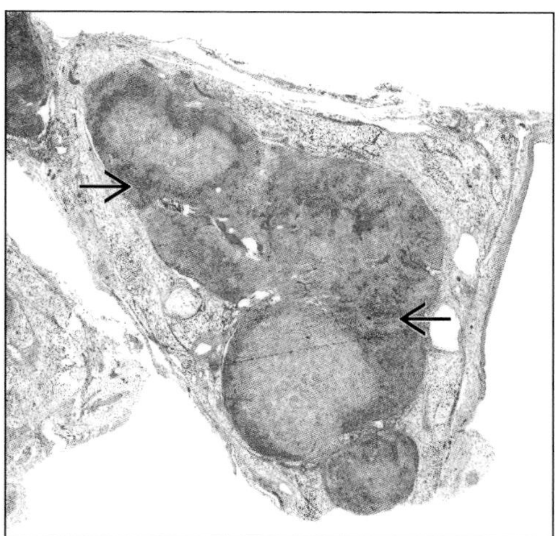
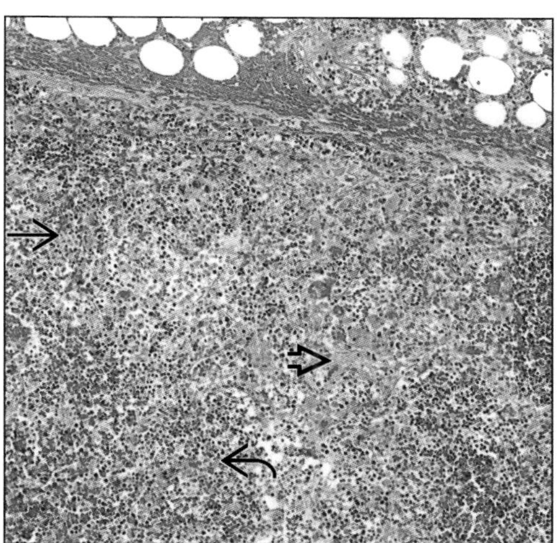

*(**Left**) This low-magnification view of an adult adrenal gland at autopsy shows diffuse hemorrhage and complete loss of the normal histoarchitecture. The patient died from severe septic shock. (**Right**) At higher magnification, hemorrhage and inflammation are apparent. There is a complete loss of recognizable adrenal cortical cells, with only a few ghost outlines remaining.*

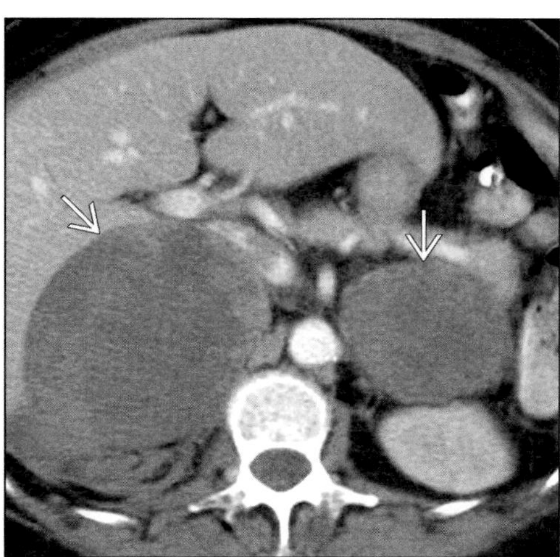
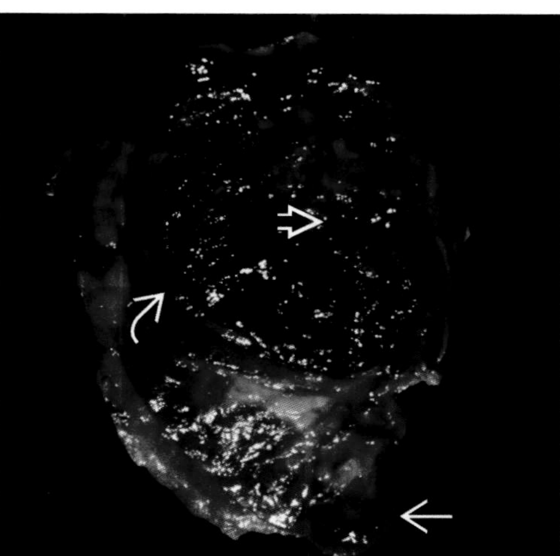

*(**Left**) This axial CT scan (antemortem) shows massive bilateral adrenal metastases from lung cancer that resulted in adrenal insufficiency. (From DI: Genitourinary) (**Right**) Metastatic lung carcinoma is shown, forming a dark hemorrhagic nodule in the adrenal gland. A thin rim of adrenal cortex is still present. The kidney (distorted by the mass) can also be seen.*

ADRENOCORTICAL EXCESS

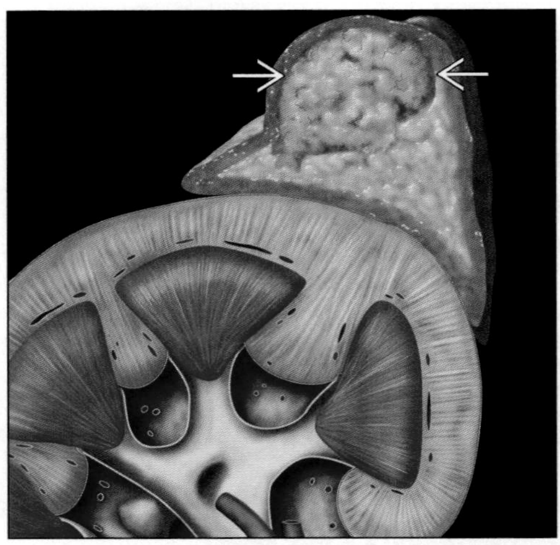

This illustration shows the location of adrenal gland atop upper pole of kidney. Note adrenal cortical adenoma ➡. Adenomas are a common cause of adrenocortical excess. (From DP: Pediatric Neoplasms.)

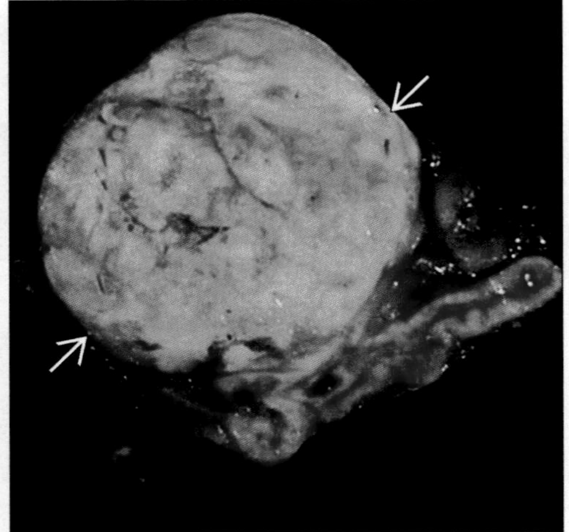

A dominant nodule ➡ of adrenal cortex is seen in a patient with adrenocortical hyperplasia. Additional, smaller nodules were scattered throughout the remaining gland. (Courtesy F. Shakil, MD.)

TERMINOLOGY

Definitions

- **Hypercortisolism**: State of glucocorticoid excess
  - Cushing syndrome
- **Aldosteronism**: State of mineralocorticoid excess
- **Adrenogenital syndrome(s)**: State of adrenal androgen excess

ETIOLOGY/PATHOGENESIS

Types

- **Hypercortisolism**
  - Can result from endogenous overproduction or exogenous sources
    - Adrenocorticotrophic hormone (ACTH)-secreting pituitary adenoma
    - Adrenal cortical hyperplasia
    - Primary adrenal neoplasms (adenoma vs. carcinoma)
    - Ectopic ACTH-producing neoplasms elsewhere in body (paraneoplastic)
- **Aldosteronism**
  - Can result from endogenous overproduction of aldosterone (primary or secondary) or, less commonly, ingestion of certain substances
    - Bilateral adrenal cortical hyperplasia
    - Primary adrenal neoplasms (cortical adenoma): Conn syndrome
    - Excessive ingestion of licorice compounds
    - Secondary causes: Renal artery stenosis, diuretic abuse
- **Adrenogenital syndrome**
  - Can result from inborn errors in enzymes involved in steroid production or from associated adrenal cortical neoplasms
    - Congenital adrenal hyperplasia (CAH) (21-hydroxylase deficiency)
    - Primary adrenal neoplasms (most typically adrenal cortical carcinoma)

CLINICAL ISSUES

Presentation

- **Hypercortisolism**
  - Fat redistribution (centripetal)
    - Moon facies, wasting of arms/legs
    - Skin changes (striae, ecchymoses)
  - Menstrual irregularity
  - Myopathy (proximal weakness)
  - Osteoporosis
- **Aldosteronism**
  - Refractory hypertension, hypokalemia
- **Adrenogenital syndrome**
  - Signs and symptoms depend on which enzyme is affected and level of altered enzyme activity
    - Absent cortisol (due to complete absence of 21-hydroxylase) → salt-wasting syndrome + virilization
  - Malignant adrenal neoplasms: Mixed picture of androgen excess ± hypercortisolism
    - Adrenal tumors associated with virilization in children are often malignant
    - Most sporadic; increased risk with Li Fraumeni, Beckwith-Wiedemann syndromes

Laboratory Tests

- Primary aldosteronism: ↑ aldosterone, ↓ renin

MACROSCOPIC FEATURES

External Exam

- Centripetal obesity with muscle wasting of extremities, moon facies, buffalo hump
- Abdominal striae, acne, ecchymoses, thinning of skin
- Hirsutism, virilization

ADRENOCORTICAL EXCESS

Key Facts

Etiology

- **Hypercortisolism**
  - ACTH-secreting pituitary adenoma
  - Adrenal cortical hyperplasia
  - Primary adrenal neoplasms (adenoma vs. carcinoma)
  - Ectopic ACTH-producing neoplasms elsewhere in body (paraneoplastic)
- **Aldosteronism**
  - Bilateral adrenal cortical hyperplasia
  - Primary adrenal neoplasms (cortical adenoma): Conn syndrome
  - Excessive ingestion of licorice compounds
  - Secondary causes: Renal artery stenosis, diuretic abuse
- **Adrenogenital syndrome**
  - CAH (21-hydroxylase deficiency)
  - Primary adrenal neoplasms (most typically adrenal cortical carcinoma)

Macroscopic Pathology

- Pituitary gland
  - ACTH-secreting adenoma in patients with Cushing syndrome
- Cardiovascular
  - Left ventricular hypertrophy, secondary to hypertension (adrenocortical excess)
- Musculoskeletal
  - Cushing myopathy (wasting), osteoporosis

- Ambiguous genitalia (fetal autopsy)

Internal Exam

- Adrenal gland
  - Assess cortical & medullary thicknesses, nodularity, masses, atrophy
    - **Adrenal cortical hyperplasia: Bilateral**, diffuse, nodular (micro- or macronodular) cortical hyperplasia
    - **Adrenal cortical adenoma: Solitary, unilateral**, cortical nodular lesion; (usually < 5 cm)
    - **Adrenal cortical carcinoma: Rare** malignant adrenal neoplasm; large, irregular, invasive massive with hemorrhage; often >100 g and > 10 cm in diameter
- Pituitary gland
  - ACTH-secreting adenoma in patients with Cushing syndrome
- Cardiovascular
  - Left ventricular hypertrophy, secondary to hypertension (adrenocortical excess)
  - Other end-organ effects of hypertension (kidneys, aorta, white matter changes)
- Musculoskeletal
  - Cushing myopathy (wasting), osteoporosis
- Exclude other solid organ malignancy (paraneoplastic syndrome)

MICROSCOPIC PATHOLOGY

Histologic Features

- Adrenal gland morphology
  - **Cortical hyperplasia** (diffuse/micro- or macronodular)
    - Hyperplasia of cortical cells seen in diffuse or nodular pattern
    - Lipid-depleted cells with compact, eosinophilic cytoplasm or lipid-rich cells
    - Occasional isolated hyperplasia of specific cortical zones may be identified
  - **Cortical adenoma**
    - Benign neoplastic proliferation of large cortical cells with abundant, pale-staining, lipid-rich, vacuolated cytoplasm
    - Round, regular nuclei typically resembling cells of zona fasciculata
    - Occasional pleomorphism ("endocrine atypia")
    - Mitosis rare or absent
    - Functioning and nonfunctioning adenomas essentially indistinguishable by morphology
  - **Cortical carcinoma**
    - Tumor cells resemble normal adrenal cortex but more pleomorphism and hyperchromasia (anaplasia)
    - Trabecular, alveolar, or solid patterns
    - Multinucleated neoplastic cells may be seen
    - Numerous mitoses (including atypical mitoses)
  - **Cortical atrophy**
    - Cortical thinning (especially zona fasciculata and reticularis)
    - Loss of cytoplasmic lipid (more eosinophilic cytoplasmic appearance)

SELECTED REFERENCES

1. Piaditis G et al: Progress in aldosteronism: a review of the prevalence of primary aldosteronism in pre-hypertension and hypertension. Eur J Endocrinol. 172(5):R191-203, 2015
2. Raff H et al: Cushing's syndrome: from physiological principles to diagnosis and clinical care. J Physiol. 593(3):493-506, 2015
3. Lloyd RV et al. Atlas of NonTumor Pathology: Endocrine Diseases (Fascicle 1). Washington DC: American Registry of Pathology and the Armed Forces Institute of Pathology. 171-257, 2002

ADRENOCORTICAL EXCESS

Gross Features

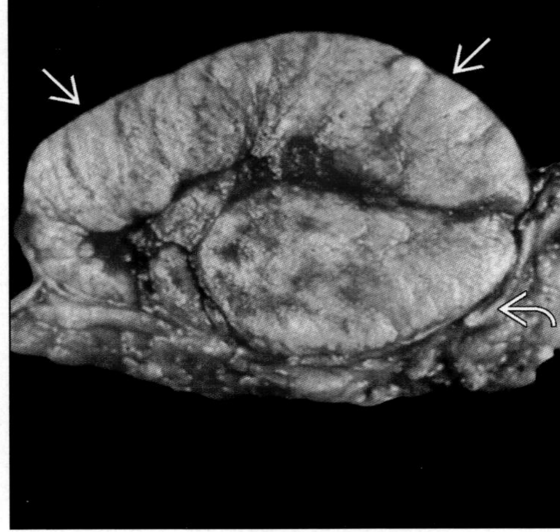

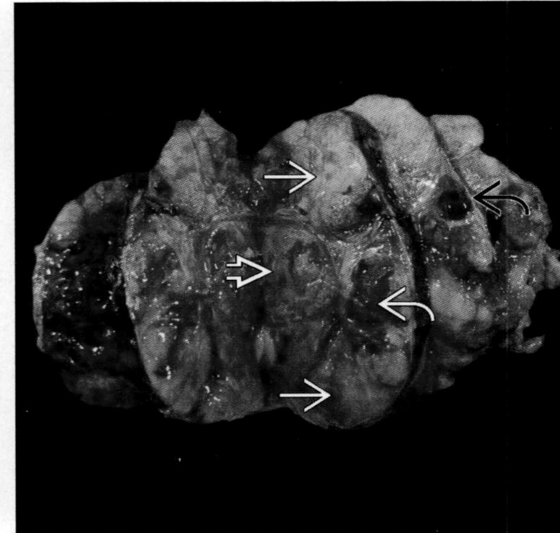

(Left) *Yellow-orange cut surface of a large, circumscribed adrenal cortical adenoma* ➔ *is seen in a patient with Cushing syndrome. Uninvolved adrenal cortex* ➔ *is atrophic. (Courtesy P. Unger, MD.)* ***(Right)*** *Large (14.5 cm) adrenal cortical carcinoma is shown. The variegated cut surface is yellow-tan and coarsely lobulated* ➔ *with areas of hemorrhage* ➔*, necrosis* ➔*, and cystic degeneration* ➔*. (Courtesy Y. Yusuf, MD.)*

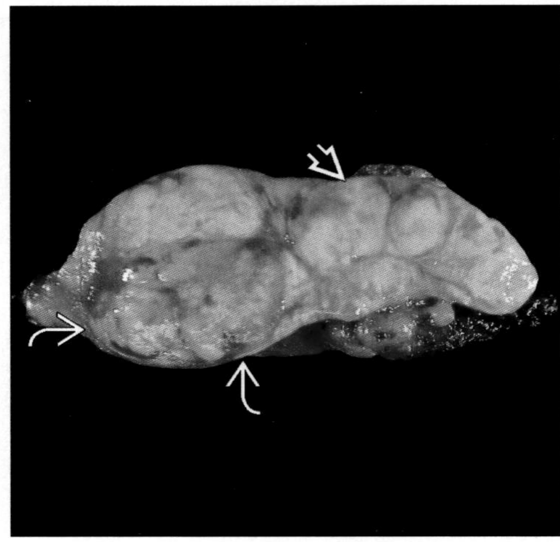

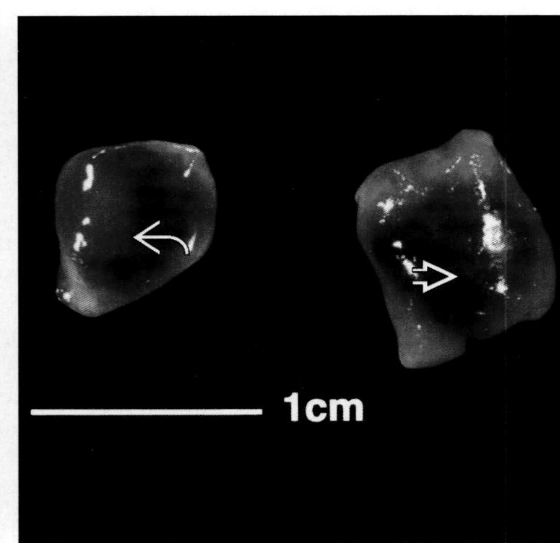

(Left) *This adrenal gland shows renal cortical macronodular hyperplasia* ➔ *with multiple cortical nodules* ➔*. Bilateral hyperplasia is seen in Cushing disease caused by pituitary adenoma. (From DP: Endocrine.)* ***(Right)*** *This pituitary gland shows a circumscribed lesion* ➔*, consistent with adenoma. ACTH-producing adenomas are often grossly hemorrhagic* ➔*. (From DP: Neuro.)*

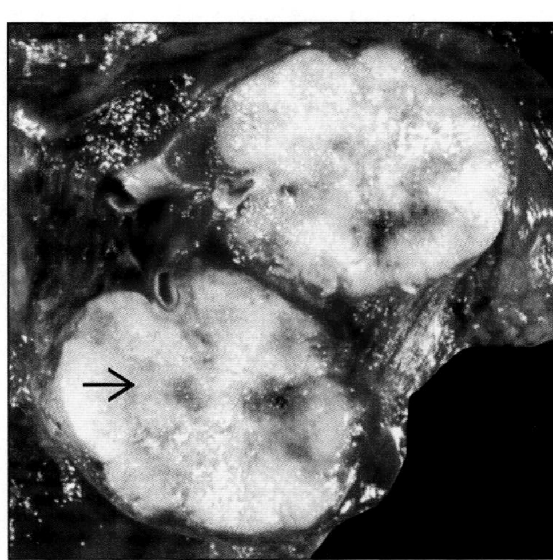

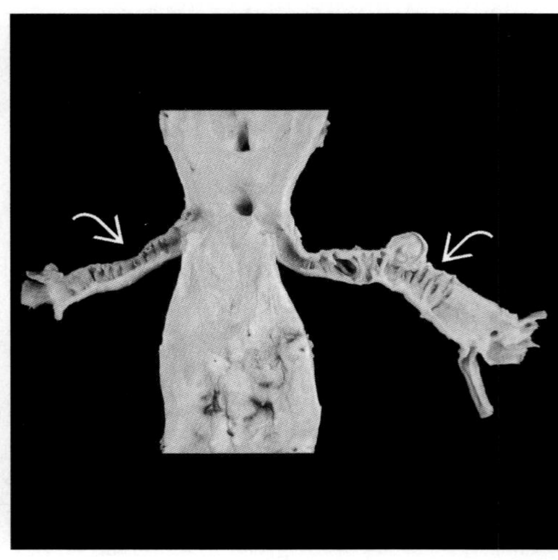

(Left) *This lung mass* ➔ *was present in a patient with metastatic lung cancer who had features of Cushing syndrome clinically. Paraneoplastic ACTH production is a potential cause of cortisol excess. (From DP: Thoracic.)* ***(Right)*** *This aortic specimen from an autopsy of a patient with bilateral renal artery stenosis shows the characteristic features of fibromuscular dysplasia* ➔*. Renal artery stenosis is a cause of secondary aldosteronism.*

Microscopic Features

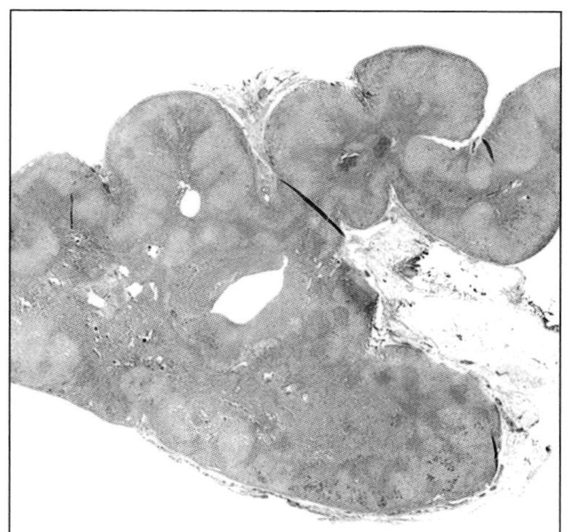

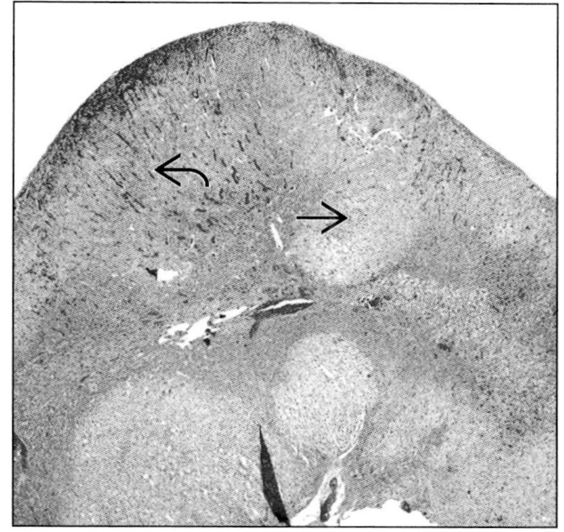

(Left) Diffuse and micronodular adrenal cortical hyperplasia is shown. In adults, cases of diffuse, bilateral adrenal cortical hyperplasia may result from an ACTH-secreting pituitary adenoma or, less commonly, by ectopic production of ACTH or CRH. *(Right)* On slightly higher magnification, nodular areas of hyperplasia show alternating areas of lipid-rich cortical cells ⇒ and more eosinophilic lipid-depleted cells ⇗.

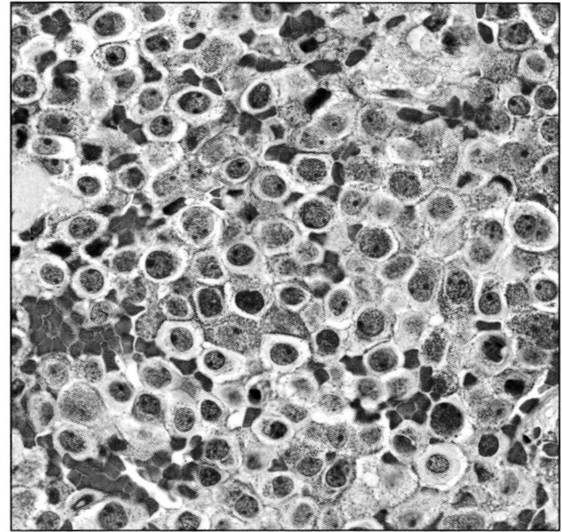

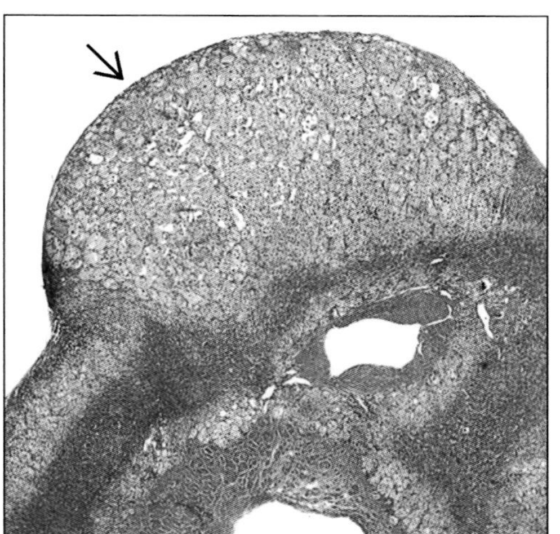

(Left) This high-power photomicrograph of a pituitary gland removed at autopsy from a patient with Cushing syndrome shows features of adenoma. There is cellular monotony. The cells form sheets rather than nests. (From DP: Neuro.) *(Right)* Cortical extrusion ⇒ in a patient with nodular adrenal cortical hyperplasia is shown. The nodule is predominantly composed of cells with abundant, pale-staining, lipid-rich cytoplasm, resembling cells of the zona fasciculata.

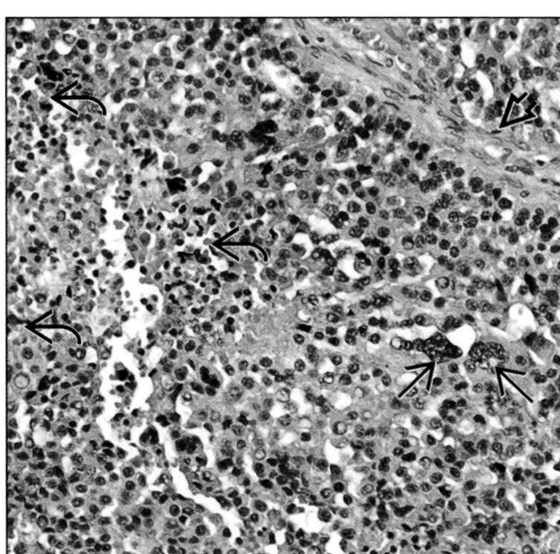

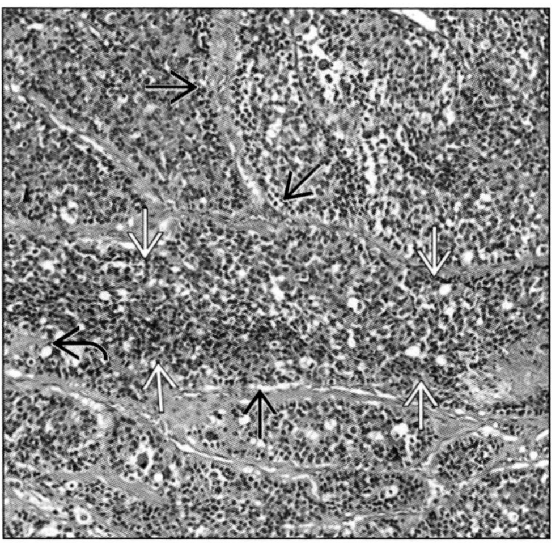

(Left) Adrenal cortical carcinoma shows pleomorphic, hyperchromatic cells with fairly compact, eosinophilic cytoplasm. Scattered cells show multilobulated nuclei ⇒. A fibrous band containing vascular channels is apparent ⇨, as is an area of necrosis ⇗. *(Right)* Adrenal cortical carcinoma shows broad trabecular growth pattern ➡ of neoplastic cells that are separated by delicate fibrous bands containing vascular channels ⇒. Areas of necrosis are apparent ⇗.

SEIZURE DISORDERS

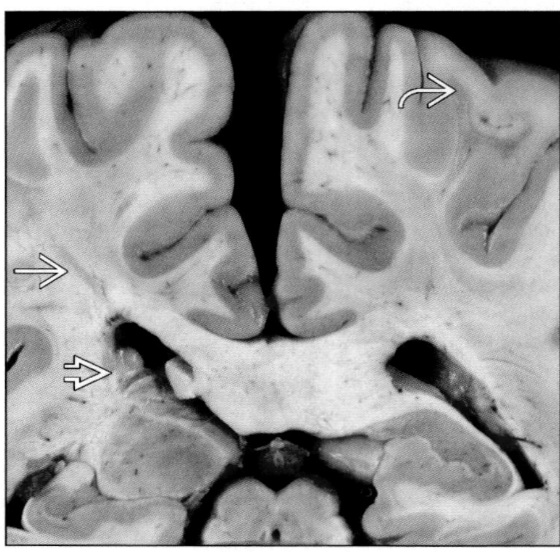

Coronal slice of brain with tuberous sclerosis (TS) is shown with cortical tuber, subcortical tuber, and subependymal nodule. (Courtesy L.C. Ang, MD.)

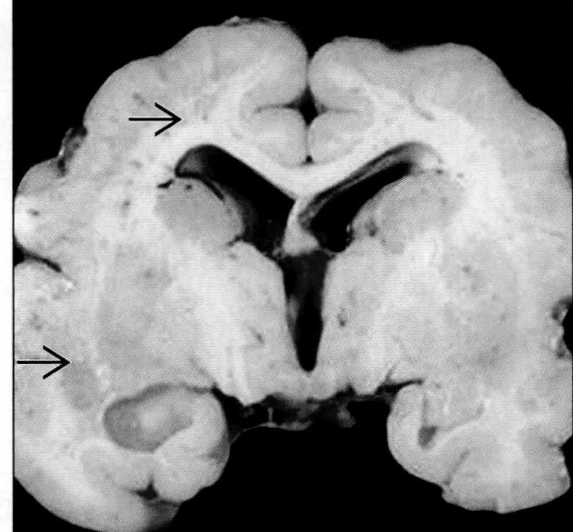

Mutation of LIS1 (neuronal migration gene) is implicated in 80% of lissencephaly, shown here. This brain demonstrates pachygyria (expanded gyri) and subcortical band heterotopia.

TERMINOLOGY

Definitions

- Seizure
  - Abnormal firing of neuron groups through uncontrolled excitation or loss of inhibition
    - Can result in disruption of consciousness, involuntary movements, vocalizations, &/or loss of continence

ETIOLOGY/PATHOGENESIS

Developmental Anomaly

- Congenital/genetic
  - Mesial temporal sclerosis (MTS)
  - Hereditary disorders: Tuberous sclerosis (TS), Sturge-Weber, mitochondrial disorders
  - Congenital: Heterotopias, cortical dysplasias, lissencephaly, polymicrogyria

Infectious Agents

- Viral
  - Herpesviridae (HSV, VZV, CMV)
  - Enterovirus
  - HIV
- Bacterial
  - Septic emboli/abscess
  - Spirochetes: Neurosyphilis, Lyme meningoencephalitis
  - Mycobacterial
- Fungal
  - Aspergillosis
  - Cryptococcal
- Parasitic
  - Protozoa: *Toxoplasma Gondii, Trypanosoma brucei, Plasmodium falciparum* (malaria)
  - Neurocysticercosis
    - Most common acquired seizure etiology in Asia, Africa, Central and South America
  - Other nematodes (*Echinococcus*, *Schistosoma*)
  - Amoeba (*Naegleria fowleri*, *Acanthamoeba* species, *Entamoeba histolytica*)
- Prion
  - Creutzfeldt-Jakob disease

Tumors/Masses

- Space occupying, mass effect

Metabolic

- Hypo-/hyperglycemia
- Hypoxemic-ischemic encephalopathy
- Ion imbalances
  - ↑ Na, ↓ Na, ↓ Ca, ↓ Mg, ↑ NH4
  - Uremia
- Eclampsia

Toxic/Drugs

- Cocaine, heroin, amphetamines
- Phencyclidine, MDMA (ecstasy)
- Tricyclic antidepressants, antihistamines, lithium
- Withdrawal from alcohol, narcotics, or barbiturates
- Organophosphates, nerve agent (VX, sarin)

Vascular

- Arteriovenous malformation (AVM) and aneurysms
- Thrombotic thrombocytopenic purpura (TTP)
- Hematomas
- Infarction (acute or old)

Trauma

- Contusions
- Hemorrhage

Alzheimer Disease

- Especially in later stages of disease

Inflammatory

- Sarcoidosis

SEIZURE DISORDERS

Key Facts

Terminology
- Abnormal firing neuron groups, either through uncontrolled excitation or loss of inhibition

Etiology
- Congenital/genetic
  - Mesial temporal sclerosis (MTS) (idiopathic)
  - Tuberous sclerosis
  - Nodular or band heterotopias
  - Cortical dysplasia
- Infections
  - Viral
  - Bacterial
  - Fungal
  - Parasitic
  - Prion
- Metabolic
  - Hypo-/hyperglycemia
  - Hypoxemic-ischemic encephalopathy
  - Ion imbalances
- Drug
  - Cocaine, heroin, amphetamines
  - Withdrawal from alcohol, narcotics, or barbiturates
- Arteriovenous malformation (AVM) and aneurysms
- Thrombotic thrombocytopenic purpura (TTP)

Clinical Issues
- Cause of death
  - Terminal seizure (e.g., status epilepticus): Diagnosis of exclusion
  - Secondary consequence (drowning, motor vehicle crash, fall)

- Rheumatoid
- Systemic lupus erythematosus

CLINICAL ISSUES

Presentation
- Simple or complex
- Partial or generalized (or secondarily generalized)
- New onset or chronic
- Note anticonvulsant use as there may be secondary neuropathological changes

Treatment
- Surgical approaches
  - Focal resection for discrete epileptogenic focus
  - Hemispherectomy for severe refractory seizures (e.g., Rasmussen, hemimeganencephaly)
  - Callosotomy (transsection of corpus callosum) for atonic seizures and to prevent secondary generalization
- Drugs
  - Clonazepam, phenobarbital, gabapentin
  - Phenytoin, carbamazepine, lamotrigine (sodium channel blockade)
  - Topiramate (inhibits effect of glutamate)

Prognosis
- Depends on etiology and individual response to treatment
- Cause of death
  - Terminal seizure (e.g., status epilepticus): Diagnosis of exclusion
  - Secondary consequence (drowning, motor vehicle crash, fall)

IMAGE FINDINGS

CT/MR
- Mass lesions
- Enhancement (e.g., in encephalitis)
- Neuronal heterotopias
- Infarction
- Hippocampal atrophy and increased T2 signal in MTS
- Malformations/anomalies
- Atrophy (Alzheimer)

Angiography
- Vasculitis, aneurysm, AVM

MACROSCOPIC FEATURES

External Exam
- Trauma from seizure
  - Contusions or lacerations to head, bite marks on tongue
- Signs of Sturge-Weber: Dark red "port-wine stain" of face, hemangioma
- Signs of TS: Pale "ash leaf" spots, leathery "shagreen patches" or reddish bumps (angiofibromas)
- Signs of intravenous drug abuse: Track marks, etc.

Internal Exam
- Thorough examination of all organs for cause of death
- Skull fractures
- Central nervous system
  - Dura and meninges
    - Hemorrhage
    - Excessive vascularity and calcifications (Sturge-Weber)
    - Meningitis (cloudy membranes)
  - Surface of brain
    - Contusions (plaques jaunes: Yellow-orange discoloration indicating old contusions), inferior frontal and temporal
    - Uncal or cerebellar tonsillar herniation
    - Congenital malformations: Porencephaly, polymicrogyria, tubers
    - Atrophy suggestive of dementias
  - Coronal 1 cm thick sections through cerebrum
    - Tumors, infarction, hemorrhage
    - Nodular or band heterotopias: Misplaced periventricular gray matter in nodules or bands

- Cortical dysplasia: Blurring of gray-white junction, expansion of gray matter
- Punctate hemorrhages: Indicative of TTP or septic emboli
- Multiple cysts: Toxoplasmosis or cysticercosis
- Hemorrhagic or necrotic temporal lobes: HSV encephalitis
- Infarction/necrosis of putamen (methanol), globus pallidus (carbon monoxide), or both (heroin, cocaine)
- Asymmetrical hippocampal atrophy: MTS
  - Parasagittal slices through cerebellum
    - Cerebellar atrophy: Long-term phenytoin use

MICROSCOPIC PATHOLOGY

Histologic Features

- Infections
  - Bacterial: Septic emboli, neutrophils and microbes, Gram stain, rim of gliosis
  - Viral: Inclusions, neuronophagia (neurons surrounded by microglia), lymphocytes
  - Fungal: Granulomas, GMS, PAS, mucicarmine (*Cryptococcus*)
- Focal cortical dysplasia/tubers
  - Disrupted cortical layering, clustering and columnar neuron arrays
  - Loss of neuron polarity and balloon neurons (giant, sometimes multinucleated neurons)
  - Tuberous sclerosis; also subependymal nodules and subependymal giant cell astrocytoma
- MTS
  - Loss of neurons and gliosis in specific areas of Ammon horn in hippocampus, with double or widened layer of dentate neurons
- Metabolic
  - Hyperammonemia/uremia: Alzheimer type 2 astrocytes (clear transparent nuclei, scant cytoplasm) abundant in basal ganglia
- Hypoxic-ischemic encephalopathy
  - Shrunken, hypereosinophilic neurons with pyknotic nuclei (especially CA1 hippocampus and Purkinje cells)
- Therapeutic complication
  - Cerebellar atrophy, loss of Purkinje cells with chronic phenytoin use

DIAGNOSTIC CHECKLIST

Clinically Relevant Pathologic Features

- Death in patient with longstanding epilepsy
  - Etiology
    - Head trauma
    - History of drug use
    - Developmental delay (perinatal hypoxia, Lennox Gastaut)
    - Systemic disease: Lupus, diabetes, malignancy, TTP, liver failure
    - Liver failure, mitochondrial disorders
    - AVM, tubers: Focal onset (partial simple)
    - MTS: Temporal lobe epilepsy (clinical)
    - Travel, immunocompetency status for infections
  - Confirm/establish cause of seizure disorder
    - Focal brain lesion (cortical dysplasia, tubers, heterotopias, vascular lesions, masses)
    - Developmental anomaly (MTS, Sturge-Weber, congenital anomalies)
    - Systemic disease (remote hypoxia, metabolic, TTP, infection)
    - Toxins/drugs (drugs of abuse, antidepressants, withdrawal symptoms)
  - Determine role of seizure disorder in cause of death
    - Signs of trauma (acute, subacute, old)
    - Secondary consequence of seizure (drowning, motor vehicle crash)
    - Therapeutic misadventure (surgical complication, medication side effect)
- Sudden death, suspected seizure-related
  - Identify substrate lesion in brain or other metabolic cause of seizure activity
  - Thoroughly exclude all other potential causes of sudden death
  - Sudden death due to epilepsy is controversial diagnosis; requires very carefully consideration and exclusion of other possible causes

Pathologic Interpretation Pearls

- Hypoxia/ischemia: "Red-dead" neurons
- Renal or hepatic failure: Alzheimer type 2 astrocytes in basal ganglia
- If recent onset of behavioral change/dementia with seizures, consider autopsy with Prion disease protocol

REPORTING CRITERIA

Cause of Seizures

- Primary seizure disorder or other cause

Cause of Death

- Whether seizure is primary cause of death or contributed to death through trauma, drowning, etc.

SELECTED REFERENCES

1. Nash TE: Parasitic diseases that cause seizures. Epilepsy Curr. 14(1 Suppl):29-34, 2014
2. Pollanen MS et al: Sudden unexpected death in epilepsy: a retrospective analysis of 24 adult cases. Forensic Sci Med Pathol. 8(1):13-8, 2012
3. Zhuo L et al: Sudden unexpected death in epilepsy: Evaluation of forensic autopsy cases. Forensic Sci Int. 223(1-3):171-5, 2012
4. Jensen L et al: Sudden death and the forensic evaluation of neurocutaneous syndromes. J Forensic Leg Med. 16(7):369-74, 2009
5. Leventer RJ et al: Malformations of cortical development and epilepsy. Dialogues Clin Neurosci. 10(1):47-62, 2008

Gross and Microscopic Features

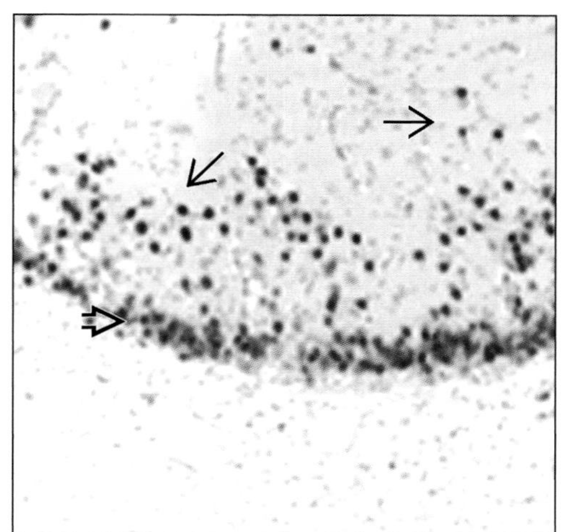

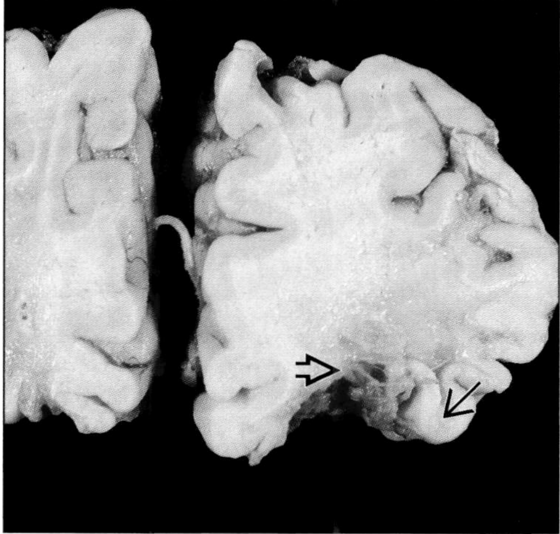

(Left) *Neu-N stains neuronal nuclei, as seen here in the dentate gyrus of the hippocampus, showing dentate dispersal (a feature of MTS) with neurons radiating out* ➙ *from the usual tight band of the dentate* ➯*. Loss of neurons in CA4 and CA1 with gliosis can also be seen.* ***(Right)*** *Old contusions are often seen where cortex abuts skull ridges as in the orbitofrontal cortex* ➯*. Note the yellow-brown discoloration of cortex (plaques jaune)* ➙ *and underlying cavitation.*

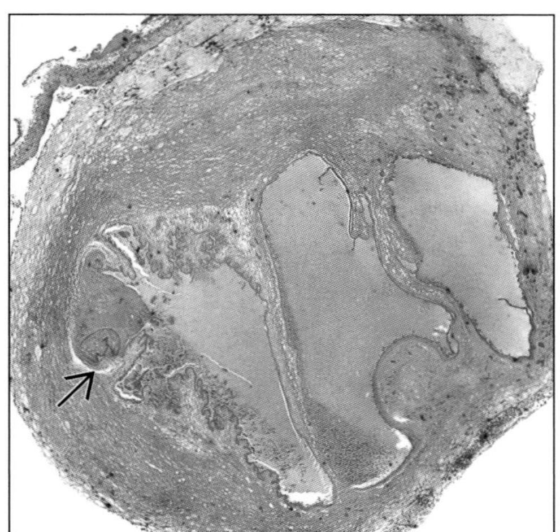

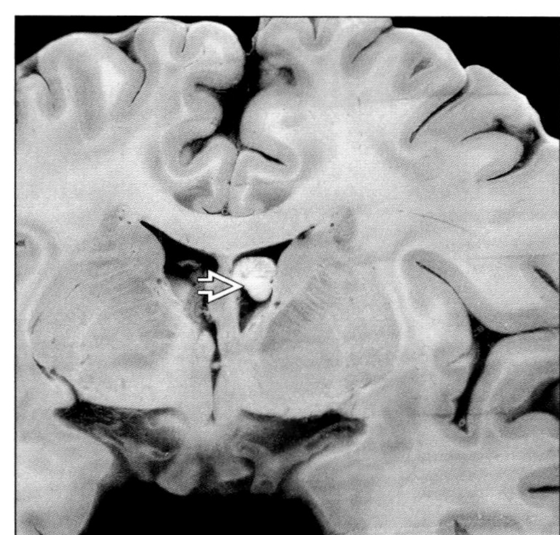

(Left) *Neurocysticercosis (T. solium) is microscopically seen with a cyst containing degenerating scolex* ➙ *on H&E. Inflammation and calcification may result with disease progression.* ***(Right)*** *Periventricular nodular heterotopia* ➯ *is shown here as a gray matter nodule protruding into the lateral ventricle. These are often associated with MTS. The appearance is similar to the subependymal nodules of tuberous sclerosis, but heterotopias are larger and rarely calcify.*

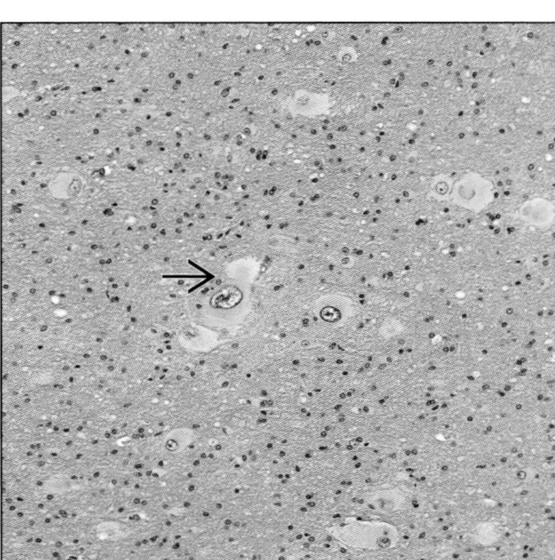

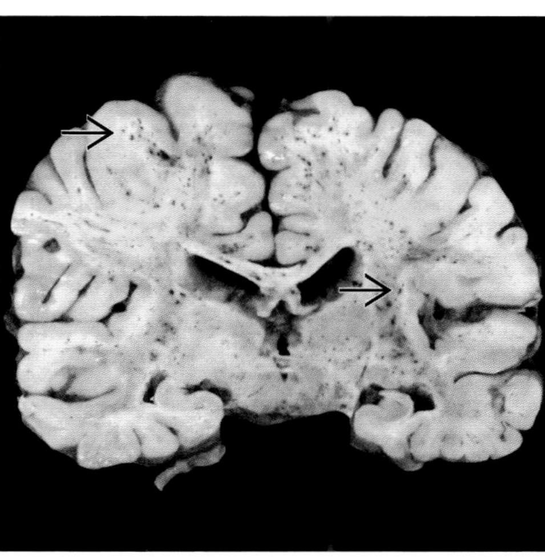

(Left) *One feature of focal cortical dysplasia is the presence of "balloon" neurons* ➙ *with large nuclei and abundant cytoplasm, as shown here on H&E.* ***(Right)*** *Thrombotic thrombocytopenic purpura in the brain manifests as multiple petechial hemorrhages* ➙ *at the gray-white junction. This disease presents with seizures and neuropsychiatric disturbances as well as renal failure, rash, and hemolytic anemia.*

SUBDURAL HEMORRHAGE

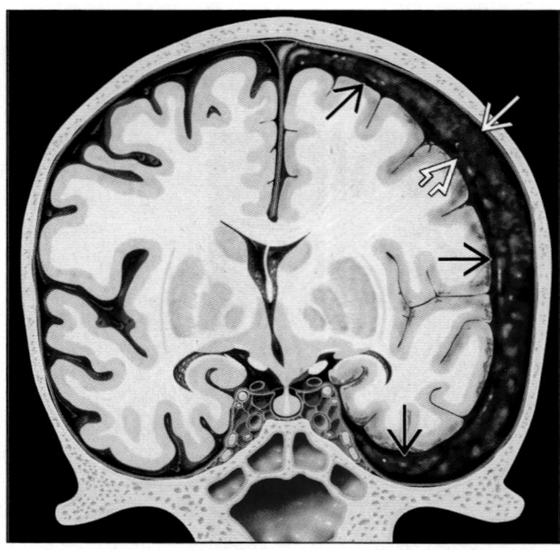

An SDH ⇒ spreads unilaterally between dura ➡ and arachnoid ➡. Dural cells form outer granulation tissue in 7-10 days. An inner neomembrane forms after 3 weeks.

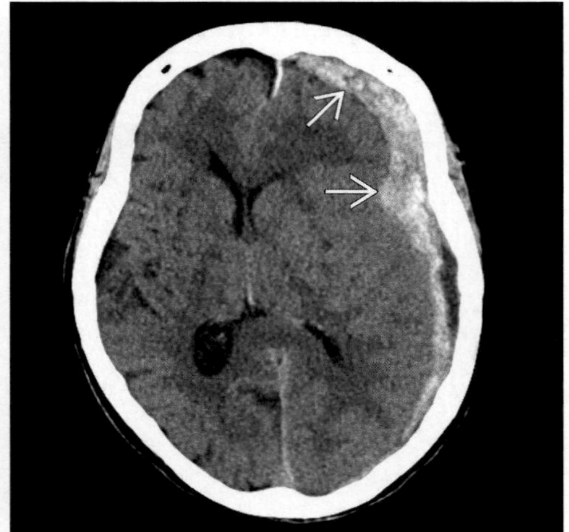

Axial CT of acute SDH in a patient post fall shows blood distribution ➡ similar to that shown in the previous image.

TERMINOLOGY

Abbreviations

- Subdural hematoma or hemorrhage (SDH)

ETIOLOGY/PATHOGENESIS

Trauma

- Severe head/spinal impact
  - Acute SDH
  - Chronic SDH
  - Often with parenchymal contusions
- Nonimpact diffuse axonal injury (DAI)
  - Acceleration/deceleration injury
  - No history of impact

Nontraumatic SDH

- Hematologic disease
- Coagulopathy
- Malignancy

Lesion Development

- Acute SDH
  - Venous (rarely arterial) blood collects between dura and outer arachnoid membrane
  - Initially clotted blood forms
- Subacute SDH
  - Clot liquefaction (over several days to 3 weeks)
- Chronic SDH
  - Granulation tissue
  - Rebleeding: Possible hematoma enlargement
  - Neomembrane visible by 3 weeks

CLINICAL ISSUES

Presentation

- History of trauma: Traumatic brain injury (TBI)
  - Assault, fall, sports injury, motor vehicle accident
- Other relevant history
  - Hematologic disease, anticoagulation, cirrhosis
  - Brain or spine surgery, intracranial malignancy
  - Alcoholism, chronic renal failure
  - Symptoms (headache, nausea, mental status change) usually gradual in onset but progressive
- Pertinent antemortem data
  - Glasgow coma score (GCS)
  - CBC, PT, aPTT, INR, D-dimer, platelet count
  - Imaging (CT or MR)
    - Fractures, hematoma, neomembrane

Treatment

- Acute SDH: Drainage → brain reexpansion
  - Twist drill or burr-hole craniostomy with catheter drainage
  - Decompressive hemicraniectomy for brain swelling
- Subacute/chronic SDH
  - Surgical craniostomy with outer membranectomy
    - Inner membranectomy avoided due to risk of brain herniation through membrane/skull defect
- Surgical complications
  - Incomplete SDH evacuation with continued symptoms
  - Rebleed (10-30%)
- Postoperative complications
  - Seizures, intracerebral hemorrhage, epidural hematoma, pneumocephalus, intracerebral abscess
    - Uncommon: Meningitis, skull osteomyelitis, acute SDH contralateral to drained chronic SDH (rapid decompression and tearing)

Prognosis

- Spontaneous resolution infrequent
- Nontraumatic SDH
  - Primary disease often dictates prognosis
- Traumatic SDH: Mortality rate ~ 50%
  - Surgery within 4 hours: Mortality rate 30-35%, functional recovery rate 55-65%

SUBDURAL HEMORRHAGE

Key Facts

Etiology
- Traumatic
  - Impact and nonimpact diffuse axonal injury (DAI)
- Hematologic disease
- Coagulopathy
- Malignancy

Clinical Issues
- Glasgow coma score (GCS)
- CBC, PT, aPTT, INR, D-dimer, platelet count
- Imaging (CT or MR)
- Fractures, hematoma, neomembrane

Macroscopic Pathology
- Acute SDH
  - Venous (rarely arterial) blood collects between dura and outer arachnoid membrane
  - Fibrinolysis → clotted to liquid blood begins
- Chronic SDH
  - Granulation tissue
  - Rebleeding: Possible hematoma enlargement
  - Neomembrane visible by 3 weeks

Microscopic Pathology
- Acute SDH
  - Intact erythrocytes, leukocytes
  - No fibrin platelet lamination
- Chronic SDH
  - Microscopically granulation tissue and hemorrhage identified as chronic SDH
  - Outer neomembrane fibrosis (variable)
  - Inflammatory cells (may include eosinophils)

  - Surgery after 4 hours: Mortality rate 65-85%, functional recovery rate 7-15%
  - Abnormal pupil light reaction on admission: ↓ survival and functional recovery rates
  - High GCS: ↑ survival and functional recovery rates
- Cause of death
  - Cerebral contusion (autonomic and metabolic dysfunction)
  - Brain swelling and herniation
  - Cerebral infarct/stroke (autonomic dysfunction)
    - Particularly right insula (cardiac dysfunction)
  - Diffuse axonal injury (sheer forces), especially brainstem

MACROSCOPIC FEATURES

Acute SDH
- Clotted blood up to several days
- Initial solid blood may resolve

Subacute SDH
- Mix of clotted blood and fluid
- Fluid by 3 weeks

Chronic SDH
- Variable-thickness neomembrane surrounding hematoma
  - Outer neomembrane adjacent to dura
  - Inner neomembrane adjacent to arachnoid
  - Central hematoma variably liquefied
- Calcified chronic SDH (armored brain)

MICROSCOPIC PATHOLOGY

Histologic Features
- Acute SDH
  - Intact erythrocytes, leukocytes
  - No fibrin platelet lamination
- Subacute SDH (stage not reliably identified by histology)
  - After 7–10 days, granulation tissue established as neomembrane
  - Microscopically granulation tissue and hemorrhage identified as chronic SDH
- Chronic SDH
  - Outer neomembrane fibrosis (variable)
  - Inflammatory cells (may include eosinophils)
  - Granulation tissue
    - Leaky macrocapillaries → spontaneous rebleeding into central hematoma
  - Inner neomembrane fibrosis (variable)
  - Hematoma between neomembranes: Degenerating blood cells and strands of fibrin
  - Fluid leakage from torn arachnoid through inner neomembrane → hygroma formation within established neomembranes

DIAGNOSTIC CHECKLIST

Pathologic Interpretation Pearls
- Important to exclude secondary causes of SDH
  - Occult metastatic malignancy microscopically
  - Amyloid angiopathy
    - Almost always associated with subarachnoid-intracerebral hemorrhage

SELECTED REFERENCES

1. Walcott BP et al: Time interval to surgery and outcomes following the surgical treatment of acute traumatic subdural hematoma. J Clin Neurosci. 21(12):2107-11, 2014
2. Sim YW et al: Recent changes in risk factors of chronic subdural hematoma. J Korean Neurosurg Soc. 52(3):234-9, 2012
3. Ma YH et al: Management of chronic subdural haematoma. Lancet. 375(9710):195; author reply 195-6, 2010
4. Wen L et al: Spontaneous rapid resolution of acute subdural hematoma after head trauma: is it truly rare? Case report and relevant review of the literature. Ir J Med Sci. 178(3):367-71, 2009
5. Love S et al: Greenfield's Neuropathology. London: Hodder Arnold, 2008

SUBDURAL HEMORRHAGE

Gross and Microscopic Features

(Left) An acute SDH ⇒ is formed of clotted blood between the dura, here seen partially reflected ⇒, and the arachnoid. The acute SDH covers most of the right dorsolateral convexity of the brain, with some temporal lobe visible ⇒. (Right) H&E stain of acute SDH reveals only intact erythrocytes and leukocytes ⇒ with no lamination that would be seen in other types of intracranial hemorrhage. A local coagulopathy is thought to prevent lamination by formed fibrin.

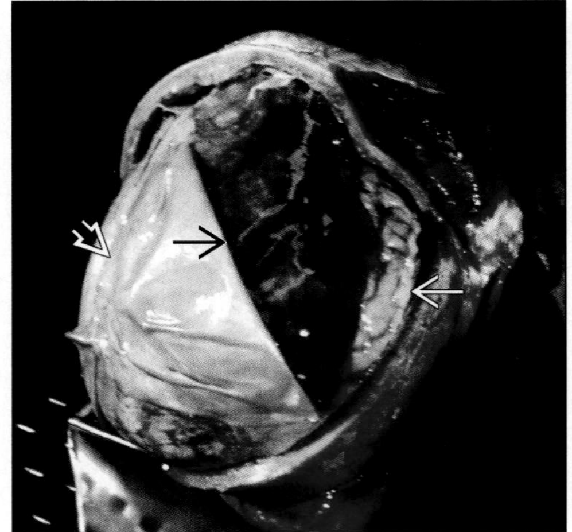

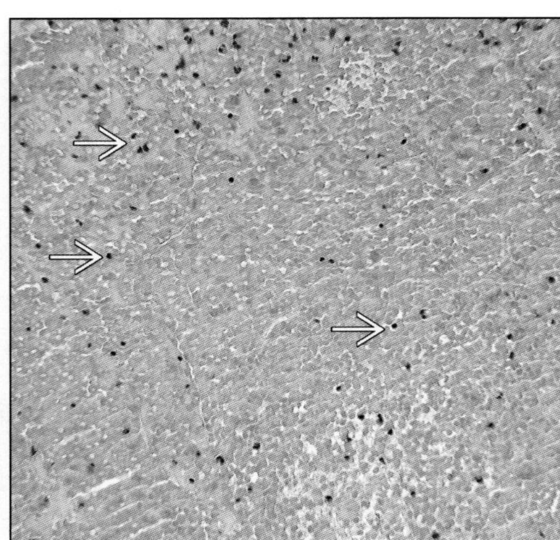

(Left) This dural cap's internal surface has a thin neomembrane of a chronic SDH ⇒ on its left side. The thinnest parts can be difficult to see. Neomembranes are adherent to the inner dura, unlike nonadherent postmortem blood collections after dissection. (Right) The left cerebrum under the chronic SDH shown at the left is compressed ⇒. Compression is not from the relatively thin neomembrane on the dural cap, but from liquefied blood that drained away during autopsy dissection.

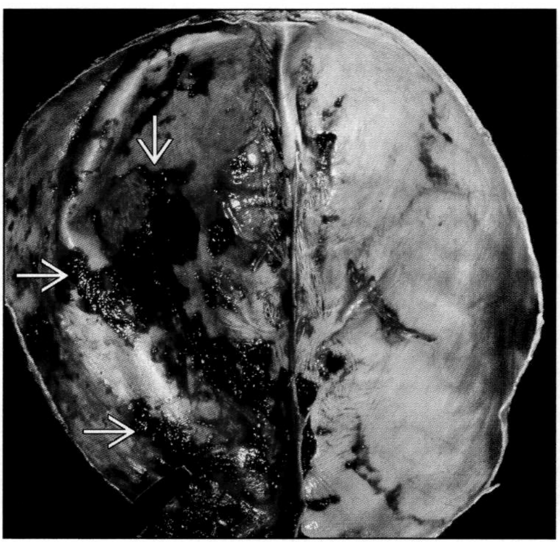

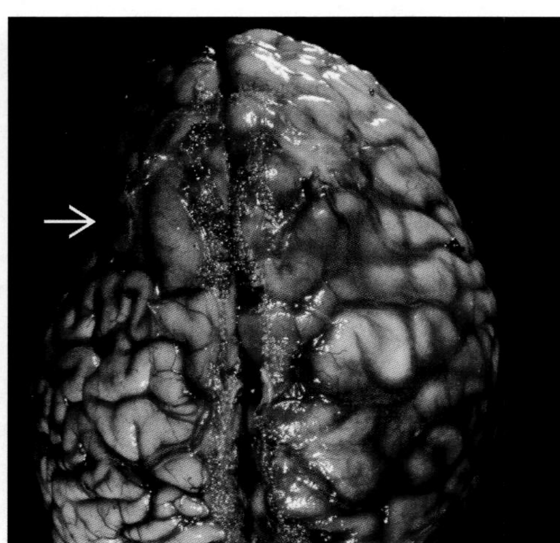

(Left) This bilateral SDH over the cerebrum ⇒ and cerebellum ⇒ resulted from traumatic skull fractures. Note how cerebral gyri and cerebellar folia are hidden by the blood external to the arachnoid ⇒. Microscopy would be needed for classification as acute or chronic. (Right) Adherent chronic SDH ⇒ (note the orange coloration often seen) is shown on the inner side of reflected dura ⇒ and also adherent over the arachnoid ⇒ in this patient with chronic myeloid leukemia.

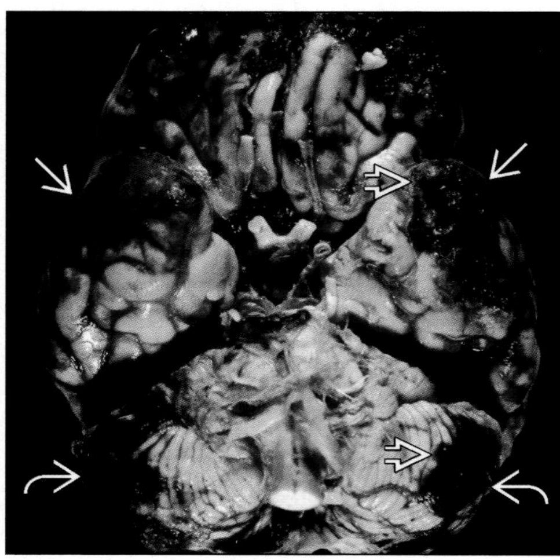

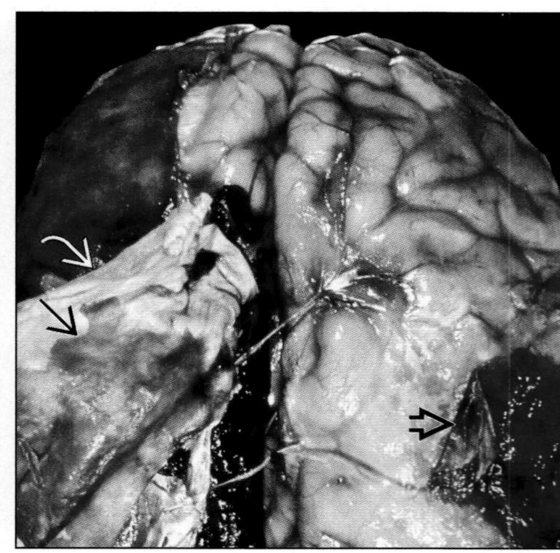

SUBDURAL HEMORRHAGE

Gross and Microscopic Features

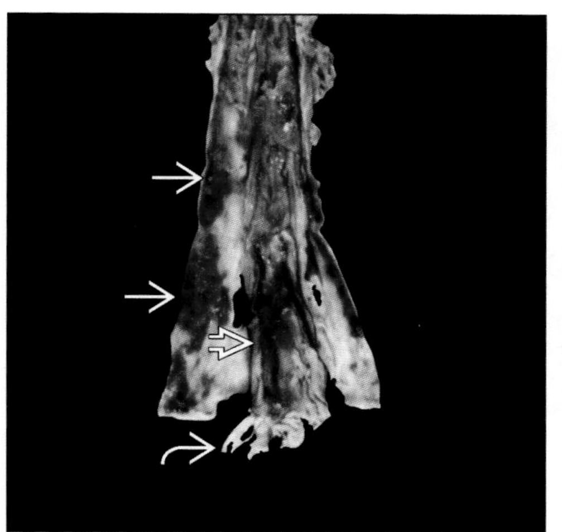

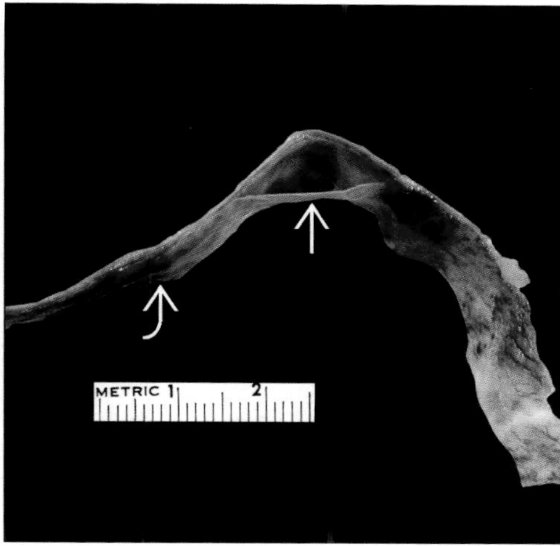

(Left) *A patient with systemic lupus erythematosus was septic and died with a coagulopathy. A patchy SDH is adherent to the inner side of the spinal dura ➡ and to the arachnoid ⇨. The cauda equina is also seen ↪.* ***(Right)*** *The neomembrane of a chronic SDH is adherent to the inner surface of this strip of the dural cap dissected for microscopic examination. One very thin area of the neomembrane ➡ has become partly dislodged during dissection. Other areas are hemorrhagic ↪.*

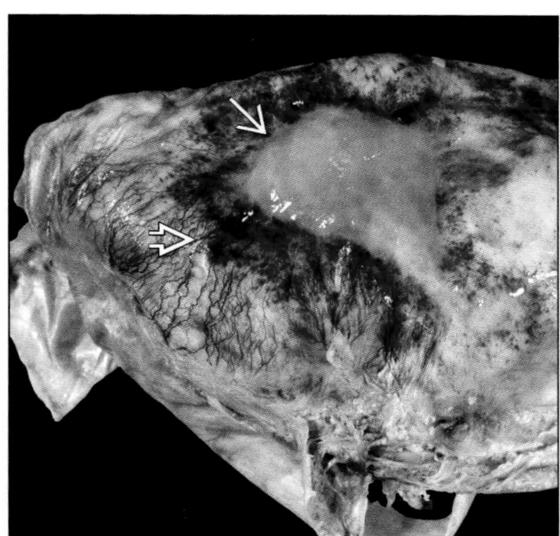

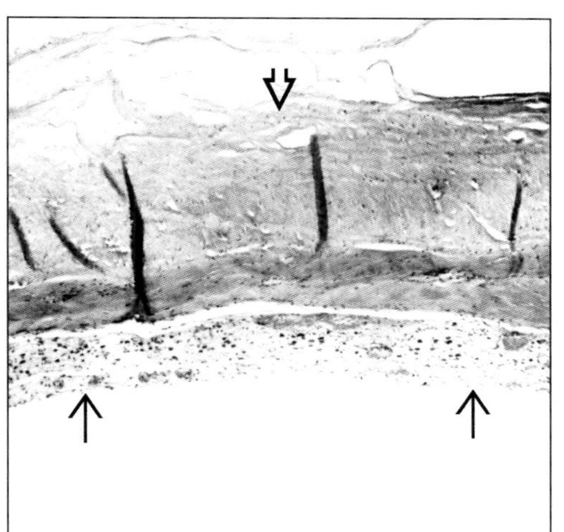

(Left) *An extensive chronic SDH on the inner surface of the dural cap is partly a thin neomembrane ➡ and partly a hygroma ⇨. The fibrous nature of the hygroma membrane is seen by the gray-white color. Fluid in hygromas leaks from breaks in the outer arachnoidal membrane.* ***(Right)*** *Low-magnification view shows dura ⇨ with a thin, loosely adherent neomembrane ➡. This chronic SDH is formed of granulation tissue that includes dilated, leaky macrocapillaries.*

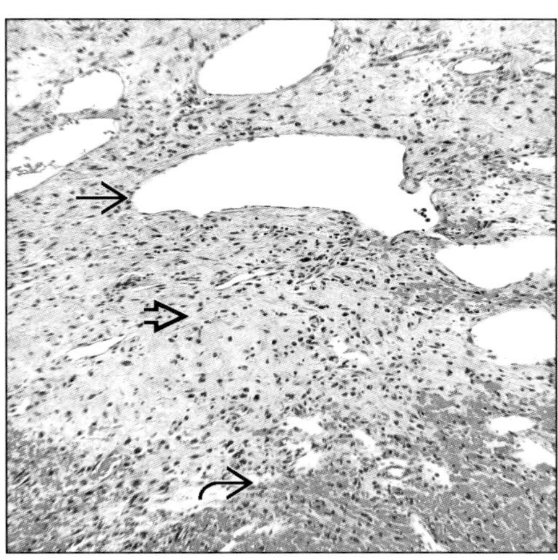

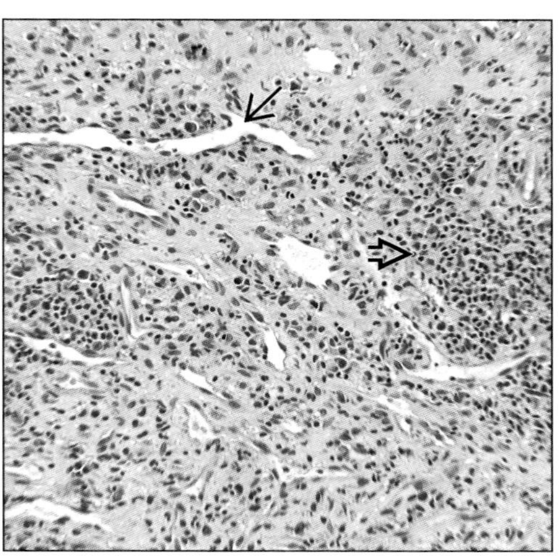

(Left) *The outer membrane of a chronic SDH is formed of granulation tissue with leaky macrocapillaries ➡ and fibrosis ⇨. The hematoma ↪ is below the outer membrane.* ***(Right)*** *The inner membrane of a chronic SDH contains dilated capillaries ➡, fibrosis, and chronic inflammation ⇨. Spontaneous resolution of a chronic SDH is not frequent. Clinical resolution below MR detection may occur, but the thin, neomembranous scar remains.*

SUBARACHNOID HEMORRHAGE

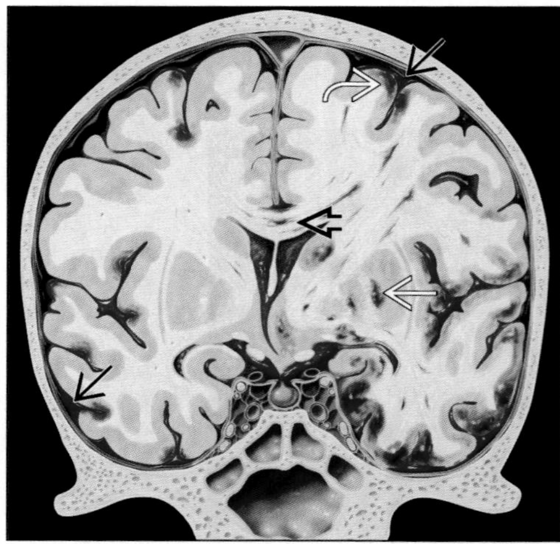

Traumatic SAH ⇒ is present as part of contusions ➡. Associated traumatic brain lesions include diffuse axonal injury in the corpus callosum ⇨ and putamen ➡ contributing to a shift of midline structures.

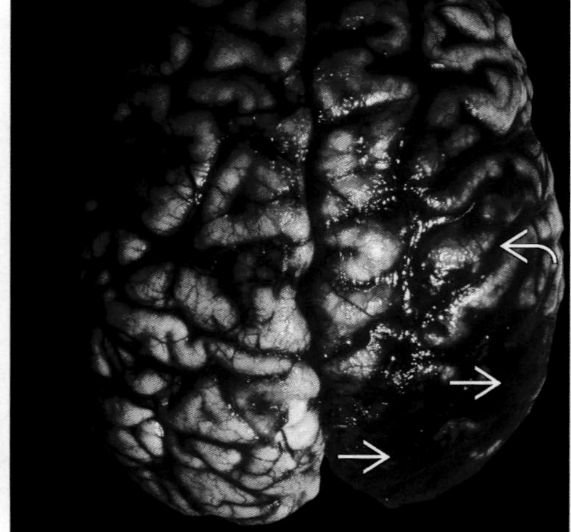

SAH was present in this patient with shock and DIC. The gyri are obscured ➡ and blood fills many of the sulci ➡ without any blood present on the external side of the leptomeninges.

TERMINOLOGY

Abbreviations

- Subarachnoid hemorrhage (SAH)

ETIOLOGY/PATHOGENESIS

Trauma

- Most common cause of SAH
  - Assault, fall, motor vehicle injury, spinal procedure

Nontraumatic

- Most common cause: Ruptured saccular (berry) aneurysm
  - Circle of Willis or posterior brain circulation
- Other vascular abnormalities
  - Vascular malformation
    - Arteriovenous (AV) malformation
    - Cavernous angioma
  - Moyamoya-like malformation
    - Children: Sickle cell disease
    - Adults: Atherosclerosis
  - AV fistula or shunt
  - Cerebral amyloid angiopathy
  - Late pregnancy/puerperium
    - Arterial aneurysm or AV malformation/fistula
    - Reversible cerebral vasoconstrictive syndrome
    - Cerebral venous sinus thrombosis

Pathogenesis

- Trauma
  - Ruptured subarachnoid vein(s)
  - Subarachnoid arterial dissection/rupture
- Nontraumatic
  - Ruptured aneurysm, vascular malformation
  - Coagulopathy
  - Vertebrobasilar artery dissection/rupture (spontaneous)
  - Hemorrhagic stroke

CLINICAL ISSUES

Presentation

- Trauma
  - Traumatic SAH → vasospasm and ischemia denote more severe injury
    - Associated lesions: Contusion, subdural hematoma, diffuse axonal/diffuse vascular injury
- Nontraumatic
  - Coagulopathy
    - Hematologic/neoplastic disease
    - Anticoagulation/antiplatelet therapy
- Headache, mental status change, neck stiffness, increased intracranial pressure
  - Significant initial bleed → "thunderclap" headache
- Complications
  - Early anoxic brain injury
    - Hypoxia, oxidative stress, inflammation
  - Delayed cerebral injury (DCI)
    - Vasospasm may occur 3-14 days post rupture, possibly late manifestation of early brain injury
    - Focal neurologic deficits, cognitive change in ≤ 50% of patients 4-12 days after rupture
  - Hydrocephalus
- Pertinent antemortem data
  - Glasgow coma scale
  - Computed tomography (CT), CT angiography, CT perfusion imaging
  - Transcranial Doppler findings for cerebral blood flow velocity
  - CBC, PT, aPTT, INR, D-dimer, platelet count

Treatment

- Saccular aneurysm
  - Surgical clipping, endovascular embolization
  - Nimodipine (calcium channel antagonist) → ↓ DCI/infarct rate; may → mild hypertension
- AV malformation

SUBARACHNOID HEMORRHAGE

Key Facts

Etiology
- Most common cause of SAH: Trauma (impact)
  - Rupture of subarachnoid veins
  - Subarachnoid arterial wall hematoma/dissection
- Nontraumatic SAH: Ruptured saccular aneurysm, vascular malformation, arteriovenous fistula, spontaneous arterial wall hematoma/dissection
- Coagulopathy (primary disease, drug-related)

Clinical Issues
- Headache, mental status change, neck stiffness, focal neurologic deficits
  - Vasospasm → neurologic deficit (variable)
  - Cerebral ischemia/infarction
- Traumatic SAH treatment: Surgical/medical approach
- Nontraumatic SAH treatment (ruptured aneurysm)
  - Surgical clipping, endovascular embolization
  - Nimodipine: Vasospasm and ischemia prevention
- Traumatic SAH prognosis: Related to associated lesions, general medical condition, autonomic compromise (e.g., ↓ cardiac function)
- Nontraumatic SAH prognosis
  - Positive effect of nimodipine
  - Cerebral infarct (poor outcome)
  - Autonomic compromise

Macroscopic Pathology
- Evidence of surgical intervention
  - Burr hole, craniotomy, hemicraniectomy
  - Catheters, ventriculoperitoneal shunt tube
  - Surgical clip, coils, stent, sponge material
- SAH over gyri, in sulci (relative amount)
- SAH filling subarachnoid cisterns (relative amount)
- Vascular rupture site, if identified

  - Staged multimodal vessel obliteration (radiation, endovascular embolization, excision)

Prognosis
- Trauma
  - Depends on extent, comorbidities, autonomic compromise (e.g., ↓ cardiac function)
- Nontraumatic
  - Saccular aneurysm rupture
    - Endovascular coils → ↓ morbidity/mortality rate compared to open surgical clip
    - Improved prognosis: Early nimodipine use
    - Poor prognosis: Infarct, vasospasm, autonomic dysfunction
- Cause of death
  - Trauma
    - Stroke, herniation
    - Autonomic compromise
    - Operative/treatment complications
  - Nontraumatic
    - Acute postrupture cerebral ischemia/infarct
    - DCI/infarcts (25% of aneurysmal rupture deaths)
    - Autonomic, metabolic dysfunction
    - Underlying disease (coagulopathy, neoplasm)

IMAGE FINDINGS

CT Findings
- Trauma
  - Intracranial blood, bony fractures
- Nontraumatic
  - Ruptured cerebral arterial aneurysm: Location and amount of blood
    - Early scan (within 24 hours of rupture)
    - Cisternal SAH amount correlates with symptomatic vasospasm
  - Enhancing intracranial/spinal lesions

MACROSCOPIC FEATURES

External Examination
- Evidence of surgical intervention
  - Burr hole, craniotomy, hemicraniectomy
  - Catheters, ventriculoperitoneal shunt tube

Internal Examination
- SAH over gyri, extending into sulci
- SAH filling subarachnoid cisterns
- Vascular rupture site, if identified
  - May be within largest SAH area (epicenter)
- Surgical clip, coils, stent, sponge material

MICROSCOPIC PATHOLOGY

Histologic Features
- Blood in subarachnoid space
  - Recent
  - Resolving (pigment-laden macrophages)
- Bleeding source
  - Ruptured saccular aneurysm
  - Vascular malformation or fistula
  - Cerebral amyloid angiopathy
- Contusion (trauma)
- Meningitis (acute/chronic inflammation)

SELECTED REFERENCES

1. Miller BA et al: Inflammation, Vasospasm, and Brain Injury after Subarachnoid Hemorrhage. Biomed Res Int. 2014:384342, 2014
2. Mrozek S et al: Biomarkers and acute brain injuries: interest and limits. Crit Care. 18(2):220, 2014
3. Lee Y et al: Current controversies in the prediction, diagnosis, and management of cerebral vasospasm: where do we stand? Neurol Res Int. 2013:373458, 2013

SUBARACHNOID HEMORRHAGE

Gross and Microscopic Features

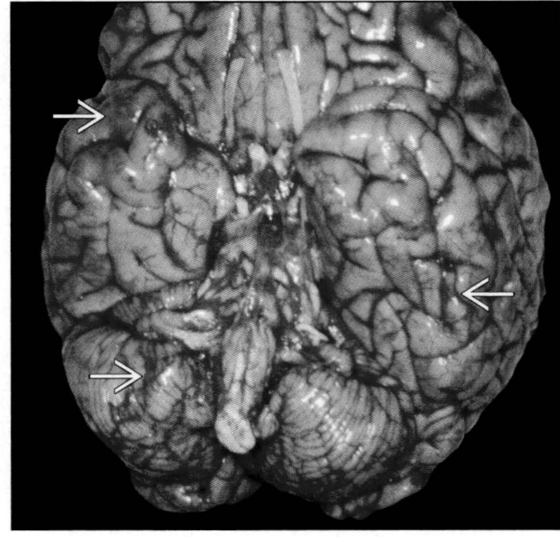

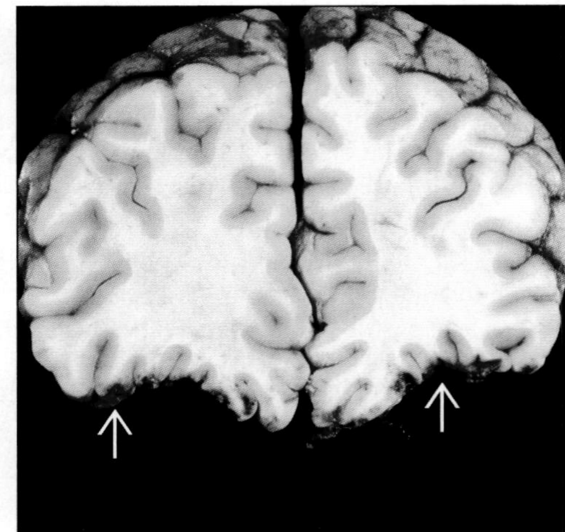

(Left) This unfixed brain has scattered, small SAH ➔. Brain sections with overlying leptomeninges taken carefully to avoid separation of cortex from leptomeninges are needed to document the SAH microscopically. *(Right)* SAH in this coronal section resulted from trauma (fall). The superficially sheared gyral crowns ➔ of the inferior frontal (orbital) cortex are obscured by neocortical hemorrhage and SAH. These are the classic finding of cortical contusions that can be confirmed microscopically.

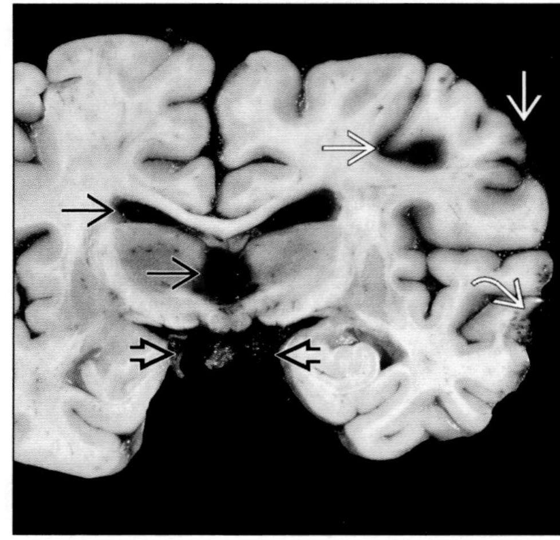

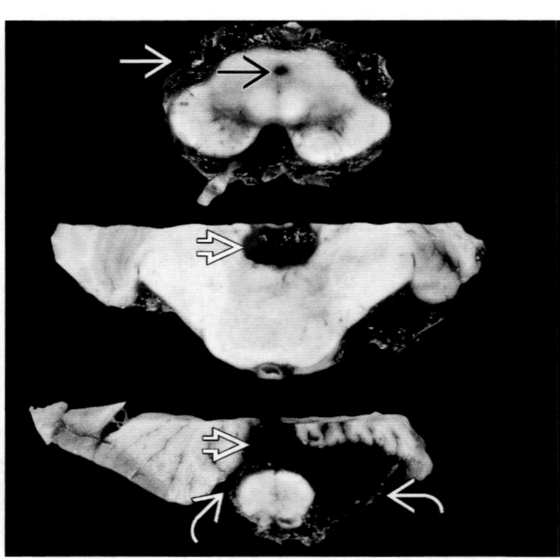

(Left) Multiple contusions ➔ with associated SAH ➔ are seen in this brain from a patient who died following a trauma. Intraventricular hemorrhage ➔ and a small subdural hematoma ➔ are also present. *(Right)* Intraventricular hemorrhage within the cerebral aqueduct ➔ and distending the 4th ventricle ➔ is seen in this traumatically injured brain. SAH is also seen extending through the foramina of Luschka ➔. SAH floods the posterior fossa ➔ and the spinal subarachnoid space.

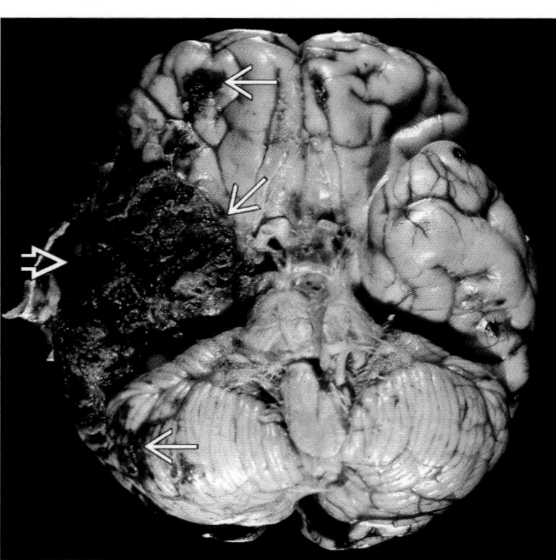

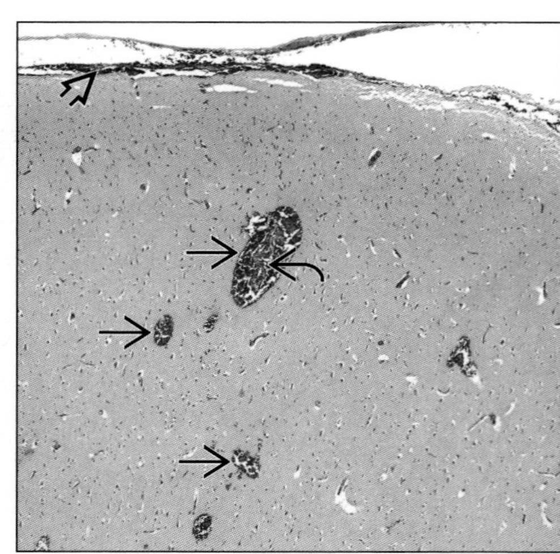

(Left) SAH ➔ is seen after a craniotomy to relieve raised intracranial pressure for a large cerebral contusion ➔. Cerebral hemorrhage and SAH now include traumatic brain injury, surgical contusion, and septic infarct. *(Right)* SAH ➔ and perivascular hemorrhages ➔ are seen in a medium-magnification photomicrograph of a recent cerebral contusion. Blood vessels ➔ within these spaces can be difficult to find.

Radiologic, Gross, and Microscopic Features

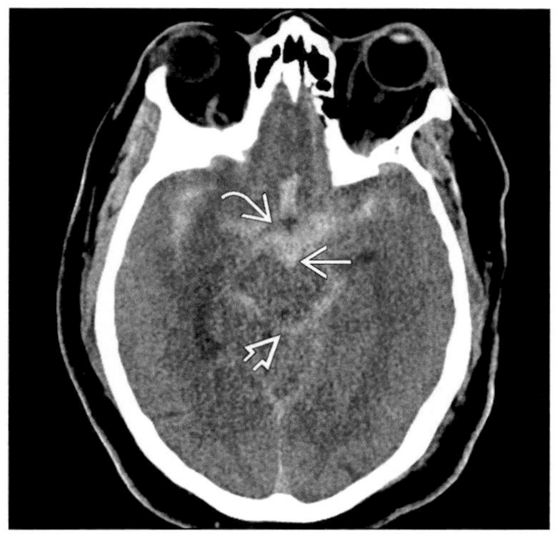

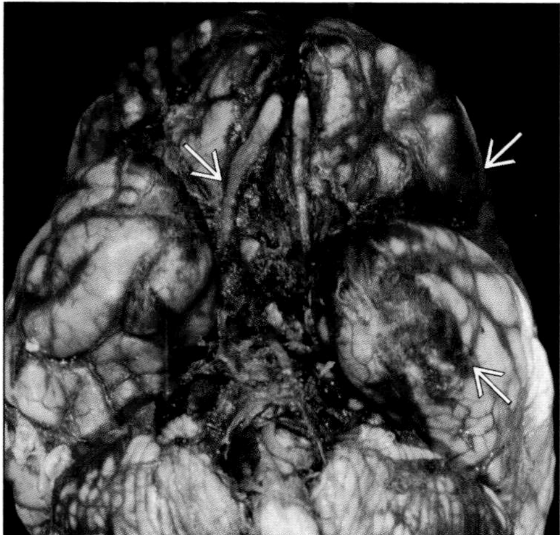

(Left) *CT shows basal cistern SAH in the suprasellar cistern ➢, interpeduncular cistern ➔, and ambient cistern ➢ following the acute rupture of a saccular aneurysm of an anterior cerebral artery. The amount of SAH in these basal cisterns is used for clinical grading of an acutely ruptured saccular aneurysm of the brain.* ***(Right)*** *Rupture of a saccular aneurysm of a branch of the left middle cerebral artery has produced SAH ➔ that is relatively concentrated around the rupture site.*

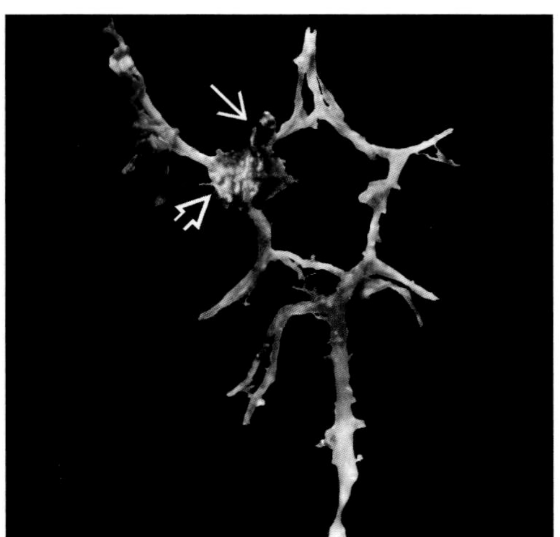

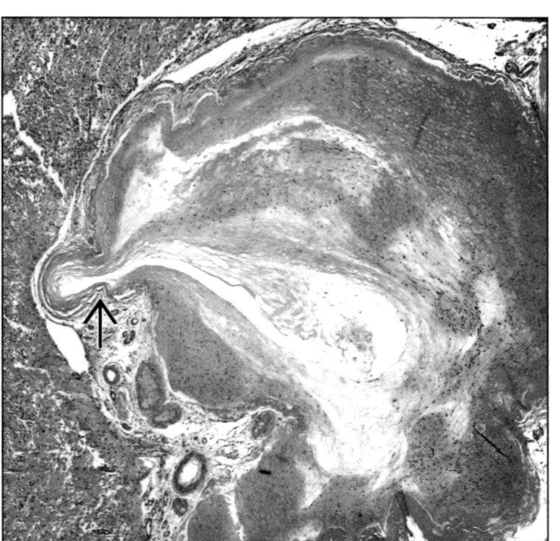

(Left) *The circle of Willis has a ruptured saccular aneurysm of the right internal carotid artery with a surgical clip ➔ placed over the rupture site. Arachnoidal fibrosis is consolidated around the rupture/ surgical site ➢.* ***(Right)*** *Leptomeningeal siderosis is helpful in identifying this small saccular aneurysm of an anterior cerebral artery, here stained with H&E. The very thin wall area ➔ may have been a site of minor blood leakage.*

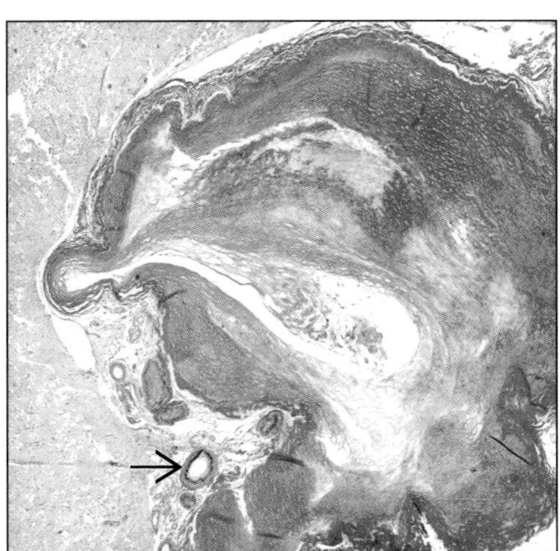

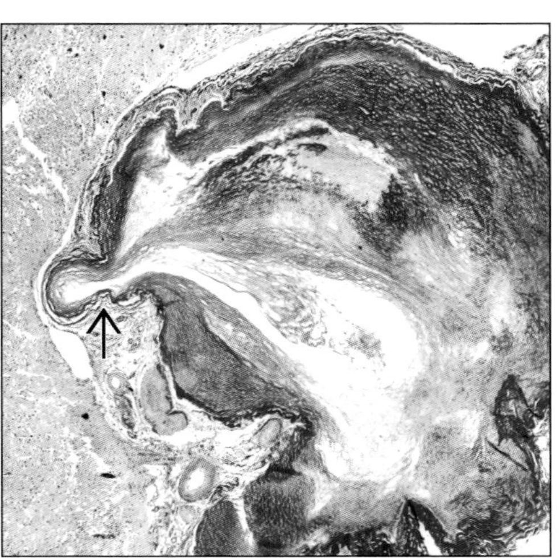

(Left) *The saccular aneurysm has no internal elastic lamina in its wall, while small adjacent normal arteries have their internal elastic lamina darkly stained with elastin stain ➔. Lack of elastin in the aneurysm allows systolic pressure to enlarge and thin the wall.* ***(Right)*** *Trichrome stain of the saccular aneurysm reveals the collagenous nature of the aneurysmal wall. Note the thin area of the wall that puts saccular aneurysms at risk of leaking and rupture to cause SAH ➔.*

STROKE

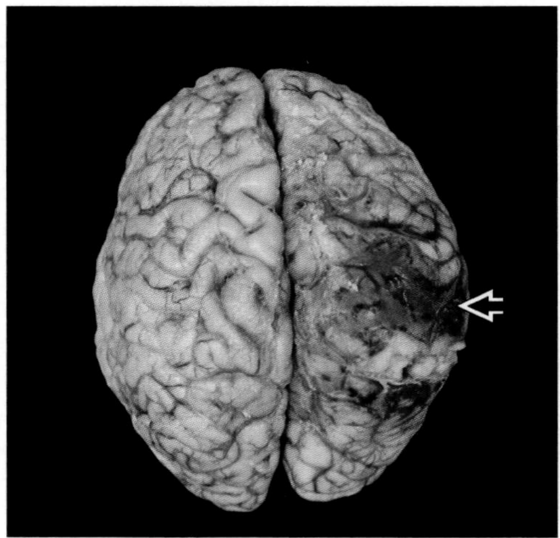

This brain removed at autopsy shows a large intraparenchymal hemorrhage ⇨ producing bulging and discoloration over much of the right hemisphere. This finding is readily apparent on external examination.

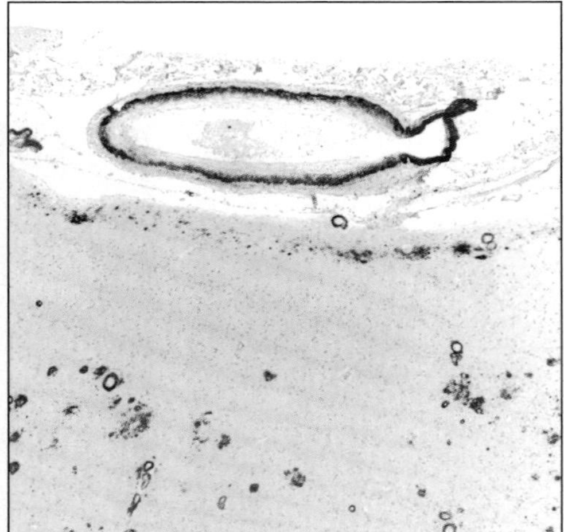

β-amyloid immunostaining in amyloid angiopathy shows accumulation in the media of cerebral blood vessels in the meninges and parenchyma. (Courtesy J. Chiaffarano, DO.)

TERMINOLOGY

Definitions

- Infarction: Ischemic necrosis due to lack of oxygenated blood
  - Lacunar infarct: Small (< 15 mm) cyst-like subcortical infarct due to small penetrating branch artery occlusion
- Hemorrhage: Extravascular accumulation of blood (may be consequence of infarction, especially embolic)
- Stroke: Cerebral damage caused by either infarction or hemorrhage

ETIOLOGY/PATHOGENESIS

Atherosclerosis/Arteriosclerosis

- Contributing factors include ↑ age, hypercholesterolemia, diabetes, smoking, hypertension
- Carotid arteries and named arteries of the cerebrovascular tree affected
- Infarction ± hemorrhage
  - Hemorrhagic infarction occurs in wedge-shaped vascular territory

Embolic Infarction

- Sources of emboli
  - Heart (mural thrombus): Atrial fibrillation, infarction, endocarditis
  - Fat: Long bone trauma
  - Plaque: Carotid artery atherosclerosis/plaque rupture

Vascular/Developmental

- Aneurysms, arteriovenous malformation, Moyamoya disease (hereditary or acquired cerebral arterial constrictions), cavernoma
- Hypertensive intracranial hemorrhage
  - Basal ganglia, cerebellum, or brainstem (intraparenchymal, no vascular territory pattern)
- Venous (cavernous sinus) thrombosis with parenchymal hemorrhage

Hereditary/Metabolic

- CADASIL (cerebral autosomal dominant arteriopathy with subcortical infarcts and leukoencephalopathy)
- Cerebral amyloid angiopathy
- Hematologic: Hyperviscosity (polycythemia), sickling, hypercoagulability

Vasculitis/Inflammatory

- Autoimmune disease (dermatomyositis, lupus, rheumatoid arthritis)
- Systemic vasculitis (ANCA-related diseases)
- Primary CNS vasculitis
- Neurosarcoidosis
- Acute hemorrhagic leukoencephalitis

Toxic/Iatrogenic

- Drugs of abuse (cocaine, amphetamines, phencyclidine)
- Overanticoagulation

Infections

- Herpes simplex encephalitis
- Infection-related vasculitis (syphilis, HIV, Lyme, Whipple, Hepatitis B and C)
- Fungal (*Aspergillus*)

Tumors

- Primary tumors (hemangioblastoma, glioblastoma)
- Metastatic (especially melanoma, renal cell carcinoma, choriocarcinoma)
- Lymphomatoid granulomatosis

Trauma

- Cortical contusion
- Infarction due to subarachnoid hemorrhage

STROKE

Key Facts

Terminology

- Infarction: Ischemic necrosis due to lack of oxygen blood flow
- Hemorrhage: Extravascular accumulation of blood (may be consequence of infarction, especially embolic)

Clinical Issues

- 10% of strokes are hemorrhagic at initial onset
- 30% of strokes (initially nonhemorrhagic) will undergo hemorrhagic transformation

Microscopic Pathology

- Acute infarction
  - Edema, red neurons, neuron "ghosts," neutrophils, vacular proliferation
- Subacute infarction
  - Macrophages, neuropil rarefaction (necrotic debris), astrocytic gliosis, calcification
- Old infarction
  - Cystic change (without fibroblasts or collagen), rare macrophages, gliosis in surrounding tissue
- Vasculitis: Transmural inflammation ± fibrinoid necrosis
- AVM: Arteries, veins, and hybrid vessels with intervening gliotic brain tissue
- Cavernoma: Back-to-back thin-walled vessels
- Amyloid angiopathy: Amorphous eosinophilic deposits

Diagnostic Checklist

- Distinguish focal ischemia (red neurons in infarct territory) from global anoxic injury (red neurons bilaterally in hippocampus, Purkinje cells)

CLINICAL ISSUES

Epidemiology

- Incidence
  - Race: Stroke more common in black patients (compared to white patients)
  - Sex: Atherosclerosis-related infarction more common in men
  - 10% of strokes are hemorrhagic at initial onset
    - Commonly seen in hypertensive hemorrhage, amyloid angiopathy, tumors, vascular malformations, and drug reactions
  - 30% of strokes (initially nonhemorrhagic) will undergo hemorrhagic transformation
    - 24 hours to 2 weeks after infarction
    - Risk factors: ↑ age, anticoagulation, larger infarction, and embolic cause
- Between ages 45-85, stroke incidence doubles each decade

Presentation

- Pertinent history: Transient ischemic attacks, trauma, malignancy, cardiac arrhythmias, anticoagulant use, drug abuse, infection/fever, endocarditis
- Symptoms localize to area of brain involved
  - Motor &/or sensory deficits: Pre/post central gyrus
  - Speech or visual disturbance: Parieto-occipital
  - Focal cognitive deficits or agnosias: Frontal
  - Cranial nerve involvement
- Decreased level of consciousness
- Multiple small subcortical infarcts may present as dementia

Laboratory Tests

- Electroencephalography (EEG) pattern may suggest herpes encephalitis
- Hypercoagulability: Serum levels of protein C, protein S, antithrombin III, factor V Leyden, lupus anticoagulant
- PT (INR), PTT
- C-ANCA, p-ANCA, rheumatoid factor, ANA

Treatment

- Surgical approaches
  - Carotid endarterectomy
  - Surgical drainage &/or placement of extraventricular drain
  - Inferior vena cava filter, cardiac septal defect repair or occluder device
- Medical approaches
  - Anticoagulation, aspirin, antiplatelet agents
  - Calcium channel blockers for vasospasm in subarachnoid hemorrhage

IMAGE FINDINGS

Ultrasonographic Findings

- Duplex (Doppler): Internal carotid artery stenosis
- Echocardiography: Vegetations and septal defects (paradoxic embolism)

CT Findings

- Acute hemorrhage: Hyperdense
- Early infarction: Edema (hypoattenuation, sulcal effacement) or hyperdensity in a vessel
- Later infarction: Hypodense
- Lacunar infarcts: Small hypodensities in basal ganglia and subcortical white matter

MR Findings

- Different MR sequences demonstrate different pathologies optimally
- Gradient echo MR: Hemorrhage hypointense
- T2 and FLAIR sequences: Infarction hyperintense
- Diffusion MR: Very early infarction
- Perfusion MR: Surrounding reversible ischemia

Angiography

- Vascular malformations, aneurysms
- Venography: Venous thrombosis
- Vasculitis: "Beading" of vessels, or tapered segmental narrowing

STROKE

MACROSCOPIC FEATURES

External Examination

- Musculoskeletal
  - Old infarction: Atrophy of unilateral limb muscles, facial asymmetry, contractures
  - Long-term immobilization → decubitus ulcers
- Trauma: Examine body for bruises and fractures, scalp for hematomas, bruising around eyes or blood in ears indicating basal skull fracture
- Needle tracks, injection sites indicating intravenous drug use
- Facies of Down syndrome or cachexia associated with Alzheimer disease (increased risk of amyloid angiopathy)

Internal Examination

- Examine heart, aorta, coronary and renal arteries, kidneys for evidence of atherosclerotic vascular disease
- Examine cardiac valves for vegetations

Gross Examination of Brain

- Surface hemorrhages, uncal or tonsillar herniation, or sulcal effacement suggesting edema
- Cut sections
  - Very early infarction: Blurring of gray-white junction and softening of tissue
  - Acute infarction: More softening, edema, discoloration, possibly hemorrhagic transformation
  - Old infarction: Cystic cavitation (lacune)
  - Acute hemorrhage: Red-brown, mass forming
  - Old hemorrhage: Cavitation with orange/yellow rim
- Atrophy (sulcal widening and gyral narrowing) → Alzheimer disease, which can coexist with amyloid angiopathy

MICROSCOPIC PATHOLOGY

Histologic Features

- Ischemic injury
  - Hypoxic-ischemic or "red" neurons
    - Shrunken, hypereosinophilic cytoplasm and dark, condensed pyknotic nuclei
    - Prominent in hippocampus (neocortex), and cerebellum (Purkinje cells)
    - Appear within 6-48 hours of ischemic injury
  - White matter infarcts: Transected axons near infarct may be seen as axonal swelling
  - Edema: Pericellular and perivascular vacuolation
- Infarction
  - Acute
    - Edema, red neurons, vascular endothelial swelling, neutrophils in 24-48 hours
  - Subacute
    - Macrophages, neuropil rarefaction, reactive astrocytes
  - Old
    - Cystic change (without fibroblasts or collagen), rare macrophages, gliosis in surrounding tissue
  - Emboli
    - Thrombus, atheroma, air, fat, septic embolus (endocarditis), cardiac myxoma, foreign material
- Vasculitis: Transmural inflammation of vessel walls ± fibrinoid necrosis
  - Composition of inflammatory infiltrate varies with etiology
- Malformations/tumors
  - AVM: Arteries, veins, and arterialized veins with intervening gliotic brain tissue
  - Cavernoma: Back-to-back thin-walled vessels
- Amyloid angiopathy: Amorphous eosinophilic deposits in media and adventitia of small and medium-sized arteries, arterioles

ANCILLARY TESTS

Histochemistry

- Congo Red
- Elastic
- Martius Scarlet Blue

Immunohistochemistry

- HSV1 and HSV2
- β-amyloid (amyloid angiopathy)
- GFAP (gliosis)

DIAGNOSTIC CHECKLIST

Clinically Relevant Pathologic Features

- Examine carotid and cerebral arteries (atherosclerosis)
- Sample hemorrhage rim for tumors, AVM, amyloid angiopathy
- Exclude cardiac septal defects, mural thrombi, vegetations

Pathologic Interpretation Pearls

- Distinguish focal ischemia (red neurons in infarct territory) from global anoxic injury (red neurons bilaterally in hippocampus, Purkinje cells)
- Uncal herniation from any cause can compress ipsilateral posterior cerebral artery, infarcting hippocampus, thalamus, occipital lobe

REPORTING CRITERIA

Location and Evolution of Infarct

- Give vascular territory of infarction and age (acute, subacute, old)

Source of Hemorrhage

- Give cause of parenchymal or subarachnoid hemorrhage and age (organization, hemosiderin within macrophages)

SELECTED REFERENCES

1. Fewel ME et al: Spontaneous intracerebral hemorrhage: a review. Neurosurg Focus. 15(4):E1, 2003
2. Garcia JH: The evolution of brain infarcts. A review. J Neuropathol Exp Neurol. 51(4):387-93, 1992

Gross and Microscopic Features

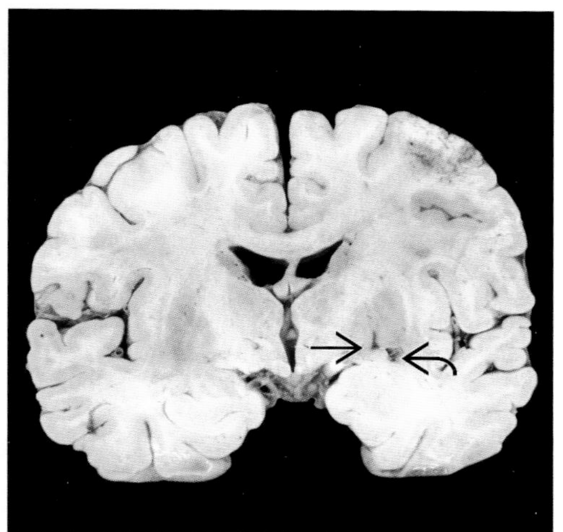

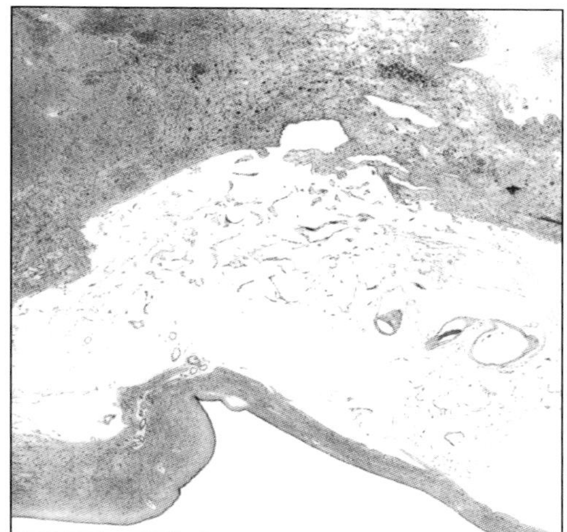

(Left) *This coronal section through a fixed brain shows old lacunar infarcts of the right putamen ⇾ and globus pallidus ⇾.* ***(Right)*** *This H&E-stained section shows an old infarction with an area of cavitation traversed by small vessels, containing residual macrophages and surrounded by gliosis.*

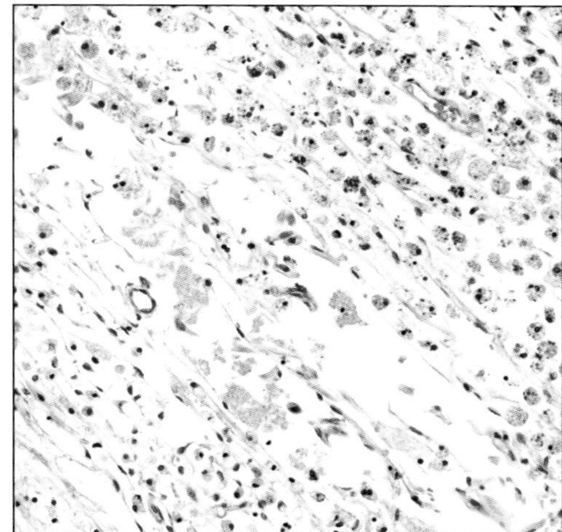

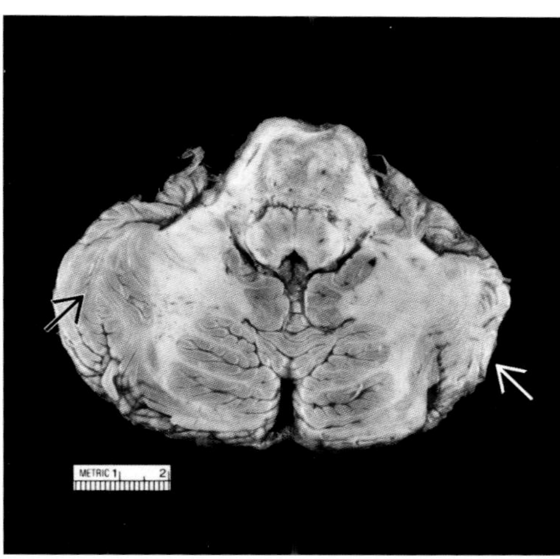

(Left) *H&E section through old/chronic hemorrhagic infarct with loss of neuropil and gliosis surrounded by hemosiderin-laden macrophages.* ***(Right)*** *This axial section of cerebellum shows old infarction in the right hemisphere ➡, characterized by atrophy, yellow discoloration, and shrinkage of the folia. The changes are apparent when compared to the opposite side ⇾.*

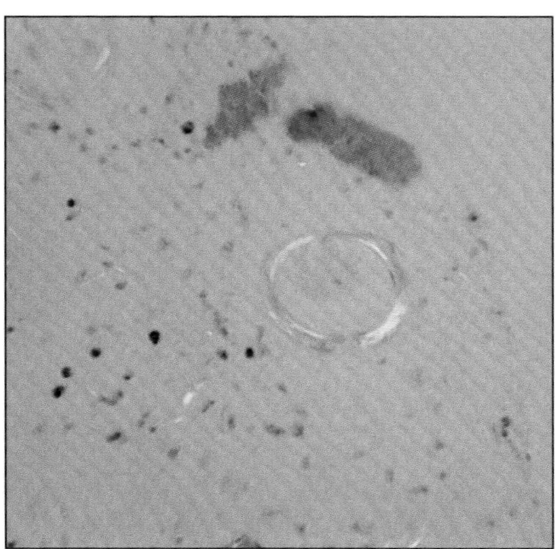

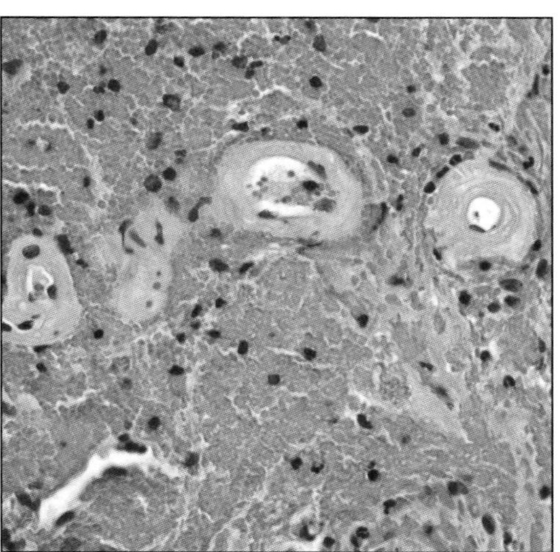

(Left) *This polarized light image of a Congo red-stained section of autopsy brain demonstrates apple-green birefringence, confirming the presence of amyloid. Amyloid angiopathy is a common cause of cerebral hemorrhage in older adults.* ***(Right)*** *This H&E-stained section of amyloid angiopathy shows vessels with eosinophilic deposits in the medial layer of arterioles with characteristic rigid round pipe shapes.*

Gross and Microscopic Features

*(**Left**) These cross sections through the occipital lobes of a fixed brain show the typical wedge-shaped or lobar hemorrhages of cerebral amyloid angiopathy. (**Right**) Red neurons ⇨ with ischemic necrosis are seen on H&E-stained sections. These neurons are shrunken, with hypereosinophilic cytoplasm and pyknotic nuclei.*

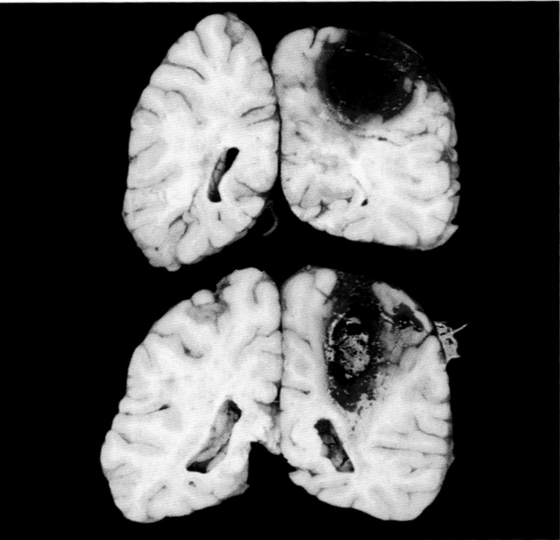

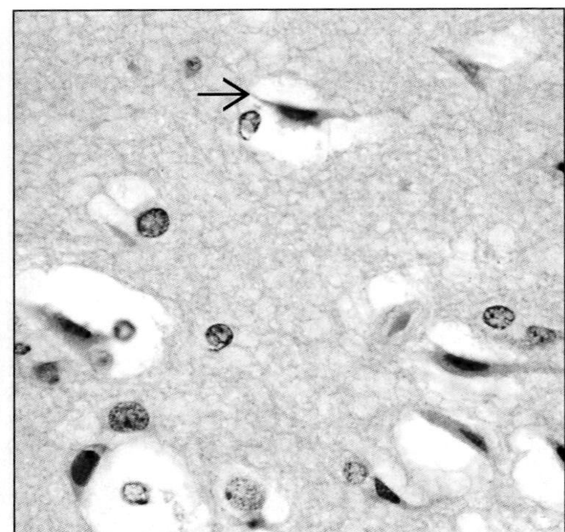

*(**Left**) This H&E/Luxol fast blue-stained section of brain adjacent to an area of acute infarction shows axonal swellings ⇨, indicating white matter tract disruption, and also shows pericellular vacuolation consistent with edema. (**Right**) This H&E-stained image of subacute infarction shows ischemic neurons ⇨, edema with pericellular vacuolization, and no significant inflammatory response.*

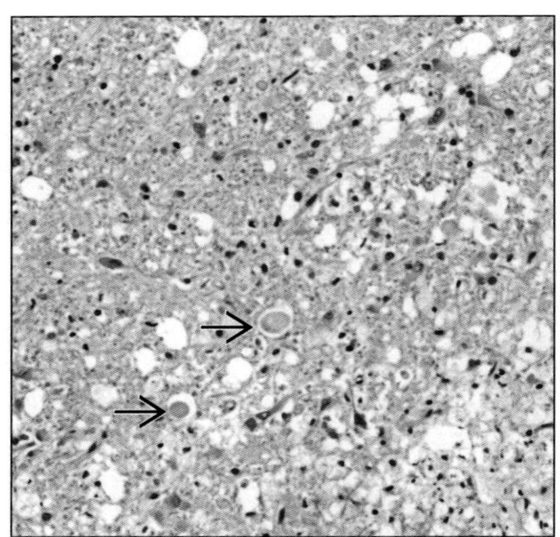

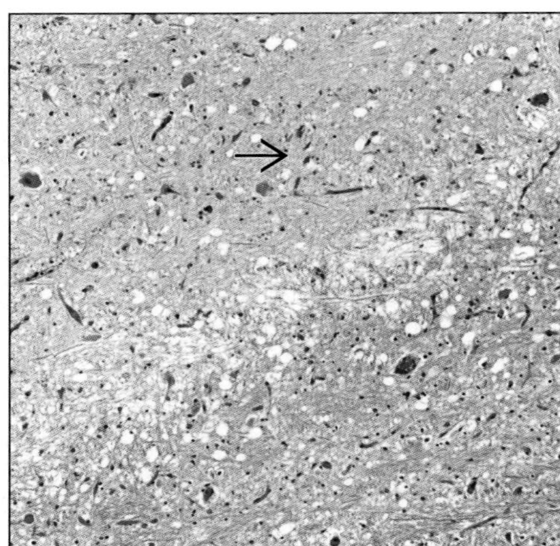

*(**Left**) Gross image of frontal lobe shows vascular malformation that is likely cavernoma (back-to-back small vessels with hemosiderin staining of surrounding parenchyma). (**Right**) This trichrome stain of a cavernoma shows back-to-back thin-walled vessels without evidence of internal elastic lamina.*

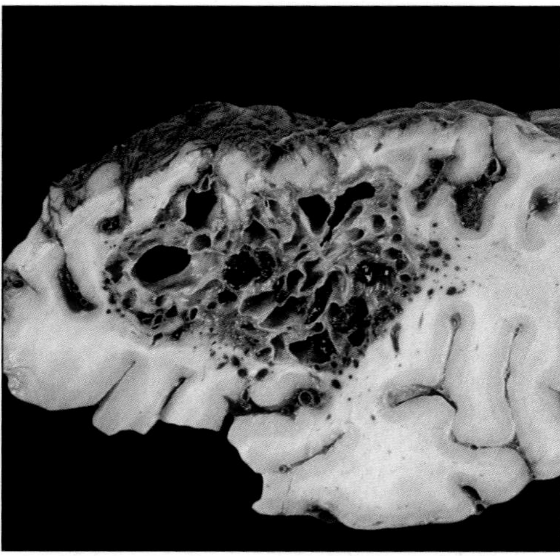

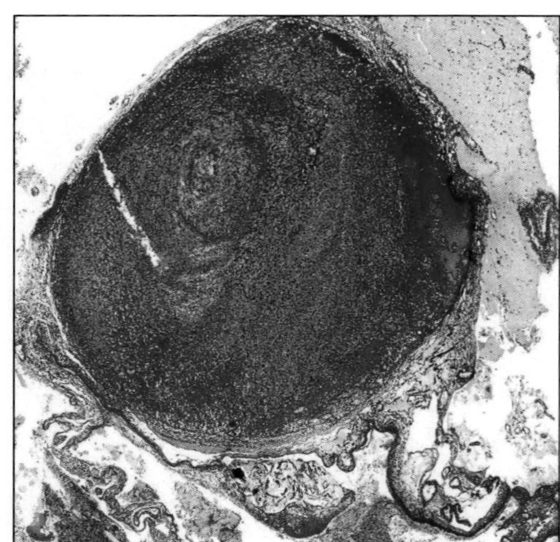

Gross and Microscopic Images

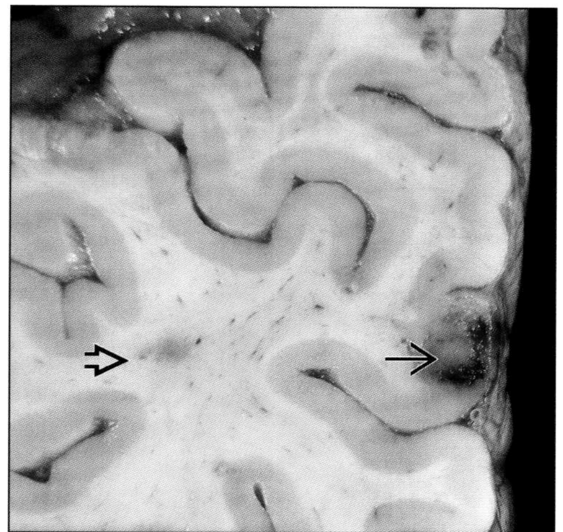

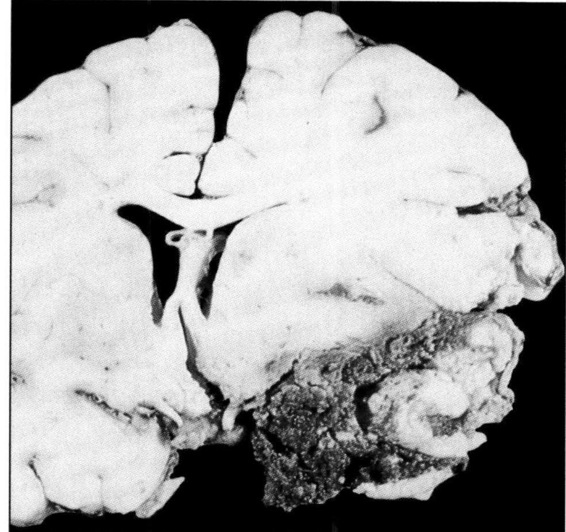

*(**Left**) Coronal section through the brain shows embolic infarction (may be septic or thromboembolic) with focal lesions at the gray-white junction ➔ and in the white matter ➲. (**Right**) This coronal section of brain with herpes encephalitis shows hemorrhagic necrosis of the right temporal lobe.*

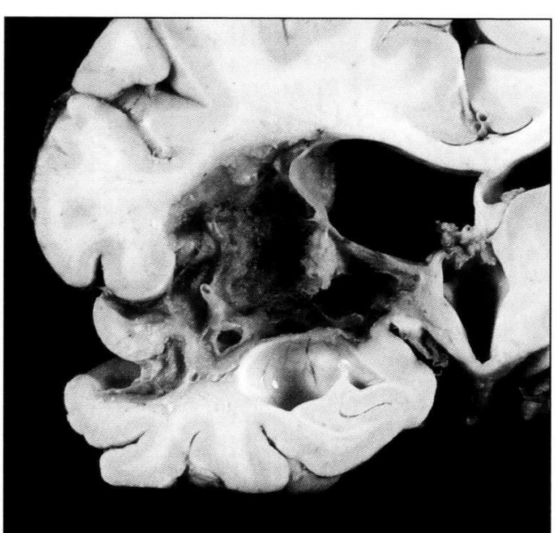

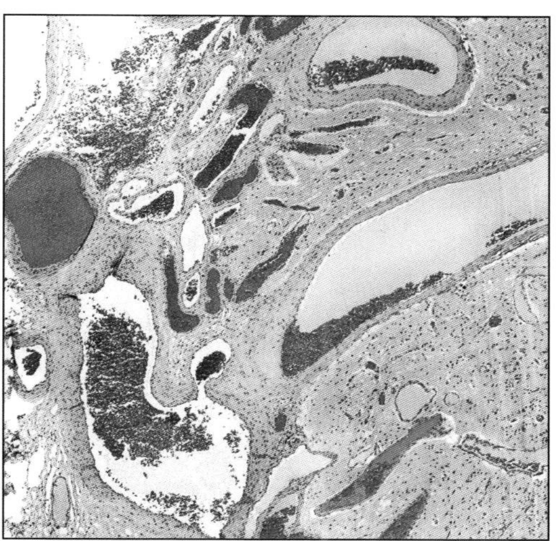

*(**Left**) Gross image shows arteriovenous malformation and surrounding hemorrhage with a collection of vessels of varying sizes. Note the enlarged lateral ventricle and 3rd ventricle, likely from hemorrhage into the ventricles. (**Right**) This H&E-stained section of an arteriovenous malformation shows vessels with varying wall thickness with intervening gliotic brain tissue between vessels (i.e., not back-to-back).*

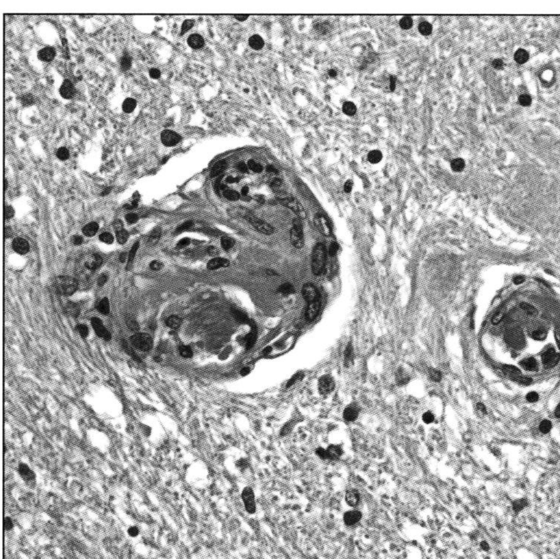

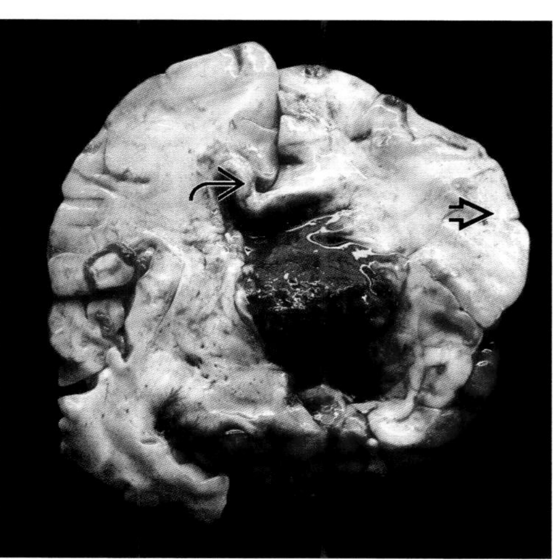

*(**Left**) H&E-stained section shows organized fibrin thrombi in small vessels, consistent with DIC or TTP. (**Right**) Coronal section of a fresh brain at autopsy shows hemorrhagic melanoma. Sulcal effacement ➲ and subfalcine herniation ➦ accompany edema of the right cerebral hemisphere.*

SECTION 2

Postoperative/Post-Interventional Death

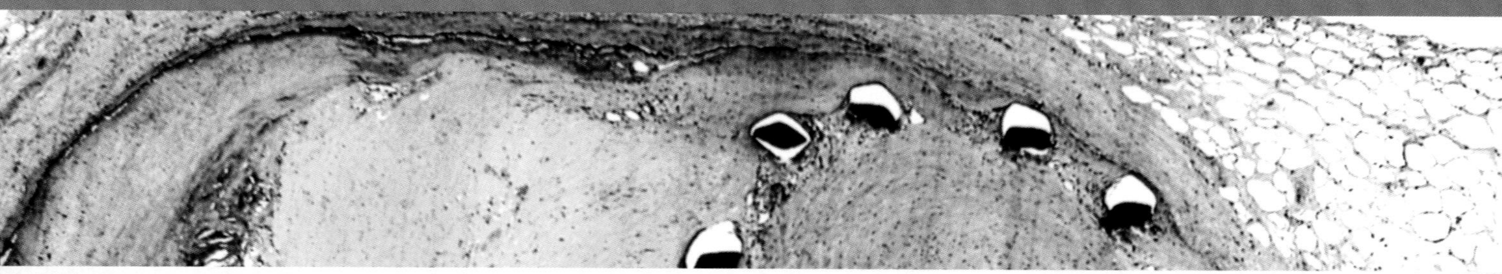

Iatrogenic

Cardiovascular

Gastrointestinal and Hepatobiliary

CNS

THERAPEUTIC COMPLICATIONS

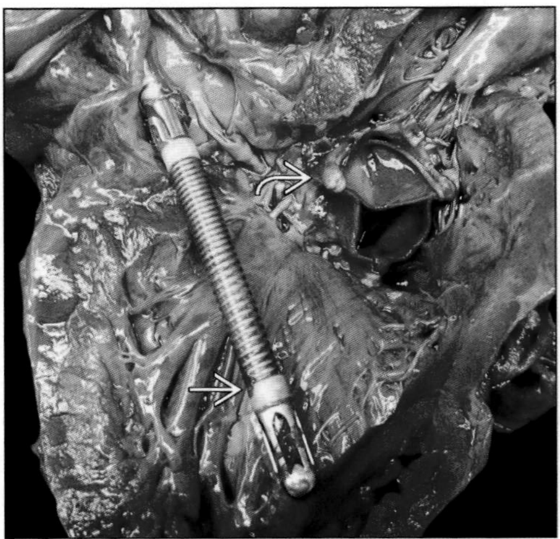

This patient who underwent a mitral valve repair with a pericardial valve ➡ could not be weaned off of bypass without the insertion of a circulatory assist device ➡. Death was considered a therapeutic complication.

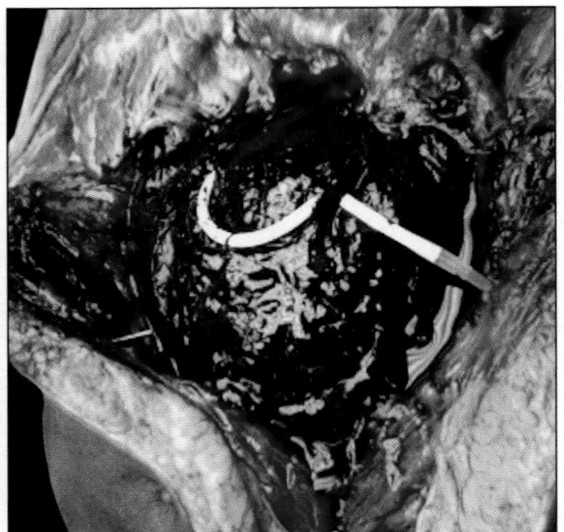

A therapeutic complication and major missed clinical diagnosis are demonstrated here in a large hematoma that surrounded a ventricular assist device generator and had been clinically diagnosed as an infection.

TERMINOLOGY

Synonyms

- Iatrogenic Injury, therapeutic misadventure
  - Semantics: "Misadventure" considered pejorative; "complication" favored

Definitions

- Therapeutic complication: Injury or adverse event caused by medical management, not underlying disease
  - May not be overtly evident at autopsy, and identification requires careful clinical pathological correlation
  - Includes medication errors as well as interventional complications
  - May not be ultimate cause of death but contributory
    - e.g., patient who had anaphylactic reaction to antibiotic but survived and ultimately died from infection; patient who had small hemothorax after central line placement (treated) but died from underlying heart failure
- Clinically unsuspected diagnoses: Distinct from therapeutic complication, refers to autopsy diagnoses that were not identified premortem and may have impacted outcome
  - Classification schema: Goldman criteria
    - Class I: Major missed diagnosis with potential for adverse outcome that would have changed clinical management
    - Class II: Major missed diagnosis without potential impact on survival that would not have changed clinical management
    - Class III: Missed minor diagnosis related to terminal disease but not causing death
    - Class IV: Other missed minor diagnosis

EXAMPLES OF THERAPEUTIC COMPLICATIONS

Surgical: Infectious, Medication, Anesthesia, Technical, Nontechnical, Thromboembolic, Transfusion-Related

- Infectious complications
  - Common: Local wound infection, postoperative pneumonia, line and urinary tract infection
    - Can progress to systemic infection and shock
    - Host and operative factors important determinants: Underlying immunosuppression, bowel surgery
- Medication complication
  - Similar to nonsurgical complication: Any adverse reaction to medication given as part of operative intervention
  - Adverse reaction usually anaphylactic
    - Pulmonary congestion and edema, sometimes laryngeal and upper airway edema, mucus plugging and hyperinflation of lungs, and petechial hemorrhages (asphyxia/anoxia)
- Anesthesia complication
  - Adverse reaction to anesthetic agents, ventilatory issues, malignant hyperthermia (MH)
    - If MH diagnosis, consider molecular testing on pre- or early postmortem blood; final report should indicate familial nature (most autosomal dominant) of disease and risk to next of kin
- Technical complication
  - Complication directly related to operation: Wound dehiscence, anastomotic leaking (e.g., bowel surgery), postoperative bleeding
- Nontechnical complication
  - Epiphenomenon of operative intervention
    - Ileus, postoperative atelectasis
    - Uncommon direct cause of death
- Thromboembolic

- Venous thromboembolism in postoperative period
  - Patient factors: Preoperative thrombophilia, obesity, underlying malignancy, hip fracture, spinal cord injury, major trauma
  - Operative factors: Major operation (thoracic or abdominal surgery with general anesthesia lasting > 30 minutes), hip or knee replacement
- Transfusion-related
  - Any operative intervention-related transfusion complication
    - Transfusion-associated circulatory overload: Pulmonary edema related to osmotic effects of transfused red blood cells leading to increased intravascular volume (2nd most common cause of transfusion related death)
    - Acute hemolytic transfusion reaction: Usually due to recipient antibodies to RBC antigens; ABO most common but may relate to other antigens; intravascular hemolysis → hemoglobinuria, acute renal failure, DIC, and occasionally death
    - Transfusion-related acute lung injury (TRALI): Uncommon reaction due to presence of anti HLA or anti leukocyte antibodies in donor plasma → leukocyte degranulation in lung and diffuse alveolar damage
  - If transfusion-related complication is noted at autopsy, consult with transfusion medicine specialists and consider collecting plasma and blood from decedent; hold any premortem blood in laboratory

Nonsurgical: Infectious, Medication, Procedure-Related (Technical or Nontechnical), Thromboembolic, Transfusion-Related

- Infectious complication: Nosocomial (hospital-acquired) infections (HAI): Infections that are associated with hospital or health care (health care-associated infection)
  - An important cause of morbidity and mortality in hospitalized patients and patients in other health care settings (nursing homes)
    - Most common nonsurgical HAI: Central line and urinary catheter-associated infection, *Clostridium difficile* infection, and methicillin-resistant *Staphylococcus aureus*
    - Other important HAI: Ventilator-associated pneumonia, hospital-acquired pneumonia, and vancomycin-resistant enterococcus
    - Autopsy identification of clinically undiagnosed HAI should be reported to hospital infection control or infectious disease team
- Medication: Any adverse reaction to administered medication
  - Can include interactions including over the counter medications and herbal medication
  - Anticoagulation therapy-related injury: Bleeding related to anticoagulation therapy
    - Gastrointestinal, retroperitoneal, cerebral
- Procedure-related technical and nontechnical
  - Technical: Complication of technical aspects of invasive but nonoperative intervention
    - e.g., pancreatitis or bleeding following endoscopic retrograde cholangiopancreatography (ERCP); coronary artery dissection during coronary angiogram
  - Nontechnical: Complication following invasive but nonoperative intervention
    - e.g., dysrhythmia or cholesterol embolization syndrome following coronary angiography
- Thromboembolic
  - Venous thromboembolism in hospital or other health care (nursing home) setting
    - Risk factors: Underlying thrombophilic (protein C or S, factor V Leiden mutation), obesity, immobility, malignancy, hormonal therapy
- Transfusion-related
  - Same complications as transfusion in operative setting

CLINICALLY UNSUSPECTED DIAGNOSES

Final Autopsy Report

- All major and minor clinically unsuspected diagnoses should be documented
- Major clinically unsuspected diagnoses should be flagged for QA review
- Minor clinically unsuspected diagnosed should also be documented and are also important as they may have impact for next of kin
  - e.g., class IV missed diagnosis of unsuspected malignancy like medullary carcinoma of thyroid may have familial implication

SELECTED REFERENCES

1. Langford NJ: Therapeutic misadventure. Med Sci Law. 50(4):179-82, 2010
2. Grzybicki DM et al. Anatomic pathology and patient safety: it's not an error: it's a diagnostic misadventure! Am J Clin Pathol. 129(1):167-8; author reply 169, 2008
3. Lau G: Perioperative deaths: a further comparative review of coroner's autopsies with particular reference to the occurrence of fatal iatrogenic injury. Ann Acad Med Singapore. 29(4):486-97, 2000
4. Pumphrey RS et al: Postmortem findings after fatal anaphylactic reactions. J Clin Pathol. 53(4):273-6, 2000
5. Goldman L et al: The value of the autopsy in three medical eras. N Engl J Med. 308(17):1000-5, 1983
6. Utting JE et al: Human misadventure in anaesthesia. Can Anaesth Soc J. 26(6):472-8, 1979
7. Therapeutic misadventure. Br Med J. 1(5594):724, 1968

THERAPEUTIC COMPLICATIONS

Gross and Microscopic Features

(Left) *Clostridium difficile enterocolitis is an important hospital-acquired infection. It has a pseudomembranous appearance with yellow nodules ⮫ overlying the mucosa. (From DP: Gastrointestinal.)* ***(Right)*** *The pseudomembranes ⇨ of Clostridium difficile enterocolitis are composed of mushrooms of mucus, acute inflammatory cells, and degenerated superficial epithelial cells. The base → of the crypts is intact. (From DP: Gastrointestinal.)*

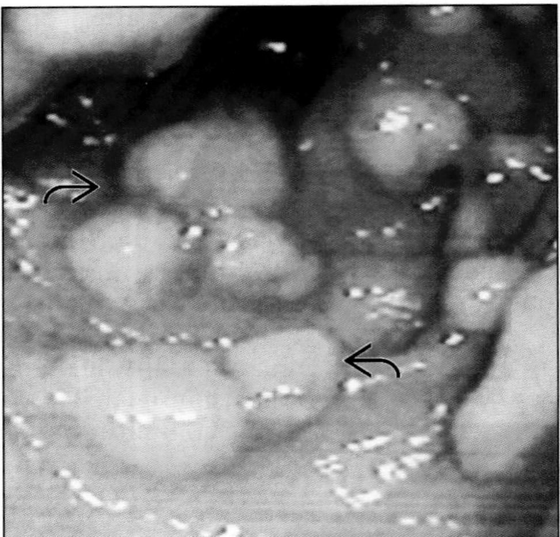

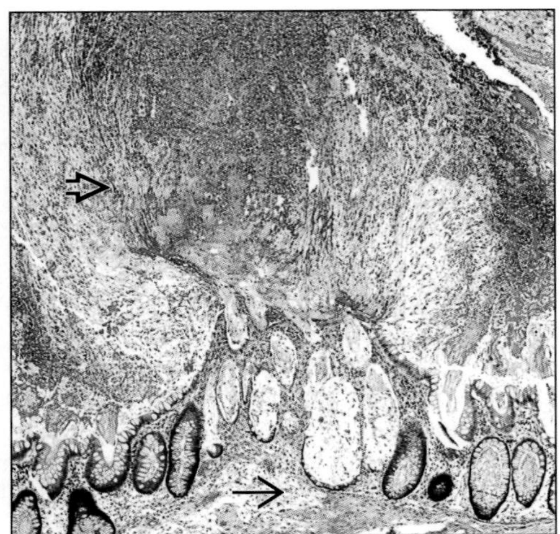

(Left) *Cirrhosis is a commonly missed clinical diagnosis and also is an important cause of medical complication, particularly Tylenol use in patients with alcoholism and cirrhosis.* ***(Right)*** *This mass of thromboemboli was found in the bifurcation of the pulmonary artery in a patient who was recently postoperative. Major surgery (thoracic or abdominal surgery with general anesthesia > 30 minutes) and hip and knee replacement surgery has a high risk of pulmonary thromboembolism.*

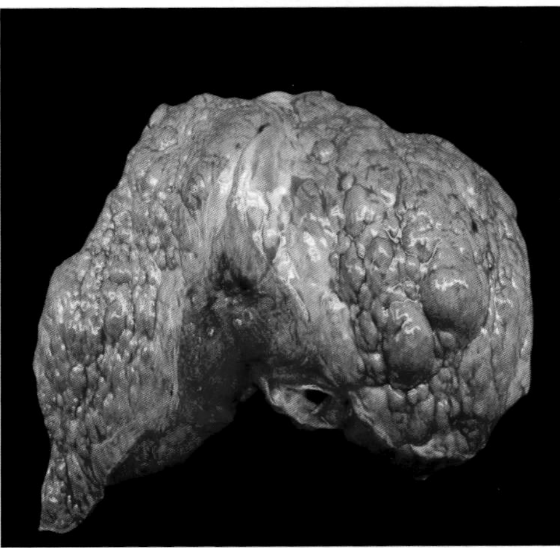

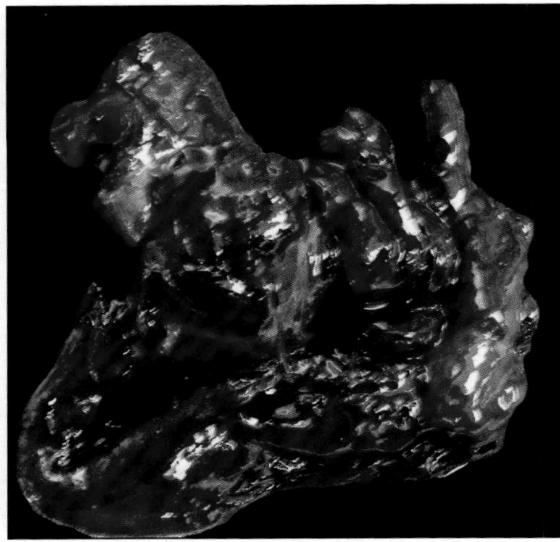

(Left) *This is an example of a patient who expired due to ascending aortic dissection with rupture ⇨ and hemothorax. The patient had undergone operative repair (sutures ⮫) and died on the table. This death would still be classified as a natural death, not therapeutic complication, due to the emergent nature of the situation and lethal nature of aortic dissection.* ***(Right)*** *Rupture of an aortic aneurysm ⮫ after stent graft repair ⇨ is a known therapeutic complication.*

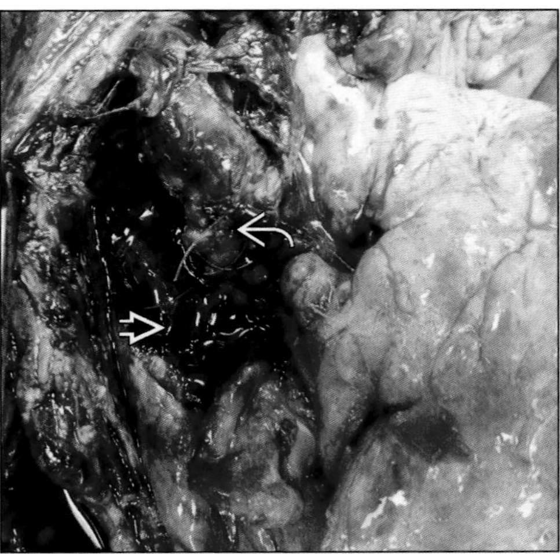

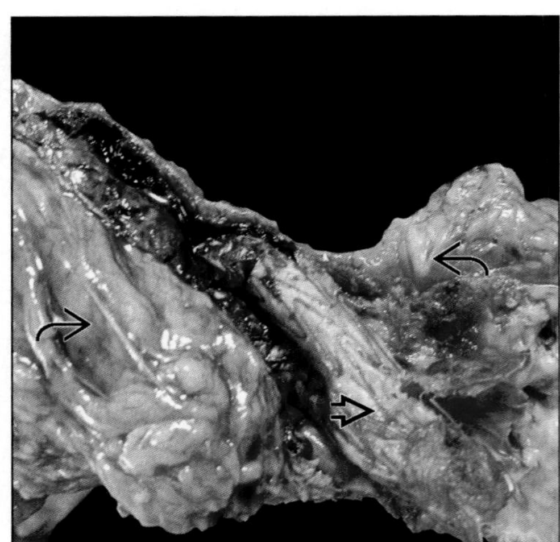

Gross and Microscopic Features

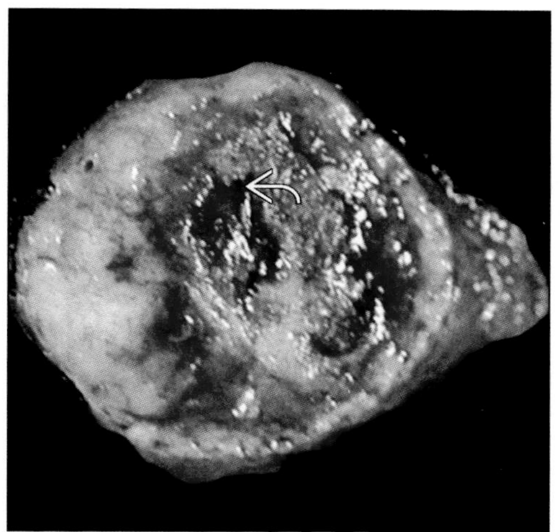

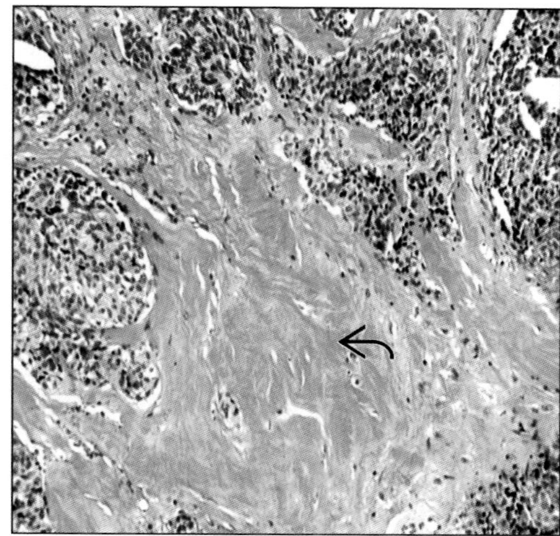

(Left) *Even a minor clinically unsuspected diagnosis like a thyroid carcinoma that has features of medullary carcinoma may have potential impact for the surviving next of kin. This thyroid demonstrates a large medullary carcinoma ➔ that has a gray-white appearance and was firm. (From DP: Endocrine.)* ***(Right)*** *The histologic features of medullary thyroid cancer are seen here with a cellular tumor with a stroma rich in amyloid ➔. (From DP: Endocrine.)*

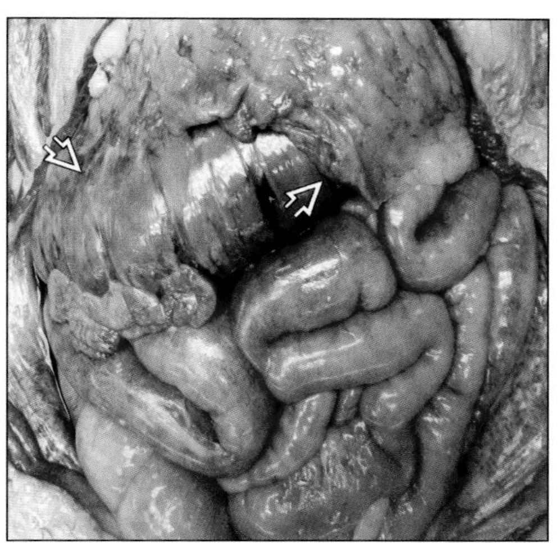

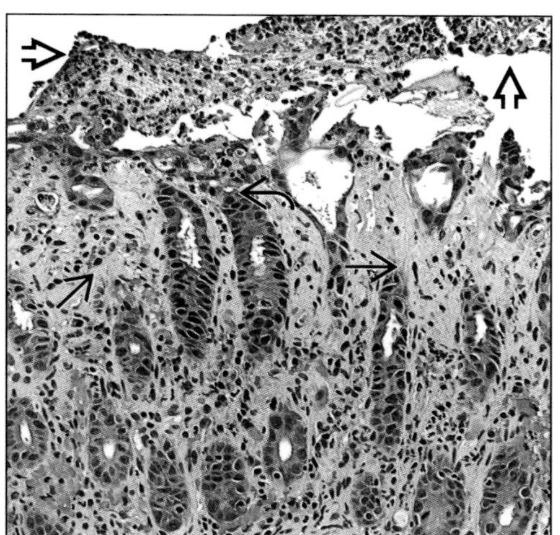

(Left) *This case demonstrates ischemic necrosis of the transverse colon ➔. This would be classified as a major missed diagnosis with potential for adverse outcome that would have changed clinical management.* ***(Right)*** *Ischemic colitis with a pseudomembrane ➔ is noted here. There is epithelial necrosis ➔ and interstitial hemorrhage and homogeneous pink appearance to lamina propria ➔. (From DP: Gastrointestinal.)*

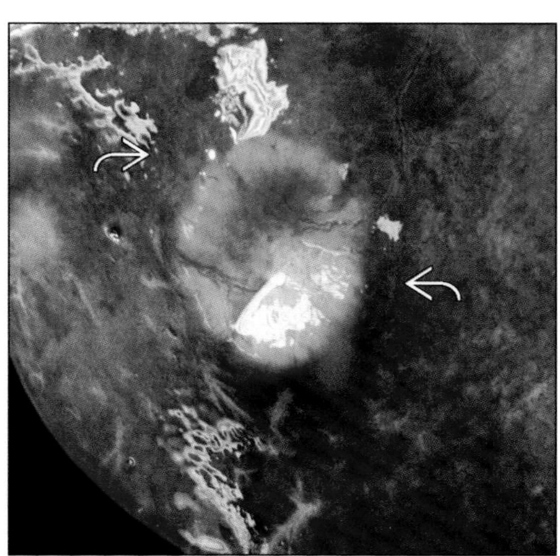

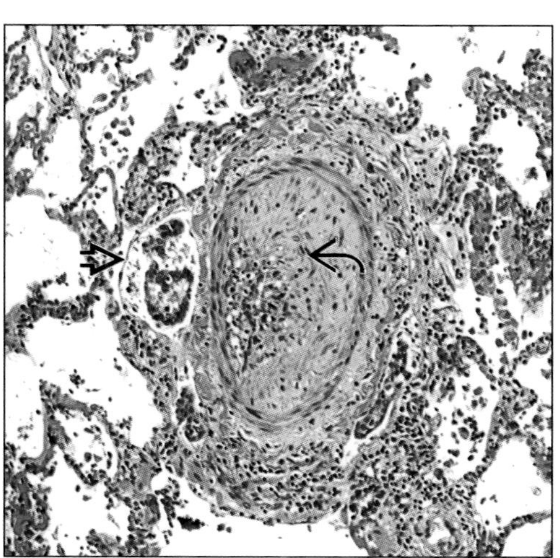

(Left) *Widely metastatic malignancy ➔ in a young boy who expired within hours of admission is not a clinically unsuspected diagnosis.* ***(Right)*** *The quick death was due to severe pulmonary hypertension caused by tumor metastasis to the lungs ➔ with associated marked intimal hyperplasia of pulmonary arteries ➔. Death was due to natural causes without clinically unsuspected diagnosis.*

CORONARY ARTERY BYPASS GRAFTING

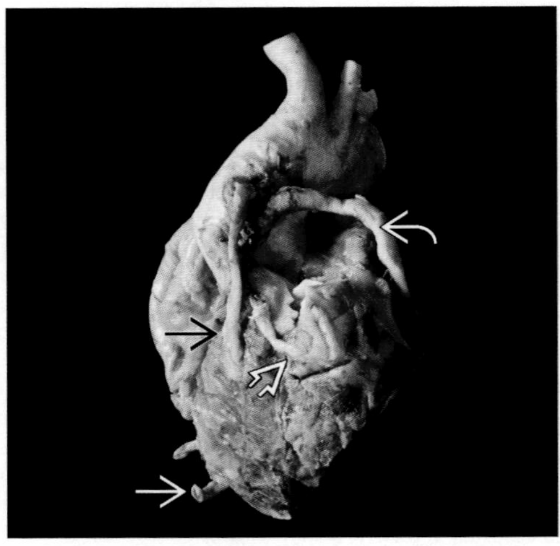

Anterior view of autopsied heart shows aortocoronary saphenous vein grafts to right coronary →, left anterior descending (LAD) →, and obtuse marginal → targets. An additional posterior descending graft → has been cut.

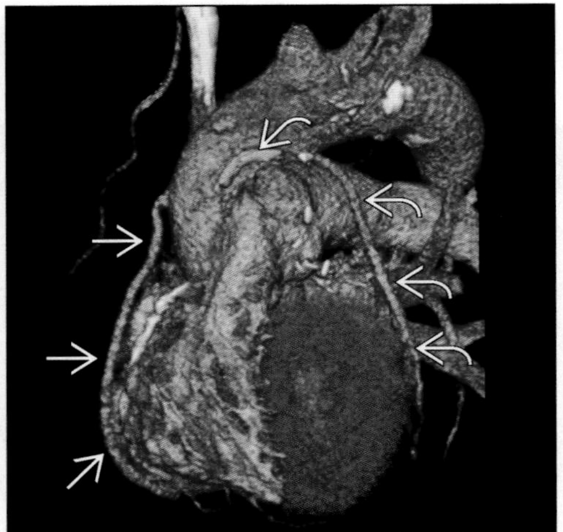

3D reconstruction CT angiogram shows bypass grafts to the posterior descending → and obtuse marginal → coronary branches. (From DI: Cardiovascular.)

TERMINOLOGY

Abbreviations

- Coronary artery bypass grafting (CABG)

CLINICAL ISSUES

Clinical Overview

- Once the primary intervention for coronary artery disease, CABG has largely been replaced by percutaneous endovascular procedures (angioplasty and stenting).
- CABG is still performed in setting of
  - Patients with coronary disease and valve disease or other need for open heart surgery
  - Left main coronary disease (given the consequences of endovascular complication in this location)
  - Certain patients with severe multifocal disease
- Patient outcomes post stenting are not better than post CABG, but stenting is obviously less invasive

Patient History Review

- Operative reports or coronary angiograms relevant to grafting targets and conduits are key to success in post-CABG heart evaluation
  - Dense pericardial adhesions may make it difficult to identify some grafts
  - Left internal mammary artery (LIMA) grafts are easily obliterated upon removal of sternal chest plate
  - Old thrombosed graft conduits may become thread-like and difficult to identify
- Mention of triple, quadruple, etc., bypass refers to number of target vessel anastomoses

Expected Graft Conduit Longevity

- Internal mammary artery graft: 90% patency at 10 years
- Saphenous vein graft (SVG): 20-30% patency at 10 years

Complications

- Early
  - "Kinking" or obstruction of graft body
  - Acute thrombosis (often due to hypercoagulability)
- Late
  - Fibrointimal proliferation and atheromatous plaques

IMAGE FINDINGS

Specimen Radiographic Findings

- Identify course of graft (clips along LIMA and SVG from graft harvesting): "Connect the dots"
- Delineate calcific plaque in native vessels and grafts
- Reveal any metallic stents

MACROSCOPIC FEATURES

General Features

- Common sources of graft conduits
  - Veins: Saphenous, gastroepiploic/inferior epigastric
  - Arteries: Internal mammary, radial
  - Scar patterns on external (skin) exam provide clues
    - Endoscopic vein harvesting may leave only subtle scars
- Common target vessels
  - Left anterior descending (LAD)
    - Ramus intermedius branch: Small branch arising at bifurcation of LAD and left circumflex (LCX) (trifurcation instead of bifurcation)
    - Diagonal branches: Primary branches of LAD serving anterior left ventricle
    - LIMA grafts almost exclusively to LAD due to anatomic constraints and adjacency
  - LCX
    - Obtuse marginal branches: Primary branches (or sometimes terminal course of LCX) serving lateral left ventricle
  - Right coronary artery (RCA)

CORONARY ARTERY BYPASS GRAFTING

Key Facts

Clinical Issues

- Operative reports or coronary angiograms relevant to grafting targets and conduits are key to success in post-CABG heart evaluation
- Internal mammary artery graft: 90% patency at 10 years
- Saphenous vein graft: 20-30% patency at 10 years
- Once the primary intervention for coronary artery disease, CABG has largely been replaced by percutaneous endovascular procedures (angioplasty and stenting)
- Patient outcomes post stenting are not better than post CABG, but stenting is obviously less invasive
- Dense pericardial adhesions may make it difficult to identify some grafts
- LIMA grafts are easily obliterated upon removal of sternal chest plate

Macroscopic Pathology

- For each bypass target vessel, document
  - Graft body: Serially sectioned with areas of plaque, thrombus, or other stenosis selected for microscopy
  - Distal anastomosis: Serial cross sectioning along axis of either native vessel or graft body
  - Distal native vessel run-off: Serial cross sectioning to evaluate potential for flow beyond target site
- Common sources of graft conduits
  - Veins: Saphenous, gastroepiploic/inferior epigastric
  - Arteries: Internal mammary, radial
- Labeling and nomenclature
  - Convention: Label graft according to target vessel and graft body type

---

      - Posterior descending: Terminal course of RCA serving posterior/inferior left ventricle
      - Posterior descending may be terminal course of LCX in ~ 10% of patients (left dominant circulation)
      - Posterolateral branch: Branch extending beyond posterior descending artery serving posterolateral left ventricle
- Sequential grafts
  - Lengthy segments of conduit may be used to supply > 1 target vessel anastomosis
  - "T" (perpendicular side-to-side) or "Y" (juxtaposed end-to-side) graft configurations
  - Each target vessel should be labeled and evaluated individually

Sections to Be Submitted

- Proximal native coronary arteries
  - All vessels should be examined per routine to document need for CABG and apparent collateral (retrograde) flow
- For each bypass target vessel, document
  - Graft body: Serially sectioned with areas of plaque, thrombus, or other stenosis selected for microscopy
  - Distal anastomosis: Serial cross sectioning along axis of either native vessel or graft body; submitted entirely
  - Distal native vessel run-off: Serial cross sectioning to evaluate potential for flow beyond target site
- Proximal anastomosis for SVG can often be inspected grossly for patency and does not routinely need to be submitted
- Decalcification often necessary prior to sectioning &/or before tissue cassette processing

MICROSCOPIC PATHOLOGY

Histologic Features

- Evaluate for plaque and thrombosis, ± recanalization
  - % stenosis, recent/organized, shallow/occlusive
- Internal mammary artery graft: Characteristic multilaminar elastic artery wall
- SVG: Single elastic layer, adventitial smooth muscle bundles
  - Arterialization
    - Distinct internal elastic lamina, intimal fibroplasia, and plaque
- Anastomosis
  - Usually elongated, "figure 8," or otherwise distorted lumen contour with part of vessel circumference made of native artery and part from graft body
  - Paired suture holes serve as useful landmarks for anastomosis ("snake eyes")

REPORTING CONSIDERATIONS

Key Elements to Report

- Report % stenosis of native target vessel, graft body, anastomosis, and distal vessel

Labeling and Nomenclature

- Convention: Label graft according to target vessel and graft body type
- Examples
  - LAD-D1-LIMA: Left internal mammary graft to 1st diagonal branch of LAD
  - LCX-OM2-SVG: Saphenous vein graft to 2nd obtuse marginal branch of LCX
  - RCA-PL-SVG: Saphenous vein graft to posterolateral branch of RCA

SELECTED REFERENCES

1. Lau GT et al: Cardiac saphenous vein bypass graft disease. Semin Vasc Med. 4(2):153-9, 2004
2. Schoen FJ: Ischemic heart disease: aortocoronary bypass grafting. In Schoen FJ: Interventional and Surgical Cardiovascular Pathology: Clinical Correlation and Basic Principles. W. B. Philadelphia: Saunders. 82-92, 1989
3. Titus JL: The heart after surgery for ischemic heart disease. Am J Cardiovasc Pathol. 1(3):339-51, 1988
4. Bulkley BH et al: Pathology of coronary artery bypass graft surgery. Arch Pathol Lab Med. 102(6):273-80, 1978

CORONARY ARTERY BYPASS GRAFTING

Gross Features

*(**Left**) This heart has had multiple cardiac procedures. External pacing wires and a left ventricular assist device inflow cannula are seen. There are also bypass grafts to the posterior descending and posterolateral coronary branches. (**Right**) This obviously dilated heart shows a sequential "T" graft with side-to-side anastomosis to the LAD (graft body mostly removed) and then continuing around to the posterolateral branch (end-to-side).*

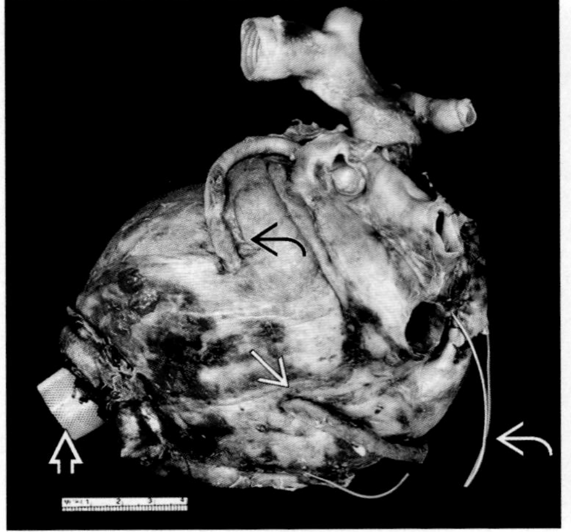

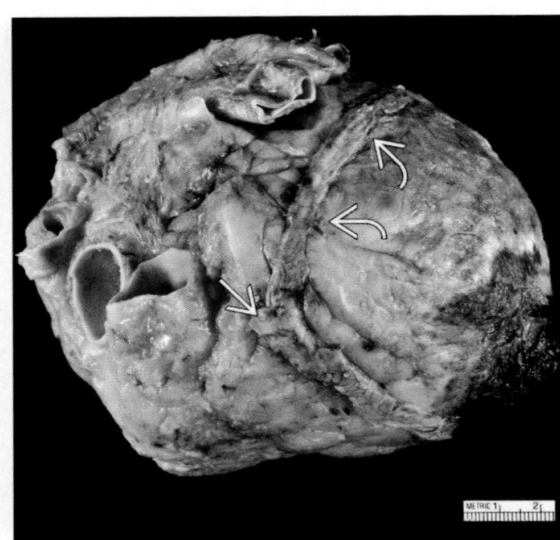

*(**Left**) This bypass graft has been dissected free from the heart. The proximal portion contains the ostium and a portion of the aorta. The distal portion includes ventricular muscle surrounding the anastomotic site. (**Right**) The distal portion of this saphenous vein graft includes a portion of the graft body. A generous tissue block is taken around the anastomotic site to avoid disrupting delicate structures. The entire anastomosis area should be sectioned and submitted.*

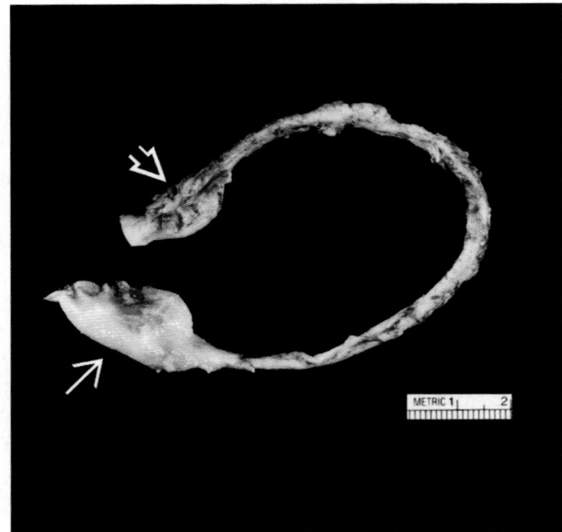

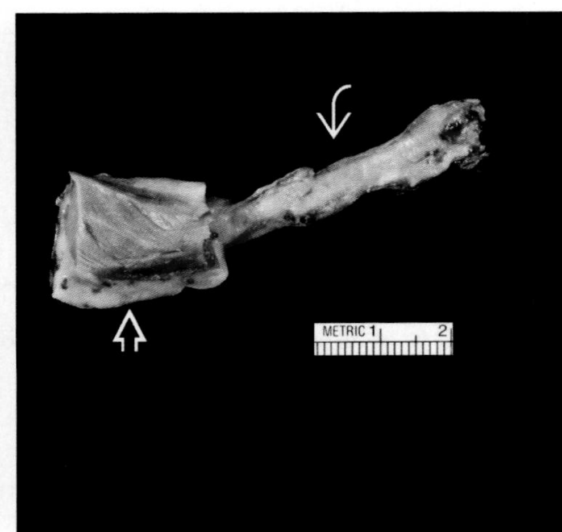

*(**Left**) Photo shows 2 separate graft anastomoses. The site can be identified by a figure 8-shaped contour. The native vessel is also seen in cross section. (**Right**) This autopsy heart specimen (shown after short-axis sectioning of the ventricles) shows 2 coronary artery bypass grafts. There is a LIMA graft to the proximal circumflex as well as a saphenous vein graft to the mid LAD.*

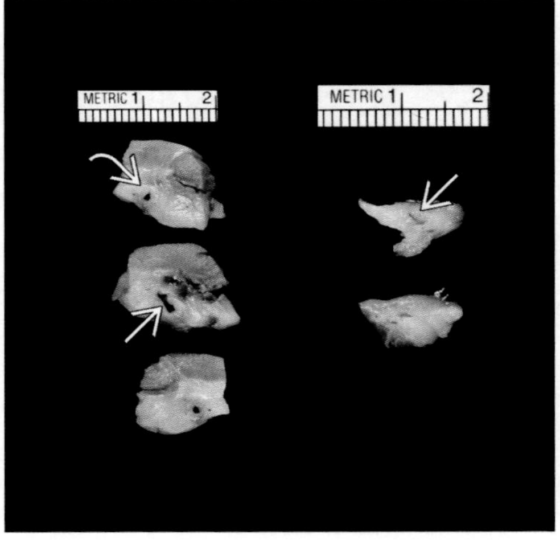

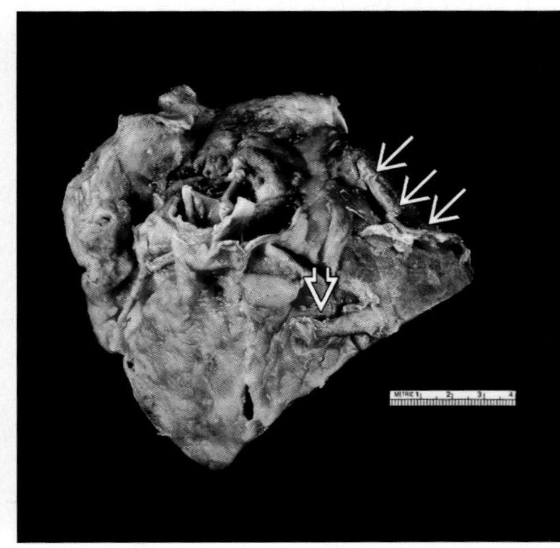

Microscopic Features

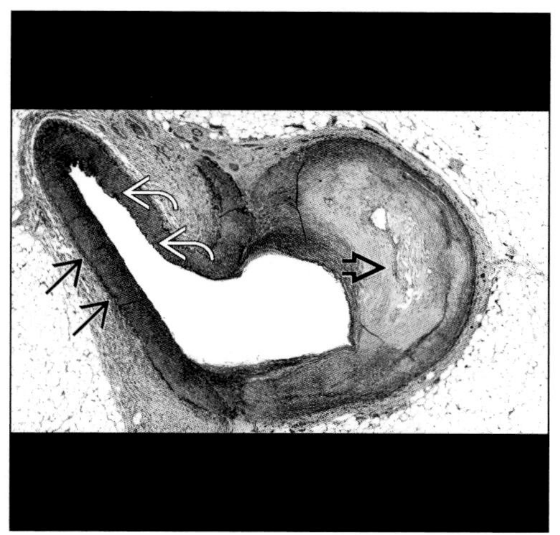

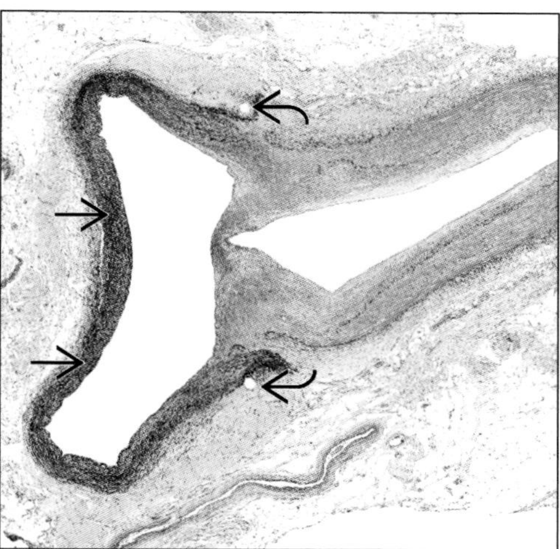

(Left) *Elastic stain section shows a muscular (radial) artery graft body characterized by distinct external and internal elastic layers. The target native vessel shows significant plaque with old plaque hemorrhage. The site is patent, without fibrous intimal ingrowth.* ***(Right)*** *Paraffin section shows a LIMA-to-LAD anastomosis. The LIMA can be identified by its characteristic multilaminar elastic wall. Paired suture holes are present at the union site.*

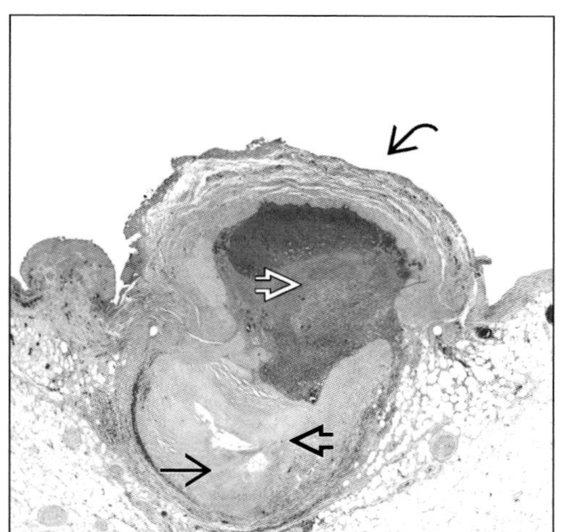

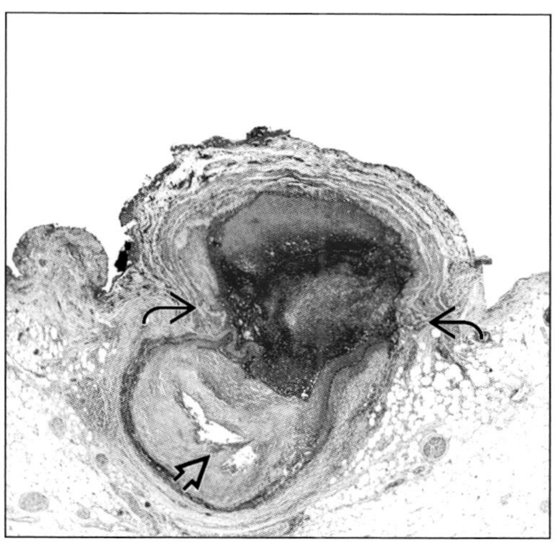

(Left) *This photomicrograph of a bypass anastomosis shows the native coronary artery with obstructive plaque forming the bottom half of the wall and the vein graft forming the top half. This graft acutely thrombosed.* ***(Right)*** *This elastic stain of the same anastomotic site illustrates how the native coronary artery can be differentiated from the vein graft by its internal elastic lamina. Suture holes are also a landmark for the anastomosis.*

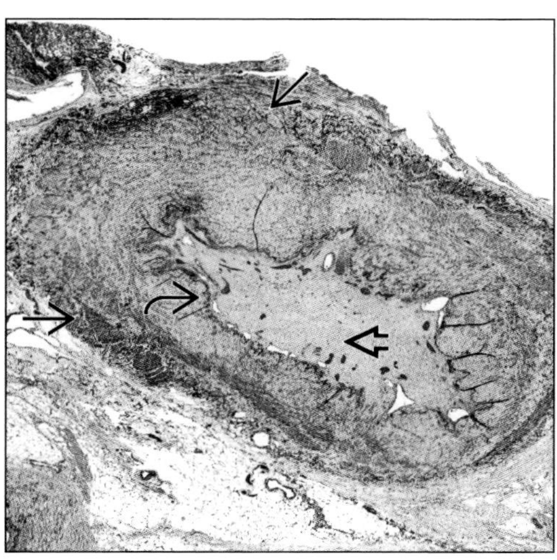

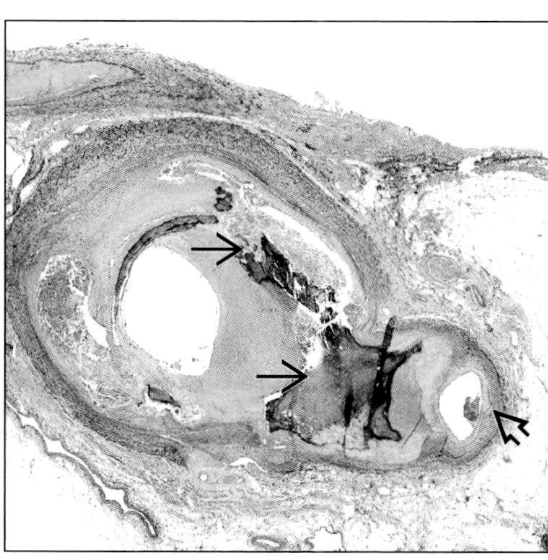

(Left) *This section of saphenous vein graft body shows old thrombotic occlusion. The vein graft has undergone "arterialization" with formation of a distinct internal elastic layer. Adventitial smooth muscle bundles confirm the venous nature of the vessel.* ***(Right)*** *This graft anastomosis site shows minor native vessel disease but severe calcific plaque involving the body and anastomotic site.*

CORONARY ARTERY STENTING

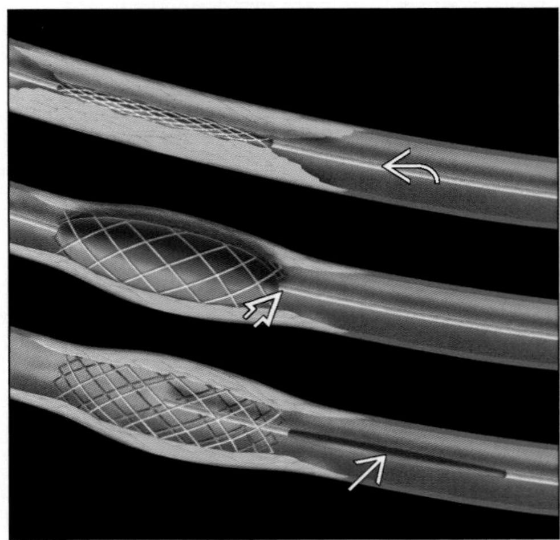

Graphic shows a deployed stent within an atherosclerotic vessel ➡, balloon inflation with dilatation of the stenotic segment ➡, and retrieval of catheter after stent placement ➡.

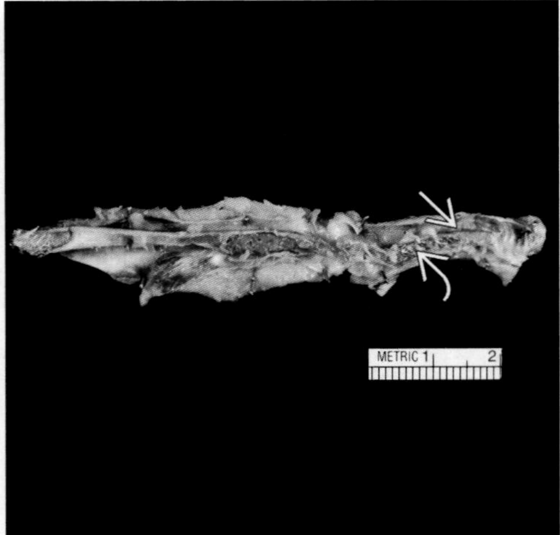

Photograph of multiple stents in a coronary artery dissected from an explanted heart shows exposed stent struts ➡ and struts enveloped in neointimal tissue ➡. This method of stent examination is not advised.

TERMINOLOGY

Definitions

- Stents are prosthetic intraluminal tubular metal scaffold devices designed to maintain lumen patency in setting of underlying intrinsic or extrinsic coronary artery disease
  - Can be deployed by inflation of balloon-tipped endovascular catheter
    - Balloon inflation disrupts vessel wall plaque and expands lumen
    - Stent holds lumen open
  - Different metals used
    - Surgical-grade stainless steel
    - Metal alloys (cobalt-chromium, platinum-chromium, nickel-titanium [nitinol])
  - May be "bare metal" or coated with drug-eluting polymers (CYPHER [sirolimus], TAXUS [paclitaxel], XIENCE V [everolimus]) designed to inhibit neointimal growth

CLINICAL IMPLICATIONS

Indications

- Primary therapy for coronary atherosclerosis
  - Revascularization therapy in acute myocardial infarction
  - Bailout procedure for abrupt or threatened artery closure due to arterial dissection or following angioplasty
- Also attempted in some cases of cardiac allograft vasculopathy

Complications

- Reocclusion/restenosis of stented coronary artery segments (in-stent restenosis) occurs in 5-30% of cases
  - Early restenosis usually results from acute thrombosis
  - Late restenosis results from concentric neointimal growth or thrombosis

MACROSCOPIC FINDINGS

External Examination

- If recent intervention, inspect percutaneous cannulation site (groin, wrist, or neck) for hematoma or vascular complication
- Other scars indicating cardiac interventions
  - Median sternotomy
  - Other thoracotomy
  - Saphenous vein or radial artery harvesting

Internal Examination

- Heart
  - Identify and carefully dissect internal mammary graft conduits, if present
  - Coronary arteries can be examined in situ or dissected free from heart
  - Care should be taken not to crush or excessively bend stented artery segments (artifactual fracturing)
  - Specimen radiograph of entire heart vs. dissected coronaries

Organ Examination

- Specimen radiographs should be used to delineate stents within cardiovascular specimens
  - Radiographs are important to assess stent expansion and determine whether stent was abnormally compressed during deployment
  - Total stented length and curvature should be documented since these correlate with risk of restenosis
  - Any apparent stent strut fractures should also be noted
- Evaluation for restenosis is made difficult by metallic stents that cannot be cut by conventional methods (scissors, scalpels, or conventional microtome blades)

- Disruption of normal histoarchitecture (especially stent-tissue interface) will occur if conventional methods are attempted
- Avoid attempts to cut through stents with scissors or scalpel
- Trim stented vessel by cutting proximal and distal to stent
- Fix stented segment in formalin prior to special handling

MICROSCOPIC FINDINGS

Methods of Stent Sectioning for Microscopy

- Plastic resin embedding and diamond or tungsten carbide blade microtomy
  - Stented vessel tissue fixed and embedded in rigid methacrylate resin (as used in transmission electron microscopy) microtomy
  - Cut using conventional microtome equipped with special blade hard enough to cut metal stents
- Diamond saw microtome
  - Stented vessel tissue fixed and embedded in plastic and cut with high-speed diamond saw with precision movement capable of cutting ~ 10 μm sections
    - Used in undecalcified bone mineral density samples
- Sawing and grinding
  - Stented vessel tissue fixed and embedded in plastic then subject to 2-stage process of sawing into ~ 100 μm sections that are mounted with adhesive to glass slide
  - Slide is then placed in sanding/grinding device that progressively erodes thick section down to < 10 μm thickness
- Reverse electroplating
  - Prior to embedding, fixed stented vessel is placed in acid-salt solution, and electrodes are connected to stent metal
  - Current is applied in such a way that stent metal dissolves by electrolysis
  - Vessel can then be sectioned with scalpel and submitted for routine paraffin sectioning

Histologic Features

- Stented artery assessments should focus on both native vessel disease and any neointimal growth within stent
  - Estimated cross-sectional area stenosis as well as plaque composition (fibrous, calcific, smooth muscle, lipid, necrosis, etc.) should be reported
- Artery sections immediately distal and proximal to stent should also be examined and reported
- Early complications
  - Rupture of thin-cap atheromas induced by balloon inflation can lead to atherothrombosis or atheroemboli
  - Lipid core penetration by struts is associated with increased acute/chronic inflammation and neointimal growth
  - Malapposition of struts relative to vessel wall
  - Fibrin and platelet aggregation is seen commonly around struts during 1st week
  - Elastic lamina disruption, a consequence of balloon inflation, is common and does not indicate vasculitis
- Late complications
  - Smooth muscle-rich neointimal proliferation may significantly occlude lumen
  - Late stent thrombosis is usually associated with malapposed struts or delayed incorporation
  - Multinucleated giant cells around struts are more common after 30 days

SELECTED REFERENCES

1. Stone JR et al: Recommendations for processing cardiovascular surgical pathology specimens: a consensus statement from the Standards and Definitions Committee of the Society for Cardiovascular Pathology and the Association for European Cardiovascular Pathology. Cardiovasc Pathol. 21(1):2-16, 2012
2. Nakazawa G et al: The pathology of neoatherosclerosis in human coronary implants bare-metal and drug-eluting stents. J Am Coll Cardiol. 57(11):1314-22, 2011
3. Bradshaw SH et al: A practical method to rapidly dissolve metallic stents. Cardiovasc Pathol. 18(3):127-33, 2009
4. Nakazawa G et al: A review of current devices and a look at new technology: drug-eluting stents. Expert Rev Med Devices. 6(1):33-42, 2009
5. Lüscher TF et al: Drug-eluting stent and coronary thrombosis: biological mechanisms and clinical implications. Circulation. 115(8):1051-8, 2007
6. Rippstein P et al: Comparison of processing and sectioning methodologies for arteries containing metallic stents. J Histochem Cytochem. 54(6):673-81, 2006
7. Farb A et al: Morphological predictors of restenosis after coronary stenting in humans. Circulation. 105(25):2974-80, 2002

Microscopic Features

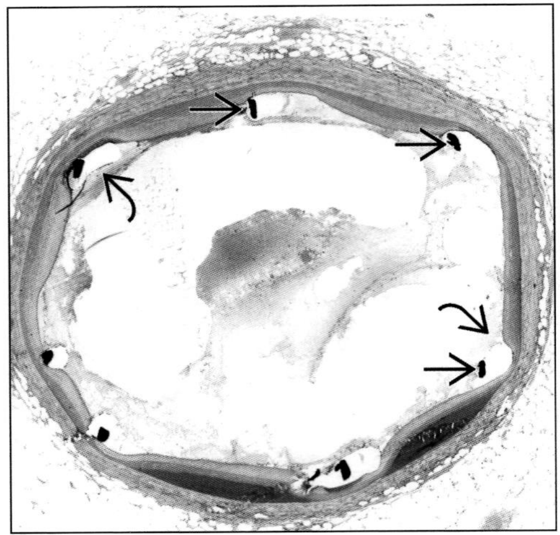

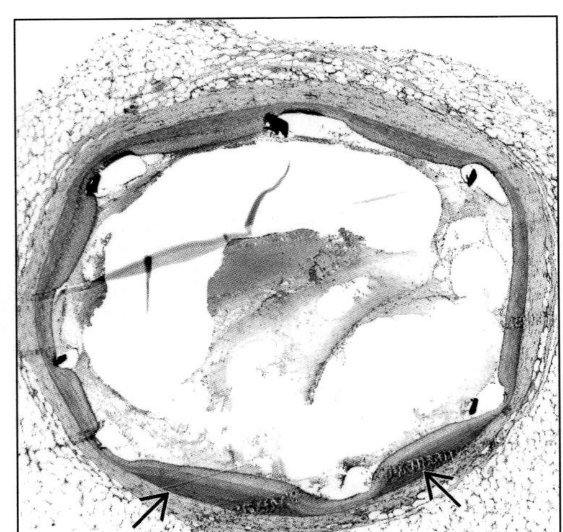

*(**Left**) Plastic-embedded cross section of a stented coronary artery from an experimental model (without atherosclerosis) demonstrates proper apposition of stent struts ⇒ to the vessel wall, causing some indentation ⇒ and polygonal distortion of the circular lumen. (**Right**) Elastic-stained section of a stented coronary artery from an experimental model highlights a small dissection in the vessel ⇒ resulting from balloon inflation during stent deployment. This is a recognized acute complication of the procedure.*

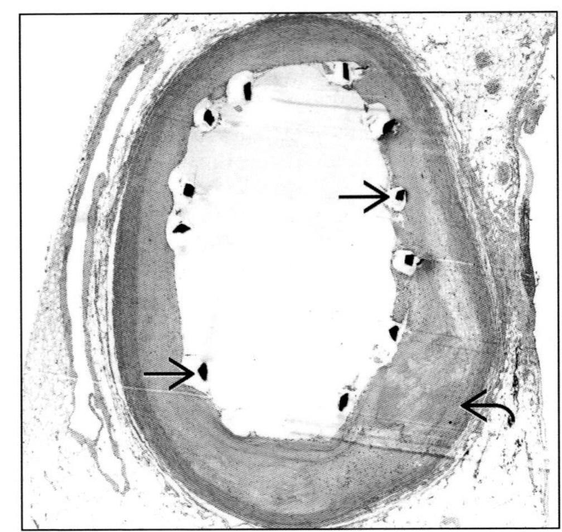

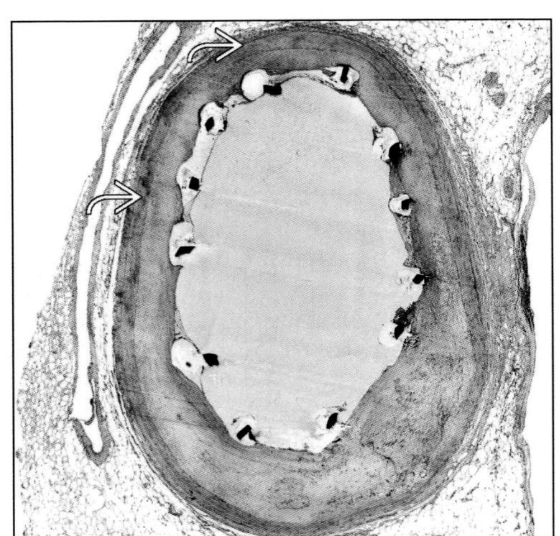

*(**Left**) Plastic-embedded cross section of a previously atherosclerotic plaque ⇒ coronary artery is shown. There has been little to no neointimal formation, suggesting that the stent was placed very recently. The stent struts ⇒ are well apposed to the wall. (**Right**) Elastic-stained plastic section of a stented coronary artery highlights the internal elastic lamina ⇒ and intimal localization of atherosclerosis and the absence of neointima formation.*

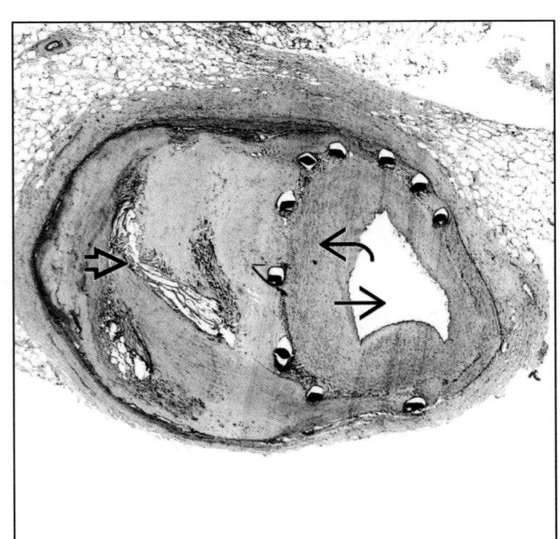

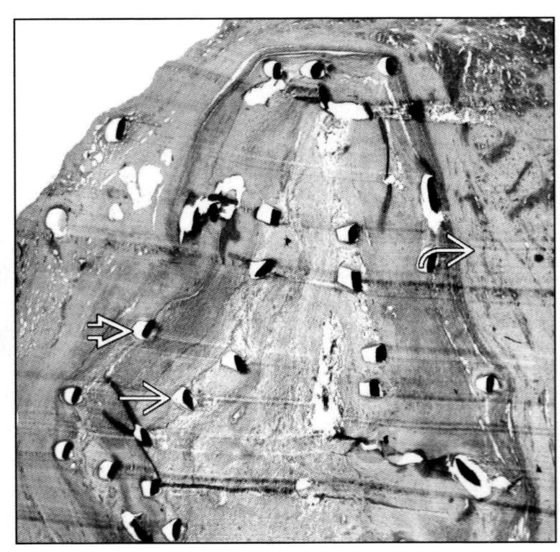

*(**Left**) Elastic-stained plastic section of a stented coronary artery shows a significant native plaque ⇒, which obstructs > 75% of the original lumen, and in-stent restenosis caused by concentric neointimal ingrowth ⇒ further restricting the lumen ⇒. (**Right**) Movat-stained plastic section shows a stent within a stent. There is a native plaque ⇒, a neointimal stenosis of the original (outer) stent ⇒, and a 2nd inner stent ⇒ that was placed later, also showing significant stenosis.*

Microscopic Features and Ancillary Techniques

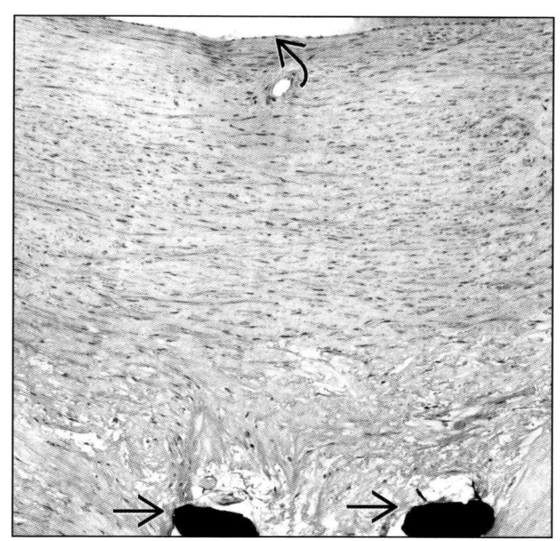

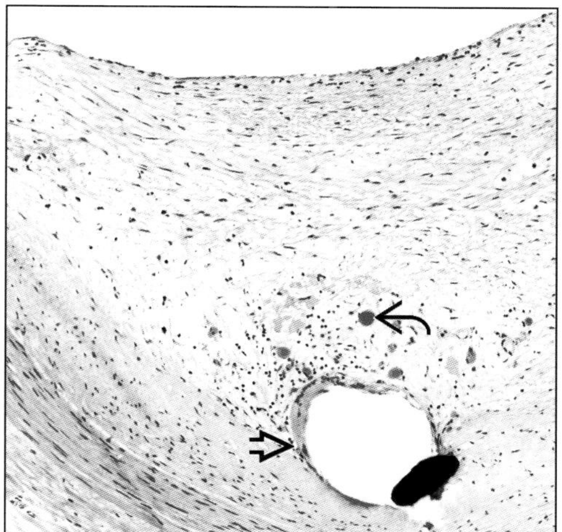

(Left) *Plastic-embedded coronary artery section shows 2 stent struts* ➙ *marking the original stented lumen boundary and substantial smooth muscle-rich neointimal ingrowth extending to the residual lumen* ➙ *at the top.* ***(Right)*** *Plastic section of stented coronary artery shows neointimal growth with neovascularization* ➙ *and inflammation* ➙ *surrounding the strut.*

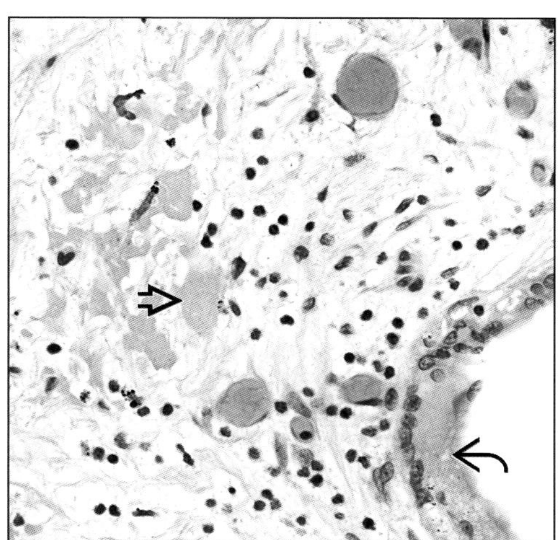

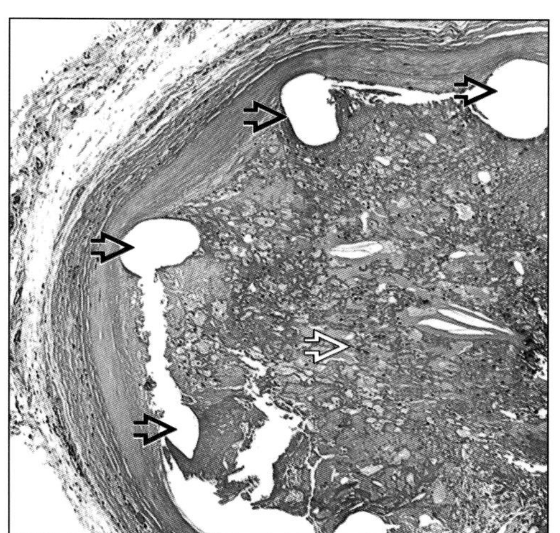

(Left) *Higher magnification of the peri-strut neointimal tissue of a stented coronary artery highlights wisps of fibrin* ➙*, sparse mononuclear cells, and a giant cell foreign body reaction* ➙*.* ***(Right)*** *Paraffin section of a stented coronary artery after reverse electroplating to remove the metallic struts shows empty "holes"* ➙*. Atherothrombosis* ➙*, which had resulted from rupture of a thin-cap soft-core plaque during stent deployment, occludes the lumen.*

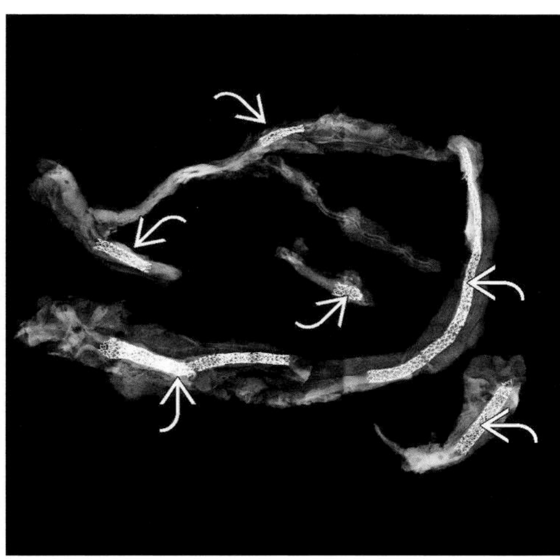

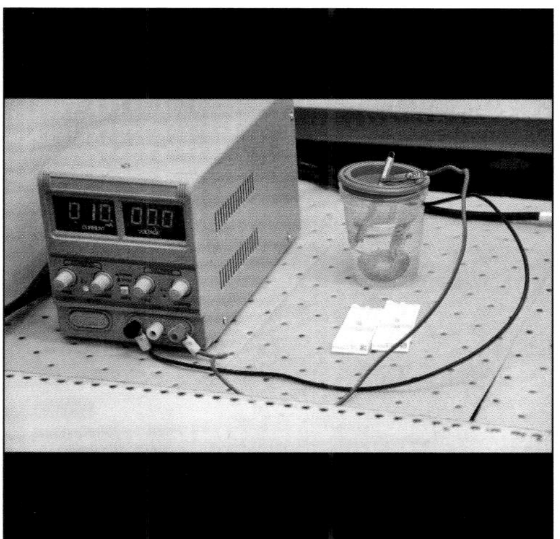

(Left) *This specimen radiograph of coronary arteries dissected free from the heart at autopsy helps facilitate further sectioning of the vessels and appropriate processing of stents* ➙*. They also allow for identification of possible stent strut fractures.* ***(Right)*** *Photograph shows an apparatus for dissolving metallic stents from coronary artery specimens using reverse electroplating. Current is applied to the stent in an artery submerged in acid-salt solution after formalin fixation.*

VALVE REPLACEMENT (INCLUDING TRANSCATHETER)

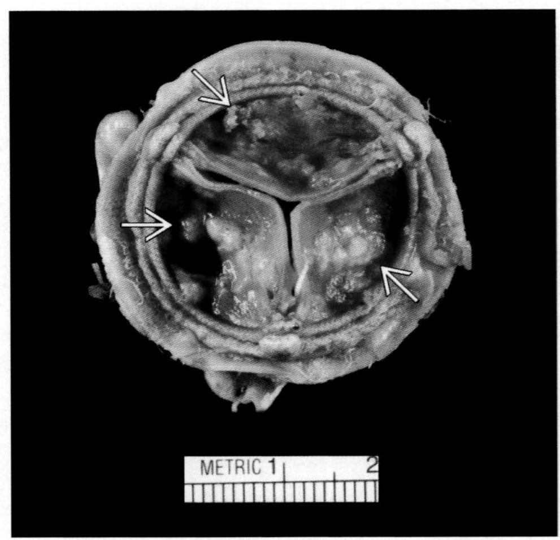

Cusp degeneration is a common cause of failure of bioprosthetic valves. Note nodular calcified deposits ➡ on the cusps of this bovine pericardial bioprosthesis, which resulted in valve stenosis.

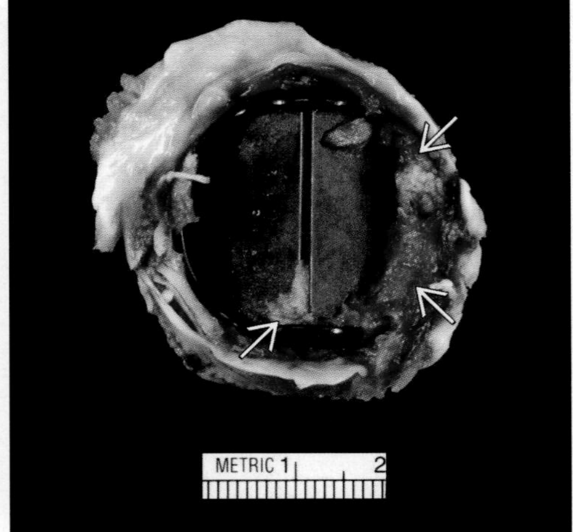

Infective endocarditis may involve prosthetic valves of any type. Here, vegetations ➡ have formed on a bileaflet mechanical valve, restricting leaflet mobility and causing severe stenosis.

TERMINOLOGY

Abbreviations

- Prosthetic valve (infective) endocarditis (PVE)
- Transcatheter aortic valve replacement (TAVR)

Major Types of Prosthetic Valves

- Mechanical
  - Ball-in-cage
  - Tilting disc
  - Bileaflet
- Bioprosthetic
  - Porcine
  - Bovine pericardial
  - Cadaveric homograft
- Catheter-deployed bioprosthetic
  - Edwards SAPIEN
  - Medtronic CoreValve
  - Medtronic Melody
  - Others
- Other devices
  - MitraClip (for percutaneous mitral valve repair)

Hemodynamic Categories of Failure

- Prosthetic valve stenosis
- Prosthetic valve regurgitation

CLINICAL ISSUES

Clinical Overview

- Selection of type of valve prosthesis driven by combination of patient factors and inherent advantages and disadvantages of each prosthesis
- Type of prosthesis will determine which complications might be seen during autopsy
- Mechanical prosthetic valves
  - Advantages: Excellent durability (most remain functional for 20-30 years)
  - Disadvantages: Require lifelong anticoagulation (risk of hemorrhage, teratogenicity in women of child-bearing age), hemolytic anemia from mechanical trauma to RBCs
- Bioprosthetic valves
  - Advantages: No anticoagulation required
  - Disadvantages: Structural deterioration common (30-35% fail within 10-15 years)
- Catheter-deployed bioprosthetic valves
  - Advantages: Less invasive (used for patients with high surgical risk), may be used when surgery is technically challenging or impossible; valve-in-valve procedures possible
  - Disadvantages: Higher risk of stroke, long-term durability unknown, numerous unique complications as outlined below

Patient History Review

- Clinical, operative, and echocardiography reports may delineate complications, anatomy, and hemodynamic abnormalities
  - Review thereof can guide postmortem evaluation of prosthetic valve

Etiology of Prosthetic Valve Failure

- Thrombosis
  - More common with mechanical valves (inadequate anticoagulation)
  - May cause stenosis &/or regurgitation
  - May be complicated by embolism and downstream infarcts
- Structural deterioration
  - Primarily involves bioprosthetic valves
  - Cusp calcification usually causes stenosis
  - Cusp tear causes regurgitation
    - Usually tear occurs at commissure
    - Results in cusp prolapse
- Paravalvular leak
  - May occur with any type of prosthetic valve
  - Results in regurgitation

VALVE REPLACEMENT (INCLUDING TRANSCATHETER)

Key Facts

Clinical Issues

- Type of prosthesis will determine which complications may be seen at autopsy
- Mechanical: Very durable, but requires anticoagulation
- Bioprosthetic: No anticoagulation, but structural deterioration common
- Catheter-deployed: Less invasive, but numerous unique complications
- Failure may cause stenosis &/or regurgitation
- Failure may affect heart, lungs, and other organs

Macroscopic Pathology

- Causes of prosthetic valve failure:
- Thrombosis (esp. mechanical valves)
- Structural deterioration (esp. bioprosthetic valves)
- Paravalvular leak (all valves)
- Pannus formation (all valves)
- Infective endocarditis (all valves)
- Incomplete expansion (catheter-deployed only)
- Suboptimal seating (catheter-deployed only)
- Other complications: Hemorrhage, embolism, infarcts, hemolytic anemia, etc.
- Autopsy performance considerations
- Submit vegetations for microbiologic cultures
- Examine prosthetic valves from both sides
- Examine for perivalvular leaks, annular abscesses
- Obtain radiographs to evaluate cusp calcification, integrity of metallic components (e.g. struts)
- Photograph abnormalities
- Evaluate for secondary cardiac/pulmonary disease
- Submit vegetations, perforations, abscesses, thrombi, and adherent tissues for microscopy

- Pannus formation
  - May occur with any type of prosthetic valve
  - Annular fibrous ingrowth causes stenosis
- Infective endocarditis
  - May occur with any type of prosthetic valve
  - Causes regurgitation if valve structures are destroyed (e.g., perforations, cusp tears) or if surrounding native tissue is involved (with valve dehiscence)
  - Causes stenosis if vegetations are large
  - Infectious agents
    - *Staphylococcus epidermidis*
    - *Staphylococcus aureus*
    - Streptococci
    - Gram-negative bacilli
    - Fungi
  - Bioprosthetic infective endocarditis
    - May involve cusps &/or sewing ring
    - Sometimes complicated by annular abscess
  - Mechanical prosthetic infective endocarditis
    - Vegetations involve sewing ring
    - Usually complicated by annular abscess
  - Annular abscess
    - May burrow, perforate, &/or cause valve dehiscence
    - May extend to involve other valves
    - High operative mortality rate
  - Septic embolism
    - May cause sterile or infected infarcts in downstream sites

Complications Specific to Catheter-Deployed Valves

- Incomplete expansion
  - Proper leaflet coaptation requires full expansion to predesigned functional circumference
  - Incomplete expansion may cause "tenting" of cusps and fixed regurgitation
  - Overexpansion rarely seen given usual calcification and sclerosis of aortic annulus in aortic stenosis
- Suboptimal seating and attachment failure
  - Proper function requires alignment at level of anatomic annulus
  - Improperly seated valves become loose and embolize distally
- Embolization of calcified debris from native cusps
  - Dislodged during balloon expansion prior to valve deployment
  - May cause strokes or infarcts in downstream organs
- Inverted orientation
  - Valve deployed via transfemoral or transapical approach; must be properly oriented in catheter sheath to prevent inverted (backward) deployment
  - Rare, but may be fatal
- Annular rupture
  - Rare, but may be fatal; due to aggressive balloon predilatation
- Coronary ostial obstruction with myocardial infarction
  - Rare; due to device itself or calcified debris from native aortic valve
- Complications specific to transapical approach
  - Hemopericardium with cardiac tamponade
  - Damage to mitral valve
  - Left ventricular pseudoaneurysm formation
  - Left ventricular arrhythmias
- Complications specific to transfemoral approach
  - Aortofemoral injury/rupture
  - Distal embolization of dislodged femoral, iliac, or aortic atherosclerotic plaque

Other Complications

- Hemorrhage
  - Primarily with mechanical valves (due to anticoagulation)
- Embolism and infarcts
  - Due to thrombosis or infective endocarditis
- Teratogenic effects
  - Primarily with mechanical valves (due to warfarin)
- Hemolytic anemia
  - Primarily with mechanical valves (due to mechanical trauma to red blood cells)

VALVE REPLACEMENT (INCLUDING TRANSCATHETER)

MACROSCOPIC FEATURES

External Examination

- If recent surgical intervention, inspect incision site for signs of infection (purulence, necrosis, dehiscence)
- If recent transcatheter intervention, inspect percutaneous cannulation site (groin, small left thoracotomy) for hematoma or vascular complication
- Other scars indicating previous cardiac interventions
  - Median sternotomy
  - Other thoracotomy
  - Saphenous vein or radial artery harvesting

Internal Examination

- Brain and other viscera
  - Evaluate for infarcts due to embolization of valve thrombus or vegetations
- Lungs
  - Evaluate for edema or other evidence of congestive heart failure due to failed valve prosthesis
- Body cavities
  - Evaluate for evidence of procedure complications (e.g., hemopericardium, hemothorax)

Organ Examination

- Heart
  - Evaluate for disease of prosthetic valve
    - Carefully remove great vessels &/or atria to expose valves ("base of heart" dissection method)
    - If vegetations or annular abscesses are present, obtain material in sterile fashion for microbiologic cultures
    - Examine prosthetic valves from both sides (inflow and outflow)
    - Examine perivalvular tissues for abnormalities (e.g., perivalvular leaks, annular abscesses)
  - Evaluate for evidence of valvular heart disease
    - Record heart weight and standard measurements: LV, RV, septal wall thicknesses; LV internal short-axis chamber diameter, RV internal short-axis chamber dimensions, annular circumferences of native valves
    - Cardiac disease may be caused by native valve disease, prosthetic valve abnormalities, or both
  - Examples of secondary cardiac effects of common valve diseases
    - Aortic stenosis: LV pressure hypertrophy **without** LV dilatation; LA dilatation; RV/RA dilatation
    - Aortic regurgitation: LV pressure and volume hypertrophy with massive 4-chamber dilatation
    - Mitral stenosis: Normal LV, massive LA dilatation, RV/RA dilatation
    - Mitral regurgitation: LV pressure and volume hypertrophy with 4-chamber dilatation
  - Evaluate for other coexisting cardiovascular abnormalities
- Specimen radiography
  - Useful to determine extent of cusp calcification
  - Useful to evaluate for strut fractures and incomplete expansion of catheter-deployed valves
- Photograph abnormalities whenever possible
  - Valuable for medicolegal and educational purposes
- At minimum, submit the following abnormalities for microscopy
  - Vegetations, cusp perforations, other features suggestive of infection
  - Annular abscesses
  - Thrombi (to evaluate for infection)
  - Any other tissue adherent to device

MICROSCOPIC PATHOLOGY

Histologic Features

- Infective endocarditis
  - Abundant thrombotic material with destruction of prosthetic valve tissue, necrosis
  - Dense neutrophilic, lymphoplasmacytic, or granulomatous inflammation
  - Microorganisms may or may not be visualized
  - Stains for microorganisms (e.g., Gram, GMS) can help, but negative result does not rule out infection
- Thrombi
  - Recent thrombi show laminated appearance, with alternating layers of RBCs/WBCs and platelets/fibrin
  - Older thrombi show organization with capillary proliferation
  - Microorganisms and dense neutrophilic inflammation are absent

SELECTED REFERENCES

1. Bourantas CV et al: Evolution of transcatheter aortic valve replacement. Circ Res. 114(6):1037-51, 2014
2. Lardizabal JA et al: The transaortic approach for transcatheter aortic valve replacement: initial clinical experience in the United States. J Am Coll Cardiol. 61(23):2341-5, 2013
3. Webb JG et al: Current status of transcatheter aortic valve replacement. J Am Coll Cardiol. 60(6):483-92, 2012
4. Lee JH et al: Prosthetic valve endocarditis: clinicopathological correlates in 122 surgical specimens from 116 patients (1985-2004). Cardiovasc Pathol. 20(1):26-35, 2011
5. Pibarot P et al: Prosthetic heart valves: selection of the optimal prosthesis and long-term management. Circulation. 119(7):1034-48, 2009
6. Siddiqui RF et al: Bioprosthetic heart valves: modes of failure. Histopathology. 55(2):135-44, 2009
7. Butany J et al: Analysis of prosthetic cardiac devices: a guide for the practising pathologist. J Clin Pathol. 58(2):113-24, 2005
8. Kent PD et al: Temporal changes in the surgical pathology of prosthetic aortic valves: a study of 157 cases spanning 26 years (1970-1995). Cardiovasc Pathol. 7(1):9-23, 1998
9. Milano A et al: Valve-related complications in elderly patients with biological and mechanical aortic valves. Ann Thorac Surg. 66(6 Suppl):S82-7, 1998
10. Cohn LH et al: Fifteen-year experience with 1678 Hancock porcine bioprosthetic heart valve replacements. Ann Surg. 210(4):435-42; discussion 442-3, 1989

Gross Findings

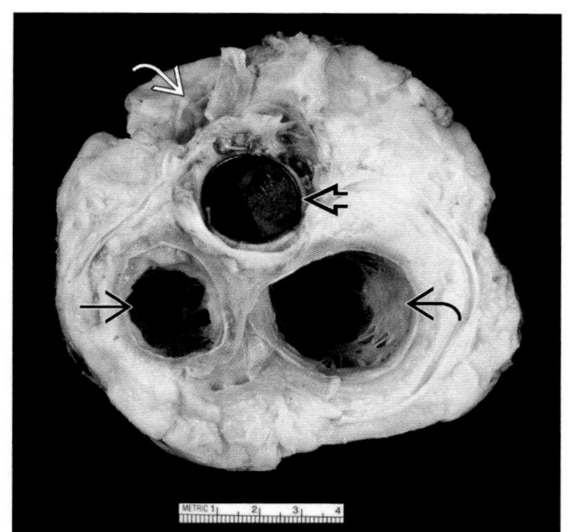

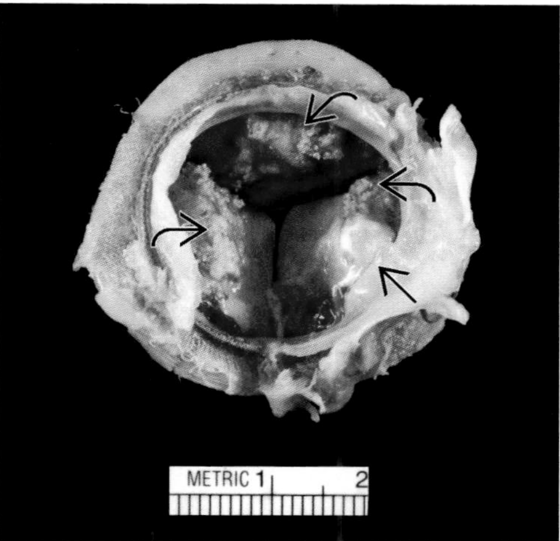

*(**Left**) Visualization of prosthetic valves is facilitated by the "base of heart" dissection method, whereby the atria are removed, revealing all four valves. Note a bileaflet mechanical prosthetic valve ⇨ in the aortic position, as well as native tricuspid ↷, mitral →, and pulmonary ➔ valves. (**Right**) Fibrocalcific degeneration of all 3 prosthetic cusps ↷ and formation of pannus → on the surface of one cusp resulted in stenosis of this bioprosthetic aortic valve.*

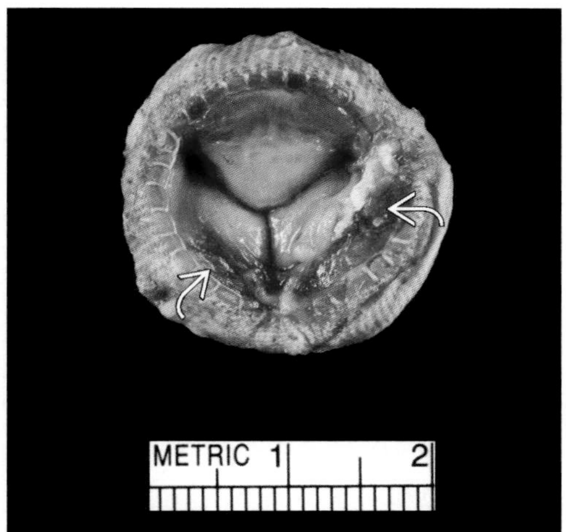

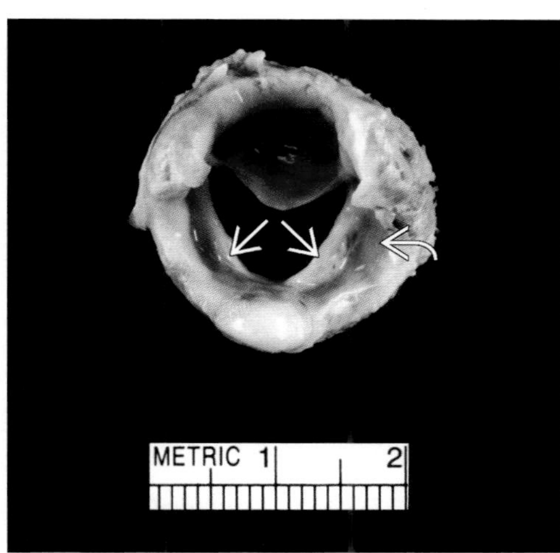

*(**Left**) Although more common on mechanical valves, thrombus ➔ may also form on the cusps of bioprosthetic valves, causing significant stenosis and potentially resulting in embolism and infarcts downstream. (**Right**) Structural degeneration is an important cause of failure of bioprosthetic valves. Here, significant fibrotic retraction ➔ of 2 cusps has resulted in torrential regurgitation of this porcine bioprosthetic valve. Also note focal pannus formation ➔ adjacent to one cusp.*

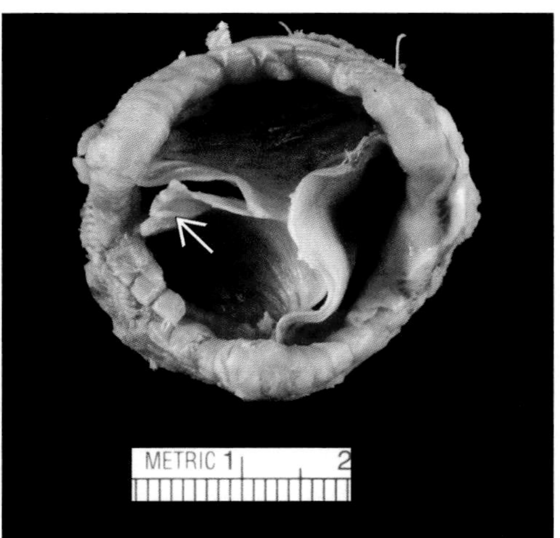

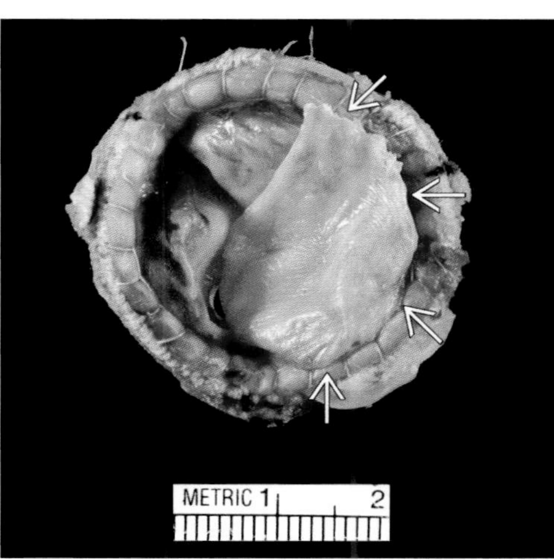

*(**Left**) Structural degeneration of bioprosthetic valves may also result in cusp tears, which usually form at commissures where mechanical strain and wear on the prosthetic cusp are greatest. Here, a large cusp tear ➔ has formed on this porcine bioprosthetic valve, resulting in severe regurgitation. (**Right**) On the reverse (inflow) side of this same valve, the extent of cusp tearing is more evident. The tear ➔ involves nearly the entire annular attachment of the involved cusp.*

Infection: Gross and Microscopic Features

(Left) *Dehiscence is an important cause of prosthetic valve failure. Here, dehiscence → of a cadaveric valved aortic homograft has resulted in formation of a perivalvular fibrotic cavity →.* **(Right)** *Infective endocarditis can involve valve prostheses of all types. Hemodynamic consequences include both regurgitation and stenosis, depending on the size of vegetation and status of the cusps. Here, vegetations → have resulted in perforation → of one cusp, causing regurgitation.*

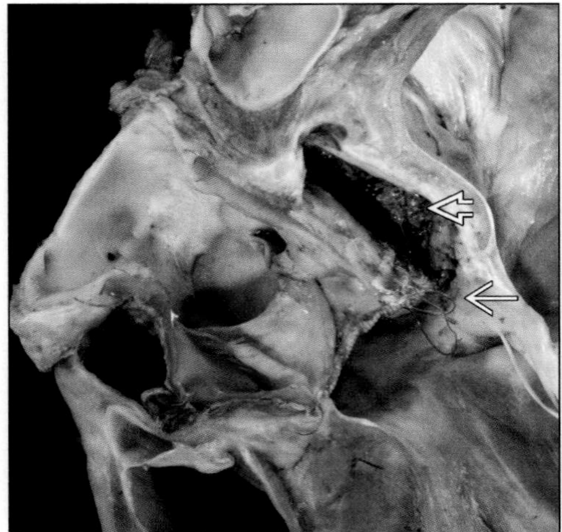

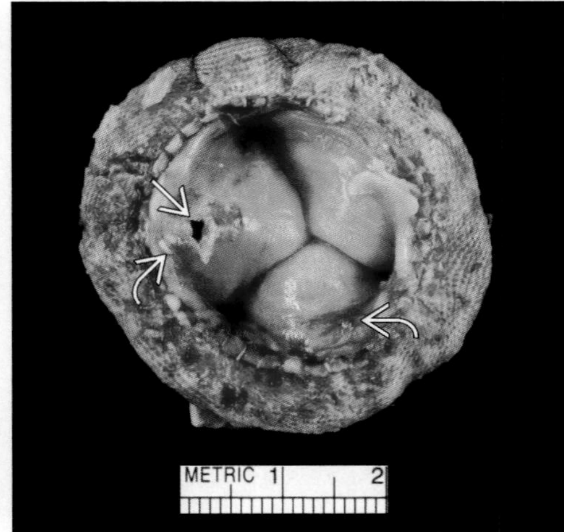

(Left) *In contrast, large infective vegetations → may obstruct the valve orifice and result in significant prosthetic valve stenosis.* **(Right)** *Infective endocarditis may also involve mechanical valves, as in this case where bulky vegetations → restrict mobility of the prosthetic leaflets, resulting in severe stenosis. Cultures and histologic sections should be obtained to confirm the infectious nature of the process and to identify the culprit microorganism.*

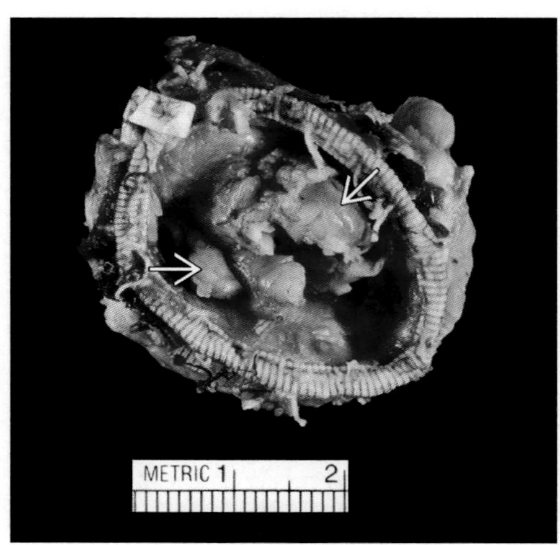

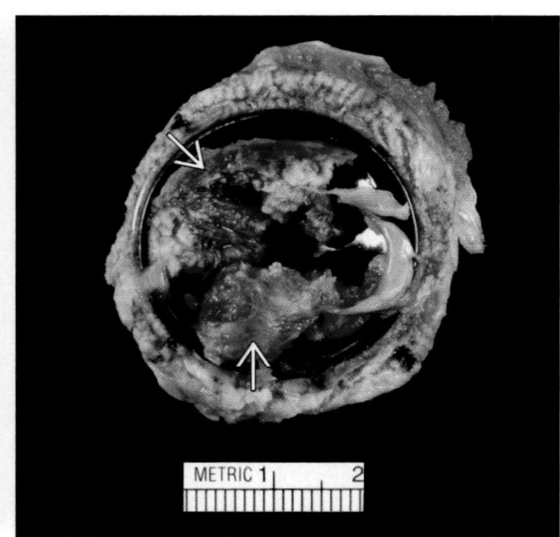

(Left) *Histologically, infective endocarditis involving a bovine pericardial bioprosthetic valve shows destruction of the cusp →, with adherent fibrin-rich thrombotic vegetation material → containing numerous irregular "fuzzy" bacterial colonies →.* **(Right)** *A tissue Gram stain highlights Gram-positive bacterial colonies within the thrombotic vegetation →, and also within the partially destroyed cusp →. Cultures confirmed the presence of Propionibacterium acnes.*

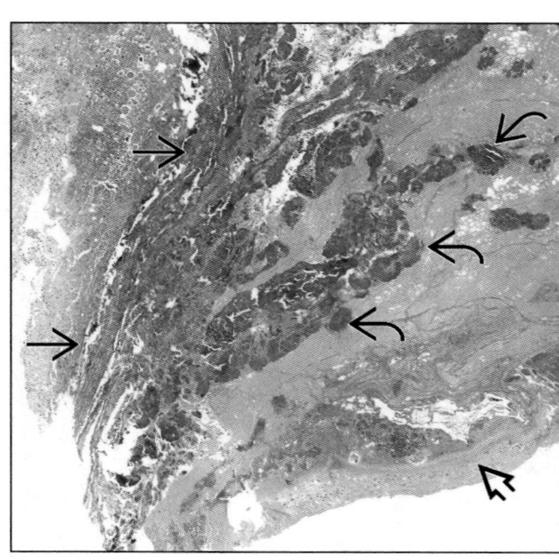

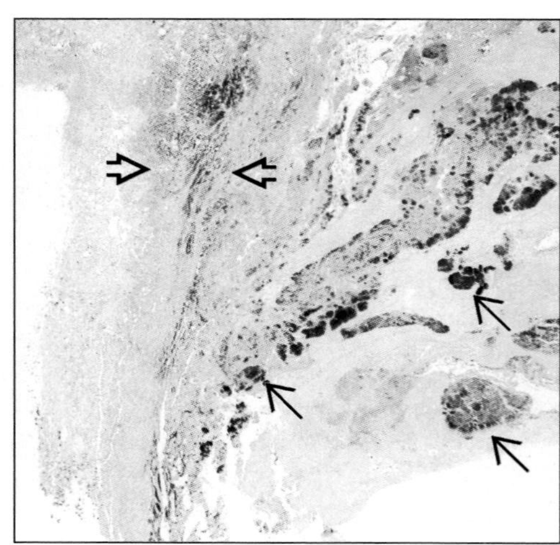

Gross Findings of Transcatheter Devices

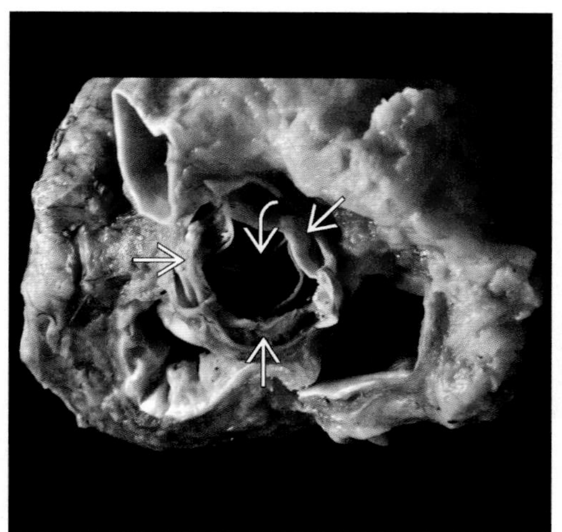

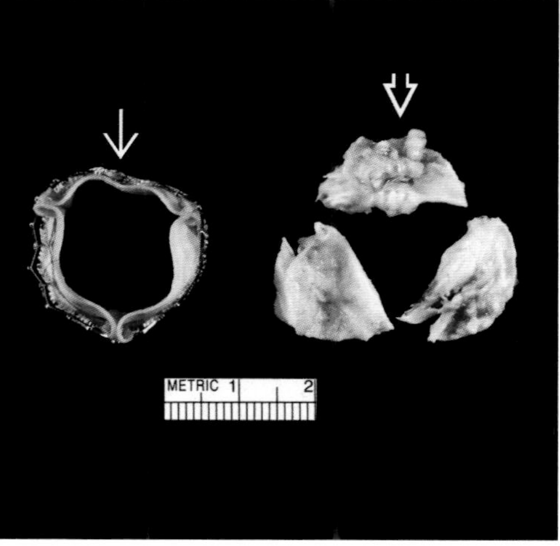

(Left) *Catheter-deployed bioprosthetic valves are positioned within a diseased valve, without surgical removal thereof. Here, the atria have been removed, revealing a catheter-deployed bioprosthesis ➔ within a diseased aortic valve. Native cusps ➔ have been pushed aside by balloon dilatation prior to deployment of the device.* ***(Right)*** *Here, a catheter-deployed SAPIEN bioprosthetic valve ➔ is displayed alongside the excised calcified aortic valve cusps ➔ that surrounded it.*

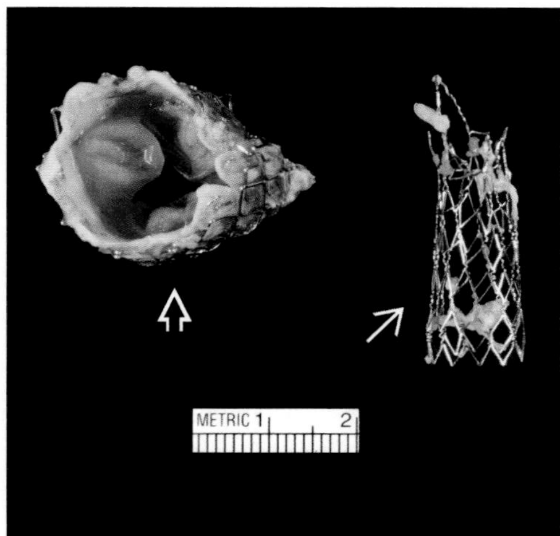

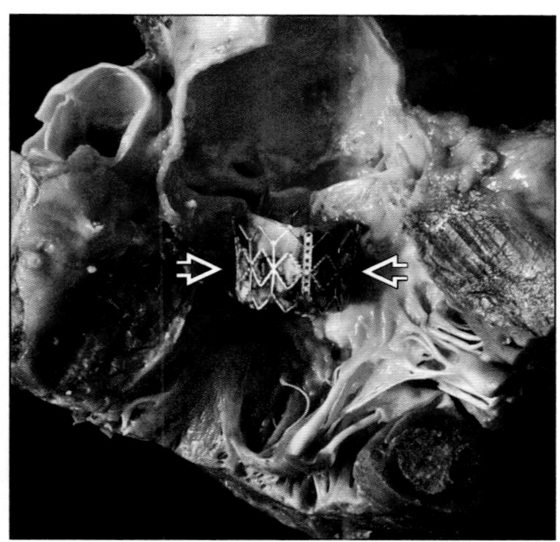

(Left) *This patient with Tetralogy of Fallot underwent stenting ➔ of the RV outflow tract and deployment of a Melody valve ➔. Devices should be assessed for deformation and strut fractures, which in this case were due to surgical removal.* ***(Right)*** *This catheter-deployed bioprosthesis ➔ was properly seated within the aortic valve annulus. Autopsy evaluation should include assessment of device position, expansion, cusp coaptation, and the potential for perivalvular leaks.*

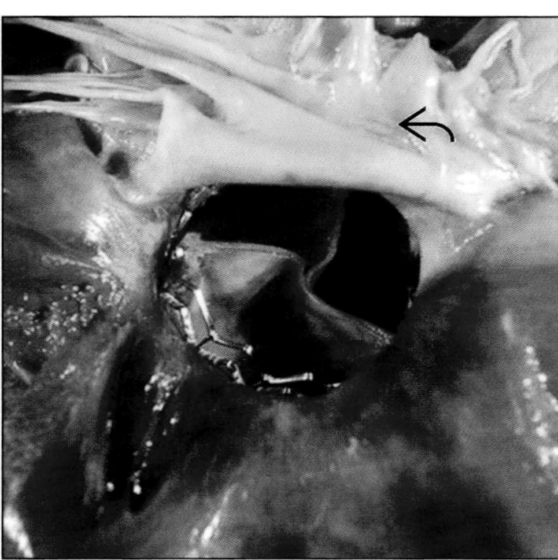

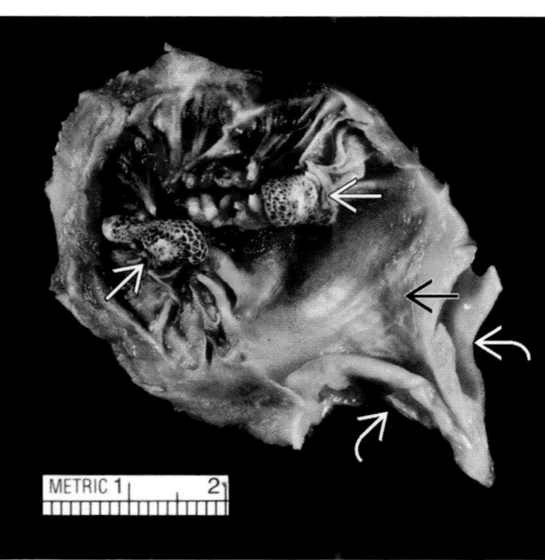

(Left) *Catheter-deployed valves may be placed transfemorally or transapically, and must be properly oriented in the catheter sheath to prevent inverted (backward) deployment, as occurred in this unfortunate fatal case. Note anterior mitral leaflet ➔.* ***(Right)*** *This mitral valve is shown from the ventricular side. Two MitraClip devices ➔ were used to fix the anterior leaflet to segments of the posterior leaflet. Note portion of aortic valve ➔ and the aortomitral continuity ➔.*

VENTRICULAR ASSIST DEVICES

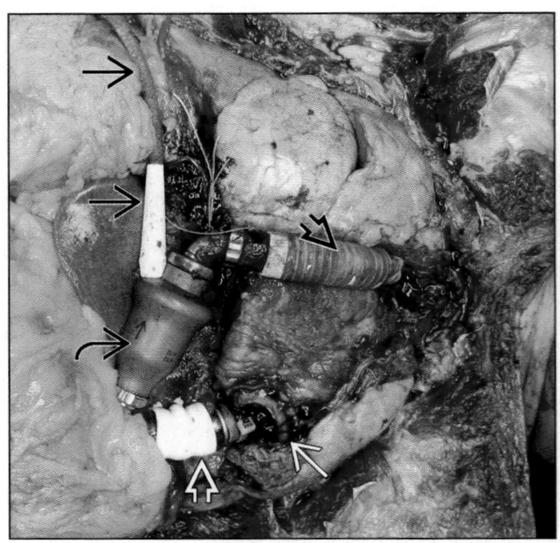

This view demonstrates all components of a HeartMate II LVAD in situ at autopsy, including the sewing ring ➡, inflow cannula ➡, pump ↷, outflow conduit ➡, and driveline →.

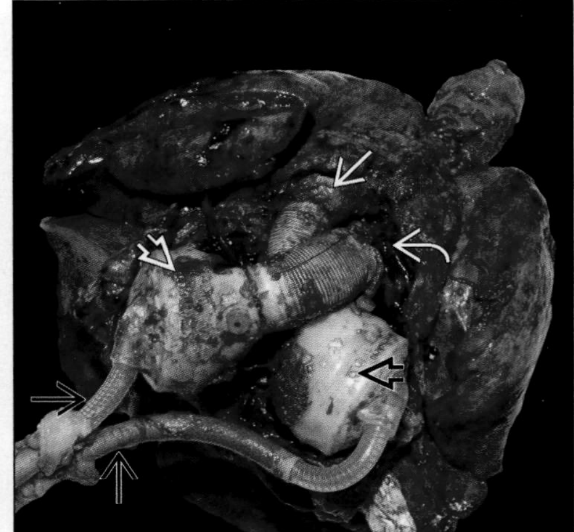

The CardioWest TAH consists of artificial right ➡ and left ➡ ventricles, connected to the atria (behind device), main pulmonary artery ➡, ascending aorta ➡, and pneumatic drivelines →.

TERMINOLOGY

Abbreviations

- Ventricular assist device (VAD)
- Left ventricular assist device (LVAD)
- Right ventricular assist device (RVAD)
- Biventricular assist device (BiVAD)
- Total artificial heart (TAH)

CLINICAL ISSUES

VADs in Clinical Practice

- Use of VADs has increased exponentially since FDA approval of HeartMate II in USA in 2008
- Support circulation during profound heart failure in 4 settings
  - Bridge to recovery: Temporary support until ventricular function is regained
    - Useful for potentially reversible cardiac conditions, such as myocarditis, postpartum cardiomyopathy
  - Bridge to transplant: Support until donor heart is available
  - Destination therapy: Provides support indefinitely (for patients who are not candidates for transplantation)
    - Increasingly becoming viable alternative to transplantation
    - Survival with VAD is expected to approach that of transplantation (10-15 years average) in the future
    - Avoids expense and complications of immunosuppression and rejection monitoring
  - Bridge to decision: Support while determining candidacy for transplantation
    - Later transitioned to either destination therapy or transplantation

VAD Applications

- LVAD most commonly used
  - Right-sided (pulmonary) circulation generally improves with "unloading" of left ventricle
- In profound right heart failure, RVAD may be used
- In biventricular failure, BiVAD or TAH may be used

Interagency Registry for Mechanically Assisted Circulatory Support (INTERMACS)

- Monitors VAD use and outcomes
- > 10,000 patients followed
- For continuous flow pumps, current actuarial survival is 80% at 1 year and 70% at 2 years

Research Opportunities

- Myocardial recovery
  - Multiple ongoing investigations exploring mechanisms of change during myocardial rest/unloading afforded by VAD support
  - Tissues commonly obtained at time of VAD implantation and at time of VAD removal (including not only at time of recovery or transplantation, but also at autopsy)

Types of VADs

- Extracorporeal
  - Pump and controller external to body (e.g., Berlin EXCOR Pediatric, BVS 5000)
  - Clinically easier to inspect circuit and replace components in event of thrombus formation
  - More invasive
  - Higher infection risk
  - Less portable
- Intracorporeal
  - Intracardiac (e.g., HeartMate II, HeartWare HVAD)
    - Direct cannulation of left ventricular apex for inflow, ascending aorta for outflow
    - Only driveline exits body
    - Lower infection risk

VENTRICULAR ASSIST DEVICES

Key Facts

Clinical Issues
- 4 main clinical settings: Bridge to recovery, bridge to transplant, destination therapy, bridge to decision
- Pros/cons of extracorporal VADs: Easier to inspect and replace components, but more invasive, carry higher infection risk, less portable
- Pros/cons of intracorporal VADs: Harder to replace components (only driveline exits body), but carry lower infection risk, are very portable
- Total artificial heart reserved for severe biventricular failure

Macroscopic Pathology
- Photograph all extracorporeal and intracorporeal components in situ
- Examine skin at site(s) of device entry for infection; obtain samples for cultures
- Inside body, evaluate device in situ for infection, malorientation of outflow conduit, etc.
- Evaluate sheath at left ventricular apex for thrombus, pannus formation
- Disassemble device and photograph components
- Open all conduits, examine blood contact surfaces for thrombus
- Confirm cannula patency
- Examine pump chamber for surface abrasions, wear
- Document serial numbers and findings

Microscopic Pathology
- Thrombus: Alternating layers of RBCs/WBCs and fibrin/platelets
- Skin at device entry site(s): Dense neutrophilic inflammation/abscesses indicate infection; perform GMS and Gram stains to identify microorganisms

    - Very portable with small battery packs and driver consoles
  - Extracardiac (Tohuku EHAM)
    - Pneumatically driven sheath placed around apex of left ventricle
    - Sheath device compresses and relaxes, mimicking cardiac massage
    - Still in developmental testing phase
  - Total artificial heart (SynCardia CardioWest)
    - Ventricles and all valves surgically removed, device sewn to atrial cuffs, and outflow cannulae anastomosed to proximal ascending aorta and main pulmonary artery
    - Only pneumatic drivelines exit body
    - FDA approved Freedom portable driver in 2014, enabling discharge from hospital
    - Reserved for patients with severe biventricular failure

MACROSCOPIC FEATURES

Photographic Documentation
- Essential for medical, legal, and educational purposes
- Photograph all extracorporeal and intracorporeal components in situ
- Photograph device components after disassembly
- Photograph thrombi, any other abnormalities

External Examination
- Examine skin at site(s) of driveline or cannula entry and exit for purulence, necrosis, erythema, and other signs of infection
- If signs of infection present, obtain samples for microbiologic culture

Internal Examination
- Evaluate device in situ for signs of infection, disconnection of components, scarring with change in orientation of outflow conduit, other abnormalities
  - Sewing ring and sheath at left ventricular apex
    - Evaluate for thrombus and pannus formation
  - Inflow cannula
  - Pump
  - Outflow conduit and anastomosis to ascending aorta
  - Driveline
- Disassemble device and examine components
  - Open all conduits and examine blood contact surfaces for thrombus
  - Confirm cannula patency
  - Examine pump chamber for surface abrasions, wear, etc. (using beam lighting and magnification or, if possible, pump disassembly)
  - Examine housings and diaphragms
- Document serial numbers and any abnormalities

MICROSCOPIC PATHOLOGY

Histologic Features
- Thrombus
  - Alternating layers of RBCs/WBCs and platelets/fibrin
  - Must be distinguished from postmortem clot, which shows heavier blood components (WBCs) settling as single layer to one side of clot, in gravity-dependent fashion
- Skin at device entry and exit sites
  - Dense neutrophilic inflammation and abscess formation indicate infection
  - Special stains (e.g., GMS and Gram) to identify and characterize microorganisms

ANCILLARY TESTS

Radiograph and CT
- Evaluate component integrity, mineralization, etc.

Scanning Electron Microscopy
- Surface topography, biofilm, platelets, fibrin, abrasions, pitting, etc.

VENTRICULAR ASSIST DEVICES

Summary of Pulsatile Flow Pump VADs

Device Name	Manufacturer	Notes
Berlin EXCOR Pediatric	Berlin Heart	Extracorporeal, pediatric applications
CardioWest	SynCardia Systems, Inc.	Total artificial heart
Thoratec pVAD II	Thoratec	Short-to-midterm support, LVAD, RVAD, or BiVAD
Novacor LVAD	Novacor	1st generation, now discontinued
BVS 5000	Abiomed	1st generation, now discontinued
HeartMate XVE	Thoratec	1st generation, now discontinued

Summary of Continuous Flow Pump Devices

Device Name	Manufacturer	Notes
HeartMate II	Thoratec	1st FDA approval, widest use in practice
HeartWare HVAD	HeartWare, Inc.	Small size allows intrapericardial implantation
Heart Assist 5	MicroMed Cardiovascular, Inc.	Direct flow sensing and management
DuraHeart	Terumo Heart, Inc.	Centrifugal flow magnetic levitation pump
2000 FlowMaker	Jarvik Heart, Inc.	Axial flow magnetically driven pump
Impella	Abiomed	Augments rather than replaces ventricle function
DeBakey Child	MicroMed Cardiovascular, Inc.	Small, intracorporeal, pediatric applications
Evaheart	Sun Medical	Centrifugal flow magnetic levitation pump
Synergy Pocket Micro-Pump	HeartWare, Inc. (formerly CircuLite, Inc.)	Size of AA battery, partial-assist of less sick patients

SELECTED REFERENCES

1. McCandless SP et al: Comparing velour versus silicone interfaces at the driveline exit site of HeartMate II devices: infection rates, histopathology, and ultrastructural aspects. Cardiovasc Pathol. 24(2):71-5, 2015
2. Blitz A: Pump thrombosis-A riddle wrapped in a mystery inside an enigma. Ann Cardiothorac Surg. 3(5):450-71, 2014
3. Cheng A et al: Comparison of continuous-flow and pulsatile-flow left ventricular assist devices: is there an advantage to pulsatility? Ann Cardiothorac Surg. 3(6):573-81, 2014
4. Diakos NA et al: Myocardial atrophy and chronic mechanical unloading of the failing human heart: implications for cardiac assist device-induced myocardial recovery. J Am Coll Cardiol. 64(15):1602-12, 2014
5. Kirklin JK et al: Sixth INTERMACS annual report: a 10,000-patient database. J Heart Lung Transplant. 33(6):555-64, 2014
6. Porepa LF et al: Destination therapy with left ventricular assist devices: for whom and when? Can J Cardiol. 30(3):296-303, 2014
7. Torregrossa G et al: SynCardia: the total artificial heart. Ann Cardiothorac Surg. 3(6):612-20, 2014
8. Xie A et al: Durability of continuous-flow left ventricular assist devices: a systematic review. Ann Cardiothorac Surg. 3(6):547-56, 2014
9. Carpenter BA et al: A brief review of ventricular assist devices and a recommended protocol for pathology evaluations. Cardiovasc Pathol. 22(5):408-15, 2013
10. Garbade J et al: Heart transplantation and left ventricular assist device therapy: two comparable options in end-stage heart failure? Clin Cardiol. 36(7):378-82, 2013
11. Peura JL et al: Recommendations for the use of mechanical circulatory support: device strategies and patient selection: a scientific statement from the American Heart Association. Circulation. 126(22):2648-67, 2012
12. Hannan MM et al: Working formulation for the standardization of definitions of infections in patients using ventricular assist devices. J Heart Lung Transplant. 30(4):375-84, 2011
13. Potapov EV et al: Managing long-term complications of left ventricular assist device therapy. Curr Opin Cardiol. 26(3):237-44, 2011
14. Rose AG et al: Pathology in patients with ventricular assist devices: a study of 21 autopsies, 24 ventricular apical core biopsies and 24 explanted hearts. Cardiovasc Pathol. 14(1):19-23, 2005

Gross Findings

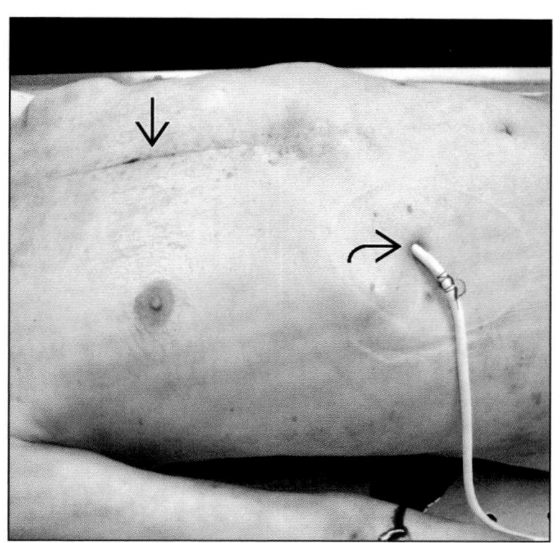

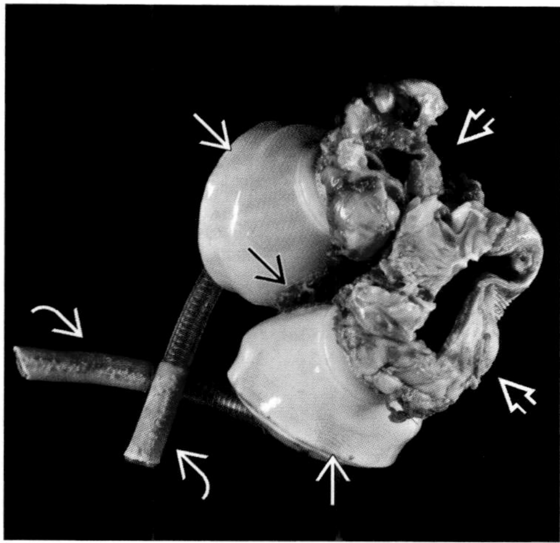

(Left) The HeartMate II LVAD is an intracorporeal device, with nearly all components inside the chest (note thoracotomy scar ➙). Only the driveline ➙ exits the body, which connects to an external driver console. This lowers the risk of infection and enables device portability. **(Right)** The CardioWest TAH is attached directly to the atria ➙ after surgical removal of the rest of the heart. Note artificial ventricles ➙, drivelines ➙, and Velcro ➙ connecting the ventricles.

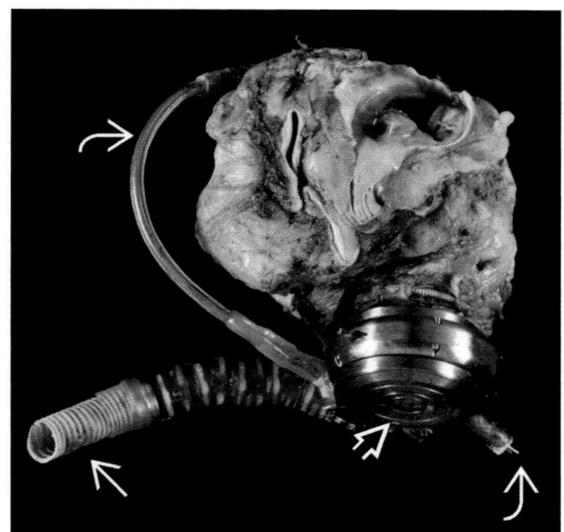

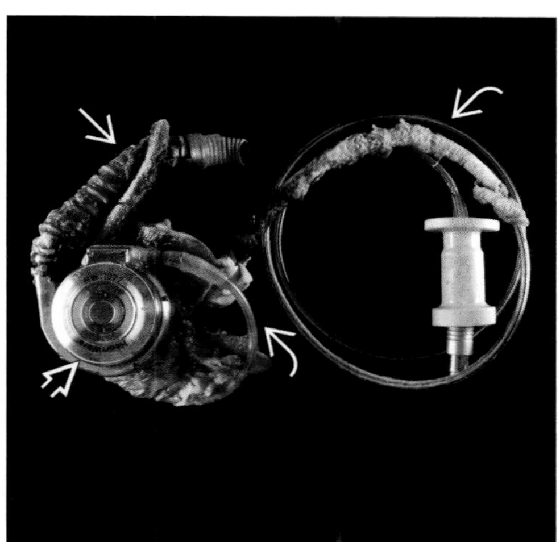

(Left) The HeartWare HVAD is implantable within the pericardium, with the pump ➙ attached directly to the left ventricular apex and the outflow conduit ➙ attached to the ascending aorta. The driveline ➙ is partially hidden under the specimen in this view. **(Right)** Here, the heart has been largely removed from the HeartWare HVAD, revealing the device's components, including the pump ➙, outflow conduit ➙, and long coiled driveline ➙ with adherent subcutaneous tissue.

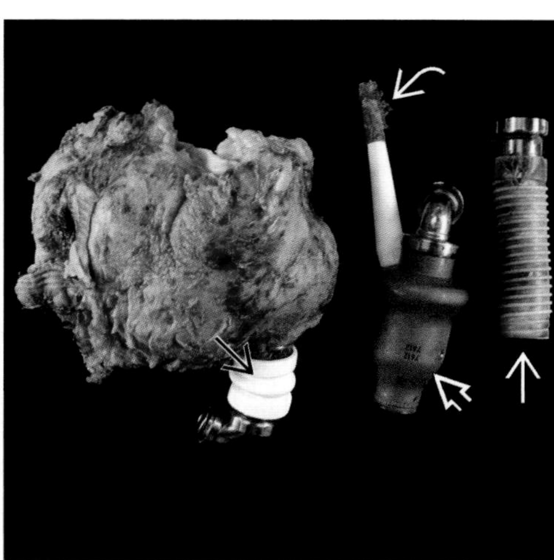

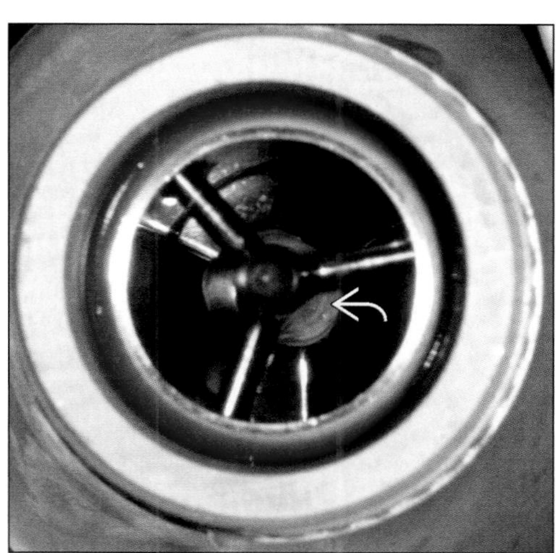

(Left) Disassembly is essential for identifying thrombi, damage, and other device abnormalities. Here, the inflow cannula ➙, pump ➙, outflow conduit ➙, and driveline ➙ of a HeartMate II LVAD are all seen. **(Right)** This view into the pump chamber of a HeartMate II LVAD demonstrates old thrombus ➙ surrounding the driveshaft above the impeller. Thrombus formation is an infrequent but important complication, and examination of VADs must include a careful search for thrombus.

THORACIC AORTIC ANEURYSM REPAIR

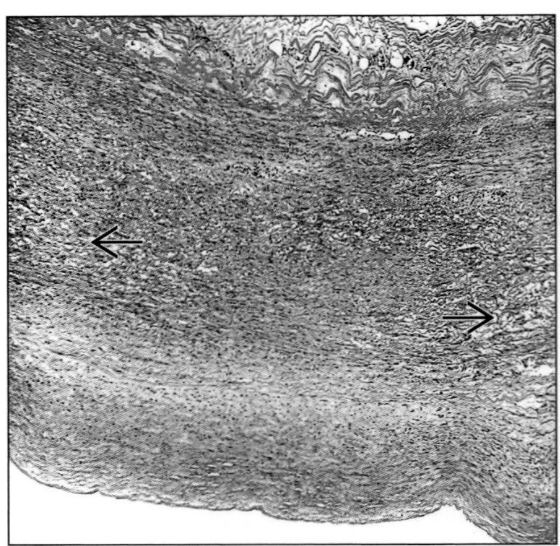

This thoracic aneurysm wall shows degenerative changes in the media. The media demonstrates loss of staining of nuclei of smooth muscle cells and increase in proteoglycans ⇨. (From DP: Cardiovascular.)

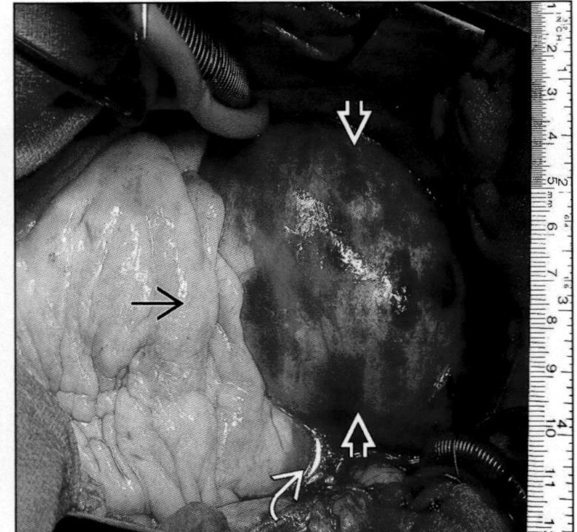

This ascending aortic aneurysm ➡ (heart ⇨, pulmonary artery ➡) required repair due to its large size. (From DP: Cardiovascular.)

TERMINOLOGY

Abbreviations

- TAA repair, TEVAR (thoracic endovascular aortic repair), OTAR (open thoracic aortic repair),

Definitions

- Aneurysm: Localized pathologic dilatation of vessel wall at least 50% > normal, true aneurysm contains all layers of vessel wall
  - Aortic size increase with age 1-2 mm/year
  - Normal ascending aorta measurements, generally < 3.5 cm; descending thoracic aorta generally < 2.5 cm

ETIOLOGY/PATHOGENESIS

Pathogenesis

- May be syndromic or nonsyndromic
- Syndromic: Marfan syndrome (fibrillin 1), vascular Ehlers Danlos, Loeys-Dietz syndrome (types 1 and 2), familial thoracic aortic aneurysm syndrome
- Nonsyndromic: 15% of patients with nonsyndromic TAA have positive family history
  - Genes associated with nonsyndromic TAA include *ACTA 2*, *MYH 11*, *TGFBRI* and *TGFBRII*
    - These genes may be associated with TGF B signaling, indicating similar pathogenesis to syndromic TAA
- Bicuspid aortic valve (BAV)
  - 1.3% of general population has BAV and 14% of patients with TAA have bicuspid aortic valve
  - Valve function may be stenotic, regurgitant, or normal, suggesting factors other than hemodynamics play a role in formation of TAA with BAV

Infection

- Historically syphilitic aortitis in tertiary syphilis was an important cause of TAA; now rare
- Proliferative endarteritis of vasa vasorum→ ischemic injury to vascular media → aneurysmal dilatation

CLINICAL ISSUES

Epidemiology

- Incidence
  - TAA incidence is 10.4/100,000 person-years

Presentation

- Usually silent until complications (dissection/rupture)
  - Risk of rupture ↑ with ↑ size; > 6 cm has 30% risk of rupture/dissection
  - Rupture presents with acute pain, hypotension/ shock
    - Pain location varies with site of aneurysm: Ascending: Anterior chest pain; arch: Neck pain; descending: Back pain between scapulae
  - Chronic pain is seen with large aneurysms due to distension and compression of surrounding structures
  - Large aneurysms may present with superior vena cava syndrome
    - First report of SVC syndrome was due to syphilitic ascending aortic aneurysm
    - Now malignancy (lung carcinoma) most common cause for SVC syndrome but 40% have benign cause
    - Syndrome caused by partial to complete obstruction to blood flow in superior vena cava ± thrombosis of vessel
    - Symptoms include dyspnea, facial swelling, facial congestion, cough, arm swelling
- Post-repair complications include
  - Shock, valvular insufficiency, stroke, embolic phenomena, ischemic myocardial, gastrointestinal and hepatic injury, acute tubular injury/necrosis, infection and ischemic spinal cord injury

THORACIC AORTIC ANEURYSM REPAIR

Key Facts

Terminology
- Aneurysm: Localized pathologic dilatation of vessel wall at least 50% > normal, true aneurysm contains all layers of vessel wall

Etiology
- May be syndromic or nonsyndromic
- Syndromic: Marfan syndrome (fibrillin 1), vascular Ehlers Danlos, Loeys Dietz syndrome (types 1 and 2), familial thoracic aortic aneurysm syndrome
- Nonsyndromic: 15% of patients with nonsyndromic TAA have positive family history
- 1.3% of general population has BAV and 14% of patients with TAA have bicuspid aortic valve

Clinical Issues
- Usually silent until complications (dissection/ rupture)
- Risk of rupture ↑ with ↑ size; > 6 cm has 30% risk of rupture/dissection
- Indications for repair: Size, growth rate, symptoms
- Endovascular repair: Fabric (polyester or PTFE)-covered metallic (nitinol, stainless steel) stent is deployed across aneurysm to exclude it from aortic blood flow leading to aneurysm thrombosis and remodeling
- Open repair: Ascending and arch repair with coronary artery and branch vessel reimplantation ± aortic valve replacement (Bentall procedure: Ascending aortic aneurysm graft with aortic valve replacement and coronary artery reimplantation)

thoracoabdominal, or descending aortic aneurysm repair

Treatment
- Surgical approaches
  - Indications for repair
    - Size, growth rate, symptoms
  - Types of repair
    - Endovascular: Fabric (polyester or PTFE)-covered metallic (nitinol, stainless steel) stent is deployed across aneurysm to exclude it from aortic blood flow leading to aneurysm thrombosis and remodeling
    - Most commonly used for descending thoracic aneurysms, ascending and aortic arch hybrid procedures (multiple grafts, combined endovascular and open procedures) used for ascending and arch repair
    - Open: Ascending and arch repair with coronary artery and branch vessel reimplantation ± aortic valve replacement (Bentall procedure: Ascending aortic aneurysm graft with aortic valve replacement and coronary artery reimplantation)

IMAGE FINDINGS

Radiographic Findings
- Postmortem chest radiograph may be valuable and reveal endovascular repair (stents visible), open repair (grafts should be visible), aortic dilatation, and pleural effusions visible

MACROSCOPIC FEATURES

External Examination
- Pallor (hemorrhagic shock from rupture), petechiae (DIC following rupture and hemorrhage), Sternotomy incision (OTAR), groin incision (TEVAR)
- Facial congestion and swelling (SVC syndrome)
- Syndromic features
  - Marfan (thin, long limbs; arm span > height; long digits; pectus excavatum)
  - Loeys-Dietz (type 1 overlaps with Marfan with craniofacial anomalies bifid uvula, cleft palate hypertelorism), type 2 with overlap with Marfan and vascular Ehlers Danlos (usually only bifid uvula, pectus, joint laxity and long digits, and bruising)
  - Vascular Ehlers Danlos (bruising, velvety translucent skin, small lax joints)

Internal Examination
- In situ documentation of graft type, segment of aorta grafted (open or endovascular), length and patency of graft, patency of branch vessels including coronary arteries in cases of ascending aneurysm, status of nongrafted aorta, presence of intramural hematoma (dissection in 15% of TAA)
  - Procure material for microbiologic culture studies if clinically indicated (suspected graft infection) immediately upon opening chest cavity
- Anastomotic integrity assessed by inspection and water infusion into aorta if concern for anastomotic integrity

Organ Examination
- Aorta and heart
  - Open aorta from distal aspect after inspecting graft and anastomoses and branch vessels
    - Section nongrafted aorta and anastomoses; Dacron graft material can be processed for histologic analysis
  - Ascending aorta: Inspect any coronary graft ostia, or coronary buttons (reimplanted native coronary ostia)
    - Coronary reimplantation or bypass may be necessary in ascending aortic repair
    - Examine coronary arteries for evidence of dissection, surgical injury
  - Inspect aortic valve from aortic aspect
    - Native valve: Cusp number (check for BAV) and coaptation, surgical injury (suture, etc.), surgical

repair (pledgeted sutures to resuspend valve cusps), vegetation
    - Bioprosthetic valve: May be part of ascending aorta replacement or separate; look for cusp integrity, thrombosis, surgical injury, vegetation
  - Heart
    - Size and weight: Dilated left ventricle with eccentric hypertrophy in aortic valve insufficiency, concentric hypertrophy with aortic stenosis and hypertension
    - Myocardial infarction: May be multifactorial: Operative stress, surgical injury, embolic, underlying coronary atherosclerosis
  - Respiratory
    - Cardiogenic pulmonary edema (congestive heart failure from aortic valve insufficiency, perioperative ischemic injury etc.)
    - Noncardiogenic pulmonary edema: Multifactorial: Operative stress, intercurrent sepsis, shock (hypovolemic from hemorrhage or cardiogenic), aspiration
    - Pneumonia: Aspiration
  - Gastrointestinal
    - Ischemic injury (shock)
  - Hepatobiliary
    - Congestion (congestive heart failure from aortic valve insufficiency), necrosis (shock liver)
    - Acute pancreatitis (uncommon complication of cardiopulmonary bypass)
  - Genitourinary
    - Acute tubular injury (operative stress, hypovolemic shock)
  - Central and peripheral nervous system
    - Spinal cord injury (ischemic) with descending aneurysm repair or arch repair with distal graft tunneled into descending aorta; examination of thoracic cord is important in these cases
    - Appearance of CNS and spinal cord infarcts varies with duration from injury, and presence or absence of hemorrhage

MICROSCOPIC PATHOLOGY

Histologic Features

- Heart and aorta
  - Anastomotic sections: Adventitial granulation tissue and fibrosis with longer duration grafts, abscess if superimposed infection
  - Aortic sections: Intramural hematoma (dissection) acute or chronic, cystic medial degeneration, smooth muscle cell loss
  - If aneurysm from syphilitic aortitis (rare), intimal proliferation of adventitial vessels (vasa vasora), plasma cell-rich inflammation and laminar necrosis of media due to ischemia
  - Heart with hypertrophy and areas of interstitial fibrosis in cases with aortic valve insufficiency, varying stages of acute and healing coagulative myocyte necrosis in cases with infarction
    - May see foreign material (suture, etc.) embolization related to surgery
- Respiratory system
  - Intraalveolar pale pink fluid (cardiogenic pulmonary edema); fibrin layering along alveolar septal walls ± evidence of organization (noncardiogenic pulmonary edema), intrabronchial and intra alveolar acute inflammation in pneumonia
    - With aspiration may see intra-airway or -alveolar gastric content or aspirated squames from oral cavity and multinucleated giant cells with chronic aspiration
- Gastrointestinal system
  - Varying severity of ischemic injury with coagulative necrosis of mucosa to serosa (severe case), submucosal vascular thrombosis, may see atheroemboli or foreign material (suture) emboli related to operative intervention and catheterization
- Hepatobiliary system
  - Centrilobular hepatocyte necrosis and congestion; larger areas of necrosis affecting entire lobule and bridging from lobule to lobule in more severe shock
  - Coagulative necrosis of pancreatic parenchyma with fibrin thrombi in vessels in bypass related acute pancreatitis
    - Usually seen in association with other shock changes such as hepatic necrosis, intestinal ischemia, and acute tubular injury
- Genitourinary system
  - Loss of brush border of distal and proximal tubular epithelial cells with coagulative necrosis in more severe cases of acute tubular injury/necrosis
- Central and peripheral nervous system
  - Cerebral infarct appearance varies with time from ischemic insult
    - 12 hours: Red neurons, vasogenic edema
    - 48 hours: Neutrophilic infiltrate begins to decrease and phagocytes increase to become prominent cell type over ensuing weeks, reactive astrocytes appear at edge of infarct
    - Spinal cord infarct will have similar features

DIFFERENTIAL DIAGNOSIS

Pseudoaneurysm

- Contained rupture of aorta with communication with vessel lumen
  - Contains hematoma surrounded by granulation tissue or fibrous tissue depending on age of pseudoaneurysm
  - Does not contain layers of vessel wall

SELECTED REFERENCES

1. Arnaoutakis DJ et al: Cohort comparison of thoracic endovascular aortic repair with open thoracic aortic repair using modern end-organ preservation strategies. Ann Vasc Surg. 29(5):882-90, 2015
2. Bicknell C et al: Aortic disease: thoracic endovascular aortic repair. Heart. 101(8):586-591, 2015

Imaging and Repair of Thoracic Aortic Aneurysms

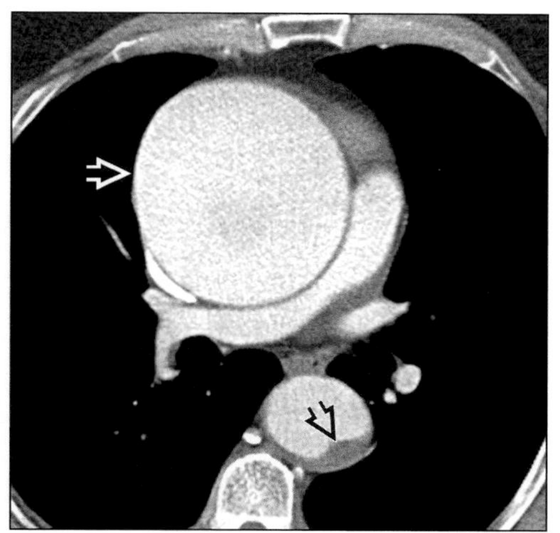

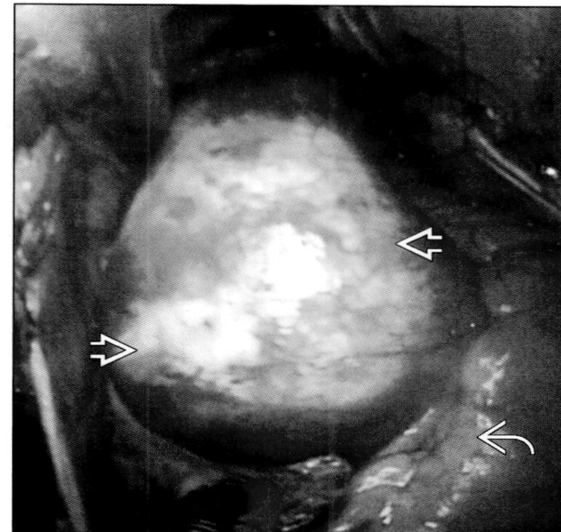

(Left) *Enhanced CT of the chest shows a large ascending aortic aneurysm* ➡*. There is atherosclerotic plaque in the descending aorta* ➡ *but the lumen is of normal caliber.* ***(Right)*** *This is an in situ view of a large ascending aortic aneurysm* ➡ *prior to repair (heart* ➡*).*

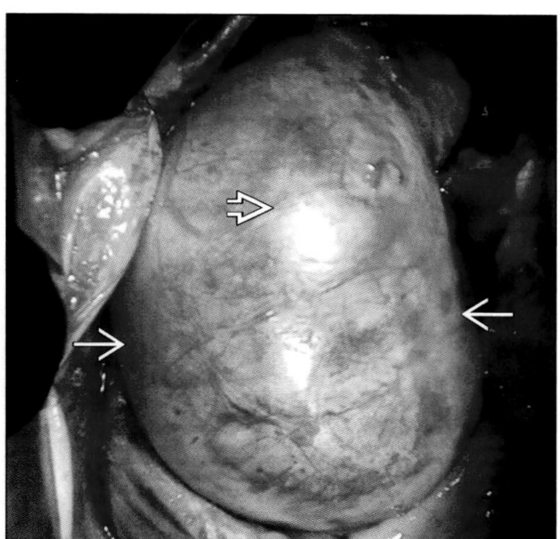

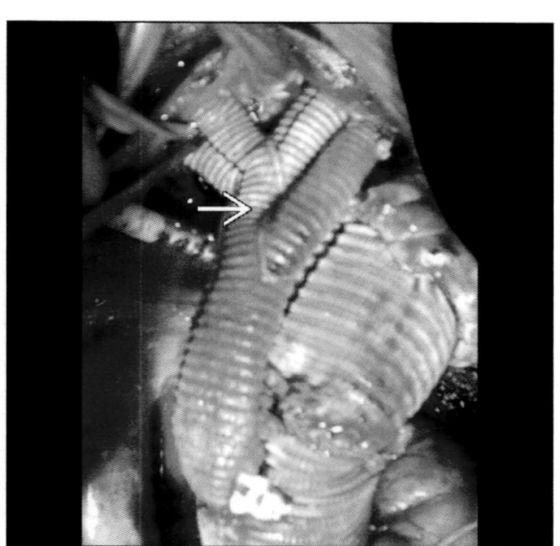

(Left) *This aortic arch is markedly dilated* ➡ *and the blue discoloration* ➡ *indicates an aortic dissection complicating this arch aneurysm.* ***(Right)*** *Aortic arch repair often includes repair of the arch vessels. Here they are replaced with grafts* ➡*. If the ostia and the proximal arch vessels are intact, the vessel-bearing portion of the arch can also sometimes be resected and attached to the arch graft, similar to coronary buttons.*

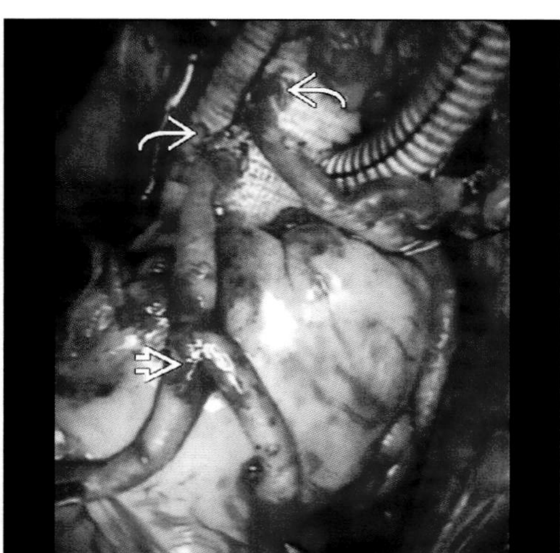

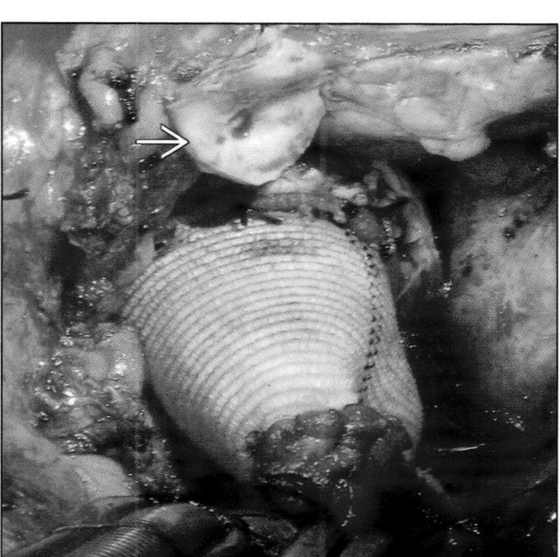

(Left) *Saphenous vein bypass grafts can be attached to ascending aortic grafts to perform a simultaneous coronary artery bypass procedure. In this case, 2 grafts are attached proximally* ➡ *and vein-to-vein Y grafts* ➡ *are used to bypass additional vessels.* ***(Right)*** *In this case of aortic root replacement, the coronary arteries are being reattached to the ascending graft as a coronary button* ➡ *that contains the coronary ostium and a portion of the surrounding aortic wall.*

Imaging and Repair of Thoracic Aortic Aneurysms

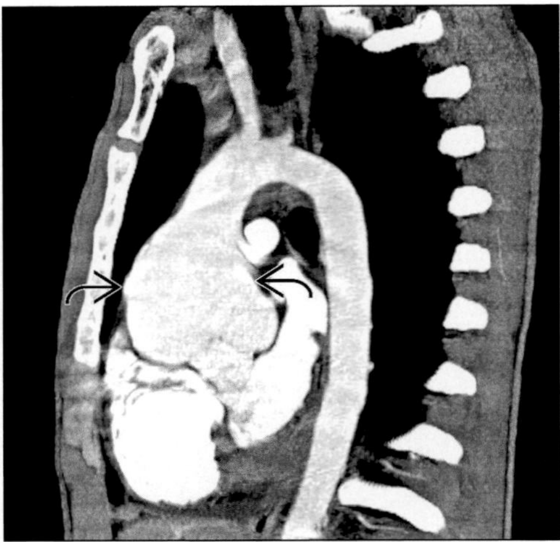

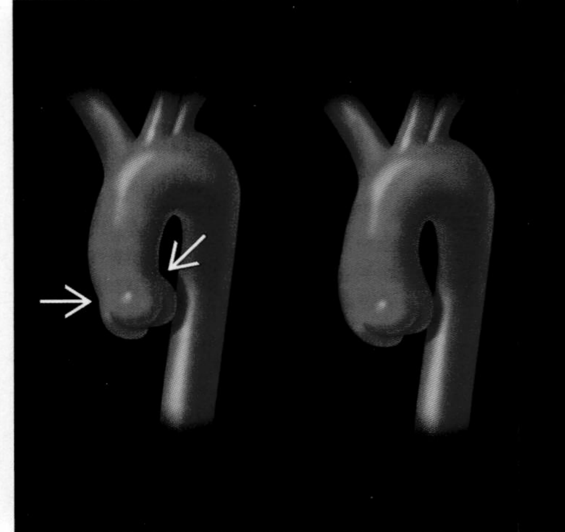

(Left) *CT angiogram in a patient with Marfan syndrome and acute chest syndrome shows the classic "tulip bulb" appearance ⇨ due to annuloaortic ectasia. Other terms describing this appearance include "onion bulb," "pear-shaped," and "Florence flask." (From DI: Cardiovascular.)* ***(Right)*** *Graphic compares a normal ascending aorta (left) with a well-defined sinotubular junction ➡ and annuloaortic ectasia with sinotubular junction effacement (right) as seen in Marfan syndrome.*

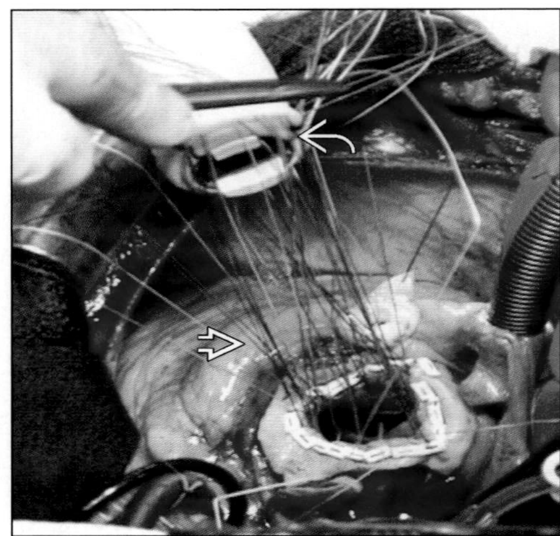

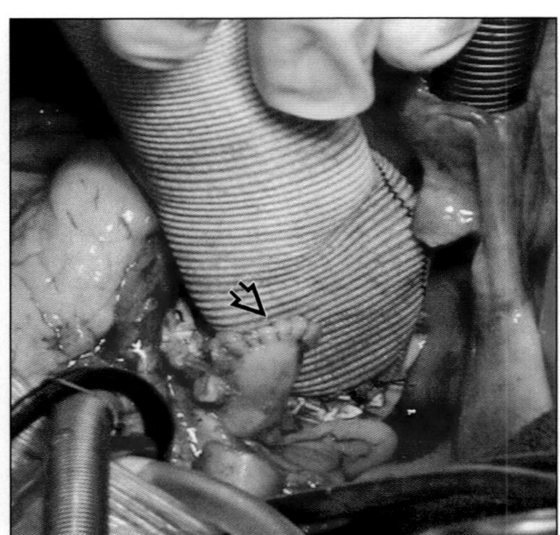

(Left) *This aortic root and ascending aortic aneurysm is being replaced with a valved conduit so the aortic valve, root, and ascending aorta are replaced simultaneously. In this photograph, the proximal suturing of the valve into the root is being performed. Multiple sutures ➡ will anastomose the sewing ring of the valve ➡ onto the root. (Courtesy J. Plate, MD & E. Pantin, MD).* ***(Right)*** *The coronary buttons ⇨ have been anastomosed to the ascending aortic graft.*

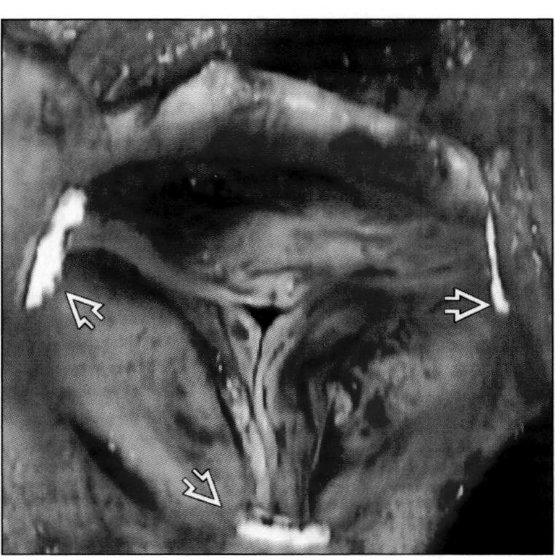

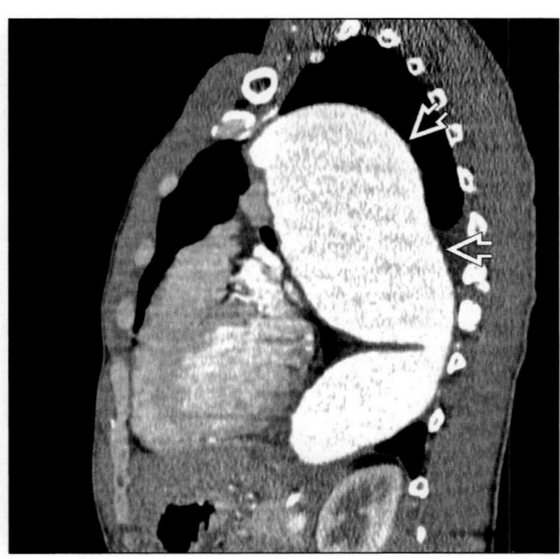

(Left) *This is the outflow view of an aortic valve that has been re-suspended with 3 commissure pledgeted sutures ➡. There is excellent coaptation of the valve cusps after resuspension.* ***(Right)*** *Sagittal reconstructed CT shows a large descending thoracic aneurysm ➡. Descending aortic aneurysms are easier to repair with endografts that ascending aneurysms. (From DI: Chest.)*

Imaging and Repair of Thoracic Aortic Aneurysms

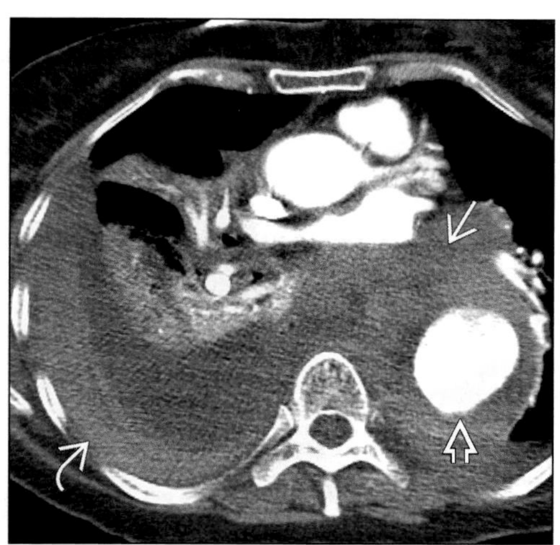

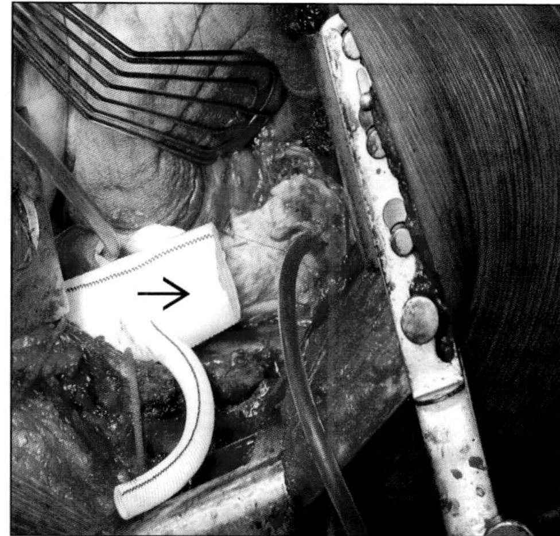

(Left) *Enhanced CT of the chest shows a large ruptured thoracic aortic aneurysm. Contrast is seen in the lumen of the aneurysm ➡, with a large amount of extravasated blood and hematoma in the mediastinum ➡ and right hemithorax ➡. (From DI: Chest.)* ***(Right)*** *This is an open repair of a descending thoracic aneurysm with a Dacron graft ➡. Repair of these aneurysms has a risk of paraplegia due to spinal cord ischemic injury. In autopsies following this type of repair, examination of the thoracic spinal cord is indicated.*

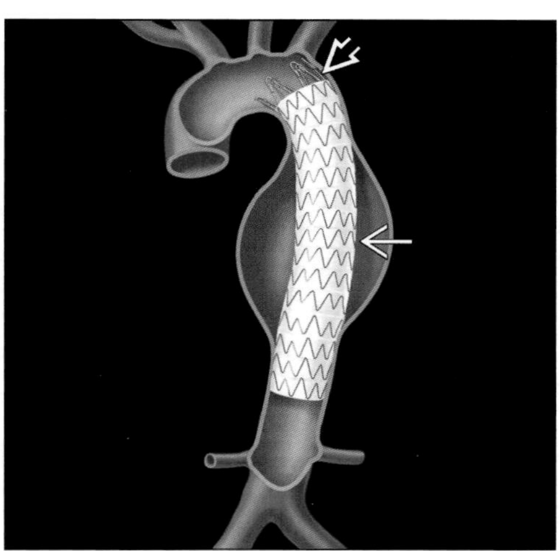

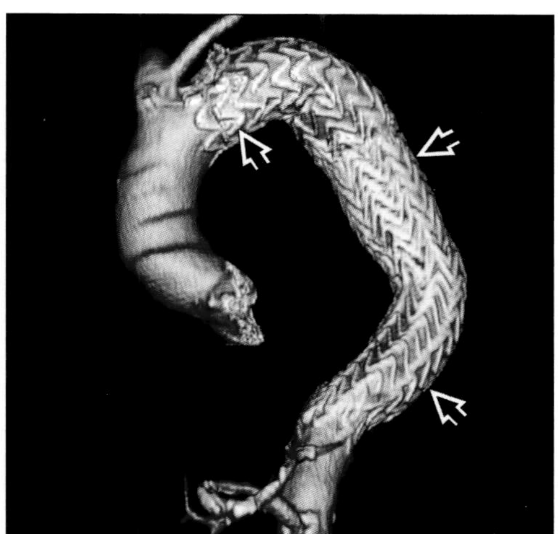

(Left) *Graphic shows a descending thoracic aneurysm repaired with an endograft. The endograft struts ➡ attach to the aortic wall. The body is composed of fabric-covered self-expanding stents ➡.* ***(Right)*** *3D reconstruction shows a thoracoabdominal aneurysm after endograft repair ➡. (From DI: Procedures.) The location of endografts should be determined by chart review, premortem imaging review &/or postmortem/ specimen imaging prior to aortic dissection to avoid iatrogenic injury to the graft.*

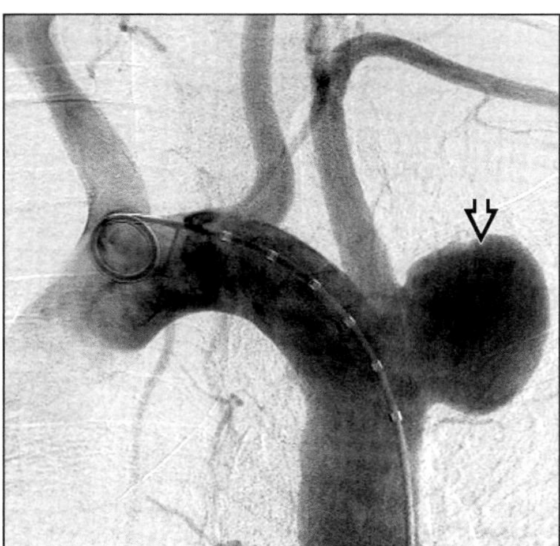

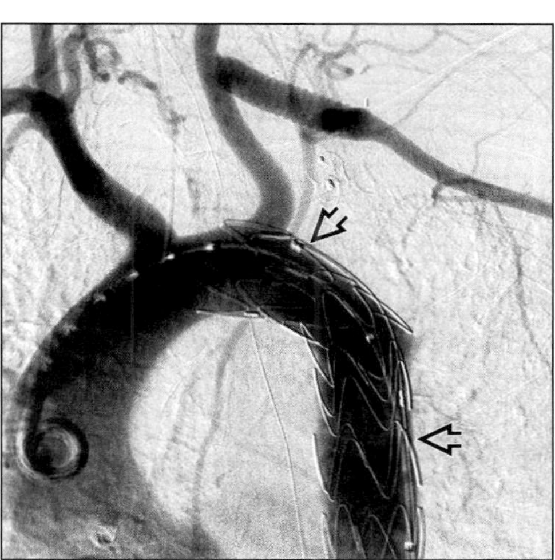

(Left) *Angiogram shows a large saccular aneurysm ➡. This is likely a pseudoaneurysm that represents a contained periaortic hematoma with retained communication to the aortic lumen.* ***(Right)*** *Angiogram in the same case is shown after endograft repair ➡. The endograft excluded the pseudoaneurysm from the aortic blood flow. (From DI: Procedures.)*

PANCREAS RESECTION

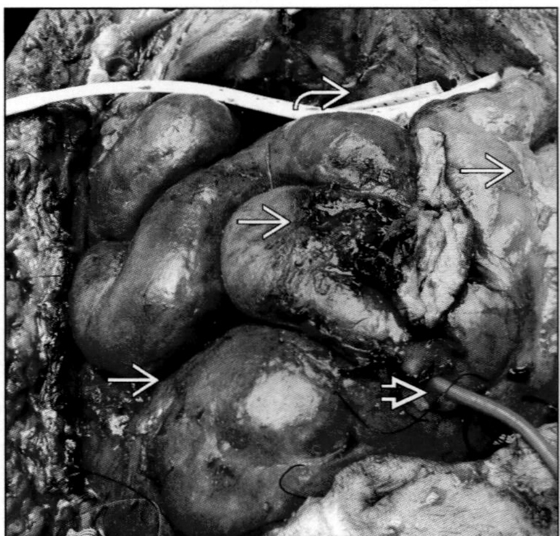

Diffuse peritonitis with green-yellow exudates ➡ covering the serosal/peritoneal surfaces occurred status post distal pancreatectomy. Jejunostomy tube ➡ and drain ➡ were in place.

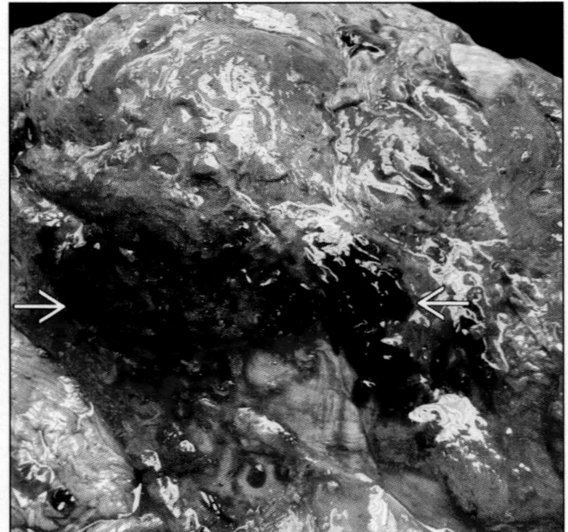

The posterior surface of the organ block in the same patient showed red-black hemorrhagic necrotic retroperitoneal soft tissue ➡ due to postoperative acute pancreatitis.

TERMINOLOGY

Definitions

- Whipple procedure (pancreaticoduodenectomy): Resection of pancreatic head and uncinate process, distal stomach, duodenum, ± proximal jejunum, ± cholecystectomy
  - Anastomoses from proximal to distal: End-to-side pancreaticojejunostomy, hepaticojejunostomy (hepatic bile duct), end-to-side gastrojejunostomy
  - Variant: Pylorus-preserving Whipple: Stomach and proximal 1st portion of duodenum are preserved with end-to-side duodenojejunostomy
- Distal pancreatectomy: Resection of body and tail of pancreas, ± splenectomy, suture/staple closure of pancreatic stump
- Central pancreatectomy: Segmental resection of isthmus or body of pancreas
  - Distal pancreaticojejunostomy with Roux-en-Y jejunojejunostomy or distal pancreaticogastrostomy (gastrointestinal tract remains intact), closure of proximal pancreatic stump
  - Usually performed for benign or premalignant/low-grade malignant tumors
  - Roux-en-Y technique: Jejunum is divided, distal pancreas anastomosed to distal end of jejunum to create Y limb, proximal jejunum anastomosed to distal jejunum
- Total pancreatectomy: Pancreaticoduodenectomy with resection of entire pancreas ± splenectomy

ETIOLOGY/PATHOGENESIS

Indications for Resection

- Malignant tumors: Pancreatic ductal adenocarcinoma, common bile duct adenocarcinoma, ampullary or duodenal adenocarcinoma, acinar cell carcinoma, pancreatic endocrine neoplasm, solid pseudopapillary neoplasm, pancreatoblastoma
- Premalignant tumors: Intraductal papillary mucinous neoplasm, mucinous cystic neoplasm
- Benign tumors: Serous or acinar cell cystic neoplasm, large duodenal adenoma
- Involvement by extrapancreatic malignancy: Gastric or colonic adenocarcinoma, metastasis (rare)
- Nonneoplastic: Chronic/autoimmune pancreatitis, pseudocyst, trauma

CLINICAL ISSUES

Presentation

- Symptoms
  - Abdominal pain, nausea, vomiting, diarrhea/steatorrhea, melena, hematemesis, dyspnea
- Signs
  - Fever, tachycardia, oliguria, hypotension, peritoneal signs, jaundice/scleral icterus, hypovolemic/septic shock
- Important elements of chart review
  - Type of operation and anastomoses performed, surgical pathology reports of resected specimens, intra-/postoperative complications ± interventions, (neo)adjuvant chemotherapy/radiation
  - Comorbidities, coagulation disorders, medications (e.g., anticoagulants, antiplatelet agents)

Laboratory Tests

- ↓ hemoglobin and hematocrit, (+) fecal occult blood
- Leukocytosis, lactic acidosis, hyperglycemia
- ↑ amylase, lipase, blood urea nitrogen, creatinine, transaminases, alkaline phosphatase, and C-reactive protein
- ↑ tumor markers (e.g., CA19-9, chromogranin-A)
- ↑ amylase or bilirubin in effusions, intraabdominal collections, or drain outputs
- (+) blood, fluid collection, wound cultures

PANCREAS RESECTION

Key Facts

Terminology
- Types of pancreas resection: Whipple procedure (pancreaticoduodenectomy), distal, central, or total pancreatectomy

Etiology
- Malignant, premalignant, or benign tumors, chronic/autoimmune pancreatitis, pseudocysts, trauma

Clinical Issues
- Complications reported in up to 50% after any type of pancreas resection
- Early complications: Pancreatic fistula/leak, bleeding, delayed gastric emptying, biliary leak, acute pancreatitis, infection, ischemia
- Early or late complications: Tumor recurrence
- Late complications: Pancreatic exocrine/endocrine insufficiency, infection

Macroscopic Pathology
- Examine upper gastrointestinal tract including remnant pancreas, biliary tract, and liver (if part of anastomosis) in situ for anastomotic leaks/strictures, fistulas
- Remove en block, then open

Diagnostic Checklist
- Immediate cause of death and how it relates to surgery
- Postsurgical complications and risk factors for developing complications
- Presence of residual/recurrent/metastatic tumor

Prognosis
- Mortality rate
  - Whipple: < 10%
  - Distal pancreatectomy: < 5%
  - Central pancreatectomy: Very low
- Causes of death
  - Pancreatic fistula/leak
  - Vascular/bleeding
  - Tumor progression
  - Infection (wound, intraabdominal, pneumonia) → sepsis
  - Acute/hemorrhagic pancreatitis, intestinal ischemia, cardiac related

Complications
- Reported in up to 50% after any type of pancreas resection
- Risk factors: Low-volume center, low-volume surgeon
- Early complications
  - Pancreatic leak/fistula: Incidence is 10-30%; can lead to bleeding or intraabdominal abscess → sepsis
    - Risk factors include soft parenchyma, obesity (fatty parenchyma), and pancreatic duct diameter < 3 mm
  - Delayed gastric emptying: Incidence is 20-50% after Whipple
  - Bleeding: Incidence is up to 20%, due to vascular injury, anastomotic ulcers/dehiscence, fistulas, pseudoaneurysms
  - Biliary complications: Incidence varies up to 10%, bile leak, cholangitis, fistulas, bile duct strictures/stenosis
  - Acute pancreatitis: Incidence is 2-3%
  - Infections: Intraabdominal, wound, or pneumonia → sepsis
  - Ischemic complications: Incidence varies; arterial stenosis, trauma, or kinking → intestinal or biliary ischemia
  - Other organ failure: Acute renal, respiratory, or liver failure; may be multifactorial
- Early or late complications
  - Tumor recurrence: Incidence varies depending on tumor type, local vs. distant
- Late complications
  - Pancreatic endocrine insufficiency → new-onset diabetes mellitus
  - Pancreatic exocrine insufficiency → steatorrhea, weight loss, vitamin deficiencies
  - Post splenectomy infection (encapsulated bacteria)

IMAGE FINDINGS

CT Findings
- Peripancreatic/intraabdominal fluid collections, ascites, hemoperitoneum, free air, intestinal obstruction
- Pulmonary infiltrates, pleural/pericardial effusions
- Masses, lymphadenopathy, evidence of metastatic disease

CT Angiography
- Identify/treat active bleeding, vascular injury, fistulas, pseudoaneurysms

Upper Gastrointestinal Series/Contrast Swallow
- Anastomotic leaks, strictures, ulcers

MACROSCOPIC FEATURES

External Examination
- Surgical interventions: Wound status, drains
- Sepsis changes: Petechiae, jaundice, acrocyanosis
- Hemorrhagic changes: Pallor

Internal Examination
- Pleural/pericardial effusions
- Ascites, hemoperitoneum, fluid collections/abscesses, peritonitis (green-yellow fibrinous peritoneal/serosal surfaces)
- Peritoneal/serosal/mesenteric tumor studding/caking, lymphadenopathy

PANCREAS RESECTION

Organ Examination

- Examine upper gastrointestinal tract including remnant pancreas, biliary tract, and liver (if part of anastomosis) in situ for anastomotic leaks/strictures, fistulas
  - Remove en block, then open
- Stomach and small intestine
  - Mucosal ulcers, anastomotic necrosis ± dehiscence and perforation, perigastric/intestinal collections, abscesses, fistulas, strictures, adhesions
  - Ischemic changes: Dusky, hemorrhagic mucosa ± ulcers, green-yellow pseudomembranes, perforations
- Remnant pancreas
  - Indurated, edematous parenchyma ± hemorrhage, necrosis, peripancreatic abscesses, pseudocysts
  - Suture/staple line dehiscence/leak
  - Masses/cystic lesions in parenchyma or pancreatic bed
- Colon: Adhesions, ischemic changes
- Extrahepatic bile ducts: Mucosal erosions/ulcers, purulent debris, stenosis/strictures, fistulas, anastomotic dehiscence
- Liver: Congestion, patchy necrosis, cholestasis, abscesses, strictures/dilatations of intrahepatic bile ducts, masses
- Vascular: Status of stents/anastomoses/ligations, stenosis/strictures, thrombosis, pseudoaneurysms, kinking
- Heart: Subendocardial/myocardial mottling, pale soft areas ± hyperemic borders, nonbacterial thrombotic endocarditis (malignancy associated)
- Lungs: Consolidation, edema/congestion, abscesses, metastatic tumor, thromboemboli
- Kidneys: Cortical pallor, medullary congestion
- Venous system: Check for thrombi, presence of IVC filter or ligation
  - "Milk" lower extremities to check for venous thrombi (free-flowing blood = nonobstructed venous system, no blood flow = venous thrombosis)

MICROSCOPIC PATHOLOGY

Histologic Features

- Stomach, small intestine, and colon
  - Mucosal erosions/ulcers, transmural inflammation ± necrosis, acute/organizing serositis, fibroinflammatory adhesions
  - Ischemic injury: Epithelial sloughing/necrosis, ulcers, hemorrhage, transmural necrosis, mucopurulent exudate (pseudomembranes), remaining crypts/glands look withered
  - Serosal/mesenteric tumor deposits
- Remnant pancreas
  - Acute inflammation, edema, hemorrhage, fat necrosis
  - Recurrent/residual tumor
- Extrahepatic bile ducts: Mucosal erosions/ulcers, inflammation, mural fibrosis, degenerative/regenerative epithelial changes
- Liver
  - Sepsis changes: Hepatocellular, canalicular, and ductular cholestasis
  - Shock changes: Centrilobular/perivenular congestion and hepatocellular necrosis
  - Acute cholangitis: Bile duct intraluminal and intraepithelial acute inflammation, ± duct rupture and portal abscesses, sinusoidal neutrophils ± lobular abscesses, parenchymal necrosis
  - Large bile duct obstruction: Portal tract edema, chronic inflammation, periportal ductular reaction with associated neutrophils, cholestasis, bile infarcts
  - Metastatic tumor
- Heart: Subendocardial/myocardial contraction band injury, coagulative necrosis, edema, hemorrhage, ± neutrophils and macrophages
- Lungs: Bronchopneumonia, abscesses, diffuse alveolar damage (alveolar hyaline membranes, neutrophils, fibrin deposition, edema), metastatic tumor, pulmonary thromboemboli
- Kidneys: Dilated tubules and tubal epithelial necrosis/sloughing (acute tubular injury)

ANCILLARY TESTS

Microbiology

- Postmortem blood, fluid collection, tissue, and wound cultures if not done premortem

DIAGNOSTIC CHECKLIST

Reporting Criteria

- Immediate cause of death and how/if it relates to surgery
- Postsurgical complications and risk factors for developing complications
- Presence of residual/recurrent/metastatic tumor and paraneoplastic effects
  - If autopsy findings change original stage of tumor, new stage should be reported
  - Correlation of postmortem and premortem tumor pathology

SELECTED REFERENCES

1. Kim JH et al: Surgical outcomes of distal pancreatectomy. Hepatogastroenterology. 60(126):1263-7, 2013
2. Lermite E et al: Complications after pancreatic resection: diagnosis, prevention and management. Clin Res Hepatol Gastroenterol. 37(3):230-9, 2013
3. Bock EA et al: Late complications after pancreaticoduodenectomy with pancreaticogastrostomy. J Gastrointest Surg. 16(5):914-9, 2012
4. Shah OJ et al: Central pancreatectomy: a new technique for resection of selected pancreatic tumors. Hepatobiliary Pancreat Dis Int. 8(1):93-6, 2009

Graphic, Gross, and Microscopic Features

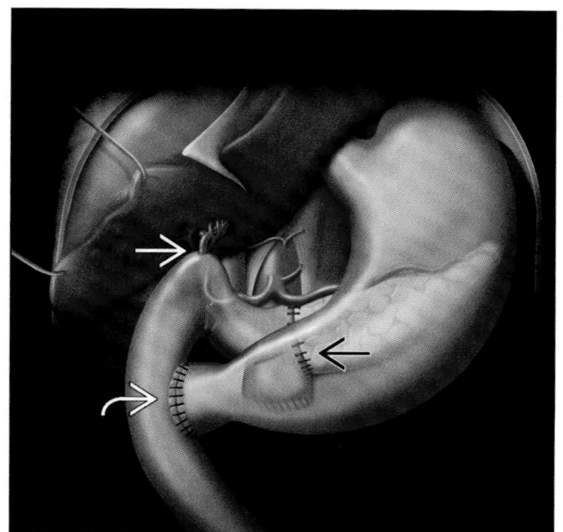

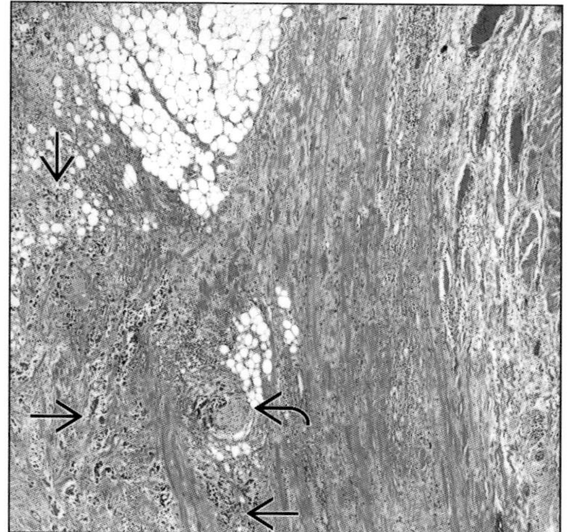

(Left) *The pylorus-preserving Whipple procedure has the following anastomoses: Remnant pancreaticojejunostomy ➙, hepatic bile duct hepaticojejunostomy ➙, and duodenojejunostomy ➙.* ***(Right)*** *Residual pancreatic ductal adenocarcinoma ➙ was identified invading the portal vein and surrounding soft tissue with perineural invasion ➙ in a patient who died 4 days after a Whipple procedure. This upstaged the original pathologic tumor stage from a pT2 to a pT4.*

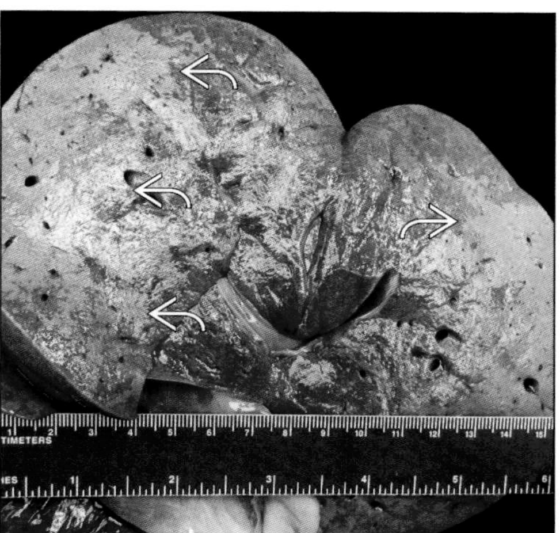

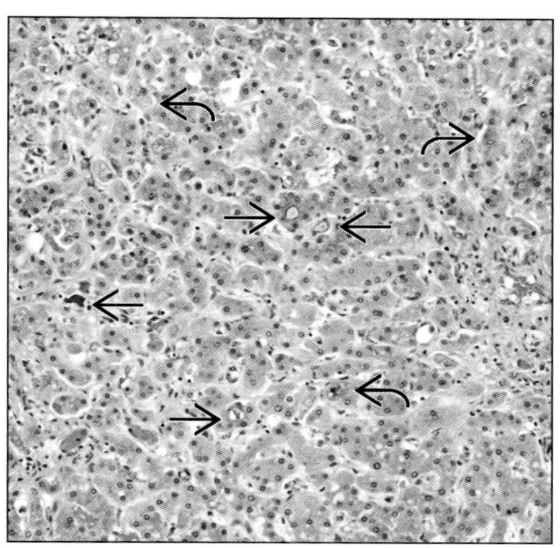

(Left) *Ischemic liver necrosis characterized by patchy pale tan soft parenchyma ➙ developed due to hemorrhagic shock secondary to rupture of a gastroduodenal artery stump pseudoaneurysm status post distal pancreatectomy.* ***(Right)*** *Sepsis changes in the liver are characterized by green-brown bile plugs ➙ in the canalicular spaces and hepatocellular cholestasis ➙. These findings were present in the patient with peritonitis and sepsis status post distal pancreatectomy.*

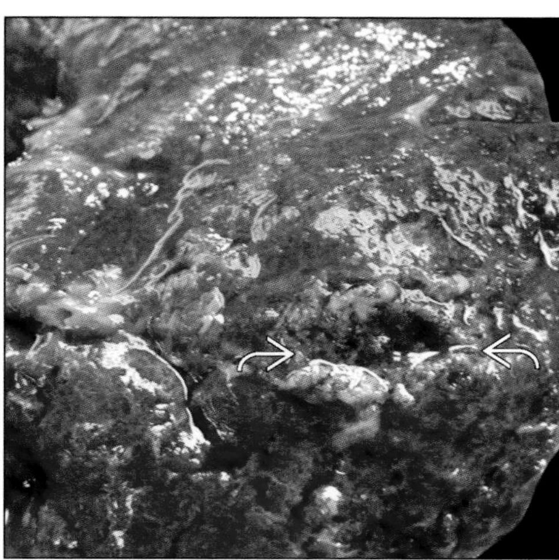

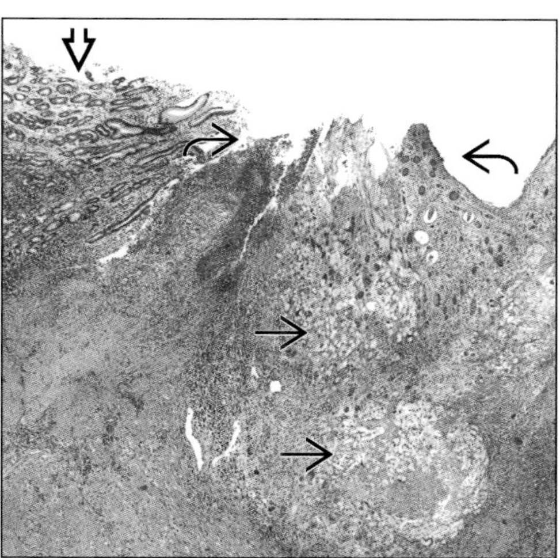

(Left) *This lung abscess ➙ was discovered at autopsy in a patient who developed postoperative pneumonia after a Whipple procedure. Postmortem culture grew Klebsiella pneumoniae.* ***(Right)*** *Section through the gastrojejunostomy site in a patient status post Whipple procedure shows a mucosal ulcer ➙, granulation tissue, and foreign body giant cell reaction to suture material ➙ at the anastomosis. Intact gastric mucosa ➙ is present on one side of the anastomosis.*

GASTRECTOMY AND ESOPHAGECTOMY

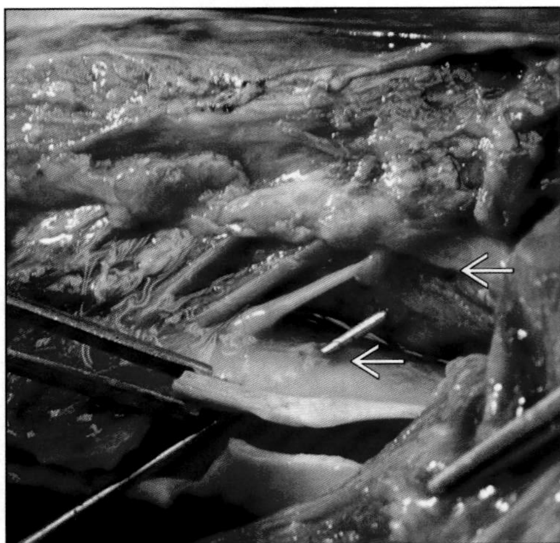

This patient died during a transhiatal esophagectomy as a result of transection of the right intercostal artery at the level of T6 as demonstrated by the probe ➡. (Courtesy J. Hon, MD.)

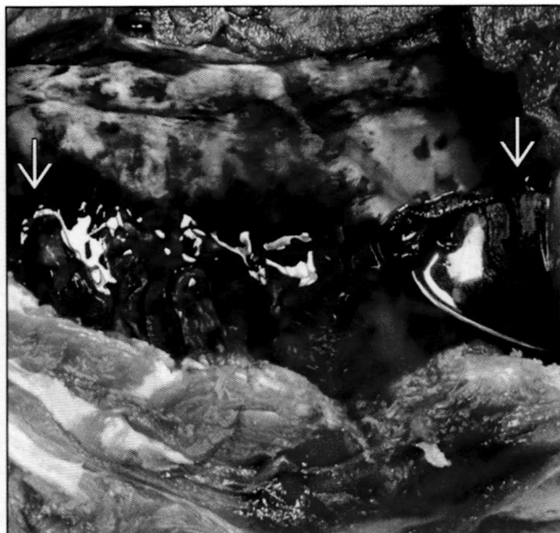

A right-sided hemothorax ➡ containing 1,700 mL of blood was found in the same patient as a result of transection of the intercostal artery at ~ 3 mm from the aortic origin.

TERMINOLOGY

Definitions

- Esophagectomy: Partial or total resection of esophagus; many different surgical approaches (transhiatal, thoracoabdominal, thoracotomy, minimally invasive, 3-hole technique)
  - ± conduit such as small intestine or colon
- Ivor Lewis esophagogastrectomy: 2-stage surgical procedure composed of subcostal abdominal incision followed by a right thoracotomy
  - Performed for tumors of distal esophagus, gastroesophageal (GE) junction, or proximal stomach
- Gastrectomy: Resection of part or all of stomach; many different surgical approaches (partial, distal, subtotal, or total resection, ± Billroth I or II or Roux-en-Y anastomosis)
- Billroth I operation (gastroduodenostomy): Anastomosis of proximal stomach directly to duodenum after distal gastrectomy
- Billroth II operation (gastrojejunostomy): Anastomosis of end of remnant stomach to side of proximal jejunum after partial or subtotal gastrectomy
- Roux-en-Y anastomosis: Anastomosis of end of remnant stomach or esophagus to a portion of jejunum with creation of a jejunojejunostomy after a partial or subtotal gastrectomy

ETIOLOGY/PATHOGENESIS

Indications for Resection

- Esophagectomy: Benign/malignant neoplasms, corrosive/peptic strictures, achalasia, perforation
- Gastrectomy: Benign/malignant neoplasms, bleeding or perforation due to peptic ulcer disease, pyloric stenosis, gastric outlet obstruction

CLINICAL ISSUES

Presentation

- Symptoms
  - Cough, dyspnea, tachypnea, chest pain, palpitations, hemoptysis
  - Nausea, vomiting, hematemesis, abdominal pain, melena
- Signs
  - Fever, tachycardia, arrhythmia, altered mental status
  - Hypotension, hypoxemia, hypovolemic/septic shock, peritoneal signs
- Important elements of chart review
  - Indication for surgery/underlying disease, comorbidities
  - Type of operation performed, intraoperative complications, postoperative course
  - Surgical pathology reports for confirmation and extent of disease

Laboratory Tests

- ↓ hemoglobin/hematocrit, (+) fecal occult blood
- Leukocytosis, lactic acidosis
- ↑ creatine kinase-MB, troponin, BUN, creatinine, amylase and lipase, (+) D-dimer
- Chylous effusion: Triglycerides > 110 mg/dL, ratio of effusion fluid to serum triglycerides > 1.0, ratio of effusion fluid to serum cholesterol < 1.0
- (+) blood, wound, fluid collection cultures (e.g., bronchial washes, effusions, abscesses)

Prognosis

- Mortality rate
  - Esophagectomy: Up to 22%, average ~ 2.5%
  - Gastrectomy: Up to 14%, average ~ 2%
- Causes of death
  - Post esophagectomy
    - Pulmonary (2/3 of postoperative deaths): Pneumonia ± aspiration due to recurrent

GASTRECTOMY AND ESOPHAGECTOMY

Key Facts

Clinical Issues
- Complications reported in up to 60% of cases following both esophagectomy and gastrectomy
- Risk factors for complications: ↑ age, procedure performed at low-volume center, male sex, comorbidities
- Mortality rate: Esophagectomy: Up to 22%, average ~ 2.5%; gastrectomy: Up to 14%, average ~ 2%
- Causes of death post esophagectomy
  - Pulmonary: Pneumonia ± aspiration, tracheoesophageal fistula, acute respiratory distress syndrome, pulmonary embolism
  - Anastomotic/conduit related: Dehiscence → mediastinitis, ischemia/necrosis → perforation
  - Cardiovascular: Myocardial infarction, atrial fibrillation/other arrhythmia
  - Others: Arterial-esophageal fistula, chylothorax, cerebrovascular accident, sepsis, multiorgan failure
- Causes of death post gastrectomy
  - Anastomotic: Dehiscence/ischemia/necrosis → intraabdominal abscess, peritonitis → sepsis
  - Intraabdominal: Ileus, intestinal obstruction, fistula formation, perforation → sepsis
  - Pulmonary: Pneumonia, acute respiratory distress syndrome, pulmonary embolism

Reporting Considerations
- Immediate cause of death and how it relates to surgery
- Other postsurgical complications
- Risk factors for developing postsurgical complications
- Presence of residual/metastatic disease

laryngeal nerve injury/other swallowing disorder/ tracheoesophageal fistula, acute respiratory distress syndrome, pulmonary embolism
    - Anastomotic/conduit related: Dehiscence → mediastinitis, ischemia/necrosis → perforation → sepsis
    - Cardiovascular: Myocardial infarction, atrial fibrillation/other arrhythmia, vascular injury
    - Chylothorax due to thoracic duct injury (rare) → protein loss → sepsis, acidosis, electrolyte abnormalities
    - Arterial-esophageal fistula
    - Others: Cerebral infarction, sepsis, multiorgan failure
  - Post gastrectomy
    - Anastomotic: Dehiscence/ischemia/necrosis → intraabdominal abscess, peritonitis → sepsis
    - Intraabdominal: Ileus, intestinal obstruction, fistula formation, perforation → sepsis
    - Pulmonary: Pneumonia, acute respiratory distress syndrome, pulmonary embolism

Complications
- Complications reported in up to 60% of cases following both esophagectomy and gastrectomy
- Risk factors for complications: ↑ age, procedure performed at low-volume center, male sex, comorbidities
- Early complications
  - Esophagectomy: Pulmonary/intrathoracic (most common), anastomotic/conduit related, cardiovascular, infection
  - Ivor Lewis procedure: Pulmonary, anastomotic, infection
  - Gastrectomy: Anastomotic (most common), intraabdominal, pulmonary, infection
- Long-term complications
  - Esophagectomy/Ivor Lewis procedure: Strictures, diaphragmatic hernia, dumping syndrome, reflux esophagitis ± Barrett esophagus → dysplasia → adenocarcinoma
  - Gastrectomy
    - Malnutrition, vitamin B12/iron deficiency → anemia, fat maldigestion → steatorrhea and fat-soluble vitamin deficiency, osteoporosis
    - Reflux esophagitis ± Barrett esophagus → dysplasia → adenocarcinoma
    - Bile reflux, remnant gastritis → remnant/stump adenocarcinoma (may be Epstein-Barr virus [EBV] associated)

IMAGE FINDINGS

CT Findings
- Pulmonary infiltrates, pleural/pericardial effusions, mediastinal fluid collections, or pneumomediastinum
- Intraabdominal abscess, free air, ascites, ileus/intestinal obstruction

Upper GI Series/Contrast Swallow
- Abnormal swallowing, anastomotic leaks, strictures, ulcers

CT Angiogram
- Identify/treat active bleeding, vascular injury, fistulas
- Pulmonary angiogram for pulmonary embolism

MACROSCOPIC FEATURES

External Examination
- Surgical interventions: Incisions, wound status, drains
- Sepsis changes: Petechiae, jaundice, acrocyanosis
- Hemorrhagic changes: Pallor

Internal Examination
- Pleural effusions, empyema, hemothorax (examine thoracic vessels in situ if present)
- Chylothorax: White, turbid, milky effusion + thoracic duct injury (examine in situ, best viewed from left side)
- Pericardial effusion
- Mediastinitis: Fibrinopurulent exudate, abscesses

GASTRECTOMY AND ESOPHAGECTOMY

- Ascites, peritonitis (green-tan fibrinous peritoneal/serosal surfaces)
- Metastatic disease, lymphadenopathy

Organ Examination

- Examine upper GI tract in situ for fistulas/anastomotic leaks: May transect cervical esophagus above anastomosis and perfuse with water/dye to assess for leaks
- Remove esophagus, stomach, duodenum ± jejunum (if part of anastomosis) en bloc, then open
  - Esophagus: Anastomotic ulcer, necrosis ± dehiscence, perforation, arterial/tracheoesophageal fistula, strictures, mucosal erythema/erosions, tan/salmon-colored mucosa (Barrett esophagus), masses
  - Stomach: Mucosal erythema/erosions, anastomotic ulcer, necrosis ± dehiscence, perforation, perigastric abscesses, fistulas, masses
  - Small and large intestine: Obstruction (functional vs. adhesions/strictures/masses), fistulas, ischemic changes (dusky, hemorrhagic mucosa ± ulcers, green-yellow pseudomembranes, perforations)
- Pancreas: Indurated, edematous pancreas ± hemorrhage, necrosis, peripancreatic abscesses, pseudocysts, fat necrosis
- Lungs: Consolidation, abscesses (R > L in cases of aspiration), edema/congestion, thromboemboli, wedge-shaped hemorrhagic infarct, fibrinous pleural exudate
- Cardiovascular: Subendocardial/myocardial mottling, pale yellow discoloration ± surrounding hyperemia (infarction), evidence of vascular injury/pseudoaneurysms/rupture
- Kidneys: Cortical pallor, medullary congestion
- Liver: Congestion, patchy necrosis, cholestasis
- Brain: Infarcts (areas of softening with tan discoloration or hemorrhage)

MICROSCOPIC PATHOLOGY

Histologic Features

- Gastrointestinal tract
  - Anastomotic mucosal ulcers, transmural acute inflammation ± necrosis, acute/organizing serositis, fibroinflammatory adhesions
  - Reflux esophagitis, Barrett esophagus, dysplasia → adenocarcinoma
  - Gastric remnant chronic gastritis/reactive gastropathy → intestinal metaplasia, dysplasia → adenocarcinoma
  - Ischemic enterocolitis: Epithelial necrosis/sloughing, mucosal ulcers, lamina propria/submucosal hemorrhage, transmural necrosis, mucopurulent exudate (pseudomembranes), "withered" crypts
  - Acute pancreatitis with neutrophils, edema, hemorrhage, adjacent fat necrosis ± calcification
- Lungs
  - Bronchopneumonia, abscesses, intraalveolar edema, fibrin deposition, hyaline membranes, foreign body giant cell reaction to food material or keratinaceous debris (aspiration)
  - Radiation pneumonitis (diffuse alveolar damage, organizing pneumonia, interstitial and alveolar fibrosis, vascular intimal fibrosis with foamy macrophages)
  - Thromboemboli ± intraalveolar hemorrhage
- Cardiovascular
  - Subendocardial/myocardial contraction band injury, coagulative necrosis, edema, hemorrhage ± neutrophils, macrophages
- Kidneys
  - Acute tubular injury/necrosis: Dilated tubules, epithelial cell sloughing/necrosis, pigmented tubular casts
- Liver
  - Shock changes: Centrilobular (perivenular) congestion ± hepatocellular necrosis without significant inflammation
  - Sepsis changes: Canalicular cholestasis, bile ductular cholestasis ± associated neutrophils
- Brain
  - Parenchymal infarcts: Vacuolization of white matter, shrunken red neurons (eosinophilic cytoplasm, pyknotic nuclei) ± neutrophils, macrophages, hemorrhage

ANCILLARY TESTS

Microbiology

- Postmortem blood, wound, tissue/fluid cultures can be performed if not done premortem

REPORTING CONSIDERATIONS

Final Report Should Include

- Immediate cause of death and how it relates to surgery
- Other postsurgical complications
- Risk factors for developing postsurgical complications
- Presence of residual/metastatic disease

SELECTED REFERENCES

1. Kim KM et al: Major early complications following open, laparoscopic and robotic gastrectomy. Br J Surg. 99(12):1681-7, 2012
2. Raymond D: Complications of esophagectomy. Surg Clin North Am. 92(5):1299-313, 2012
3. Schieman C et al: Patterns of operative mortality following esophagectomy. Dis Esophagus. 25(7):645-51, 2012
4. Smith JK et al: National outcomes after gastric resection for neoplasm. Arch Surg. 2007 Apr;142(4):387-93. Erratum in: Arch Surg. 144(7):634, 2009
5. Atkins BZ et al: Reducing hospital morbidity and mortality following esophagectomy. Ann Thorac Surg. 78(4):1170-6; discussion 1170-6, 2004
6. Wang CS et al: Resectable gastric cancer: operative mortality and survival analysis. Chang Gung Med J. 25(4):216-27, 2002
7. Karl RC et al: Factors affecting morbidity, mortality, and survival in patients undergoing Ivor Lewis esophagogastrectomy. Ann Surg. 231(5):635-43, 2000

Gross and Microscopic Findings

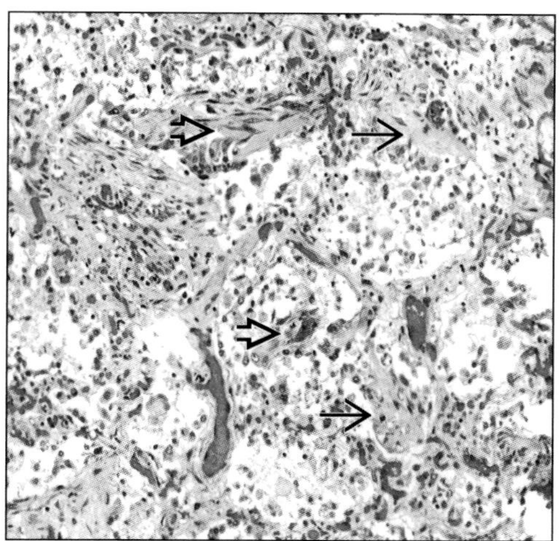

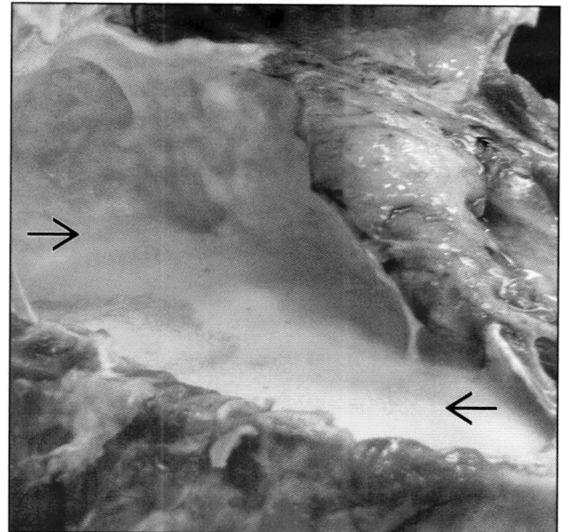

(Left) *Radiation pneumonitis in a patient who was irradiated for esophageal carcinoma is characterized by features of diffuse alveolar damage with intraalveolar fibrin ➡ and inflammation as well as fibroblastic foci with reactive atypia of pneumocytes and fibroblasts ➡.* ***(Right)*** *Chylothorax is a rare complication of esophagectomy, characterized by a turbid, milky, yellow-white effusion ➡ and occurs as a result of thoracic duct injury. (Courtesy R. Irvine, MD.)*

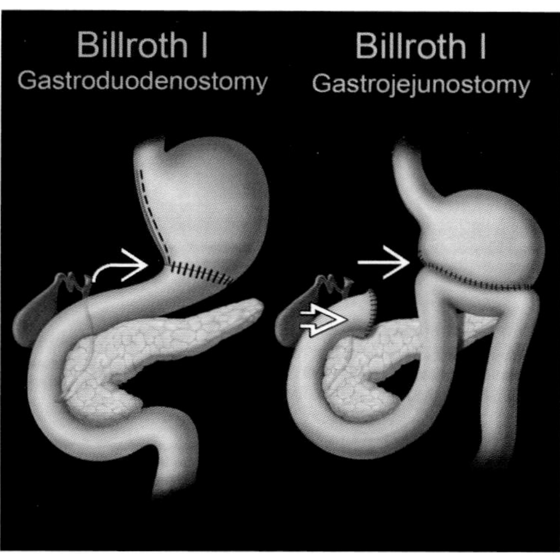

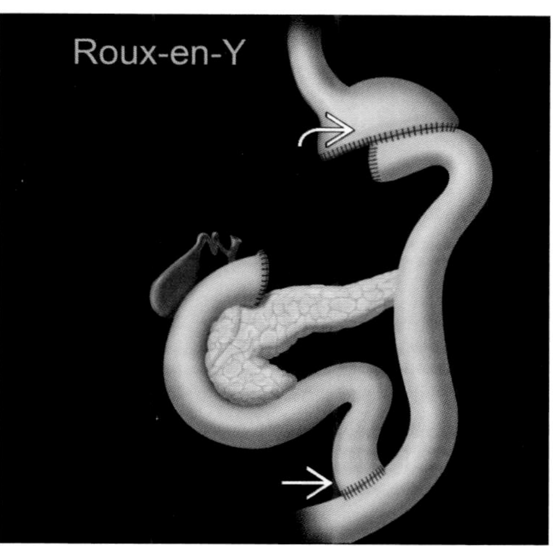

(Left) *The proximal stomach is connected directly to the duodenum ➡ in the Billroth I anastomosis and is connected to the jejunum ➡ with closure of the proximal duodenum ➡ in the Billroth II anastomosis after partial gastrectomy.* ***(Right)*** *The esophagus or proximal stomach is connected to a portion of divided jejunum ➡, and the other end of the proximal jejunum is reconnected to the distal jejunum ➡, creating a "Y" shape in the Roux-en-Y anastomosis after gastrectomy.*

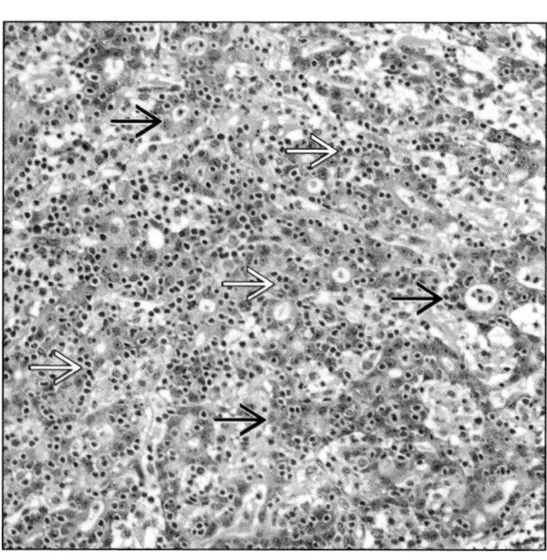

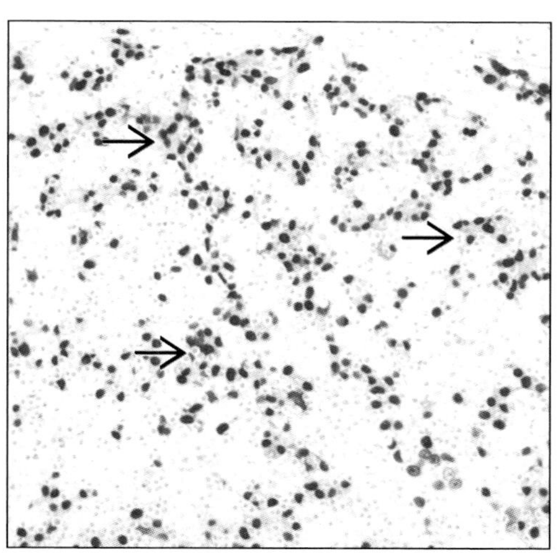

(Left) *Gastric remnant adenocarcinoma composed of poorly formed tubules ➡ with numerous tumor-infiltrating lymphocytes ➡ (gastric carcinoma with lymphoid stroma) was present near the gastroenteric anastomosis in a patient status post partial gastrectomy 40 years prior for peptic ulcer disease.* ***(Right)*** *In situ hybridization for EBV (EBER) is positive (red) in tumor cell nuclei ➡ and negative in lymphocytes in this EBV-associated gastric remnant carcinoma with lymphoid stroma.*

BARIATRIC SURGERY

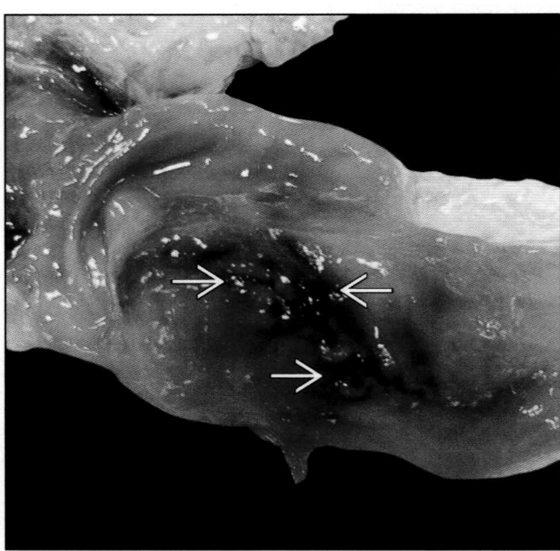

This residual sleeve of stomach shows mucosal necrosis along the staple line ➡ with associated dehiscence and leak, status post laparoscopic sleeve gastrectomy. (Courtesy R. Irvine, MD.)

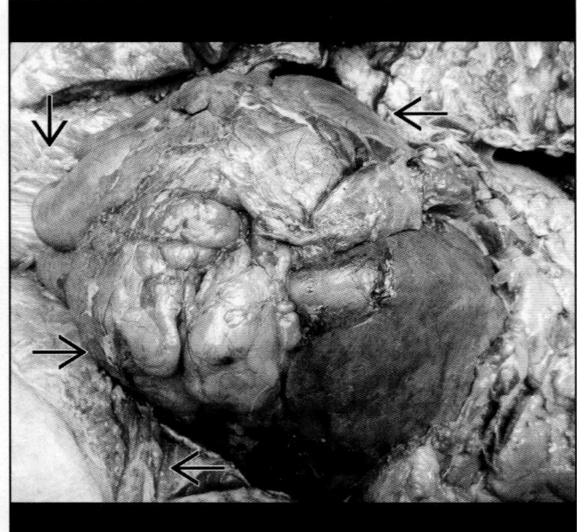

Peritonitis characterized by a greenish exudate ➡ covering the peritoneal and abdominal organ serosal surfaces was due to a leak status post laparoscopic sleeve gastrectomy.

TERMINOLOGY

Definitions

- Morbid obesity: Body mass index (BMI) ≥ 40 kg/m² or BMI ≥ 35 kg/m² with associated comorbidities
- Types of bariatric surgery: Restrictive vs. both restrictive and malabsorptive
  - Restrictive procedures
  - Gastric banding
    - Laparoscopic adjustable gastric banding: Band wrapped around entire stomach to create pouch; adjustable and reversible; continuity of gastrointestinal tract remains intact
    - Vertical banded gastroplasty: Gastric pouch and "window" (defect through both anterior and posterior walls) created with staples; band wraps around pouch through window to restrict pouch
  - Laparoscopic sleeve gastrectomy: Vertical resection of lateral portion (~ 80%) of stomach to create thin residual "sleeve"
  - Restrictive and malabsorptive procedures
  - Roux-en-Y gastric bypass
    - Stomach is divided proximally to create a small pouch, which is connected directly to a segment of jejunum (Roux limb)
    - Remaining bypassed stomach with attached duodenum and proximal jejunum is stapled closed proximally
    - Jejunojejunostomy creates "Y" intersection
  - Biliopancreatic diversion: Not commonly performed
    - Partial distal gastrectomy and closure of duodenal stump
    - Small bowel divided between ligament of Treitz and ileocecal valve with Roux-en-Y gastroenterostomy of proximal gastric pouch to distal portion of small bowel
    - Biliopancreatic limb (duodenum and proximal small bowel) anastomosed to distal small bowel
    - Modification: Duodenal switch procedure: Vertical sleeve gastrectomy (in lieu of partial distal gastrectomy for preservation of antrum and pylorus) combined with duodenoenterostomy

CLINICAL ISSUES

Epidemiology

- Incidence
  - Incidence of morbid obesity in USA: 2-5%
  - Incidence of complications of bariatric surgery: Up to 20% depending on procedure; average: 6-10%

Presentation

- Symptoms: Abdominal pain, nausea, vomiting, dysphagia, hematemesis, melena, chest pain, dyspnea
- Signs: Tachycardia, tachypnea, arrhythmia, hypotension, altered mental status
- Important elements of chart review
  - Underlying comorbidities: Diabetes mellitus, coronary artery disease, hypertension, obstructive sleep apnea, obesity hypoventilation syndrome, cirrhosis, dyslipidemia, cholelithiasis
  - Type of operation performed, intraoperative complications, postoperative course, interventions performed for complications, concurrent surgical procedures (e.g., herniorrhaphy, cholecystectomy)

Laboratory Tests

- Leukocytosis, lactic acidosis, ↑ blood urea nitrogen and creatinine (sepsis)
- ↑ C-reactive protein, lactate, and B-type natriuretic peptide (BNP)
- ↓ hemoglobin and hematocrit, (+) fecal occult blood, (+) D-dimer
- ↓ serum iron, ferritin, transferrin saturation, and reticulocyte count; ↑ total iron binding capacity (iron deficiency)

BARIATRIC SURGERY

Key Facts

Terminology
- Types of bariatric surgery: Gastric banding (vertical banded gastroplasty vs. laparoscopic adjustable gastric banding), laparoscopic sleeve gastrectomy, Roux-en-Y gastric bypass, biliopancreatic diversion

Clinical Issues
- Incidence of morbid obesity in USA: 2-5%
- Incidence of complications of bariatric surgery: Up to 20% depending on procedure; average 6-10%
- Risk factors for complications: Male sex, older age, higher preoperative BMI, diabetes mellitus, pulmonary hypertension, low hospital case load, prolonged operation time, open surgery
- Overall mortality: ~ 0.05-5%
- Common causes of death: Pulmonary embolism, sepsis, arrhythmia, hemorrhage
- Early complications
  - Deep vein thrombosis, pulmonary embolism, gastrointestinal ulcers/hemorrhage/ischemia, small bowel obstruction, adhesions, fistulas, strictures, arrhythmia
  - Sepsis due to wound infection, anastomotic leak/dehiscence, intraabdominal abscess
  - Hemorrhagic shock due to iatrogenic vascular injury, pseudoaneurysms
  - Complications related to band

Macroscopic Pathology
- Evaluate upper gastrointestinal tract in situ for fistulas and anastomotic leaks
- Note location and status of band, if present
- Remove esophagus, stomach, and small bowel (if part of anastomosis) en bloc, then open

- Megaloblastic anemia (B12 and folate deficiency), microcytic hypochromic anemia (iron deficiency)
- (+) blood, wound, fluid collection (e.g., abscesses, ascites, effusions) cultures

Prognosis
- Overall mortality: ~ 0.05-5%
- Mortality rate by procedure: Banding < sleeve gastrectomy < Roux-en-Y bypass < biliopancreatic diversion
- Common causes of death: Pulmonary embolism, sepsis, arrhythmia, hemorrhage

Complications
- Risk factors for complications
  - Male sex, older age, higher preoperative BMI, diabetes mellitus, pulmonary hypertension
  - Low hospital case load, prolonged operative time, open vs. laparoscopic surgery
- Early complications
  - Deep vein thrombosis (DVT), pulmonary embolism, gastrointestinal ulcers/hemorrhage/ischemia, small bowel obstruction, adhesions, fistulas, strictures, arrhythmia
  - Sepsis due to wound infection, anastomotic leak/dehiscence, intraabdominal abscess
  - Hemorrhagic shock due to iatrogenic vascular injury, pseudoaneurysms
  - Complications related to band: Pressure necrosis of stomach, erosions, reflux, band/port infection, band slippage/migration, tube or port disconnection → small bowel obstruction, perforation
- Late complications
  - Vitamin deficiencies: Folate, iron, B12, fat-soluble vitamins
  - Protein-calorie malnutrition
  - Adhesions/strictures → obstruction
  - Reflux esophagitis → Barrett esophagus → dysplasia/adenocarcinoma

IMAGE FINDINGS

Ultrasonographic Findings
- Duplex ultrasound for DVT

CT Findings
- Ascites, intraabdominal abscess, abdominal free air, intestinal obstruction, pleural/pericardial effusions, pulmonary infiltrates
- CT pulmonary angiography for pulmonary embolism

Upper GI Series/Contrast Swallow
- Anastomotic leaks, strictures, ulcers, evidence of band dislocation/slippage

CT Angiogram
- Identify/treat active bleeding, vascular injury, pseudoaneurysms, fistulas

MACROSCOPIC FEATURES

External Examination
- Surgery-related: Wound status, drains, incisional hernias, cutaneous fistulas
- Obesity-related: ↑ weight (record weight and height to calculate BMI at postmortem), decubitus ulcers, venous stasis, striae, excess skin folds after significant weight loss
- Sepsis changes: Petechiae, jaundice, acrocyanosis
- Shock changes: Pallor (also related to anemia)

Internal Examination
- Ascites, peritonitis (green fibrinous exudates on peritoneal/serosal surfaces), hemoperitoneum

Organ Examination
- Evaluate upper gastrointestinal tract in situ for surgically altered anatomy, fistulas, and anastomotic/staple line leaks
  - May perfuse esophagus with water or dye to assess for leaks

BARIATRIC SURGERY

- Note location and status of band and associated connecting tube and port, if present
- Remove esophagus, stomach, and small bowel (if part of anastomosis) en bloc
  - Esophagus: Mucosal erythema, erosions, tan/salmon-colored mucosa (Barrett esophagus)
  - Stomach: Mucosal erosions/ulcers, anastomotic ulcers/dehiscence ± perforation, perigastric abscesses, fistulas
  - Small and large intestine: Obstruction, strictures, fistulas, adhesions, perforations, ischemic changes (dusky red-black mucosa ± ulcers, tan-green pseudomembranes), thrombi in mesenteric vessels
- Obesity-related findings
  - Atheromas in pulmonary arteries (pulmonary hypertension)
  - Cardiomegaly, biventricular hypertrophy and dilatation (obesity cardiomyopathy)
  - Right ventricular hypertrophy and dilatation (cor pulmonale: May relate to associated obstructive sleep apnea), concentric left ventricular hypertrophy (hypertension), ± atrial dilatation
  - Hepatomegaly, yellow fatty cut surface (obesity-related ± metabolic syndrome), cirrhosis (due to nonalcoholic fatty liver disease)
  - Cholelithiasis (obesity ↑ risk)
- Surgery-related findings
  - Pulmonary thromboemboli, wedge-shaped hemorrhagic infarct, fibrinous pleural exudate, consolidation/congestion
  - Evidence of vascular injury/pseudoaneurysms
  - Legs can be "milked" for DVT once organs are removed
- Shock/sepsis changes
  - Subendocardial/myocardial mottling, tan-yellow soft areas ± hyperemic borders (if sepsis or hemorrhagic complications have caused myocardial ischemia)
  - Liver: Congestion and necrosis (shock), cholestasis (sepsis)
  - Kidneys: Cortical pallor, medullary congestion (shock)

MICROSCOPIC PATHOLOGY

Histologic Features

- Gastrointestinal tract
  - Anastomotic ulcers, transmural inflammation ± necrosis, acute/organizing serositis, fibroinflammatory adhesions
  - Ischemic enterocolitis: Epithelial necrosis/sloughing, mucosal ulcers, hemorrhage, transmural necrosis, remaining crypts are "withered," mucopurulent exudate (pseudomembranes)
    - ± mesenteric arterial thrombi, atherosclerosis
  - Reflux esophagitis, Barrett esophagus → dysplasia → adenocarcinoma
- Obesity-related findings
  - Pulmonary vessels with medial hypertrophy, intimal hyperplasia/fibrosis, plexiform arteriopathy with capillary tufts forming web that spans lumen (pulmonary hypertension)
  - Fat within right ventricle without fibrosis, myocyte hypertrophy (obesity cardiomyopathy)
  - Hepatic steatosis, steatohepatitis ± fibrosis, cirrhosis
  - Cholecystitis, cholesterolosis
  - Renal diabetic or hypertensive changes (↑ risk with obesity)
- Surgery-related findings
  - Pulmonary artery thromboemboli ± recanalization, intraalveolar hemorrhage
- Shock/sepsis changes
  - Bronchopneumonia, abscesses, intraalveolar edema, or alveolar hyaline membranes with edema and inflammation (i.e., diffuse alveolar damage)
  - Subendocardial/myocardial contraction band injury, coagulative necrosis, edema, hemorrhage ± neutrophils, interstitial fibrosis/scar
  - Canalicular, hepatocellular, and ductular cholestasis (sepsis)
  - Centrilobular congestion ± hepatocellular necrosis (shock)
  - Dilated renal tubules, epithelial sloughing (i.e., acute tubular injury/necrosis)

ANCILLARY TESTS

Microbiology

- Postmortem blood, wound, fluid collection, and tissue cultures if not done premortem

REPORTING CRITERIA

Final Report Should Include

- Immediate cause of death and how it relates to surgery
- Other postsurgical complications
- Risk factors for developing complications

SELECTED REFERENCES

1. Benotti P et al: Risk factors associated with mortality after Roux-en-Y gastric bypass surgery. Ann Surg. 259(1):123-30, 2014
2. Fryer E et al: Postmortem examination in the morbidly obese. Histopathology. 64(2):200-10, 2014
3. Anderson B et al: Biliopancreatic diversion: the effectiveness of duodenal switch and its limitations. Gastroenterol Res Pract. 2013:974762, 2013
4. de la Matta-Martín M et al: Perioperative morbi-mortality associated with bariatric surgery: from systematic biliopancreatic diversion to a tailored laparoscopic gastric bypass or sleeve gastrectomy approach. Obes Surg. 22(7):1001-7, 2012
5. Kirshtein B et al: Bariatric emergencies for non-bariatric surgeons: complications of laparoscopic gastric banding. Obes Surg. 20(11):1468-78, 2010
6. Cummings PM et al: Postmortem findings in morbidly obese individuals dying after gastric bypass procedures. Hum Pathol. 38(4):593-7, 2007

Gross and Microscopic Features

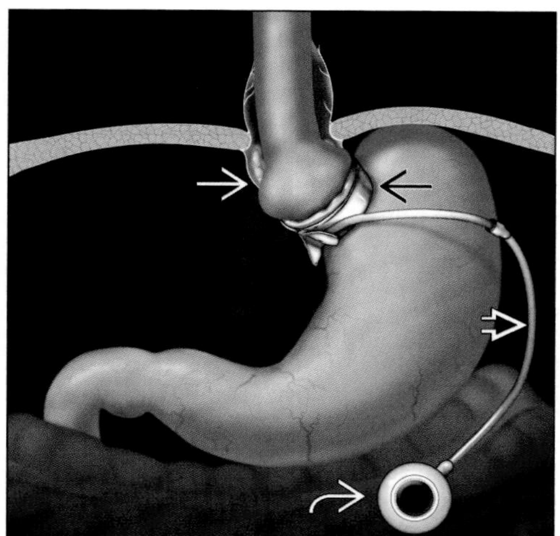

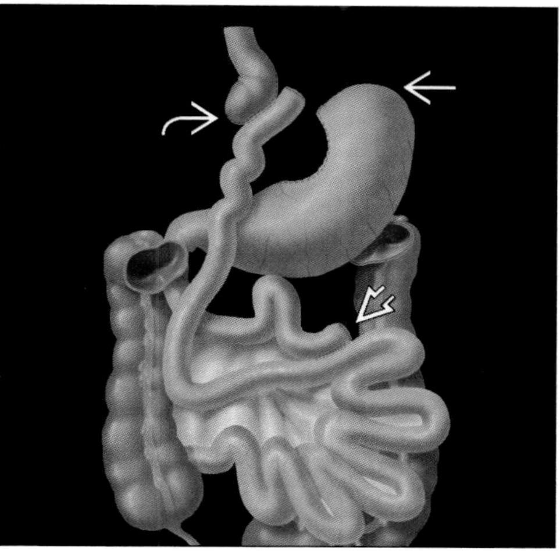

(Left) A band ⇒ is wrapped around the proximal stomach to create a small pouch ➡ in the laparoscopic adjustable gastric banding procedure. A connecting tube ➡ attaches to a port ➡ to inflate/deflate band. ***(Right)*** A small pouch of stomach is connected to a segment of jejunum (Roux limb) ➡, and the remaining portion of stomach with duodenum and proximal jejunum is closed proximally ➡. A jejunojejunostomy ➡ creates the "Y" intersection in a Roux-en-Y gastric bypass.

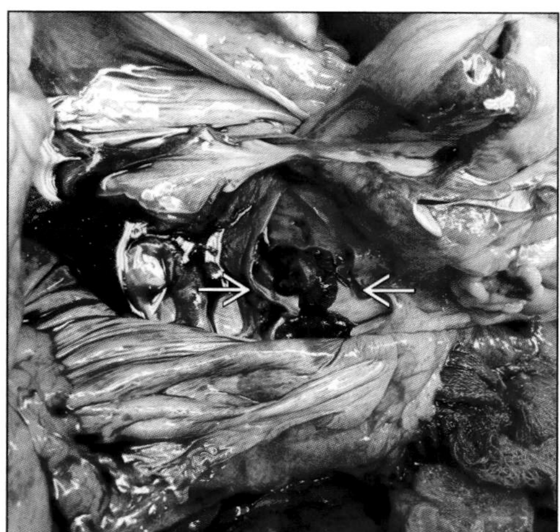

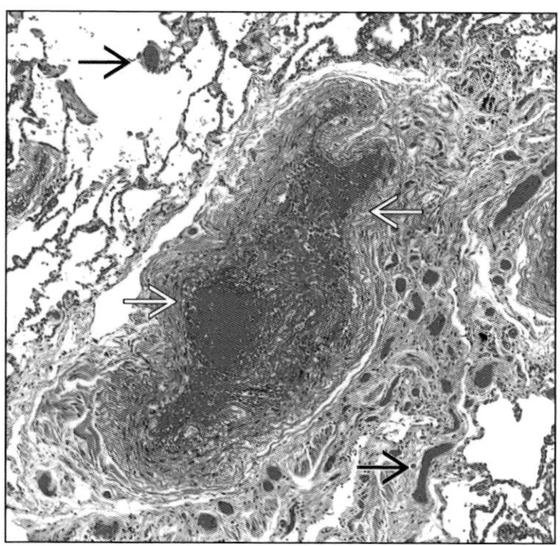

(Left) A saddle embolus ➡ in the pulmonary artery bifurcation was the cause of death status post Roux-en-Y gastric bypass surgery. ***(Right)*** Sections through the lung in a patient with pulmonary embolism after gastric bypass surgery show organizing thromboemboli ➡ in the arteries with associated vascular congestion ⇒.

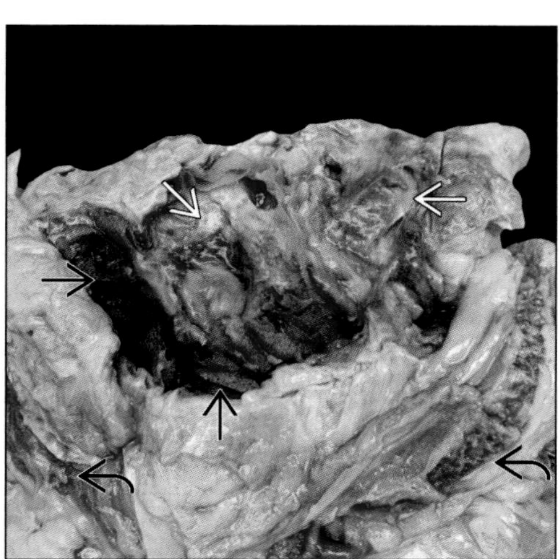

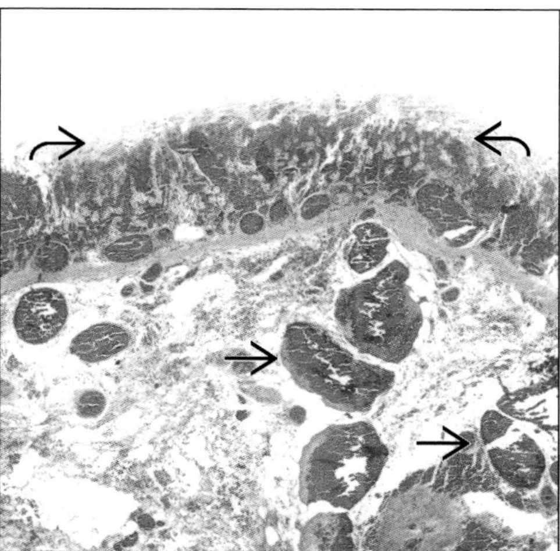

(Left) The anterior abdominal wall contained a mesh ⇒ with purulent exudate ➡ in a patient with a chronically infected incisional herniorrhaphy wound, status post open gastric bypass surgery. Loops of small bowel ⇒ were entrapped in adhesions around the mesh. (Courtesy M. Nagar, MD.) ***(Right)*** The remnant (excluded) stomach showed ischemic mucosal necrosis ⇒ with vascular congestion ⇒ as a result of adhesions to the reduced gastric pouch in the same patient.

CENTRAL NERVOUS SYSTEM TUMORS

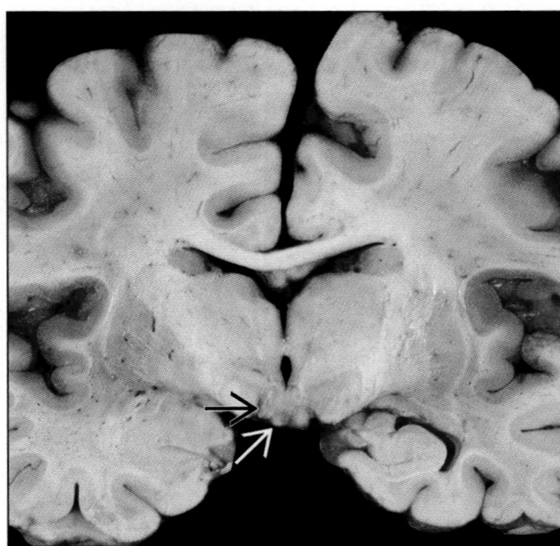

A young adult died with a pilocytic astrocytoma (WHO grade I) in the hypothalamus ⇨. There was local infiltration into the mammillary bodies ➡, which are becoming obscured, and into the optic chiasm.

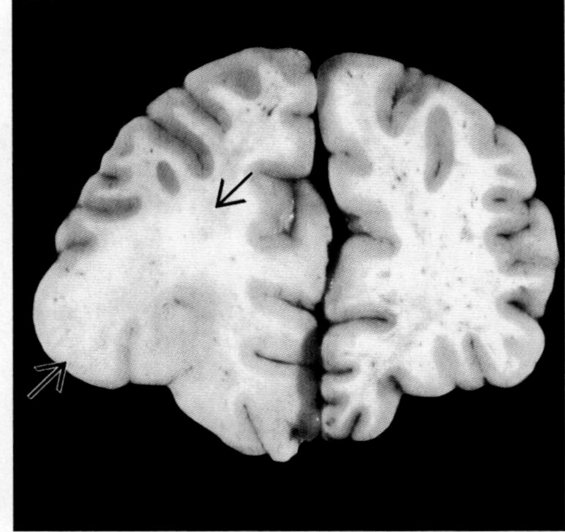

A low-grade infiltrating glioma is seen in the left frontal lobe ⇨. A previously well young man with sudden malaise lost consciousness and fell to his death. Autopsy revealed a large oligodendroglioma (WHO grade II).

TERMINOLOGY

Scope

- Brain tumors in adults, including incidental, 1st discovered at autopsy, or post-therapy settings

ETIOLOGY/PATHOGENESIS

Familial

- 5%, most syndromic
- Neurofibromatosis type 1 and type 2, Li-Fraumeni, von Hippel-Lindau, and Turcot syndromes
- Nonsyndromic
  - Tend to be high grade
  - Usually few cases in consecutive generations
  - Low risk of more family members developing glioma

Sporadic

- No clear causative associations

Post Radiation Tumors

- Meningiomas
- Parenchymal gliomas

Metastatic Brain Tumors

- Lung, breast, skin (melanoma), kidney, colon

CLINICAL ISSUES

Epidemiology

- Diffusely infiltrating astrocytomas (> 60% of primary brain tumors)
  - Diffuse astrocytoma (WHO grade II)
  - Anaplastic astrocytoma (WHO grade III)
  - Glioblastoma (WHO grade IV)
    - > 50% of all astrocytomas
- Meningiomas
  - ~ 30% of intracranial tumors
- Metastatic brain tumors
  - 14-22%

Presentation

- Headache, nausea/vomiting, behavior change, fatigue, seizure, hemorrhage

Natural History

- Local effects and progression
  - Infiltration, pressure on vital brain centers
    - Fatal pressure on brainstem, upper spinal cord
  - Intratumoral hemorrhage; massive can be fatal
  - Intracranial and occasionally spinal dissemination
- Cause of death (gliomas)
  - Low-grade gliomas
    - Progression to high-grade glioma, involvement of brainstem, death from other illnesses
  - High-grade gliomas; often multifactorial
    - Herniation (subfalcial, transtentorial, tonsillar)
    - Death in postoperative period
    - Severe systemic illness (coagulopathy/pulmonary embolus, myocardial infarct, infection/sepsis)
  - Sudden death (true sudden death rare)
    - 3rd ventricle colloid cyst at foramina of Monro
    - High-grade astrocytoma, oligodendroglioma

Treatment

- Resection, steroids, radiation, chemotherapy
- Complications
  - Immunosuppression
  - Infections
    - Bacterial
    - Viral

MACROSCOPIC FEATURES

Surgical Sites

- Inspect surgical incision site(s)

CENTRAL NERVOUS SYSTEM TUMORS

Key Facts

Clinical Issues

- Diffusely infiltrating astrocytomas (> 60% of primary brain tumors)
  - Glioblastoma (grade IV); > 50% of astrocytomas
- Local effects and progression
  - Infiltration, pressure on vital brain centers
  - Fatal pressure on brainstem, upper spinal cord
  - Intracranial and occasionally spinal dissemination
- Cause of death: Low-grade glioma
  - Progression to high-grade glioma, brainstem involvement, death from other illnesses
- Cause of death: High-grade glioma
  - Herniation (subfalcial, transtentorial, tonsillar)
  - Death in postoperative period
  - Severe systemic illness (coagulopathy/pulmonary embolus, myocardial infarct, infection/sepsis)
  - Massive intratumoral hemorrhage
- Sudden death
  - 3rd ventricle colloid cyst at foramina of Monro
  - High-grade gliomas

Reporting Considerations

- Correlation with clinical reports
  - Extent of tumor, including further tumor spread
  - Histology consistent with radiation necrosis
- Associated conditions and complications
  - Herniations, secondary hemorrhage
  - Hypoxic changes, infarcts
  - Familial tumor: Syndromic, non-syndromic
  - Radiation-induced tumor
- Unexpected tumor, incidental to cause of death
  - Meningioma(s), colloid cyst of 3rd ventricle, subependymoma, hamartoma, lipoma

---

  - State of wound closure: Inflamed, purulent, healed, sutures, staples
  - Ventricular drainage tubes: Number, location
  - Operative site, including hemorrhage, herniation
    - Fungus cerebri: Swollen brain protruding through craniotomy site

Calvarial and Brain Examination

- Calvaria: Modify calvarial removal as required (e.g., posthemicraniectomy)
- Dura: Surgical site, grafts, neomembrane, tumor attachment
- Brain: Generally no modification to routine removal and sectioning

Glioma

- Low grade (WHO I-II)
  - Solid (diffuse glioma), or cystic (pilocytic astrocytoma); homogeneous
    - Possible subtle effacement, obscuring gray-white junction (not well demarcated)
- High grade (WHO III-IV)
  - Solid (anaplastic glioma, many glioblastomas) or cystic (glioblastoma), heterogeneous, variegated (gray-white, yellow or tan necrosis/hemorrhage)
  - Thick infiltrated corpus callosum and fornix
  - Spread to opposite hemisphere ("butterfly glioma")
  - Invaded ventricular space, local dural attachment

Ependymoma

- Soft, well demarcated, associated with ventricles

Meningioma

- Firm, lobulated, dural based

Metastatic Tumors

- Single or multiple masses (small or large)
- Usually develop at gray-white junction

Therapy-Related Changes

- Extensive necrotic or little visible tumor, hemorrhage

Tumor-Associated Findings

- Midline shift
- Herniation: Subfalcial, uncal, tonsillar
- 2° occipital infarct, brainstem hemorrhage

MICROSCOPIC PATHOLOGY

Histologic Features

- Glioma
  - Astrocytic, oligodendroglial, mixed
  - High-grade (anaplastic) features
    - Hypercellularity, pleomorphism
    - Mitoses ≥ 6/10 HPF
    - Vascular endothelial hyperplasia
    - Necrosis
- Meningioma
  - Majority are WHO grade I: Typical meningioma
  - Atypical meningioma (WHO II): Necrosis, small-cell appearance, prominent nucleoli, loss of lobularity (3 of 4 required); or mitoses ≥ 4/10 HPF alone; or brain invasion alone
  - Anaplastic meningioma (WHO III): Mitoses ≥ 20/10 HPF; usually necrosis and marked pleomorphism
- Metastasis
  - Morphology, immunohistochemistry
  - History to suggest primary
  - Autopsy examination of other organs
- Radiation necrosis
  - Vessel wall hyaline thickening, fibrinoid necrosis, endothelial proliferation, thrombosis
  - Extravasated fibrin, telangiectases, necrosis, gliosis, calcifications

SELECTED REFERENCES

1. Brat D, et al: Protocol for the Examination of Specimens From Patients With Tumors of the Brain/Spinal Cord. Northfield: College of American Pathologists. 2013
2. Louis D et al: WHO Classification of Tumours of the Central Nervous System. Geneva: WHO Press, World Health Organization. 2007

CENTRAL NERVOUS SYSTEM TUMORS

Gross Brain Tumor Features

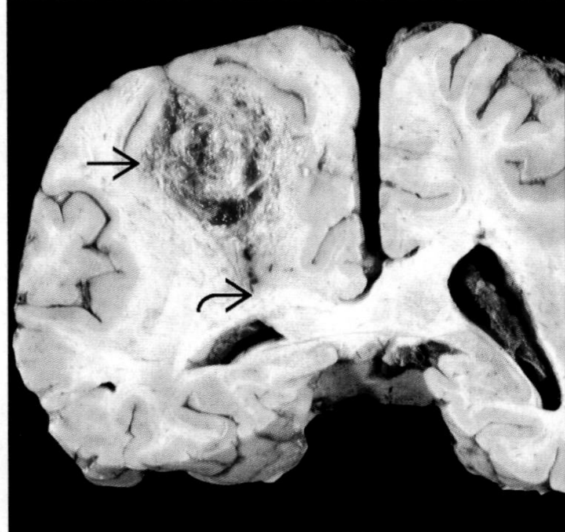

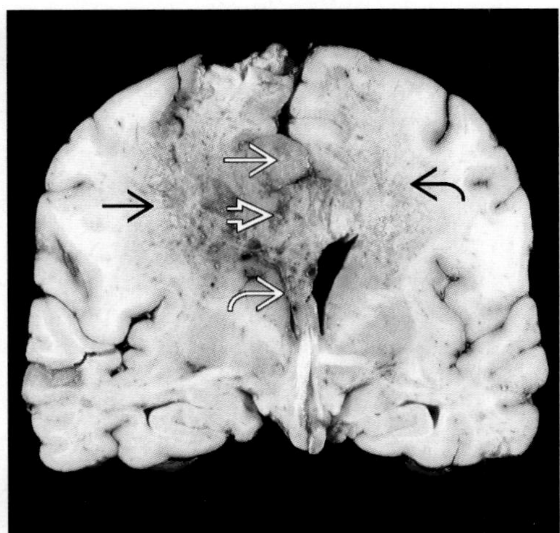

(Left) *This coronal section of the cerebral hemispheres shows the classic appearance of a glioblastoma with central necrosis extending to the splenium of the corpus callosum.* ***(Right)*** *A glioblastoma in the left frontal lobe thickens and obscures the body of the corpus callosum. The tumor crosses to the right frontal lobe. This appearance is termed "butterfly glioma." The columns of the fornix are also infiltrated. A left cingulate gyrus (subfalcial) herniation under the falx is present.*

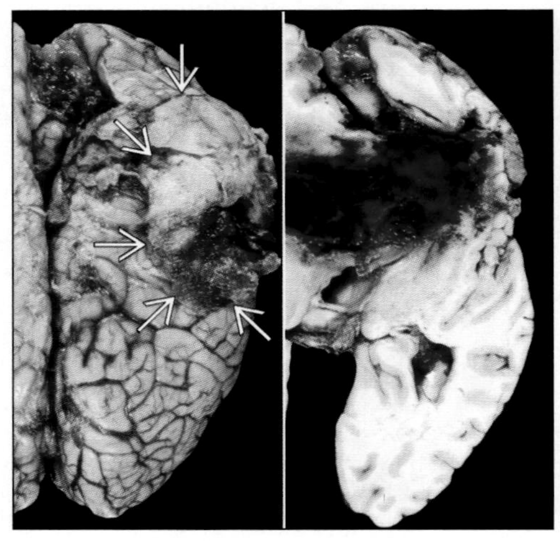

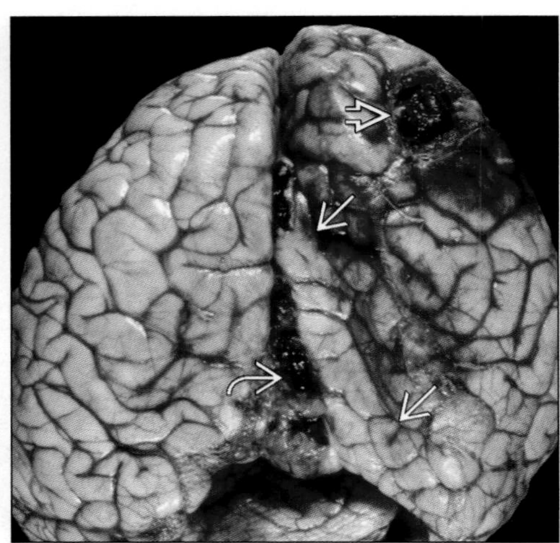

(Left) *A glioblastoma with massive postoperative hemorrhage herniated through the surgical site of the skull (fungus cerebri), seen externally and in axial section. Decompressive hemicraniectomy prevents this disastrous complication of surgery for tumor, infarct, or other significant lesion causing an expanding brain.* ***(Right)*** *There is a large postoperative subfalcial herniation. The operative site for this high-grade glioma and the area over the body of the corpus callosum show substantial hemorrhage.*

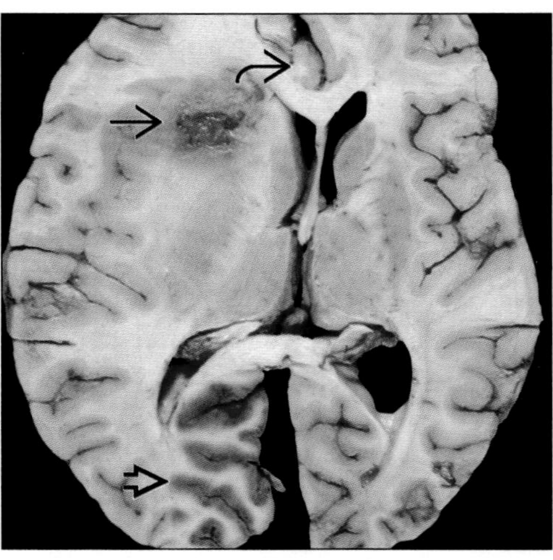

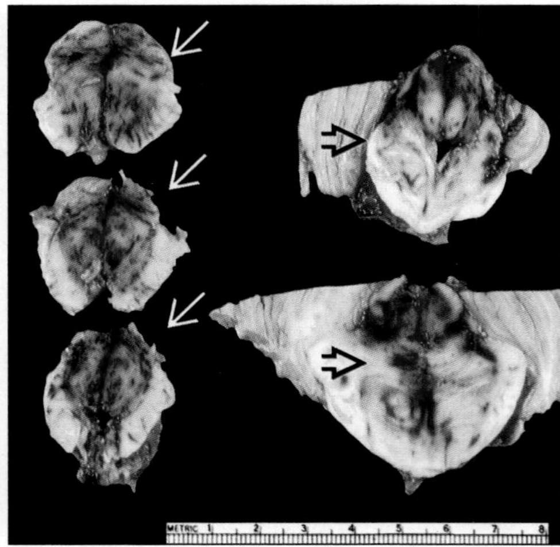

(Left) *This left frontal lobe glioblastoma caused a midline shift and cingulate herniation. An uncal herniation (not see here) compressed the left posterior cerebral artery leading to a secondary medial occipital lobe hemorrhagic infarct.* ***(Right)*** *Uncal herniation from the tumor itself or from a complication such as a large hemorrhage can push the brainstem caudally, pulling on blood vessels and causing this mostly midline secondary brainstem hemorrhage of the midbrain and pons.*

Gross and Microscopic Brain Tumor Features

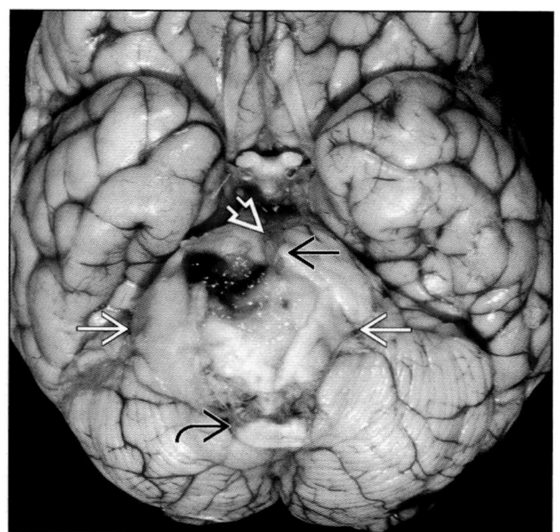
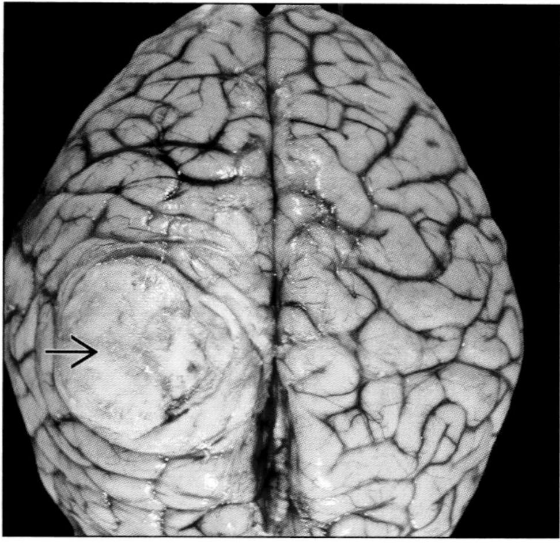

(Left) *A brainstem glioblastoma encircles the basilar artery by exophytic tumor* → *growing anteriorly from the pons. Rostral basilar artery is seen* → *. Pons is expanded* → *. Tumor also infiltrates the medulla* → *, which is widened.* ***(Right)*** *The dural cap was removed from this left frontoparietal meningioma (WHO grade I)* → *. The tumor's growth over a long period of time depressed the dorsolateral brain tissue so that when the tumor was removed, a large defect was found. No brain infiltration had occurred.*

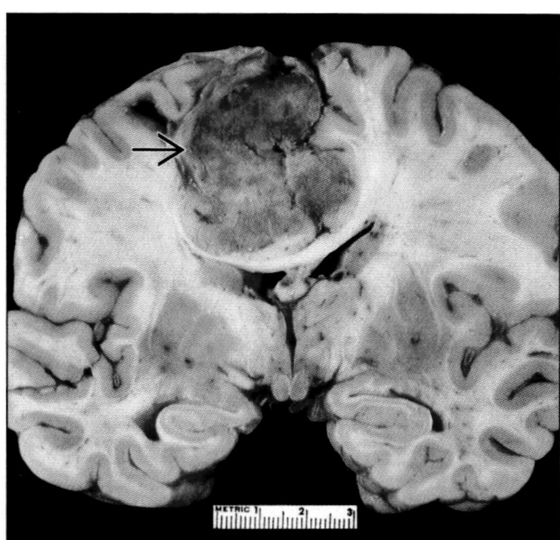

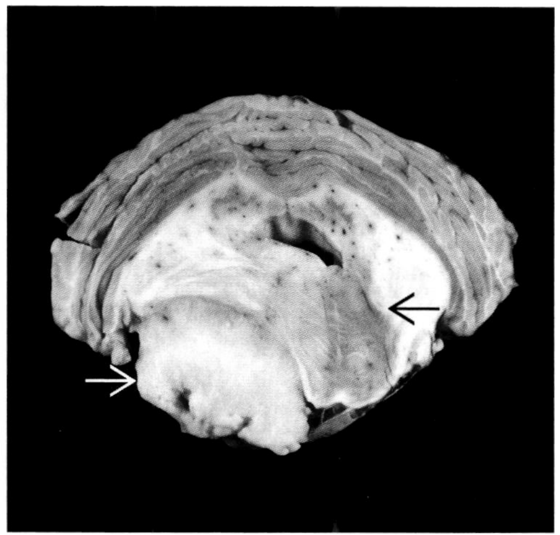

(Left) *This dura-based (falx cerebri) meningioma (WHO grade I)* → *was biopsied or partially resected 35 years previously. The actual remote procedure was not available at autopsy. The patient died of longstanding cardiac disease.* ***(Right)*** *A meningioma (WHO grade I)* → *causes devastating brainstem compression in this axial section. The pons* → *is compressed and deviated to the right by the meningioma. Pontine compression can cause cardiorespiratory compromise.*

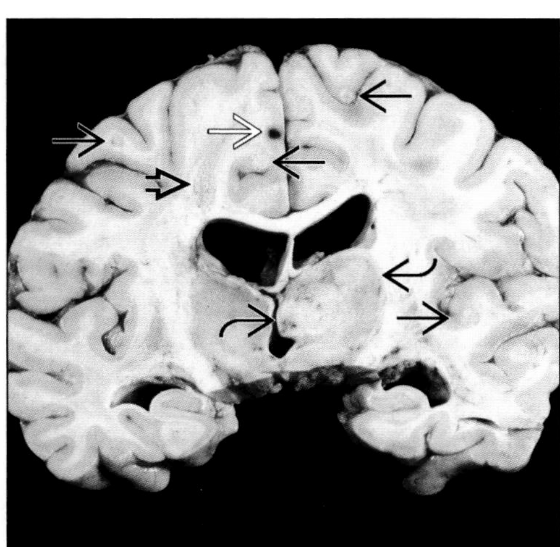
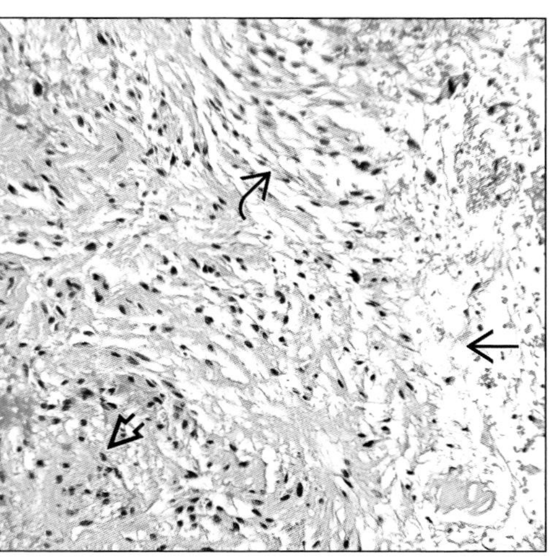

(Left) *Multiple metastases of a pulmonary adenocarcinoma are at or near the gray-white junction* → *. One neocortical metastasis is hemorrhagic* → *, and another metastatic deposit is in white matter* → *. Large, confluent metastases expand the area of the right thalamus* → *.* ***(Right)*** *A pilocytic astrocytoma (WHO grade I) is biphasic, with compact* → *and loose regions* → *required for diagnosis. Pilocytic tumor cells (hair-like) are thin and elongated with small nuclei* → *.*

CENTRAL NERVOUS SYSTEM TUMORS

Microscopic Brain Tumor Features

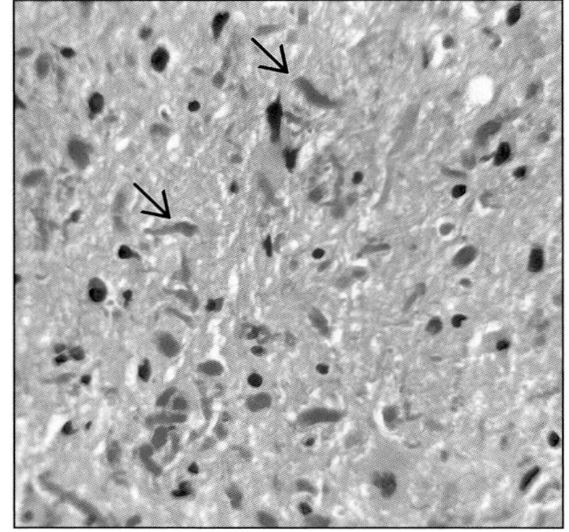

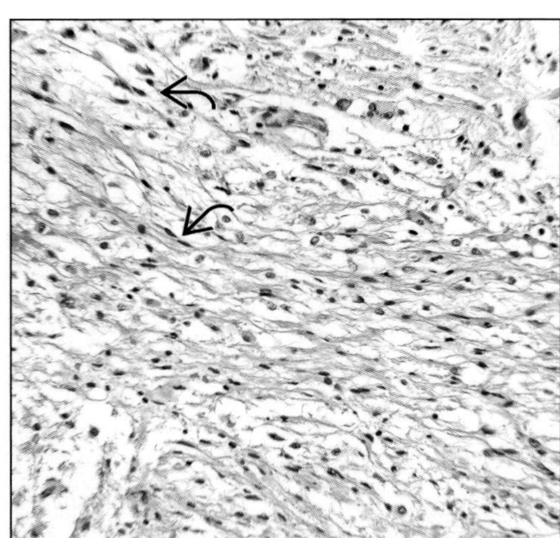

(Left) *Pilocytic astrocytomas usually have brightly eosinophilic Rosenthal fibers* → *in compact regions. Rosenthal fibers, although not required or specific, are characteristic of childhood and adult pilocytic astrocytomas.* ***(Right)*** *This is a diffuse fibrillary astrocytoma (WHO grade II) of the lower medulla and upper cervical spinal cord (cervicomedullary low-grade tumor). The elongated astrocytoma cells resemble normal fibrillary astrocytes* ↷*. There are no compact regions.*

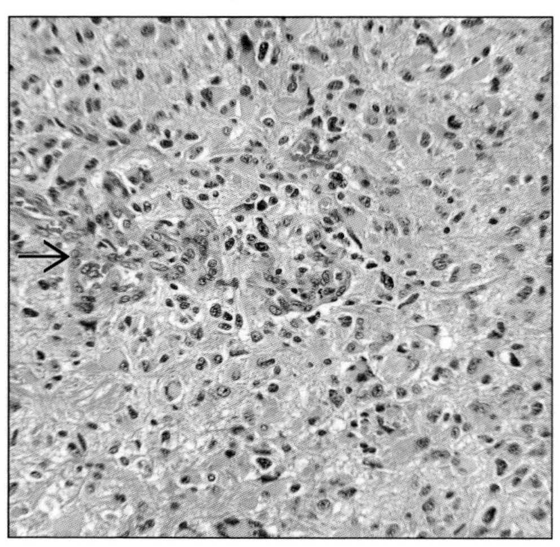

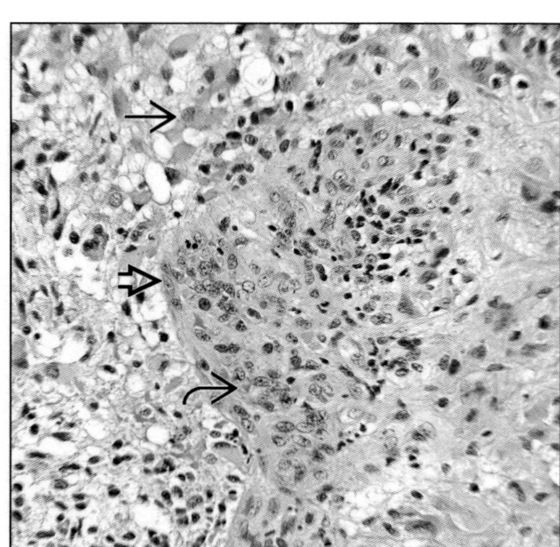

(Left) *Anaplastic astrocytoma (WHO grade III) is more pleomorphic than the fibrillary astrocytoma. Vascular endothelial hyperplasia* → *is a high-grade feature.* ***(Right)*** *Glioblastoma (WHO grade IV) usually has at least some enlarged astrocytic tumor cells* → *in routine stains, but glioblastoma cells may be mostly poorly differentiated. There is both vascular endothelial hyperplasia, seen here as a glomeruloid vascular structure* ⇨ *with multiple small lumina containing red cells* ↷ *and at least focal necrosis (not seen here).*

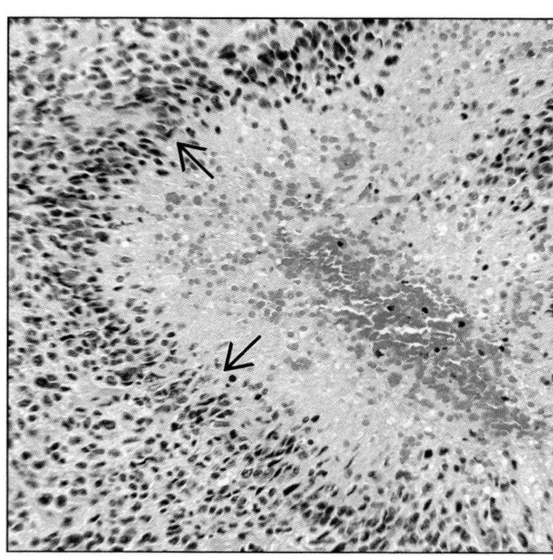

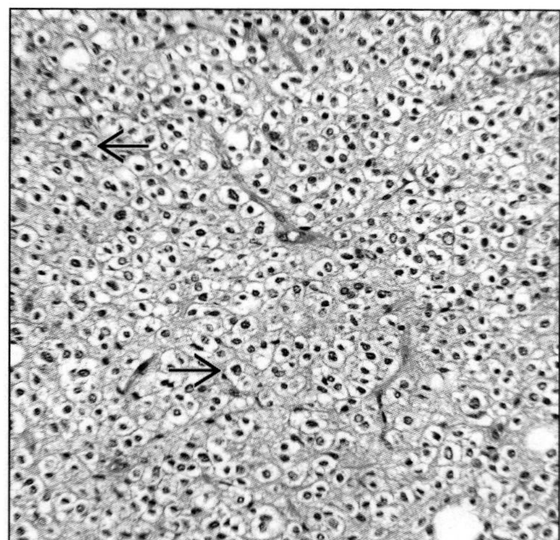

(Left) *Glioblastomas may have a crowded layer of (pseudopalisading) cells* → *around necrosis, with the crowded tumor cells presumably migrating from the central anoxic area (center of necrosis often contains a thrombosed microvessel).* ***(Right)*** *Oligodendroglioma (WHO grade II) cells have optically empty cytoplasm* → *(fried egg or honeycomb appearance) and delicate capillaries. Cytoplasmic clearing is an artifact of delayed fixation. Nuclei are mostly round but some are oval.*

Microscopic Brain Tumor Features

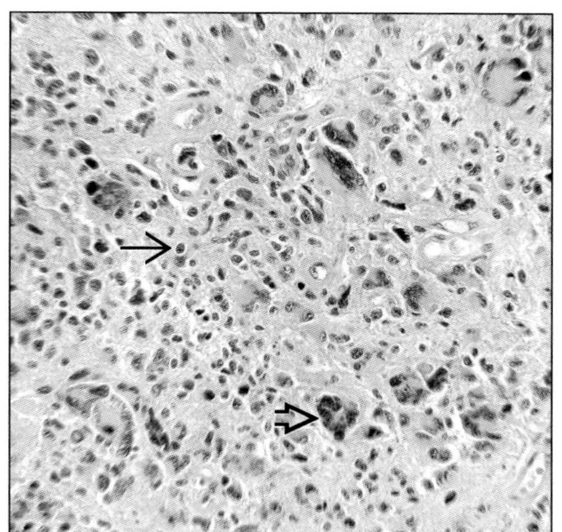
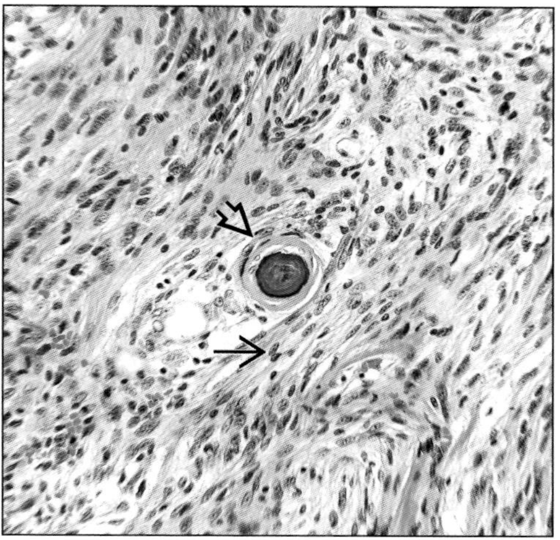

(Left) *Anaplastic oligoastrocytoma (WHO grade III) has oligodendroglioma ➔ and astrocytoma cells ➲, with a high mitotic rate &/or vascular endothelial hyperplasia.* ***(Right)*** *Meningiomas have spindle cells and are dural based. Most are WHO grade I (seen here), with cells in small ➔ or large fascicles, and lobules of syncytial-appearing and whorled cells may be seen. Psammoma bodies ➲ are characteristic.*

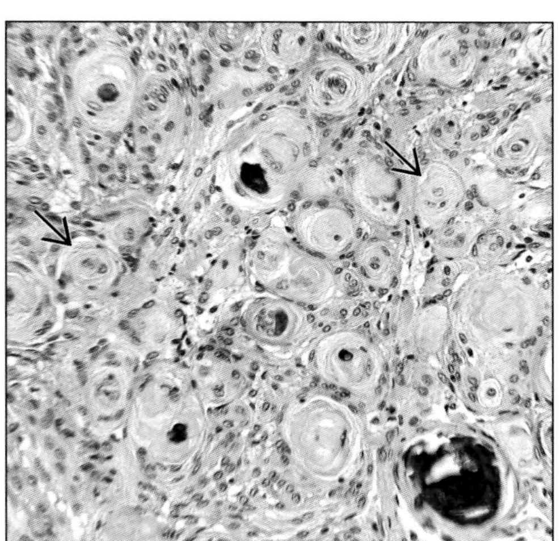
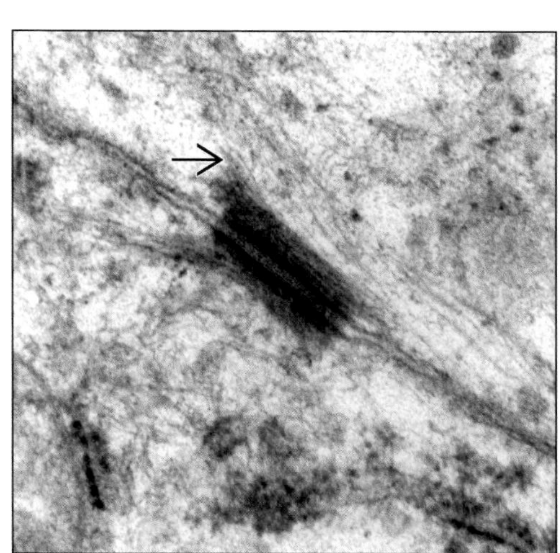

(Left) *Small, tight, cellular whorls ➔ are often seen in meningiomas. Psammoma bodies may be small or large.* ***(Right)*** *This desmosome-type junctional complex with tonofilaments ➔ extending from it aids in meningioma diagnosis. The differential diagnosis of an intracranial spindle cell tumor is schwannoma, which lacks junctional complexes but has basement membranes. Meningiomas do not have basement membranes around their cells.*

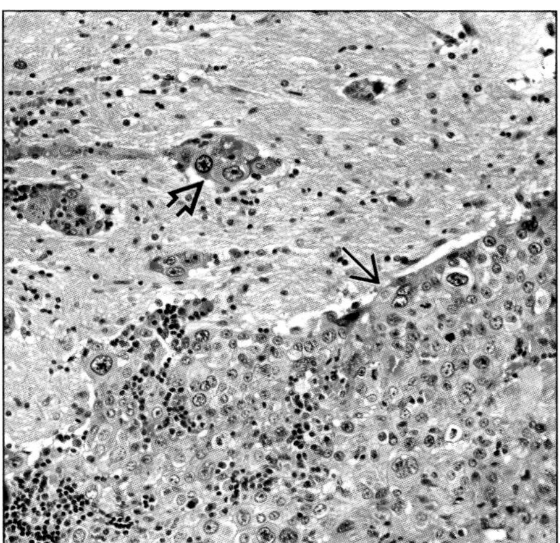
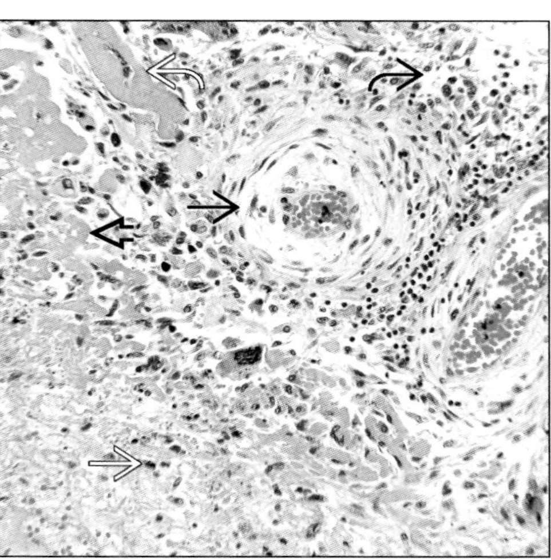

(Left) *Metastatic adenocarcinoma has a "pushing" margin at the brain interface ➔. Perivascular infiltration ➲ is also typical.* ***(Right)*** *Radiation necrosis in this patient with a treated glioblastoma manifests as necrosis ➚, vascular wall thickening ➔, fibrin exudation ➲, and vascular fibrinoid necrosis ➚. Old hemorrhage in the tissue is evidenced by hemosiderin pigment ➔.*

CEREBRAL ANEURYSM AND VASCULAR MALFORMATION

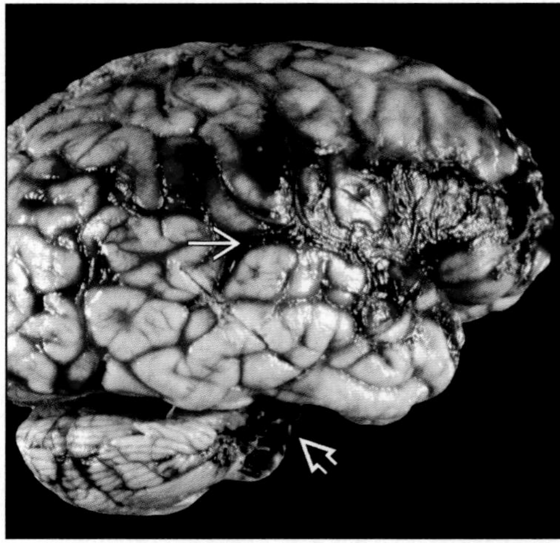

Subarachnoid hemorrhage around the sylvian fissure ➡ suggests the location of the ruptured right middle cerebral artery aneurysm. Some subarachnoid blood has also settled over the brainstem ➡.

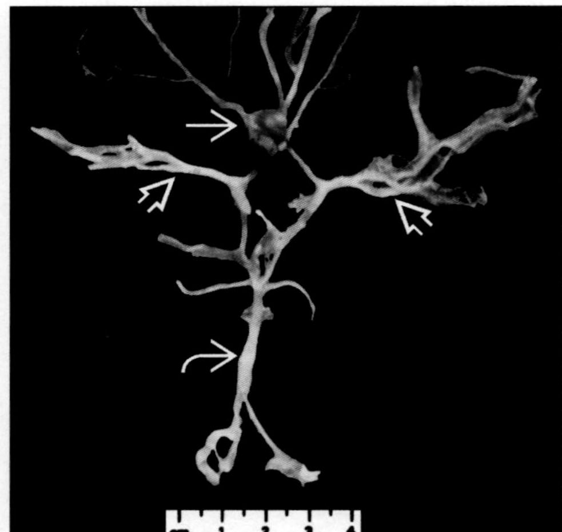

A ruptured anterior communicating artery aneurysm ➡ is seen on the circle of Willis, with arachnoidal tissue dissected away. The middle cerebral arteries ➡ and basilar artery ➡ are indicated.

TERMINOLOGY

Abbreviations

- Arteriovenous malformation (AVM)

ETIOLOGY/PATHOGENESIS

Developmental Aneurysms

- Saccular, "berry," or congenital (although rarely present at birth) aneurysms
- Lacks medial smooth muscle layer, precluding formation of internal elastic lamina
  - Internal elastic lamina provides tensile strength
  - Systolic blood pressure enlarges wall over time into saccular aneurysm
- Usually at bifurcations (circle of Willis)
- Distal aneurysms (not at bifurcation) mostly cerebellar
- AVM-associated aneurysms (↑ hemodynamic instability): Alter prognosis, management

Acquired Aneurysms

- Vascular wall damage, repair
  - Trauma (pseudoaneurysm): Often near dural free edge
  - AVM-associated acquired aneurysms
  - Spheroidal (early) or fusiform (late alteration)
- Intrinsic vascular wall weakness
  - Genetic predisposition
    - Vascular Ehlers-Danlos syndrome
    - Sickle cell anemia
- Vertebrobasilar dolichoectasia (arteriopathy)
  - Mostly older males; hypertension association
  - Juvenile cases (rare)
    - Connective tissue disorders, sickle cell disease
- Mycotic (infective) aneurysms
  - Usually 2° to bacterial endocarditis
  - Fungal infection (very rare)

Vascular Malformations

- Blood vessel hamartomas
  - Most cases sporadic
- Genetic background; some cases
  - Osler-Weber-Rendu disease
  - Sturge-Weber disease
- AVM
  - Arterial feeder systolic pressure directly enters abnormal veins
  - Affected vessels leak → blood pigment, gliosis
  - Rupture not inevitable but may be fatal
- Cavernous angioma
  - Focally thin walls in large abnormal vessels may rupture
- Capillary hemangioma
  - Usually incidental finding
- Telangiectasia (telangiectases)
  - 4-12% of vascular malformations
- Venous malformation
  - Frequent, usually incidental finding
  - Low pressure, rupture infrequently
  - Vein of Galen aneurysmal malformation
    - Infrequent; may cause high-output cardiac failure
- Dural arteriovenous fistula or shunt
  - Direct connection between dural artery and brain/spinal cord blood vessels
    - Leak or sudden rupture into neural parenchyma
  - Foix-Alajouanine syndrome or venous congestive myelopathy
    - Reflux of dural arterial blood into spinal cord venous drainage

CLINICAL ISSUES

Presentation

- Developmental (saccular) aneurysms
  - Autopsy prevalence rate 1-5%
  - Annual rupture rate < 2%

CEREBRAL ANEURYSM AND VASCULAR MALFORMATION

Key Facts

Etiology

- Developmental aneurysms
  - Termed saccular, "berry," or congenital aneurysms (rarely appear at birth)
  - Lacks medial smooth muscle layer, precluding formation of internal elastic lamina
- Vertebrobasilar dolichoectasia (arteriopathy)
  - Focally dilated basilar artery, mostly older men
  - Longstanding case may form fusiform aneurysm
- Vascular malformations
  - AVM: No capillary bed; may cause seizures, prone to rupture
  - Cavernous angioma, prone to rupture
  - Capillary hemangioma
  - Telangiectasia (telangiectases)
  - Venous malformation, minor to extensive
  - Dural arteriovenous fistula or shunt; potential for major clinical hemorrhage

Clinical Issues

- Subarachnoid or intraparenchymal hemorrhage, seizure disorder, fatal rupture
- Medical treatment (antiepileptics), open surgery, endovascular thrombosis-promoting procedures

Macroscopic Pathology

- Aneurysm rupture often obscured by blood; multiple aneurysms common
- Common incidental finding (aneurysm, vascular malformation)

Microscopic Pathology

- Developmental aneurysmal wall characteristic
- Malformed vessels in AVM

    - Up to 80% do not rupture (incidental)
  - Can be incidental on imaging report for other investigations
  - Subarachnoid hemorrhage (major presentation)
    - Headache, mental status change, neck stiffness, focal neurologic deficits, acute brain injury
  - Subdural hematoma (rare)
  - Distal embolization (rare)
- Acquired aneurysms
  - Infrequent, may be 2° to larger problem (e.g., connective tissue disorder)
  - Vertebrobasilar dolichoectasia
    - 10% symptomatic
    - Brain ischemia, cranial nerve or brainstem compression, cerebellar symptoms, obstructive hydrocephalus, fatal rupture
- AVM
  - Prevalence: 18/100,000 adults
    - Autopsy prevalence rate: 1-4%
    - Clinical imaging incidental rate: 0.05%
  - Lifetime bleeding risk: 17-90%
    - Depends on size, location (e.g., deep), venous drainage, associated aneurysm, previous bleed
  - Presentation with rupture
    - Hemorrhage (50%)
    - Seizure (25%)
    - Headache (25%)
    - Focal neurologic deficits
  - Unruptured (present 2x as commonly as ruptured)
    - 1st hemorrhage fatality rate: 15-18%
    - After 1st rupture, 4-34% rerupture risk: Higher for deep brain location or deep venous drainage
    - Overall morbidity/mortality estimates uncertain
  - Associated developmental or acquired aneurysm in 3-16%
  - Worse prognosis if large or eloquent area (brainstem, thalamus, hypothalamus, motor or sensory [parietal, visual] cortex)
  - Better prognosis for small AVM (≤ 3 cm)
  - Angiographically occult AVM: < 3 cm or thrombosed
    - Annual bleeding risk: < 1%
- Cavernous angioma
  - Subarachnoid/intraparenchymal bleed with rupture
- Capillary hemangioma
  - Symptoms if size increase → tissue pressure
- Telangiectases and venous malformations
  - Commonly incidental
- Dural arteriovenous fistula or shunt
  - Leak or sudden rupture into neural parenchyma

Treatment

- Surgical approaches
  - AVM or cavernous angioma extent &/or vascular supply may limit or prevent surgical approach
- Aneurysm
  - Small (< 7 mm) aneurysms: Small rupture potential, traditionally observed, but increasingly embolized
  - Surgical clipping (open): Larger aneurysms
  - Endovascular embolization (coils, stent-assisted coils, pipeline embolization mesh)
- AVM
  - Staged multimodality, for vessel obliteration
    - Stereotactic (focused) irradiation (radiosurgery)
    - Endovascular embolization (polymer, glue)
    - Excision; may follow radiation, embolization
  - Observation: Active treatment ↑ harm if unruptured; case dependent
  - Brainstem AVM: Single-mode less harmful

Prognosis

- Developmental aneurysms
  - Subarachnoid hemorrhage
    - Mortality rate 45%; most deaths in 1st week
    - Reduced mortality (13-35%) in centers with higher case numbers
    - Rebleed ↑ untreated or treated mortality rate
  - Morbidity/mortality factors
    - Acute brain injury: Vasospasm, hypoxia, infarcts
    - Rebleed risk: Older patient, size > 10 mm, blood pressure > 160 mm Hg, poor initial clinical status
    - Morbidity/mortality rate after endovascular coiling lower than after surgical clipping

CEREBRAL ANEURYSM AND VASCULAR MALFORMATION

    - Coil-packed ruptured aneurysm rebleed rate ~ 1% higher compared to clipping
    - Complications: Seizures, SIADH, hydrocephalus
  - Cause of death
    - Subarachnoid hemorrhage sequelae (acute brain injury)
    - Treatment complications in 1st postoperative year
    - Pneumonia, organ failure (cardiopulmonary)
    - Intracerebral hemorrhage (rare)
- AVM
  - Associated aneurysm(s) ↓ prognosis
    - Unruptured with associated aneurysm: 7% annual hemorrhage risk
  - Hemorrhage risk ↓ over time
  - Radiation ↑ rebleed risk for large AVM
  - Embolization alone ↑ hemorrhage risk for 1 year
  - Brainstem AVM prognosis favorable
  - Seizure risk same with drugs or surgery
  - Combined therapy compounds treatment-related risk
  - Hemorrhage risk until full obliteration (many years)
  - Cause of death
    - Intracerebral hemorrhage, herniation
    - Treatment complications, seizures
    - Operative complication

Pertinent Antemortem Data

- CBC, PT, aPTT
- Computed tomography (CT), reconstructed computed tomography angiogram (CTA)
- Magnetic resonance imaging (MRI)
- Conventional angiography
- Operative and radiation therapy report(s)

MACROSCOPIC FEATURES

Aneurysm

- Incidental in some autopsies, usually circle of Willis
  - May be multiple, occasionally symmetrical
- Rupture with subarachnoid hemorrhage
  - Clip, coils, stent, mesh visible or palpable, if used
  - Blood often obscures aneurysm
    - Aneurysm usually at epicenter of hemorrhage
    - Dissect away blood and cerebral tissue as needed
    - May require multiple samples from hemorrhage to locate aneurysm microscopically
    - With no organ retention permitted, remove some blood and fix area(s) likely to contain aneurysm
    - Postmortem cerebral angiography for location (brain edema may interfere by vascular collapse)

Vascular Malformation

- Common incidental finding
  - Usually venous anomaly or telangiectasia
    - Occasionally, only old blood pigment or vague discoloration grossly
- Inoperable AVM or cavernous angioma
  - Often large; in brainstem, may be small
  - Often at least a few vessels over 1 mm in diameter
  - Old blood pigment, firm surrounding gliosis
- Post-treatment lesion
  - Variable appearance
    - Residual vessels often grossly apparent
    - Embolized polymer in AVM, may migrate past malformed vessels

MICROSCOPIC PATHOLOGY

Histologic Features

- Aneurysm
  - Fraying and loss of internal elastic lamina at aneurysm neck
  - Collagenous tissue in sac wall, no smooth muscle
  - Rupture site, if seen, often in sac dome
    - Fragile fibrin plug (rarely found)
- Dolichoectasia
  - Smooth muscle atrophy, fragmented internal elastic lamina
- Vascular malformations
  - Back-to-back vessel walls in part or entirely
    - Wall thickness from capillary-like to very thick
    - Types prone to rupture have arterial feeder &/or some thin vessel walls
  - AVM
    - No capillary bed; intervening parenchyma present
    - Old blood pigment, calcification/bone, gliosis
  - Cavernous angioma
    - Large abnormal vessels, no intervening parenchyma
    - Old blood pigment, gliosis
  - Capillary hemangioma
    - Small thin-walled vessels, little if any intervening parenchyma
  - Telangiectasia
    - Loosely clustered or scattered very thin-walled, dilated branches
    - Wall: Endothelium, some pericytes
  - Venous malformation
    - Variable; very thin vessel walls (focally endothelium and little adventitia) to very thick
    - Rare: 1 anomalous vein
  - Dural arteriovenous fistula or shunt
    - Enlarged arterialized subarachnoid veins, thickened elastic laminae
    - Venous congestive myelopathy: Enlarged subarachnoid veins and small, dilated, thick-walled spinal cord vessels; spinal cord congestion and hemorrhage, gray matter necrosis

SELECTED REFERENCES

1. Bradac O et al: Treatment for brain arteriovenous malformation in the 1998-2011 period and review of the literature. Acta Neurochir (Wien). 155(2):199-209, 2013
2. Karamanakos PN et al: Risk factors for three phases of 12-month mortality in 1657 patients from a defined population after acute aneurysmal subarachnoid hemorrhage. World Neurosurg. 78(6):631-9, 2012
3. McNulty ML et al: Management of unruptured intracranial aneurysms and arteriovenous malformations. Am J Ther. 18(1):64-9, 2011
4. Love S et al: Greenfield's Neuropathology. 8th ed., vol. 1. London: Edward Arnold, 2008

Gross and Angiographic Features

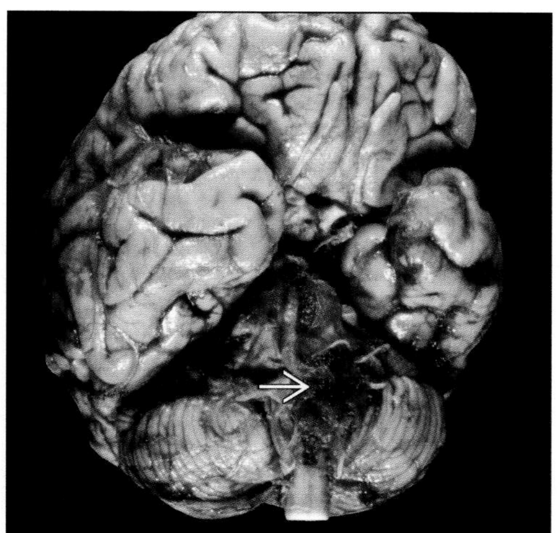

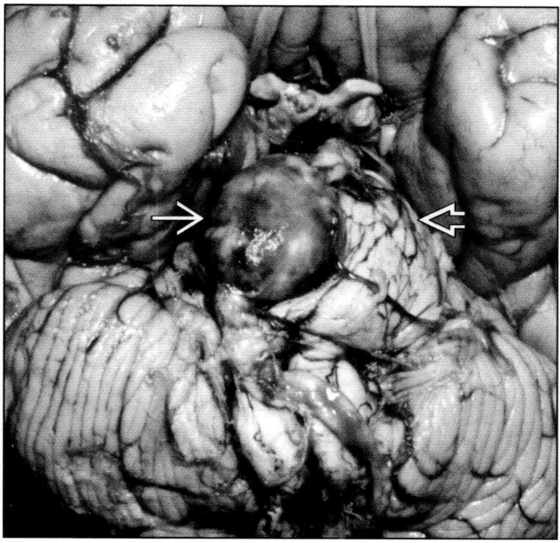

(Left) *Subarachnoid hemorrhage* ➡ *covers a ruptured distal aneurysm of the left posterior inferior cerebellar artery. An infarct in the medulla causes the Wallenberg syndrome.* ***(Right)*** *Basilar artery dolichoectasia* ➡ *pushed the basis pontis laterally* ⇨*. These spheroidal dilations become fusiform later. They can cause cardiorespiratory failure from pontine compression. Dolichoectasia ("long dilated") has hypertension, trauma, genetic, and AVM associations.*

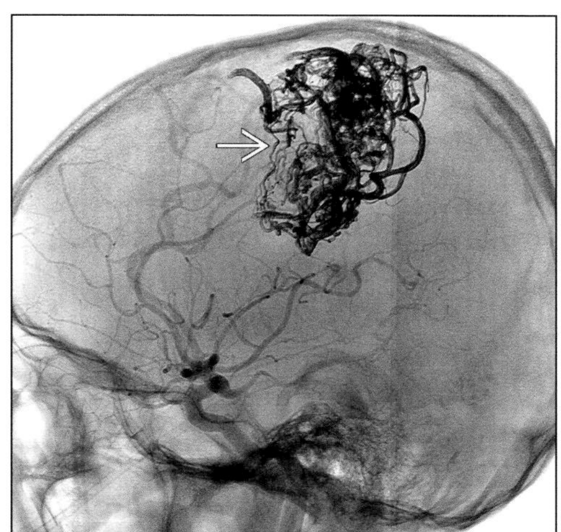

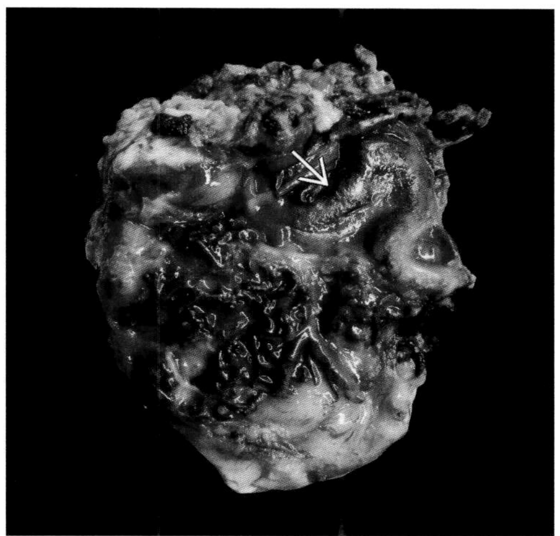

(Left) *Onyx injected into the feeding artery of a large frontoparietal AVM* ➡ *has high attenuation so that its distribution is clearly seen in this cerebral angiogram.* ***(Right)*** *Onyx, a viscous black polymer mixture, fills all vascular sizes in this cerebral AVM photographed in the surgical suite after excision. The dark, somewhat firm polymer is seen through the relatively thin (for size) abnormal vascular walls* ➡*. (Courtesy G. Gupta, MD.)*

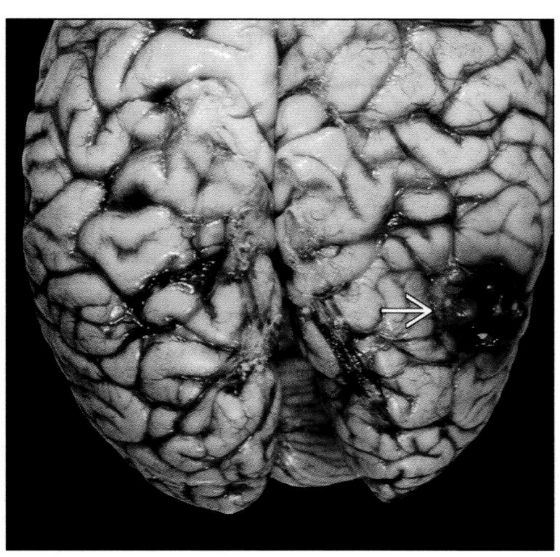

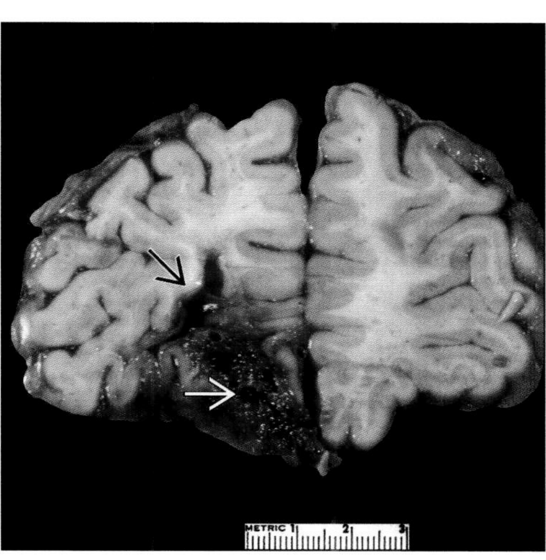

(Left) *A patient with a chronic seizure disorder had an AVM of the right occipital lobe* ➡*. No surgical procedure was performed on it, but a seizure was thought to have contributed to death.* ***(Right)*** *This patient with a chronic seizure disorder had a right medial frontal orbital AVM. Several abnormal vessels are large and easily seen* ➡*. Blood leakage and perhaps small ruptures resulted in a cavity in the white matter with blood-stained walls* ➙*.*

CEREBRAL ANEURYSM AND VASCULAR MALFORMATION

Gross, Angiographic, and Microscopic Features

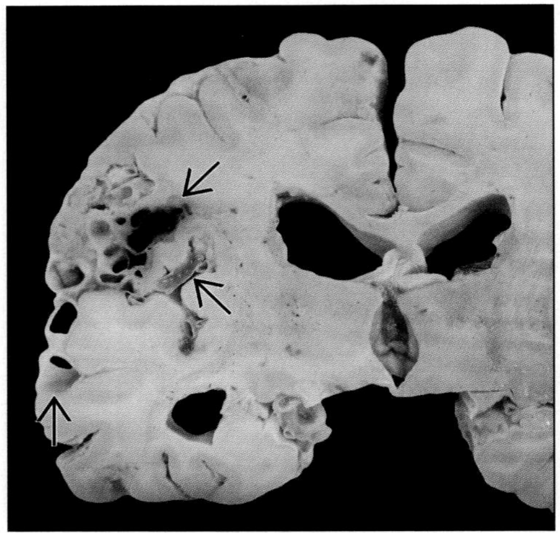

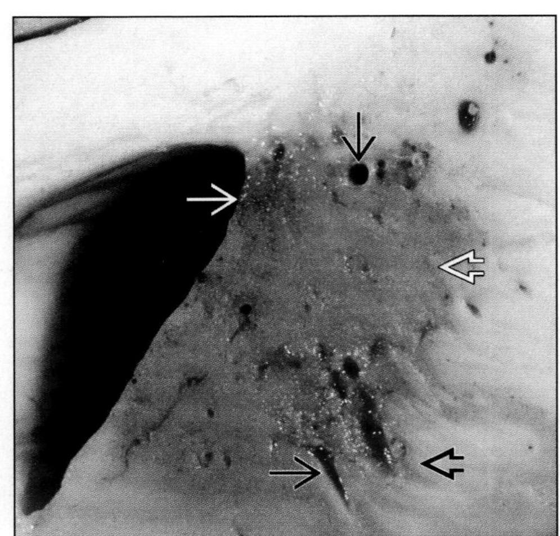

(Left) *Very wide-bore, back-to-back venous structures make up this extensive, inoperable cavernous angioma ➡ that was present in several coronal cerebral sections and was the cause of death.* ***(Right)*** *Like many vascular malformations in the brain, this is a composite vascular malformation in the right corpus striatum, including the head of the caudate nucleus ➡ and the internal capsule ➡. An area of telangiectasia ➡ is a classic punctate patch. Large venous channels ➡ are in the same general vascular distribution.*

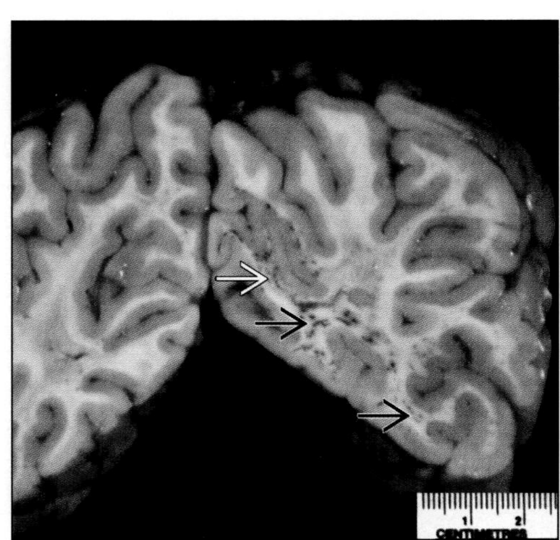

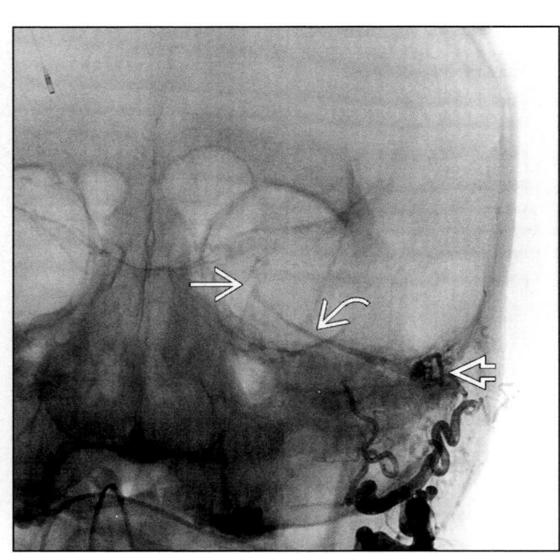

(Left) *A typical incidental venous malformation with a wide distribution is in the right occipital white matter ➡ with little cortical involvement ➡.* ***(Right)*** *This angiogram shows a dural arteriovenous fistula ➡ draining upward from the left transverse sinus ➡ into the basal ganglia ➡. Most intracranial dural arteriovenous fistulas originate in association with a dural venous sinus. The patient presented with basal ganglia hemorrhage and was treated by Onyx and intravascular glue embolization.*

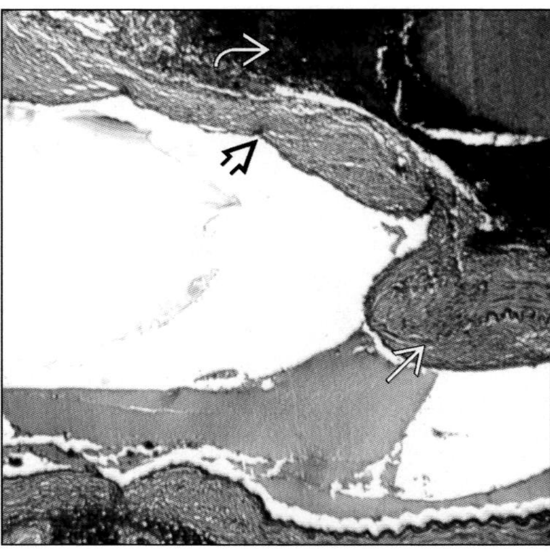

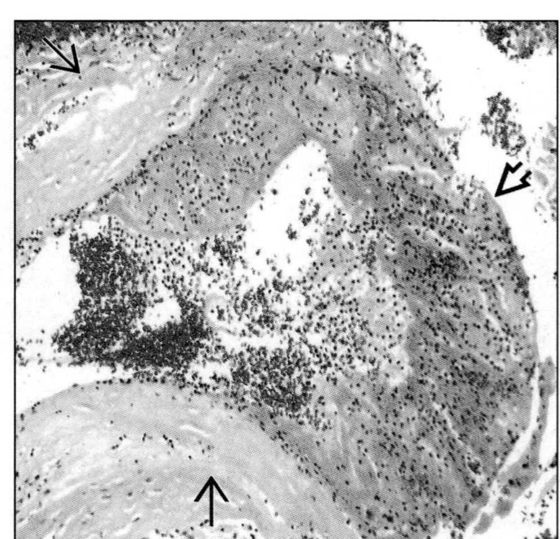

(Left) *H&E stain of a middle cerebral artery shows a normal, wavy internal elastic lamina that ends at the aneurysmal neck ➡. The aneurysmal wall is irregular and fibrotic ➡. Subarachnoid blood ➡ surrounds the sac that is intact in this field.* ***(Right)*** *The fibrous wall of a saccular aneurysm ➡ is seen where the rupture site is filled by a delicate fibrin (and cellular) plug ➡ or fibrin net. The fibrin net is thought to be disrupted easily by blood flow, and this may be the cause of acute rebleeding prior to interventional therapy.*

Microscopic Features

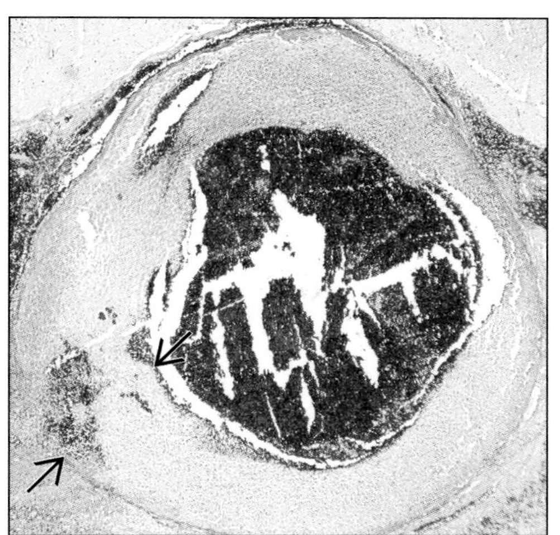

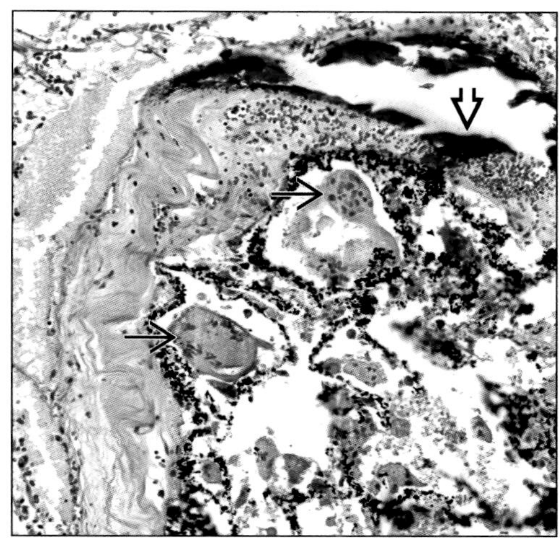

(Left) *This mycotic aneurysm, seen in cross section with H&E stain at low magnification, arose from a bacterial infection of the arterial wall. The wall is replaced by acute inflammatory cells and tissue debris* ⇨*, predisposing to rupture.* ***(Right)*** *A dilated AVM channel has an irregular wall with focal calcification* ⇨*. The lumen was embolized with Onyx polymer seen as discrete, black particles that promote thrombosis. Foreign-body giant cells* ⇨ *can respond to Onyx, as seen here.*

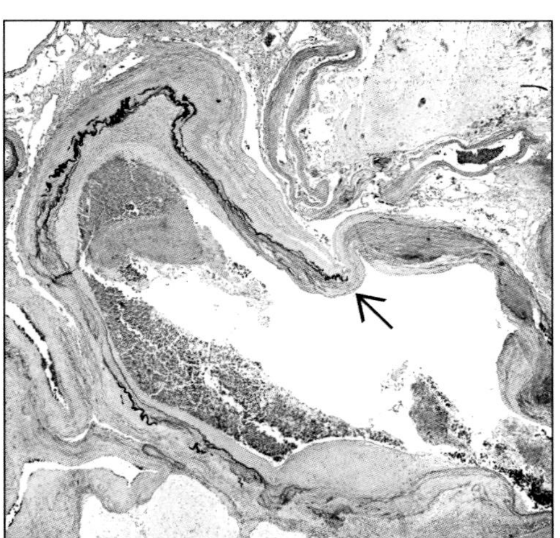

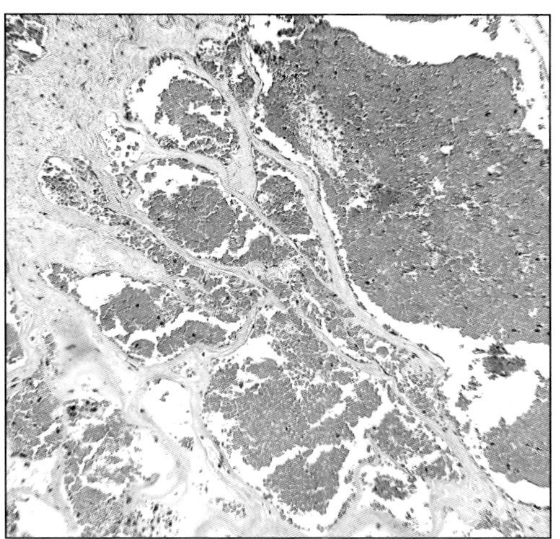

(Left) *Elastin stain (blue-black) at low magnification shows the reduplicated internal elastic lamina of an AVM artery ending* ⇨ *at the transition directly into a dilated, irregular vein. Systolic pressure acts directly on the venous wall.* ***(Right)*** *A cavernous angioma in the medulla, seen at medium magnification, has back-to-back dilated vessels with variable wall thickness, without intervening parenchyma. Focal dystrophic ossification and old blood pigment were present.*

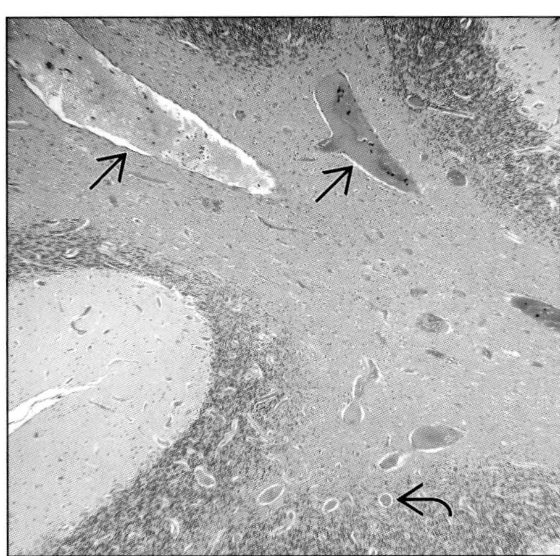

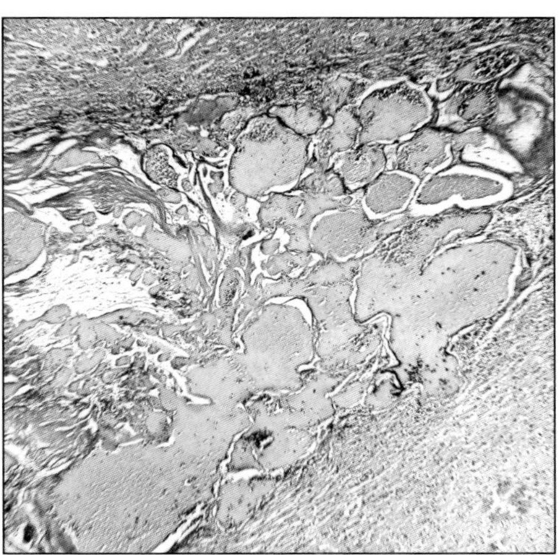

(Left) *An extensive incidental cerebellar telangiectatic malformation, seen in part at low magnification, is formed of many very thin-walled, dilated, small* ⇨ *and large vessels* ⇨ *with scant adventitia. The abnormal vascular tree has scattered branches.* ***(Right)*** *This small, incidental capillary hemangioma of back-to-back, dilated, thin-walled, capillary-like vessels in cerebral white matter is seen at low magnification. Capillary-like refers to the thin walls, not the wide lumina.*

SECTION 1

Transplantation

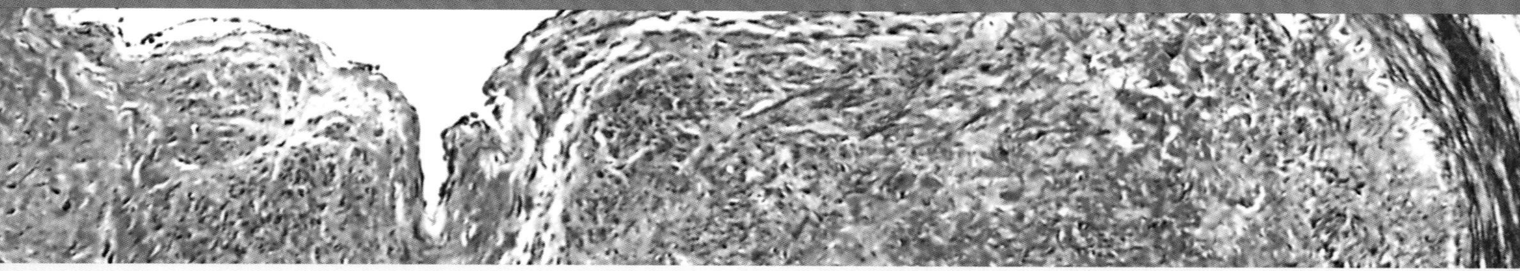

HEART TRANSPLANT

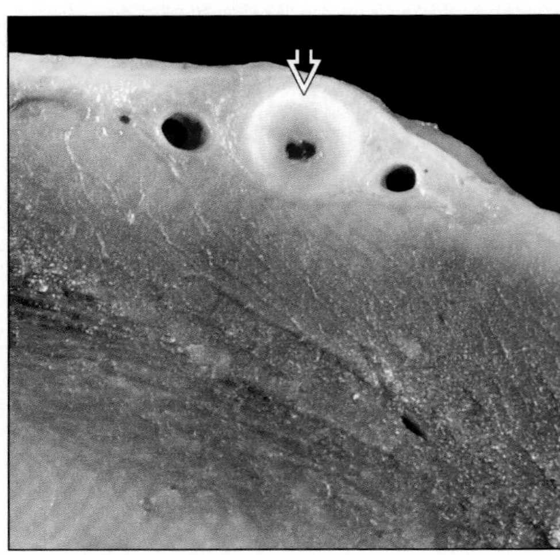

This autopsy heart from a patient with cardiac transplantation shows severe cardiac allograft vasculopathy with near complete occlusion of the left anterior descending artery ⮚.

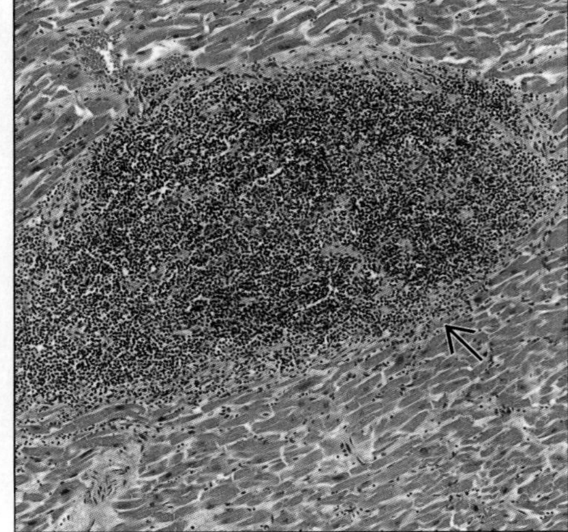

This photomicrograph shows a well-demarcated lymphoid aggregate deep in the myocardium ⮕. This most likely represents "deep" Quilty effect, a clinically insignificant and enigmatic finding in cardiac allografts.

TERMINOLOGY

Synonyms

- Antibody-mediated rejection (AMR): Humoral rejection, vascular rejection
- Cardiac allograft vasculopathy (CAV): Transplant coronary artery disease, transplant vasculopathy, allograft arteriopathy, transplant arteriosclerosis

ETIOLOGY/PATHOGENESIS

Cellular Rejection (CR)

- T-cell-mediated host response to allografted heart stimulated by "foreign" human leukocyte (HLA) and other antigens expressed in graft tissue
  - Class I antigens (HLA-A, -B, and -C) are constitutively expressed on most cells in heart, especially vascular endothelium
  - Class II antigens (HLA-DP, -DQ, and -DR) are constitutively expressed on vascular endothelium, resident macrophages
  - Presentation of antigen occurs to T cells directly or indirectly via antigen-presenting cells (APCs) and endothelial cells
- T-cell antigen stimulation leads to graft injury
  - Activated T cells produce proinflammatory cytokines
  - Activated CD8-positive cytotoxic T cells participate in cytotoxic killing of graft myocytes
  - Activated T cells activate B cells and can stimulate donor-specific antibody production

Antibody-Mediated Rejection

- Antibody-mediated host response to allografted heart with damage from complement activation and antibody dependent cellular cytotoxicity
  - Antibody binding to capillary antigen presented by endothelium activates endothelial signaling and cell activity
  - Antibody binding initiates complement cascade
  - Complement split products and other chemoattractants lead to macrophage aggregation within injured vessels

Cardiac Allograft Vasculopathy

- Arterial narrowing due to concentric intima thickening by proliferating smooth muscle cells and fibroblasts, leading to chronic ischemia with secondary myocyte changes and interstitial fibrosis
- Proposed mechanisms include
  - Immunologic
    - Ongoing endothelial injury (such as with persistent or repetitive AMR)
    - Increased T-helper cell activity
    - HLA mismatch
  - Nonimmunologic
    - CMV infection
    - Coagulation cascade and fibrin deposition
    - Traditional atherosclerotic risk factors

CLINICAL ISSUES

Epidemiology

- Incidence
  - Most rejection episodes occur within 6 months post transplant
  - ~ 30% of recipients have some rejection during 1st year post transplant
  - Cellular and antibody-mediated rejection (AMR) can occur simultaneously
  - CAV incidence post transplant
    - 8% at 1 year
    - 20% at 3 years
    - 30% at 5 years
    - 50% at 10 years

HEART TRANSPLANT

Key Facts

Etiology
- Cellular rejection
  - T-Cell mediated host response to allografted heart stimulated by "foreign" human leukocyte (HLA) and other antigens expressed in graft tissue
- Antibody-mediated rejection
  - Antibody-mediated host response to allografted heart with damage with complement activation
- Cardiac allograft vasculopathy
  - Arterial narrowing due to concentric intima thickening by proliferating smooth muscle cells and fibroblasts

Clinical Issues
- Most rejection episodes occur within 6 months post transplant

Macroscopic Pathology
- Rejection
  - May appear grossly normal
- Cardiac allograft vasculopathy
  - Epicardial and intramyocardial artery involvement

Microscopic Pathology
- Cellular rejection
  - Perivascular/interstitial mononuclear inflammation
  - Myocyte damage in association with mononuclear inflammation
- Antibody-mediated rejection
  - Capillary endothelial cell swelling and injury
  - Positive staining for complement (C4d and C3d)
- Cardiac allograft vasculopathy
  - Marked concentric intima thickening

Presentation
- Asymptomatic presentation is most common
- Symptoms occur only with moderate or severe ACR and include symptoms associated with heart failure
- Risk factors associated with cellular rejection (CR)
  - Noncompliance with immunosuppressive regimen
  - Diarrhea, vomiting interfering with medication absorption
  - Infections
  - Untoward effects/interference of other medications
  - Drastic changes in weight
- Risk factors associated with AMR
  - Young, female
  - Multiparity
  - Presensitization (panel reactive antibody or single antigen bead)
  - Previous transplantation
  - Multiple transfusions

Treatment
- Options
  - Cellular rejection
    - Mild rejection (ISHLT 1R) may resolve spontaneously (~ 85%)
    - Pulse corticosteroids or modification of baseline calcineurin inhibitor dose
    - Anti-thymocyte globulin
  - Antibody-mediated rejection
    - Corticosteroids, augmented immunosuppressives
    - Rituximab, bortezomib
    - Plasmapheresis
  - Cardiac allograft vasculopathy
    - Stents, mTOR inhibitors to stop progression

IMAGE FINDINGS

General Features
- Echocardiography
- Angiography
  - Cardiac allograft vasculopathy

MACROSCOPIC FEATURES

External Examination
- Median sternotomy
- Other scars
  - Coronary bypass grafting (harvest sites)
  - Ventricular assist device, driveline exit site
  - Chest tubes
- Congestive heart failure
  - Edema
  - Ascites
  - Hepatomegaly
- Sepsis/DIC
  - Petechiae, ecchymoses

Rejection
- Myocardial mottling, global
- May appear grossly normal

Cardiac Allograft Vasculopathy
- Epicardial and intramyocardial artery involvement
- Vein involvement
- Subendocardial ischemic changes
- Interventions (e.g., stenting)

Complications
- Infection (pneumonia, urinary tract, abscess, meningitis, pyelonephritis)
- Malignancy (masses, metastases, lymphadenopathy, splenomegaly)
- Medication toxicity (cushingoid features, nephrosclerosis, adrenal atrophy)

Biopsy Sites
- Right ventricle apical trabeculations
- Predominantly septal, but may be on free wall aspect as well

HEART TRANSPLANT

MICROSCOPIC PATHOLOGY

Cellular Rejection

- Perivascular/interstitial mononuclear inflammation, predominantly composed of activated lymphocytes and macrophages
- Myocyte damage in association with mononuclear inflammation
  - Damage is not myocyte necrosis but rather encroachment of inflammatory cells into myocyte borders leading to architectural distortion
- In severe ACR, neutrophils, &/or eosinophils may be present; such rejection is usually mixed with AMR
- Grading
  - International Society of Heart Lung Transplantation (ISHLT) 2004 grading schema intended for biopsy, but may be applied loosely (1R, 2R, 3R)
  - Alternatively, descriptive diagnosis of severity could be given (mild/moderate/severe; focal/diffuse, etc.)

Antibody-Mediated Rejection

- Histopathology
  - Capillary endothelial cell swelling and injury
  - Interstitial edema, hemorrhage
  - Adherence of macrophages to endothelium
  - Severe cases show edema, hemorrhage, karyorrhexis, vasculitis, and thrombi
  - Occasional neutrophils, eosinophils
- Immunopathology
  - Positive staining for complement (C4d and C3d)
  - CD68 positive intravascular macrophages

Cardiac Allograft Vasculopathy

- Epicardial coronary arteries
  - Marked concentric intima thickening
  - Smooth muscle cell proliferation
  - Intimal inflammatory cells
  - Variable lipid, foamy macrophages
- Intramyocardial arteries
  - Myointimal proliferative changes
  - Endothelialitis
  - Perivascular fibrosis
- Myocardium
  - Subendocardial sarcoplasmic vacuolization
  - Myocyte hypertrophy, interstitial fibrosis
  - Rare infarct like changes

Other Conditions

- Post-transplant lymphoproliferative disorder
  - EBV-positive lymphoproliferation
  - Polyclonal/polymorphous or monoclonal (lymphoma-like)
- Infections
  - CMV
  - Toxoplasma
  - Chagas
- Recurrent amyloid

Quilty Effect

- Nodular subendocardial lymphoid aggregates
  - Well circumscribed, rounded
  - May extend or be seen deep to endocardium as well
- Must be distinguished from CR
- Prominent capillary vascularity within lymphoid aggregates
- B cells admixed in lymphoid aggregate

Biopsy Sites

- Fibrosis with entrapped myocytes and variable amount of mononuclear inflammation

"Harvesting" or Perioperative Ischemic Damage (for Fresh Transplants)

- Mixed infiltrate and coagulation necrosis secondary to perfusion-related damage to myocardium
- Resolves in 1st weeks post transplant

ANCILLARY TESTS

Immunohistochemistry

- CD3, CD20, may be used to rule out post-transplant lymphoproliferative disorder and Quilty effect
- C4d to assess AMR (frozen tissue for immunofluorescence, or else paraffin immunohistochemistry methods)
- CD68 to identify intravascular macrophages, which would support diagnosis of AMR

SELECTED REFERENCES

1. Berry GJ et al: The 2013 International Society for Heart and Lung Transplantation Working Formulation for the standardization of nomenclature in the pathologic diagnosis of antibody-mediated rejection in heart transplantation. J Heart Lung Transplant. 32(12):1147-62, 2013
2. Kittleson MM et al: Antibody-mediated rejection. Curr Opin Organ Transplant. 17(5):551-7, 2012
3. Kobashigawa J et al: Report from a consensus conference on antibody-mediated rejection in heart transplantation. J Heart Lung Transplant. 30(3):252-69, 2011
4. Lu WH et al: Diverse morphologic manifestations of cardiac allograft vasculopathy: a pathologic study of 64 allograft hearts. J Heart Lung Transplant. 30(9):1044-50, 2011
5. Tan CD et al: Update on cardiac transplantation pathology. Arch Pathol Lab Med. 131(8):1169-91, 2007
6. Marboe CC et al: Nodular endocardial infiltrates (Quilty lesions) cause significant variability in diagnosis of ISHLT Grade 2 and 3A rejection in cardiac allograft recipients. J Heart Lung Transplant. 24(7 Suppl):S219-26, 2005
7. Stewart S et al: Revision of the 1990 working formulation for the standardization of nomenclature in the diagnosis of heart rejection. J Heart Lung Transplant. 24(11):1710-20, 2005
8. Rowan RA et al: Pathologic changes in the long-term transplanted heart: a morphometric study of myocardial hypertrophy, vascularity, and fibrosis. Hum Pathol. 21(7):767-72, 1990

Microscopic Features

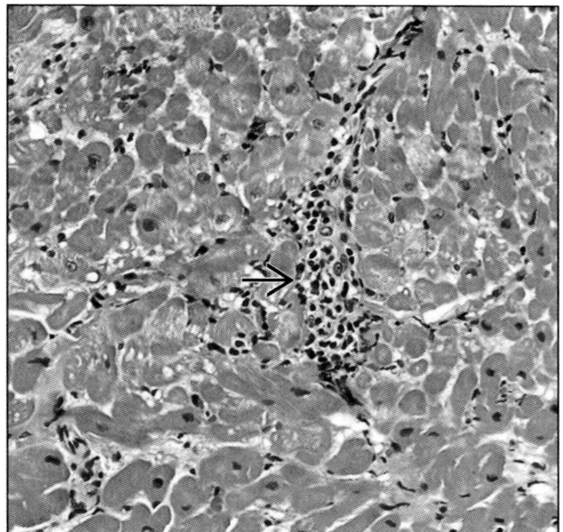
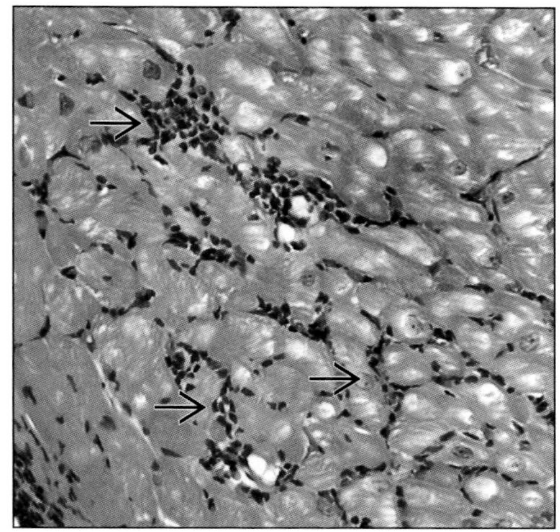

(Left) *This photomicrograph from a cardiac allograft at autopsy shows a small perivascular lymphocytic infiltrate ⇨, without obvious myocyte injury. This would be consistent with mild cellular rejection.* ***(Right)*** *A more diffuse lymphocytic infiltrate ⇨ is seen in this cardiac allograft at autopsy. There is still no obvious or definite myocyte injury, so it would be considered mild. The ISHLT grading system is intended for biopsies, and caution should be taken when applying this to autopsy.*

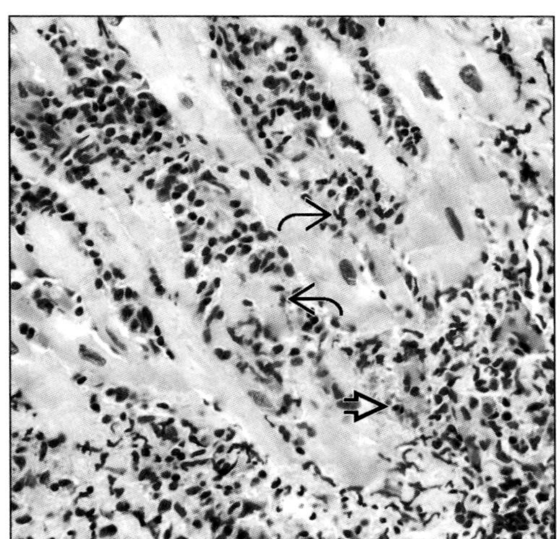
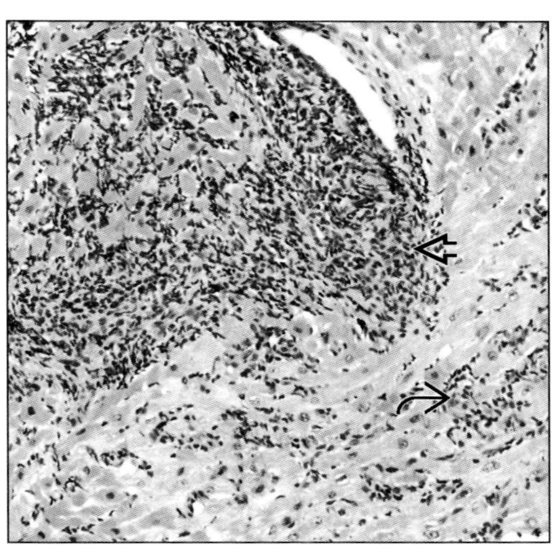

(Left) *This photomicrograph of a heart allograft at autopsy shows a lymphoid inflammatory infiltrate with rare eosinophils ⇨, associated with multifocal myocyte injury ⇨, consistent with more severe rejection. Clinical correlation would be needed to determine the role of rejection in the cause of death.* ***(Right)*** *This allograft heart at autopsy also showed marked perivascular infiltrate ⇨ with several foci of myocyte injury ⇨, consistent with severe rejection.*

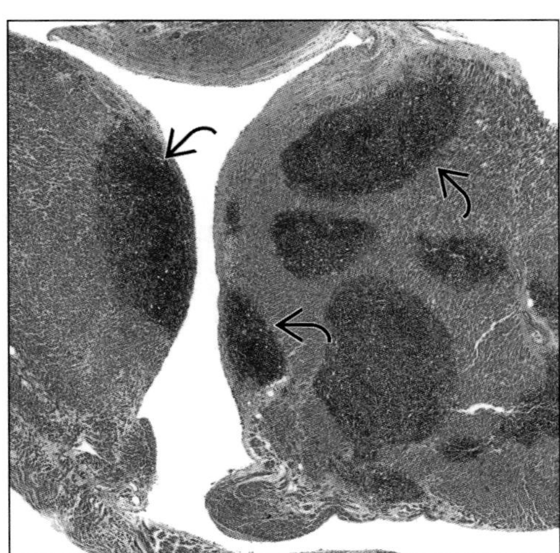
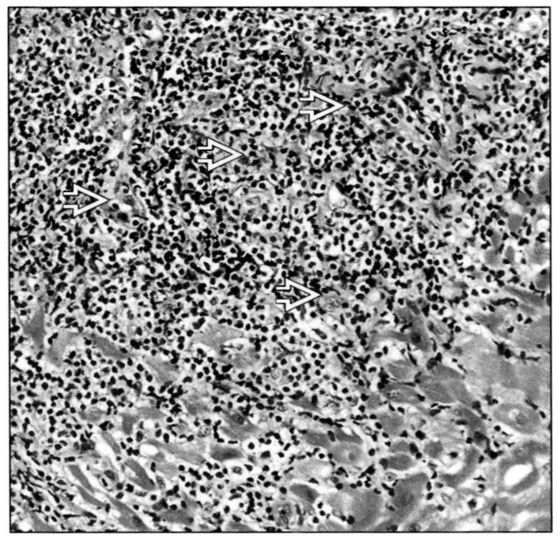

(Left) *This photomicrograph shows trabecular myocardium from the right ventricle of a transplant heart at autopsy. There are rounded lymphoid aggregates ⇨ without interstitial extension, consistent with Quilty effect.* ***(Right)*** *At higher magnification, Quilty effect shows proliferating capillaries ⇨. This is helpful in the differential diagnosis with cellular rejection.*

Microscopic Features

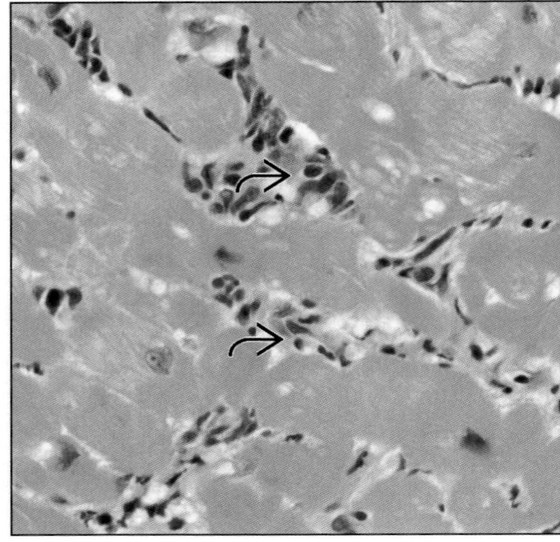

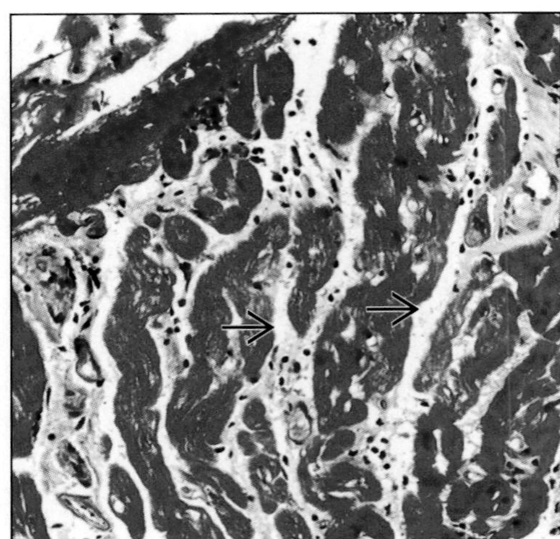

(Left) *This high-power photomicrograph of cardiac transplant myocardium at autopsy shows prominent intravascular mononuclear cells, a hallmark of antibody-mediated rejection. Immunostaining for complement (C4d, C3d) &/or macrophages (CD68) should be performed to complete the diagnostic workup.* ***(Right)*** *This trichrome stain shows another feature prominent in antibody-mediated rejection: Interstitial edema. The capillaries also show intravascular mononuclear cells.*

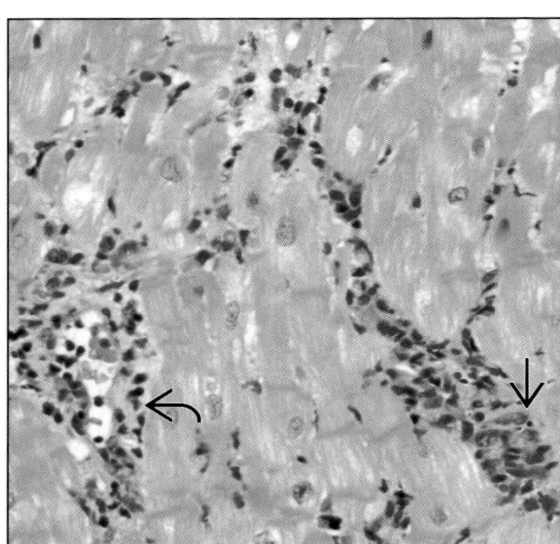

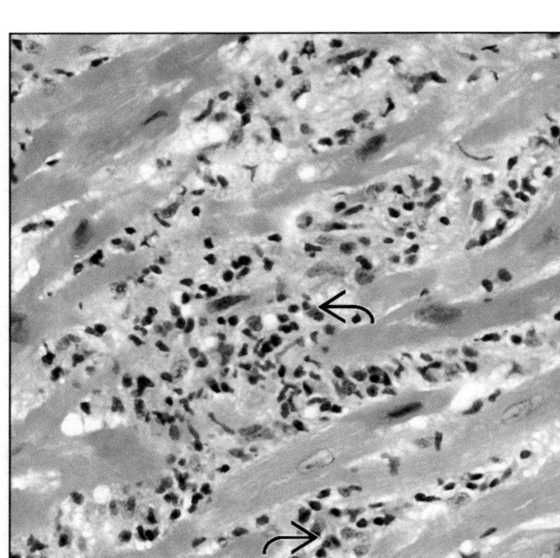

(Left) *This high-magnification view of transplant myocardium at autopsy shows more severe venular changes with transmural mononuclear inflammation and focal karyorrhectic debris. Complement stains were positive in this case.* ***(Right)*** *In severe rejection, it can be difficult to distinguish cellular rejection features from those of severe antibody-mediated rejection. Several eosinophils are seen in this case of severe rejection. Complement staining is helpful in cases like this.*

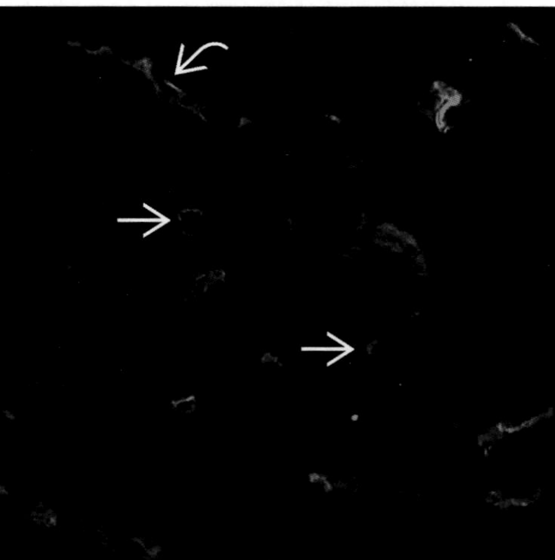

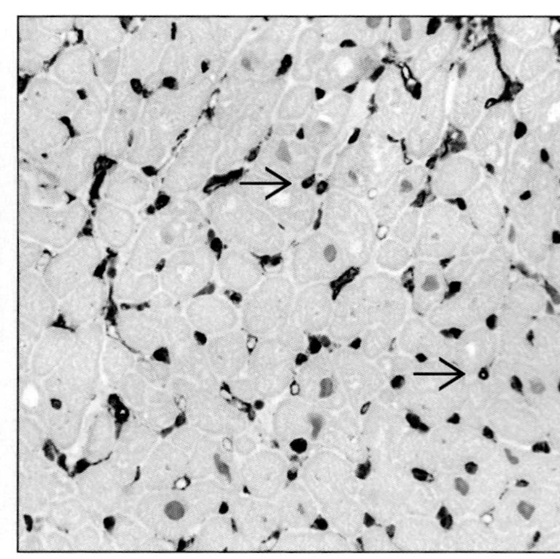

(Left) *Immunofluorescence staining of this cardiac allograft at autopsy is positive for C4d deposition. Capillaries are seen in cross section and longitudinal section.* ***(Right)*** *C4d staining can also be performed using immunohistochemistry techniques in paraffin sections at autopsy. The capillaries are strongly and diffusely positive. The staining is crisp, linear, and circumferential, all features that are helpful in excluding false-positive artifact staining.*

Artifacts Confused With Acute Rejection

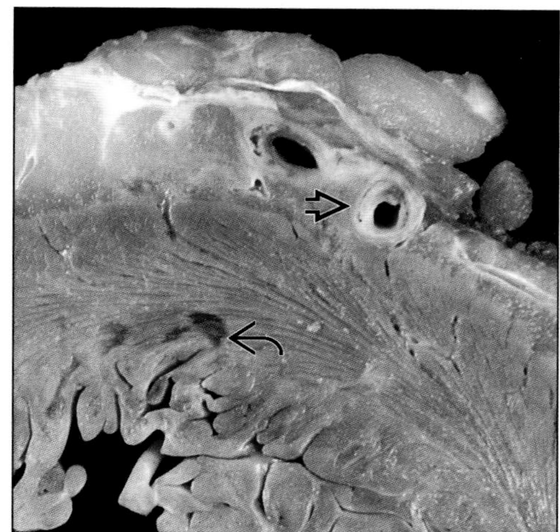

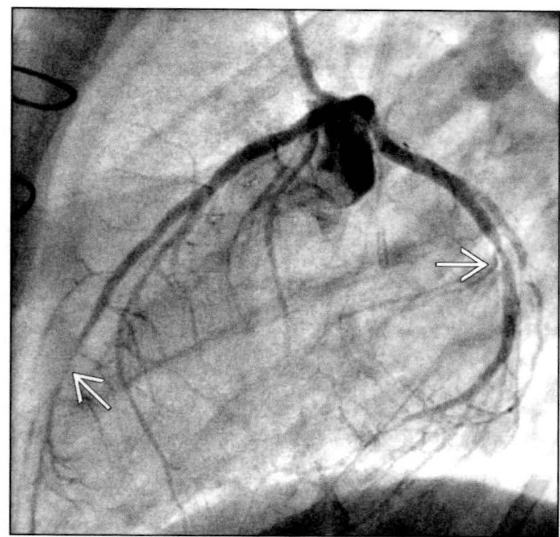

(Left) *This epicardial coronary artery from a transplanted heart at autopsy shows significant allograft vasculopathy ➩. There are also small, depressed, old subendocardial infarctions ↪ in the territory of this artery.* ***(Right)*** *This angiogram in a cardiac transplant patient shows areas of tapered narrowing ➡, consistent with graft vasculopathy. Since this is only a "luminogram," the degree of cross-sectional stenosis is likely to be greater than anticipated based on the angiogram.*

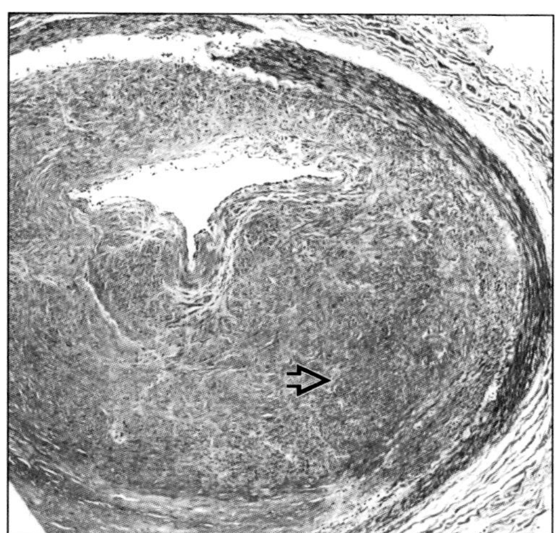

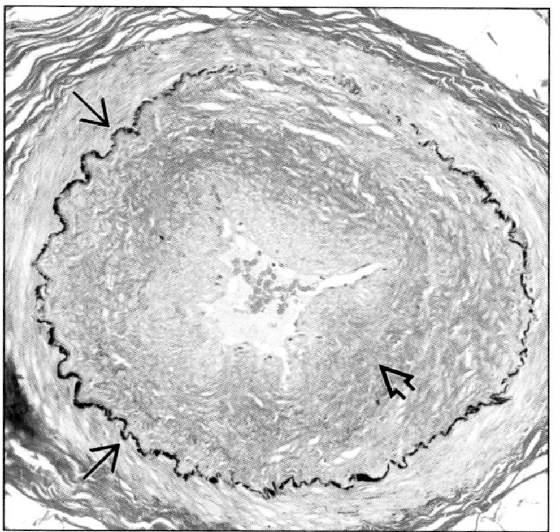

(Left) *This low-power photomicrograph of an epicardial coronary artery from an allograft heart at autopsy shows near complete luminal occlusion. The intima has been expanded by smooth muscle cells and collagen ➩.* ***(Right)*** *This elastic stain highlights the internal elastic lamina →. The narrowing of this artery is due to an increase in collagen ➩ and proliferating vascular smooth muscle cells in the intimal layer (inside the internal elastic lamina).*

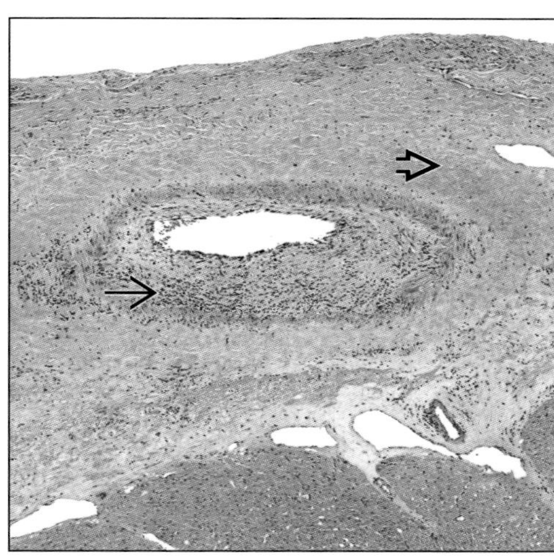

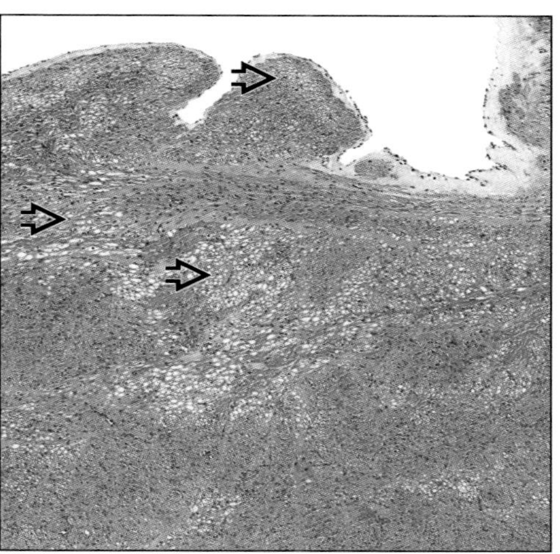

(Left) *This epicardial branch coronary artery from a transplanted heart at autopsy also shows inflammation, largely confined to the intima →. There is also an unusual amount of epicardial fibrosis ➩.* ***(Right)*** *Prominent subendocardial myocyte vacuolization change ➩ is seen in this allograft with cardiac allograft vasculopathy. This finding suggests ongoing chronic ischemia leading to "hibernating" myocardium.*

LUNG TRANSPLANT

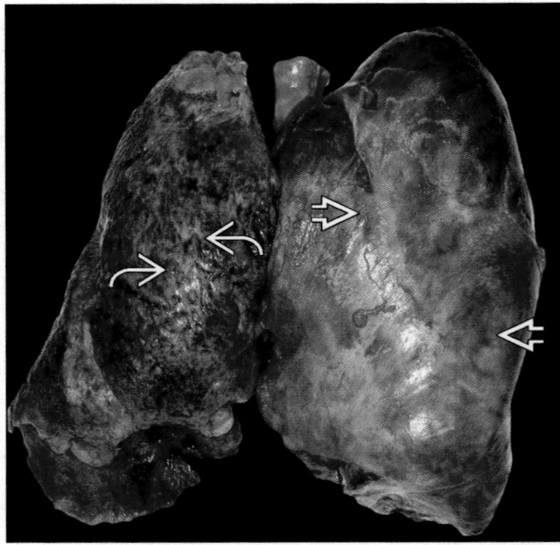

This SLT case shows the right native lung with interstitial fibrosis denoted by a cobblestone appearance and a left allograft with postsurgical pleural adhesions and thickening from other complications.

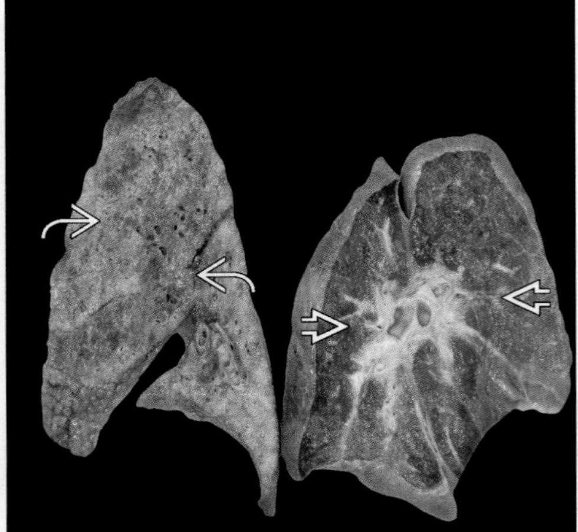

This right native lung shows interstitial fibrosis, and the left allograft has only mild peribronchial fibrosis. The patient died 2 months post transplant with severe pseudomembranous colitis and sepsis.

TERMINOLOGY

Abbreviations

- Orthotopic lung transplant (OLT), single lung transplant (SLT), bilateral lung transplant (BLT), living donor lobar lung transplantation (LDLLT)

ETIOLOGY/PATHOGENESIS

Pathogenesis of Complications Following Lung Transplantation

- Primary graft dysfunction (PGD): Multifactorial, mild to severe injury to allograft occurring within 72 hours of transplantation
  - Incidence of severe PGD ~15-35%
    - ↑ early morbidity and mortality, ↑ length of mechanical ventilation and hospital stay, ↑ short- and long-term mortality, ↑ risk of bronchiolitis obliterans syndrome (BOS)
  - Clinically progressive hypoxemia with radiographic infiltrates without other identifiable causes
    - Exclusion criteria: Cardiogenic pulmonary edema, pneumonia and aspiration, hyperacute cellular rejection, and pulmonary venous obstruction
  - Pathogenesis not completely understood; inflammatory and immunological repair responses appear to be key controlling mechanisms following ischemia and reperfusion
    - Donor-inherent, donor-acquired, recipient, and operative variables have all been identified
- Infectious disease
  - Lung transplant compromises normal host defenses (e.g., cough and mucociliary clearance), leaving recipients more susceptible than other solid organ transplant recipients to infections
  - CMV and other DNA viruses; community-acquired respiratory viruses; bacterial, nontuberculous mycobacterial, and fungal infections must all be considered
    - Bacterial infections are most common in 1st few weeks post transplant
    - Most infections occur within 3 months to 1 year post transplant, but ↑ lifelong risk due to immunosuppression
    - Cytomegalovirus (CMV) donor-recipient matching and viral prophylaxis; has not eliminated risk for CMV pneumonia
    - *Aspergillus* and *Candida* species most common fungal infections, involving bronchial anastomotic site &/or lung
- Anastomotic complications
  - Pulmonary arterial or venous obstruction is rare but has high mortality
    - Intraoperative pressure gradient measurement and transesophageal echocardiography have improved outcomes
    - Early signs include unexplained hypoxia, particularly with pulmonary hypertension
  - Airway complications
    - Airway complications estimated to cause 2-5% of mortalities
    - 6 major types: Anastomotic necrosis and dehiscence, infection, excessive endoluminal granulation tissue formation, bronchomalacia, bronchial stenosis, bronchial fistulae
- Acute cellular rejection (ACR) and antibody-mediated rejection (AMR)
  - At least 1/3 of lung transplant patients have acute rejection within 1 year post transplantation
  - Acute rejection rarely a direct cause of death but ↑ risk for subsequent BOS and may ↑ susceptibility to infection when immunosuppression intensified
    - Patients present with fever, cough, dyspnea, and radiographic infiltrates in which major differential diagnosis is infection
- Chronic lung allograft dysfunction (CLAD) and BOS

LUNG TRANSPLANT

Key Facts

Clinical Issues

- Graft failure and mortality rates for lung transplantation exceed those of most other solid organ transplants
- Major post-transplant complications likely to be encountered at autopsy
  - Primary graft dysfunction
  - Infectious disease
  - Anastomotic complications
  - Airway complications
  - Rejection (acute &/or chronic)
  - Malignancy
- Most infections occur within 3 months to a 1 year post transplant, but persistent lifelong risk due to immunosuppression
- Major long-term mortality mostly attributable to infection &/or chronic lung allograft failure

Macroscopic Pathology

- Evaluate anastomotic sites
- Procure fresh tissue for ancillary studies
- Examine allograft and native lung (if present) for evidence of consolidation, hemorrhage, and masses

Microscopic Pathology

- Variable histologic and sometimes nonspecific findings such as pulmonary edema, hemorrhage, and diffuse alveolar damage, requiring clinical correlation
- Special stains should be used to exclude infection and to assess chronic airway rejection

  - Main limitation to better long-term survival; pathogenesis poorly understood
  - Recent International Society for Heart and Lung Transplantation (ISHLT) data: Incidence of BOS 48% at 5 years post transplant and 76% at 10 years
  - Patients present with cough, dyspnea, and irreversible decrease in pulmonary function tests over time
- ↑ malignancy risk due to preexisting risk factors (such as smoking) and immunosuppression
  - Incidence: 13% between 5 and 10 years post transplant
  - Malignancies include skin cancer, post-transplant lymphoproliferative disorder, lung cancer, and other common solid organ tumors
- Recurrence of nonneoplastic native disease
- Hyperacute cellular rejection
  - Rare complication that occurs during or shortly after transplantation due to preformed donor-specific antibodies (DSAs) that react immediately with lung allograft
  - Characterized by neutrophilic margination, vasculitis, fibrinoid necrosis, vascular thrombosis, and infarction

CLINICAL ISSUES

Epidemiology

- Incidence
  - 2014 ISHLT Registry data includes > 47,000 adult lung transplant recipients and > 3,700 heart-lung transplant recipients
  - Major indications for lung transplantation
    - Chronic obstructive pulmonary disease (COPD), idiopathic pulmonary fibrosis (IPF), primary arterial hypertension (PAH), cystic fibrosis
  - SLT is used most frequently for COPD and IPF
  - BLT is used in diseases such as cystic fibrosis and sarcoidosis where incidence of coexistent infection is high
  - Both SLT and BLT have been used in treatment of pulmonary arterial hypertension
- Age
  - Lung transplantation successful in pediatric and adult patients with nonneoplastic lung disease
  - Older patients (> 65) undergoing lung transplant has ↑, although data indicate that ↑ age may negatively impact long-term outcomes and ↑ incidence of certain post-transplant complications such as malignancy

Prognosis

- In USA, adult lungs have been allocated according to lung allograft score (LAS) since 2005
  - LAS has reduced transplant wait list deaths, but data suggests that the practice has resulted in higher post-transplant mortality
- Graft failure and mortality rates for lung transplantation exceed those of most other solid organ transplants
- Short-term outcomes have markedly improved with current 3-month survival 90% and 1-year survival ~ 80%
- 5-year survival rate is ~ 50% and 10-year survival rate is ~ 30%
  - Major long-term mortality attributable to infection &/or chronic lung allograft failure

MACROSCOPIC FEATURES

External Examination

- Surgical techniques vary for single and bilateral lung transplants
  - Single lung: Lung with worst function replaced or right lung if equal lung dysfunction
    - Incision usually from beneath the shoulder blade across chest to sternum
  - Bilateral lung
    - Incision usually from axilla to sternum to opposite axilla (clamshell)

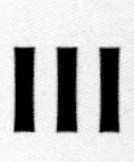

LUNG TRANSPLANT

- Thoracotomy sites/scars should be inspected for signs of dehiscence or infection
- Chest tubes and endotracheal tubes and vascular access lines assessed for appropriate placement, as they are present
- Signs of complications of transplantation and chronic lung disease
  - Sepsis: Petechiae, jaundice
  - Chronic hypoxia: Clubbing of fingers (hypertrophic osteoarthropathy)

Internal Examination

- Depending on post-transplant interval and history of postoperative complications, lungs may or may not be densely adhesed to chest wall
- Inspect mediastinum and pleura for evidence of fistulae or infection

Organ Examination

- Identify and inspect anastomotic sites (mainstem bronchi, pulmonary artery, and pulmonary veins)
  - Note that pulmonary venous anastomosis is indirect and accomplished by recipient left atrium to donor left atrium sutures
  - Particular attention should be paid to bronchial anastomotic site(s)
    - Site(s) may be grossly characterized as well healed, with granulation tissue, necrosis limited to mucosa or extending through wall, or signs of infection
- Following procurement of fresh tissue for culture or other ancillary studies such as immunofluorescence, lungs should be inflated with formalin for overnight fixation
- Examine allograft and native lung (if present) for evidence of consolidation, hemorrhage, or masses
- Other organs: Features of shock (hepatic necrosis, acute tubular injury, ischemic bowel), complications of therapy (renal scarring and hypertensive heart disease [calcineurin inhibitor therapy]), pseudomembranous colitis (antibiotics)

MICROSCOPIC PATHOLOGY

Histologic Features

- Acute T-cell-mediated cellular rejection (ACR)
  - Based on extent of perivascular and interstitial lymphocytic infiltrates ± acute lung injury
  - There may also be component of airway inflammation
- Antibody-mediated rejection (AMR)
  - Diagnosis of exclusion and requires comprehensive serologic, microbiologic, and pathologic correlation
  - Histologic features nonspecific: Acute lung injury and neutrophilic infiltration of alveolar capillaries
  - C4d immunohistochemical staining is used, but it is difficult to interpret and has poor sensitivity
- Chronic rejection
  - Eccentric submucosal fibrosis or obliterative scarring of small airways (bronchiolitis obliterans)
  - Distal airway narrowing results in more proximal bronchiectasis
  - Extensive sampling may be necessary in addition to trichrome and elastin stains to better highlight obliterated airways
- Aspiration is common in lung transplant patients
  - Scattered multinucleated giant cell or granulomas are occasionally seen as incidental finding
- Infection is always within differential diagnosis and should be rigorously excluded
- Primary graft dysfunction
  - Diffuse alveolar damage without evidence of infection or other etiology
- Other organs
  - Kidney: Calcineurin inhibitor toxicity: Nodular hyaline arteriolosclerosis of arterioles (chronic), "foamy" cytoplasm of proximal tubular epithelial cells (acute), thrombotic microangiopathy
  - Shock changes: Ischemic necrosis of organs
  - Infection: Viral inclusions (CMV, HSV, adenovirus) in organs and tissues, suppurative inflammation (bacterial and fungal), and granulomatous inflammation (mycobacteria)

ANCILLARY TESTS

Immunofluorescence

- Portion of lung may be frozen for C4d staining; paraffin immunohistochemistry for C4d also may be performed

Microbiology

- Cultures, histochemistry, immunohistochemistry, in situ hybridization, and molecular studies for infection, as indicated

REPORTING CRITERIA

Transplantation Cause of Death

- Directly related to or a known complication
  - Specify type of transplant (single or bilateral) and time elapsed since allograft transplant
  - Findings directly related to transplantation
    - Rejection
    - Infection, particularly in association with immunosuppression
    - Drug toxicity
    - Anastomotic complications
- Unrelated to transplantation, if appropriate

SELECTED REFERENCES

1. Todd JL et al: Update in lung transplantation 2013. Am J Respir Crit Care Med. 190(1):19-24, 2014
2. Wallace WD et al: Update on pathology of antibody-mediated rejection in the lung allograft. Curr Opin Organ Transplant. 19(3):303-8, 2014
3. Yusen RD et al: The registry of the International Society for Heart and Lung Transplantation: thirty-first adult lung and heart-lung transplant report--2014; focus theme: retransplantation. J Heart Lung Transplant. 33(10):1009-24, 2014

Lung Allograft Pathology at Autopsy

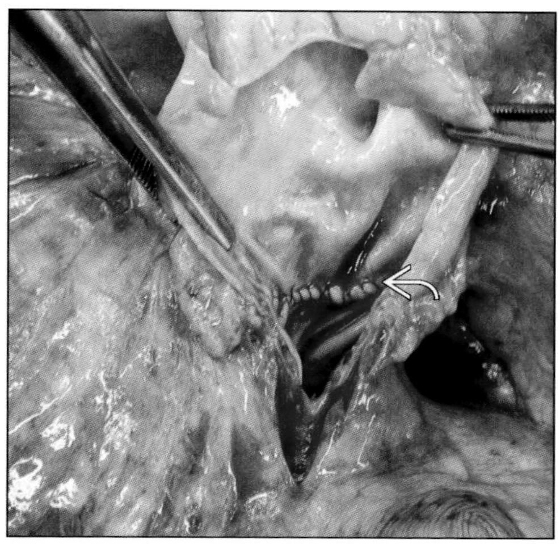

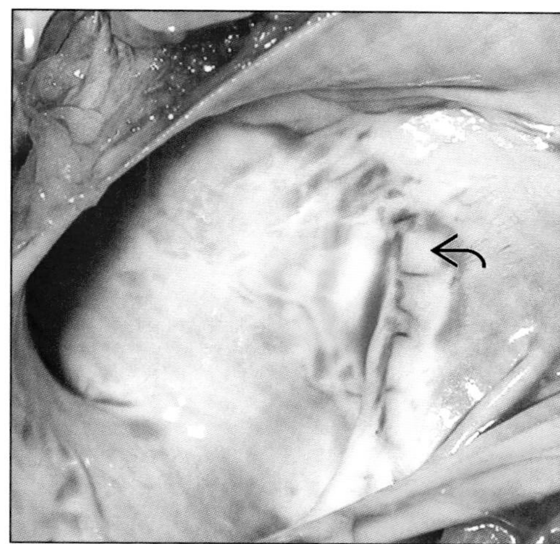

(Left) *This gross photograph shows an intact suture line* ➡ *at the pulmonary arterial anastomosis.* ***(Right)*** *This gross photograph shows an intact suture line* ➡ *at the left atrial anastomotic site. Tan-white endocardium now covers the blue suture material.*

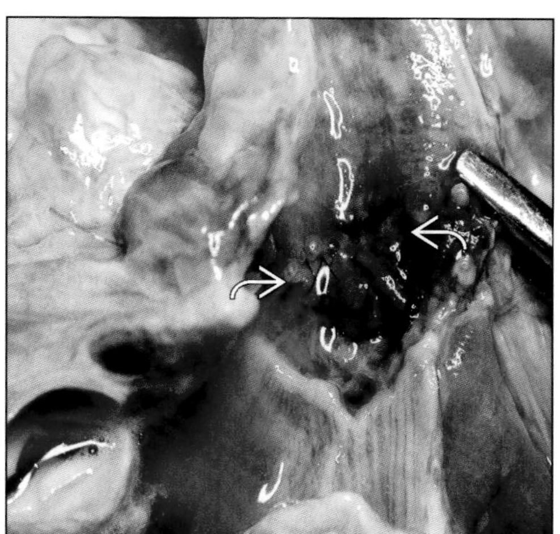

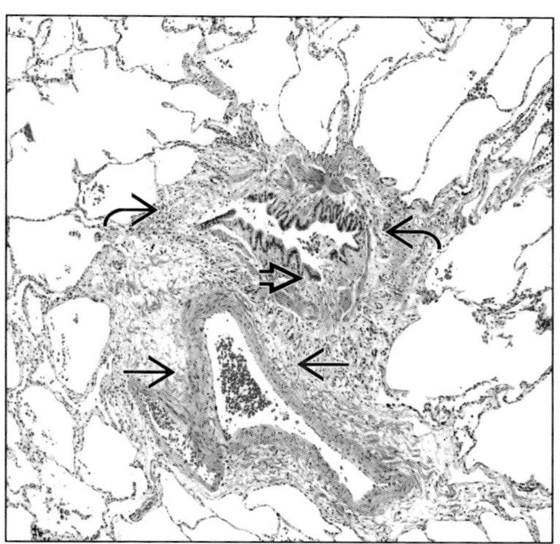

(Left) *The bronchial anastomosis is particularly susceptible to complications. This patient developed a necrotizing infection at the anastomotic site* ➡*, which led to fatal bleeding into the airway.* ***(Right)*** *Note the reduced caliber of the airway* ➡ *in comparison to its companion vessel* ➡ *in this example of chronic allograft rejection. This is due to scar tissue forming in the submucosa of the small airway* ➡*.*

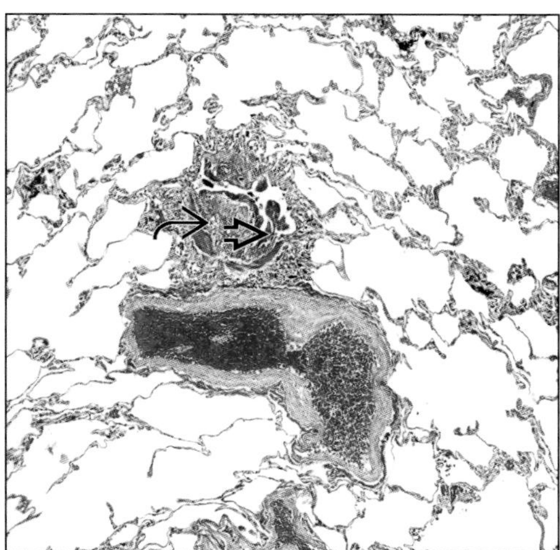

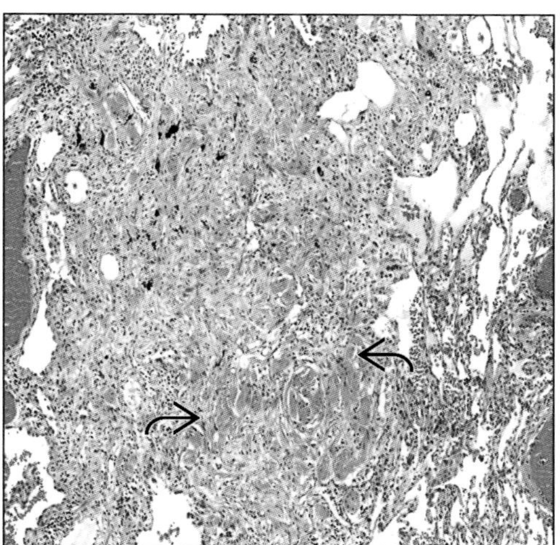

(Left) *This trichrome stain of chronic allograft rejection helps to highlight the submucosal fibrosis* ➡ *in the small airway. The epithelium* ➡ *is intact but protruding into the lumen of the airway due to the submucosal fibrosis.* ***(Right)*** *In this image of chronic allograft rejection, this airway lumen has been completely obliterated by fibrosis. The residual mural smooth muscle remains* ➡*.*

KIDNEY TRANSPLANT

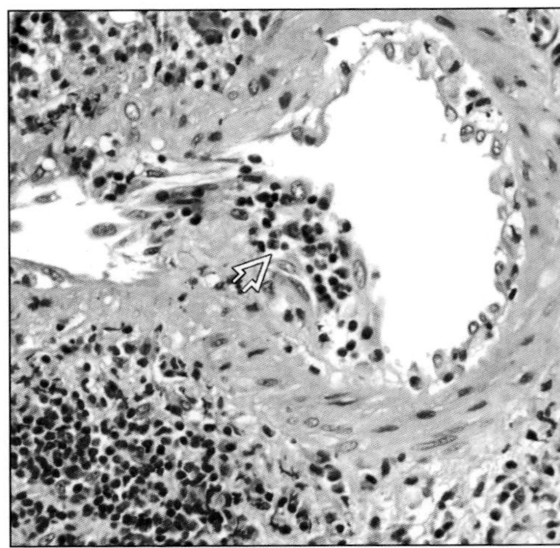

Artery shows endothelial swelling and lifting with intima infiltration by mononuclear cells (endothelialitis) ➪ involving > 25% of the lumen, consistent with acute rejection Banff type IIA.

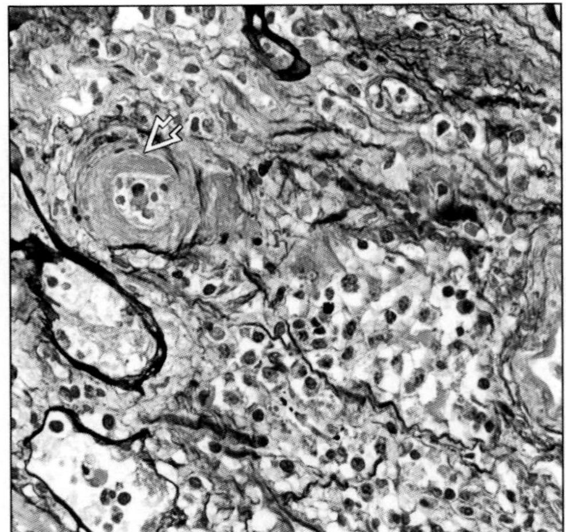

Arteriole shows fibrinoid necrosis of the wall ➪ in this case of acute rejection. Fibrinoid necrosis or transmural inflammation are features of rejection Banff type III.

TERMINOLOGY

Synonyms

- Kidney allograft

Definitions

- Allograft implantation for treatment of end-stage renal disease (ESRD)
  - Allograft types
    - Living, related
    - Living, unrelated
    - Deceased

ETIOLOGY/PATHOGENESIS

Diseases Leading To Kidney Transplant

- Glomerular diseases: 12-16% of patients with chronic renal failure (CRF)
- Hypertensive nephrosclerosis: 29-38% of patients with CRF
- Diabetic nephropathy: ~ 50% of patients with CRF and ≥ 1/3 of patients in dialysis
- Polycystic kidney disease: ~ 3% of patients with CRF

CLINICAL ISSUES

Epidemiology

- Incidence
  - Antibody-mediated rejection (AMR)
    - Hyperacute rejection in < 0.5% of transplants
    - Acute antibody-mediated rejection ~ 25% of acute rejection episodes
  - Acute T-cell-mediated rejection episode occurs in 5-10% of kidney transplants in 1st year post transplant
  - Chronic cellular rejection major cause of long-term allograft failure
  - Drug toxicity
    - Calcineurin inhibitor: Thrombotic microangiopathy 2-5%, chronic toxicity 60-70% at 2 years
  - Infections
    - BK nephropathy present in ~ 5% of kidney transplanted patients on tacrolimus and mycophenolate mofetil
  - Recurrence of primary disease
    - Membranous glomerulopathy: 30%
    - IgA nephropathy: 13-50%
    - Membranoproliferative glomerulonephritis type 1: 20-50%
    - Dense deposit disease: > 80%
    - Lupus nephritis: Up to 30%
    - Focal segmental glomerulosclerosis: 20-40%
    - Diabetic nephropathy : > 50%
  - Most common de novo glomerular disease
    - Membranous nephropathy: 0.5-9% of allografts
    - Focal segmental glomerulosclerosis: 10-20% of allografts
    - Anti-glomerular basement membrane disease: 3-5% of Alport patients allografts
  - Post-transplant lymphoproliferative disease <1%

Presentation

- Early complications
  - Allograft rejection
    - Hyperacute rejection: At implantation, allograft becomes cyanotic and flaccid within minutes of anastomosis; no urine production; fever; thrombocytopenia; intravascular hemolysis
    - Acute AMR: Rapid development of graft failure after initial period of good function; elevation of creatinine; reduced urine output
    - Acute cellular rejection: Most common type of rejection; occurs 1-6 weeks post transplant, but may develop even years post transplant; elevation of creatinine; urine output reduction
- Late complications

KIDNEY TRANSPLANT

Key Facts

Terminology
- Allograft implantation for treatment of ESRD

Etiology
- Glomerular diseases constitute 12-16% of patients with chronic renal failure (CRF)
- Hypertensive nephrosclerosis is 29-38% cause of CRF
- Diabetic nephropathy in ~ 50% of patients with CRF and ≥ 1/3 of patients in dialysis
- Polycystic kidney disease in ~ 3% of patients with CRF

Clinical Issues
- Living donor median survival: 18.5 years
- Deceased donor median survival: 9.8 years
- Causes of death: Infection (most common), cardiovascular complications, malignancy
- Episodes of acute cellular and antibody-mediated rejection significantly reduce allograft lifetime
- Clinical manifestations are nonspecific, and many different pathologic processes may be found

Microscopic Pathology
- In early post-transplant period, acute T-cell and antibody-mediated rejection are most common
- In late post-transplant period, different pathologic changes may be present and may overlap
  - Chronic T-cell rejection
  - Chronic antibody-mediated rejection
  - Drug toxicity
  - Recurrence or "de novo" glomerular diseases
  - Infections
  - Post transplant lymphoproliferative disorder

- Chronic cellular rejection: Progressive renal failure, proteinuria, hypertension
- Chronic AMR: Progressive renal failure, proteinuria, hypertension
- Drug toxicity
  - Calcineurin inhibitor: Renal dysfunction; acute or chronic
  - MTOR inhibitor: Delayed graft function, acute renal failure, proteinuria
- Infections
  - BK nephropathy: Acute renal failure, hemorrhagic cystitis, ureteral obstruction
  - Acute pyelonephritis: Acute renal failure, fever, pyuria, bacteriuria
- Recurrence of primary disease
  - Glomerulonephritis: Proteinuria may be in nephrotic or nonnephrotic range, hematuria, decline of renal function
- De novo glomerular diseases
  - Proteinuria may be in nephrotic or nonnephrotic range, hematuria, decline of renal function
- Post-transplant lymphoproliferative disorder
  - Malaise, weight loss, fever, abdominal mass, hepatocellular or pancreatic dysfunction, central nervous system disease

Prognosis
- Living donor median survival: 18.5 years
- Deceased donor median survival: 9.8 years
- Causes of death: Infection (most common), cardiovascular complications, malignancy
- Episodes of acute cellular and antibody-mediated rejection significantly reduce allograft lifetime
- Recurrent glomerular diseases may cause graft loss at variable time intervals, usually slower than primary disease
- BK nephropathy may cause graft loss (13-100% at 3 years); poorer prognosis with marked interstitial fibrosis and tubular atrophy at diagnosis

MACROSCOPIC FEATURES

External Examination
- Allograft kidney may be palpated in right/left iliac fossa
- Surgical scar may be evident in right/left iliac fossa
- In some cases, > 1 allograft may be present

Organ Examination
- Hyperacute rejection
  - Parenchyma is purple-blue with soft, flaccid consistency
  - Hemorrhagic infarction and swelling
  - Large and medium-sized artery thrombi
- Acute AMR
  - Enlarged and swollen graft
  - Focal hemorrhage and infarcts
- Acute cellular rejection
  - Enlarged and swollen graft
  - Pale or with mottled hemorrhagic appearance in more severe forms
  - Kidney rupture may occur
- Chronic rejection
  - Small shrunken kidney

MICROSCOPIC PATHOLOGY

Histologic Features
- Hyperacute rejection
  - Early features
    - Endothelial swelling & necrosis
    - Neutrophilic margination within peritubular and glomerular capillaries
    - Microthrombosis in capillaries, arterioles, and small arteries
    - Tubular necrosis
  - Late features
    - Interstitial hemorrhage
    - Neutrophilic inflammation
    - Intravascular thrombosis
    - Cortical and medullary necrosis

KIDNEY TRANSPLANT

- Acute AMR
  - Early features
    - Neutrophilic margination in glomerular and peritubular capillaries
    - Tubular necrosis
  - Late features
    - Endothelial injury
    - Microvascular thrombosis
    - Mesangiolysis
    - Larger arteries with transmural arteritis
    - Interstitial edema and mononuclear inflammation
- Acute cellular rejection
  - Interstitial mononuclear inflammation and edema
    - Inflammation may include variable numbers of plasma cells and eosinophils
  - Tubulitis involving nonatrophic tubules
  - Acute tubular injury
  - Endothelialitis (mononuclear cells underneath endothelium) present in more severe type of cellular rejection, most common in larger arteries
  - Transmural inflammation and arteriolar or arterial fibrinoid necrosis in most severe cases
- Chronic cellular rejection
  - Global &/or segmental glomerulosclerosis
  - Interstitial mononuclear inflammatory infiltrate in scarred and nonscarred areas
  - Interstitial fibrosis with nonspecific pattern
  - Tubular atrophy and tubulitis in atrophic and nonatrophic tubules
  - Arteries with intimal fibrosis, foamy cells, and mononuclear inflammation in intima
- Chronic AMR
  - Transplant glomerulopathy
    - Duplication of capillary basement membrane
    - Negative immunofluorescence
    - Electron-dense deposits are not identified
  - Transplant arteriopathy
    - Fibrous intimal thickening with infiltrating lymphocytes &/or monocytes
  - Peritubular capillaritis characterized by presence of mononuclear cells within peritubular capillaries
- Drug toxicity
  - Calcineurin inhibitor, acute toxicity
    - Functional toxicity without morphologic changes
    - Isometric vacuolization in tubular epithelial cells
    - Thrombotic microangiopathy
  - Calcineurin inhibitor, chronic toxicity
    - Secondary segmental glomerulosclerosis
    - Interstitial fibrosis and tubular atrophy with striped pattern
    - Arterioles and most distal portions of interlobular arteries affected by nodular hyaline deposits in smooth muscle cells with beaded circular pattern
- Infections
  - BK nephropathy
    - Pleomorphic interstitial inflammation: Lymphocytes, plasma cells, eosinophils, and neutrophils
    - Viral cytopathic changes: Nuclear enlargement, nuclear inclusions with ground-glass appearance
- Glomerular diseases recurrent or de novo show morphology similar to primary disease
  - Immunofluorescence and electron microscopy examination are necessary for diagnosis
  - Knowledge of primary disease leading to end-stage renal disease is indispensable for classification of glomerular lesions

ANCILLARY TESTS

Immunohistochemistry

- SV40 immunohistochemical stain necessary to confirm BK polyomavirus nephropathy
- CMV stain
- C4d by immunohistochemistry can be used when no frozen tissue is available

Immunofluorescence

- Hyperacute rejection
  - C3, C4d in capillaries, arterioles and small arteries; fibrin staining in microvasculature
- Acute and chronic AMR
  - C4d(+) in peritubular capillaries
- Glomerular diseases
  - Panel of IgG, IgA, IgM, C3, C1q, light chains, and albumin should be performed when there is history of proteinuria and cause of end-stage renal disease was glomerulonephritis

Electron Microscopy

- Transmission
  - Electron dense deposits can be identified and confirm diagnosis of glomerular diseases recurrent or de novo
  - Multilamellation of peritubular capillaries is characteristic of chronic AMR
  - Transplant glomerulopathy is characterized by expansion of lamina rara interna by electron-lucent material

REPORTING CONSIDERATIONS

Banff Classification

- Background
  - Classification is currently based on light microscopy, immunofluorescence, or immunohistochemistry and, in some cases, electron microscopy
    - Diagnostic categories defined by semiquantitative scores
    - Opportunity to add other modalities, e.g., gene expression
  - Refinement occurs through biannual open meetings to reach consensus on additions/changes based on published, confirmed evidence
  - Widely used in drug trials
- Sample adequacy is 7 glomeruli and 2 arteries and should be noted

Banff Categories

- **Category 1: Normal**
- **Category 2: Antibody-mediated rejection (C4d[+])**
  - Requires acute or chronic tissue injury or inflammation, evidence of antibody interaction

with tissue (usually C4d in peritubular capillaries [PTC]), and circulating antibodies reactive to donor endothelium
  - Acute antibody-mediated rejection
    - I: Acute tubular injury
    - II: Peritubular &/or glomerular capillary inflammation (neutrophils), ± thrombi
    - III: Arterial involvement by transmural arteritis, &/or arterial fibrinoid necrosis and medial smooth muscle necrosis with inflammatory infiltrate in vessel
  - Chronic antibody-mediated rejection
    - Chronic tissue injury includes GBM duplication without immune complex deposition (transplant glomerulopathy), PTC basement membrane multilamination (usually seen by electron microscopy), transplant arteriopathy, and interstitial fibrosis and tubular atrophy
    - Often manifested by mononuclear cells in PTC (capillaritis) &/or glomeruli (transplant glomerulitis)
  - Hyperacute rejection
    - Usually due to preformed antibody, e.g., antibodies to HLA or ABO antigens
  - C4d deposition without evidence of active rejection
- **Category 3: Borderline or suspicious for acute cellular rejection**
- **Category 4: T-cell-mediated rejection**
  - Requires > i1 and ≥ t2 or > v0; C4d negative for pure T-cell-mediated rejection
  - Acute T-cell-mediated rejection
    - IA: Interstitial inflammation (> 25% of unscarred cortex) and foci of moderate tubulitis (> 4 mononuclear cells per tubular cross section)
    - IB: Interstitial inflammation (> 25% of unscarred cortex) and foci of severe tubulitis (> 10 mononuclear cells per tubular cross section)
    - IIA: Mild to moderate intimal arteritis (< 25% of luminal area) (v1)
    - IIB: Severe intimal arteritis (> 25% of luminal area) (v2)
    - III: Transmural arteritis &/or fibrinoid necrosis of medial smooth muscle (v3)
  - Chronic active T-cell-mediated rejection
    - Chronic allograft arteriopathy (arterial intimal fibrosis with mononuclear cell infiltration in fibrosis, formation of neointima)
- **Category 5: Interstitial fibrosis and tubular atrophy, no evidence of any specific etiology**
  - Use only when etiology of IF/TA is unknown
  - Formerly known as chronic allograft nephropathy (CAN)
- **Category 6: Other**
  - Changes considered not due to rejection
    - Calcineurin inhibitor toxicity, polyomavirus infection, and others

Caveats

- Biopsies may meet criteria for ≥ 2 diagnoses
- Detailed criteria established only for rejection categories
- Reproducibility of certain categories and features is limited

Banff Scoring Categories

- **Interstitial inflammation (i)**
  - Mononuclear inflammation in nonfibrotic areas; excludes subcapsular cortex and perivascular infiltrates
    - i0: < 10% of nonfibrotic cortex
    - i1: 10-25%
    - i2: 26-50%
    - i3: > 50%
  - Do not include fibrotic areas in denominator
- **Tubulitis (t)**
  - Mononuclear cells in tubules; for longitudinal sections count per 10 tubular epithelial nuclei
    - t0: No mononuclear cells in tubules
    - t1: Foci with 1-4 cells/tubular cross section
    - t2: Foci with 5-10 cells/tubular cross section
    - t3: Foci with > 10 cells/tubular cross section
  - Need at least 2 foci of tubulitis to be present
- **Vascular inflammation (v)**
  - Mononuclear cells in intima or media of arteries or medial necrosis
    - v0: No arteritis
    - v1: Intimal arteritis in < 25% of lumen (minimum = 1 cell, 1 artery)
    - v2: Intimal arteritis in ≥ 25% of lumen in ≥ 1 artery
    - v3: Transmural arteritis &/or medial smooth muscle necrosis (fibrinoid necrosis)
- **Glomerulitis (g)**
  - % of glomeruli with increased mononuclear cells in capillaries
    - g0: No glomerulitis
    - g1: < 25% of glomeruli
    - g2: 25-75% of glomeruli
    - g3: > 75% of glomeruli
- **Interstitial fibrosis (ci)**
  - % of cortex with fibrosis
    - ci0: ≤ 5%
    - ci1: 6-25%
    - ci2: 26-50%
    - ci3: > 50%
- **Tubular atrophy (ct)**
  - % of cortex with atrophic tubules
    - ct0: 0%
    - ct1: ≤ 25%
    - ct2: 26-50%
    - ct3: > 50%
- **Arterial fibrointimal thickening (cv)**
  - % of narrowing of lumen of most severely affected artery
    - cv0: 0%
    - cv1: ≤ 25%
    - cv2: 26-50%
    - cv3: > 50%
  - Note if lesions characteristic of chronic cellular rejection are present (inflammatory cells in intima, foam cells, breaks in internal elastica or lack of fibroelastosis in intima)
- **Transplant glomerulopathy (cg)**

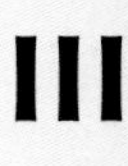

- % of glomerular capillary loops with duplication of GBM in most affected glomerulus
  - cg0: < 10%
  - cg1: 10-25%
  - cg2: 26-50%
  - cg3: > 50%
- **Mesangial matrix increase (mm)**
  - % of glomeruli with mesangial increase, defined as > 2 mesangial cells in width in at least 2 glomerular lobules
    - mm0: 0%
    - mm1: ≤ 25%
    - mm2: 26-50%
    - mm3: > 50%
- **Arteriolar hyalinosis (ah)**
  - Circumferential or noncircumferential (focal) hyaline
    - ah0: No arterioles with hyaline
    - ah1: 1 arteriole with noncircumferential hyaline
    - ah2: ≥ 1 arteriole with noncircumferential hyaline
    - ah3: ≥ 1 arteriole with circumferential hyaline
  - Note if peripheral nodules are present
- **Peritubular capillary inflammation (ptc)**
  - % of cortical PTC with neutrophils or mononuclear cells
    - ptc0: < 10% PTC with cells
    - ptc1: > 10% with < 5 cells/PTC
    - ptc2: > 10% with 5-10 cells/PTC
    - ptc3: > 10% with > 10 cells/PTC
  - Note whether only mononuclear cells, < 50% neutrophils, or > 50% neutrophils
- **C4d score in PTC (C4d)**
  - % of PTC with C4d deposition scored in at least 5 HPF
    - C4d0: 0%
    - C4d1: 1-9%
    - C4d2: 10-50%
    - C4d3: > 50%
  - Note technique used (frozen vs. paraffin)
- **Total inflammation (ti)**
  - Includes all cortical inflammation, even subcapsular, perivascular, nodular, and fibrotic areas
    - ti0: < 10% of cortex
    - ti1: 10-25%
    - ti2: 26-50%
    - ti3: > 50%

REPORTING CRITERIA

Required Final Report Elements

- Cause of death and how it may relate to transplantation
- Presence of complications, rejection, recurrent disease, de novo disease, malignancy

SELECTED REFERENCES

1. de Kort H et al: The role of electron microscopy in renal allograft biopsy evaluation. Curr Opin Organ Transplant. Epub ahead of print, 2015
2. Kozakowski N et al: The diffuse extent of peritubular capillaritis in renal allograft rejection is an independent risk factor for graft loss. Kidney Int. Epub ahead of print, 2015
3. Haas M et al: Banff 2013 meeting report: inclusion of c4d-negative antibody-mediated rejection and antibody-associated arterial lesions. Am J Transplant. 14(2):272-83, 2014
4. Haas M: Chronic allograft nephropathy or interstitial fibrosis and tubular atrophy: what is in a name? Curr Opin Nephrol Hypertens. 23(3):245-50, 2014
5. Naesens M et al: The histology of kidney transplant failure: a long-term follow-up study. Transplantation. 98(4):427-35, 2014
6. Mengel M et al: Banff 2011 Meeting report: new concepts in antibody-mediated rejection. Am J Transplant. 12(3):563-70, 2012
7. Sellarés J et al: Understanding the causes of kidney transplant failure: the dominant role of antibody-mediated rejection and nonadherence. Am J Transplant. 12(2):388-99, 2012
8. Racusen LC et al: The pathology of chronic allograft dysfunction. Kidney Int Suppl. (119):S27-32, 2010
9. Boldorini R et al: Kidney and urinary tract polyomavirus infection and distribution: molecular biology investigation of 10 consecutive autopsies. Arch Pathol Lab Med. 129(1):69-73, 2005
10. Michalak G et al: Infectious complications after simultaneous pancreas-kidney transplantation. Transplant Proc. 37(8):3560-3, 2005
11. Sanromán Budiño B et al: Autopsy-determined causes of death in solid organ transplant recipients. Transplant Proc. 36(3):787-9, 2004
12. Gill JS et al: Mortality after kidney transplant failure: the impact of non-immunologic factors. Kidney Int. 62(5):1875-83, 2002
13. Porazko T et al: Causes of death among cadaver kidney graft recipients between 1983 and 2000. Transplant Proc. 34(6):2066-7, 2002
14. Racusen LC et al: The Banff 97 working classification of renal allograft pathology. Kidney Int. 55(2):713-23, 1999

Microscopic Features

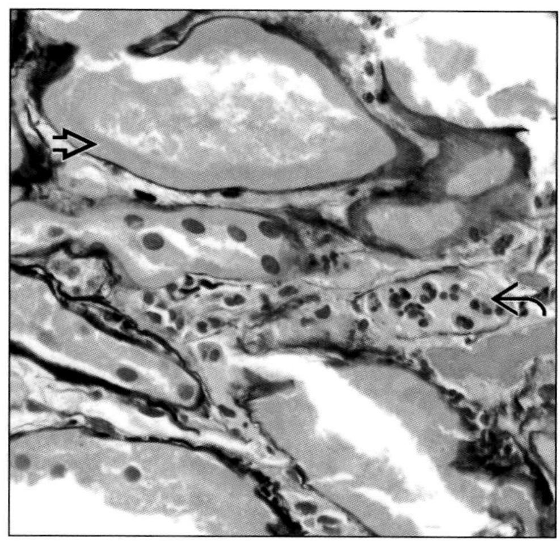

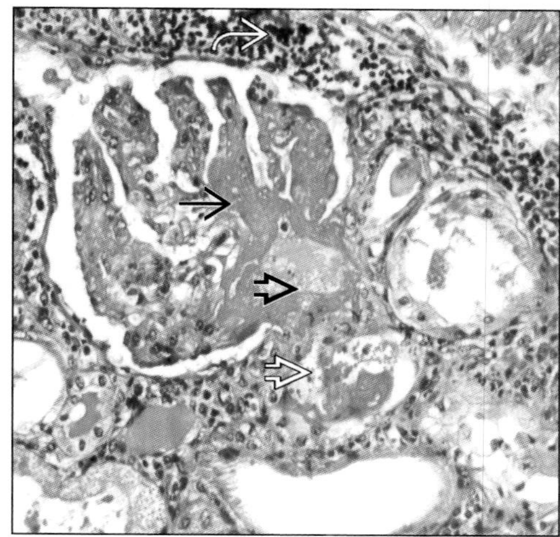

(Left) *Early histologic features of hyperacute rejection shown in this section include margination of neutrophils in peritubular capillaries ➔ and tubular epithelial cell necrosis ➔.* ***(Right)*** *In hyperacute rejection, the glomerular capillaries can be involved by microthrombosis ➔. In this case, there is also a thrombus at the glomerular vascular pole ➔. In the adjacent interstitium, edema and mild inflammation are seen ➔. The tubules show epithelial injury ➔.*

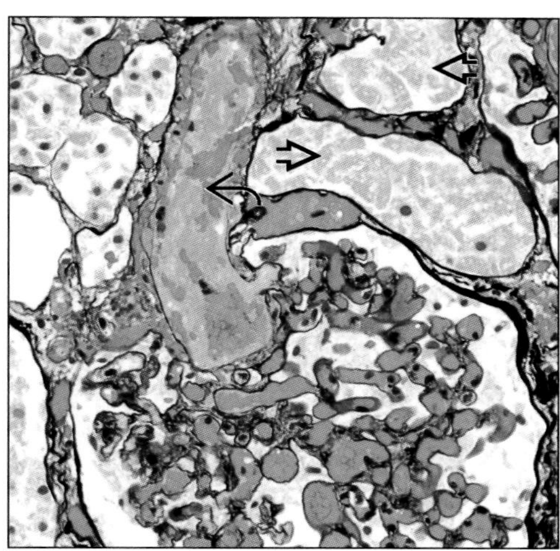

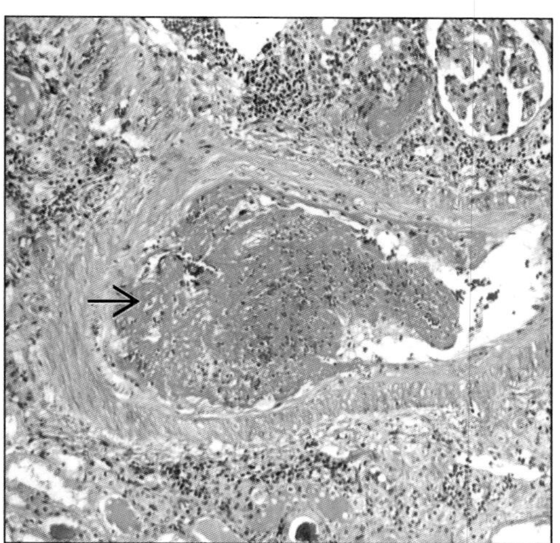

(Left) *In hyperacute rejection, microthrombosis in capillaries and arterioles ➔ can be seen in early phase, leading to glomerular ischemic changes. Acute tubular necrosis ➔ is also shown in this case.* ***(Right)*** *H&E-stained section shows a large artery nearly completely occluded by a fibrin thrombus ➔ in a case of hyperacute rejection. This process occurs immediately or within the 1st hours post transplant. The kidney is usually lost.*

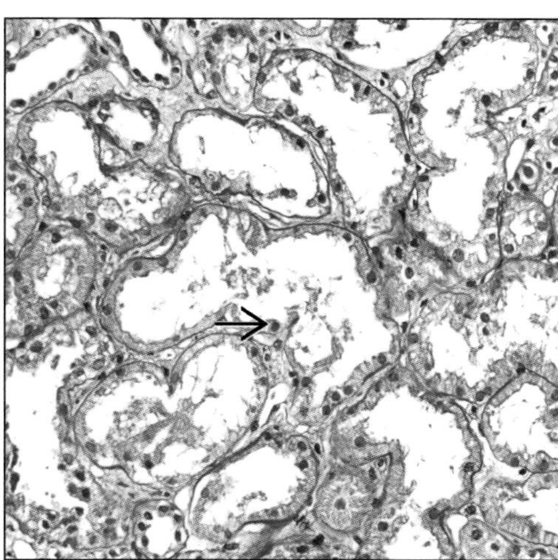

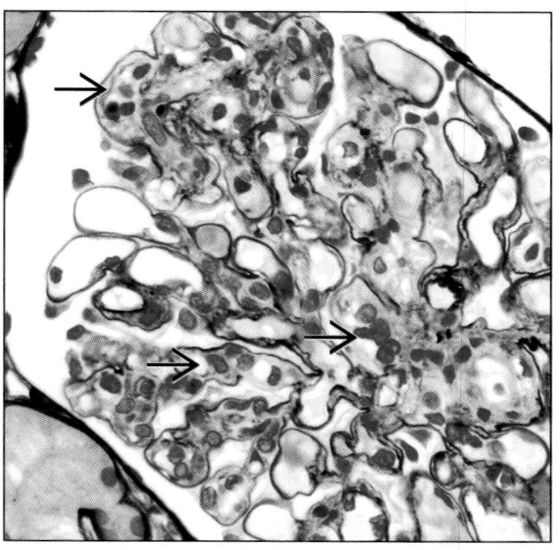

(Left) *Acute tubular injury can occur as a manifestation of antibody-mediated rejection, and it is characterized by sloughing off of epithelial cell lining ➔. Positive C4d and donor-specific antibody are necessary for diagnosis.* ***(Right)*** *Transplant glomerulitis is a morphologic finding indicative of acute antibody-mediated rejection. There is accumulation of mononuclear cells in glomerular capillary lumina ➔. Endothelial swelling can also be present.*

Microscopic Features

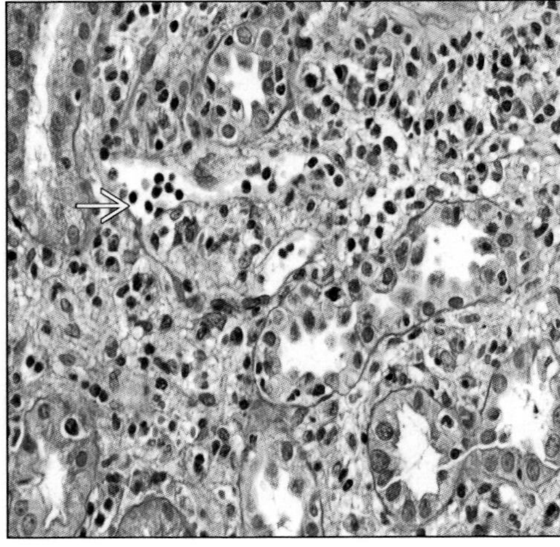

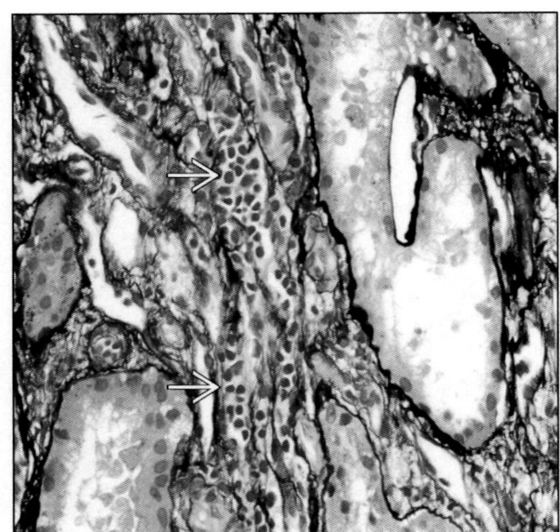

(Left) *Peritubular capillaritis is characterized by mononuclear cells within peritubular capillaries ➡. This finding is a reliable marker of antibody-mediated rejection. In this case, there are > 10 mononuclear cells, which would correspond to Banff ptc3.* ***(Right)*** *On silver stain, the basement membranes of the peritubular capillaries are highlighted, facilitating their identification. This is an example of marked peritubular capillaritis ➡.*

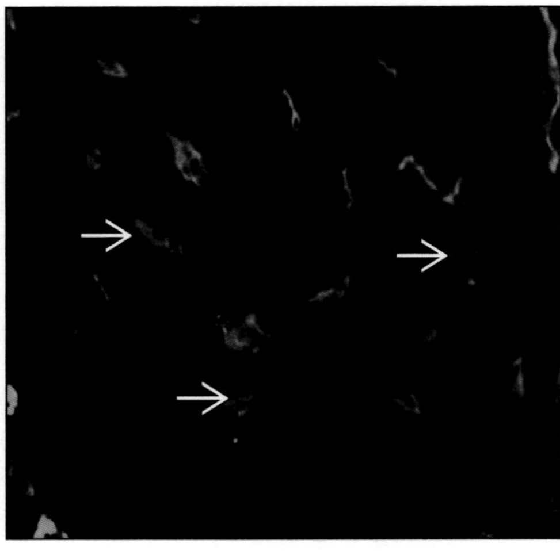

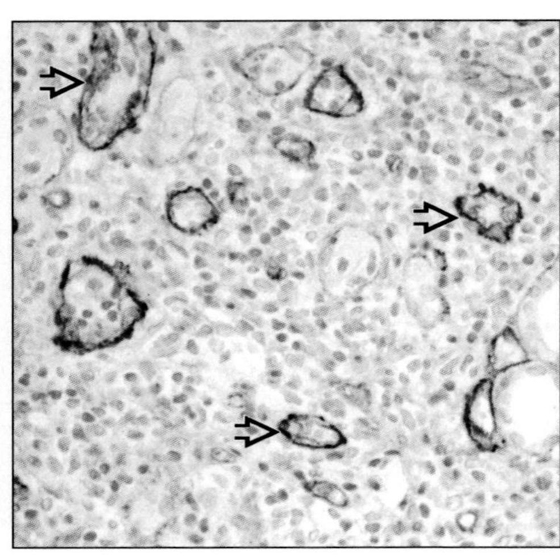

(Left) *C4d immunofluorescence staining highlights the peritubular capillaries ➡ that appear as circles when transversely sectioned with bright linear staining. This finding supports antibody-mediated rejection. Immunofluorescence is a more sensitive method for diagnosis.* ***(Right)*** *C4d immunohistochemical stain can be performed if frozen tissue is not available. Although less sensitive, this method is useful for diagnosis of AMR. Linear staining in the PTCs ⇨ is seen.*

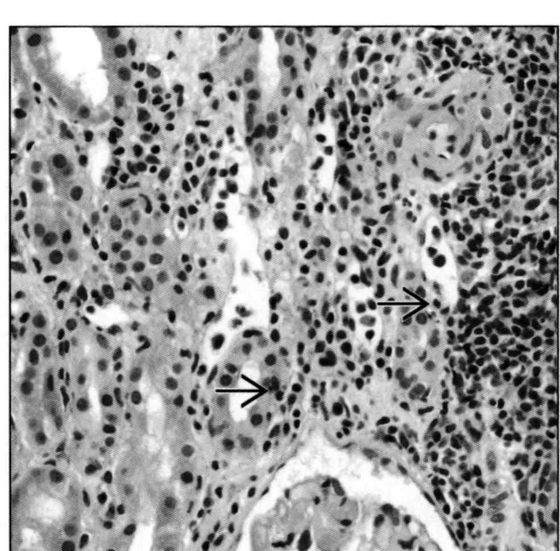

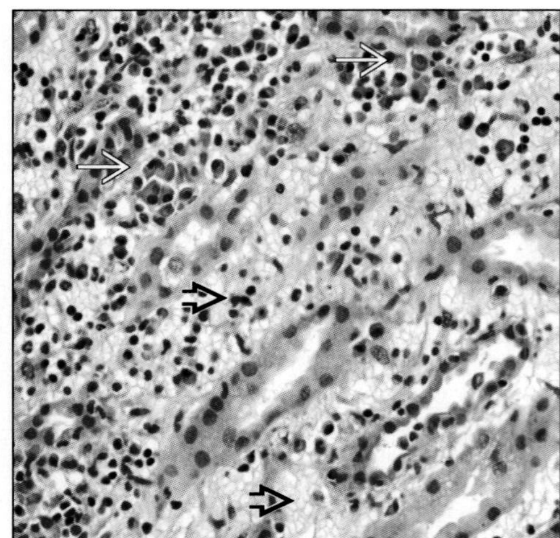

(Left) *Acute T-cell-mediated rejection occurs commonly during the 1st year post transplant. Mononuclear interstitial inflammation with tubulitis ➡, tubular injury, and interstitial edema are characteristic. Banff scoring for tubulitis in this case is t2.* ***(Right)*** *In some cases of T-cell-mediated rejection, the predominant cell in the inflammatory infiltrate is the plasma cell ➡. In this case, significant interstitial edema is also seen ⇨.*

Gross and Microscopic Features

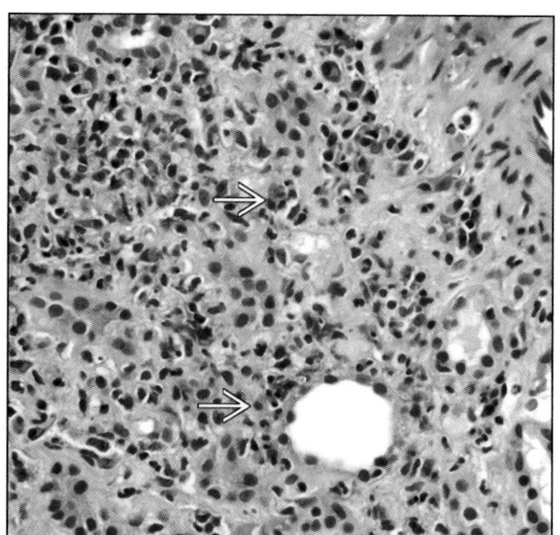
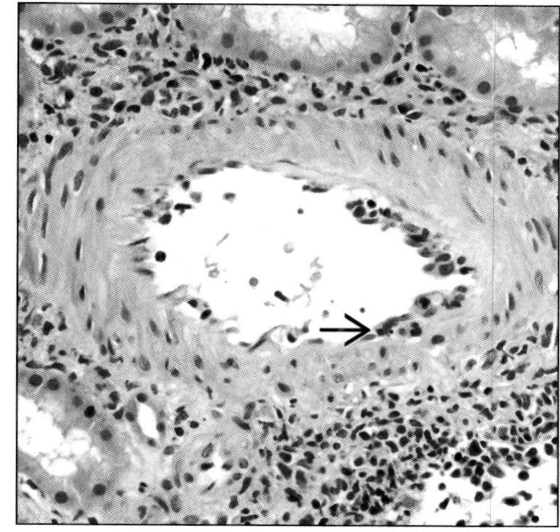

(Left) In some cases of acute T-cell-mediated rejection, the inflammatory infiltrate may contain numerous eosinophils ➡ admixed with mononuclear cells. It may not be possible, in this setting, to differentiate T-cell-mediated rejection from acute interstitial nephritis. ***(Right)*** *Endothelialitis is a finding indicative of a more severe T-cell-mediated rejection. It is characterized by inflammatory cells underneath the endothelium ➡. This is an example of Banff IIA.*

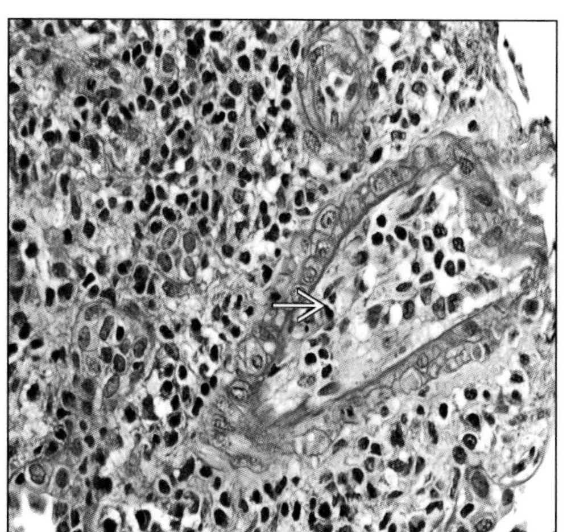
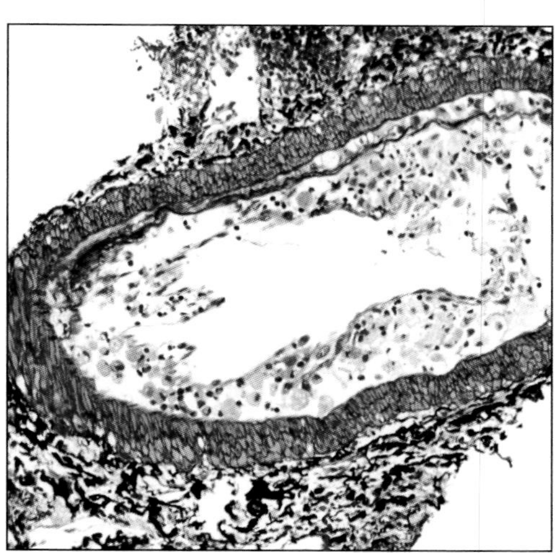

(Left) *In more severe cases of cellular rejection, endothelialitis with lifting of endothelial cells with subintimal lymphocytes ➡ can be identified. This case corresponds to Banff IIB with involvement of > 25% of the lumen.* ***(Right)*** *This case of T-cell-mediated rejection Banff IIB shows on silver stain a large artery with lifting of the endothelium and presence of inflammatory cells and some foamy macrophages involving nearly completely the artery circumference.*

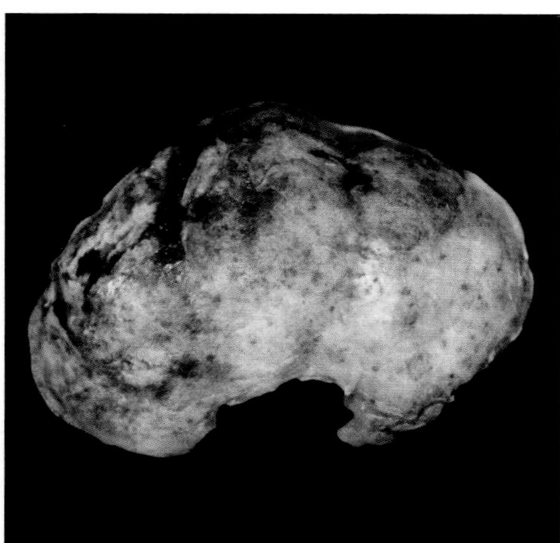
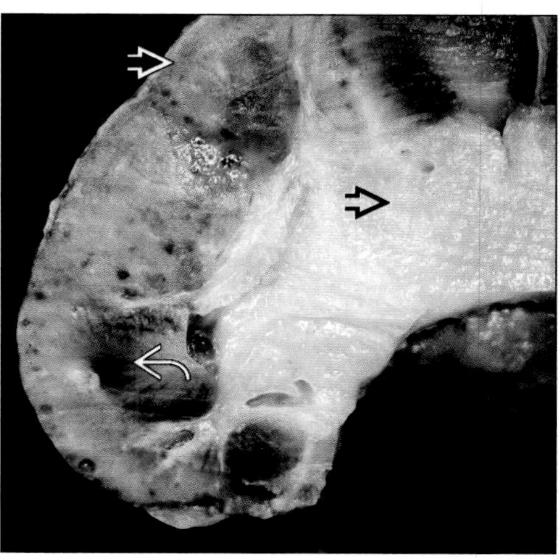

(Left) *This specimen is from a transplant patient who died from a cardiovascular event 8 years post transplant. Immunosuppression had been withdrawn due to allograft failure. The external surface is covered by a white connective tissue, and there are areas of hemorrhage.* ***(Right)*** *On cut surface, the allograft shows thinned cortex ➡ and medullary congestion ➡. The pyelocaliceal system is not dilated, but increase in adipose tissue is seen at the hilum ➡.*

Microscopic Features

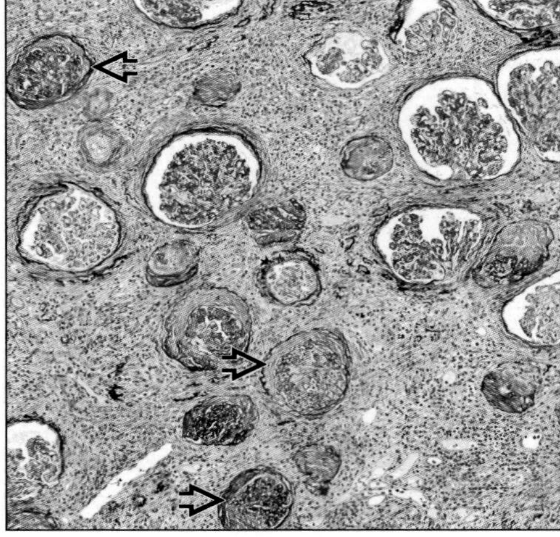

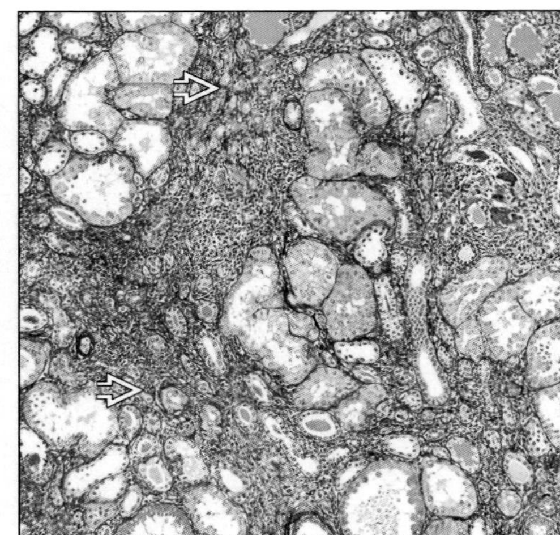

(Left) *Section from failed allograft 8 years post transplant shows several globally sclerosed glomeruli ➩, which is a nonspecific finding. There is interstitial fibrosis and tubular loss. Inflammatory infiltrate is also present.* ***(Right)*** *In allografts with chronic injury, interstitial fibrosis and tubular atrophy ➩ are common findings. They usually do not show any specific pattern, and chronic inflammatory infiltrate accompanies these changes.*

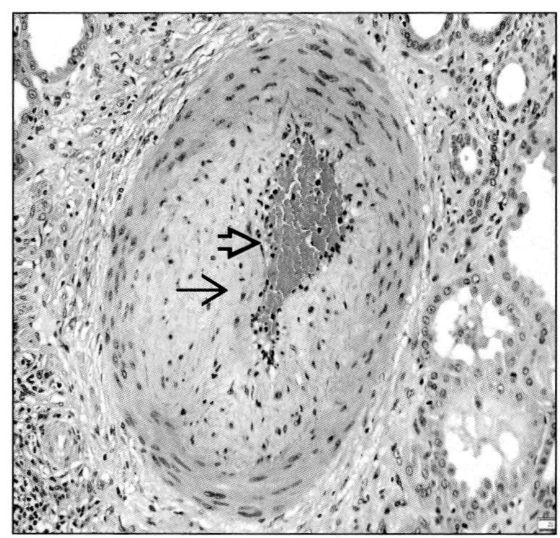

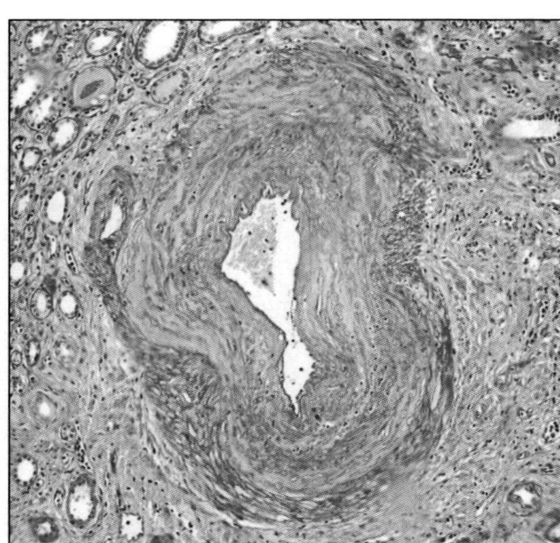

(Left) *In chronic active allograft vasculopathy, there is concentric intimal proliferation in the arteries → with associated subintimal lymphocytes ➩.* ***(Right)*** *In an advanced case of chronic cellular rejection, the arteries show marked intima proliferation with no significant inflammatory cells. It may be difficult to differentiate from changes due to hypertension; however, no significant elastic duplication is seen, which is most characteristic of hypertensive arteriosclerosis.*

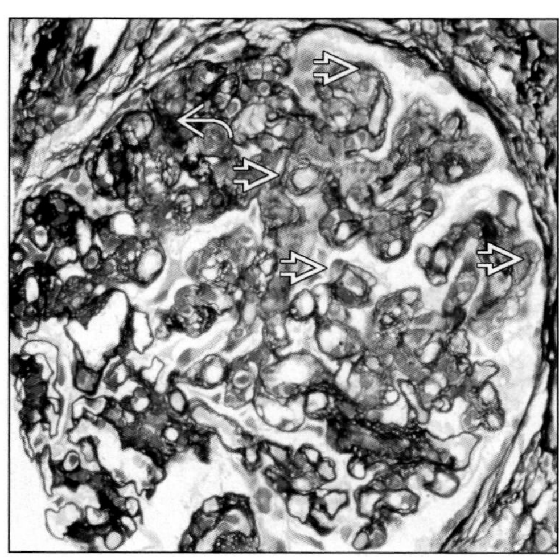

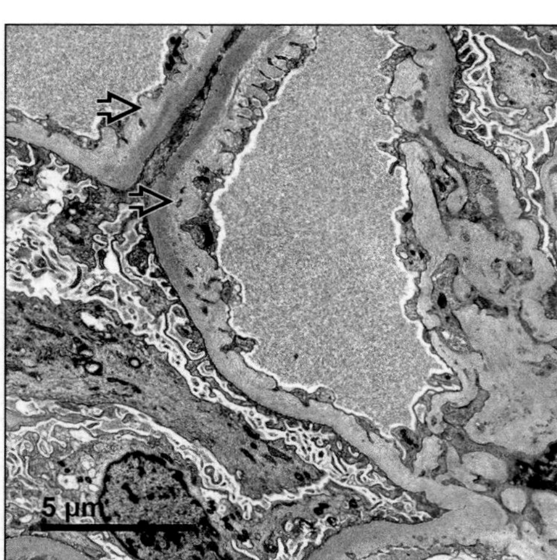

(Left) *Transplant glomerulopathy is characterized by "double contours" in the capillary walls ➩. The Banff scoring is performed in the most affected glomerulus. This case corresponds to Banff cg3. There is also segmental sclerosis ➩.* ***(Right)*** *Electron microscopy examination confirms diagnosis of transplant glomerulopathy. In early stage, there is expansion of the subendothelial space by electron lucent material ➩. These features should be differentiated from other causes of TMA.*

Microscopic Features

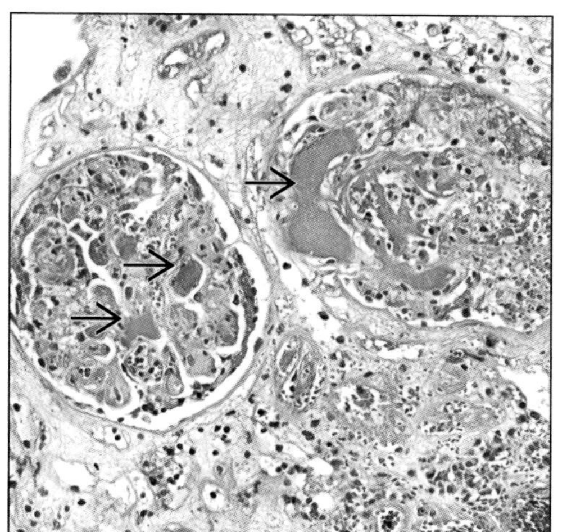

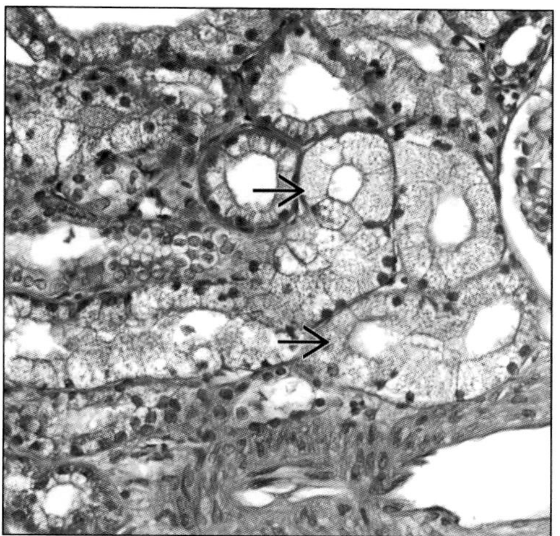

(Left) *Drug toxicity is a complication that can cause allograft failure. Acute features of calcineurin inhibitors toxicity can manifest as thrombotic microangiopathy. In this case, there are numerous fibrin thrombi in glomerular capillaries ⇒.* ***(Right)*** *Tubular isometric vacuolization ⇒ is nonspecific and can be seen in intravenous immunoglobulin therapy, contrast media, and osmotic agent-induced nephropathy and is also a manifestation of acute CNI toxicity, seen here.*

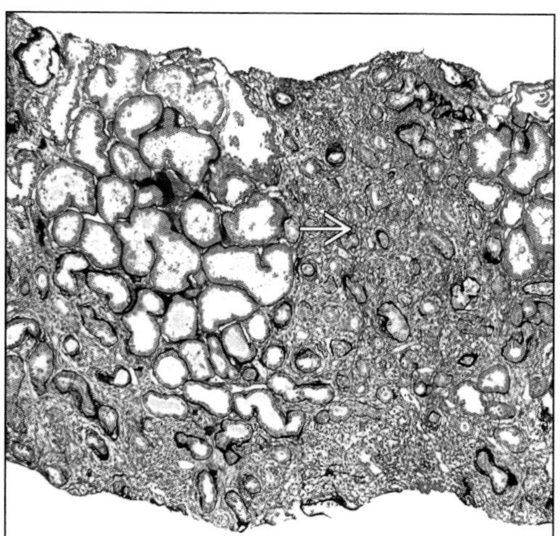

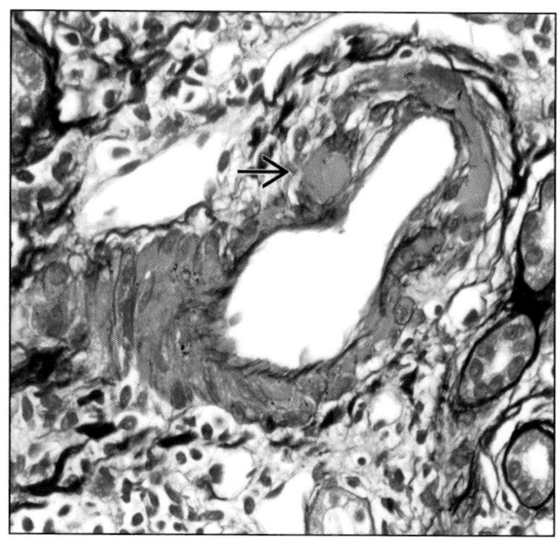

(Left) *Striped tubular atrophy and fibrosis ➡, a pattern of alternating atrophic and nonatrophic parenchyma, might arise secondary to narrowing of small arterioles/ arteries along the medullary ray. The findings are seen in several ischemic conditions, including hypertension, calcineurin inhibitor toxicity, etc.* ***(Right)*** *Nodular hyalinosis of an interlobular artery ⇒ can be seen in chronic calcineurin inhibitor toxicity.*

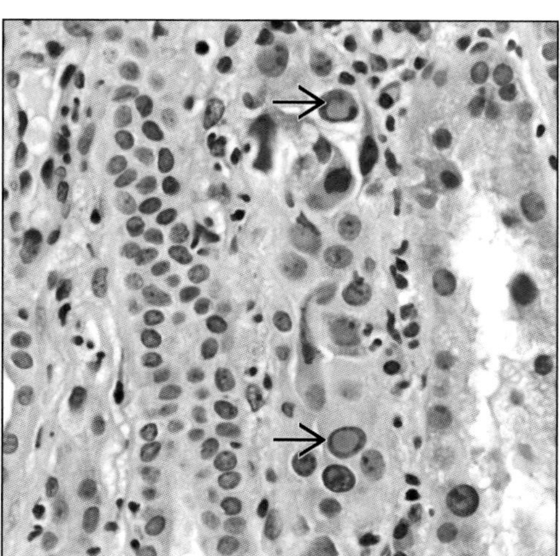

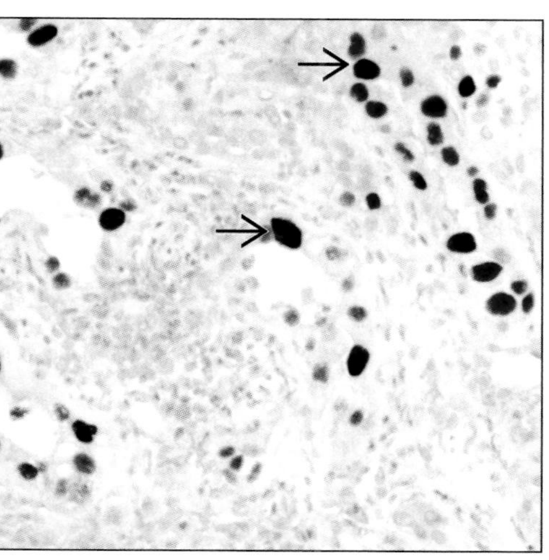

(Left) *BK polyomavirus nephropathy is a complication seen in solid organ transplants. It occurs in 5-10% of kidney allografts. It usually manifests 12-18 months post transplant. The characteristic findings are the basophilic, glassy-appearing nuclear inclusions ⇒, and a mixed interstitial inflammatory infiltrate.* ***(Right)*** *Polyomavirus can be demonstrated in tissue section by immunohistochemistry. The infected cells show nuclear staining ⇒.*

LIVER TRANSPLANT

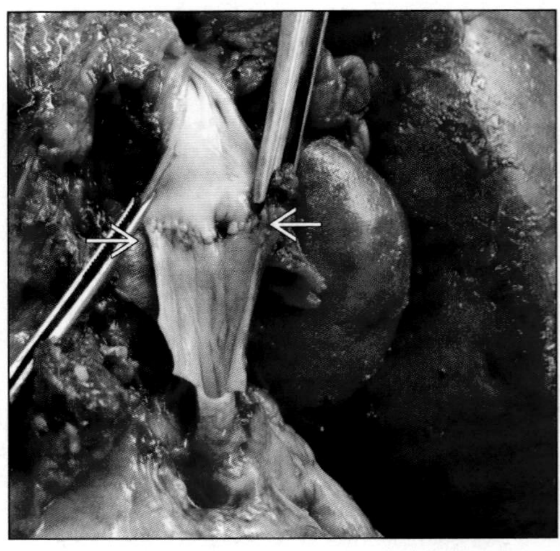

This dissection shows an intact hepatic artery anastomosis ➔ status post liver transplant. (Courtesy P. Lento, MD.)

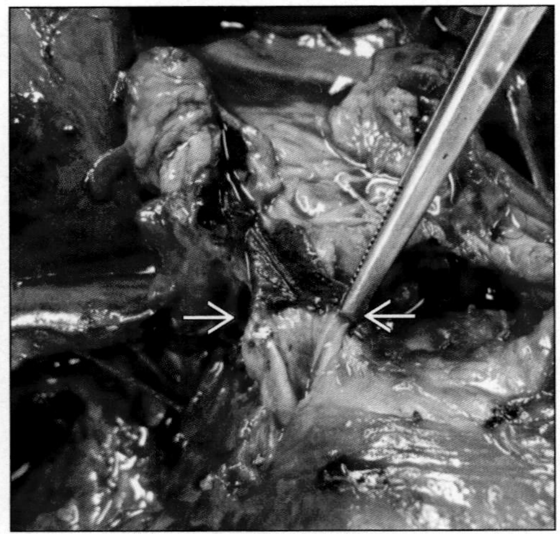

This dissection shows an intact bile duct anastomosis ➔ status post liver transplant. (Courtesy P. Lento, MD.)

TERMINOLOGY

Definitions

- Deceased donor liver transplantation: Replacement of native liver with an allograft liver from a nonliving/ cadaveric donor
- Living donor liver transplantation: Replacement of native liver with a portion of liver from a living donor (usually a relative)

ETIOLOGY/PATHOGENESIS

Reasons for Liver Transplantation

- Chronic liver failure (most common)
  - Chronic viral hepatitis C (most common), hepatitis B ± D, alcoholic liver disease, nonalcoholic steatohepatitis (NASH), autoimmune hepatitis (AIH)
  - Biliary diseases: Primary biliary cirrhosis (PBC), primary sclerosing cholangitis (PSC), extrahepatic biliary atresia (most common reason in children)
- Acute liver failure
  - Drug/toxin induced (acetaminophen most common), acute viral hepatitis A, B ± D or E, AIH, Budd-Chiari syndrome
- Metabolic diseases
  - Diseases that cause liver injury
    - Wilson disease, α-1-antitrypsin deficiency, hemochromatosis
  - Diseases that do not cause liver injury
    - Ornithine carbamoyltransferase deficiency, protein C deficiency, familial amyloidosis
- Neoplasms
  - Hepatocellular carcinoma (HCC) (usually in setting of cirrhosis)
  - Rare: Cholangiocarcinoma, hepatocellular adenomatosis, epithelioid hemangioendothelioma, hepatoblastoma, metastatic neuroendocrine tumor (NET)

Pathogenesis of Complications

- Early complications
  - 1° graft dysfunction/nonfunction: 2-20%, hours to days post transplant, multifactorial, preservation/ reperfusion injury
  - Hyperacute/acute humoral rejection: Rare, hours to weeks, preformed (hyperacute) or de novo antidonor antibodies
  - Acute (cellular) rejection: 20-40%, days to months, T-cell-mediated immune injury
  - Fibrosing cholestatic hepatitis: Rare, 1-3 months, type of recurrent hepatitis B or C, rapidly progressive graft failure
- Early or late complications
  - Infection: 60-80%, bacterial > viral > fungal (*Aspergillus* and *Candida* most common)
  - Biliary: 10-25%, early leak/strictures, late strictures 2° to hepatic artery thrombosis/chronic rejection ± superimposed infection
  - Hepatic artery thrombosis: 2-10%, most common vascular complication
    - Early → graft ischemic injury, late → ischemic bile duct injury → necrosis, superinfection, and stricture
  - Portal vein thrombosis: Rare, early → graft dysfunction, late → portal hypertension
  - Hepatic vein/IVC obstruction: Rare, kinking, stricture, or thrombosis may → venous outflow obstruction and Budd-Chiari syndrome
  - Disease recurrence: Hepatitis C: > 90%; hepatitis B: < 10%; AIH: 20-30%; PBC: 10-30%; PSC: 20-25%; HCC: 30-50%
- Late complications
  - Chronic rejection: 2-3%, months to years, immune-mediated irreversible injury to arteries, veins, bile ducts
  - Nodular regenerative hyperplasia: Up to 80%, may be incidental or → portal hypertension

LIVER TRANSPLANT

Key Facts

Etiology
- Early complications: Primary graft dysfunction/nonfunction, hyperacute/acute rejection, fibrosing cholestatic hepatitis
- Early or late complications: Infection, biliary complications, vascular thrombosis, disease recurrence
- Late complications: Chronic rejection, de novo disease, nodular regenerative hyperplasia

Clinical Issues
- Important elements of chart review: Reason for/type of transplantation, findings in explanted liver, postoperative course, episodes of rejection, comorbid conditions
- Causes of death: Infection (most common), technical failure/intraoperative complications, liver/graft failure, cardiovascular/respiratory failure, multiorgan failure, malignancy
- 15% mortality rate within 1st year

Macroscopic Pathology
- Sections to submit
  - Gross lesions/masses
  - Central and peripheral parenchyma
  - Hepatic artery, portal vein, vena cava, and bile duct anastomoses
  - Deep hilum to include vessels, bile ducts, nerves

Diagnostic Checklist
- Cause of death and how it relates to transplantation
- Presence of post-transplantation complications, recurrent disease, de novo disease, malignancy
- Risk factors for complications

  - De novo disease: Viral hepatitis, AIH, NASH, neoplasia (immunosuppression-related: Post-transplant lymphoproliferative disorder [PTLD], Kaposi sarcoma, skin cancer)

CLINICAL ISSUES

Epidemiology
- ~ 6,200 liver transplants performed in USA in 2012
- Current 5-year survival ~ 70%
- Rate of retransplantation: Up to 20%, commonly due to primary nonfunction, rejection, hepatic artery thrombosis, or disease recurrence

Presentation
- Fever, abdominal pain, jaundice, fatigue, ascites (nonspecific presentation related to many transplant-related complications)
- Important elements of chart review
  - Reason for and type of transplantation, preexisting donor lesions (degree of steatosis), findings in explanted liver
  - Operative note with anastomosis details, postoperative course, episodes of rejection, results of postoperative/protocol liver biopsies
  - Immunosuppressive/other drugs, comorbid conditions

Laboratory Tests
- ↑ transaminases, alkaline phosphatase, bilirubin, viral RNA/DNA levels, α-fetoprotein
- ↑ prothrombin and partial thromboplastin times, international normalized ratio (INR)
- Leukocytosis, thrombocytopenia, ↓ total serum complement (humoral rejection)
- (+) blood, wound, tissue cultures, (+) new viral titers
- ↓ immunosuppressive drug levels (rejection)

Prognosis
- 15% mortality rate within 1st year
- Causes of death: Infection/sepsis (most common), technical complications, liver/graft failure, cardiovascular/respiratory failure, multiorgan failure, malignancy

IMAGE FINDINGS

Radiographic Findings
- CT scan/MR: Cirrhosis, masses, evidence of portal hypertension (ascites, collateral vessel formation, splenomegaly)
- Angiography: Diagnostic (thrombosis, pseudoaneurysm, stenosis) and therapeutic
- Cholangiography: Diagnostic (stenosis/stricture, leaks) and therapeutic (stents)

MACROSCOPIC FEATURES

Sections to Be Submitted
- Liver: Gross lesions/masses, central/peripheral parenchyma, hepatic artery, portal vein, vena cava, and bile duct anastomoses, deep hilum to include vessels, bile ducts, nerves
- Other organs: Representative sections and sections of any gross pathology

External Examination
- Scleral icterus, jaundice, abdominal varices
- Surgical interventions (wound, drains)
- Ascites (fluid wave), cachexia (malignancy), cutaneous lesions (squamous cell carcinoma), palpable lymph nodes (PTLD), bruises (allograft liver failure)
- Hirsutism, central obesity and striae (iatrogenic Cushing syndrome [steroid therapy])

Internal Examination
- Ascites, pleural/pericardial effusions, metastatic disease

Organ Examination
- Liver
  - Probe and open each of the 4 anastomoses

- Hepatic artery: Usually donor hepatic artery to celiac trunk, open celiac trunk from posterior → past splenic artery → past gastroduodenal artery to anastomosis
- Vascular grafts may be present, depending on anatomical variations
- Biliary (2 types): Common bile duct to common bile duct anastomosis or Roux-en-Y hepatojejunostomy (examine before removing intestines)
- Note presence of sludge, stones, necrosis, stenosis
- Portal vein (may be beneath celiac trunk) and upper/lower inferior vena cava
- Note thrombosis, kinking, strictures
  - Cirrhosis, nodules, necrosis, masses, hemorrhage
- Other organs
  - Gastric/esophageal varices, esophagitis/gastroenteritis/colitis ± ulcers, splenomegaly
  - Lung consolidation/abscesses, targetoid lung lesions with central hemorrhage/necrosis (fungal infection), cystitis, meningoencephalitis
  - Renal cortical pallor and medullary congestion, myocardial mottling, ischemic bowel (shock)

MICROSCOPIC PATHOLOGY

Histologic Features

- Hepatic findings
  - Preservation/reperfusion injury: Centrilobular/perivenular hepatocyte ballooning, necrosis, apoptosis, ± cholestasis
  - Hyperacute/humoral rejection: Sinusoidal and intravascular fibrin deposition, congestion, hemorrhagic necrosis, (+) immunostain for C4d in portal stroma/vessels and sinusoids
  - Acute (cellular) rejection: Triad of mixed portal inflammation (including large activated lymphocytes), bile duct injury with inflammatory cell infiltration, venular endotheliitis
  - Hepatic artery thrombosis: Geographic infarction/coagulative necrosis, ± neutrophils, portal tracts usually spared, ± subsequent ischemic large bile duct injury → necrosis/ulcers/superinfection
  - Vena cava/hepatic vein thrombosis/occlusion (venous outflow obstruction/Budd-Chiari syndrome): Severe perivenular/midzonal congestion, sinusoidal dilatation ± necrosis
  - Portal vein thrombosis: May be normal or parenchymal atrophy, nodularity, mild portal fibrosis
  - Bile duct obstruction: Portal tract edema, periportal ductular reaction with neutrophils, ± cholestasis, feathery degeneration of hepatocytes, bile infarcts, bile lakes, secondary biliary cirrhosis
    - Ischemic cholangiopathy: Features of duct obstruction, ulcers/necrosis of large ducts ± superinfection, ± secondary sclerosing cholangitis
  - Chronic rejection: Bile duct injury, ductopenia, occlusive foam cell arteriopathy ± intimal hyperplasia, fibrous obliteration of veins, perivenular cholestasis
  - Fibrosing cholestatic hepatitis: Periportal/perisinusoidal fibrosis, hepatocyte ballooning, cholestasis, ± inflammation
  - Nodular regenerative hyperplasia: Hyperplastic regenerative nodules alternating with compressed atrophic hepatocytes (reticulin stain), **no** fibrosis
  - Recurrent disease: Hepatitis or cirrhosis related to primary disease
  - Neoplasia: Recurrent from 1° neoplasia or de novo (PTLD, other malignancies)
  - Opportunistic infection: Cytomegalovirus (CMV), herpes simplex virus (HSV), adenovirus, fungal
- Other organs
  - Shock: Myocardial infarction, acute tubular necrosis
  - Infection: Pneumonia, abscesses ± central necrosis/hemorrhage, diffuse alveolar damage, inflammation/infection of gastrointestinal tract, brain/meninges
  - Exogenous steroid effect: Adrenal gland atrophy

ANCILLARY TESTS

Immunohistochemistry

- (+) hepatitis B surface and core antigens, CMV, HSV, adenovirus
- (+) C4d in humoral rejection

In Situ Hybridization

- EBER (PTLD, infection)

Special Stains

- Routine liver stains (reticulin, trichrome, iron)
- Elastic: Arterial intimal thickening and portal vein fibrous occlusion in chronic rejection
- Gram, fungal, acid-fast bacillus stains

DIAGNOSTIC CHECKLIST

Final Report Should Include

- Cause of death and how it relates to transplantation
- Presence of post-transplantation complications, recurrent disease, de novo disease, malignancy
- Risk factors for complications

SELECTED REFERENCES

1. Ayva EŞ et al: Pathological findings of liver allografts evaluated at autopsy. Exp Clin Transplant. 12 Suppl 1:120-5, 2014
2. Hubscher SG et al: Transplantation pathology. In Burt A et al: MacSween's Pathology of the Liver. Edinburgh New York: Churchill Livingstone/Elsevier. 853-933, 2012
3. Alqahtani SA et al: Adult liver transplantation in the USA. Curr Opin Gastroenterol. 27(3):240-7, 2011
4. Nichols L: Autopsy evaluation of transplant recipients. In Collins KA et al: Autopsy Performance & Reporting. Northfield, IL: College of American Pathologists, 205-17, 2003
5. Markin RS et al: Main autopsy findings in liver transplant patients. Mod Pathol. 2(4):339-48, 1989

Gross and Microscopic Findings After Liver Transplantation

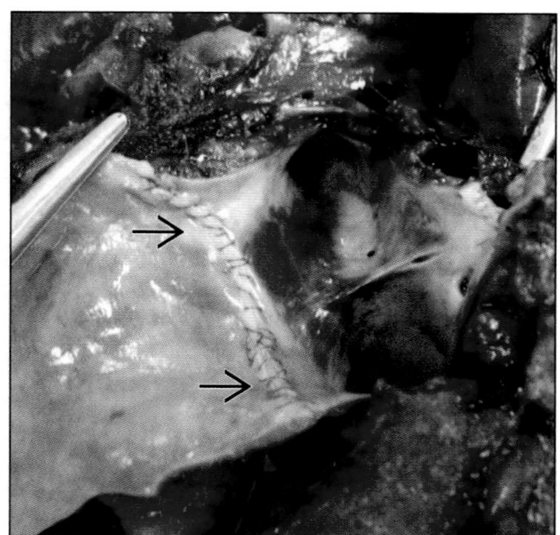

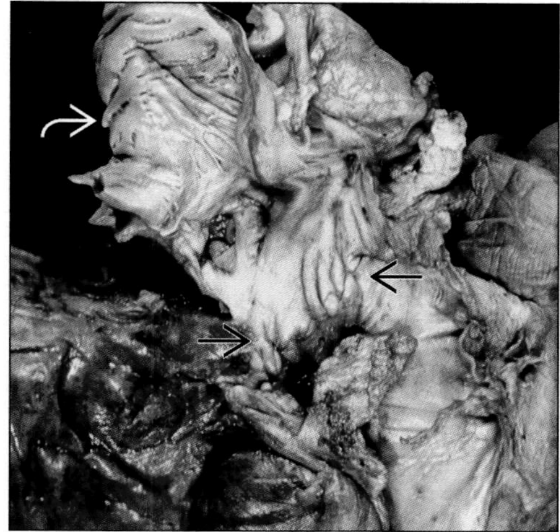

(Left) *This dissection shows an intact portal vein anastomosis ➔ as it exits the hilum of the donor liver. (Courtesy P. Lento, MD.)* ***(Right)*** *This dissection shows an intact inferior vena cava anastomosis ➔ distal to the point of entry into the right atrium ➔. (Courtesy D. Rubin, MD.)*

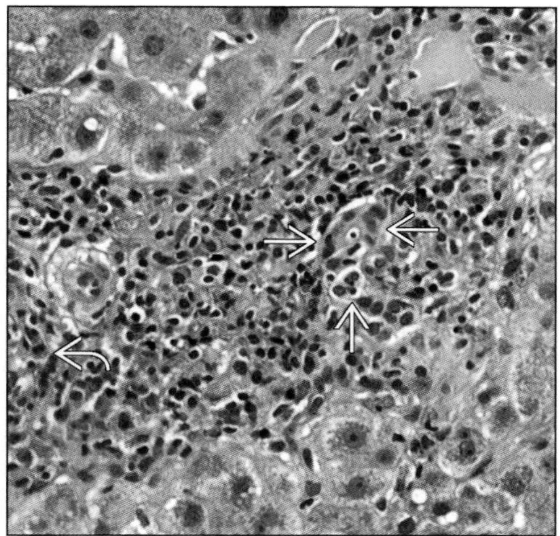

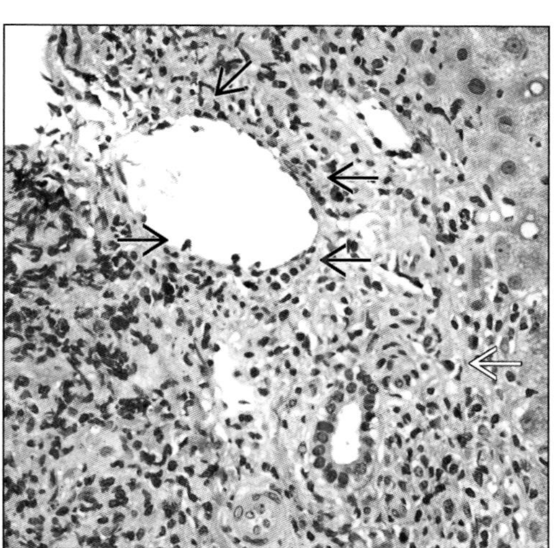

(Left) *This portal tract shows changes of acute cellular rejection, including inflammation composed of lymphocytes and eosinophils ➔, and an injured bile duct ➔ with nuclear pleomorphism and lymphocytes infiltrating the epithelium.* ***(Right)*** *In addition to lymphocytes and eosinophils ➔ that are characteristic of acute cellular rejection, this portal tract also shows mild endotheliitis ➔ with subendothelial inflammation and endothelial cell tufting into the lumen.*

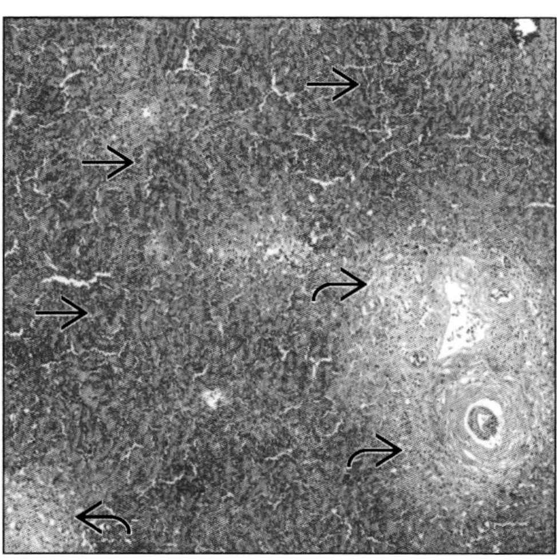

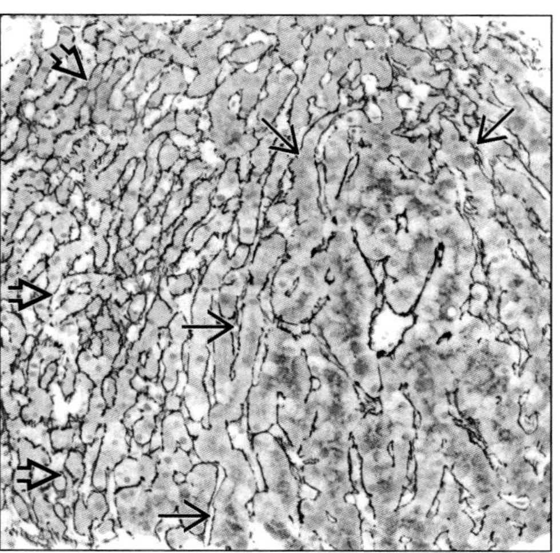

(Left) *These changes of severe parenchymal congestion and associated hepatocellular necrosis ➔ are the sequelae of venous outflow obstruction caused by thrombosis of a hepatic vein. The immediate periportal region is preserved ➔.* ***(Right)*** *This reticulin stain highlights a nodule of hyperplastic hepatocytes ➔ surrounded by cords of compressed atrophic hepatocytes ➔ that are characteristic of nodular regenerative hyperplasia.*

Gross and Microscopic Findings After Liver Transplantation

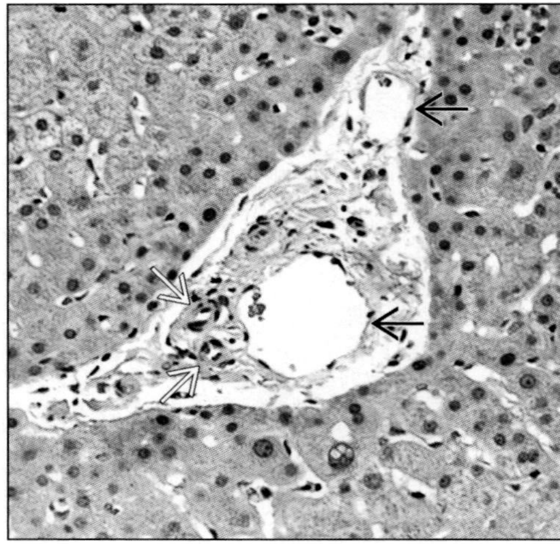

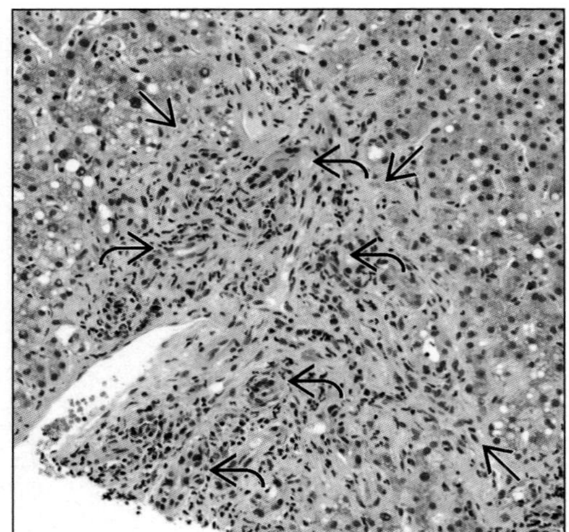

(Left) *This portal tract shows hepatic arteriole ➡ and portal venule ⇨ branches without an accompanying bile duct, indicative of ductopenia. Ductopenia is a histologic feature of chronic rejection. (Courtesy M. Fiel, MD.)* ***(Right)*** *This portal tract shows the triad of large bile duct obstruction that may be seen in stenosis, strictures, and ischemic injury: Portal tract edema ⇨ with "blurring" of the interface, bile ductular reaction ↗, and associated neutrophils.*

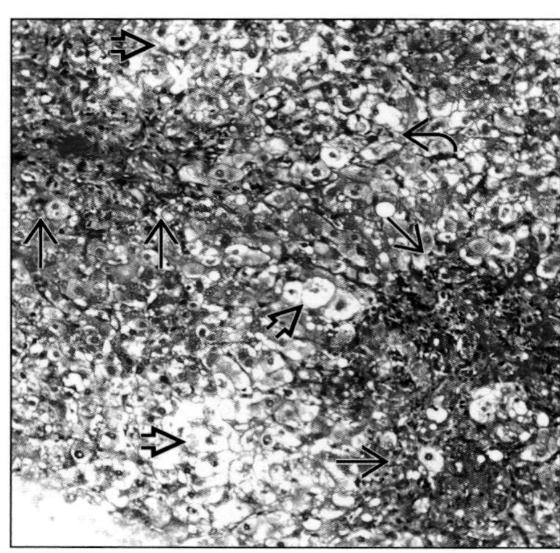

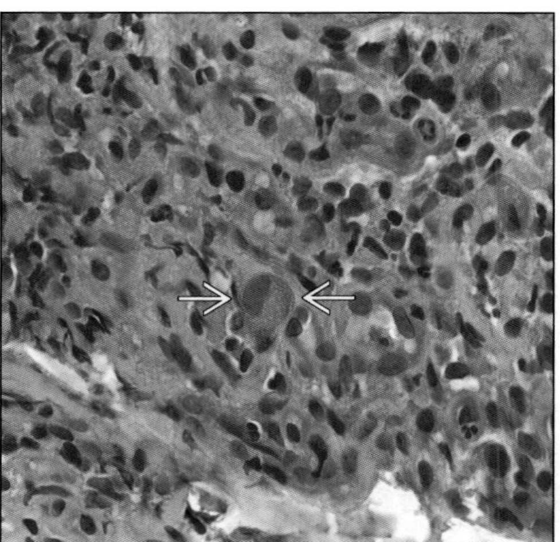

(Left) *Fibrosing cholestatic hepatitis is characterized by periportal and sinusoidal fibrosis ⇨, ballooning of hepatocytes ⇨, and cholestasis ↗. (Courtesy M. Fiel, MD.)* ***(Right)*** *This section from a colon ulcer bed shows nuclear and cytoplasmic inclusions ➡ characteristic of cytomegalovirus in an immunosuppressed patient status post transplant.*

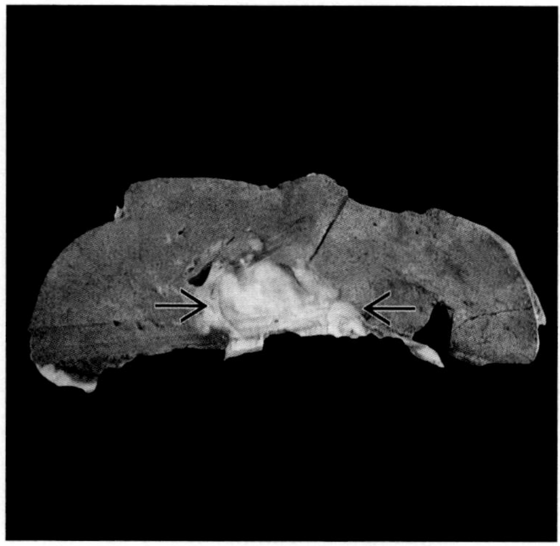

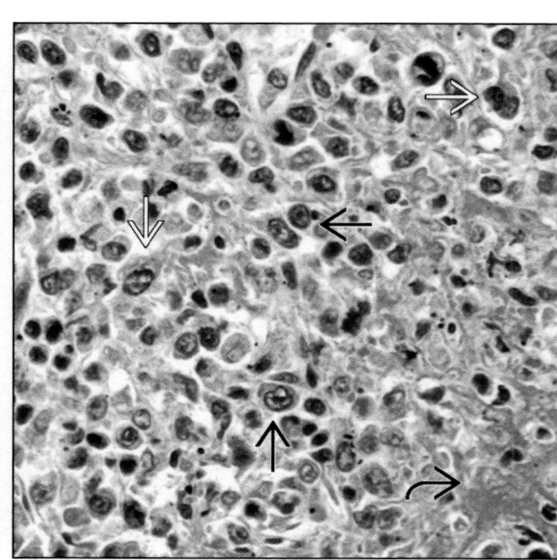

(Left) *Post-transplant lymphoproliferative disorder (PTLD) developed in a patient status post transplant for familial amyloidosis. This section of the transplanted liver shows a large necrotic mass ⇨. (Courtesy P. Lento, MD.)* ***(Right)*** *The mass is composed of large atypical plasma cells ➡ and lymphocytes ⇨ with necrosis ↗ consistent with PTLD, polymorphic type, with monoclonal plasma cells. (Courtesy P. Lento, MD.)*

Gross and Microscopic Findings After Liver Transplantation

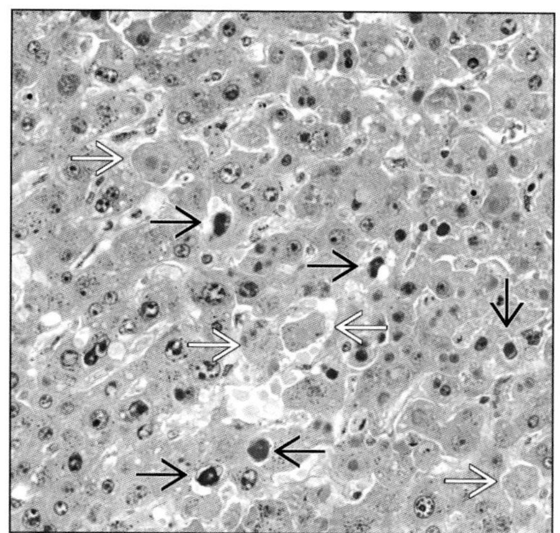
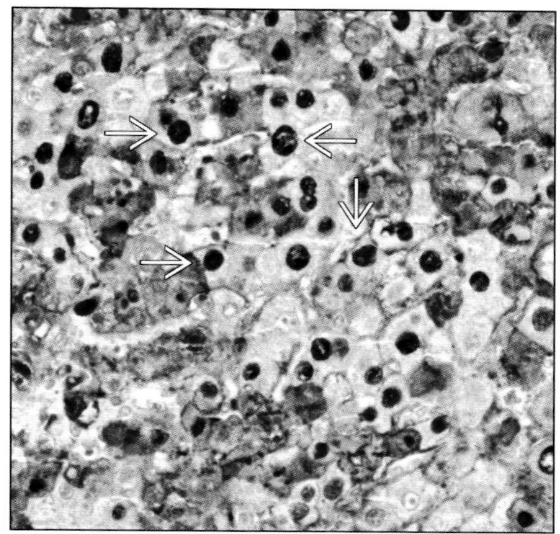

***(Left)** Adenovirus infection in the liver often occurs in the setting of immunosuppression and is characterized by basophilic smudgy intranuclear inclusions and patchy hepatocellular necrosis. **(Right)** Immunostain for adenovirus is positive in the nuclei of infected hepatocytes.*

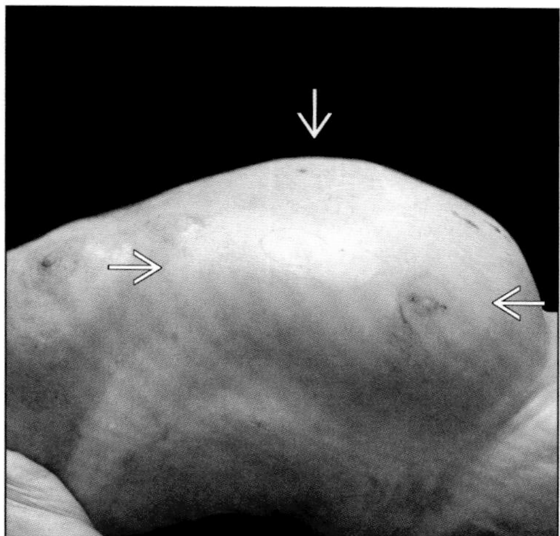
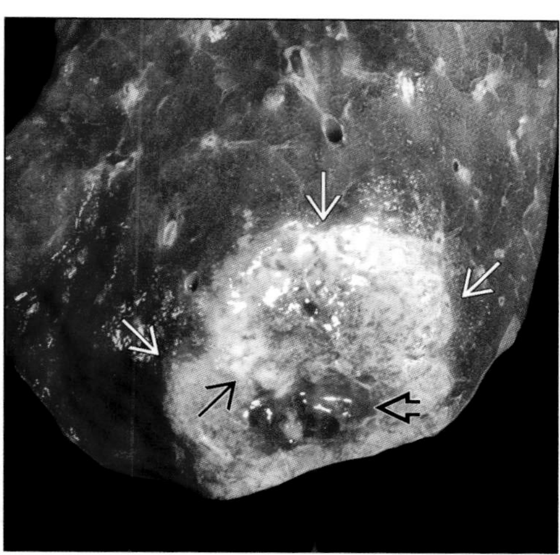

***(Left)** Massive ascites developed in a patient with cirrhosis due to recurrent hepatitis C infection. **(Right)** This section of lung shows a well-circumscribed "targetoid" mass lesion with central necrosis and hemorrhage typical of fungal infection in an immunosuppressed patient status post transplant.*

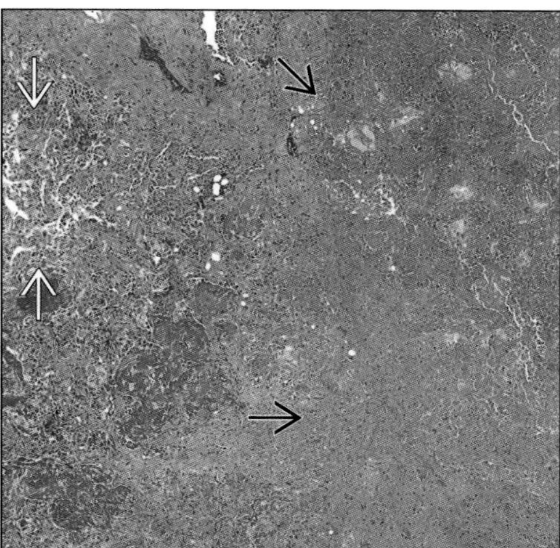
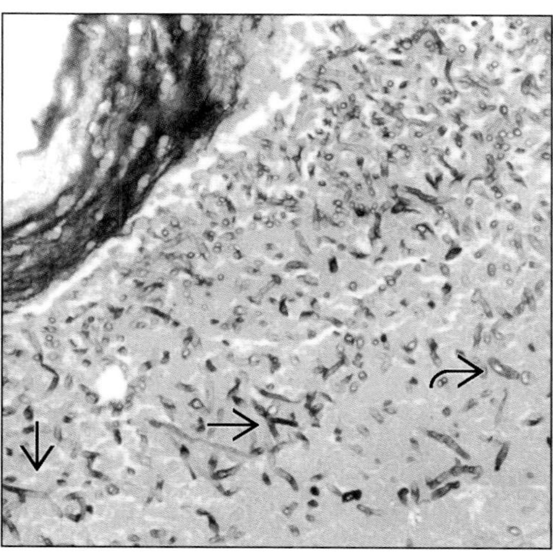

***(Left)** Sections through a targetoid mass lesion in the lung of an immunosuppressed patient status post transplant reveal large areas of necrosis and inflammation filling the alveolar spaces. **(Right)** GMS stain performed on areas of necrosis show numerous septate hyphae with acute angle branching and a bulbous appearance, consistent with Aspergillus species. Cultures grew Aspergillus fumigatus.*

PANCREAS TRANSPLANT

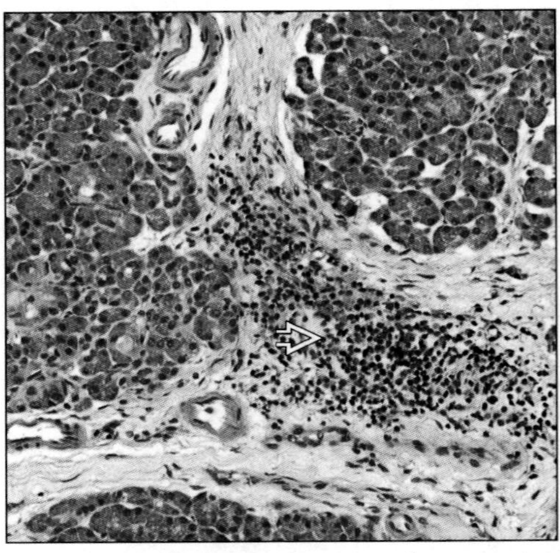

Pancreas allograft section shows septal mononuclear inflammation ⇨ without acinar or vessel involvement. The cells do not show blastic appearance. This case would be classified as indeterminate for acute rejection.

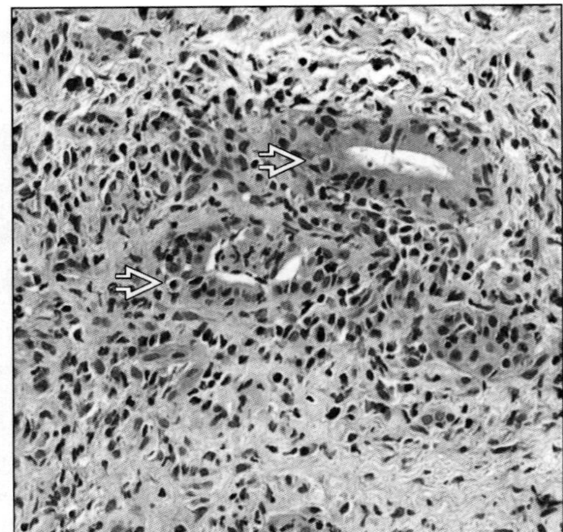

Pancreas allograft section shows mixed septal inflammatory infiltrate and ductitis ⇨ consistent with mild acute T-cell-mediated rejection (Banff grade I).

TERMINOLOGY

Synonyms

- Pancreas allograft

Definitions

- Pancreas allograft implantation from deceased donor for treatment of diabetes mellitus type 1 or type 2
- Types of pancreas transplants
  - Simultaneous pancreas/kidney (SPK)
  - Pancreas after kidney (PAK)
  - Pancreas transplant alone (PTA)

ETIOLOGY/PATHOGENESIS

Reasons for Pancreas Transplantation

- Diabetes mellitus type 1 with kidney failure
- Diabetes mellitus type 2, insulin-dependent with kidney failure

Pathogenesis of Complications

- Technical
  - Allograft thrombosis most common complication and cause of graft loss (~ 16.4% with enteric drainage); risk factors include old donor age, long cold ischemia time, poor surgical technique
  - Infection 1-5%; bacterial, viral, fungal
  - Anastomotic leak: 0.5-2%
  - Pancreatitis
  - Peritonitis chemical or bacterial
  - Bleeding
- Early immunological
  - Hyperacute rejection rare event with current HLA testing
  - Acute T-cell-mediated rejection (ACR)
  - Acute antibody-mediated rejection (AMR)
- Late immunological
  - Chronic rejection/graft sclerosis

CLINICAL ISSUES

Presentation

- Thrombosis of allograft will manifest as acute abdomen and graft dysfunction
- Acute T-cell or antibody-mediated rejection
  - Usually asymptomatic
  - Serum amylase/lipase levels increase
  - Hyperglycemia
- Chronic rejection
  - Gradual deterioration in graft function
  - Reduction of urine amylase levels
  - Hyperglycemia needing insulin treatment
  - Risk factors: Episodes of early acute cellular rejection, type of allograft PTA and PAK, HLA mismatch, CMV infection, younger recipient

Treatment

- Drugs
  - Immunosuppression with calcineurin inhibitors, mycophenolate mofetil, mTOR inhibitors

Prognosis

- SPK survival at 1 year: 86%; immunological loss rate: 1.8%; half life: 13 years
- PAK survival at 1 year: 80%; immunological loss rate: 3.7%; half life: 8 years
- PTA survival at 1 year: 78%; immunological loss rate: 6.0%; half life: 8 years

IMAGE FINDINGS

Ultrasonographic Findings

- Doppler ultrasound useful for identification of vascular complications

CT Findings

- Peripancreatic collections, hematomas, lymphoceles, abscesses can be identified

PANCREAS TRANSPLANT

Key Facts

Terminology
- Pancreas allograft implantation from deceased donor for treatment of diabetes mellitus type 1 or type 2

Clinical Issues
- Thrombosis of allograft will manifest as acute abdomen and graft dysfunction
- Acute T-cell or antibody-mediated rejection may be asymptomatic or show elevation of amylase/lipase or hyperglycemia
- Chronic rejection manifest with progressive deterioration of graft function

Macroscopic Pathology
- Autopsy should be performed as soon as possible to minimize effects from autolysis in graft
- Sections to be submitted
- Cross section of large vessels
- Several sections from parenchyma to include medium and small vessels
- Include any area that appears different from normal parenchyma
- Save a sample frozen if C4d is performed by immunofluorescence

Microscopic Pathology
- Allograft thrombosis
- Pancreatitis
- Hyperacute rejection
- Acute T-cell-mediated rejection
- Acute antibody-mediated rejection
- Chronic rejection
- Other histologic findings

- Small shrunken mass in case of chronic rejection

MACROSCOPIC FEATURES

General Features
- Autopsy should be performed as soon as possible to minimize effects from autolysis in graft

External Examination
- In abdomen, scar from surgery should be identified

Internal Examination
- Graft location and any peripancreatic collection noted
- Attention to vascular anastomotic sites to identify injury in vessels and thrombosis
- Examination for leaks in other anastomotic sites

Organ Examination
- Gross examination
  - Graft should be carefully examined and prosected intact with duodenum and enteric or bladder anastomoses
- Sections to be submitted
  - Cross section of large vessels
  - Several sections from parenchyma to include medium and small vessels
  - Include any area that appears different from surrounding parenchyma
  - Save a frozen piece if C4d is to be performed by immunofluorescence
- Other studies
  - Cultures should be taken if abscess is identified

MICROSCOPIC PATHOLOGY

Histologic Features
- Allograft thrombosis
  - Parenchymal necrosis
  - Interstitial hemorrhage
- Pancreatitis
  - Neutrophils are the most prevalent inflammatory cell in the infiltrate affecting exocrine pancreas in acute pancreatitis
  - In chronic pancreatitis perilobular and ductal fibrosis with mononuclear inflammation and atrophy of exocrine glands
- Hyperacute rejection (rare)
  - Fibrinoid necrosis of arteries/veins
  - Vascular thrombosis
  - Parenchymal necrosis
  - Deposit of IgG/C3 in vessel walls
- Acute T-cell-mediated rejection
  - Mild/grade I
    - Septal mononuclear inflammatory infiltrate with features of activation (blastic lymphocytes, eosinophils)
    - Venulitis
    - Ductitis
    - Perineural inflammation
    - Focal acinar inflammation
  - Moderate/grade II
    - Multifocal acinar inflammation (≥ 3 foci/lobule) with single cell acinar cell injury and dropout
    - Minimal intimal arteritis: Scattered mononuclear cells in intima or muscularis without endothelial reaction
  - Severe/grade III
    - Severe multifocal/confluent acinar inflammation with focal or diffuse multicellular acinar cell injury/necrosis
    - Moderate intimal arteritis: Mononuclear cells in intima with endothelial injury, fibrin leakage, coating neutrophils &/or macrophages
    - Arteritis: Complete or partial circumferential necrosis due to transmural inflammatory infiltrates
- Acute antibody-mediated rejection
  - Interacinar capillaritis with neutrophil margination
- Chronic rejection
  - Perilobular & ductal fibrosis
  - Acinar atrophy

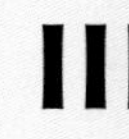

PANCREAS TRANSPLANT

Banff Schema for Grading Pancreas Allograft Rejection

Category	Pathologic Findings
Normal	Absent inflammation or inactive inflammation not involving vessels, ducts, or acini; no fibrosis or acinar atrophy or injury
Indeterminate	Active septal inflammation not fulfilling criteria of mild cellular rejection
Cell-mediated rejection	Mild/grade I: Active septal inflammation with venulitis, ductitis or perineural inflammation, focal acinar inflammation (2 foci maximum and minimal or absent acinar injury; moderate/grade II: Multifocal (not confluent) acinar inflammation, acinar injury and drop-out &/or minimal arteritis; severe/grade III: Diffuse acinar inflammation with focal or diffuse acinar cell necrosis &/or moderate arteritis &/or transmural arteritis; chronic active: Chronic allograft arteriopathy
Antibody-mediated rejection	C4d positive, confirmed donor specific antibodies and graft dysfunction; hyperacute rejection: Immediate graft necrosis (≤ 1 h); accelerated AMR: Graft necrosis occurring hours or days post transplant; acute AMR: No histologic findings, neutrophilic or mononuclear capillaritis, thrombosis, vasculitis, parenchyma necrosis
Chronic allograft rejection/graft sclerosis	Mild/grade I: Fibrosis in < 30% with irregular acinar contours, normal central areas; moderate/grade II: Fibrosis > 30-60% involving peripheral acini and central areas; severe/grade III: Fibrosis > 60% with isolated areas of acinar tissue &/or islets
Other histologic diagnosis	Pancreatitis, viral infection, ischemic injury, recurrent autoimmune disease, post-transplant lymphoproliferative disorder

  - Ductal ectasia
  - Mononuclear inflammatory infiltrate
  - Atrophy or disruption of islets
  - Arteriopathy with concentric narrowing
- Other histologic findings
  - Post-transplant ischemic pancreatitis: Neutrophilic inflammation, foamy macrophages in septa or involving acini in severe cases, fat necrosis, hemorrhage, edema
  - Bacterial/fungal infections: Variable, acute, chronic, purulent, necrotizing, granulomatous
  - Cytomegalovirus pancreatitis: Septal, acinar patchy chronic inflammation with cytopathic changes in acinar, endothelial or stromal cells
  - Recurrent autoimmune disease: Mononuclear inflammation involving islets, no inflammation in later stages after loss beta cells

ANCILLARY TESTS

Immunohistochemistry

- C4d should be performed when AMR is suspected

Immunofluorescence

- C4d should be performed when AMR is suspected

Special Stains

- Trichrome for evaluation of fibrosis
- Gram, AFB, and GMS in cases of infections

REPORTING CRITERIA

Final Report Should Include

- Cause of death and how it relates to transplantation
- Presence of post-transplant complications, de novo diseases, rejection, malignancy

SELECTED REFERENCES

1. Watson CJ: The current challenges for pancreas transplantation for diabetes mellitus. Pharmacol Res. Epub ahead of print, 2015
2. de Kort H et al: Diagnosis of early pancreas graft failure via antibody-mediated rejection: single-center experience with 256 pancreas transplantations. Am J Transplant. 14(4):936-42, 2014
3. Haas M et al: Banff 2013 meeting report: inclusion of c4d-negative antibody-mediated rejection and antibody-associated arterial lesions. Am J Transplant. 14(2):272-83, 2014
4. Weems P et al: Pancreas transplantation in type II diabetes mellitus. World J Transplant. 4(4):216-21, 2014
5. Niederhaus SV et al: Acute cellular and antibody-mediated rejection of the pancreas allograft: incidence, risk factors and outcomes. Am J Transplant. 13(11):2945-55, 2013
6. Yates A et al: Imaging pancreas transplants. Br J Radiol. 86(1030):20130428, 2013
7. Drachenberg CB et al: Guidelines for the diagnosis of antibody-mediated rejection in pancreas allografts-updated Banff grading schema. Am J Transplant. 11(9):1792-802, 2011
8. Drachenberg CB et al: Banff schema for grading pancreas allograft rejection: working proposal by a multi-disciplinary international consensus panel. Am J Transplant. 8(6):1237-49, 2008
9. Takahashi H et al: Analysis of acute and chronic rejection in multiple organ allografts from retransplantation and autopsy cases of multivisceral transplantation. Transplantation. 85(11):1610-6, 2008
10. Humar A et al: Chronic rejection: the next major challenge for pancreas transplant recipients. Transplantation. 76(6):918-23, 2003
11. Drachenberg CB et al: Pancreas transplantation: the histologic morphology of graft loss and clinical correlations. Transplantation. 71(12):1784-91, 2001

Microscopic Features

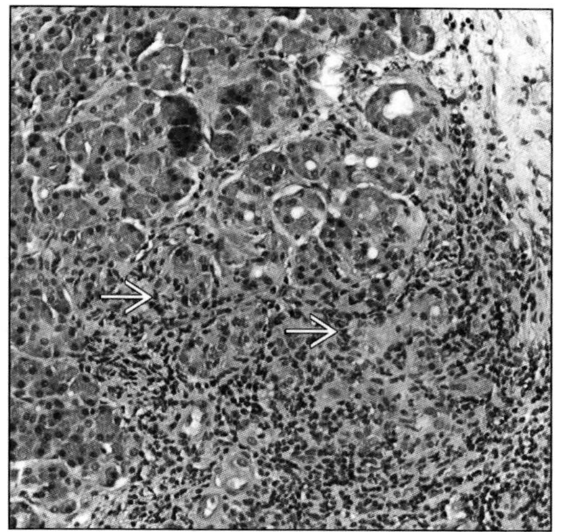

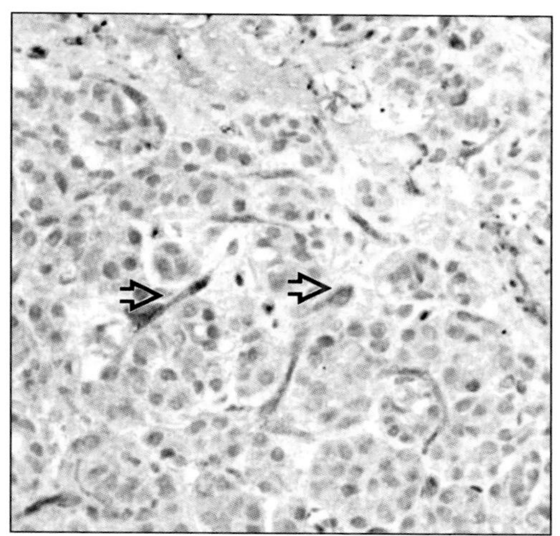

(Left) *Acute cell-mediated rejection is characterized by mixed inflammatory infiltrate initially involving septa and venules that in more severe cases extends to the acini* ➡*, as is shown in this case of moderate (Banff grade II) rejection. There is associated acinar epithelial injury.* ***(Right)*** *Antibody-mediated rejection can occur in pancreas allografts, and positive peri acinar capillaries* ➲ *for C4d by immunofluorescence or immunohistochemical stain is required for diagnosis as well as positive DSA.*

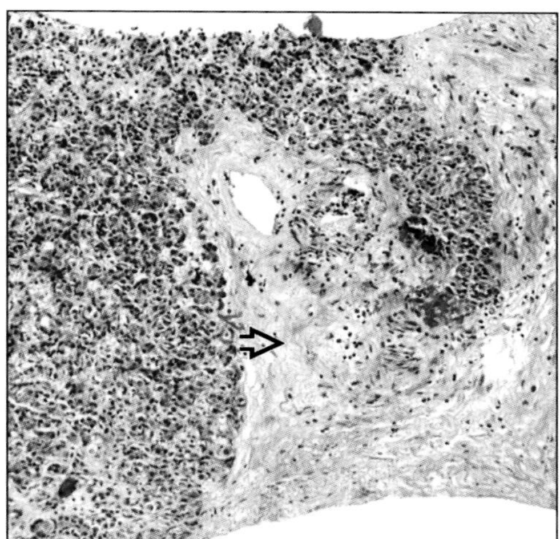

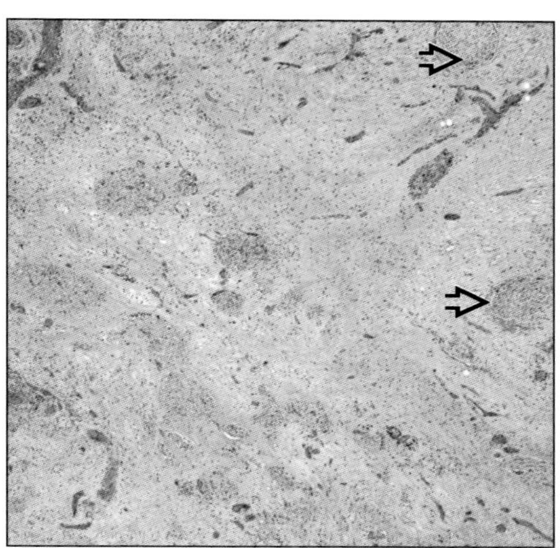

(Left) *Trichrome stain of a pancreas allograft highlights areas of fibrosis* ➲*. There is exocrine parenchyma still uninvolved by fibrous tissue. In this case, the extent of fibrosis was approximately 50%, which is consistent with moderate chronic allograft rejection (Banff grade II).* ***(Right)*** *Pancreas allograft section shows marked fibrosis (graft sclerosis) consistent with severe chronic rejection (Banff grade III) with only scattered islets* ➲ *still preserved.*

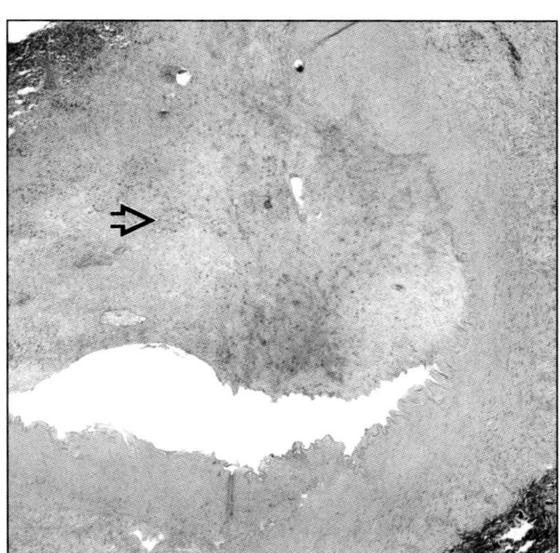

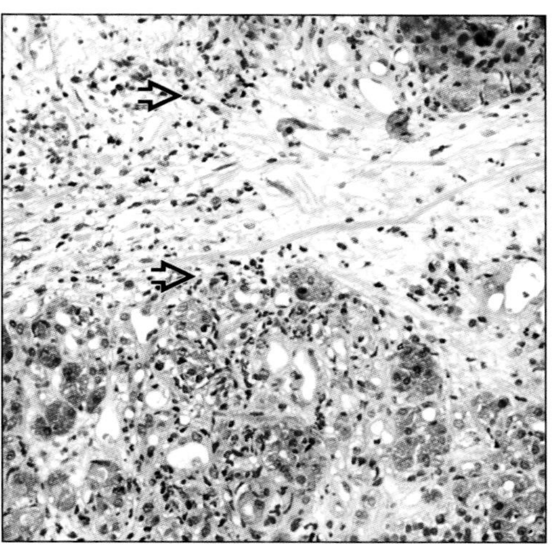

(Left) *Pancreas allograft section of a large artery shows allograft vasculopathy characterized by concentric intima fibrous thickening* ➲*. These features are similar to other graft arteriopathy occurring in other solid organ transplants.* ***(Right)*** *Pancreatitis is a complication that may affect the pancreas allograft and has to be differentiated from cellular rejection. The inflammatory cells in pancreatitis are mainly neutrophils that may be placed in septi and involving acini* ➲*.*

BONE MARROW TRANSPLANT

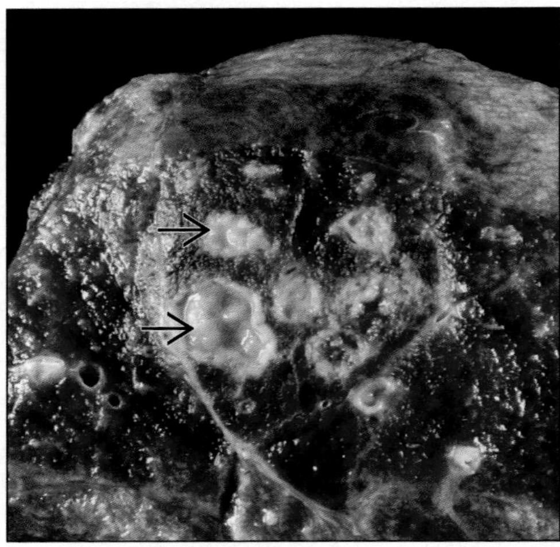

Pus-filled cavitary lesions are seen in the right upper lobe lung ➔ of a patient with recent bone marrow transplantation. Fungal hyphae consistent with Aspergillus were seen microscopically.

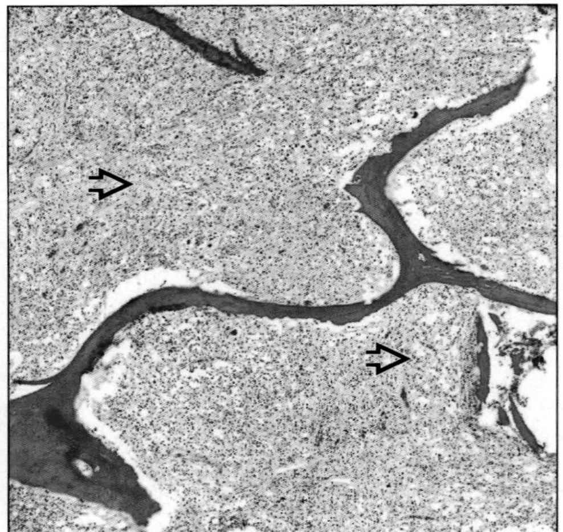

Autopsy photomicrograph of the vertebral marrow in a patient with recent bone marrow transplant shows decreased cellularity and serous atrophy of the marrow fat ➢, indicating incomplete engraftment.

TERMINOLOGY

Abbreviations

- Bone marrow transplantation (BMT)

Synonyms

- Hematopoietic stem cell transplantation (HSCT)

Definitions

- Intensive medical therapeutic procedure, undertaken in phases
  - Harvesting: Hematopoietic stem cells collected from peripheral blood using apheresis
    - Autologous: Harvested from self
    - Allogeneic: Harvested from another person (HLA matched)
  - Conditioning: Diseased bone marrow is eradicated by chemotherapy &/or radiation (myeloablation)
  - Transplantation: Hematopoietic stem cells infused, engraft in bone marrow to repopulate immune system

ETIOLOGY/PATHOGENESIS

Bone Marrow Transplantation Indications

- Leukemia
- Myelodysplasia
- Lymphoma
- Aplastic anemia
- Sickle cell disease, thalassemia
- Immune deficiency syndromes
- Inherited metabolic disorders

CLINICAL ISSUES

Assessing Engraftment

- Review antemortem complete blood count
  - Previous bone marrow biopsies (if available)
  - Molecular chimerism studies

Recurrent Hematolymphoid Disease (Relapse)

- Leukemia
  - Blast %, comparison to primary
- Lymphoma
  - Staging (nodal, extranodal, bone marrow)
  - EBV infection (post-transplant lymphoproliferative disorders)

Graft-vs.-Host Disease (GVHD)

- Skin: Rash, eczematous plaques
  - Face, trunk, palms, and soles most common
- GI tract
  - Watery diarrhea
- Liver
  - Cholesteatotic hepatitis

Infectious Complications

- Immunocompromised host
  - Incomplete granulocyte &/or lymphocyte engraftment
  - Change in adaptive immunity repertoire
  - Immunosuppressive drugs (to prevent rejection and GVHD) in allogeneic transplants
- Opportunistic infections
  - Fungal
    - Angioinvasive *Aspergillus*
    - *Cryptococcus*
    - *Mucor*
  - Mycobacterial
    - *Mycobacterium avium* complex
    - Miliary tuberculosis
  - Viral
    - CMV, HSV, VZV
  - Parasitic
    - *Toxoplasma*
- Nosocomial infections
  - Methicillin-resistant *Staphylococcus aureus*

BONE MARROW TRANSPLANT

Key Facts

Terminology
- Sources of hematopoietic stem cells
  - Autologous: Harvested from self
  - Allogeneic: Harvested from another person (HLA matched)

Clinical Issues
- Engraftment
  - Review antemortem complete blood count
  - Previous bone marrow biopsies (if available)
  - Molecular chimerism studies

Macroscopic Pathology
- Infectious complications
  - Postmortem culture of any pus or drainage
  - Opportunistic infections
- Graft-versus-host disease (GVHD)
  - Skin samples (taken along "Y" incision lines), intestinal samples, liver sections

Microscopic Pathology
- Engraftment
  - Assess marrow for cellularity and trilineage hematopoiesis
- Relapsed disease
  - Leukemia, lymphoma, plasma cell dyscrasia
- Infectious complications
  - Fungal, viral, parasitic, and bacterial
  - Special stains (Gram, MS, AFB)

Grading of Graft-vs.-Host Disease

Skin	GI tract (Often not possible to accurately grade due to autolysis)	Liver
Grade I: Focal or diffuse vacuolar change at dermal-epidermal junction	Grade I: Single cell apoptosis of crypt epithelium	(No accepted grading scheme)
Grade II: Epidermal spongiosis with apoptotic keratinocytes	Grade II: Destruction of single crypts or glands with apoptotic crypt abscesses	Bile duct epithelial cell damage with minimal inflammation or duct loss
Grade III: Subepidermal clefting, more spongiosis, and more dyskeratotic keratinocytes	Grade III: Focal mucosal necrosis with ulceration	Epithelial cell vacuolization and attenuation
Grade IV: Complete epidermal detachment with extensive epidermal necrosis	Grade IV: Diffuse mucosal necrosis with denudation	Ductopenia

- Vancomycin-resistant *Enterococcus*

MACROSCOPIC FEATURES

External Examination
- Venous infusion catheters and ports
  - Signs of infection
- Skin lesions
  - Petechiae, ecchymoses (coagulopathy, sepsis, DIC)
  - Abscesses, cellulitis
- Bulky adenopathy

Internal Examination
- Bone marrow sampling (for engraftment/relapse evaluation)
  - Expressed from individual ribs after chest plate removed
    - Compress bone 1-2 cm from cut surface and scrape extruded marrow into fixative
  - Cancellous bone from vertebral bodies or sternum
    - Sliced thin with vibrating saw and decalcified before processing
  - Flow cytometry usually limited value due to low viability postmortem
- Hematolymphoid organs
  - Splenomegaly, splenic infarction
  - Lymph nodes
    - Hilar, retroperitoneal, mesenteric, pelvic
- GVHD
  - Skin samples (taken along "Y" incision lines), intestinal samples, liver sections
- Infectious complications
  - Gross purulence, abscesses in organs, body cavities, psoas muscle
  - Postmortem culture of any pus or drainage

MICROSCOPIC PATHOLOGY

Histologic Features
- Engraftment/relapse
  - Assess marrow for cellularity and trilineage hematopoiesis
  - Lymph nodes
    - Overall cellularity, follicles and germinal centers
  - Spleen histology
    - Red pulp (cords and sinuses)
    - White pulp cellularity, germinal centers
  - Extramedullary hematopoiesis
    - Liver, kidneys, lungs, lymph nodes

SELECTED REFERENCES

1. Seftel MD et al: High rate of discordance between clinical and autopsy diagnoses in blood and marrow transplantation. Bone Marrow Transplant. 40(11):1049-53, 2007
2. Al-Saidi F et al: Relationship between premortem and postmortem diagnosis in critically ill bone marrow transplantation patients. Crit Care Med. 30(3):570-3, 2002

BONE MARROW TRANSPLANT

Microscopic Features

*(**Left**) A hilar lymph node sampled at autopsy 1 week after bone marrow engraftment shows retained lymph node architecture with a capsule ⇨ and intact trabecular sinuses ⇨. However, there is a paucity of lymphocytes and no follicles are seen. There is also considerable autolysis. (**Right**) This oil immersion field of the bone marrow shows a potential complication of bone marrow transplantation, hemophagocytic syndrome. The macrophage cytoplasm is filled with erythrocytes ⇨.*

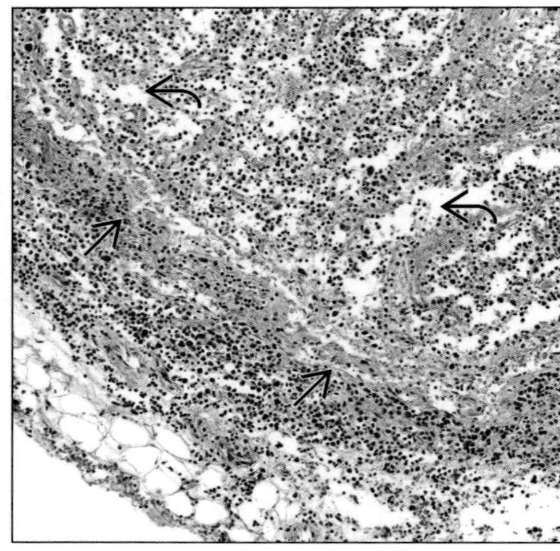

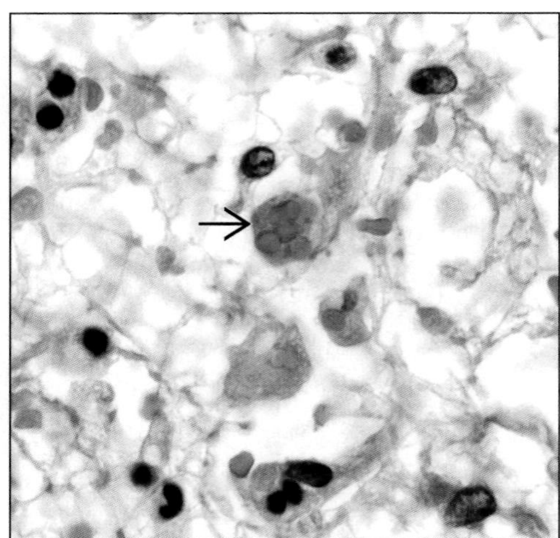

*(**Left**) Features of graft-versus-host disease are seen in this skin sample. There is interface dermatitis with satellite cell necrosis characterized by apoptotic keratinocytes ⇨ with adjacent lymphocytes ⇨. (From DP: Nonneoplastic Dermatopathology.) (**Right**) This autopsy lung section from a patient with bone marrow transplant several months ago shows features of recurrent diffuse large B-cell lymphoma ⇨. This is recognizable despite significant autolysis in the lung.*

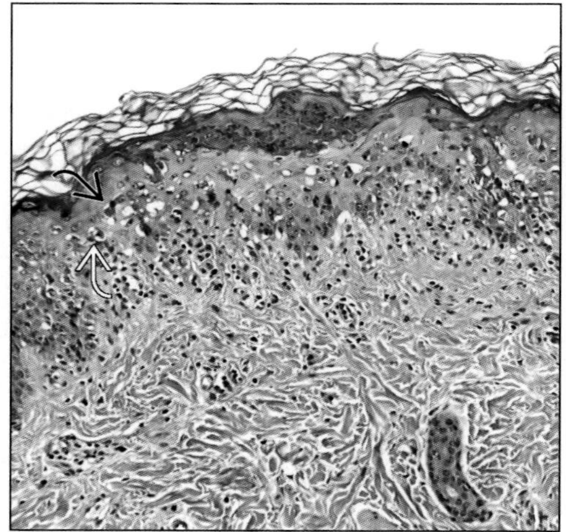

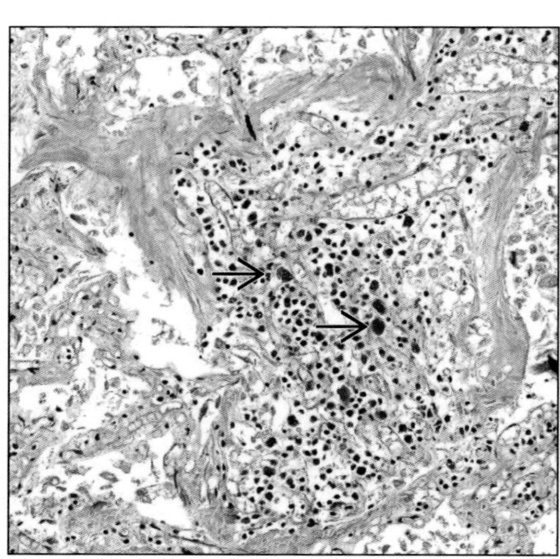

*(**Left**) Recurrent large cell lymphoma is seen in the kidney of this bone marrow transplant patient. Despite the autolysis of tubules ⇨ and glomeruli ⇨, atypical hyperchromatic lymphocytes ⇨ are apparent in the lymphomatous infiltrate. (**Right**) Myriad Cryptococcus neoformans organisms ⇨ are seen in this glomerulus of a patient with immunosuppression for graft-versus-host disease following bone marrow transplantation. Note the virtual absence of inflammation.*

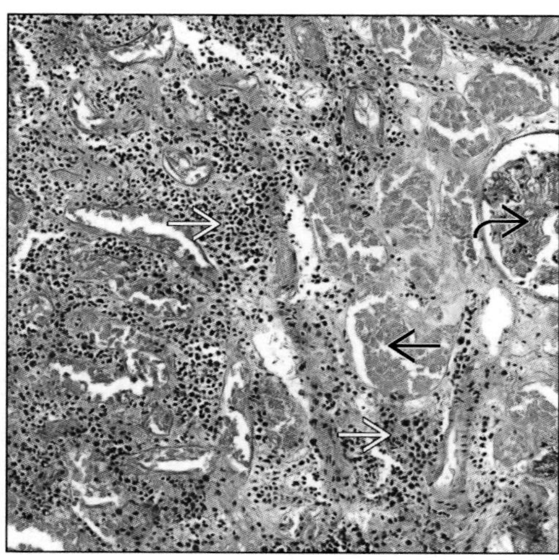

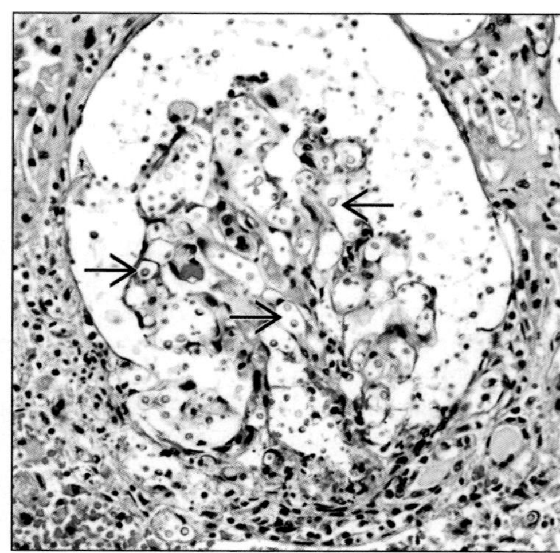

Microscopic Features

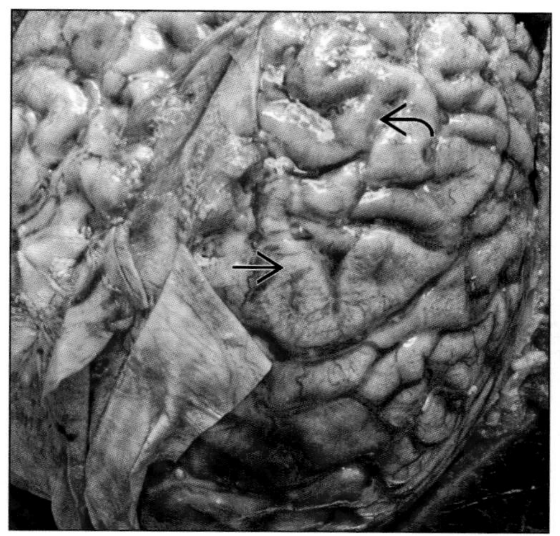

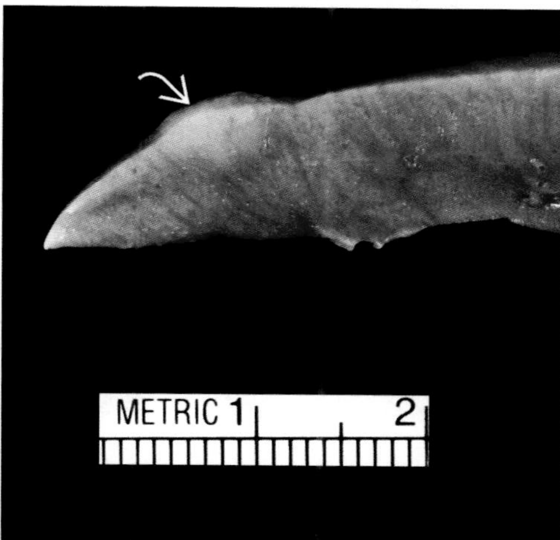

(Left) After removing the calvarium of this bone marrow patient, clouding of the meninges ⇒ and purulence in the sulci ⇒ were apparent. Meningitis was confirmed histologically. (Right) Wedge section of the kidney from a bone marrow transplant patient autopsy shows a nodular focus ⇒ of recurrent lymphoma (confirmed histologically).

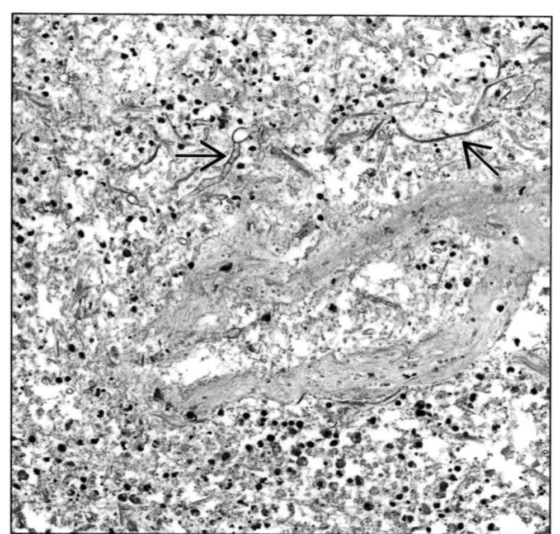

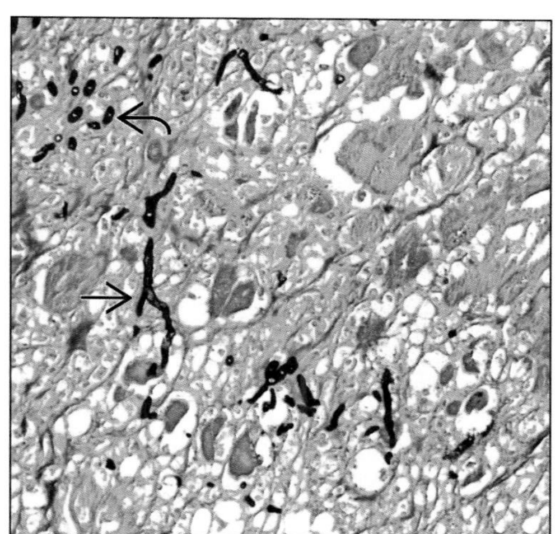

(Left) Fungal hyphae with 45° angle branching ⇒ consistent with Aspergillus species can be seen by H&E in this autopsy lung sample from a bone marrow transplant patient. (Right) Silver staining highlights the morphology of the fungal elements. Cross sections of the hyphae ⇒ can be seen, along with characteristic 45° angle branching ⇒ of Aspergillus species.

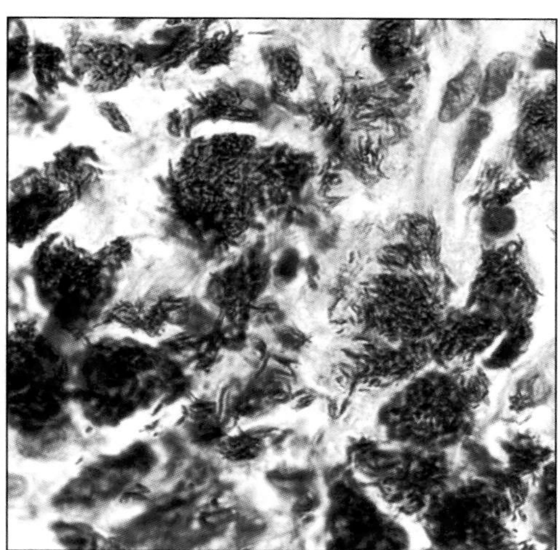

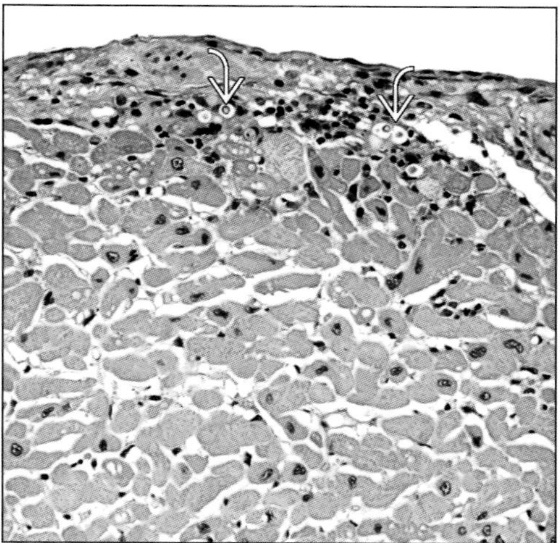

(Left) Acid-fast stain shows innumerable positive-staining thread-like bacilli within macrophages in a lymph node. Several mycobacterial species can give this appearance in immunocompromised patients, with the avium intracellulare group being most common. (From DP: Gastrointestinal.) (Right) Autopsy heart section shows myocarditis with encapsulated yeast forms ⇒ morphologically consistent with Cryptococcus.

DECEASED DONOR AUTOPSY

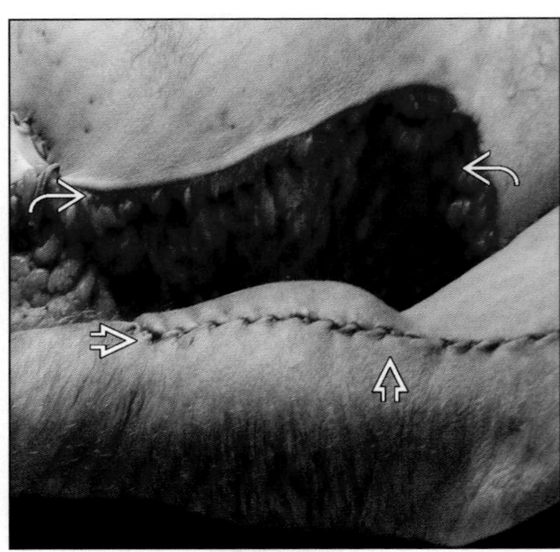

This large area of excised skin ➡ from an organ and tissue donor should not be mistaken for trauma. There is also an incision from long bone and tendon retrieval ⇨.

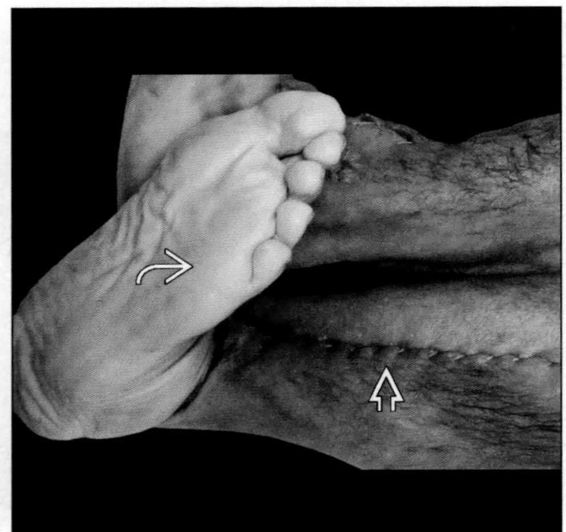

These feet are awkwardly oriented ➡ due to the removal of the long bones of the leg. The lower portion of the long incision that ran the length of the leg is visible ⇨. This should not be mistaken for trauma.

TERMINOLOGY

Definitions

- There are special considerations when performing an autopsy on organ &/or tissue donors
- Deceased donor
  - Individual whose next of kin (or through premortem indications) consents to organ &/or tissue donation
    - Organ donors are most often declared brain dead (donation after brain death [DBD]): Kidneys, heart, lungs, liver, pancreas, intestine
    - Patients may also donate some organs after circulatory (cardiac) death (DCD): Kidneys (most frequent), infrequently liver and lung
    - Tissue donors may be DCD: Heart valves, skin, bone, tendon
  - Eyes and corneas are often donated
    - Corneas transplanted, eyes often used for research
  - Donation consent does not mean autopsy consent
    - Next of kin of deceased donors who die a natural death must complete separate autopsy consent
    - Donors who die an unnatural death are sent to local medical examiner for investigation
- Organ procurement organization (OPO)
  - Local organizations certified by center for Medicare and Medicaid service (CMS) to evaluate potential donors and arrange for recovery and transport of transplanted organs

CLINICAL ISSUES

Laboratory Tests

- Local OPO will screen donors extensively for potentially transmissible disease and for markers of organ function prior to donation
  - OPO can provide that data to pathologist responsible for autopsy

MACROSCOPIC FEATURES

External Examination

- Remarkable for effects of organ and tissue donation
  - Abdominal and chest incisions from organ donation procedure
  - Linear incisions along extremities in bone donation
    - Awkward orientation of boneless extremity (do not mistake for trauma)
  - Large areas of extraction of skin and dermis by dermatome
    - Rectangular areas of loss of skin with exposed soft tissue and fat
    - Do not mistake for trauma
  - Eye caps used following eye donation
    - Plastic cups shaped like eyeballs that are placed in eye socket and have corrugated outer edge to hold eyelid in place
    - Difficult to open eyelid when eye cap is in place
    - Data regarding appearance of eye and conjunctiva can be retrieved from local eye bank

Internal Examination

- Note all donated organs

Organ Examination

- Remaining organs examined as per complete autopsy
- Try to determine underlying cause of death
  - Most commonly related to CVA, subarachnoid hemorrhage, intracerebral hemorrhage, brain tumor without metastasis, hypoxia
  - Drug overdose, head trauma cases would be examined by medical examiner
- Identify features related to brain death: Will vary with duration of brain death and pre-donation physiologic alterations
  - Mottling of subendocardial (myocardial ischemia related to vasoconstriction)

DECEASED DONOR AUTOPSY

Key Facts

Terminology

- Organs usually procured in brain dead donors: Kidneys, heart, lungs, liver, pancreas, intestine
- Some organs rarely used after circulatory (cardiac) death (DCD): Kidneys (most frequent), infrequently liver and lung

Macroscopic Pathology

- Brain death usually: CVA, subarachnoid hemorrhage, intracerebral hemorrhage, brain tumor without metastasis, hypoxia
- Identify features related to brain death: Pulmonary edema, visceral ischemia, disseminated intravascular coagulation
    - Increased weight and increased fluid in lungs (pulmonary edema)
    - Intestinal ischemia (visceral hypoperfusion)
    - Petechiae, hemorrhages (disseminated intravascular coagulation)
    - Adrenal gland stress response: ACTH secreted during stress response causes lipid depletion in adrenal gland
        - Grossly adrenal cortex loses yellow color

MICROSCOPIC PATHOLOGY

Histologic Features

- Subendocardial myocardial coagulative necrosis ± myocyte necrosis with contraction bands
- Intraalveolar pink fluid (pulmonary edema)
- Coagulative necrosis of bowel mucosa (intestinal ischemia)
- Centrilobular hepatic necrosis (visceral ischemia)
- Coagulative necrosis or degenerative changes of tubular epithelial cells of kidney (intestinal hypoperfusion)
- Lipid depletion in cells of zona fasciculata of adrenal cortex (stress response)

DIFFERENTIAL DIAGNOSIS

Brain Death: Primary vs. Secondary Effects

- May be difficult to distinguish hypoperfusion changes due to brain death from pre-brain death physiologic instability
- Correlation with clinical history may help distinguish timing of organ alterations

REPORTING CRITERIA

OPO Notification

- Findings of potential clinical impact to any organ or tissue recipients must be reported to OPO as soon as recognized
    - Included but not limited to malignancy and infection
- All reports are shared with OPO
    - Highlight any information of potential impact to donor family (potentially heritable diseases, community acquired communicable disease, etc.)

SELECTED REFERENCES

1. Lipshutz GS et al: Death from donor-transmitted malignancy despite emergency liver retransplantation. Liver Transpl. 9(10):1102-7, 2003
2. Keating MR et al: Transmission of invasive aspergillosis from a subclinically infected donor to three different organ transplant recipients. Chest. 109(4):1119-24, 1996

IMAGE GALLERY

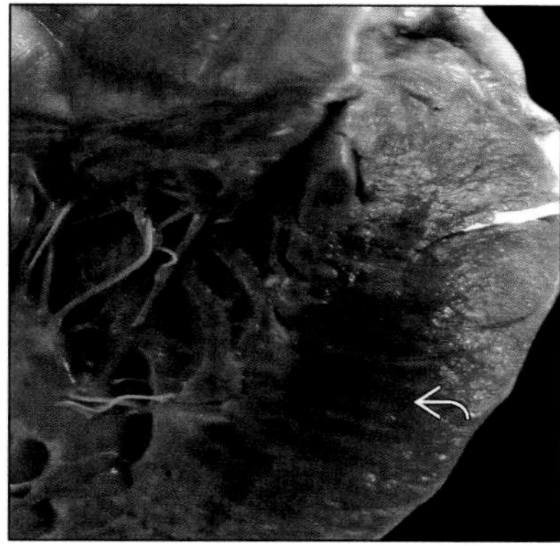

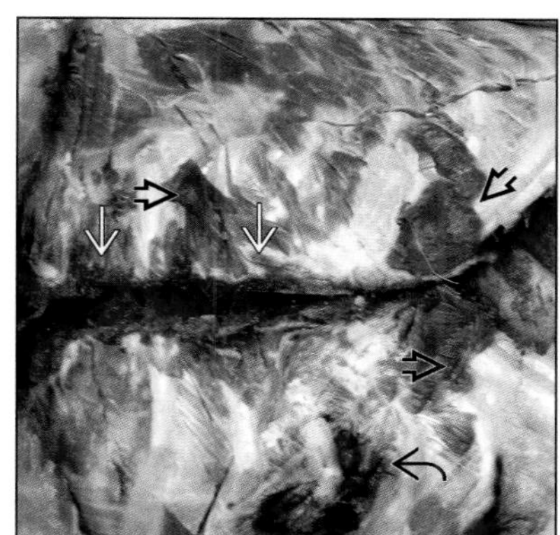

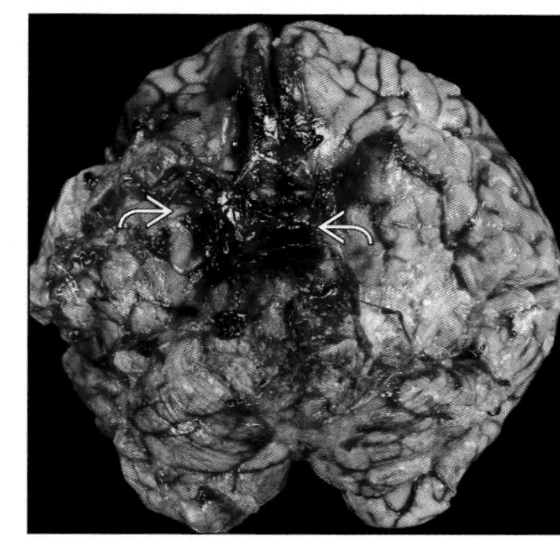

(Left) *The cause of death in this tissue donor was an acute myocardial infarction ➡. It is important to note any possible communicable/ transmissible diseases during donor autopsies.* ***(Center)*** *This unsutured sternal incision ➡ was the consequence of thoracic organ donation. There is also soft tissue hematoma ⇨ present from resuscitation. The muscle ⇨ appears brown as a consequence of embalming prior to autopsy.* ***(Right)*** *The cause of death for this donor was intracerebral hemorrhage that extends into subarachnoid space ➡.*

SECTION 2

Infection-Related Death

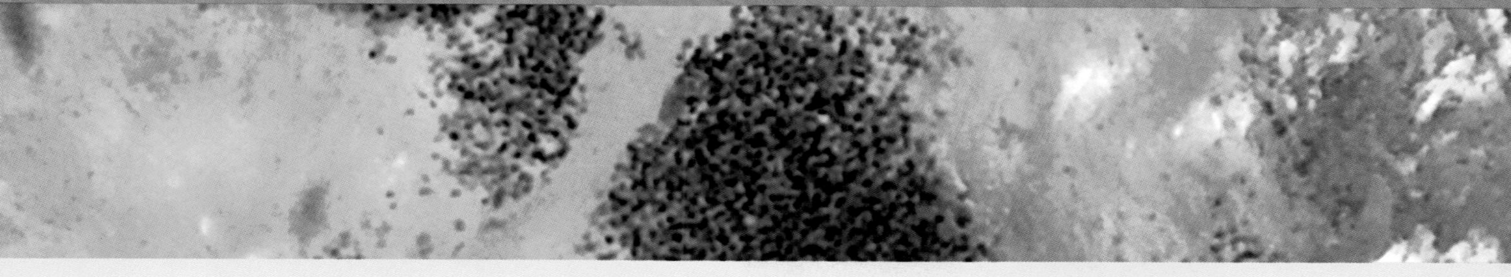

Systemic Infection/Sepsis Overview

Organ System Infection

HIV/AIDS

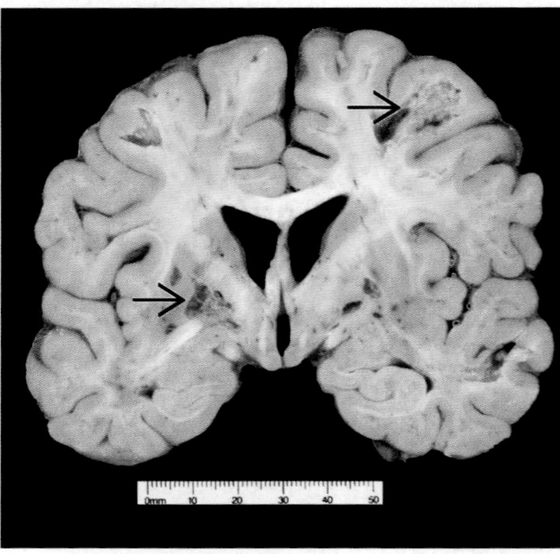

This coronal section of brain was taken from a patient with CNS Toxoplasma gondii. Note the areas of cystic necrosis ➡ in the cortex and basal ganglia.

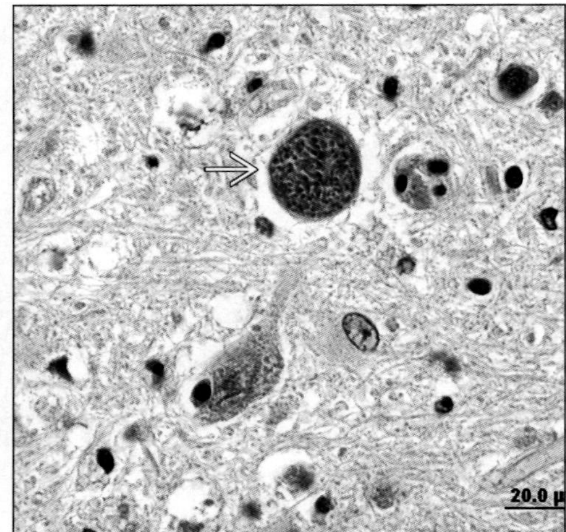

This H&E histologic section of brain was taken from a patient with Toxoplasma gondii. A cyst ➡ containing numerous bradyzoites is seen.

TERMINOLOGY

General Features of AIDS Pathology

- Loss of cell-mediated immunity
  - Opportunistic infection
    - Most common cause of death
    - Often reactivation of latent infection
  - Virus-associated neoplasms
  - ↑ likelihood of disseminated disease
- Autopsy often reveals unexpected findings
  - Minimal gross findings (e.g., poorly formed or absent granulomas for fungi and mycobacteria)
  - Minimal inflammatory response despite numerous organisms
  - Cultures, special stains, and sampling of grossly normal tissue are essential
- Complications of highly active antiretroviral therapy (HAART)
  - Immune reconstitution inflammatory syndrome (IRIS): Sudden worsening of symptoms with onset of therapy and rebound of CD4 count
  - Coronary artery disease

MACROSCOPIC FEATURES

Pulmonary Manifestations

- Fungi
  - Diffuse or patchy areas of dark red, airless lung
  - *Pneumocystis jirovecii*: **Most common opportunistic infection in AIDS patients**
  - *Cryptococcus neoformans*: Diffuse or miliary patterns
  - *Histoplasma capsulatum*: Endemic areas (Mississippi and Ohio River valleys)
    - Classic histoplasma granuloma: Cut section shows concentric lamellae
    - Disseminated cases lack granulomas
  - *Coccidioides immitis*: Mostly in endemic, arid areas (Southwestern USA)
- Mycobacteria: (*Mycobacterium avium* complex [MAC], less frequently *Mycobacterium tuberculosis* MTB); other species more unusual
  - Often miliary rather than cavitary/granulomatous
  - Stains and cultures are crucial
- Other bacteria
  - Bacterial pneumonia common in AIDS autopsies
    - Particularly encapsulated organisms (e.g., Pneumococcus, *Haemophilus influenzae*)
- Viruses
  - Cytomegalovirus (CMV)
    - Often coinfection (e.g., with *Pneumocystis*)
    - Patterns: 1-3 cm necrotic nodules, ARDS pattern
    - Gross changes can be subtle
  - Herpes simplex virus (HSV) and varicella zoster virus (VZV)
    - Variable inflammatory response; may be necrotizing
- Tumors
  - Kaposi sarcoma (KS)
    - Lungs: Hemorrhagic lesions
    - Airways: Raised red to purple plaques

Cardiovascular Manifestations

- Coronary artery disease
  - In part from metabolic effects of antiretroviral medications
- Dilated cardiomyopathy: Mechanism unknown
- Infections: *Toxoplasma gondii*, fungi, CMV, mycobacteria
  - Often part of disseminated infections
- Tumors: KS and lymphoma

Gastrointestinal Manifestations

- Fungi
  - *Candida albicans*
    - White plaques, discrete or confluent, on inflamed mucosa
    - Typically oral and esophageal
  - *Histoplasma*: Hepatosplenomegaly

Key Facts

Terminology

- HIV/AIDS is 6th leading cause of death worldwide and is 2nd leading cause of death in low income countries (WHO 2012 data)
- Autopsies on AIDS patients require meticulous attention to personal protection
  - Respiratory precautions
  - Double gloving
  - Splash protection
- Opportunistic infections are most common cause of death
- Impaired immune response may dramatically alter gross and microscopic findings
  - Gross findings may be minimal; histologic sampling of grossly normal tissue is essential
  - Histologic changes may be minimal and granulomas may be poorly formed or absent
  - Histochemical stains, immunoperoxidase, and culture can dramatically increase diagnostic yield
- Besides opportunistic infections, patients with AIDS are at increased risk for disseminated bacterial infections
- Viral-associated tumors can be seen in AIDS patients
  - Kaposi sarcoma
  - Lymphoma, particularly CNS lymphoma and primary effusion lymphoma
  - Condylomas and squamous cell carcinoma of oral cavity and anorectum
- Antiretroviral therapy is highly effective but carries certain risks (IRIS, increased risk of coronary artery disease)

- Mycobacteria
  - MAC
    - Typically in small bowel with minimal gross change (mild villous blunting)
    - Can involve liver; less often stomach and colon
- Other bacteria: *Salmonella*, *Shigella*, *Campylobacter*
  - Significantly higher risk for enteric bacterial infections
- Viruses
  - CMV
    - Variable mucosal changes: From minimal changes to ulceration with hemorrhage
    - Typically in colon (especially distal) and esophagus (especially distal)
    - Esophagus: Linear and oval ulcers
  - HSV
    - Typically esophageal
    - First vesicles, then punched out shallow ulcers surrounded by normal mucosa
- Parasites
  - *Cryptosporidium*: In 10-20% of diarrheal stool samples from AIDS patients
    - Minimal gross changes: Mild villous blunting
    - Rarely associated with acalculous or gangrenous cholecystitis
- Tumors
  - KS: Submucosal red macules or violaceous nodules

Lymph Nodes and Bone Marrow

- Persistent generalized lymphadenopathy seen early in disease course
- Fungi
  - *Cryptococcus*, *Histoplasma*, and *Coccidioides*: Lymphadenopathy and marrow involvement
- Mycobacteria
  - MAC: May involve lymph nodes and marrow; gross changes often subtle
- Tumor
  - KS: May involve lymph nodes
  - Lymphoma: Usually B-cell non-Hodgkin, often high grade
  - Primary effusion lymphoma: Associated with HHV-8

Central Nervous System

- Parasites
  - *Toxoplasma gondii*: **Most common CNS opportunistic pathogen**
    - Necrotic, abscess-like lesions, often multiple, predominantly in gray matter
  - Fungi
    - *Cryptococcus*: Meningoencephalitis; destructive lesions, sometimes gelatinous
  - Mycobacteria
    - MTB: Miliary lesions; MAC rarely produces gross lesions
  - Viruses
    - CMV: May produce no gross lesions
    - HSV: Lesions may be diffuse (typically frontotemporal in immunocompetent patients)
  - Tumors
    - Lymphoma: 90% EBV-associated diffuse large B-cell lymphoma; also Burkitt lymphomas, T-cell lymphomas
- Vacuolar myelopathy
- Progressive multifocal leukoencephalopathy

Skin

- Viruses
  - HSV and VZV: Vesicular skin lesions; VZV lesions may be diffuse rather than dermatomal
  - HPV: From condylomas to squamous cell carcinoma of oral cavity and anorectum
- KS
  - Pink to violet patches, plaques, angiomatoid nodules
  - Distribution in AIDS patients: Arms, oral mucosa, trunk, face, soles

MICROSCOPIC PATHOLOGY

Histologic Features

- Pulmonary
  - *Pneumocystis jerovicii*

HIV/AIDS

- H&E: Foamy, pink, refractile intraalveolar fluid; sparse inflammation
- GMS stain: Spherical, crescentic, and cup-shaped organisms, 5-7 µm

- *Cryptococcus neoformans*
  - H&E: Variable inflammation; ± granulomas
  - PAS or GMS stain: 4-6 µm yeast with doubly refractile walls and narrow-based budding
  - Mucicarmine to highlight capsule
- *Histoplasma capsulatum*: Granulomas may be poorly formed or absent
  - H&E: Variable inflammation; often subtle foamy histiocytic infiltrate
  - PAS or GMS stain: 2-5 µm oval to round budding yeast; may be inside histiocytes
- *Coccidioides immitis*
  - H&E: Affected areas can show a rim of eosinophilia
  - PAS and GMS stain: Large (30-60 µm) spherules full of 2-5 µm spherules; hyphae with barrel-shaped arthroconidia
- Mycobacteria: Granulomas may be poorly formed or absent
  - MTB: Often miliary with necrosis
  - MAC: Often just subtle infiltrate of foamy macrophages; special stains crucial
  - AFB stain: Typically intracellular, red bacilli; usually 3-5 µm long by 0.2-0.6 µm wide
- Other bacteria
  - May have typical histology of bacterial pneumonia with intraalveolar acute inflammation
  - Severely immunosuppressed patients may have cavitary lesions
- CMV
  - Variable patterns (necrotic nodules, interstitial pneumonitis, diffuse alveolar damage)
  - H&E: CMV-infected cells: Enlarged (25-50 µm) cells, single "owl's-eye" 20 µm nuclear inclusion, multiple 1-3 µm cytoplasmic inclusions
  - Immunoperoxidase stains helpful
- KS
  - Distribution: Pleural, bronchovascular bundles, interlobular septa
  - H&E: Typically spindled cells with slit-like space containing extravasated red cells
  - Immunoperoxidase: Positive for CD34, factor VIII antigen, HHV8

- Gastrointestinal
  - *Candida albicans*
    - H&E: Acutely inflamed, eroded mucosa
    - GMS and PAS: Yeast (2-7 µm) and pseudohyphae
  - MAC
    - H&E: Infiltrate of foamy macrophages
    - AFB stain: Typically intracellular, red bacilli; usually 3-5 µm long by 0.2-0.6 µm wide
  - CMV: Immunoperoxidase very helpful
    - CMV cytopathic changes in stromal, endothelial and glandular cells **at ulcer base**
  - HSV: Immunoperoxidase very helpful
    - Esophagus: Infected squamous cells **at ulcer periphery**
    - H&E: Typical cytopathic changes: Multinucleated giant cells, ground glass nuclei, nuclear molding, nuclear inclusions
    - Consider VZV if immunostains negative for HSV
  - *Cryptosporidium*
    - H&E: Faint 2-4 µm oval to round oocysts on epithelial cell surfaces
    - Kinyoun, Giemsa, and PAS positive
- Lymph nodes and bone marrow
  - Persistent generalized lymphadenopathy: Reactive changes with florid follicular hyperplasia
  - Fungi and mycobacteria
    - H&E: Necrotizing granulomas, poorly formed granulomas, or histiocytic infiltrate without granulomas
    - Special stains are essential
- Central nervous system
  - *T. gondii*
    - H&E: Necrotizing encephalitis, arteritis, thrombosis; organisms at periphery of necrotic zone
    - Wright or Giemsa: Tachyzoites; 3-4 µm ovals or crescents, dark blue cytoplasm and eccentric nucleus
    - Cysts: Up to 40 µm with numerous bradyzoites

SELECTED REFERENCES

1. Guimarães LC et al: Morphological changes in the digestive system of 93 human immunodeficiency virus positive patients: an autopsy study. Rev Inst Med Trop Sao Paulo. 54(2):89-93, 2012
2. Fuster V et al: Hurst's the Heart. 13th ed. New York: McGraw Hill New York, 2011
3. Singer EJ et al: Neurologic presentations of AIDS. Neurol Clin. 28(1):253-75, 2010
4. Fenoglio-Preiser CM et al. Gastrointestinal Pathology, an Atlas and Text. 3rd ed. Philadelphia: Lippincott, Williams and Wilkins, 2008
5. Wormser GP: AIDS and Other Manifestations of HIV Infection. 4th ed. Amsterdam: Elsevier, 2004
6. Masliah E et al: Changes in pathological findings at autopsy in AIDS cases for the last 15 years. AIDS. 14(1):69-74, 2000

Gross and Microscopic Features

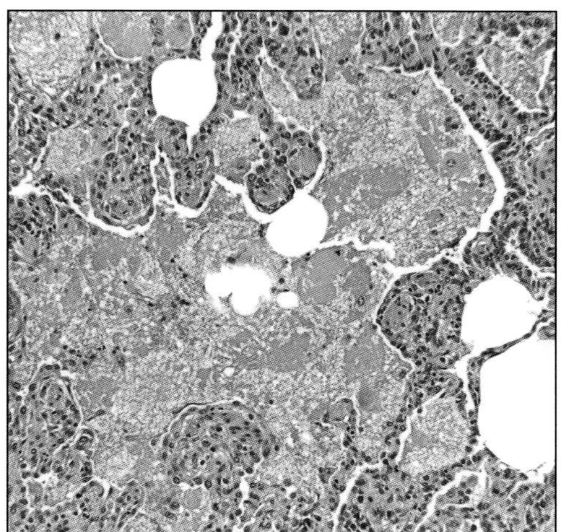

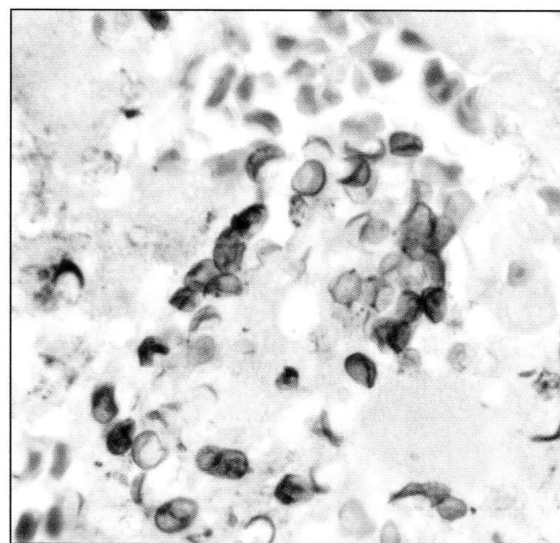

*(**Left**) H&E histologic section of lung infected with Pneumocystis jerovicii shows the mild inflammatory infiltrate and foamy, eosinophilic intraalveolar fluid. Organisms are typically not discernible without special stains. (**Right**) Histologic section from lung with pneumocystis is shown by GMS. With the silver stain, the organisms appear as circular, crescentic, and cup-shaped gray to black 5 μm cysts.*

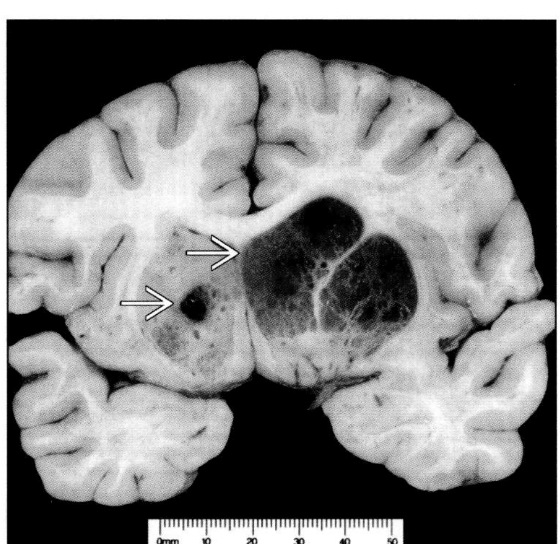

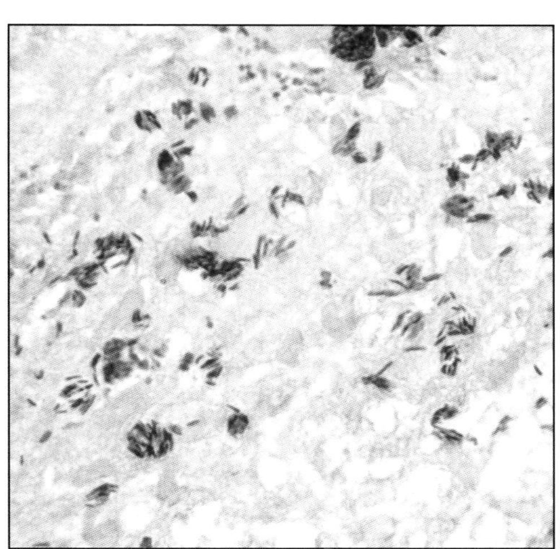

*(**Left**) This coronal section of brain is taken from a patient dying with CNS cryptococcus. Destructive, cystic lesions ➡ appear in the basal ganglia. Cryptococcus produces a thick polysaccharide capsule, and the gross lesions may appear gelatinous, as in this case. (**Right**) Image shows an acid-fast stain of small bowel with MAC. AIDS patients often cannot form granulomas. Routine H&E sections may show only foamy histiocytes, but acid-fast stains will show numerous organisms.*

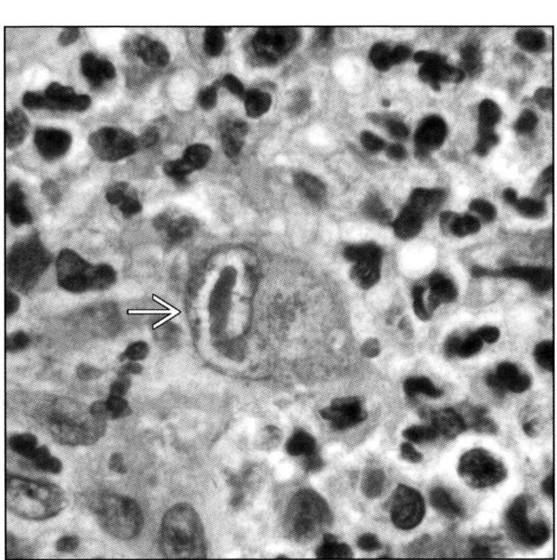

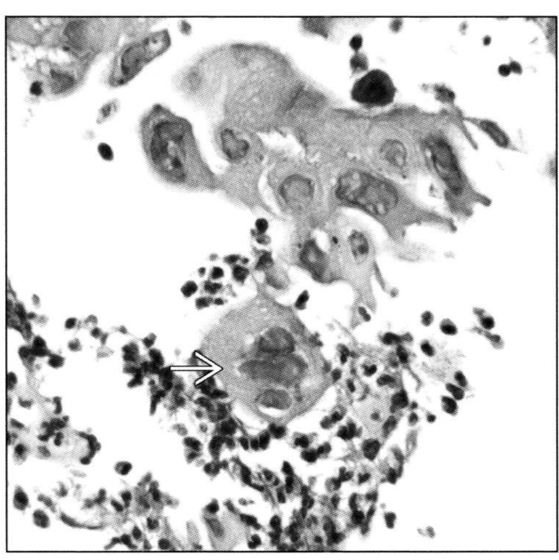

*(**Left**) Typical viral cytopathic effect of cytomegalovirus (CMV) is shown on H&E ➡. Note the large size (compared to surrounding inflammatory cells) of the infected cell, its prominent "owl's-eye" intranuclear inclusion, and the smaller intracytoplasmic inclusions. (**Right**) HSV-infected cells from esophagus are shown on H&E. A cell with typical herpetic viral cytopathic effect ➡ can be seen. The affected cell is enlarged and multinucleated with "ground-glass" nuclei and nuclear molding.*

SHOCK AND SEPSIS

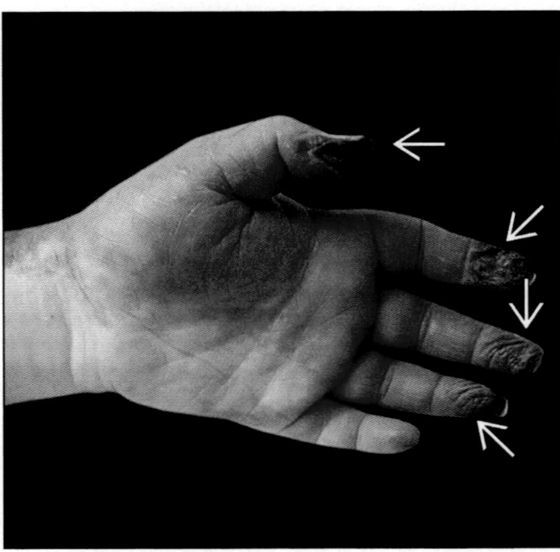

This image shows ischemic necrosis of the fingertips ➡ with proximal edema and erythema as a result of prolonged, severe shock.

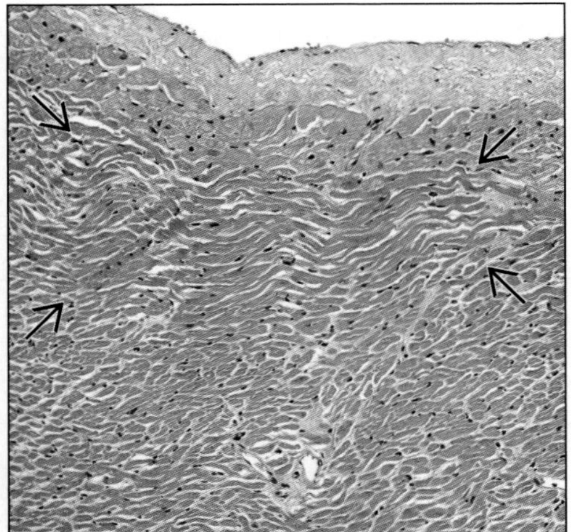

The subendocardium in this autopsy heart section shows early ischemic changes of hypereosinophilia and wavy myocytes ➡ due to prolonged shock (demand ischemia).

TERMINOLOGY

Abbreviations

- Systemic inflammatory response syndrome (SIRS)
- Multiple organ dysfunction syndrome (MODS)

Synonyms

- MODS: Multi-organ failure, multiple systems organ failure

Definitions

- Shock: Inability to meet cellular metabolic requirements due to global hypoperfusion from inadequate circulating blood or plasma volume
- MODS: Physiologic dysfunction of ≥ 2 organ or physiologic systems not directly related to primary cause of shock
  - e.g., acute tubular injury and coagulopathy following cardiogenic shock due to acute myocardial infarction
- SIRS: Systemic activation of innate immune response, regardless of cause, clinically manifested as 2 or more of the following
  - Temperature > 38°C or < 36°C; heart rate (HR) > 90 beats/min; hyperventilation (respiratory rate > 20 breaths/min or $PaCO_2$ < 32mmHg); white blood cell (WBC) count > 12,000/μL or < 4,000/μL or 10% bands
- Sepsis: Probable or documented infection plus SIRS manifestations
- Severe sepsis: Sepsis plus infection-induced organ dysfunction, tissue hypoperfusion, or hypotension
  - Organ dysfunction: Altered mental status, generalized edema, acute lung injury, acute renal injury, oliguria, edema, coagulopathy, hyperbilirubinemia, hyperglycemia, ileus, thrombocytopenia
  - Tissue hypoperfusion: Lactate > 1mmol/L, ↓ capillary refill, or mottling
  - Hypotension: Systolic blood pressure (BP) < 90mmHg or mean arterial pressure < 70mmHg
- Septic shock: Sepsis plus hypotension persisting despite administration of adequate fluid resuscitation
- Stigmata of shock: Nonspecific pathologic findings reflecting pattern of organ injury due to tissue hypoperfusion

ETIOLOGY/PATHOGENESIS

Causes of Shock

- Hypovolemic: Massive loss of blood or plasma volume
  - e.g., hemorrhage, burns, massive vomiting or diarrhea, anaphylaxis
- Cardiogenic: Inability of heart to pump blood due to intrinsic failure (e.g., infarction, arrhythmia, cardiomyopathy) or external factors (e.g., cardiac tamponade, pulmonary embolism, tension pneumothorax)

Pathogenesis of Shock

- Initial phase: ↓ tissue perfusion → sympathetic nervous system activation → ↑ HR, ↑ myocardial contractility, ↑ arterial & venous tone; activation of renin-angiotensin system → BP maintained with blood preferentially shunted to heart & brain
- Progressive phase: ↓ BP & tissue perfusion → global tissue hypoxia, ↑ lactic acid, ↓ pH → arteriolar dilation, venous constriction, ↑ capillary permeability → loss of intravascular volume → organ dysfunction
- Irreversible phase: Refractory hypotension, multiple system organ failure, and death

Causes of SIRS

- Overwhelming microbial infection or release of microbial toxins
  - Deaths due to sepsis: Gram negative bacteria > Gram positive bacteria > fungal >> opportunistic bacteria & fungi, viruses

SHOCK AND SEPSIS

Key Facts

Terminology
- Shock: Inability to meet cellular metabolic requirements due to inadequate circulating blood or plasma volume
- MODS: Physiologic dysfunction of ≥ 2 organ or physiologic systems not directly related to primary cause of shock
- SIRS: Systemic activation of innate immune response, regardless of cause
- Sepsis: Probable or documented infection plus SIRS manifestations

Etiology
- Shock: Hypovolemic, cardiogenic, systemic inflammation
- SIRS: Sepsis, massive tissue injury, metabolic derangements, malignancy, neurologic trauma

Macroscopic Pathology
- Evidence of specific cause of shock
- Macroscopic stigmata of shock: e.g., diffuse petechia, pallor, edema, serosal effusions, "nutmeg" liver

Microscopic Pathology
- Shock: Diffuse vascular congestion, hemorrhage, fibrin thrombi of microvasculature involving any organ system
- Sepsis: Evidence of primary infection, septic emboli to any organ, widespread bacterial overgrowth
- Microscopic stigmata of shock: e.g., subendocardial demand ischemia, diffuse alveolar damage, hepatic centrilobular hemorrhagic necrosis, acute tubular necrosis

- Tissue injury: Massive trauma, severe burns, surgery, ischemia/reperfusion injury, transplant rejection, pancreatitis, erythroderma
- Metabolic: Thyroid storm, acute adrenal insufficiency
- Therapy related: Blood products, granulocyte-macrophage colony-stimulating factor, anesthesia-related malignant hyperpyrexia, neuroleptic malignant syndrome, opiates, benzodiazepines
- Malignancy: Lymphoma, tumor lysis syndrome
- Neurologic: Subarachnoid hemorrhage

Predisposing Factors to SIRS
- Inherited or acquired defects in innate or adaptive immune system
- Age (↑ risk neonates & elderly)

Pathogenesis of SIRS
- Systemic activation of innate immune response
  - Activation of neutrophils, monocytes/macrophages, & endothelium
    - Early phase: Excessive pro-inflammatory cytokines release → vasodilation, edema
    - Late phase: Diminished innate immune function → diminished adaptive immune function
  - Pro-oxidant state: ↑ reactive oxygen & nitrogen species, ↓ free radical scavengers → vasodilation, edema
  - Pro-coagulation state: Complement, coagulation cascade, & endothelial activation → disseminated intravascular coagulation (DIC)
  - → metabolic derangements, organ dysfunction, and shock

CLINICAL ISSUES

Epidemiology
- SIRS: Most critically ill patients meet criteria
- Sepsis: Most common cause of death in noncoronary intensive care unit (ICU)
  - 600,000 cases annually in USA
  - Incidence and number of deaths increasing in USA and worldwide

Presentation
- Shock: Varies with etiology; most common clinical manifestations are hypotension, tachycardia, cyanosis, and evidence of organ dysfunction
- Sepsis: Most common primary sites of infection (in ↓ frequency) are lung, bloodstream, abdomen, skin and soft tissue, urinary tract, and central nervous system

Treatment
- Shock: Identify and treat underlying cause
- Sepsis: Supportive therapy only

Prognosis
- Mortality rate of shock: Varies according to severity and etiology
- Mortality rate of sepsis:
  - Average: 20-30%; range: 5-50%
  - Varies according to predisposing factors, degree of organ dysfunction, type and site of infectious agent

Clinical Organ Dysfunction Scoring Systems
- Commonly used scoring systems for assessing severity of illness and predicting mortality in ICU patients
  - General prognostication scores: Acute physiology and chronic health evaluation (APACHE), simplified acute physiology score (SAPS), mortality probability models (MPM)
  - Organ dysfunction scores: Sequential organ failure assessment (SOFA), multiple organ dysfunction score (MODS), logistic organ dysfunction system (LODS)

IMAGE FINDINGS

Radiographic Findings
- Lungs: Diffuse bilateral infiltrates ("white out")

Ultrasonographic Findings
- Heart: Systolic and diastolic ventricular dysfunction

SHOCK AND SEPSIS

 ○ Low ejection fraction is predictor of mortality in septic shock

CT Findings

- Brain: Hypodensities in bilateral watershed areas progressing to whole brain edema
- Other: Evidence of specific underlying cause of shock &/or sepsis

MACROSCOPIC FEATURES

External Examination

- Extensive petechia &/or ecchymoses
- Pallor of conjunctiva &/or nailbeds
- Cyanosis of distal extremities
- Severe peripheral edema
- Jaundice

Internal Examination

- Evidence of specific cause of shock such as massive acute myocardial infarction, gastrointestinal hemorrhage, perforated viscus with fecopurulent exudate
- Macroscopic stigmata of shock
  - Soft tissue edema &/or hemorrhage
  - Serous effusions
  - Brain: Diffuse cerebral swelling ± uncal or cerebellar herniation
  - Lungs: Firm, heavy, wet ± hemorrhage, frothy fluid within airways
  - Heart: Epicardial &/or endocardial petechia, acute subendocardial ischemia
  - Liver: Mottled cut surface ("nutmeg" appearance)
  - Pancreas: Fat saponification
  - Gastrointestinal tract: Serosal and mucosal petechia, mucosal erosions
  - Kidneys: Cortical pallor with medullary congestion

MICROSCOPIC PATHOLOGY

Histologic Features

- Shock: Diffuse vascular congestion, hemorrhage, fibrin thrombi of microvasculature involving any organ system
- Sepsis: Evidence of primary infection (e.g., acute bronchopneumonia, meningitis), septic emboli to any organ (highly specific), widespread bacterial overgrowth disproportional to postmortem interval

Organ Examination

- Microscopic stigmata of shock
  - Brain: Hypoxic nerve cell change, cerebritis (sepsis)
  - Heart: Subendocardial ischemia (demand ischemia)
  - Lungs: Alveolar edema, capillary congestion, diffuse alveolar damage
  - Liver: Centrolobular hemorrhagic necrosis, canalicular or ductal cholestasis, steatosis
  - Gastrointestinal tract: Submucosal hemorrhages, erosions, or ulcerations
  - Kidneys: Acute tubular necrosis, pigmented casts (hemoglobin, myoglobin, or bile)
  - Spleen: Acute splenitis, congestion
  - Bone marrow: Reactive hypercellularity
  - Adrenal glands: Cortical cell lipid depletion, microscopic foci of hemorrhage within cortex

ANCILLARY TESTS

Histochemistry

- GMS (Gomori methenamine silver)
- Gram

Laboratory Tests

- Supporting evidence of organ dysfunction (if antemortem samples not available)
  - e.g., troponin level, CBC, chemistry panel
- Postmortem blood cultures: High false positive rate due to agonal bacteremia, postmortem bacterial transmigration
  - Positive postmortem blood cultures should correlate with gross and histologic evidence of infection

Specialty Consultation

- Centers for Disease Control and Prevention Infectious Diseases Pathology Branch
  - Provides important information and guidelines related to transport of pathology materials and clinical samples for ancillary testing

SELECTED REFERENCES

1. Centers for Disease Control and Prevention: Specimen Submission Guidelines. http://www.cdc.gov/ncezid/dhcpp/idpb/specimen-submission/index.html. Updated May 7, 2015. Accessed June 22, 2014
2. Dellinger RP et al: Surviving Sepsis Campaign: international guidelines for management of severe sepsis and septic shock, 2012. Intensive Care Med. 39(2):165-228, 2013
3. Orsini J et al: Microbiological profile of organisms causing bloodstream infection in critically ill patients. J Clin Med Res. 4(6):371-7, 2012
4. Vincent JL et al: Clinical review: scoring systems in the critically ill. Crit Care. 14(2):207, 2010
5. Neely WA et al: Septic shock: clinical, physiological, and pathological survey of 244 patients. Ann Surg. 173(5):657-66, 1971

Gross, Radiographic, and Microscopic Features

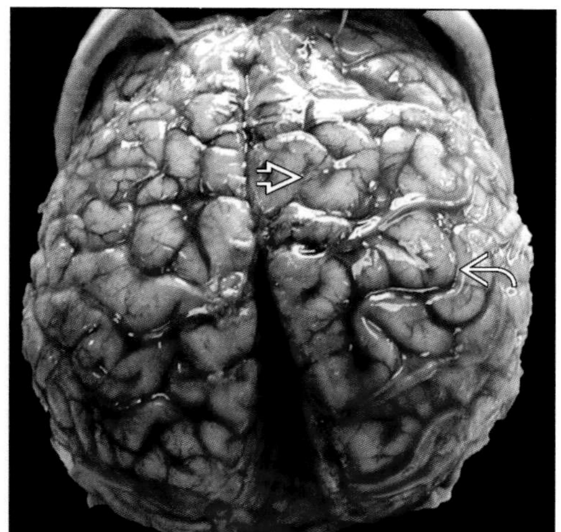

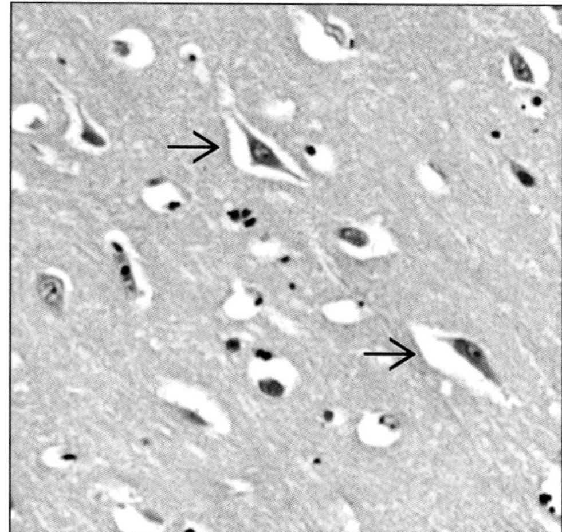

(Left) *At autopsy, this brain demonstrated severe cerebral edema with swollen, flattened gyri* ➪ *and narrowed sulci* ➪*. Cerebellar tonsil herniation was also present (not shown).* ***(Right)*** *This is the cerebrum of the same patient with diffuse hypoxic nerve cell change* → *. The neurons are shrunken and triangular.*

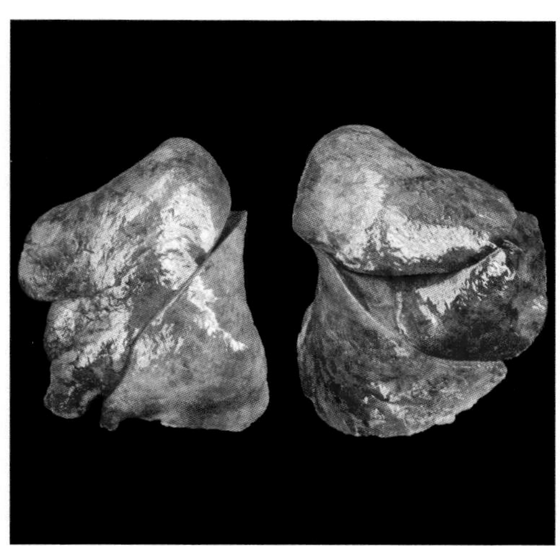

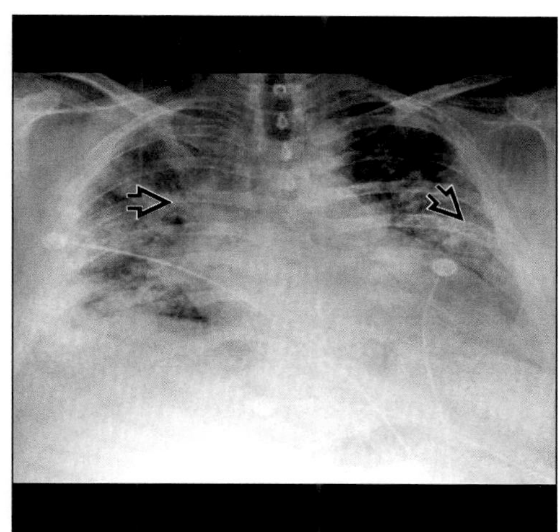

(Left) *These lungs from a patient dying of H1N1 influenza were profoundly edematous and congested (weight was 4x upper limit normal). There was widespread diffuse alveolar damage of 1 week duration present microscopically.* ***(Right)*** *This chest x-ray of the same patient demonstrates diffuse bilateral infiltrates* ➪ *(white-out). The costovertebral angles and cardiac silhouette are difficult to visualize due to the infiltrates.*

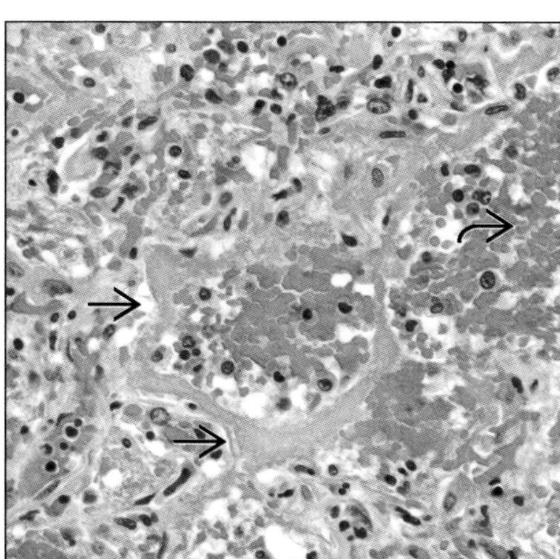

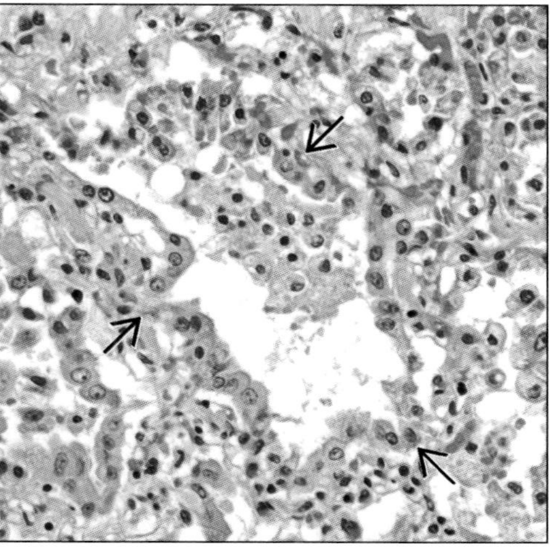

(Left) *The microscopic features of diffuse alveolar damage of less than 1 week duration are shown here, including hyaline membrane formation* → *and intra-alveolar hemorrhage* ➪*.* ***(Right)*** *Diffuse alveolar damage of greater than 1 week duration is seen in this image, with resolution of the acute changes with extensive type II pneumocyte hyperplasia along the alveoli* → *. Marked interstitial fibrosis may result as well (not shown here).*

SHOCK AND SEPSIS

Gross and Microscopic Features

__(Left)__ Diffuse petechiae of the skin are a frequent finding in patients dying of shock due to terminal coagulopathy. __(Right)__ The visceral and parietal serosa also frequently demonstrated petechial hemorrhages in coagulopathy associated with shock and sepsis.

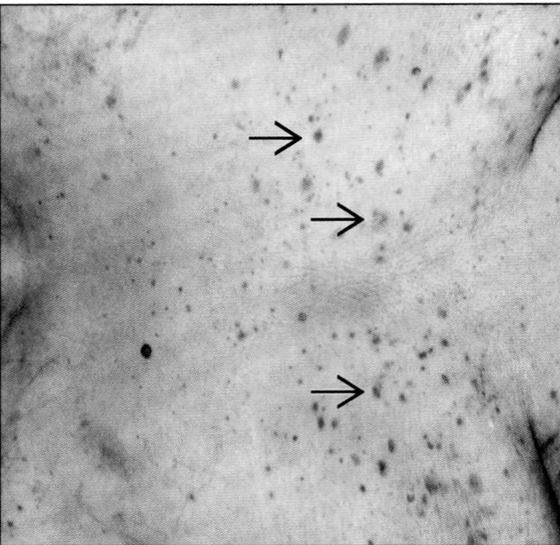

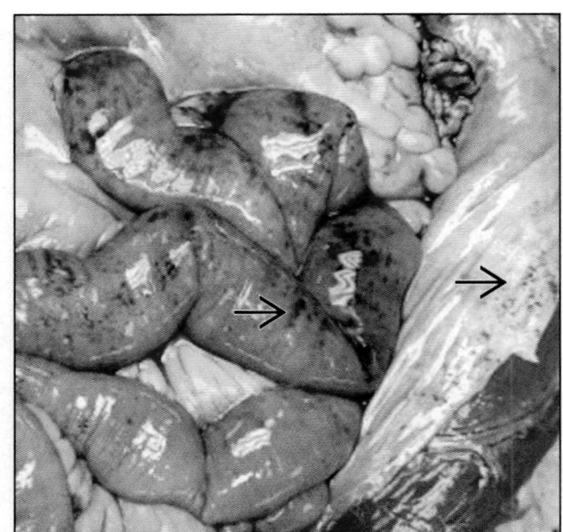

__(Left)__ This pancreas contained numerous thrombi of the microvasculature in a patient dying of disseminated intravascular coagulation. Other organs involved included the heart, lungs, and adrenal glands. An uninvolved, patent venule is also shown for comparison. __(Right)__ This autopsy heart, opened through the tricuspid valve to view the right atrium and ventricles, shows multiple friable vegetations on the closing surface and cords of the valve (bacterial endocarditis).

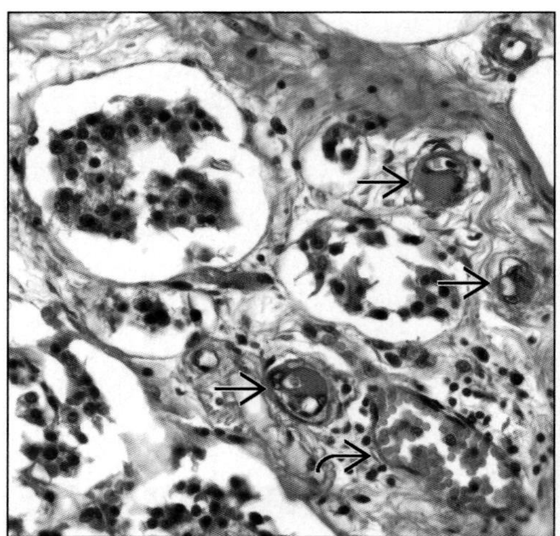

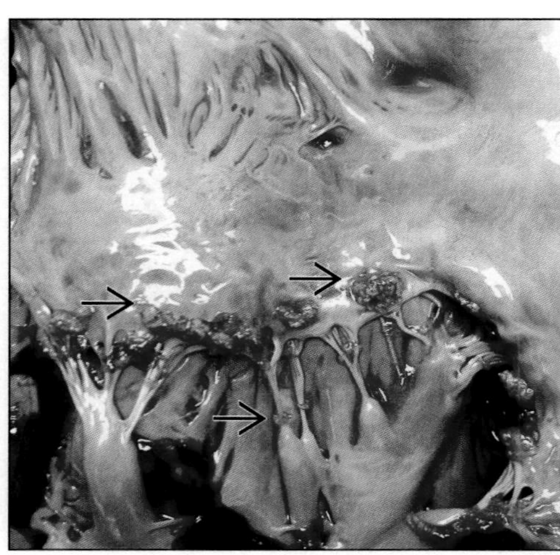

__(Left)__ This photomicrograph of the heart with a right atrial subendocardial abscess shows neutrophilic inflammation and bacterial colonies. Normal myocardium is seen at the lower left for reference. __(Right)__ This photomicrograph of the lung from the same patient with right atrial abscess shows a septic embolus in a pulmonary artery branch.

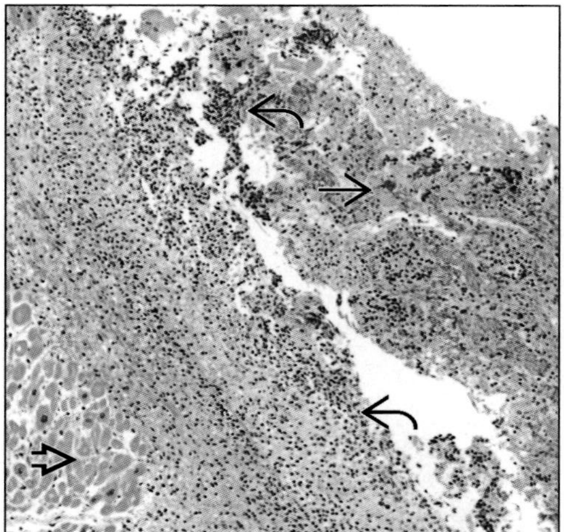

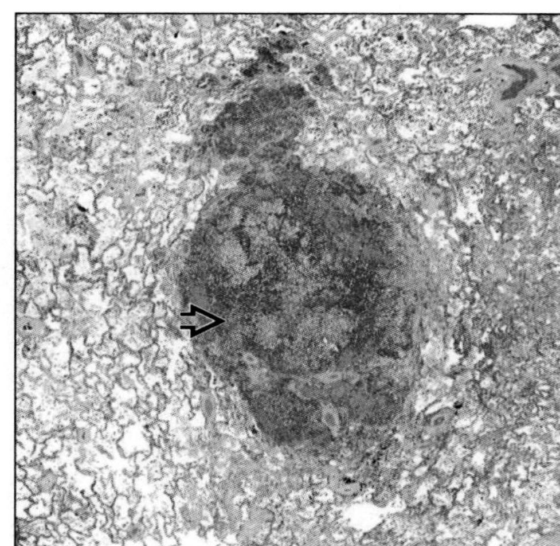

Gross and Microscopic Features

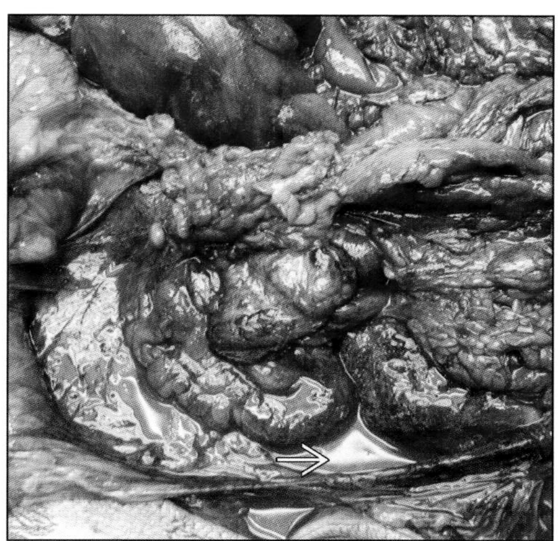
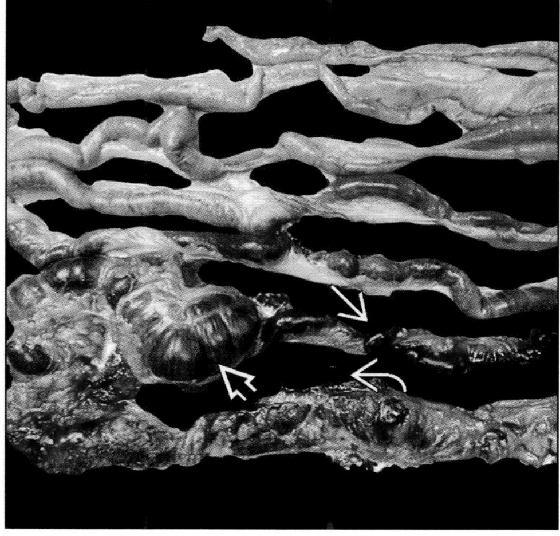

(Left) A perforation in the small bowel in this patient caused acute peritonitis with fecopurulent fluid ➡ within the peritoneal cavity, ultimately leading to septic shock and death. *(Right)* The dark black discoloration of the distal small bowel ➡ and colon ➡ is due to a massive lower gastrointestinal bleed, which caused the patient to exsanguinate. The lumen contained dark liquid blood ➡.

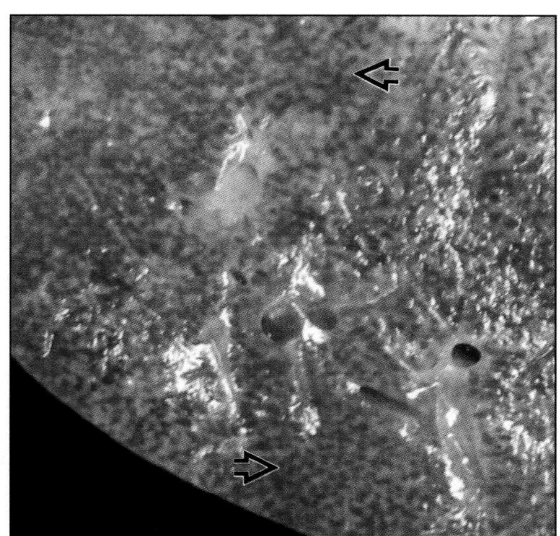
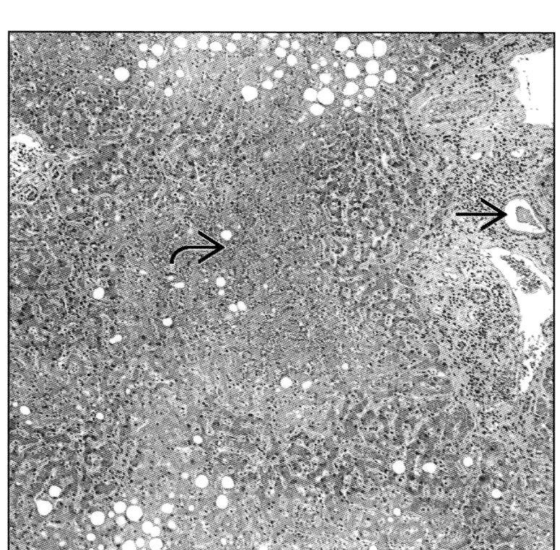

(Left) The variegated, "nutmeg" ➡ appearance of the cut surface of the liver is due to passive congestion from a lack of adequate forward flow blood circulation. *(Right)* This photomicrograph from the same liver shows centrilobular hemorrhagic necrosis ➡ and ductal cholestasis ➡ microscopically.

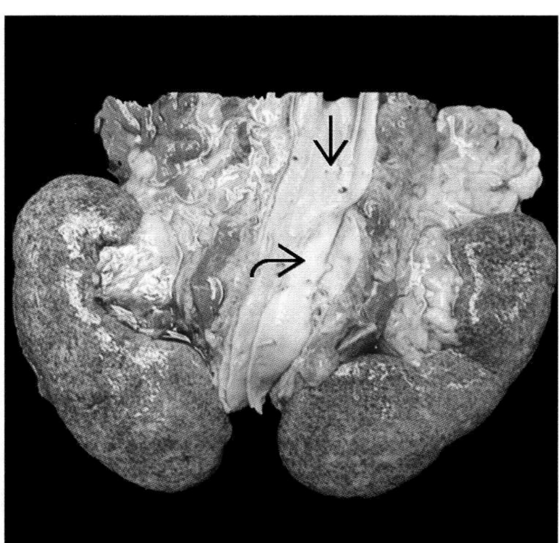
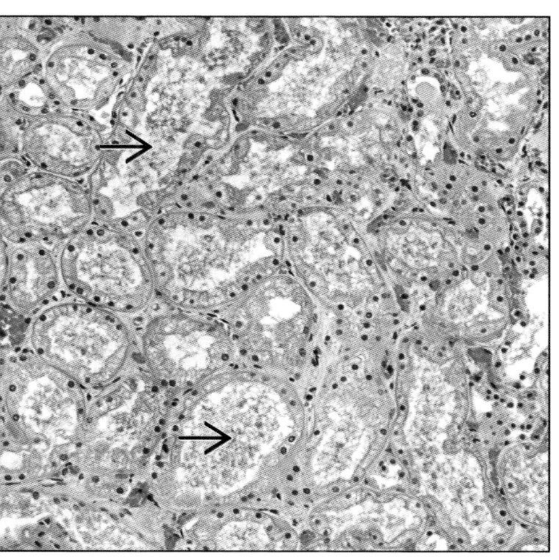

(Left) These severely mottled kidneys are from a patient dying of hemorrhagic shock due to a dissecting aortic aneurysm originating in the thoracic aorta. The true lumen ➡ and false lumen ➡ of the aorta are shown, with a medial flap separating them. *(Right)* This kidney shows acute tubular necrosis (ATN) with dilated proximal tubules ➡. Autolysis often precludes definitive evaluation of the nuclear and cytoplasmic changes of ATN.

BRONCHOPNEUMONIA

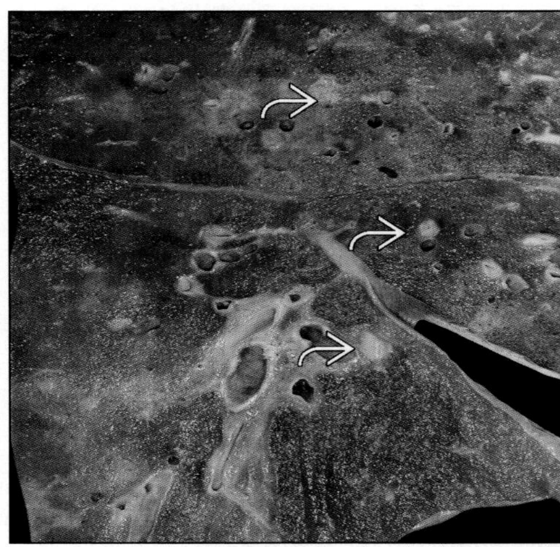

This gross photograph of a lung shows bronchopneumonia with foci of consolidation centered on the airway ➔ and often most pronounced in the basilar regions.

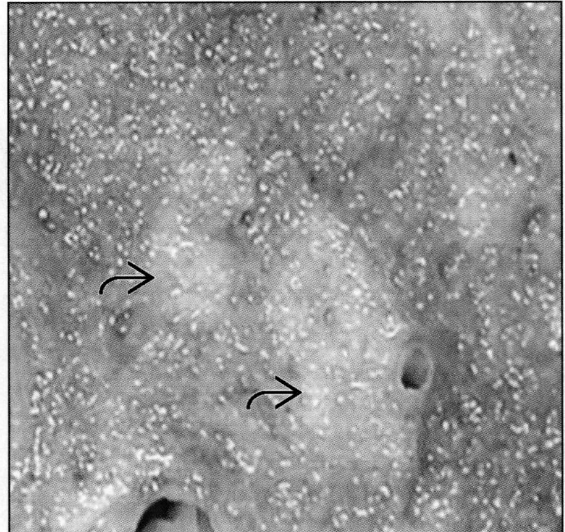

Foci of bronchopneumonia are typically 1-3 cm in diameter and poorly circumscribed ➔.

TERMINOLOGY

Definitions

- Pneumonia is classified by specific etiologic agent; however, if no pathogen can be isolated, clinical setting in which infection occurs is used as a guide for therapy
  - Community-acquired pneumonia (CAP): Pneumonia acquired outside of health care setting
    - Most common type of pneumonia
    - ↑ incidence in winter
    - ~ 20% of patients with CAP will require hospitalization
    - Up to 50% of CAP have no pathogen identified
    - Atypical Pneumonia: Old terminology for CAP with milder symptoms, scant sputum, and lack of response to penicillin
  - Hospital-acquired pneumonia: Acquired while in hospital for another illness (synonym: Nosocomial pneumonia)
    - Patients tend to be sicker due to underlying illness
    - ↑ risk of antibiotic-resistant bacteria
  - Health care-associated pneumonia: Acquired in a nonhospital health care setting such as nursing home, dialysis center, outpatient clinic
- Pathologic definition of bronchopneumonia is based on anatomic distribution of acute inflammatory changes
  - Pathologic changes can be appreciated grossly as patchy foci of airway-centered consolidation with intervening areas of normal lung parenchyma (lobular distribution)
    - This lobular pattern is in contrast to lobar pneumonia, which is consolidation of an entire lobe
  - Pathologic changes can be appreciated microscopically as foci of airway-centered inflammation with contiguous involvement of peribronchial/peribronchiolar alveolated parenchyma

ETIOLOGY/PATHOGENESIS

Pathogenesis

- Microorganisms reach lung by 4 basic mechanisms
  - Inhalation
  - Aspiration (primarily from a previously colonized oropharynx)
  - Hematogenous spread
  - Direct extension from an adjacent focus of infection
- In most circumstances, pathologic entity of bronchopneumonia is result of inhalation and aspiration
- Endotracheal tube placement further compromises host defenses by impairing mucociliary function, injuring mucosa, and allowing secretions to pool
- More likely in patients with other comorbidities
- More common in patients with an impaired immune response (due to immunosuppressive medications, underlying immunodeficiency disease, or critical illness)
- More common with a large inoculum (such as occurs with massive aspiration)
- More common in patients with genetic differences, which are a focus of ongoing research
- A preceding viral pneumonia increases susceptibility to bacterial pneumonia

Infectious Agents

- Bacteria
  - Gram positive: *Staphylococcus aureus, Streptococcus pneumoniae* (most common cause of lobar pneumonia)
  - Gram negative: *Haemophilus influenzae, Moraxella catarrhalis, Escherichia coli, Legionella pneumophila, Pseudomonas aeruginosa, Klebsiella pneumoniae*

BRONCHOPNEUMONIA

Key Facts

Terminology

- Pathologic definition of bronchopneumonia based on anatomic distribution of acute inflammatory changes
- Distribution can be appreciated grossly as patchy foci of airway-centered consolidation with intervening areas of normal lung parenchyma (lobular distribution)
- Lobular pattern is in contrast to lobar pneumonia (consolidation of an entire lobe)
- Pneumonia is classified by specific etiologic agent

Etiology

- Most often result of inhalation of microorganisms or aspiration
- A preceding viral pneumonia increases susceptibility to secondary infection (bronchopneumonia)
- Nosocomial pneumonia is leading cause of death from hospital-acquired infection
- Gram-negative organisms predominate in ICU-acquired infections and ventilator-associated pneumonia

Macroscopic Pathology

- May involve 1 or multiple lobes and is frequently bilateral
- Most pronounced changes often in basilar regions

Microscopic Pathology

- Airway-centered acute inflammation with contiguous involvement of peribronchial/peribronchiolar alveolated parenchyma
- Focal or extensive organization may be present

- Gram-negative organisms predominate in ICU-acquired infections and ventilator-associated pneumonia, particularly *P. aeruginosa*, *Acinetobacter baumannii*, and Enterobacteriaceae
- Viruses and fungal organisms can cause bronchopneumonia, mainly in immunocompromised patients
  - Herpes viruses, *Candida* spp, and *Aspergillus* spp most common
- Agents associated with community-acquired "atypical pneumonia" include
  - Bacteria: *Mycoplasma pneumoniae*, *Legionella* spp., *Chlamydia* spp., *Coxiella burnetii*
  - Viruses: Respiratory syncytial virus, adenovirus, and influenzas A and B
- Progressive primary pulmonary tuberculosis can resemble an acute bacterial pneumonia

CLINICAL ISSUES

Epidemiology

- Incidence
  - Only a small percentage of those patients requiring hospitalization for CAP will die, usually of complications related to pneumonia (such as empyema, meningitis, or endocarditis) or because of a debilitated state
    - Nosocomial pneumonia: 2nd most common cause of nosocomial infection and leading cause of death from hospital-acquired infection
  - Mechanical ventilation is the leading risk factor for development of nosocomial pneumonia
- Age
  - Very young and elderly are more susceptible than other patient populations

Presentation

- Shortness of breath, fever, productive cough, malaise, and pleuritic chest pain

Laboratory Tests

- Check premortem sputum and blood culture results
- Elevated WBC with left shift and ↑ bands (low WBC in patients who have underlying neutropenia and sometimes with severe infection)
- Thrombocytopenia, elevated fibrin degradation products (sepsis, DIC)
- Cold agglutinins: Not specific for Mycoplasma but if high titer cold agglutinin (> 1:64) in CAP = high likelihood of mycoplasma
- Increased liver function tests and elevated creatinine (organ system injury from sepsis/shock) and lactic acid (shock)
- Serologic evidence of infection: Paired sera to look for antibodies to *Mycoplasma*, *Chlamydia* influenza A and B, adenovirus, and respiratory syncytial virus
  - Being replaced by more specific and rapid PCR techniques for organism isolation
- Legionella urine antigen test

Prognosis

- Patients with healthcare-acquired pneumonia (HCAP) typically have a worse clinical course and outcome than those of patients with CAP
- Patients developing necrotizing pneumonia usually have concomitant medical illness, most common being diabetes mellitus and alcohol abuse

IMAGE FINDINGS

Radiographic Findings

- Multifocal, heterogeneous opacities distributed along course of airways and centered in distal airways

MACROSCOPIC FEATURES

External Examination

- Signs of treatment: Endotracheal tube, chest tube (empyema, parapneumonic effusion), central and peripheral intravenous lines

BRONCHOPNEUMONIA

- Chest radiograph prior to autopsy may indicate placement of endotracheal tube, chest tube, presence of effusion, empyema, central line placement
- Follow radiologic safety precautions: Leave room during x-ray procedure if performed in autopsy suite
- Signs of sepsis/shock: Petechiae (DIC), jaundice, pallor

Internal Examination

- Acute pleuritis and fibrinous adhesions may be present in addition to frank empyema
- Fresh lung and spleen tissue should be procured for microbiology cultures before excessive organ manipulation
  - Culture technique: Use sterile equipment (scalpel, forceps), sterilize pleural or capsular surface of organ with either heat (hot spatula or scalpel blade used to sear surface) or iodine and alcohol decontamination of surface
    - Use sterile container for transport to microbiology lab
  - Follow safety precautions if using heat source, check with safety engineers prior to using, and use flame retardant gloves
  - Use universal precautions for all pneumonia autopsies: Personal protective equipment and particulate respirators
- Look for evidence of bacteremic dissemination to other organs

Organ Examination

- Respiratory System: Bronchopneumonia may involve 1 or multiple lobes and is frequently bilateral
  - Most pronounced changes are often in basilar regions
  - Foci of consolidation are centered on airway and are typically 1-3 cm in diameter, poorly circumscribed, and yellow to gray-red in color
    - Consolidation is best appreciated following formalin perfusion
  - Foci of consolidation can expand to near confluence, thereby mimicking lobar pneumonia
    - Gross description should include distribution of consolidated areas as well as complications of pneumonia, such as prominent necrosis (necrotizing pneumonia) and abscess formation
    - Section adequately to document distribution of disease, areas of necrosis or abscess, and noninvolved lung parenchyma
- Other organs
  - Sepsis/shock changes: Pallor of renal cortex (acute tubular injury), softening of liver (shock liver), Ischemic bowel (shock)
  - Disseminated Infection: Vegetations on cardiac valves, disseminated abscesses
  - Cause for underlying immunosuppression: Malignancy, transplantation, etc.

MICROSCOPIC PATHOLOGY

Histologic Features

- Respiratory system
  - Acute bronchitis: Neutrophil-rich suppurative exudate within lumen, and mucosal ulceration/ necrosis
  - Acute pneumonia involving peribronchial/ peribronchiolar alveolated parenchyma
    - Neutrophil-rich intraalveolar fibrinous exudate and active capillary congestion
  - Depending on time course of infection and effectiveness of therapy, focal or extensive organization may be present
    - It is not uncommon in patients with a protracted hospital course to see evidence of multiple episodes of infection, with acute inflammation in 1 region and more advanced organizing pneumonia in others
    - Organizing pneumonia: Polypoid accumulation of granulation tissue in alveolar spaces, ducts, and sometimes in bronchioles

ANCILLARY TESTS

Histochemistry

- Tissue gram, silver, PAS, mucicarmine or acid-fast/ modified acid-fast stains as appropriate

Immunohistochemistry

- Immunohistochemical stains for microorganisms as appropriate

In Situ Hybridization

- In situ hybridization for microorganisms as appropriate

Microbiology

- Tissue culture procured in sterile fashion
- Molecular diagnostic tests, as appropriate

DIFFERENTIAL DIAGNOSIS

Processes That Mimic Gross Consolidation

- Pulmonary hemorrhage
- Diffuse alveolar damage

SELECTED REFERENCES

1. DiBardino DM et al: Aspiration pneumonia: A review of modern trends. J Crit Care. Epub ahead of print, 2014
2. Wunderink RG et al: Community-acquired pneumonia. N Engl J Med. 370(19):1863, 2014
3. Nair GB et al: Nosocomial pneumonia: lessons learned. Crit Care Clin. 29(3):521-46, 2013
4. Peleg AY et al: Hospital-acquired infections due to gram-negative bacteria. N Engl J Med. 362(19):1804-13, 2010

Gross and Microscopic Features

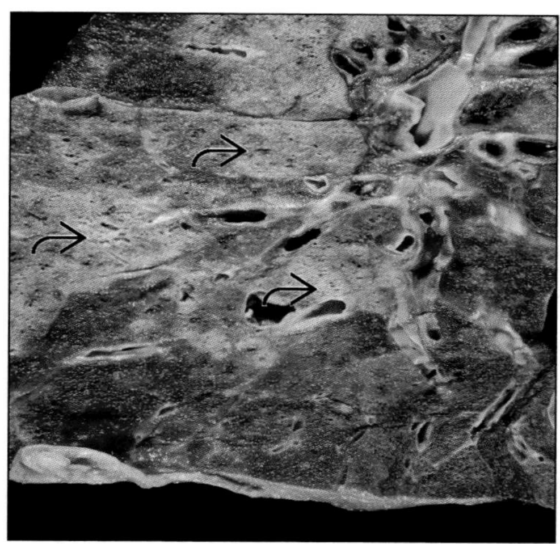

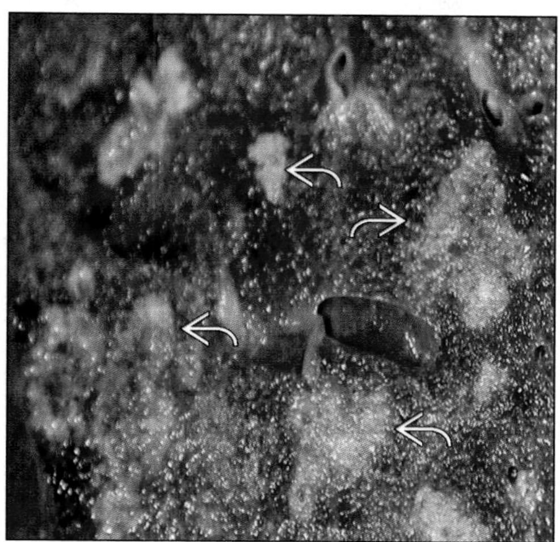

(Left) More confluent areas of bronchopneumonia are pictured here ➩. These areas are paler than the surrounding parenchyma and will feel firmer than the adjacent lung tissue on palpation (consolidation). **(Right)** Gross image shows fungal bronchopneumonia ➩ (Aspergillus spp.). Aspergillus is vasoinvasive and although not demonstrated here, may show a targetoid appearance with consolidation surrounding a central thrombosed vessel.

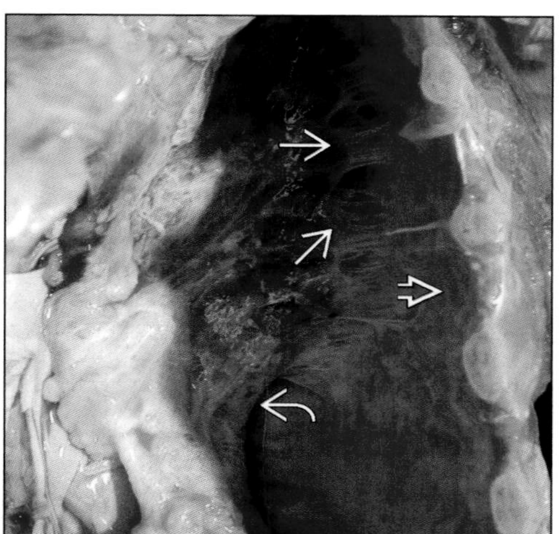

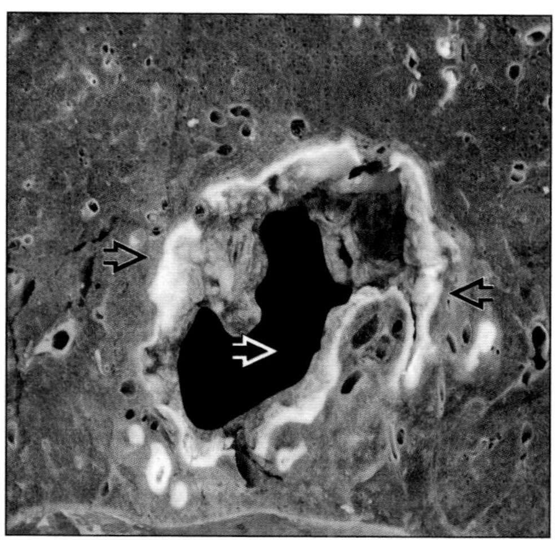

(Left) Fibrinous pleural adhesions are illustrated in this gross image of a patient who had pneumonia with a parapneumonic effusion. The fibrinous strands ➡ coursing between visceral ➩ and parietal ➡ pleura are easily disrupted, as opposed to fibrous adhesions. **(Right)** Abscess cavity formation is a major complication of bronchopneumonia. The necrotic material in the center ➡ has fallen out and we see the edge of the cavity surrounded by white fibrous tissue ➡.

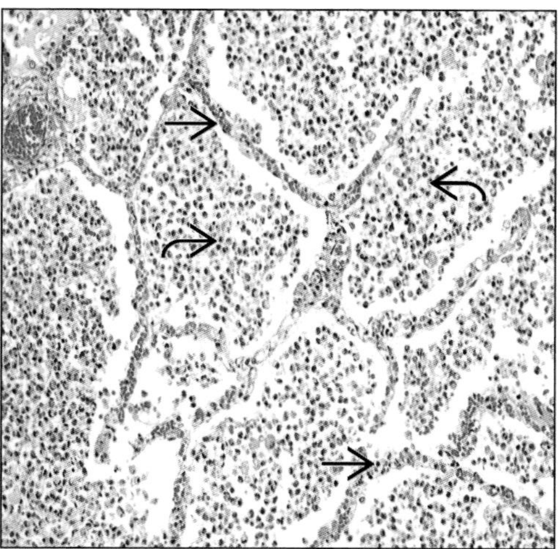

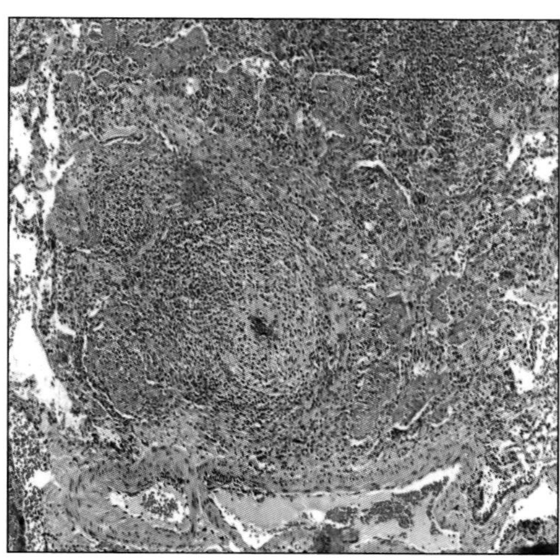

(Left) Neutrophils and fibrin ➩ fill the alveolar spaces in this example of acute pneumonia with congestion ➡. **(Right)** This example of acute pneumonia was ultimately culture-proven as Mycobacterium tuberculosis. Note the single giant cell in the center but the lack of a well-organized granulomatous response in an early primary infection. Universal precautions must be used during autopsies on patients with pneumonia.

INFECTIVE ENDOCARDITIS

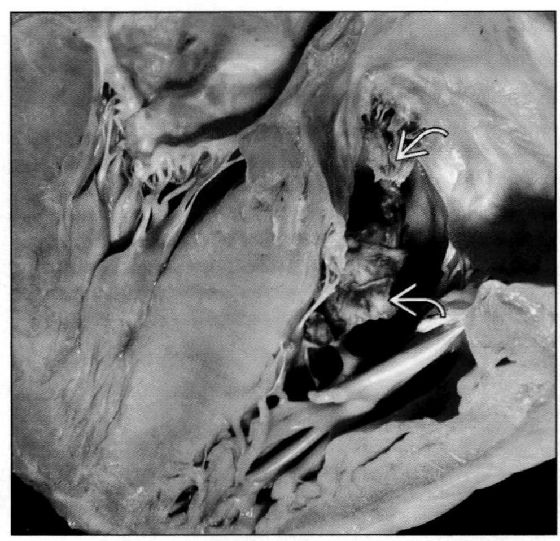

This autopsy heart shows a large pedunculated vegetation ➜ involving the tricuspid valve. The vegetation appears to arise at a septal leaflet commissure.

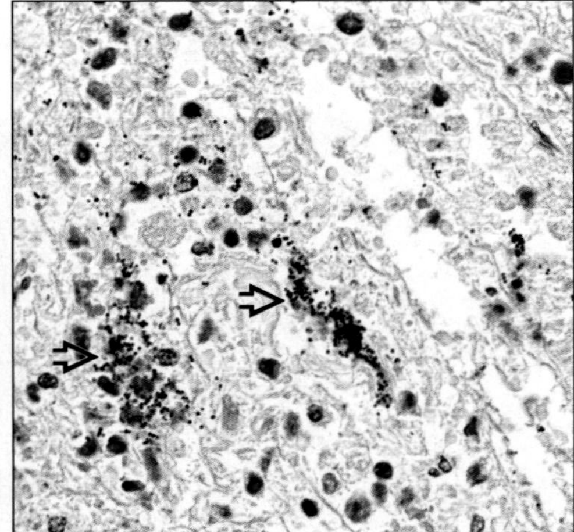

A tissue Gram stain from this vegetation shows gram-positive cocci ➜, the most common type of bacteria seen in endocarditis. Necrotic debris, fibrin, and inflammation are also seen.

TERMINOLOGY

Definitions

- Inflammation of endocardium (typically refers to infections on valve surfaces)

ETIOLOGY/PATHOGENESIS

Infectious Agents

- *Staphylococcus aureus* (31%)
- *Streptococcus viridans* (17%)
- Coagulase-negative staphylococci (11%)
- Enterococci (11%)
- Other streptococci (12%)
- Gram-negative HACEK (*Haemophilus*, *Aggregatibacter*, *Cardiobacterium*, *Eikenella*, and *Kingella* species) (2%)
- Gram-negative non-HACEK (2%)

Risk Factors

- Microbe portal of entry
  - Intravenous drug abuse
  - Indwelling catheter
  - Hemodialysis
  - Dental procedure
- Valve surface damage
  - Degenerative
  - Congenital
  - Rheumatic

CLINICAL ISSUES

Presentation

- 3-10 episodes per 100,000 person-years
- Mean age: 51-65 years
- M > F 1.2-2.5:1
- Hospital mortality rate 9.6-26%
- Acute
  - Distant septic emboli
  - Acute valvular insufficiency
- Subacute
  - Duke criteria
    - Positive blood culture (2 separate draws)
    - Positive imaging study (vegetation by echocardiogram, abscess by CT, etc.)
    - Minor criteria: Predisposition, fever, emboli, glomerulonephritis

Treatment

- Antibiotic therapy (intravenous) often followed by surgery several weeks later

Prosthetic Valve Endocarditis

- More common in people whose native valves had infective endocarditis
  - Often with same organism
- Commonly occurs within 2 years of replacement (incidence 1-6%)
- Presentation
  - Paravalvular leak
  - Valve sewing ring abscess
  - Dehiscence
  - Obstructive vegetation

IMAGE FINDINGS

Echocardiography

- Vegetations
- Regurgitant jets (Doppler)
- Abscesses
- Prosthetic valve dehiscence

MACROSCOPIC FEATURES

External Examination

- Splinter hemorrhages under fingernails

INFECTIVE ENDOCARDITIS

Key Facts

Terminology
- Infective endocarditis: Inflammation of endocardium (typically refers to infections on valve surfaces)

Etiology
- *Staphylococcus aureus* (31%)
- *Streptococcus viridans* (17%)
- Microbe portal of entry
  - Intravenous drug abuse, dental procedure
- Valve surface damage
  - Degenerative, rheumatic, congenital

Clinical Issues
- 3-10 episodes per 100,000 person-years
- Mean age: 51-65 years
- M > F (1.2-2.5:1)
- Hospital mortality rate 9.6-26%

Macroscopic Pathology
- Vegetations
  - Fleshy, soft, clot-like, friable
  - Septic emboli and infarcts (brain, spleen, kidneys, liver)

Microscopic Pathology
- Vegetations
  - Acute: Fibrin, platelets, neutrophils, microorganisms
  - Subacute: Granulation tissue, fibroblasts, collagen, plasma cells, absent microbes
- Valve annulus abscess
- Myocardial abscess

Top Differential Diagnoses
- Nonbacterial thrombotic endocarditis

- Janeway lesions: Flat macules, especially on hands and feet
- Osler nodes: Red raised lesions of hands and feet
- Conjunctival hemorrhage

Heart Findings
- Vegetations
  - Typically atrial aspect of atrioventricular valves and ventricular aspect of semilunar valves
  - Fleshy, soft, clot-like, friable
- Ruptured cordae
- Leaflet perforation
- Cusp aneurysm (old healed endocarditis)
- Infraction (septic emboli to coronary arteries)
- Perivalvular (ring) abscess

Extracardiac Findings
- Septic emboli and infarcts (brain, spleen, kidneys, liver)
- Mycotic (pseudo) aneurysms
- Glomerulonephritis (endocarditis-associated postinfectious type)
- Secondary infection of abdominal aortic aneurysm

MICROSCOPIC PATHOLOGY

Histologic Features
- Vegetations
  - Acute: Fibrin, platelets, neutrophils, microorganisms
  - Subacute: Granulation tissue, fibroblasts, collagen, plasma cells, absent microbes
- Tendinous cord and leaflet destruction, erosion
- Valve annulus abscess
- Myocardial abscess

DIFFERENTIAL DIAGNOSIS

Nonbacterial Thrombotic Endocarditis
- Fibrin, platelets, without bacteria or purulent inflammation
- Typically, small, dotting closing surfaces of leaflets
- Specific types
  - Marantic: Associated with malignancy
  - Libman-Sacks: Associated with lupus, other autoimmune disease

SELECTED REFERENCES

1. Erdozain JG et al: Cardiac valve replacement in patients with antiphospholipid syndrome. Arthritis Care Res (Hoboken). 64(8):1256-60, 2012
2. Asopa S et al: Non-bacterial thrombotic endocarditis. Eur J Cardiothorac Surg. 32(5):696-701, 2007
3. Aryana A et al: Nonbacterial thrombotic endocarditis with recurrent embolic events as manifestation of ovarian neoplasm. J Gen Intern Med. 21(12):C12-5, 2006
4. Edoute Y et al: Cardiac valvular vegetations in cancer patients: a prospective echocardiographic study of 200 patients. Am J Med. 102(3):252-8, 1997
5. Lopez JA et al: Nonbacterial thrombotic endocarditis: a review. Am Heart J. 113(3):773-84, 1987
6. Deppisch LM et al: Non-bacterial thrombotic endocarditis: clinicopathologic correlations. Am Heart J. 92(6):723-9, 1976
7. MACDONALD RA et al: The significance of nonbacterial thrombotic endocarditis: an autopsy and clinical study of 78 cases. Ann Intern Med. 46(2):255-73, 1957
8. Allen AC et al: The morphogenesis and significance of degenerative verrucal endocardiosis (terminal endocarditis, endocarditis simplex, nonbacterial thrombotic endocarditis). Am J Pathol. 20(6):1025-55, 1944

INFECTIVE ENDOCARDITIS

Gross Features

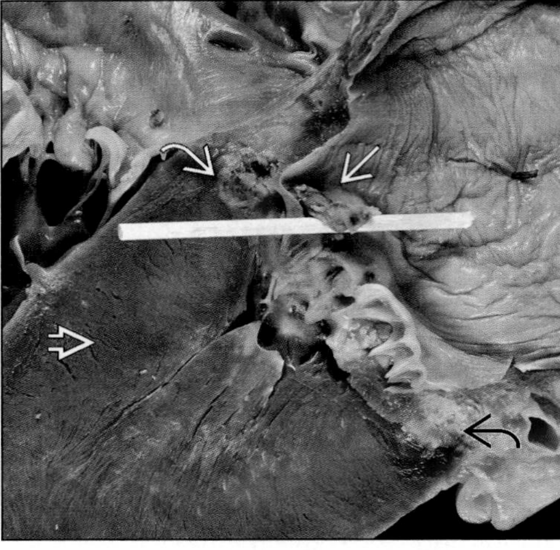

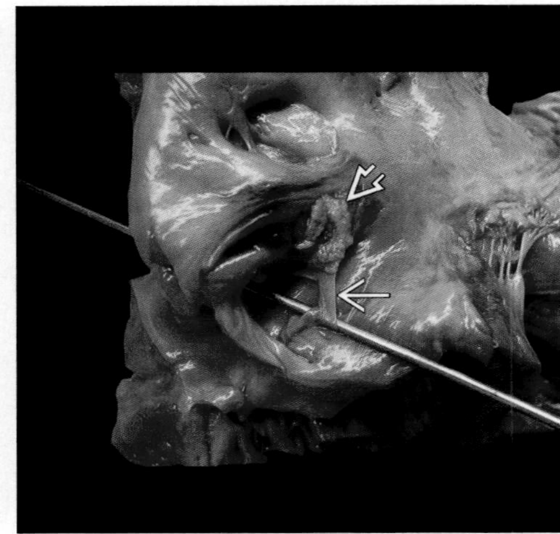

(Left) *This autopsy heart shows a friable vegetation ➡ associated with the mitral valve. Significant left ventricular hypertrophy ➡ and mitral annular calcification ➡ are also present in this elderly person (unrelated to endocarditis).* ***(Right)*** *Endocarditis can involve other nonvalvular endocardial surfaces also, such as this right atrial vegetation ➡ associated with an infected catheter tip. The metal probe passes under the thebesian valve of the coronary sinus ostium ➡.*

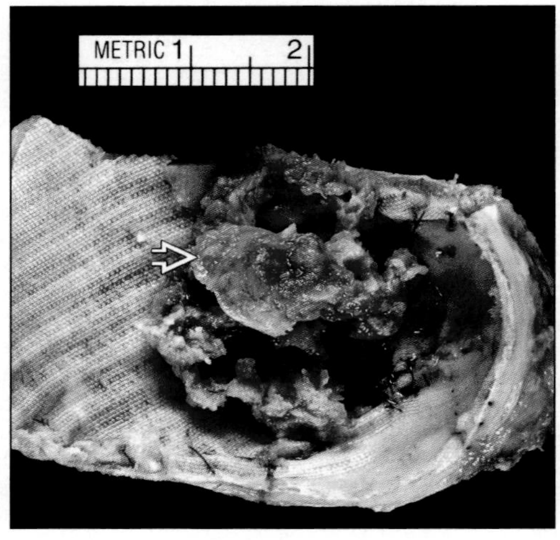

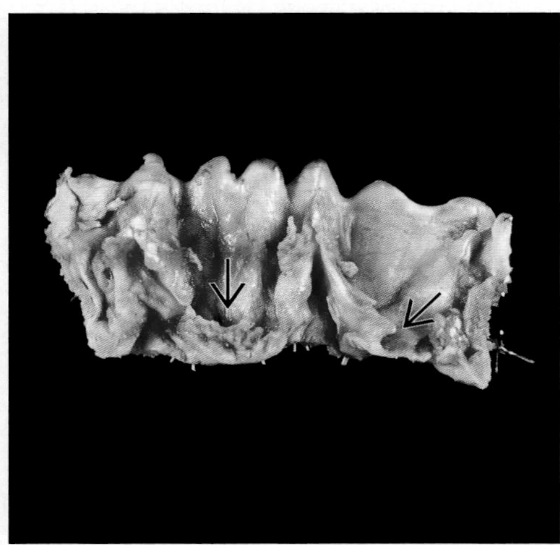

(Left) *Endocarditis can also involve prostheses, such as this valved conduit specimen. The texture of the vegetation ➡ is similar to thrombus and is often crumbly and friable. Embolic potential of masses like this is obvious.* ***(Right)*** *The leaflets ➡ of this Melody valve prosthesis have been perforated and eroded by active endocarditis. The cusp edges show fleshy, friable, pink vegetative material.*

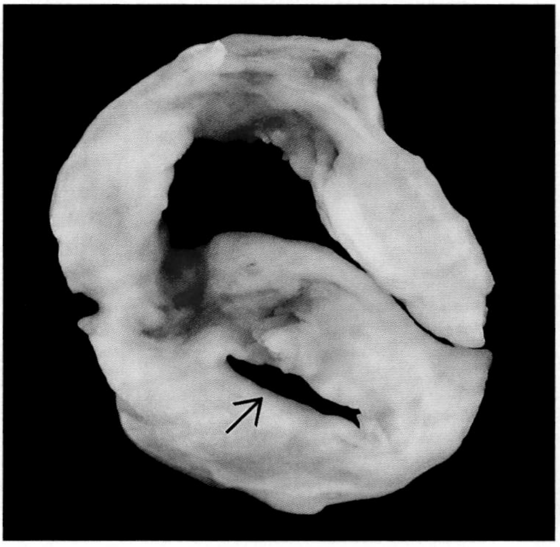

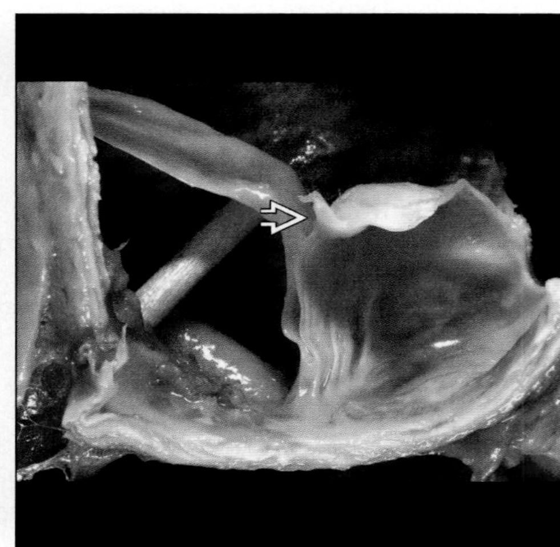

(Left) *This congenitally malformed aortic valve was secondarily infected. Old healed endocarditis has resulted in persistent leaflet perforation ➡ that would have resulted in significant valvular incompetence. The leaflet shows significant thickening due to fibroelastosis, consistent with postinflammatory disease.* ***(Right)*** *Lambl excrescences ➡, as seen on this aortic valve cusp, are normal anatomic variants and should not be mistaken for endocarditis.*

Microscopic Features

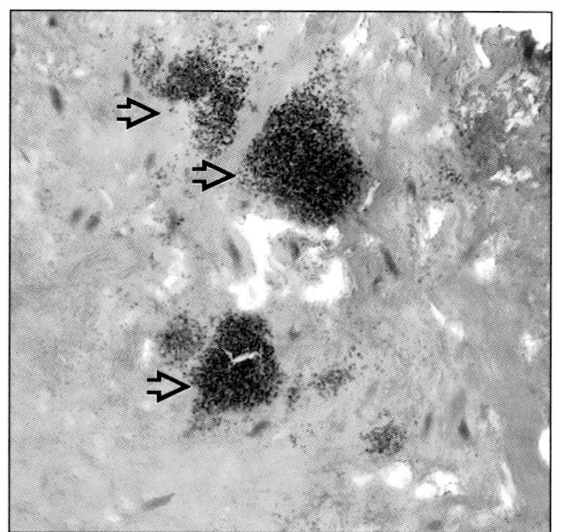

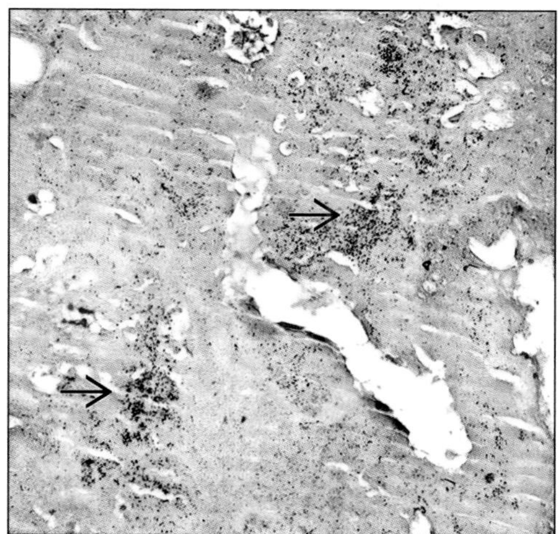

(Left) *"Colonies" or clusters of bacterial organisms ⇨ can often be seen well on the H&E stain alone in active endocarditis. Gram staining is needed to assess the Gram reaction. After prolonged antibiotic treatment, they may be harder to appreciate.* ***(Right)*** *Tissue Gram staining is helpful in narrowing the diagnosis to a particular class of microbes (in this case, gram-positive cocci →). Organisms are more likely to be identified in the absence of antibiotic treatment.*

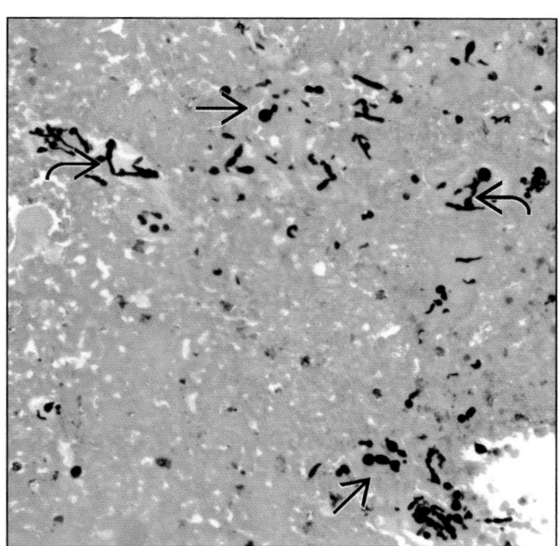

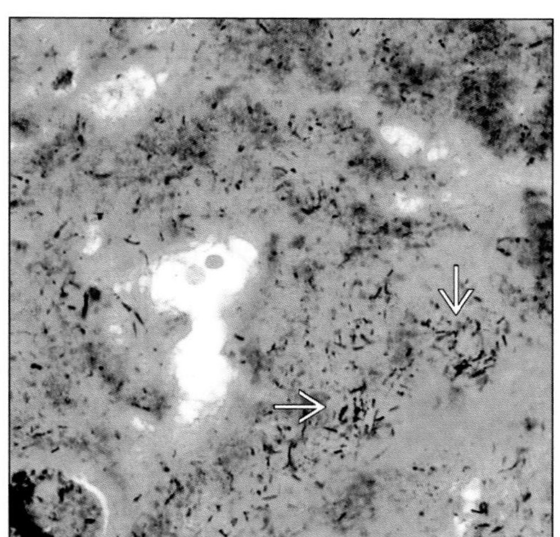

(Left) *Fungal endocarditis is most commonly due to Candida species. The yeast forms in Candida infections show both budding → and pseudohyphae ↪. Candida vegetations are typically very bulky and obstructive.* ***(Right)*** *This tissue Gram stain of an endocarditis vegetation demonstrates gram-positive rods →, such as may be seen in infections due to Erysipelothrix or Nocardia.*

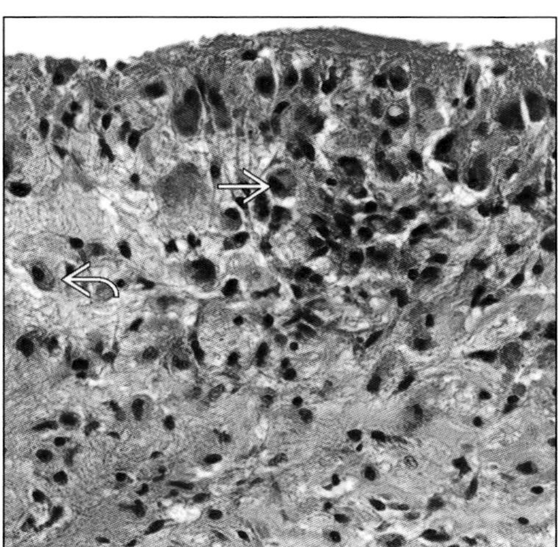

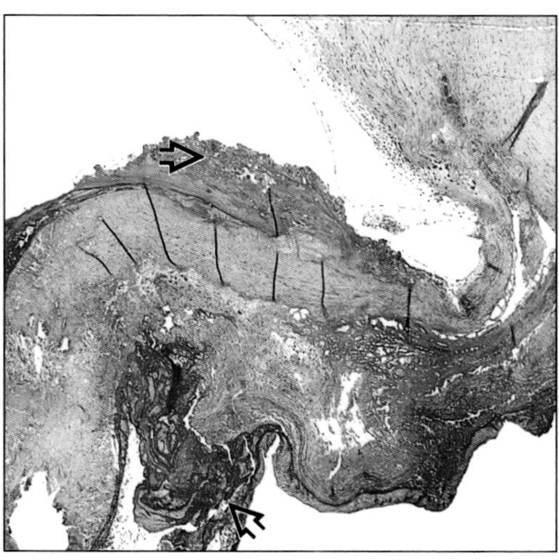

(Left) *In cases of subacute or healing endocarditis, there may be a predominance of plasma cells → and macrophages ↪ rather than neutrophils. Organisms are rarely present at this stage of endocarditis.* ***(Right)*** *This elastic-stained mitral leaflet shows vegetative material ⇨ on both sides of the valve. Classically, endocarditis is destructive and disrupts the normal trilaminar architecture of the valves. Evidence of destruction persists after healing and may be a helpful clue.*

CLOSTRIDIUM DIFFICILE ENTEROCOLITIS

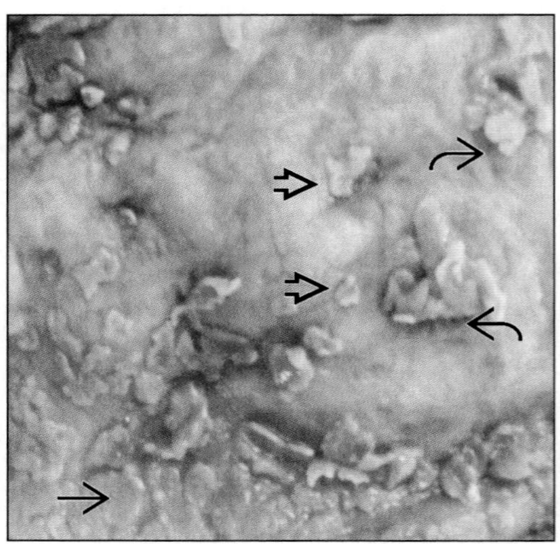

This colonic mucosa is covered with small ⇨ to confluent ⇨ pseudomembranes. They are green-yellow and focally lift off of the mucosal surface ⇨.

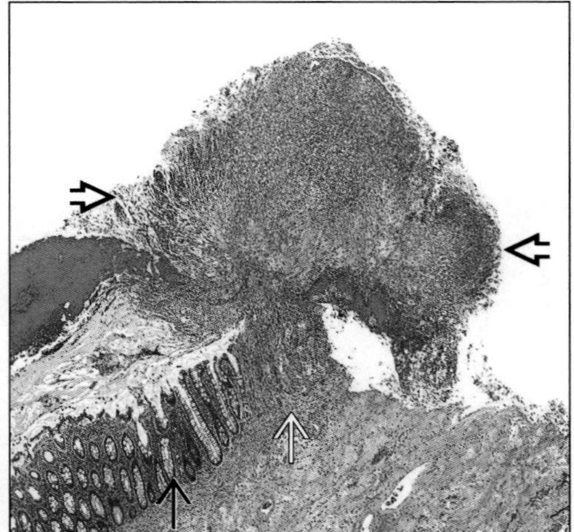

A pseudomembrane ⇨ of Clostridium difficile enterocolitis is classically mushroom shaped. Abrupt transition from normal ⇨ to affected ➡ mucosa is also characteristic.

TERMINOLOGY

Synonyms

- Pseudomembranous enterocolitis or colitis, *Clostridium difficile*-associated disease (CDAD), antibiotic or clindamycin-associated colitis

Definitions

- Colitis due to toxins of *C. difficile* organism

ETIOLOGY/PATHOGENESIS

Infectious Agents

- *C. difficile*
  - Anaerobic gram-positive spore-forming bacterium
    - Dormant spore form resistant to antibiotics/heat; may remain in environment for months to years
    - Vegetative (nondormant), toxin-producing form
    - Fastidious; "difficile" derived from difficulty growing organism in culture

Pathogenesis

- Altered gut flora → colonization (usually nosocomial), fecal-oral
  - Host factors + organism virulence → disease
- Disease due to effects of toxins A and B
  - A: Enterotoxin: Marked fluid exudation from bowel
  - B: Cytotoxin: Affects actin polymerization
- Hypervirulent NAP-1 strain
  - ↑ virulence ↑ renal failure ↑ toxic megacolon

CLINICAL ISSUES

Epidemiology

- Incidence
  - Age-adjusted death rate: 2.4/100,000 in standard population (2011)
    - ↑ 9.1% from 2010
  - 17th leading cause of death in patients ≥ 65 years of age (2011)
- Age
  - More common in older individuals (≥ 60 years)
- Risk factors
  - Age, hospitalization (prolonged or intensive care unit), prior CDAD, current or prior antibiotic use, underlying severe illness, immunosuppression (solid organ and bone marrow transplant patients susceptible to severe disease), bypass of gastric acid (medications or enteral feeds)

Presentation

- Diffuse watery diarrhea, abdominal pain, fever
- Acute renal failure, sepsis, and shock progressing to death
- Uncommon extraintestinal symptoms
  - Large joint arthritis, osteomyelitis, and splenic abscess

Laboratory Tests

- Leukocytosis and elevated creatinine
- Electrolyte disturbances (dehydration), ↓ albumin (protein-losing enteropathy), ↑ lactate (septic shock)
- Enzyme immunoassay for toxins A and B and PCR for *C. difficile* toxin gene

IMAGE FINDINGS

Radiographic Findings

- Nodular haustral thickening
- Dilated colon, ileus, pneumatosis (severe disease)

CT Findings

- Thickened bowel wall (most common finding), mild pericolonic stranding

CLOSTRIDIUM DIFFICILE ENTEROCOLITIS

Key Facts

Etiology
- Altered gut flora → colonization (usually nosocomial), fecal-oral
- Host factors + organism virulence → disease
- Disease due to effects of toxins A and B
  - A: Enterotoxin: Marked fluid exudation from bowel
  - B: Cytotoxin: Affects actin polymerization

Macroscopic Pathology
- Changes due to prolonged severe diarrhea, colitis, and protein-losing enteropathy
- Dehydration changes (skin tenting, sunken eyes), raw-appearing anal tissue with possible tissue breakdown, often with decubitus ulcer
- Distended abdomen
- Generalized edema (anasarca)

Microscopic Pathology
- Patchy process involving clusters of crypts surrounded by normal-appearing mucosa
  - Dilated crypt erupts into bowel lumen as pseudomembrane
  - Epithelial cells lining involved crypts are necrotic
  - Inflammation is superficial in crypts and pseudomembrane
- Pseudomembrane composed of mucus, neutrophils, fibrin and necrotic epithelium
- Severe disease has mucosal necrosis and deep mural inflammation
- Other organ changes
  - Sepsis-related acute tubular injury, patchy hepatic necrosis

MACROSCOPIC FEATURES

External Examination
- Sepsis changes: Petechiae, secondary acrocyanosis, jaundice
- Surgical intervention: Laparotomy incision ± ostomy
- Changes due to prolonged severe diarrhea and colitis and protein-losing enteropathy
  - Dehydration (skin tenting, sunken eyes), raw-appearing anal tissue with possible tissue breakdown, possible decubitus ulcer
  - Distended abdomen, anasarca

Internal Examination
- Serous ascites (protein loss), fibrinopurulent ascites (toxic megacolon, perforation)
- Dusky, dilated colon (if toxic megacolon)
- Surgical bowel anastomosis ± ostomy

Organ Examination
- Bowel wall edema; mucoid, liquid, sometimes blood-speckled bowel content
- Green-yellow pseudomembranes
  - 2-10 mm in early disease
  - Confluent, with ulcerated mucosa, severe disease
- Splenic abscess: Rare extraintestinal manifestation
- Pallor of renal cortex (acute tubular injury), patchy hepatic necrosis (shock)

MICROSCOPIC PATHOLOGY

Histologic Features
- Patchy process: Affected crypts, intervening normal-appearing mucosa
- Dilated crypt erupts into bowel lumen as pseudomembrane
- Epithelial cells lining involved crypts are necrotic
- Inflammation is superficial in crypts and pseudomembrane
  - Pseudomembrane composed of mucus, neutrophils, fibrin, and necrotic epithelium
- Lamina propria intact (no ischemia)
- Severe disease: Mucosal necrosis and deep mural inflammation
- Other organs: Acute tubular necrosis, patchy hepatic necrosis, subendocardial ischemia, heart failure (usually underlying coronary artery/ischemic heart disease)

DIFFERENTIAL DIAGNOSIS

Pseudomembranous Colitis
- Nonantibiotic drug-induced colitis (chlorpropamide, NSAIDs)
- Colitis caused by other organisms: Verotoxin-producing *Escherichia coli*, *Staphylococcus aureus*

REPORTING CRITERIA

Final Report
- Presence of *C. difficile* colitis (after ruling out other causes of pseudomembranous colitis), severity of disease, associated findings (shock, etc.)
  - State whether it was cause of death, contributing factor, or incidental
- Risk factors for developing disease
  - Severe underlying illness, transplantation, clinical history of prior antibiotic therapy
- Implication of finding
  - Unsuspected disease in hospitalized patient warrants institutional infection control notification to avoid spread of disease

SELECTED REFERENCES

1. Hurley BW et al: The spectrum of pseudomembranous enterocolitis and antibiotic-associated diarrhea. Arch Intern Med. 162(19):2177-84, 2002
2. Totten MA et al: Clinical and pathological spectrum of antibiotic-associated colitis. Am J Gastroenterol. 69(3 Pt 1):311-9, 1978

CLOSTRIDIUM DIFFICILE ENTEROCOLITIS

Clostridium difficile Colitis and Ischemic Colitis

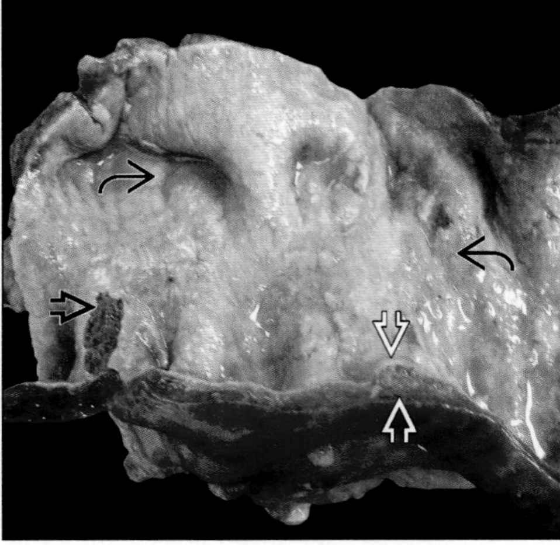

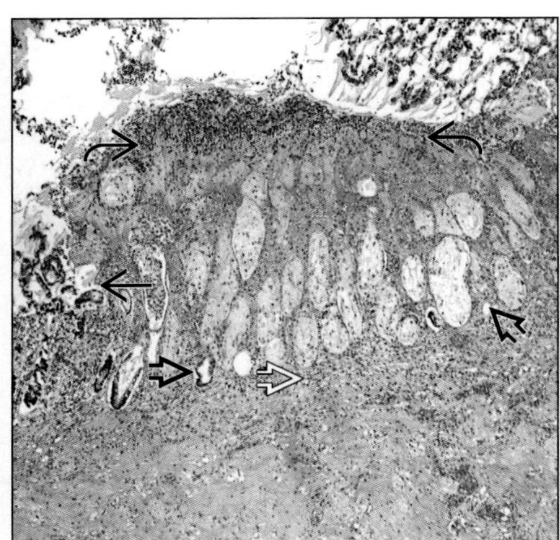

(Left) *The green-yellow pseudomembrane ➩ in this colon is confluent. Only focal ulcerated mucosa is visible ➩. The bowel wall is thickened and edematous ➩.* ***(Right)*** *Pseudomembranous colitis is patchy, involving small clusters of crypts ➩ with epithelial cell necrosis and overlying necrotic debris of pseudomembrane ➩ with abrupt transition to normal glands ➩. There is limited inflammation in the lamina propria ➩.*

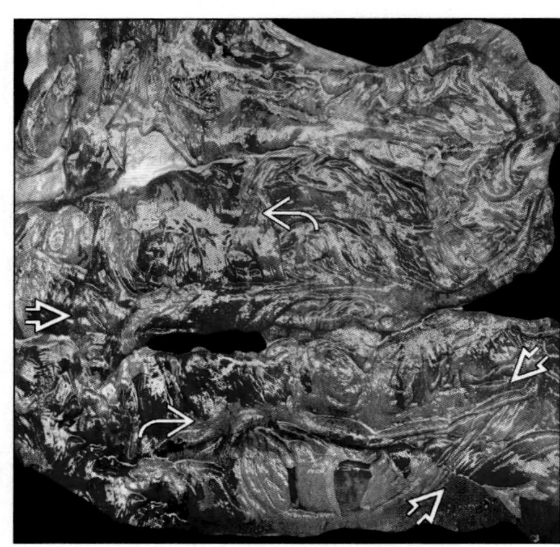

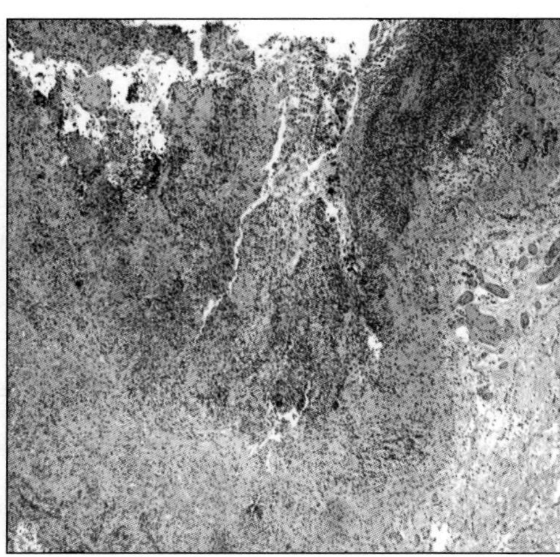

(Left) *The pseudomembranes ➩ on the mucosal surface of this colon are well demarcated and arise in the setting of ischemic colitis. The mucosa between the pseudomembranes is dusky ➩, and histology showed ischemic colitis.* ***(Right)*** *At low power, ischemic colitis shows more involvement of the submucosa with edema and inflammation and necrosis in severe cases and is much more cellular than pseudomembranous colitis.*

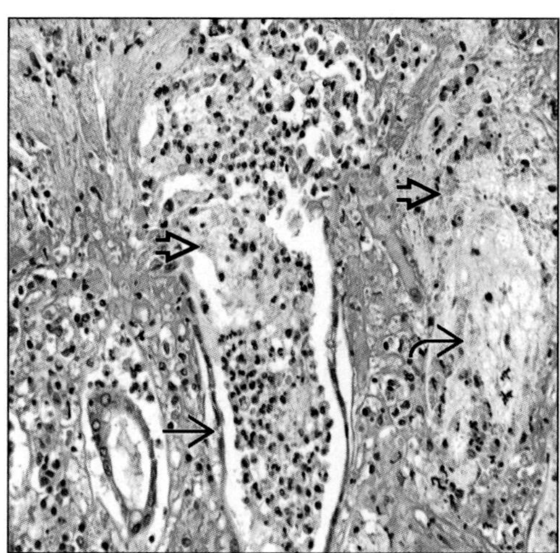

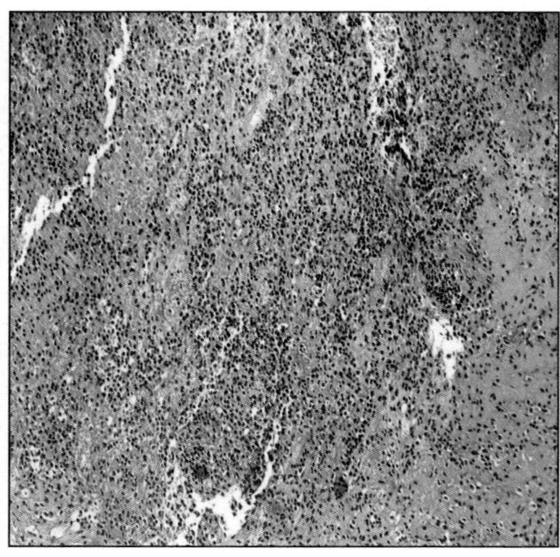

(Left) *Necrotic debris ➩ erupts into bowel lumen from dilated crypts. The crypt in the center is lined by attenuated cells ➩, and the crypt on the right ➩ demonstrates epithelial necrosis.* ***(Right)*** *The mucosa in ischemic colitis loses glandular architecture as opposed to pseudomembranous colitis where mucin-distended glands can still be identified even when the epithelium is necrotic, except in severe cases.*

Severe C. diff Colitis and Other Organ Changes

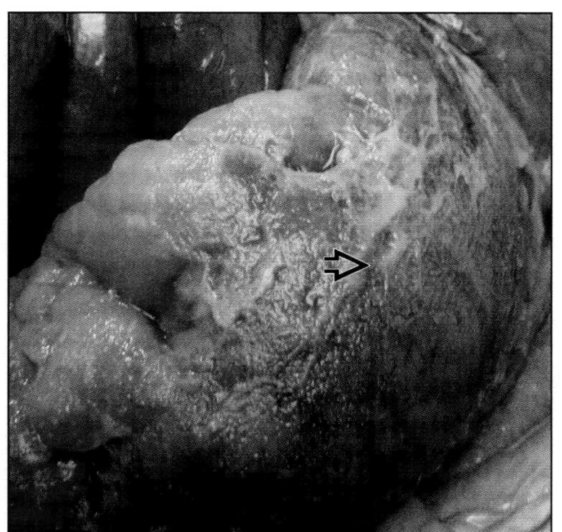

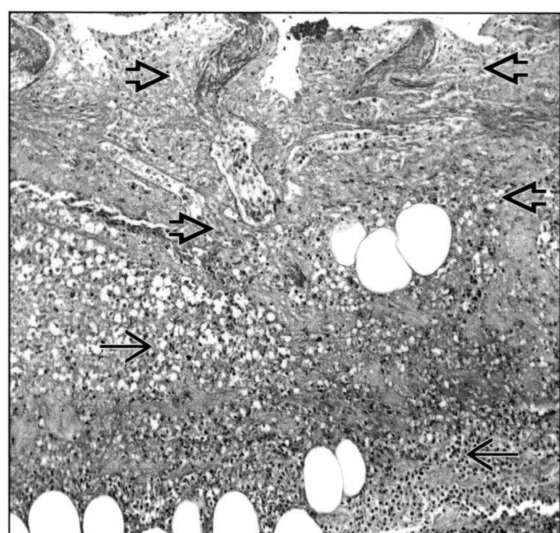

(Left) *This dilated and dusky-appearing ascending colon is evolving toward toxic megacolon in a patient with known Clostridium difficile infection. Note the fibrinopurulent exudate on the serosal surface ➪ indicating transmural inflammation or perhaps even perforation.* ***(Right)*** *In severe disease (toxic megacolon), the mucosa becomes necrotic ➪ and inflammation extends more deeply though the wall ➔, as in ischemic colitis.*

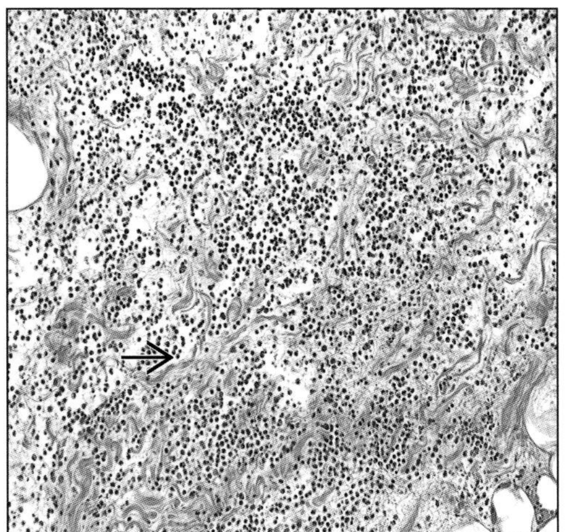

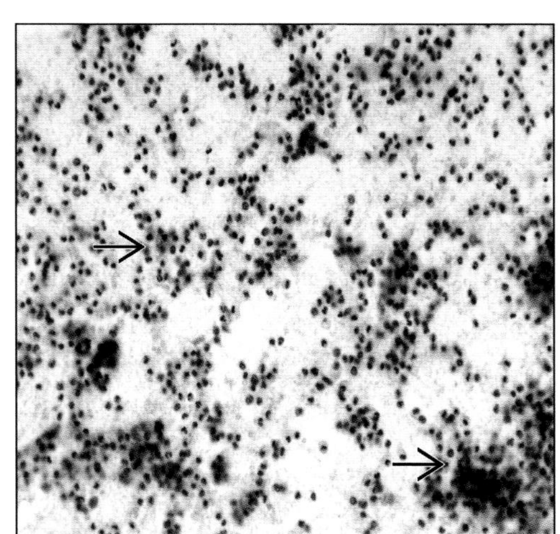

(Left) *This higher power view shows the acute inflammation ➔ expanding the submucosa in a case of toxic megacolon.* ***(Right)*** *This cell block preparation of ascitic fluid in a case of toxic megacolon contains innumerable polymorphonuclear leukocytes ➔.*

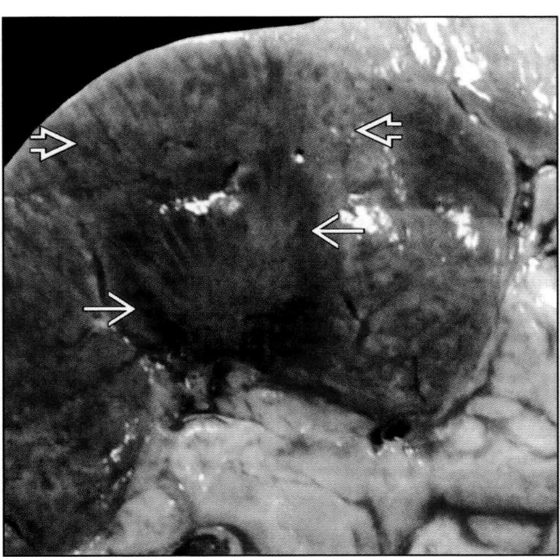

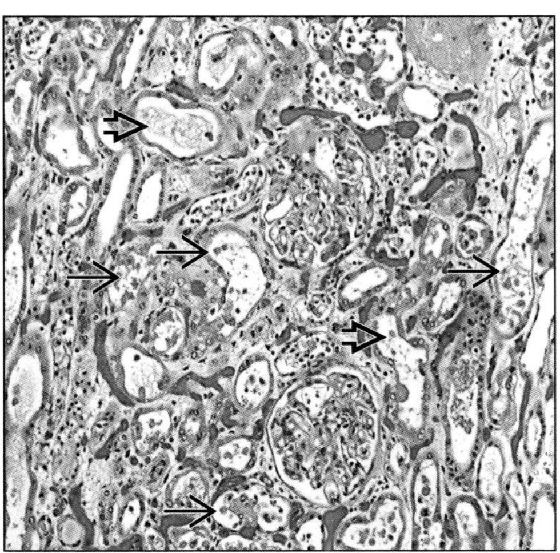

(Left) *Cortical pallor ➪ and a congested medulla ➔ are apparent grossly in a kidney with acute tubular injury.* ***(Right)*** *Acute tubular injury has dilated tubules ➪ due to flattening of the epithelium, and cellular debris is noted in the tubular lumen ➔.*

VIRAL HEPATITIS

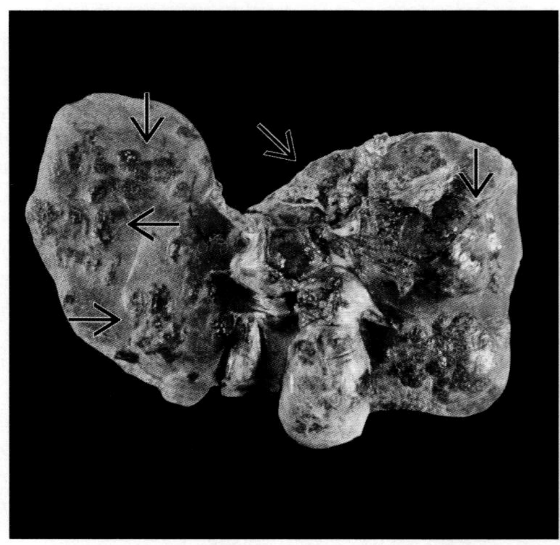

This liver with green discoloration due to cholestasis shows areas of necrosis ➔ and capsular irregularity that is typically seen in fulminant viral hepatitis. (Courtesy of D. Rubin, MD.)

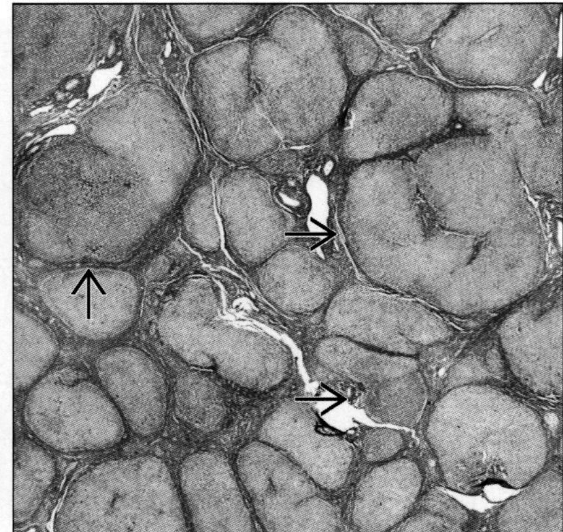

A trichrome stain highlights fibrous bands surrounding regenerative nodules ➔ in this liver with cirrhosis due to chronic hepatitis C infection.

ETIOLOGY/PATHOGENESIS

Hepatotropic Viruses

- Hepatitis A (HAV), B (HBV), C (HCV), D (HDV), and E (HEV)

Systemic Viruses

- Herpes virus group
  - Risk factors: Immunocompromised states, especially HIV, pregnancy, and neonatal period, rare in immunocompetent hosts
  - Herpes simplex virus (HSV): Disseminated infection often fatal
  - Cytomegalovirus (CMV): May cause infectious mononucleosis-like syndrome in immunocompetent
  - Epstein-Barr virus (EBV): Infectious mononucleosis with liver involvement, lymphoproliferative disorders, and hemophagocytic syndrome (usually fatal)
  - Varicella zoster virus (VZV)
  - Human herpesvirus 6 (HHV-6): May cause hemophagocytic syndrome
- Viral hemorrhagic fevers (VHF)
  - 4 families of RNA viruses: Filovirus (e.g., Marburg and Ebola), flavivirus (e.g., yellow fever, dengue), arenavirus (e.g., Argentine, Bolivian, Lassa, etc.), and bunyavirus (e.g., Rift Valley fever, hantavirus)
  - Life cycles involve humans, primates, rodents, bats, mosquitos, and ticks; also nosocomial spread
  - Severity and mortality vary, not all infected patients develop disease
  - Hemorrhage due to abnormal vascular regulation/damage → capillary leakage → effusions, edema, hemorrhage → disseminated intravascular coagulation (DIC), hepatic/organ necrosis, shock
- Other viruses that rarely affect liver
  - Adenovirus, enterovirus, parvovirus

CLINICAL ISSUES

Epidemiology

- Incidence
  - Hepatotropic viruses
    - HAV: ~ 2,800 acute infections in USA (2011)
    - HBV: ~ 18,000 acute infections in USA (2011), ~ 1 million chronic infections
    - HCV: ~ 16,500 acute infections in USA (2011), ~ 3 million chronic infections
    - HDV: Rare in US, ~ 5% of HBV carriers
    - HEV: Clinical hepatitis rare in USA; seroprevalence may be higher
  - Viral hemorrhagic fever
    - Rare in USA, endemic viruses include dengue and Sin Nombre viruses

Presentation

- Fever, jaundice, abdominal pain, nausea, vomiting, anorexia, fatigue, arthritis, pruritis, hematuria
- Maculopapular, urticarial, purpural, or vesicular/pustular rash, neurologic symptoms
- Cough, dyspnea, hemoptysis (pneumonitis), chest pain and palpitations (myocarditis)
- Headache, neck stiffness, photophobia, seizures (meningoencephalitis)
- Petechial rash, epistaxis, melena, hematemesis, conjunctival bleeding, shock (VHF)
- Important elements of chart review
  - Travel, food consumption, sexual history, history of injection drug use, blood transfusions, tattoos/piercings, other blood/body fluid exposures, immunosuppression, sick contacts

Laboratory Tests

- ↑ transaminases, bilirubin, ammonia, and α-fetoprotein, + viral hepatitis antibodies/RNA/DNA, + other viral serologies/RNA/DNA

Key Facts

Etiology
- Hepatotropic viruses: Hepatitis A, B, C, D, and E
- Herpes virus group: HSV, CMV, EBV, VZV, HHV-6
- Viral hemorrhagic fevers: Yellow fever, dengue fever, Ebola, hantavirus, etc.

Clinical Issues
- Important elements of chart review: Travel, food consumption, and sexual history, history of injection drug use, blood transfusions, tattoos/piercings, blood/body fluid exposures, immunosuppression

Macroscopic Pathology
- Acute hepatitis: Hepatomegaly, cholestasis, necrosis, regenerative nodules, hemorrhage
- Chronic hepatitis: Hepatomegaly or atrophy, cirrhosis, masses

Microscopic Pathology
- Acute hepatitis (HAV, HBV ± HDV, HCV, HEV): Lobular inflammation, acidophil bodies, variable necrosis, swollen hepatocytes, lobular disarray, cholestasis, variable portal inflammation
- Chronic hepatitis (HBV ± HDV, HCV, rarely HEV): Portal inflammation, variable interface and lobular activity, fibrosis, cirrhosis, ± siderosis, dysplastic nodules, hepatocellular carcinoma

Reporting Considerations
- Final report should include: Type of viral hepatitis, extent of hepatic disease, associated extrahepatic findings, whether the virus was the cause of death or a contributing factor

  - Postmortem blood testing for HBV and HCV antibodies and PCR has been shown to work
  - Consider postmortem viral testing in cases of unknown liver injury
- ↑ blood urea nitrogen and creatinine, proteinuria, hematuria, hypocomplementemia, + serum cryoglobulins
- Thrombocytopenia, anemia, lymphocytosis, prolonged prothrombin and partial thromboplastin times
- ↑ C-reactive protein and erythrocyte sedimentation rate, pancytopenia, hemophagocytosis on blood smear

Prognosis
- ~ 25% chronic HBV and HCV infection will → cirrhosis/chronic liver failure → ↑ risk of hepatocellular carcinoma (HCC)
  - Coinfection with HIV accelerates liver damage by HBV and HCV
- Mortality of acute viral hepatitis varies, higher in immunocompromised

MACROSCOPIC FEATURES

External Examination/Autopsy Safety
- Jaundice, scleral icterus, abdominal distension, pitting edema, anasarca, caput medusae, spider angiomas (liver failure/portal hypertension)
- Maculopapular, purpural, urticarial, pustular, vesicular rashes (viral exanthems)
- Pallor (shock), petechiae, gangrene, and mucocutaneous hemorrhage (DIC)
- Universal precautions mandatory in setting of necrotic or cirrhotic liver, always consider HIV coinfection

Internal Examination
- Ascites

Organ Examination
- Liver
  - Acute/fulminant hepatitis: Hepatomegaly, edematous capsule, green discoloration (cholestasis), necrosis ± atrophy with wrinkled capsule and regenerative nodules if extensive, hemorrhagic foci
  - Chronic hepatitis: Hepatomegaly or atrophy, cirrhosis (usually macronodular), masses (HCC usually softer than surrounding nodules and vary in color ± necrosis)
- Other organs
  - Necrosis/hemorrhage (DIC)
  - Gastrointestinal tract: Ulcers, inflammation, gastric/esophageal varices
  - Lungs: Consolidation, edema
  - Kidneys: Cortical pallor and medullary congestion (shock), atrophic with granular subcapsular surface (chronic glomerulonephritis)
  - Spleen: Splenomegaly

MICROSCOPIC PATHOLOGY

Histologic Features
- Liver
  - Acute hepatitis (HAV, HBV ± HDV, HCV, HEV): Lobular inflammation, acidophil bodies, necrosis (spotty, confluent, bridging, submassive), swollen hepatocytes, lobular disarray ± parenchymal collapse, cholestasis, variable portal inflammation
    - Specific findings in HAV: Periportal/interface inflammatory activity and necrosis, + plasma cells, perivenular cholestasis without inflammation/necrosis
  - Chronic hepatitis (HBV ± HDV, HCV, rarely HEV): Chronic hepatitis (portal inflammation) with variable interface and lobular inflammatory activity, variable fibrosis, cirrhosis, ± siderosis, HCC
    - HBV: Ground-glass hepatocytes (cytoplasmic inclusions containing HBV surface antigen), "sanded" nuclei (pale pink inclusions containing HBV core antigen)

VIRAL HEPATITIS

Summary of Hepatotropic Viruses

Virus	Genome and Classification	Mode of Transmission	Type of Hepatitis	Extrahepatic Manifestations
Hepatitis A	Single-stranded RNA, picornavirus	Fecal-oral	Acute, usually mild; may be protracted, relapsing, or fulminant	Acute pancreatitis, thrombocytopenia, cryoglobulinemia (rare)
Hepatitis B	Incomplete double-stranded DNA, hepadnavirus	Parenteral, sexual, perinatal	Acute with recovery ± reactivations, rarely fulminant, carriers without chronic hepatitis, chronic ± exacerbations	Glomerulonephritis, serum sickness-like syndrome, polyarteritis nodosa, Guillain-Barré syndrome, cryoglobulinemia
Hepatitis C	Single-stranded RNA, hepacivirus	Parenteral; sexual and perinatal are less common	Chronic, rarely acute	Glomerulonephritis, cryoglobulinemia, lichen planus, autoimmune diseases ± cytopenia, porphyria cutanea tarda, insulin resistance
Hepatitis D	Single-stranded RNA (defective), deltavirus	Parenteral and sexual, only occurs with coinfection or superinfection with hepatitis B	May clear with clearance of hepatitis B (coinfection), chronic ± exacerbations and rarely fulminant (superinfection)	N/A
Hepatitis E	Single-stranded RNA, hepevirus	Fecal-oral	Acute, fulminant in pregnancy, chronic in immunosuppressed	Acute pancreatitis, aplastic anemia, neurologic diseases, acute thyroiditis, glomerulonephritis

        - HDV: Same as HBV but usually more severe activity and necrosis
        - HCV: Lymphoid aggregates ± germinal centers in portal tracts, acidophil bodies, ± steatosis, ± mild bile duct injury
        - Rarely fibrosing cholestatic hepatitis in immunocompromised with HBV or HCV (periportal/perisinusoidal fibrosis, cholestasis, little/no inflammation)
    - Nonhepatotropic viral hepatitis
        - HSV: Geographic coagulative necrosis ± inflammation, purple glassy intranuclear inclusions with chromatin margination ± clear halo and multinucleation
        - CMV: Intranuclear inclusions with clear halo, intracytoplasmic basophilic granules, ± microabscesses, infectious mononucleosis-like syndrome (lymphocytes in sinusoids, no inclusions), neonatal giant cell hepatitis
        - EBV: Diffuse sinusoidal lymphocytic infiltrates
        - VZV: Variable necrosis, little inflammation, intranuclear inclusions
        - HHV-6: Nonspecific lobular inflammation
    - Viral hemorrhagic fevers
        - Most appear similar with perivenular or mid-zonal necrosis without inflammation or cholestasis, ± steatosis, ballooned hepatocytes
- Other organs
    - Esophageal/gastrointestinal ulcers ± viral inclusions
    - Pneumonitis, myocarditis ± viral inclusions
    - Glomerulonephritis, acute tubular injury/necrosis
    - DIC: Widespread microthrombi ± hemorrhage and ischemic necrosis, schistocytes in peripheral blood

ANCILLARY TESTS

Immunohistochemistry

- HBV surface and core antigens, HDV antigen, HSV, CMV, VZV, HHV-6, adenovirus, parvovirus, enterovirus
- Some VHFs: Dengue ([+] in Kupffer cells), Lassa, Ebola

In Situ Hybridization

- EBER for EBV

Special Stains

- Trichrome to evaluate fibrosis/staging
- Iron stain for siderosis
- Reticulin stain to evaluate sinusoidal architecture and presence of parenchymal collapse

REPORTING CRITERIA

Final Report Should Include

- Type of viral hepatitis, extent of hepatic disease, associated extrahepatic findings, whether virus was the cause of death or a contributing factor

SELECTED REFERENCES

1. Dalton HR et al: Hepatitis E. Curr Opin Infect Dis. 26(5):471-8, 2013
2. Paessler S et al: Pathogenesis of the viral hemorrhagic fevers. Annu Rev Pathol. 8:411-40, 2013
3. Eriksen MB et al: Postmortem detection of hepatitis B, C, and human immunodeficiency virus genomes in blood samples from drug-related deaths in Denmark*. J Forensic Sci. 54(5):1085-8, 2009
4. Amarapurkar DN et al: Extrahepatic manifestations of viral hepatitis. Ann Hepatol. 1(4):192-5, 2002

Microscopic Findings in Viral Hepatitis

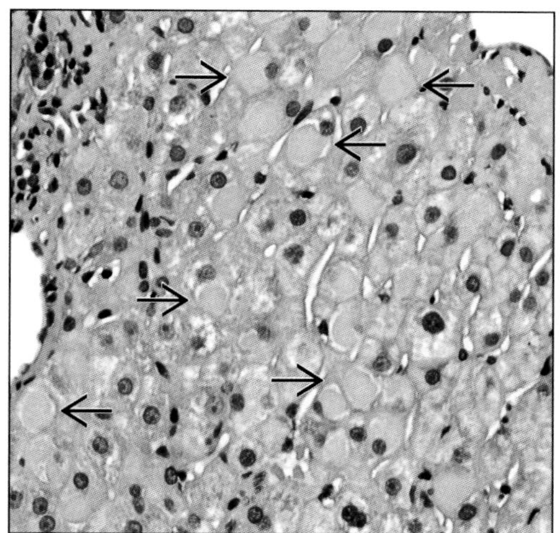

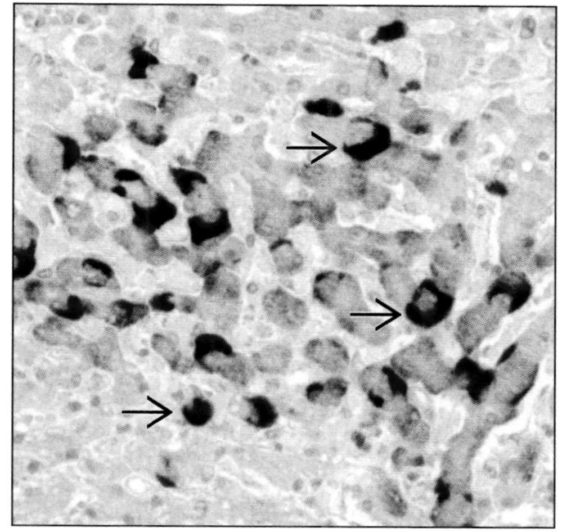

(Left) *Ground-glass hepatocytes as seen in hepatitis B infection are characterized by homogeneous pink intracytoplasmic "glassy" inclusions ⇨, often surrounded by a clear halo. These inclusions contain hepatitis B surface antigen.* ***(Right)*** *Immunohistochemical stain for hepatitis B surface antigen (HBsAg) is positive ⇨ in the cytoplasmic inclusions of the ground-glass hepatocytes.*

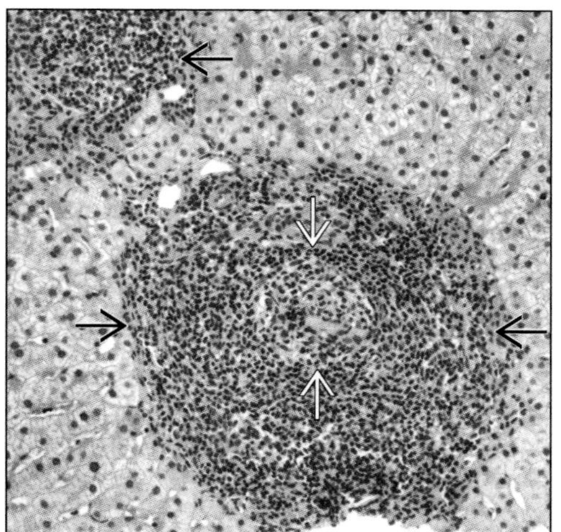

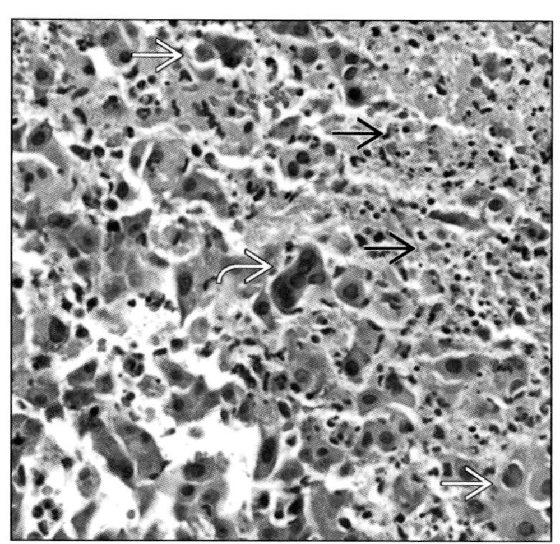

(Left) *Lymphoid aggregates in portal tracts ⇨ are characteristic of chronic hepatitis C infection. Occasionally, the aggregates contain reactive germinal centers ➡.* ***(Right)*** *Herpes simplex virus (HSV) hepatitis is associated with irregular areas of necrosis ⇨. Scattered viable hepatocytes show glassy intranuclear inclusions ➡ with chromatin margination and multinucleation ➦, which are characteristic of herpes virus infection.*

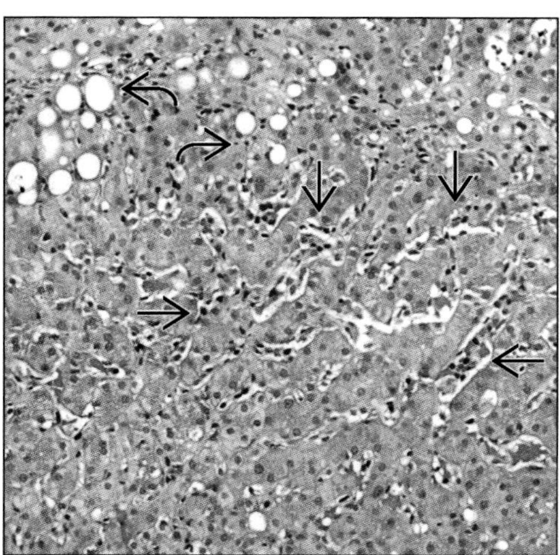

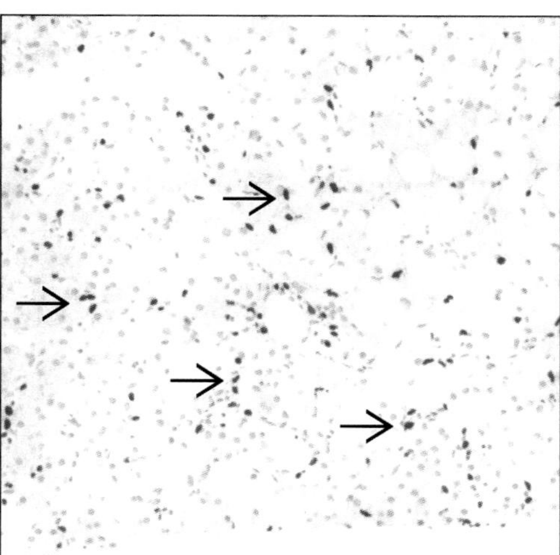

(Left) *This liver shows diffuse sinusoidal lymphocytic infiltrates ⇨ without significant necrosis that is characteristic of Epstein-Barr virus (EBV) hepatitis. Patchy steatosis ⇨ may also be present.* ***(Right)*** *In situ hybridization for EBV (EBER) is positive in the nuclei of numerous lymphocytes that infiltrate the sinusoidal spaces ⇨ in this case of EBV hepatitis.*

UROSEPSIS

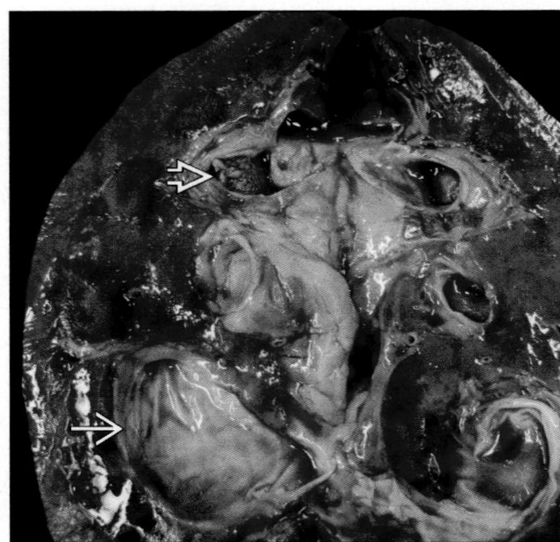

This bisected kidney shows hydronephrosis with dilated calyces ➡ and a kidney stone ➡. Nephrolithiasis is the most common cause of urinary obstruction in young adult patients.

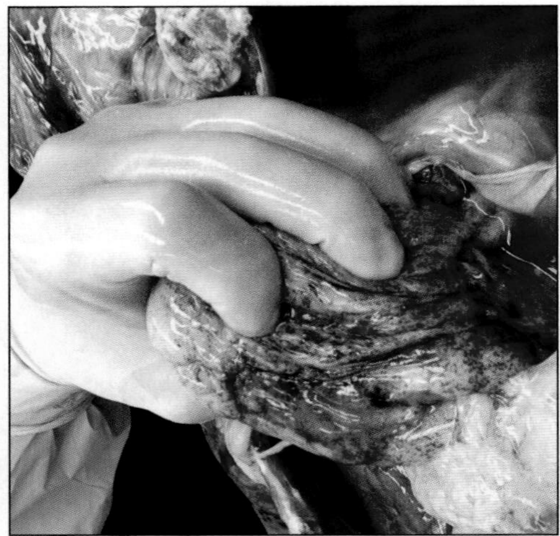

The heart in this patient with urosepsis and disseminated intravascular coagulation (DIC) shows epicardial petechial hemorrhages as well as pleural and pericardial effusions.

TERMINOLOGY

Definitions

- Sepsis: Systemic inflammatory response syndrome (SIRS) caused by infection
- Urosepsis: Sepsis as a result of a complicated urinary tract infection
    - ~ 25% of sepsis
- Complicated cystitis/pyelonephritis: Infection of bladder/upper urinary tract and kidney associated with condition that increases possibility of treatment failure
    - Diabetes, pregnancy, urinary obstruction, catheters, instrumentation, stones, anatomic abnormality

ETIOLOGY/PATHOGENESIS

Infectious Agents

- Enteric gram-negative rods, e.g., *Escherichia coli, Klebsiella, Enterobacter, Proteus*
- *Pseudomonas*
- Enterococci
- Fungi, especially *Candida albicans* and *Candida glabrata*

Ascending Infections

- Most common
- Fecal contamination of urethra → urethritis → cystitis → pyelonephritis
- Enterococci, especially in hospitalized/institutionalized patients with urinary catheters

Blood-Borne Infections

- Much less common
- *Staphylococcus aureus*: From skin/soft tissue infection or aortic bacterial endocarditis
    - Pyelonephritis, often with abscess formation
- *Mycobacterium tuberculosis* (MTB)
    - Complication of disseminated pulmonary TB
    - Clinical picture UTI with negative bacterial cultures

CLINICAL ISSUES

Clinical Presentations

- Cystitis: Dysuria, urinary frequency, urinary urgency
- Pyelonephritis
    - Same as cystitis, plus fever, costovertebral angle tenderness
- Urosepsis
    - Complicated urinary tract infection, SIRS, multiorgan failure, disseminated intravascular coagulation (DIC)

Risk Factors

- Urinary obstruction
    - Congenital
        - Strictures: Ureteral or urethral
        - Polycystic kidney disease
    - Acquired
        - Calculi: Most common cause of obstruction in young adults
        - Prostatic hyperplasia: Most common cause of obstruction in older men
        - Tumors
        - Pregnancy: Some degree of hydroureter/hydronephrosis is normal in pregnancy
        - Complication of radiation therapy
- Instrumentation
    - Urethral catheter, ureteral stent, nephrostomy
- Impaired voiding
    - Neurogenic bladder
    - Cystocele/prolapse
    - Vesicoureteral reflux
- Metabolic disorders
    - Diabetes (especially atypical pathogens)
    - Nephrocalcinosis

UROSEPSIS

Key Facts

Terminology

- Urosepsis is defined as SIRS in setting of complicated urinary tract infection
- Accounts for 25% of all cases of sepsis
- Certain groups are at increased risk of urosepsis
  - Patients with abnormal urinary tract anatomy
  - Patients with urinary tract catheters/hardware or history of urinary tract procedure
  - Patients with certain underlying conditions: Diabetes, sickle cell, neurogenic bladder
- Usually result of ascending infection
  - Most often gram-negative enteric bacteria
  - Enterococci: In institutional settings in catheterized patients
- Secondary involvement of urinary tract by bloodstream infection is less common
  - Typically *Staphylococcus aureus*
- Urinary tract findings
  - Obstructive lesions: Extrinsic tumors, prostatic enlargement, bladder distension and trabeculation, hydroureter, hydronephrosis
  - Inflammatory urinary tract changes: Cystitis, pyelonephritis, renal abscess
- Findings associated with sepsis
  - Changes of disseminated intravascular coagulation: Petechiae, ecchymoses, microthrombi
  - Anasarca, effusions
  - Diffuse alveolar damage
  - Changes of septic organ injury and failure

MACROSCOPIC FEATURES

External Examination in Sepsis

- Edema (anasarca)
  - Capillary leak (SIRS)
  - Aggressive intravenous fluid therapy
- Petechial hemorrhages (DIC)

Internal Examination

- Urethral obstruction
  - Bladder distension and trabeculation
  - Prostate enlargement
- Ureteral obstruction
  - Obstructing lesion (e.g., tumor)
  - Hydroureter: Dilated and sometimes tortuous
  - Hydronephrosis: Thinned parenchyma and compressed papillae are signs of chronicity
- Nephrolithiasis

Organ Examination

- Urinary Tract: Possible findings
  - Acute pyelonephritis
    - Cortical abscesses: Especially with nephrolithiasis or reflux
    - Renal papillae with yellow streaks
  - Renal papillary necrosis
    - Diabetics and patients with sickle cell
  - Cystitis
    - Hyperemic, boggy mucosa with cloudy urine

MICROSCOPIC PATHOLOGY

Histologic Features

- Evidence of local inflammation/infection
  - Acute pyelonephritis
    - Abscesses with destruction of tubules
    - Acute inflammation with neutrophil casts
    - Glomeruli usually spared
  - Cystitis
- Evidence of systemic inflammatory response/ coagulopathy
  - Disseminated intravascular coagulation
    - Widely scattered microthrombi
  - Evidence of ischemic organ injury
  - Diffuse alveolar damage

ANCILLARY TESTS

Histochemistry

- Gram stain of fresh tissue
  - Less reliable in postmortem tissue
  - Nonviable gram positive organisms may appear gram negative
- Special stains for bacteria in formalin fixed, paraffin-embedded tissue
  - Brown-Brenn or Brown-Hopp stain: Gram positive organisms blue, gram negative organisms red, nuclei red, background yellow
    - Alternatives: Taylor stain, Lisa stain
- Special stains for fungi in formalin-fixed, paraffin-embedded tissue
  - GMS, PAS

Bacterial Cultures

- Not necessary if positive premortem cultures
- Low yield in patients on broad spectrum antibiotics
- Blood and splenic cultures to prove systemic infection
- Urine cultures only diagnostic if they match blood or splenic cultures

Molecular Testing

- Molecular microbiology in formalin-fixed, paraffin-embedded tissue
  - Probes for species specific DNA sequences for prokaryotic ribosomes

SELECTED REFERENCES

1. Kalra OP et al: Approach to a patient with urosepsis. J Glob Infect Dis. 1(1):57-63, 2009
2. Annane D et al: Septic shock. Lancet. 365(9453):63-78, 2005

UROSEPSIS

Gross and Histologic Features

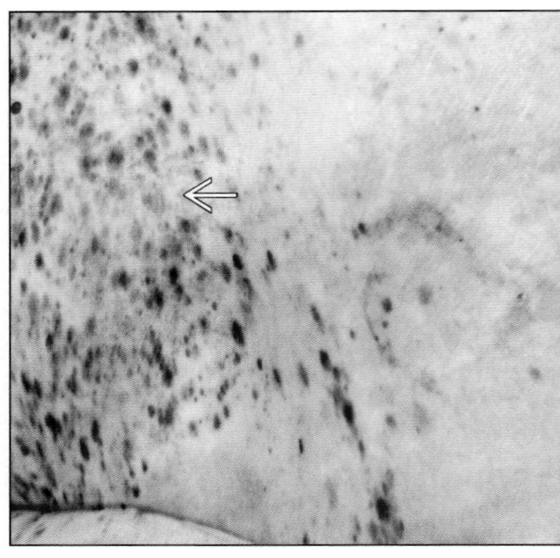

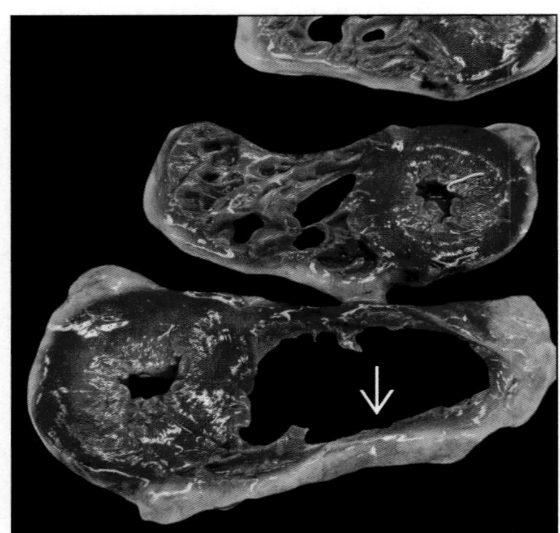

(Left) *These petechial skin hemorrhages ➡ in a patient with urosepsis are one manifestation of DIC. DIC is characterized by diffusely scattered microthrombi and diffuse petechial hemorrhages in the skin as well as mucosal and serosal surfaces.* ***(Right)*** *These cross sections of ventricles from a patient dying from sepsis and multiple organ dysfunction syndrome show a markedly dilated right ventricle ➡. The patient also showed hepatic necrosis and anasarca.*

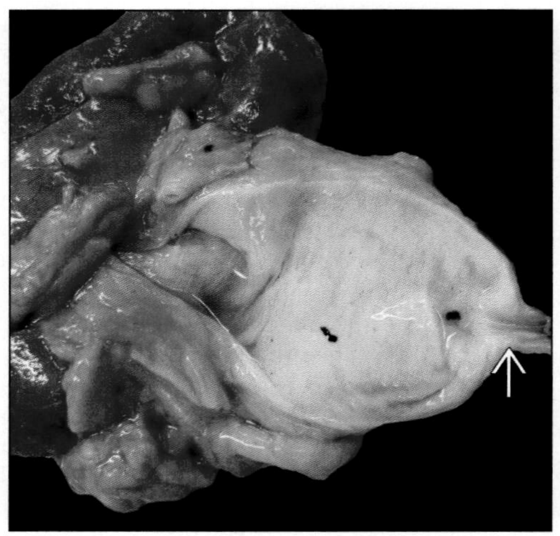

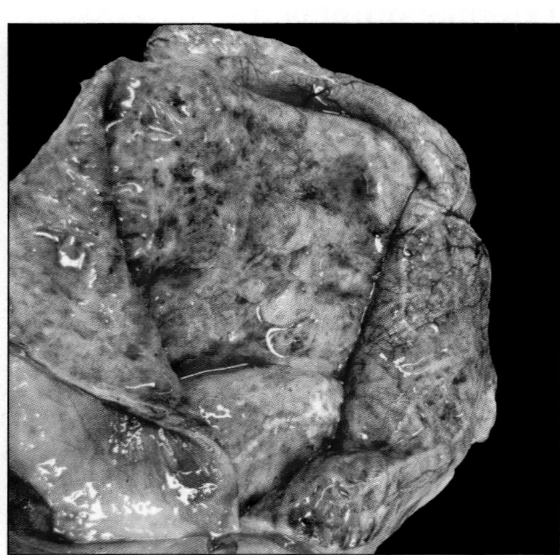

(Left) *Gross image shows an abrupt transition from hydroureter on the left to normal diameter ureter on the right ➡. The ureter was compressed by a tumor. Abnormal anatomy, reflux, obstruction, and stones increase the risk of urinary tract infection.* ***(Right)*** *The congested mucosa and tan-yellow exudate indicate acute cystitis. The trabeculation suggests chronic urethral obstruction. Prostatic hyperplasia with urethral obstruction is a common risk factor for urosepsis in older men.*

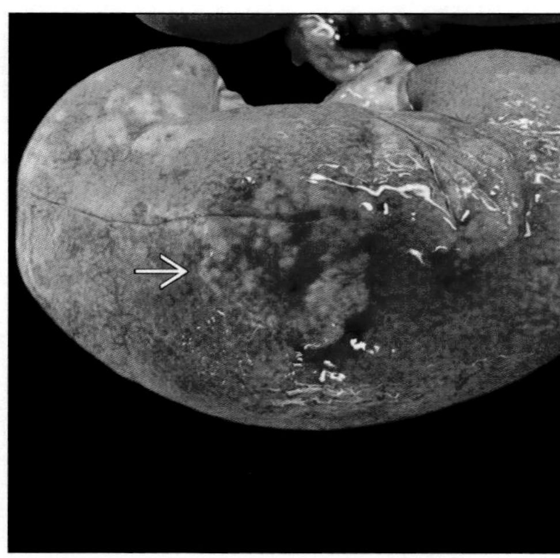

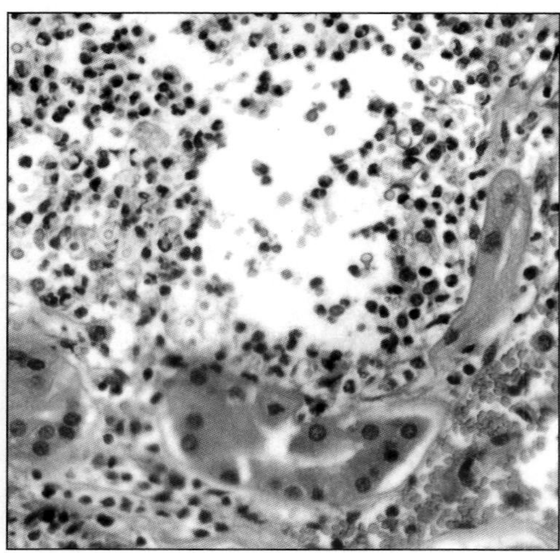

(Left) *Scattered tan-yellow cortical abscesses ➡ with hyperemic, red borders can be seen in this case of acute pyelonephritis. Renal abscesses are more common in patients with nephrolithiasis or vesicoureteral reflux.* ***(Right)*** *Necrotizing acute inflammation can be seen in this section taken from a renal abscess. Although most commonly the result of ascending enteric infections, this can also be seen with hematogenously spread Staphylococcus aureus.*

Histologic and Microbiologic Features

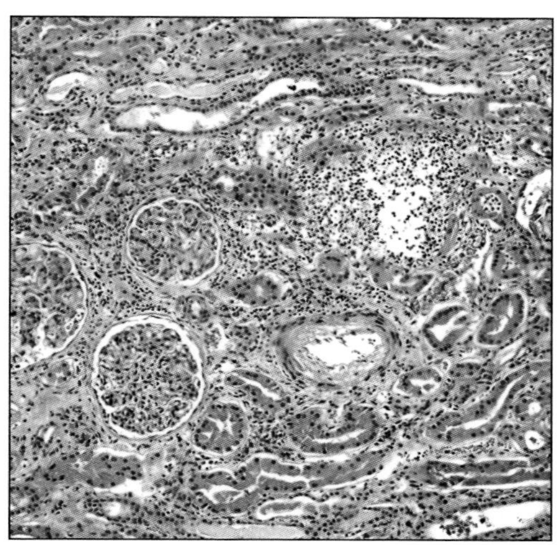

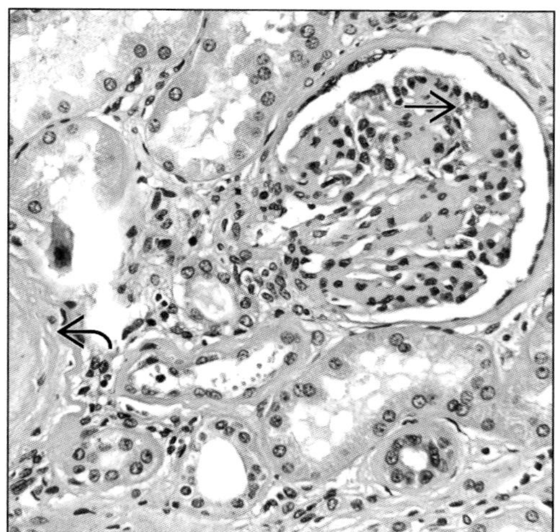

(Left) *Pyelonephritis is characterized by interstitial acute inflammation with sparing of the glomeruli. Neutrophils may fill the tubules and result in neutrophil casts seen on urinalysis.* ***(Right)*** *This section shows the nodular glomerulosclerosis* ➔ *and sclerotic glomeruli* ➔ *characteristically seen in the kidneys of diabetic patients. Diabetics are at increased risk for complicated urinary tract infections and urosepsis and may have infections with unusual organisms.*

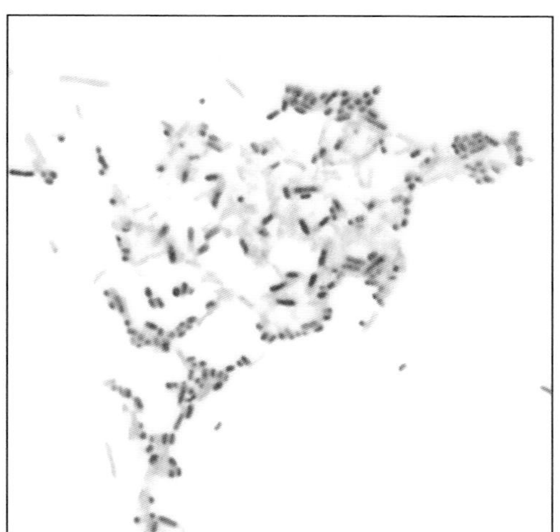

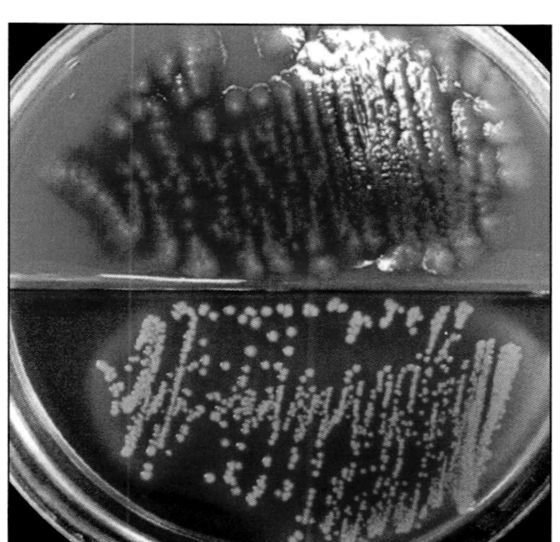

(Left) *The thick gram-negative rods seen in this Gram stain are typical of organisms like E. coli and other enterics, which cause urinary tract infections. Other common causative gram-negative rods include Proteus, Klebsiella, and Enterobacter.* ***(Right)*** *This blood agar/MacConkey agar biplate shows the characteristic appearance of Escherichia coli, the most common cause of urosepsis.The majority of cases of urosepsis are caused by ascending infections with enteric organisms.*

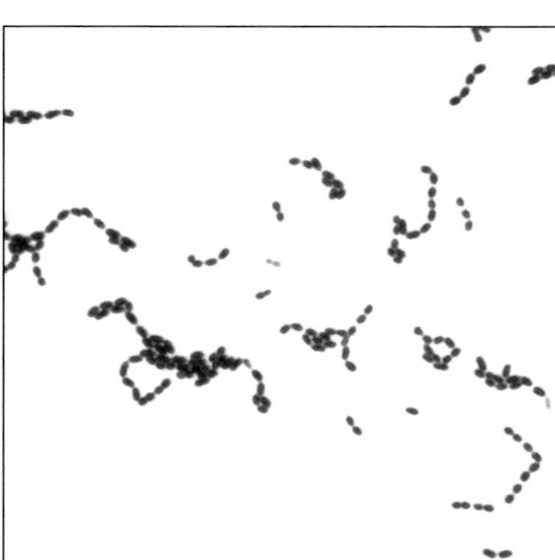

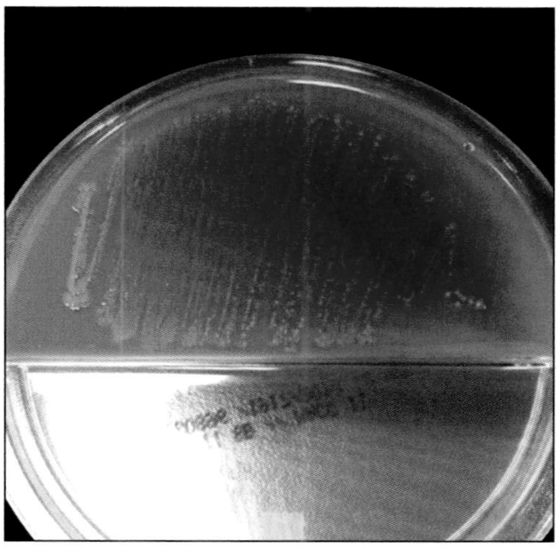

(Left) *Enterococcus, a Gram-positive coccus that grows in chains, is a particularly important cause of hospital-acquired urinary tract infections. Risk factors include urinary catheterization, older age, severe underlying illness, and prior antibiotic therapy.* ***(Right)*** *Enterococci grow only on the blood agar portion of a biplate and not on MacConkey agar, which selects for gram-negatives. A significant fraction of hospital-acquired enterococci are multiply drug resistant.*

SECTION 3

Neoplasia-Associated Death

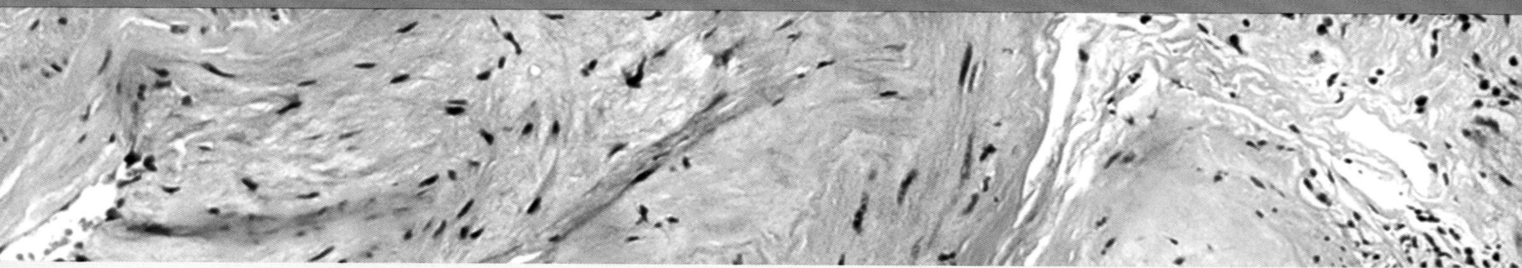

NEOPLASIA-ASSOCIATED DEATH

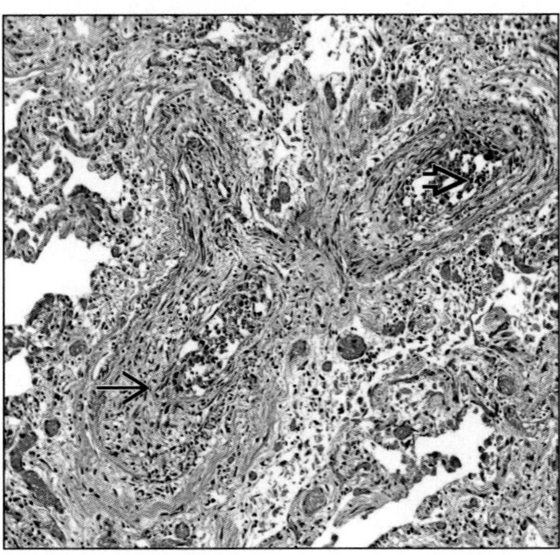

This patient had an occult malignancy at autopsy that had metastasized to the pulmonary arteries and caused thrombosis with organization ➡. Tumor cells can be seen in the organizing thrombus ➢.

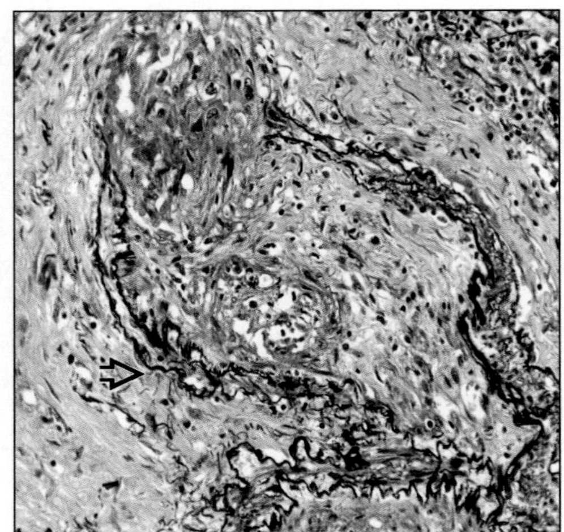

An elastic stain demonstrates the disrupted elastic lamina ➢ of the artery in this case with organizing tumor thromboemboli.

TERMINOLOGY

Direct Tumor Effects

- Mass effect
  - Respiratory: Bronchial obstruction and postobstructive pneumonia
  - Gastrointestinal tract: Obstruction → malnutrition, intestinal ischemia, etc.
  - CNS: May cause brain swelling and herniation
  - SVC syndrome: Obstruction to blood flow in superior vena cava (most commonly due to malignancy [usually lung])

Paraneoplastic Effects

- Paraneoplastic syndromes (PNS) are systemic effects of tumors not due to metastatic disease
  - 2 main mechanisms for PNS: Secreted tumor product and immunologic cross reactivity between tumor and normal tissues
  - May not cause death but contributes to death; is clue to underlying malignancy
  - Neurological, endocrine, dermatologic, hematologic manifestations most common
    - Neurological: Limbic encephalitis, paraneoplastic cerebellar degeneration; Lambert-Eaton syndrome and myasthenia gravis; autonomic neuropathy and subacute sensory neuropathy
    - Dermatologic: Dermatomyositis, acanthosis nigricans, paraneoplastic pemphigus
    - Endocrine: Syndrome of inappropriate antidiuretic hormone secretion (SIADH), Cushing syndrome, hypoglycemia, carcinoid syndrome (flushing, diarrhea, and bronchospasm)
    - Hematologic: Eosinophilia, granulocytosis, thrombocytosis, pure red cell aplasia (thymoma, leukemias/lymphomas, and myelodysplastic syndromes)
    - Amyloidosis (AL) and myeloma cast nephropathy: Secretion of light chains by myeloma may cause extracellular deposits as amyloid fibrils or light chain cast nephropathy

Morbidity and Mortality Associated With Tumor Therapy

- Tumor lysis syndrome: Metabolic derangement seen with lysis of large numbers of tumor cells usually seen 48-72 hours after initial treatment of non-Hodgkin lymphoma and leukemias
  - Hyperuricemia, hyperkalemia, hyperphosphatemia, hypocalcemia
  - Usually acute renal failure due to uric acid nephropathy and nephrocalcinosis
- Graft-vs.-host disease (GVHD): Immune-mediated disease following allogeneic bone marrow or (rarely) solid organ transplantation
  - In setting of neoplasia, GVHD usually follows allogeneic stem cell or bone marrow transplantation
  - 3 criteria for GVHD to occur: Immune competent graft, disparate (nonidentical) recipient, immunocompromised recipient
  - Systemic disease most often affecting skin, liver, and gastrointestinal tract
- Infection
  - Bacterial and fungal infections are major complication of tumor therapy with attendant immunosuppression
- Radiation injury
  - Effects of ionizing radiation include mucosal necrosis (early) to fibrosis (late); diffuse alveolar damage and fibrosis of lungs; skin erythema (early) to depigmentation and fibrosis (late); lymph node fibrosis

Thrombophilia

- Very common, often lethal complication of malignancy, multifactorial in etiology: Host response to tumor, tumor effects, and therapy

NEOPLASIA-ASSOCIATED DEATH

Key Facts

Terminology

- Paraneoplastic syndromes (PNS) are systemic effects of tumors not due to metastatic disease
  - 2 main mechanisms for PNS: Secreted tumor product and immunologic cross-reactivity between tumor and normal tissues
- Tumor lysis syndrome: Metabolic derangement usually seen 48-72 hours after initial treatment due to massive lysis lymphoma/leukemia cells
- Graft-vs.-host disease (GVHD): Immune-mediated disease following allogeneic stem cell transplantation
  - 3 criteria for GVHD to occur: Immune competent graft, disparate (nonidentical) recipient, immunocompromised recipient
- Manifestations of thrombophilia in malignancy
  - Trousseau syndrome: Often associated with pancreatic adenocarcinoma and other mucinous adenocarcinomas
  - Venous thromboembolism
  - Migratory thrombophlebitis: Recurrent venous thrombosis that changes location (migratory) often affecting superficial veins
  - Nonbacterial thrombotic endocarditis (NBTE): Sterile thrombi usually along closing edge of valves; can embolize
- Thrombotic microangiopathy (TMA): Usually related to cancer therapy

  - Host response: Acute phase reactants, inflammation, necrosis, hemodynamic disturbances
  - Tumor: Secretion of factors by tumor cells that promote coagulation, angiogenesis, fibrinolysis and inflammation; direct tumor interaction with endothelial cells, platelets, and leukocytes stimulating their procoagulant properties
  - Tumor therapy: Direct injury to endothelial cells (radiation therapy, bleomycin, anti-VEGF, thalidomide, gemcitabine), hormonal therapy (tamoxifen)
- Venous thromboembolism (15% of cancer patients have thrombotic complication)
- Migratory thrombophlebitis: Recurrent venous thrombosis that moves (migratory) and affects superficial veins at uncommon sites (e.g., arms and chest wall)
  - Often associated with mucinous adenocarcinoma
  - Commonly referred to as Trousseau syndrome or Trousseau sign of malignancy
- Nonbacterial thrombotic endocarditis (NBTE): Sterile thrombi usually along the closing edge of valves; can embolize and rarely may cause death
- Thrombotic microangiopathy (TMA): Usually related to cancer therapy, including bone marrow transplantation

MACROSCOPIC FEATURES

External Examination

- Signs of potential underlying malignancy
  - Dermatologic: Acanthosis nigricans
    - Thickened, hyperpigmented skin, axilla, and neck
  - Dermatomyositis/polymyositis
    - Purple (heliotrope) rash on upper eyelids, erythematous rash on upper body (face, neck, back, chest, and shoulders)
  - Paraneoplastic pemphigus
    - Blistering disease with superficial vesicles and bullae that rupture easily leaving erythematous base, mucosal involvement common
  - SVC syndrome: Facial plethora and congestion, upper extremity swelling
- Signs of therapy
  - Port-a-cath: Permanent intravenous lines with subcutaneous port in subcutaneous tissue of chest (usually left sided)
  - GVHD skin changes
    - Acute GVHD: (within 100 days of transplant) erythematous macules characteristically on palms and soles
    - Chronic GVHD: (after 100 days) lichenoid plaques or scleroderma- like changes

Organ Examination

- Primary tumor
  - Size and extent, regional lymph node, and organ metastases or document no residual tumor
  - Document prior therapy (resections, radioactive seeds)
- Thrombophilic complications
  - Pulmonary thromboembolism (PTE) is most lethal thrombotic complication of neoplasia and associated therapy
  - Thrombotic microangiopathy may not have gross findings but may show small petechial hemorrhages in renal cortex
- Infectious complications
  - Respiratory
    - Pneumonia (viral, bacterial, and fungal) characterized by areas of consolidation: Fungal pneumonia often with targetoid areas of central necrosis with surrounding hemorrhage due to vasculotropic nature of many fungal infections
    - Diffuse congestion and consolidation: Diffuse alveolar damage (infection/shock)
  - Gastrointestinal
    - Ulcerative infection from virus (punched-out ulcers: HSV, shallow ulcers: CMV), candidal infection (pseudomembranes), neutropenic enterocolitis (segmental ulceration, inflammation of terminal ileum, cecum, and ascending colon [a.k.a. typhlitis])

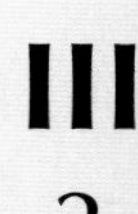

NEOPLASIA-ASSOCIATED DEATH

- Direct tumor complications
  - Mass effects
    - CNS: Brain swelling with enlargement of gyri and effacement of sulci; tonsillar herniation of cerebellar tonsils through foramen magnum is lethal
    - SVC syndrome: Tumor (usually lung primary) surrounds superior vena cava ± thrombosis
  - Hemorrhage and extensive necrosis
    - Extensive hemorrhage into tumor may extend into body cavity (e.g., peritoneal hemorrhage with hepatocellular tumors) → shock
    - Extensive necrosis of large amounts of tumor such as leukemias and lymphomas may be associated with tumor lysis syndrome
- Graft-vs.-host disease
  - Ulcerations and edema in gastrointestinal tract and cholestatic-appearing liver
- Paraneoplastic syndromes
  - Carcinoid syndrome
    - Carcinoid tumor either metastatic from intestine to liver/lung or primary ovarian carcinoid (vasoactive amines that → carcinoid syndrome are inactivated by liver and lung)
    - Cardiovascular: Plaques form along endocardial surface of right heart and tricuspid and pulmonic valves, pulmonary artery

MICROSCOPIC PATHOLOGY

Histologic Features

- Primary tumor, determine type, extent (stage), and differentiation (grade)
- Thrombotic complications
  - PTE: Thromboembolus should have layered fibrin and red blood cells; presence of tumor cells indicates tumor thrombus
  - NBTE: Small (1-5 mm) fibrin thrombi loosely attached to closing edge of valve (usually left heart), without associated inflammatory response
    - Strong association with mucinous adenocarcinoma
  - Thrombotic microangiopathy: Kidney most frequently affected
    - Diffuse endothelial swelling, arteriolar and capillary thrombi, thickened glomerular capillary walls (subendothelial debris and fibrin)
- Tumor lysis syndrome
  - Best seen in kidney: Acute tubular injury with urate crystal deposition and calcinosis (calcification of tubular cells, tubular basement membrane, and calcified tubular casts)
- PNS: Neurologic
  - Limbic encephalitis: Perivascular inflammation, some neuronal loss and microglial nodules in anterior and medial temporal lobe
  - Paraneoplastic cerebellar degeneration: Destruction of Purkinje cells, gliosis, mild inflammation
- PNS: Dermatologic
  - AN: Epidermis and dermal papillae undulate (peaks and valleys), variable hyperplasia, basal cell hyperpigmentation and hyperkeratosis
  - Paraneoplastic pemphigus: Suprabasal acantholytic blister, immunofluorescence with anti-IgG shows staining of plasma membrane of epidermal cells
- PNS: Other
  - Amyloidosis: Extracellular deposition of hyaline material that stains with congo red and shows apple-green birefringence; immunofluorescence will demonstrate isolated light chain, usually lambda
  - Carcinoid syndrome: Plaques within cardiovascular system composed of smooth muscle cells in mucopolysaccharide-rich matrix without changes to underlying endocardial tissue
- Graft-vs.-host disease
  - Epidermal and mucosal epithelial apoptosis with associated, usually mild lymphocytic infiltrate
  - Liver: Bile duct inflammation (early), bile duct epithelial degenerative change (late), bile duct loss (late), cholestasis
- Radiation injury
  - Vascular injury: Endothelial swelling and occasionally necrosis (early); intimal fibrosis (late)
  - Interstitial fibrosis often containing atypical cells with prominent nucleoli and giant cell formation

REPORTING CRITERIA

Tumor Classification, Staging, and Grading in Final Report

- Most commonly staging system is TNM: T = tumor, N = lymph nodes, M = metastatic disease
- Prefix "a" indicates diagnosis at autopsy (e.g., aT3N1M1)

Quality Assurance

- Compare tumor type, grading, and staging to prior pathology reports; address discrepancies

SELECTED REFERENCES

1. Deng A et al: Venous thromboembolism in cancer patients. Hosp Pract (1995). 42(5):24-33, 2014
2. Phan M et al: Primary venous thromboembolism prophylaxis in patients with solid tumors: a meta-analysis. J Thromb Thrombolysis. 38(2):241-9, 2014
3. Connolly GC et al: Cancer-associated thrombosis. Hematology Am Soc Hematol Educ Program. 2013:684-91, 2013
4. Jones LM et al: Cardiovascular disease among breast cancer survivors: the call for a clinical vascular health toolbox. Breast Cancer Res Treat. 142(3):645-53, 2013

Infectious & Paraneoplastic Complications of Malignancy

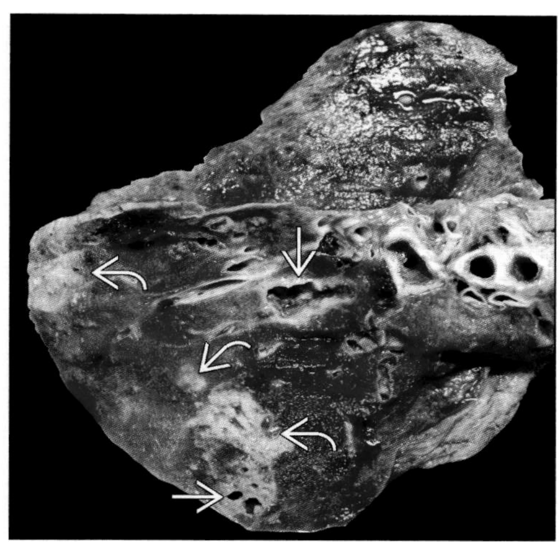

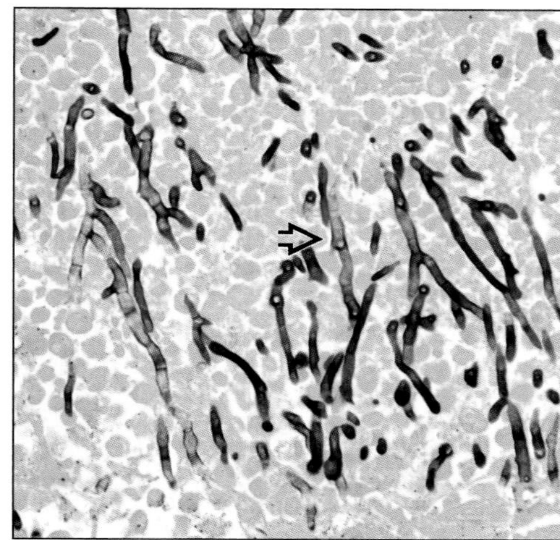

(Left) This lung demonstrates fungal pneumonia with multiple areas of consolidation ➦ and abscess formation with necrosis ➡. (From DP: Transplant.) ***(Right)*** *A GMS stain reveals the presence of septate hyphae ⇨ that branch at acute angles consistent with aspergillosis. (From DP: Transplant.)*

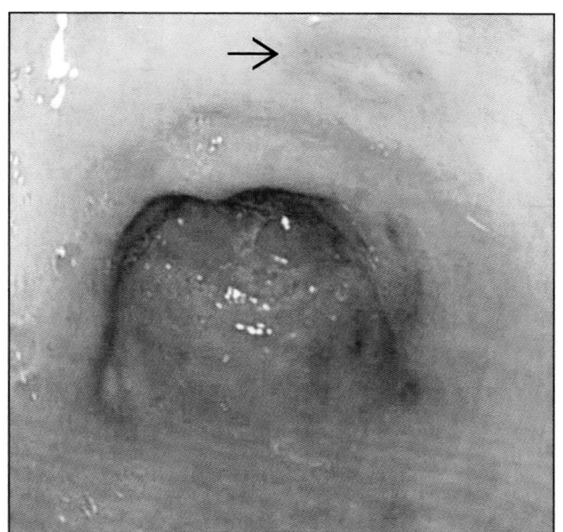

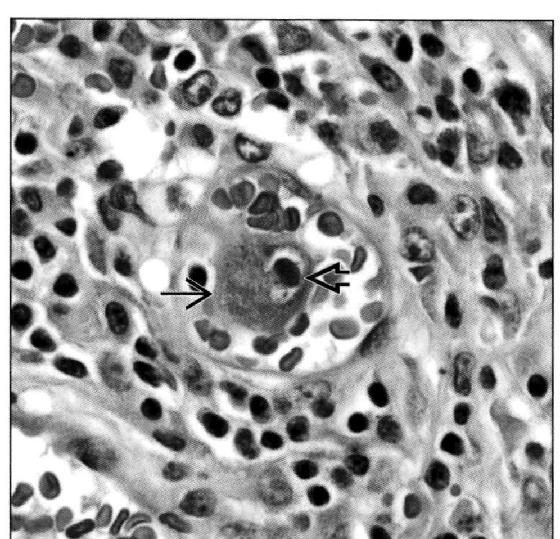

(Left) *The ulcers caused by cytomegalovirus are shallow ➙ as opposed to the punched-out ulcers of herpes simplex virus. (From DP: Endoscopic.)* ***(Right)*** *Cytomegalovirus inclusion in an endothelial cell is shown. There is an intranuclear "owl's-eye" basophilic inclusion surrounded by an area of clearing ⇨ and smaller intracytoplasmic basophilic inclusions ➙. (From DP: Kidney.)*

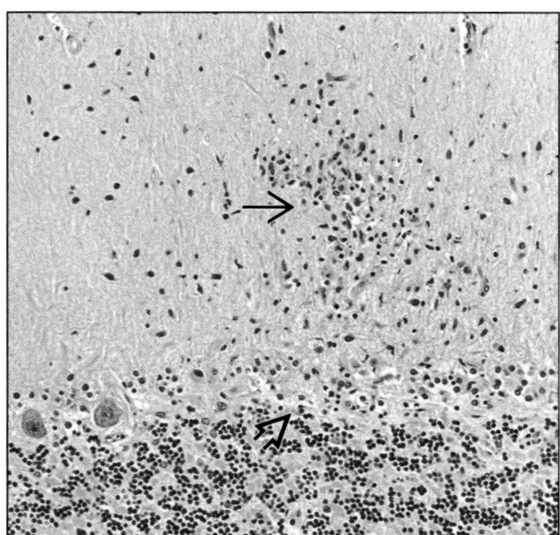

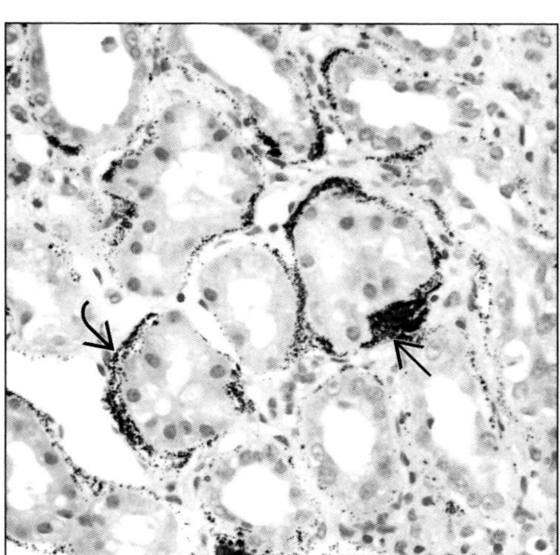

(Left) *In paraneoplastic cerebellar degeneration, perivascular inflammation ➙ and Purkinje cell loss ⇨ are noted. (From DP: Neuro.)* ***(Right)*** *This von Kossa stain for calcium phosphate demonstrates staining of the tubular basement membranes ➙ and interstitium ➦ in a case of nephrocalcinosis. (From DP: Kidney.)*

NEOPLASIA-ASSOCIATED DEATH

Malignancy, General Features

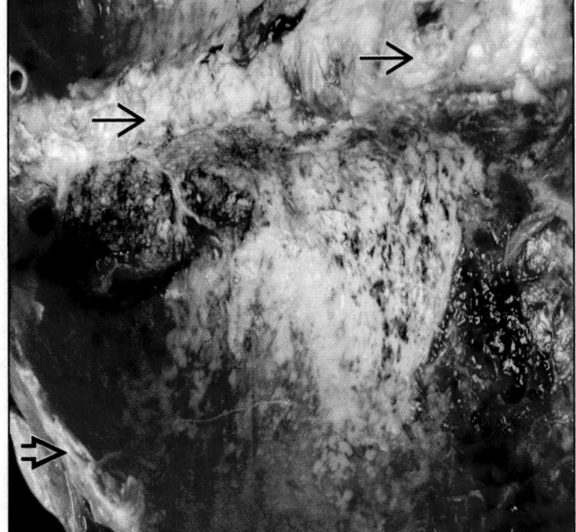

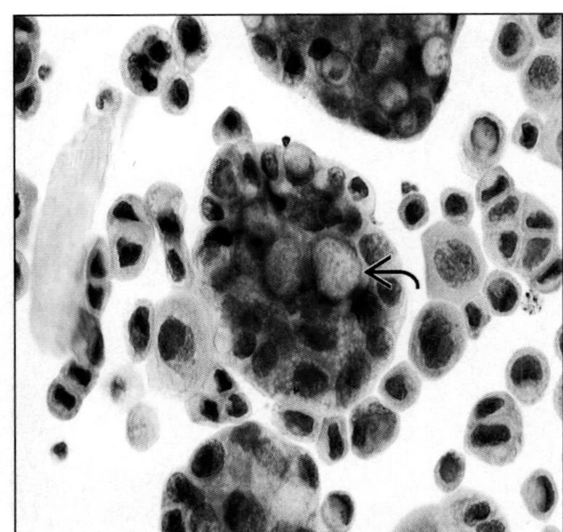

(Left) *This parietal pleural surface on the right chest (thoracic vertebrae ⇒, ribs ⇒) is red and granular due to recent instillation of tetracycline for pleurodesis for malignant pleural effusion.* ***(Right)*** *Cytology of the pleural fluid revealed clusters of malignant cells (high nuclear to cytoplasmic ratio, nuclear pleomorphism) with intracytoplasmic mucin vacuoles ⇒ consistent with lung adenocarcinoma. Cytology of postmortem material-like effusions can yield diagnostic information. (From DP: Cytopathology.)*

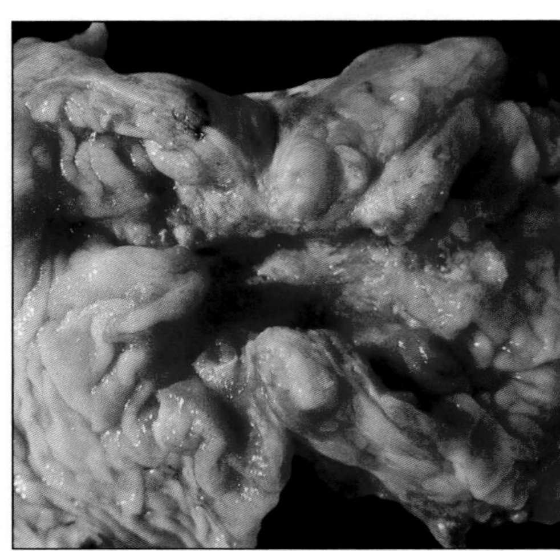

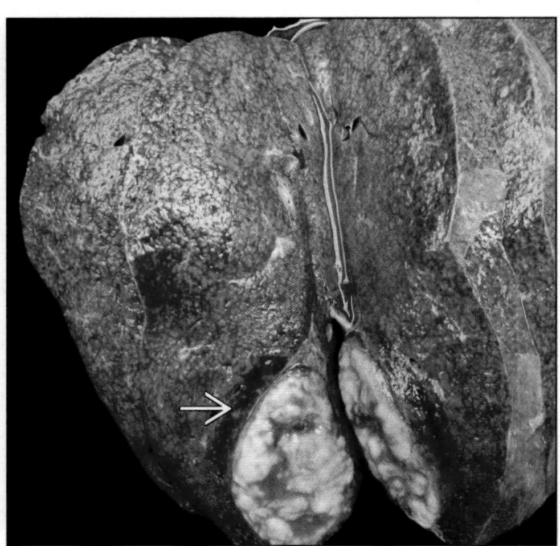

(Left) *Tumor mass effects include obstruction. This colon cancer has a "napkin ring" patten causing colonic obstruction. This tumor would be measured and the transmural invasion documented to stage it according to TNM staging system. (From DP: Endoscopic.)* ***(Right)*** *Limited metastatic disease to the liver in a colon cancer, as shown here ⇒, would be recorded as an M1a (metastasis confined to 1 organ or site).*

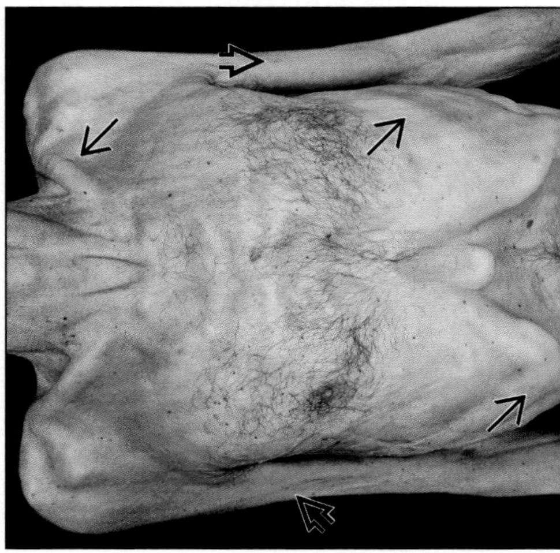

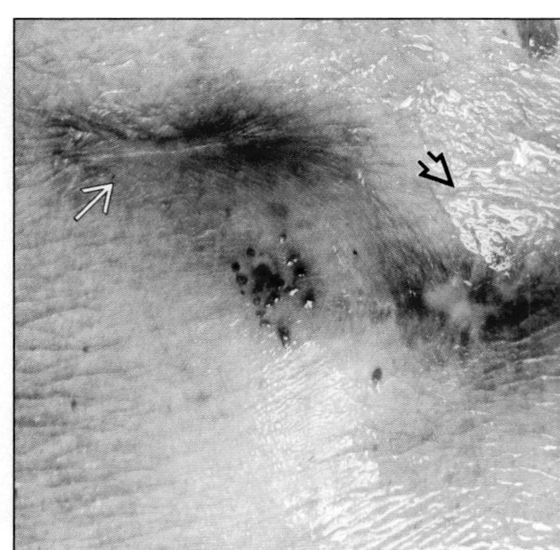

(Left) *Marked cachexia with severe loss of adipose tissue and muscle mass as noted here by prominent bony protrusions ⇒ and marked muscular atrophy ⇒ is common in malignancy and felt to be due to effects of TNFα on metabolism.* ***(Right)*** *This scar ⇒ is associated with a port-a-cath reservoir ⇒ on the anterior chest wall of a patient with malignancy. These devices must be checked for placement and any associated infection at autopsy of patients with malignancy.*

Therapeutic Complications

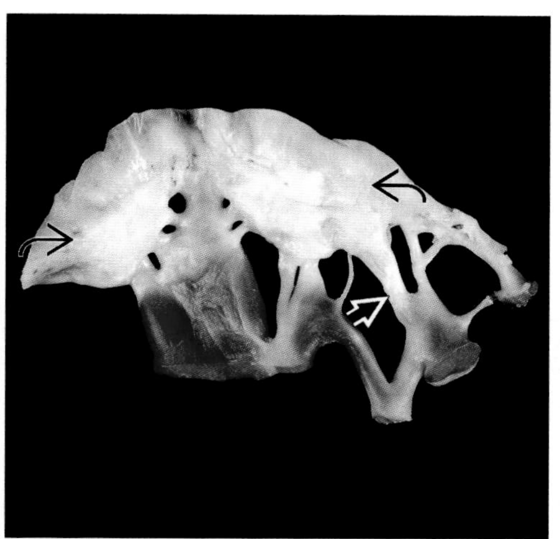

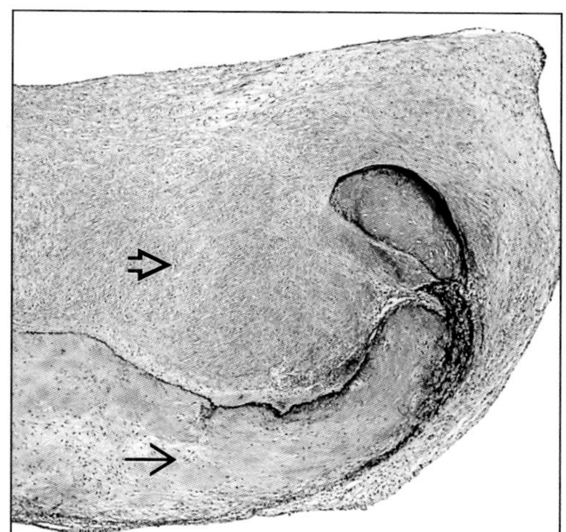

(Left) *This resected atrioventricular valve shows the characteristic plaques of carcinoid valve disease. They lay over the valvular leaflet ⇨ as well as chordae tendinea ➡. (From DP: Cardiovascular.)* ***(Right)*** *An elastic stain reveals the carcinoid plaque to be devoid of elastic tissue ⇨, which is limited to the valve tissue →. There is no injury to the underlying valve tissue. The plaque is comprised of smooth muscle cells in a matrix rich in acid mucopolysaccharides. (From DP: Cardiovascular.)*

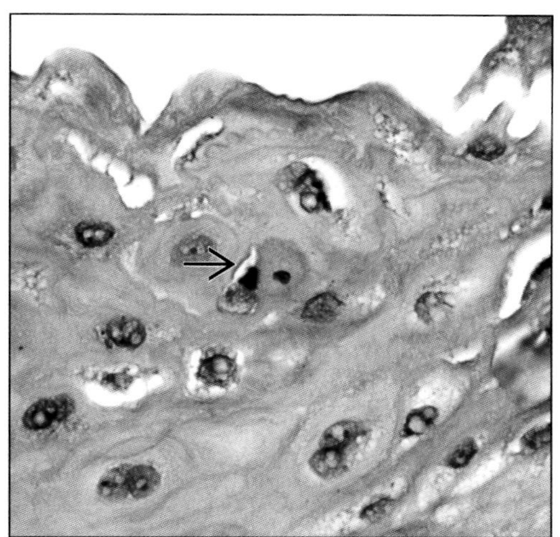

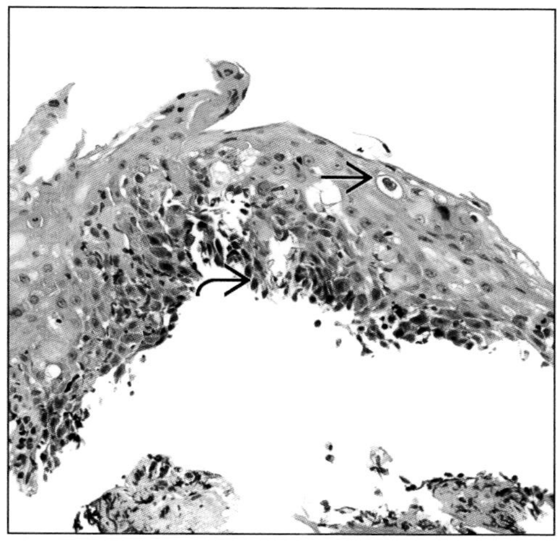

(Left) *Histologically, there were scattered apoptotic squamous cells in the epithelium →. (From DP: Endoscopic.)* ***(Right)*** *With more severe graft-vs.-host disease, there is more extensive epithelial apoptosis → that can progress to frank necrosis and ulceration. Lymphocytic inflammation is present ⇨. (From DP: Endoscopic.)*

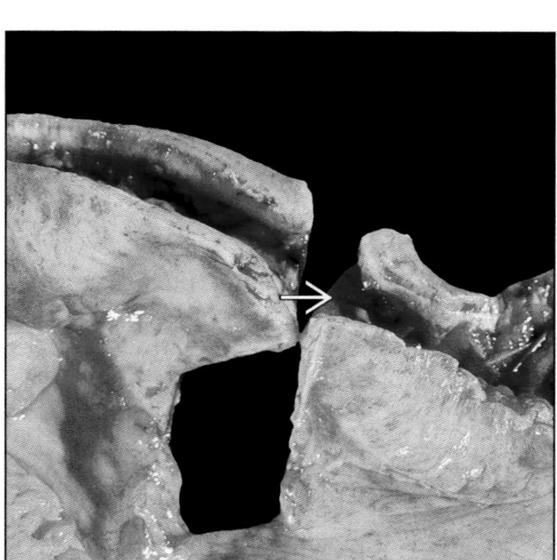

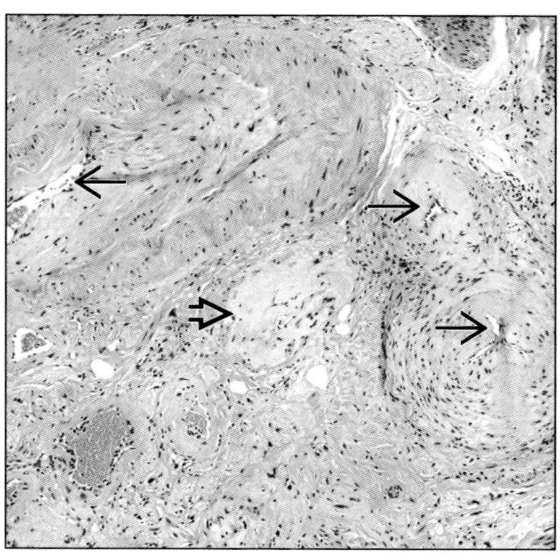

(Left) *This small bowel was resected due to obstruction following radiation therapy for gynecologic malignancy. The bowel wall is markedly thickened ➡ due to fibrosis. (From DP: Endoscopic.)* ***(Right)*** *Radiation therapy leads to marked intimal fibrosis of the arteries → and may lead to complete obstruction of the lumen ⇨. (From DP: Endoscopic.)*

DEATH DUE TO PARANEOPLASTIC EFFECT

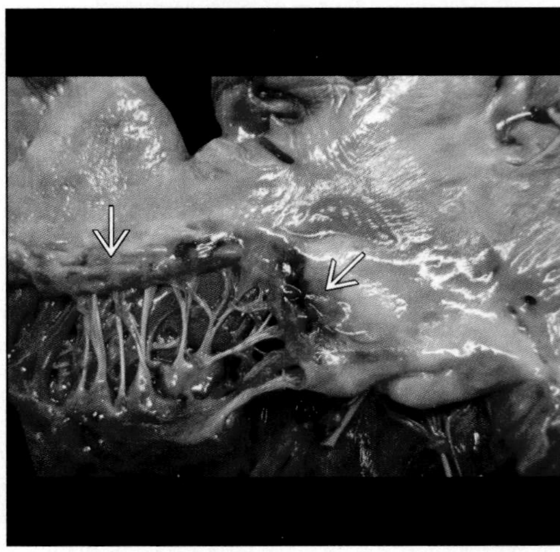

Marantic endocarditis is also known as nonbacterial thrombotic endocarditis. Note the small valve vegetations ➡, a result of a tumor-associated hypercoagulable state.

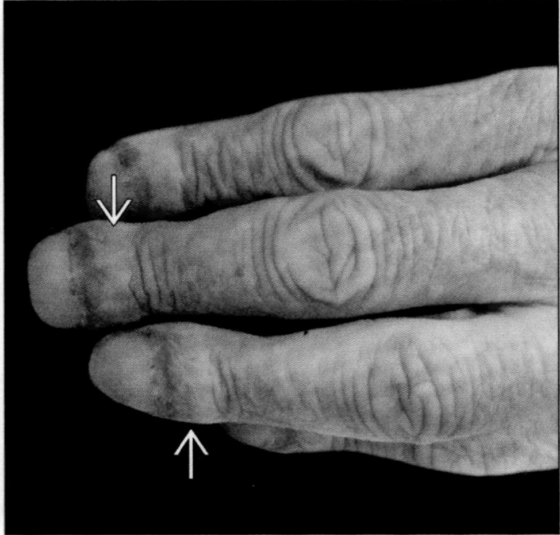

Hypertrophic osteoarthropathy is characterized in part by by digital clubbing. Widening of the distal phalanx ➡ is due to collagen deposition and capillary proliferation.

TERMINOLOGY

Definitions

- Paraneoplastic syndromes
  - Remote effects (signs and symptoms) produced by tumor
  - Not related to mass effect, invasion, obstruction, or metastasis
  - Definition excludes infections, nutritional effects, and complications of therapy
  - Often precede malignant diagnosis

ETIOLOGY/PATHOGENESIS

Commonly Associated Tumors

- Lung
  - Particularly small cell lung carcinoma (SCLC)
- Hematolymphoid
- Breast
- Ovary
- Kidney

Mechanisms

- Tumor-produced humoral factors: Hormones, cytokines, enzymes, precursors, etc.
  - e.g., neuroendocrine tumors of pancreas
- Altered immune response: Cross-reactive antitumor antibodies
  - e.g., onconeural antibodies

CLINICAL ISSUES

Epidemiology

- Incidence
  - Overall incidence estimated at 1-20% of malignancies
    - Likely represents an underestimate
  - Incidence for some specific tumor types
    - 5% of cases of small cell lung cancer
    - 10% of cases of lymphoma, myeloma
    - 10-40% of cases of renal cell carcinoma
- Age
  - Later in life (median: 6th decade)
- Gender
  - Women with SCLC have increased risk of paraneoplastic encephalomyelitis
  - Gender distribution in other clinical scenarios uncertain
- Hormone-producing tumors especially may be part of an inherited syndrome
  - Multiple endocrine neoplasia type 1
  - von Hippel-Lindau disease
  - Neurofibromatosis type 1
  - Tuberous sclerosis

Presentation

- General
  - Most of these syndromes may also be seen in absence of a tumor
    - Clinicopathologic correlation is essential
  - Paraneoplastic syndrome may be 1st sign of malignancy
  - Some paraneoplastic syndromes will resolve with successful tumor treatment
    - Typically true of endocrine paraneoplastic syndromes
  - Other paraneoplastic syndromes may persist despite tumor treatment
    - Especially true of immune-mediated and neurologic paraneoplastic syndromes
- Cutaneous
  - Dermatomyositis
    - Heliotrope facial rash
    - Periorbital edema
    - Erythematous papules on extensor surfaces of joints (Gottron sign)
    - Progressive proximal muscle weakness

DEATH DUE TO PARANEOPLASTIC EFFECT

Key Facts

Terminology

- Paraneoplastic syndromes are remote effects of tumors, not related to invasion, metastasis, or obstruction
- Typically produced by 1 of 2 mechanisms
  - Tumor-elaborated substance (hormones, cytokines, enzymes, etc.)
  - Cross-reacting antitumor antibodies (especially in neuromuscular paraneoplastic syndromes)
- Clinical syndrome of a paraneoplastic syndrome may present before or after diagnosis of underlying tumor
- Demonstration of paraneoplastic syndromes may be challenging
  - Occur in an estimated 1-20% of cases of malignant tumors
  - Tumors may be occult and small
  - Clinical presentations are often nonspecific and may be seen unassociated with tumors
- Clinicopathologic correlation is essential
  - Review clinical records, including laboratory and imaging results, carefully
  - Perform a diligent external examination
  - Perform a thorough gross and histologic examination
  - Sample thoroughly for histology
- Almost any tumor may be associated, but most common are lung (especially small cell carcinoma), hematolymphoid, kidney, breast, and ovary

  - Erythema nodosum
  - Melanosis cutis
    - Gray discoloration of skin distant from primary tumor
    - May be diffuse or localized
    - No associated tumor cells
  - Acanthosis nigricans
    - Strong association with malignancy
    - Velvety, gray-black epidermal hyperplasia
    - Most typically in skin folds (axillary, inguinal)
    - Strong association with malignancy
  - Syndrome of Leser-Trelát
    - Sudden eruption of numerous seborrheic keratoses
    - Existing seborrheic keratoses may increase in size
    - May be associated with acanthosis nigricans
  - New nonpigmented lanugo hair
  - Acquired ichthyosis
  - Necrolytic migratory erythema
    - Often associated with glucagon-producing tumors (e.g., pancreatic neuroendocrine tumor)
  - Sweet syndrome
  - Scleroderma
- Neuromuscular
  - Lambert-Eaton myasthenia
    - Proximal muscle weakness
    - Often SCLC
  - Myasthenia gravis
    - Antibodies directed toward neuromuscular acetylcholine receptors
    - Muscle weakness
    - Associated with thymoma (15% of cases)
  - Subacute sensory neuronopathy
    - Most often with SCLC
  - Opsoclonus-myoclonus: Disordered ocular motility and multifocal myoclonus
    - Pediatric patients: Associated with neuroblastoma
    - Adult patients: Especially breast and gynecologic cancer
  - Cerebellar degeneration: Diplopia, vertigo, gait disturbances, nystagmus, dysarthria
  - Encephalomyelitis
  - Limbic encephalitis: Rapid-onset mental status changes and seizures, antibody mediated
- Gastrointestinal
  - Zollinger-Ellison syndrome
    - Result of gastrin-producing tumors (e.g., pancreatic neuroendocrine tumors)
    - Gastroduodenal ulcers as well as ulcers in atypical locations
    - Refractory to standard therapy
- Orthopedic
  - Hypertrophic osteoarthropathy
    - Digital clubbing, arthralgias, and ossifying periostitis
  - Tumor-related osteomalacia
    - Bone pain, hypophosphatemia, phosphaturia, low vitamin D
    - May be caused by tumor-produced fibroblast growth factor 23 (FGF23)
    - Mesenchymal hyperphosphaturic tumors, lung cancer, multiple myeloma, prostate cancer; often small tumors
- Metabolic/endocrine
  - Hypercalcemia
    - Tumor-associated parathyroid hormone production
    - Squamous cell carcinoma of lung
    - Renal cell carcinoma (15-20%)
  - Syndrome of inappropriate antidiuretic hormone production (SIADH)
    - Tumor-produced ADH, often by SCLC (75%)
    - Rarely non-small cell lung cancer, head and neck cancer, esthesioneuroblastoma
    - Euvolemic hyponatremia; may be associated with seizures and mental status changes
  - Hypoglycemia
    - Insulin-producing tumors (e.g., pancreatic neuroendocrine tumors)
  - Cushing syndrome
    - Result of tumor-produced adrenocorticotrophic hormone (ACTH)
    - SCLC most common

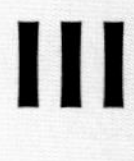

DEATH DUE TO PARANEOPLASTIC EFFECT

- Rarely, thyroid, adrenal, thymic, or pancreatic tumors
- Carcinoid syndrome
  - Episodic cutaneous flushing, watery diarrhea
  - May produce endocardial and valvular changes
  - Neuroendocrine tumor production of vasoactive peptides
  - Typically midgut neuroendocrine tumors with liver metastasis
  - 10% of cases associated with bronchial neuroendocrine tumors
  - 1% pancreatic neuroendocrine tumors
- Hematologic
  - Migratory thrombophlebitis (Trousseau syndrome)
    - Classically seen with gastrointestinal adenocarcinomas, but may be seen with many other types
  - Marantic endocarditis
    - Result of tumor-associated hypercoagulable state
    - May produce emboli and ischemic symptoms
    - Most commonly with adenocarcinoma of lung or pancreas
  - Erythrocytosis
    - Tumor-produced erythropoietin, often by renal cell carcinomas (1-8%)
    - Less commonly: Hepatocellular carcinoma, Wilms tumor, cerebellar hemangioblastoma, sarcomas
  - Eosinophilia
    - Hodgkin disease and mycosis fungoides

Laboratory Tests

- Tumor-secreted substances
  - Can be used clinically as tumor markers
  - Carcinoid syndrome
    - Elevated 24-hour urine 5-HIAA
- Tumor-associated antibodies
  - Antineuronal antibodies
    - Anti-Hu: Tumor-associated cerebellar degeneration and encephalomyelitis
    - Anti-Yo: Tumor-associated cerebellar degeneration, especially with ovarian or breast tumors
  - Anti-acetylcholine receptor antibody: Myasthenia gravis
  - Anti-voltage-gated calcium channel antibodies
    - Lambert-Eaton myasthenic syndrome
- Electrolytes
  - SIADH
    - Hyponatremia, hypo-osmolality, urine sodium > 40 mEq/L
  - Tumor-related osteomalacia
    - Hypophosphatemia, hyperphosphaturia, low vitamin D

MACROSCOPIC FEATURES

External Examination

- General
  - Tumor-associated cachexia
    - Body mass index
    - Estimation of adipose tissue: Thickness of abdominal pannus
    - Muscle wasting
  - Digital clubbing: Hypertrophic osteoarthropathy
  - Cushing syndrome
    - Truncal obesity, dorsocervical fat ("buffalo hump"), cutaneous striae, hirsutism, bruising
- Skin
  - Document appearance and distribution of lesions
  - Consider biopsy, but not of hands or face
  - Consequences of tumor-related pruritus
    - Linear excoriations
    - Related skin infections

Internal Examination

- Thorough examination and sampling essential
- Underlying tumor may be inconspicuous
  - Examine breasts
  - Run entire gastrointestinal tract
  - Thorough sectioning of pancreas

Organ Examination

- Carcinoid syndrome-related heart disease
  - Fibrous endocardial fibrous plaques on valve leaflets and cardiac chambers
  - Right heart more often than left heart

MICROSCOPIC PATHOLOGY

Histologic Features

- Paraneoplastic cerebellar ataxia
  - Loss of Purkinje cells
  - Lymphocytic inflammation
- Tumor-related osteomalacia
  - Tumors often small and inconspicuous
  - Spindle and giant cell pattern
- Marantic endocarditis
  - Valve vegetations composed of fibrin and platelets
  - Typically lack inflammatory cells and microorganisms

SELECTED REFERENCES

1. Ito T et al: Pancreatic neuroendocrine tumors: clinical features, diagnosis and medical treatment: advances. Best Pract Res Clin Gastroenterol. 26(6):737-53, 2012
2. Pelosof LC et al: Paraneoplastic syndromes: an approach to diagnosis and treatment. Mayo Clin Proc. 85(9):838-54, 2010
3. Dalmau J et al: Paraneoplastic syndromes of the CNS. Lancet Neurol. 7(4):327-40, 2008
4. Rees JH: Paraneoplastic syndromes: when to suspect, how to confirm, and how to manage. J Neurol Neurosurg Psychiatry. 75 Suppl 2:ii43-50, 2004
5. Boyce S et al: Paraneoplastic dermatoses. Dermatol Clin. 20(3):523-32, 2002
6. Palapattu GS et al: Paraneoplastic syndromes in urologic malignancy: the many faces of renal cell carcinoma. Rev Urol. 4(4):163-70, 2002

Gross and Histologic Features

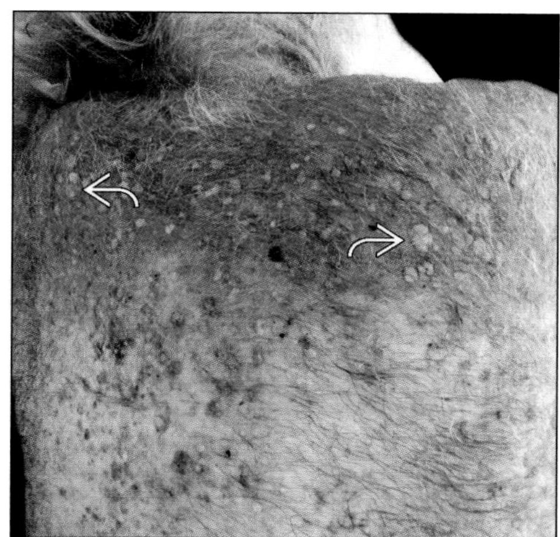

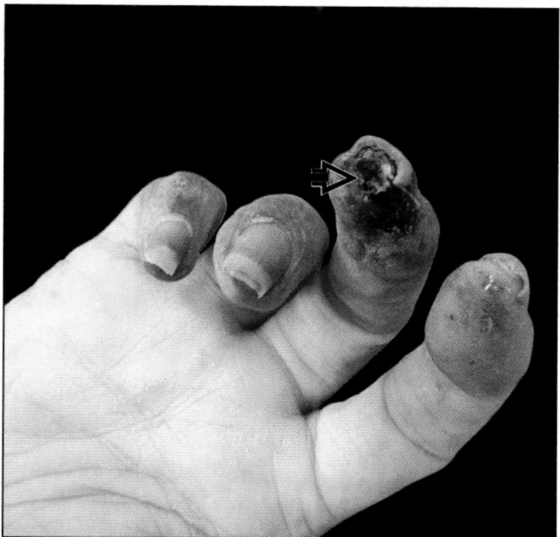

(Left) *Lester-Trelát sign refers to the sudden appearance of multiple new seborrheic keratoses ➡ and the rapid increase in size of existing seborrheic keratoses.* ***(Right)*** *This patient with scleroderma has characteristic digital ulcers ➡. Scleroderma and systemic lupus are associated with increased risk of malignancy (this patient had lung carcinoma). Some scleroderma patients also have tumor-directed antibodies that cross-react with RNA polymerase.*

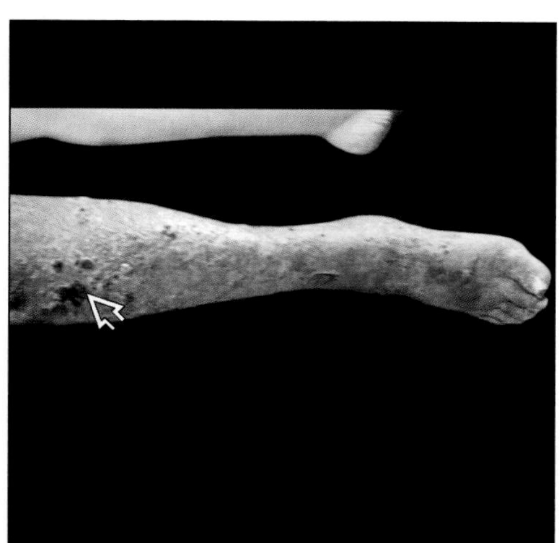

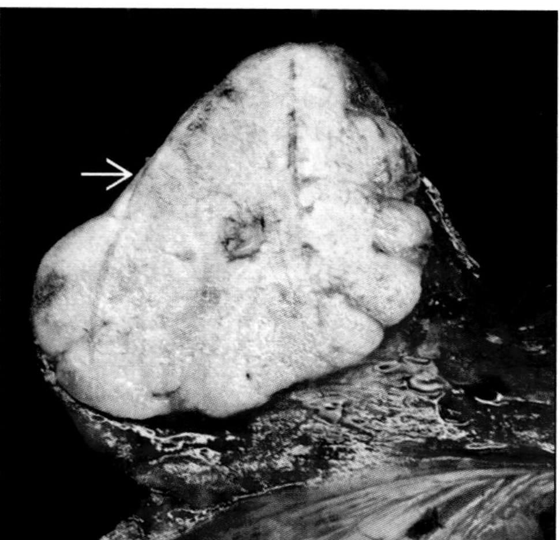

(Left) *Melanosis cutis (diffuse or localized) is the deposition of melanin pigment in skin ➡ not directly affected by melanoma and is usually seen in advanced cases.* ***(Right)*** *Neuroendocrine tumors (NET), especially small cell lung cancers, are particularly likely to be associated with paraneoplastic syndromes. In addition to producing biologically active peptides, they may be associated with antineuronal antibodies. The cut surface ➡ of a NET of the lung is seen.*

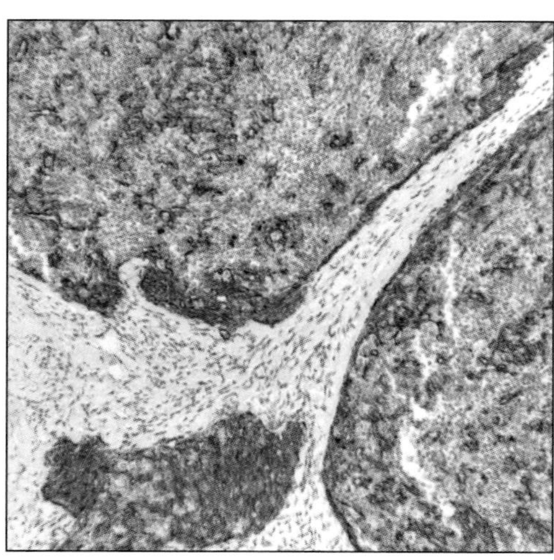

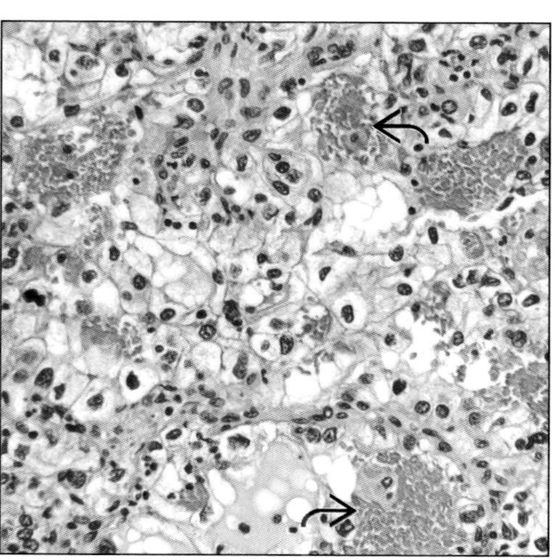

(Left) *Thymoma is associated with myasthenia gravis in 15% of cases. This section of thymoma stained with CK5/6 shows the characteristic nodularity and biphasic nature of the tumor (the background cells are T cells).* ***(Right)*** *This clear cell renal cell carcinoma (RCC) shows characteristic chicken-wire vascularity ➡. RCC is associated with a paraneoplastic syndrome (such as polycythemia or hypercalcemia) in 10-40% of cases. Some RCCs produce renin and can result in hypertension.*

SECTION 4

Other Common Hospital Death

CHRONIC OBSTRUCTIVE PULMONARY DISEASE

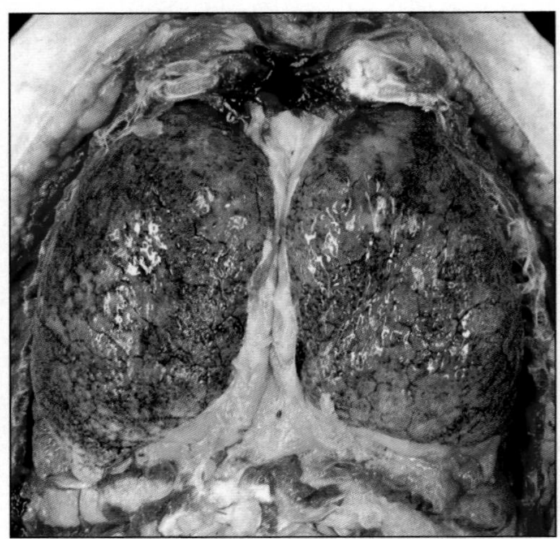

These emphysematous lungs, shown in situ, are hyperinflated and obscure the heart. Note the anthracotic pigment.

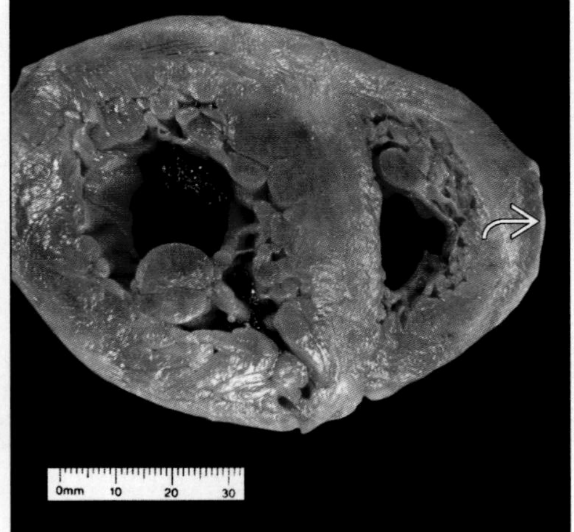

Chronic cor pulmonale is shown. Cross section of the ventricles reveals marked right ventricular hypertrophy ➢. The right and left ventricle are virtually the same thickness.

TERMINOLOGY

Abbreviations

- Chronic obstructive pulmonary disease (COPD)

Definitions

- Pulmonary lobule
  - Composed of respiratory bronchiole, alveolar ducts, and alveoli
    - Gas exchange unit of lung
  - Terminal bronchiole: Final portion of conducting system
- COPD: Group of airway diseases causing dyspnea and characterized by airflow limitation, with considerable overlap between them
  - Emphysema: Defined anatomically
    - Abnormal, permanent enlargement of airspaces distal to terminal bronchioles
    - Accompanied by destruction of airspace walls
    - No obvious component of fibrosis
  - Chronic bronchitis: Defined clinically
    - Chronic productive cough for 3 months in 2 successive years
    - Often have repeated respiratory tract infections
  - Asthma: **Not all authors include asthma as part of COPD;** early on there is no fixed anatomic lesion
    - Chronic airway disorder with variable and recurring episodes of dyspnea and wheezing
    - Inflammation (often eosinophilic), mucus production, bronchoconstriction
    - Longstanding, severe cases can develop fixed airway changes similar to chronic bronchitis
  - **Many patients with COPD show elements of both chronic bronchitis and emphysema**

ETIOLOGY/PATHOGENESIS

Developmental Anomaly

- Congenital α-1-antitrypsin deficiency
  - Emphysema and cirrhosis
    - Early onset of onset of emphysema
    - Panacinar pattern of emphysema
    - Sometimes family history of emphysema
  - ~ 1-5% of COPD patients
  - Mutations in *SERPINA1* gene; autosomal recessive
    - α-1-antitrypsin produced in liver
    - Protects against protease activity

Environmental Exposure

- Cigarette smoking
  - 80% of COPD patients in USA have smoking history
    - But < 20% of smokers develop COPD
    - 20% of COPD patients are never smokers
    - Other unidentified genetic and environmental factors must be involved
  - Amount and duration of cigarette smoking contribute to severity
- Biomass fuel use for heating and cooking
  - Wood &/or dung
  - Particularly in developing world
- Workplace inhaled irritants
  - Agricultural: Organic dusts
  - Industrial: Metallic fumes (e.g., cadmium, aluminum)
  - Mining: Coal, heavy metals
- Air pollution
  - COPD more common in urban settings than rural

CLINICAL ISSUES

Epidemiology

- Incidence
  - 5% of USA population affected

CHRONIC OBSTRUCTIVE PULMONARY DISEASE

Key Facts

Terminology

- COPD: Spectrum of pulmonary diseases that produces dyspnea and is characterized by airflow limitation
  - Emphysema: Airspace destruction distal to terminal bronchioles without significant fibrosis
  - Chronic bronchitis: Productive cough for 3 months in 2 successive years without other explanation
  - Asthma: Episodic dyspnea and wheezing with inflammation, mucus production, and inflammation (eosinophilic)
  - Considerable clinical and pathological overlap between these
- 3rd leading cause of death in USA
- Cigarette smoking is most important etiologic agent in USA
  - Other inhaled irritants (industrial particulates, agricultural dusts, biomass fuel) are also implicated
  - α-1-antitrypsin is a rare cause of emphysema and hepatic cirrhosis
- Autopsy suggestions
  - Consider checking for pneumothorax before opening thorax
  - Look for changes of chronic cor pulmonale, right ventricular hypertrophy
  - Look for evidence of right heart failure & associated changes (hepatosplenomegaly, ascites)
  - Look for evidence of pulmonary hypertension
  - If emphysema is accompanied by hepatic cirrhosis, consider α-1-antitrypsin deficiency

---

  - 3rd most common cause of death in USA
    - 120,000 deaths per year
- Age
  - Considerable overlap between emphysema and chronic bronchitis
    - Chronic bronchitis: 40-45 years
    - Emphysema: 50-75 years
- Gender
  - Historically more prevalent in men
  - Increased incidence in women in last 2 decades
    - Possibly result of increased cigarette smoking, which peaked in women 10 years later than in men
    - Women have more severe symptoms with same cigarette exposure
  - Women: ↑ exposure to biomass cooking fuels in developing world
  - 80% of never-smokers with COPD are women
- Asthma
  - Increases risk for emphysema and chronic bronchitis
  - True even after correction for smoking history

Presentation

- Typical emphysema: "Pink puffer"
  - Thin
  - Pulmonary hyperinflation
  - Normal or near normal PaO2, normal or ↓ PCO2: No cyanosis
    - Destruction of airspaces **and** associated capillaries
    - Little ventilation/perfusion (VQ) mismatch
  - Less often show signs of right-sided heart failure
- Typical chronic bronchitis: "Blue bloater"
  - Heavy
  - ↓ PAO_2, ↑ PCO_2: Cyanosis
    - Airway obstruction by mucus; no loss of capillaries
    - Marked VQ mismatch
  - Cor pulmonale with edema and signs of right heart failure
  - Prone to sleep apnea
- "Pink puffer" and "blue bloater" are extremes of clinical spectrum
  - Most COPD patients have elements of both
- Asthma
  - Episodic occurrence of dyspnea and wheezing
    - Known allergic or other types of triggers in some patients
  - Reversible spontaneously or with treatment
    - No characteristic fixed anatomic defect early in disease course

Laboratory Tests

- Abnormal spirometry
  - ↓ FEV1: Forced expiratory volume (FEV) in 1 second
    - Typically < 80% of predicted
  - ↓ FEV1/FVC: FEV1 as a fraction of total forced vital capacity
    - Typically < 0.7
  - Obstruction to airflow caused by increased airway resistance and airway collapse
- Polycythemia and ↑ hemoglobin and hematocrit in hypoxemic patients
- EKG: Right ventricular hypertrophy in patients with cor pulmonale

IMAGE FINDINGS

Radiographic Findings

- Plain films are not sensitive; symptomatic patients may have normal chest films
- Emphysema
  - Hyperinflated lungs
  - Flattened diaphragms
  - Large retrosternal air space
- Chronic bronchitis
  - Nonspecific changes
  - Increased bronchial markings and cardiomegaly

CT Findings

- High-resolution CT much more sensitive than plain films for emphysema
  - Can distinguish patterns of emphysema

CHRONIC OBSTRUCTIVE PULMONARY DISEASE

- However, 20% of pathologically proven cases show negative CT scans
- Chronic bronchitis
  - Bronchial wall thickening and enlarged vessels

MACROSCOPIC FEATURES

External Examination

- Barrel chest: ↑ anteroposterior (hyperinflation)
- Prominent accessory muscles of respiration and angle of Louis
- Cyanosis (but not typically clubbing)
- Edema in those with right heart failure
- Yellow discoloration of fingertips in smokers
- Changes secondary to "tripod posture" (sitting forward with elbows on thighs or tabletop)
  - Dahl sign: Symmetrical slanted calluses or discolorations on thighs
  - Calluses on forearms or olecranon bursitis
- Skin changes in patients on chronic steroids
  - Thin, easily torn skin with bruising

Internal Examination

- Body cavities
  - Pneumothorax should be considered in patients with emphysema
    - Incise pleura under water seal prior to opening thorax
  - Ascites in patients with right heart failure
- Hyperinflated lungs obscure heart
- Anthracotic mediastinal lymph nodes

Organ Examination

- Lungs
  - Emphysema
    - Bullous emphysema: Airspaces > 1 cm; often apical
  - Chronic bronchitis
    - Mucus in airways
  - Asthma
    - Hyperinflated lungs; may show impressions from ribs
    - Tenacious mucus plugs in bronchi and bronchioles
- Heart: Cor pulmonale
  - Right ventricular hypertrophy in chronic cor pulmonale
    - Acute cor pulmonale (e.g., in pulmonary embolus or ARDS) characterized by right ventricular dilatation
  - Pulmonary arteries may show evidence of pulmonary hypertension
    - Yellow atherosclerotic plaques
- Liver
  - Hepatomegaly and centrilobular congestion ("nutmeg liver") in patients with heart failure
  - Cirrhosis in patients with α-1-antitrypsin deficiency
- Spleen
  - Splenomegaly in patients with heart failure

MICROSCOPIC PATHOLOGY

Histologic Features

- Emphysema: Destruction of airspaces; 3 patterns with much overlap
  - Centriacinar
    - Affects terminal bronchiole with relative sparing of peripheral respiratory lobule
    - Most pronounced in apices of upper lobes and superior segments of lower lobes
    - Most common type
    - Most strongly associated with cigarette smoking
  - Panacinar
    - Affects entire respiratory lobule
    - Most pronounced in lung bases
    - Can be associated with α-1-antitrypsin deficiency and methylphenidate injection
  - Paraseptal
    - Most pronounced in subpleural locations including lung fissures
    - Can lead to bullous formation and pneumothorax
- Chronic bronchitis
  - Hyperplasia of peribronchial mucus glands
    - Reid index: Ratio of thickness of mucus gland layer to thickness of bronchial wall from basement membrane to cartilage
    - Normally < 0.4
    - Increased in chronic bronchitis
  - Goblet cell metaplasia of bronchial epithelium
  - Peribronchial chronic inflammation
  - Bronchiolar mucus and exudate
- Asthma
  - Thickened bronchial basement membrane
  - Bronchial edema and inflammation
    - Inflammation typically eosinophil rich
  - Enlarged bronchial mucus glands
  - Bronchial smooth muscle hypertrophy
- Liver
  - Centrilobular congestion with heart failure
  - α-1-antitrypsin deficiency
    - Cirrhosis, cholestasis, cholangitis
    - **Periportal globules of PAS positive material** (accumulated α-1-antitrypsin in hepatocyte endoplasmic reticulum)

SELECTED REFERENCES

1. Aryal S et al: Influence of sex on chronic obstructive pulmonary disease risk and treatment outcomes. Int J Chron Obstruct Pulmon Dis. 9:1145-1154, 2014
2. Kim V et al: Chronic bronchitis and chronic obstructive pulmonary disease. Am J Respir Crit Care Med. 187(3):228-37, 2013
3. Nussbaumer-Ochsner Y et al: Systemic manifestations of COPD. Chest. 139(1):165-73, 2011
4. Silva GE et al: Asthma as a risk factor for COPD in a longitudinal study. Chest. 126(1):59-65, 2004
5. Tomashefski JF Jr et al: The bronchopulmonary pathology of alpha-1 antitrypsin (AAT) deficiency: findings of the Death Review Committee of the national registry for individuals with Severe Deficiency of Alpha-1 Antitrypsin. Hum Pathol. 35(12):1452-61, 2004

Gross and Microscopic Images

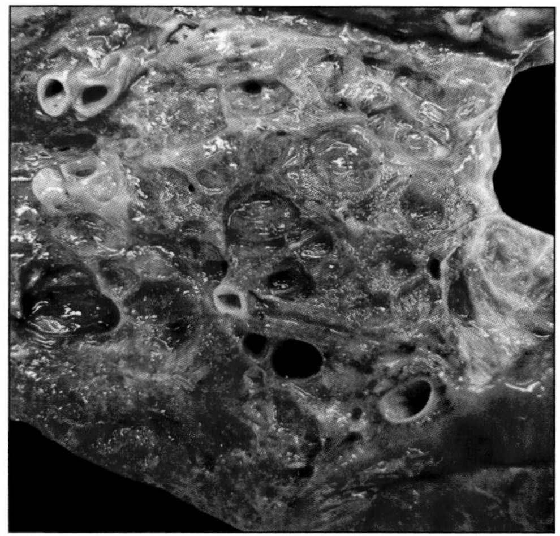

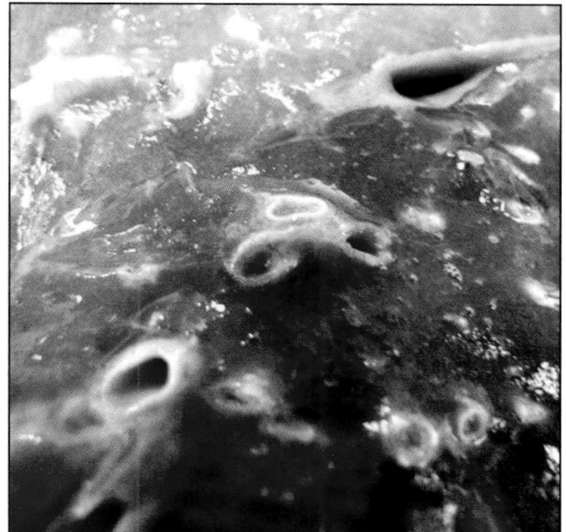

(Left) *The cut surface of this lung shows markedly dilated airspaces in the case of emphysema.* ***(Right)*** *A close-up view of the cut surface of lung shows prominent bronchi projecting slightly above the surface of the lung tissue like tent poles.*

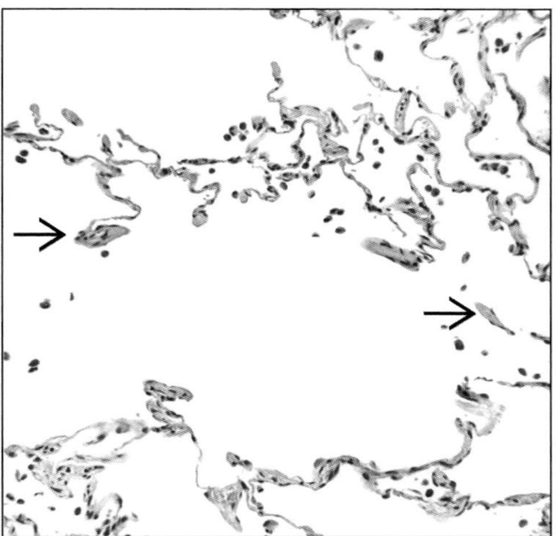

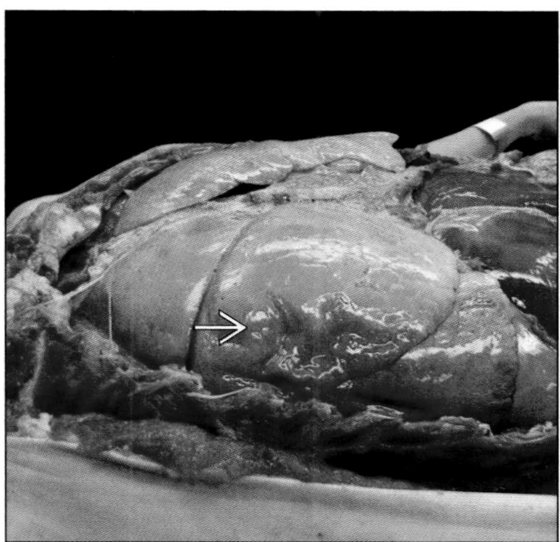

(Left) *Histologic section of emphysematous lung shows abnormally large alveoli with alveolar septa that appear to float or end blindly with club-like tips* ➔*.* ***(Right)*** *This in situ photograph of a patient dying of an acute asthmatic episode shows hyperinflated lungs with rib impressions* ➔*. Note the tan-pink color and lack of anthracotic pigment.*

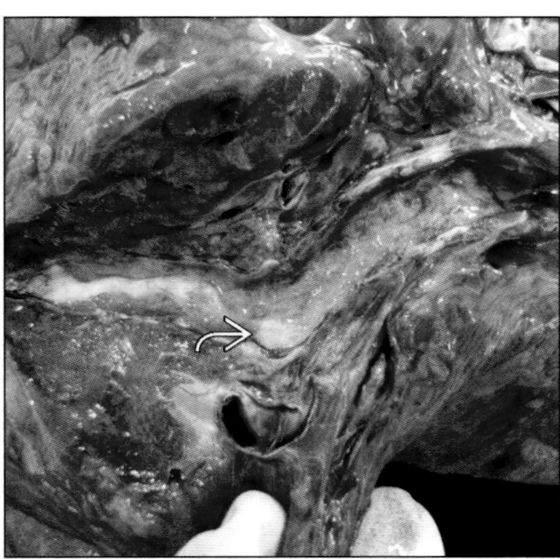

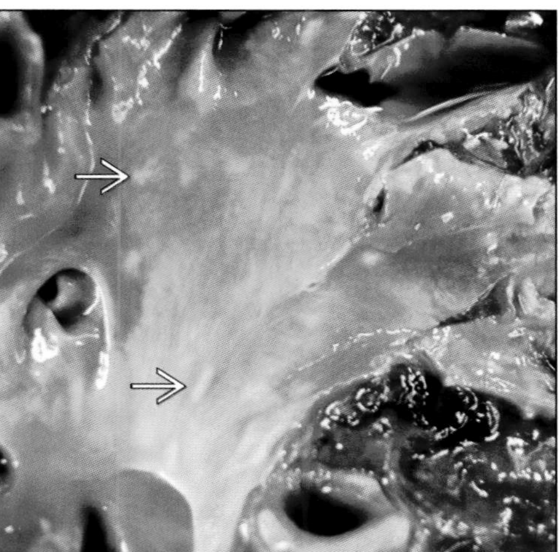

(Left) *This lung was taken from a patient who died during an acute asthmatic episode. The bronchial tree is opened to show copious, thick mucus* ➔*.* ***(Right)*** *Close-up view of an opened pulmonary artery shows yellow atherosclerotic plaques* ➔*, an indication of pulmonary hypertension. COPD with cor pulmonale is a common cause of pulmonary hypertension.*

VENTILATOR DEPENDENT RESPIRATORY FAILURE

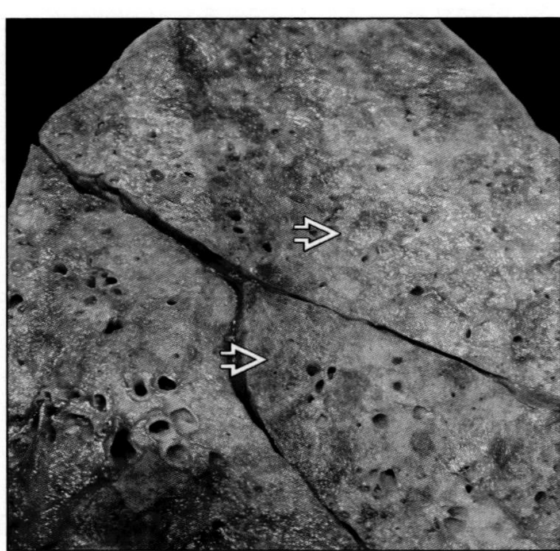

Gross photograph shows organizing diffuse alveolar damage in a patient with connective tissue disease and prolonged mechanical ventilation. The lung shows tan areas of consolidation ➡.

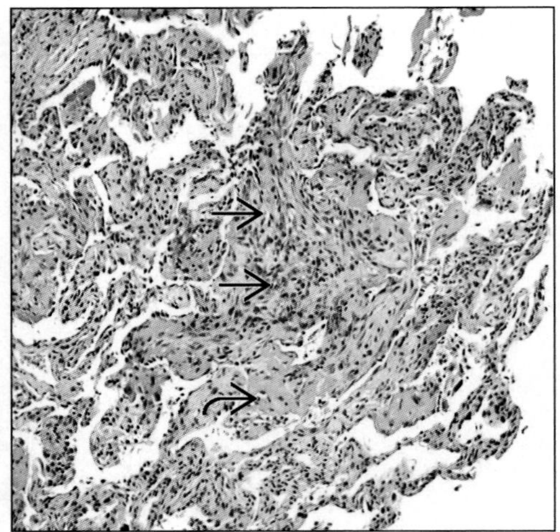

Organizing diffuse alveolar damage is shown histologically, with diagnostic features of residual hyaline membranes ➡ and fibroblastic proliferation ➡.

TERMINOLOGY

Abbreviations

- Ventilator-dependent respiratory failure (VDRF)

Definitions

- Failure to wean from mechanical ventilation after a defined period of time
  - Autopsied hospital population includes those who die while on mechanical ventilation and those who die shortly after terminal extubation or discontinued mechanical ventilation
- Ventilator-induced lung injury refers to histologic findings associated with mechanical ventilation: Hyaline membranes, increased vascular permeability, pulmonary edema, and inflammatory cell infiltrates
  - Note that these findings are characteristic of diffuse alveolar damage related to any number of initiating etiologies that may have led to need for mechanical ventilation
    - It is therefore difficult to separate out cause(s) leading to mechanical ventilation from effects of treatment
- 1994 American-European Consensus Conference on ARDS set forth clinical criteria for acute lung injury (ALI) and acute respiratory distress syndrome (ARDS) in order to provide a more uniform approach for further study (a.k.a. the Berlin Definition)
  - From a histologic perspective, patients with clinical evidence of acute lung injury most often have histologic pattern of diffuse alveolar damage
    - However, other histologic patterns may be seen, including acute fibrinous and organizing pneumonia (AFOP), acute eosinophilic pneumonia, and diffuse hemorrhage with capillaritis
    - These criteria were revised in 2012 to stratify ARDS into 3 grades
    - Term ALI was retained only for research purposes and not for clinical stratification
- Centers for Disease Control and Prevention has introduced new surveillance definitions for ventilator-associated event that include all complications severe enough to result in sustained increases in ventilatory support
  - Ventilator-associated infectious complications are included in this definition as are other complications such as excess fluid administration and adverse effects of opioid administration

ETIOLOGY/PATHOGENESIS

Pathogenesis

- Purpose of mechanical ventilation is to provide adequate gas exchange while resting respiratory muscles
- Ventilator strategies designed to reduce lung injury have been shown to decrease mortality in patients with ARDS; however, as is well known, morality is high, particularly in some groups of patients
- In a patient who dies with clinical diagnosis of ventilator-dependent respiratory failure, there are 4 major etiologic categories that may influence autopsy findings and may be superimposed on each other
  - Initial inciting event that led to lung injury
  - Frequent occurrence of what are now termed ventilator-associated events (VAEs)
  - Direct effects of ventilator-induced lung injury
  - Other comorbid conditions such as cardiac disease or liver failure, as well as others
- Regional lung overdistension is a critical factor in ventilator-induced lung injury
  - Ventilation at high lung volumes results in alveolar rupture, air leaks, and barotrauma (pneumothorax, pneumomediastinum, and subcutaneous emphysema)

VENTILATOR DEPENDENT RESPIRATORY FAILURE

Key Facts

Terminology
- Ventilator-dependent respiratory failure (VDRF) is failure to wean from mechanical ventilation after a defined period of time

Etiology
- 4 major etiologic categories to consider in VDRF
  - Initial inciting event that led to lung injury
  - Superimposed ventilator-associated complications such as infection
  - Direct effects of ventilator-induced lung injury
  - Other comorbid conditions

Clinical Issues
- Most common cause of VDRF is an acute lung injury superimposed on severe chronic disease

Macroscopic Pathology
- Gross findings correlate with stage of diffuse alveolar damage
- Mechanical ventilation may result in alveolar rupture, air leaks, and barotrauma (pneumothorax, pneumomediastinum, and subcutaneous emphysema)

Microscopic Pathology
- Diffuse alveolar damage is the most common pattern associated with VDRF
- Infection, either as a primary etiology or as a ventilator-associated complication, should be rigorously excluded with special stains and ancillary microbiology studies

  - Overdistension may also result in pulmonary edema, although exact mechanism is not completely understood
  - Even at low lung volumes, there are effects caused by repetitive opening and closing of airways and respiratory units, effects on surfactant function, regional hypoxia, and intracellular/inflammatory mediators

CLINICAL ISSUES

Presentation
- Most common cause of VDRF is an acute lung injury superimposed on severe chronic disease
  - It is possible for underlying chronic disease to be undiagnosed or obscured by the acute presentation
    - Particularly true of older patients with pulmonary fibrosis in whom fibrosis may have been insidious in onset until time of an acute exacerbation
  - A major clinical goal (and in some instances a postmortem examination goal) is to define or exclude underlying chronic disease
- De novo acute lung injury, occurring as either a primary respiratory disease or in setting of multiorgan system dysfunction, is also common and can also result in VDRF
- Other patients are ventilator dependent as a consequence of neuromuscular disorders or chest wall trauma

Prognosis
- Even when normalization of arterial blood gases is achieved by mechanical ventilation, many patients die while on mechanical ventilation
- Ventilator strategies designed to reduce lung injury have been shown to decrease mortality in patients with ARDS
- Causes of mortality
  - Barotrauma
  - Oxygen toxicity
  - Hemodynamic compromise
- Both ventilator-associated conditions and infection-related ventilator associated conditions are associated with prolonged mechanical ventilation and hospital death

MACROSCOPIC FEATURES

External Examination
- If present, tracheostomy site should be examined for evidence of bleeding or infection
- Other intensive monitoring devices are often present

Internal Examination
- If present, appropriate positioning of endotracheal tube and chest tubes should be documented

Organ Examination
- Lungs should be weighed prior to formalin inflation
  - It is not uncommon for combined lung weights to exceed 1,500 g
  - Lung weights generally correlate with severity of respiratory failure and presence of diffuse alveolar damage
- Tracheal, mucosal, and mural changes consistent with prolonged intubation
  - Pressure necrosis (mucosal ulceration and cartilage degeneration)
  - Section to exclude infection (viral, bacterial, and fungal infections such as *Aspergillus* or *Candida* most likely)
- Important chronic diseases that may have contributed to ventilator dependence and that can be anatomically characterized include upper airway obstruction, obstructive lung disease, pulmonary fibrosis, ischemic cardiomyopathy, and direct traumatic (central or peripheral) neuromuscular injury
  - Contributing factors that may be difficult to define anatomically but that can be supported by clinical history include critical illness neuromuscular abnormalities, metabolic or endocrine disorders, and therapy effects

- Following fixation of lung, careful attention should be paid to the possibility of underlying chronic lung disease
  - In addition to characterizing acute changes and excluding infection, sections should be taken of more fibrotic areas
  - Gross findings correlate with stage of diffuse alveolar damage
  - In early phase, lungs are firm, heavy, and have a relatively homogeneous dark red appearance
  - In later phase, lungs are very heavy with irregular areas of dense consolidation and fibrosis
  - If patient was maintained on mechanical ventilation for a long period of time, there will be progressive fibrosis that may result in some "cobblestoning" of pleural surface
  - Extensive peripheral cyst formation consistent with honeycombing is a finding that suggests possibility of underlying chronic fibrotic lung rather than acute interstitial pneumonia (AIP)
- Evidence of mechanical ventilation such as pulmonary interstitial emphysema and small cysts as well as more consequential findings such as pneumothorax

MICROSCOPIC PATHOLOGY

Histologic Features

- Diffuse alveolar damage (DAD) is the most common pattern associated with VDRF
  - Criteria for the diagnosis of DAD include the presence of hyaline membranes in addition to at least 1 of the following
    - Intraalveolar edema, type 1 alveolar cell necrosis, type 2 alveolar pneumocyte hyperplasia covering denuded alveolar-capillary membrane, interstitial fibroblastic/myofibroblastic proliferation of fibroblasts, or organizing interstitial fibrosis
- Other histologic patterns that resemble clinical picture of ARDS and VDRF but are not associated with classic DAD histopathology include bacterial or viral pneumonia, diffuse interstitial pneumonia, pulmonary hemorrhage, or tumor infiltration
- Less common histologic patterns associated with acute lung injury
  - Acute eosinophilic pneumonia is often recognized clinically and treated appropriately with good response
    - It is therefore a very uncommon cause of VDRF
    - Once steroid treatment is instituted, it may be very difficult to identify eosinophils
  - Alveolar hemorrhage should be considered where there is marked coarse hemosiderin and capillaritis
  - Acute fibrinous and organizing pneumonia is characterized by diffuse intraalveolar fibrin balls as opposed to classic hyaline membranes
- Acute interstitial pneumonia (AIP) also should be considered within differential diagnosis of diffuse alveolar damage and VDRF
  - AIP is an idiopathic interstitial lung disease that is clinically characterized by sudden onset of dyspnea and rapid development of hypoxemic respiratory failure that requires prolonged mechanical ventilation
  - Definition excludes patients with ARDS that can be attributed to an identifiable cause as well as patients with underlying fibrotic lung disease or systemic disorders known to be associated with lung involvement, e.g., connective tissue disease
  - Many patients describe a URI/viral-like prodrome and a nonproductive cough
    - This prodrome may precede shortness of breath by 1 week to 2 months
  - Autopsy sections usually show enlarged and remodeled airspaces that resemble the honeycomb change of UIP and reflect progressive disease, but fibroblastic proliferation along with collagen deposition should still be conspicuous within walls of air spaces

DIAGNOSTIC CHECKLIST

Pathologic Interpretation Pearls

- Diffuse alveolar damage, often in different phases, is a common finding
- Possibility of infection should be rigorously evaluated with special stains and ancillary microbiology studies
- Identify underlying chronic disease(s) that may have contributed to ventilator dependence

SELECTED REFERENCES

1. Lewis SC et al: Risk factors for ventilator-associated events: a case-control multivariable analysis. Crit Care Med. 42(8):1839-48, 2014
2. Slutsky AS et al: Ventilator-induced lung injury. N Engl J Med. 370(10):980, 2014
3. ARDS Definition Task Force et al: Acute respiratory distress syndrome: the Berlin Definition. JAMA. 307(23):2526-33, 2012
4. Ambrosino N et al: The difficult-to-wean patient. Expert Rev Respir Med. 4(5):685-92, 2010
5. Beasley MB: The pathologist's approach to acute lung injury. Arch Pathol Lab Med. 134(5):719-27, 2010
6. Wunsch H et al: The epidemiology of mechanical ventilation use in the United States. Crit Care Med. 38(10):1947-53, 2010
7. Bernard GR et al: The American-European Consensus Conference on ARDS. Definitions, mechanisms, relevant outcomes, and clinical trial coordination. Am J Respir Crit Care Med. 149(3 Pt 1):818-24, 1994

Gross and Microscopic Features of VDRF and Underlying Lung Pathology

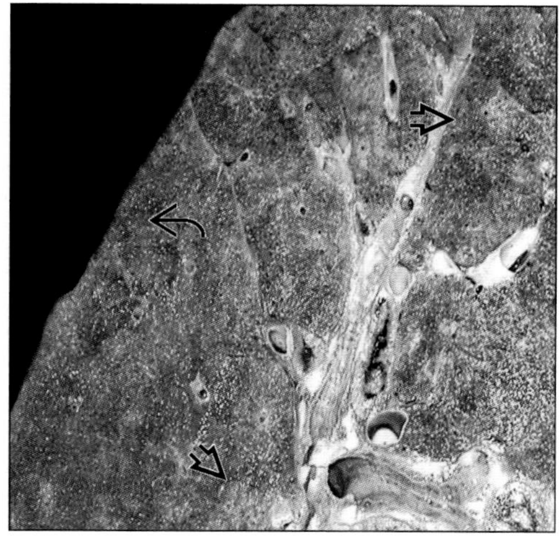

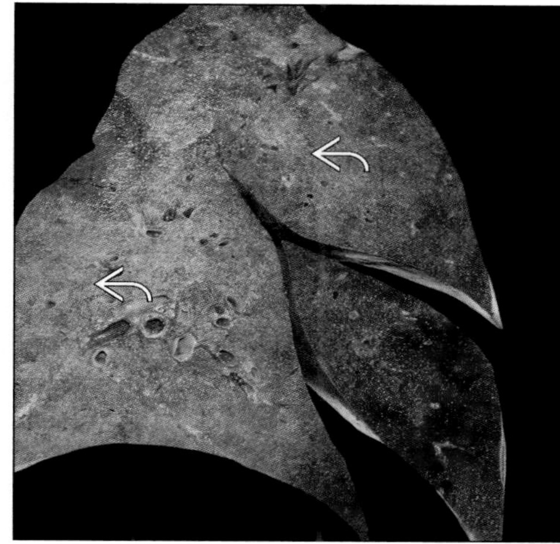

(Left) Gross image shows organizing diffuse alveolar damage with tan areas of consolidation ⇨ and some more preserved lung parenchyma ⇨. (Right) This lung demonstrates organizing diffuse alveolar damage in a mechanically ventilated patient who also received extracorporeal membrane oxygenation (ECMO). The parenchyma is diffusely consolidated ⇨ and red brown in appearance.

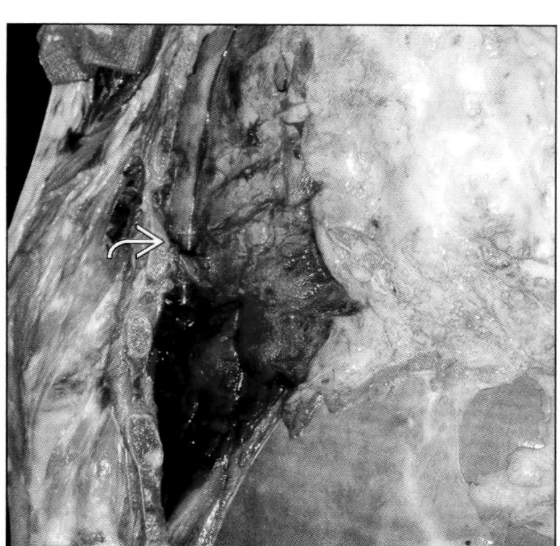

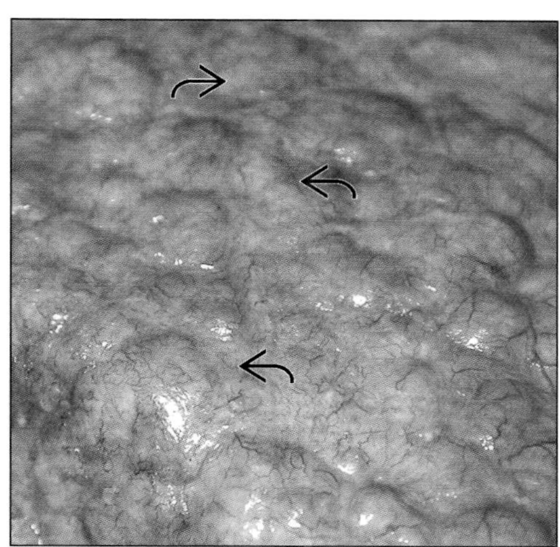

(Left) Gross image shows diffuse alveolar damage in a patient who had a prolonged course of mechanical ventilation and the additional complication of a chest tube in the oblique fissure ⇨. (Right) The extensive cobblestoning of the pleural surface ⇨ of this lung from a patient with VDRF indicated underlying pulmonary fibrosis.

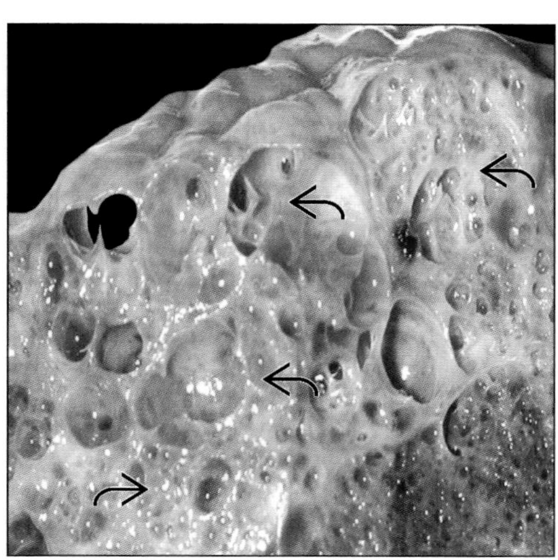

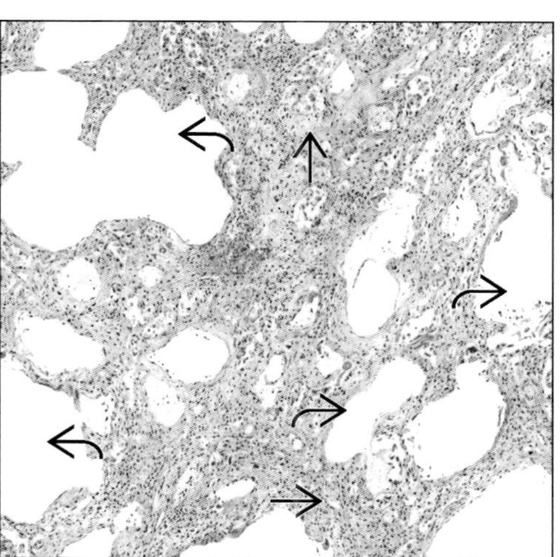

(Left) The cut surface of this lung shows honeycombing ⇨ in a patient with underlying pulmonary fibrosis and ventilator dependent respiratory failure. (Right) This patient with VDRF had acute interstitial pneumonia with diffusely enlarged and remodeled airspaces ⇨. There is conspicuous fibroblastic proliferation and collagen deposition within the alveolar walls ⇨.

CHRONIC LIVER FAILURE

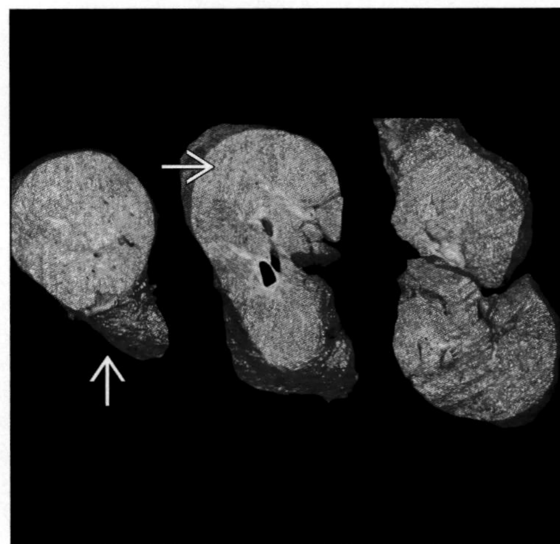

The cut surface of this liver with micronodular cirrhosis due to alcoholic liver disease shows innumerable small nodules ➡ ≤ 3 mm in diameter. (Courtesy D. Rubin, MD.)

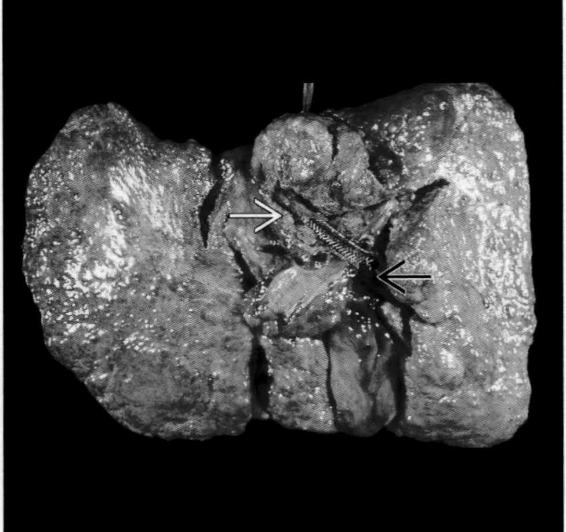

This cirrhotic liver has an intact transjugular intrahepatic portosystemic shunt (TIPS) between the middle hepatic vein ➡ and the right portal vein ⇨. (Courtesy D. Rubin, MD.)

TERMINOLOGY

Abbreviations

- Chronic liver failure (CLF)

Definitions

- Liver dysfunction due to diseases that cause progressive destruction and regeneration of parenchyma over weeks to years, leading to fibrosis, disruption of the vascular architecture, and cirrhosis

ETIOLOGY/PATHOGENESIS

Common Etiologies of CLF/Cirrhosis

- Alcoholic liver disease
  - CLF in 15-20% of chronic heavy alcoholics
  - Women ↑ susceptibility and mortality
- Chronic viral hepatitis infection
  - CLF in ~ 25-30% of chronic hepatitis C and hepatitis B ± D
  - Rarely hepatitis E in immunosuppressed
- Nonalcoholic fatty liver disease (NAFLD)
  - ~ 30% of general population, CLF in ~ 20% with steatohepatitis
  - Associated with diabetes mellitus, dyslipidemia, obesity, drugs (e.g. amiodarone, corticosteroids, tamoxifen)
- Autoimmune hepatitis
  - Females > males; ~ 30% with cirrhosis at time of diagnosis
- Biliary diseases
  - Primary biliary cirrhosis (PBC)
    - Females >> males; CLF in ~ 15% at 5 years
  - Primary sclerosing cholangitis (PSC)
    - Males > females; 60-80% have inflammatory bowel disease
    - ~ 15% with cirrhosis at time of diagnosis; ↑ risk of cholangiocarcinoma
  - Secondary biliary cirrhosis
    - Chronic large duct obstruction by tumors, stones, strictures, parasites, extrahepatic biliary atresia
- Metabolic disorders
  - Hemochromatosis
    - Primary/hereditary: Many types of mutations with variable penetrance; most common is C282Y *HFE* mutation, usually autosomal recessive
    - Secondary: Due to multiple blood transfusions, chronic hemolysis, enteral/parenteral overload, cirrhosis of any cause
  - Wilson disease
    - Copper accumulation due to mutations in *ATP7B* gene; autosomal recessive
  - α-1-antitrypsin (A1AT) deficiency
    - Accumulation of abnormal A1AT protein → cirrhosis and emphysema; autosomal recessive
- Drug/toxin-induced injury
  - Steatohepatitis (e.g., methotrexate, estrogens)
  - Chronic hepatitis (e.g., antibiotics, doxorubicin)
  - Immune-mediated hepatitis (e.g., statins, minocycline)
  - Chronic cholestasis (e.g., total parenteral nutrition, antibiotics)
- Venous outflow obstruction
  - Chronic outflow obstruction due to hepatic vein thrombosis (Budd-Chiari syndrome), congestive heart failure, constrictive pericarditis

Pathogenesis of Complications of CLF/Cirrhosis

- Portal hypertension (HTN)
  - Present in nearly all cirrhotics, due to increased resistance to portal blood flow secondary to scarring, distortion of vascular architecture, formation of intrahepatic shunts, and endothelial dysfunction
  - → collateral vessel formation → esophageal/gastric varices, portal hypertensive gastropathy, caput

CHRONIC LIVER FAILURE

Key Facts

Terminology

- Chronic liver failure: Result of liver disease that causes progressive destruction and regeneration of parenchyma over weeks to years, leading to fibrosis, disruption of vascular architecture, and cirrhosis

Etiology

- Alcoholic/nonalcoholic fatty liver disease
- Chronic viral hepatitis infection, autoimmune hepatitis
- Biliary diseases: Primary biliary cirrhosis, primary sclerosing cholangitis
- Metabolic disorders: Wilson disease, hemochromatosis, α-1-antitrypsin deficiency
- Drug/toxin-induced injury
- Venous outflow obstruction

Clinical Issues

- Complications: Portal hypertension, ascites, encephalopathy, hepatorenal syndrome, hepatopulmonary syndrome, spontaneous bacterial peritonitis, hepatocellular carcinoma, portal vein thrombosis, coagulopathy

Macroscopic Pathology

- Cirrhosis (micronodular, macronodular, or mixed), masses

Microscopic Pathology

- Cirrhosis: Regenerative nodules of hepatocytes surrounded by fibrous bands without central veins

Top Differential Diagnoses

- Acute liver failure

medusae, and splenomegaly → hypersplenism and thrombocytopenia

- Ascites (due to portal HTN + splanchnic vasodilation)
  - Refractory (diuretic-resistant) treated with transjugular intrahepatic portosystemic shunt (TIPS) or peritoneovenous shunt
  - Spontaneous bacterial peritonitis (SBP): Infection of ascites fluid → sepsis
- Hepatic encephalopathy
  - ~ 70% of cirrhotics, ↓ in neuropsychiatric function caused by ↑ toxins produced by intestinal bacteria in portal venous blood
  - Due to inability of hepatocytes to metabolize toxins and to portosystemic shunting (varices or TIPS procedure)
- Hepatocellular carcinoma: Risk varies by cause of cirrhosis (higher in hepatitis B and C infection)
- Hepatorenal syndrome (portal HTN + splanchnic vasodilation + Na + retention + renal vasoconstriction): Incidence ~ 8% of cirrhotics → renal failure
  - Type 1 hepatorenal syndrome: Rapid deterioration of renal function usually precipitated by SBP
  - Type 2 hepatorenal syndrome: Remains stable for longer; usually associated with refractory ascites
- Hepatopulmonary syndrome: ~ 4-50%, hypoxemia due to intrapulmonary arteriovenous dilatations leading to ventilation/perfusion mismatch, diffusion-perfusion defects, and shunting of blood from pulmonary arteries to veins
- Portal vein thrombosis: ~ 15-25%, due to stasis or infection; can worsen portal HTN
- Hyperestrogenemia → spider angiomas, palmar erythema, gynecomastia, hypogonadism
- ↓ synthetic function: Hypoalbuminemia → edema, coagulopathy → bleeding, protein malnutrition → cachexia

CLINICAL ISSUES

Epidemiology

- Incidence
  - Cirrhosis is 9th leading cause of death in USA

Presentation

- Abdominal pain, anorexia, fatigue, pruritus, fever, arthralgia, weight loss, easy bruising/bleeding, dyspnea
- Jaundice, ↑ abdominal girth, osteoporosis, mental status changes, asterixis, oliguria
- Important elements of chart review: History of alcohol use, intravenous drug use, blood/body fluid exposure, medications, family history of liver disease, comorbid conditions

Laboratory Tests

- ↑ transaminases, bilirubin, alkaline phosphatase, gamma-glutamyl transferase, alpha-fetoprotein
- Hyperammonemia, hypoalbuminemia, hyperglycemia, hyponatremia, ↑ serum creatinine, ↓ creatinine clearance
- ↑ prothrombin and partial thromboplastin times, ↑ international normalized ratio, thrombocytopenia
- Serum ascites albumin gradient > 1.1 g/dL; > 250 polymorphonuclear cells/mm³ in ascites fluid (SBP)
- (+) blood, urine, ascites fluid cultures
- (+) viral hepatitis titers/DNA/RNA
- (+) antinuclear and anti-smooth muscle antibody (autoimmune hepatitis type 1); + anti-liver kidney microsomal and anti-liver cytosol type 1 antibody (autoimmune hepatitis type 2), ↑ IgG
- (+) antimitochondrial antibody and ↑ IgM (PBC); (+) perinuclear antineutrophil antibodies (p-ANCA) (PSC)
- ↑ fasting transferrin saturation, ferritin, iron-binding capacity (hemochromatosis)
- ↓ serum A1AT levels; ↓ serum ceruloplasmin, ↑ urine copper, and hemolytic anemia (Wilson disease)

CHRONIC LIVER FAILURE

Prognosis

- Annual mortality ranges from 1-57% depending on level of decompensation
- Mortality of complications
  - Bleeding esophageal/gastric varices 30-day mortality ~ 15-20%
  - Hepatic encephalopathy 1-year mortality ~ 64%
  - Type 1 hepatorenal syndrome: Almost all die within 10 weeks
  - Type 2 hepatorenal syndrome: Median survival: 3-6 months
  - Infection: Most common types are SBP, urinary tract infections, pneumonia, skin infections; 30% die within 1 month, another 30% die within 1 year
  - Coagulopathy → massive gastrointestinal bleeding: Death within weeks to months
  - HCC 5-year mortality ~ 10-50%

IMAGE FINDINGS

Radiographic Findings

- Hepatic atrophy, hepatomegaly, nodularity, fatty change, masses
- Evidence of portal hypertension: Splenomegaly, collateral vessel formation, hepatofugal flow in portal vein, ascites

Cholangiography

- Bile duct stenosis, strictures, stones, masses
- "Beading" due to strictures and dilatations and "pruned tree" appearance due to ↓ intrahepatic branching (PSC)

MACROSCOPIC FEATURES

External Examination

- Scleral icterus, jaundice, spider angiomas, palmar erythema, prominent periumbilical vessels (caput medusae), bronze skin (hemochromatosis)
- Gynecomastia, temporal wasting, finger clubbing, cyanosis
- Evidence of interventional/surgical procedures

Internal Examination

- Ascites, pleural/pericardial effusions

Organ Examination

- Liver
  - Hepatomegaly, yellow greasy cut surface, green discoloration, masses ± necrosis
  - Nodules surrounded by fibrous tissue: Micronodular (≤ 3 mm), macronodular, or mixed
  - Congested "nutmeg" liver, thrombi in hepatic or portal veins
  - Dilated bile ducts ± fibrotic walls, stenosis, inspissated bile, mucosal ulcers, chole-/hepatolithiasis
  - Status of TIPS: Shunt between branch of hepatic and portal vein
- Gastrointestinal tract
  - Esophageal/gastric varices (dilated, engorged submucosal vessels), erosions, ulcers
  - Portal hypertensive gastropathy ("mosaic"-appearing friable gastric mucosa with vascular ectasia), hemorrhagic gastritis
  - Pancreas: Firm fibrotic atrophic parenchyma, dilated ducts, ± stones, pseudocysts
- Lungs: Small vessel dilatations, emphysema, consolidation
- Other organs
  - Cardiomegaly (systemic or pulmonary hypertension), cardiomyopathy (alcohol/hemochromatosis)
  - Testicular atrophy and gynecomastia (hyperestrogenism)
  - Splenomegaly (portal hypertension), bile nephrosis (green-yellow-appearing kidneys, especially medulla)
  - Cerebral and cerebellar atrophy (chronic alcoholism)

MICROSCOPIC PATHOLOGY

Histologic Features

- Hepatic findings
  - Cirrhosis: Regenerative nodules of hepatocytes surrounded by fibrous bands **without** central veins, ± dysplastic nodules, HCC
    - Biliary-type cirrhosis: "Jigsaw puzzle"-like with irregular nodules surrounded by edematous bands of fibrous tissue seen in PBC, PSC, and secondary biliary cirrhosis
    - Venocentric-type cirrhosis: Central vein to central vein fibrosis with sparing of portal tracts
  - Alcoholic liver disease
    - Steatosis, steatohepatitis (ballooning degeneration of hepatocytes, ± necrosis and pericellular inflammation), neutrophilic infiltrates, Mallory-Denk bodies, ± cholestasis
    - Foamy degeneration (microvesicular steatosis), sclerosing hyaline necrosis (perivenular necrosis + fibrosis)
    - Pericellular fibrosis, usually micronodular cirrhosis
  - Chronic viral hepatitis C infection: Lymphoid aggregates in portal tracts, variable interface and lobular inflammatory activity, naked acidophil bodies, macronodular or mixed cirrhosis
  - Chronic viral hepatitis B ± D infection: Chronic hepatitis, variable interface and lobular inflammatory activity, ground-glass hepatocytes, "sanded" nuclei, macronodular or mixed cirrhosis
  - NAFLD: Steatosis, steatohepatitis (mainly lymphocytes ± neutrophils), ± Mallory-Denk bodies, ± glycogenated nuclei, perivenular/pericellular fibrosis
  - Autoimmune hepatitis: Portal and interface lymphoplasmacytic infiltrates, ± perivenular inflammation/necrosis, hepatocyte rosettes
  - Metabolic disorders
    - Hemochromatosis: Hepatocellular iron deposition (begins in zone 1), bile duct iron deposition, ± portal inflammation and fibrosis → cirrhosis, Kupffer cell siderosis (usually secondary hemochromatosis)

- Wilson disease: Variable portal inflammation, periportal ductular reaction, steatosis, periportal glycogenated nuclei, Mallory-Denk bodies, hepatocellular copper accumulation (focal/patchy)
- A1AT deficiency: Eosinophilic periodic acid-Schiff with diastase (PAS-D)-resistant globules in periportal hepatocytes ([+] immunostain for A1AT), ± steatosis, portal lymphocytic infiltrates

- PBC
  - Nonsuppurative granulomatous destructive cholangitis (florid duct lesion)
  - Associated portal inflammation ± plasma cells and eosinophils, variable interface activity, ductular reaction
  - Cholate stasis ("feathery" degeneration of hepatocytes), ductopenia
- PSC
  - Portal inflammation, periportal ductular reaction, "onion-skin" concentric periductal fibrosis
  - Inflammation, degenerative changes, and atrophy of bile ducts, "fibro-obliterative" lesions (bile ducts replaced by whorls of fibrous scar tissue), ductopenia
  - Large ducts with ulcers, xanthogranulomatous inflammation, and fibrous scars, biliary intraepithelial neoplasia (BilIN), cholangiocarcinoma
- Secondary biliary cirrhosis
  - Features of large bile duct obstruction (portal tract edema, periportal ductular reaction, associated neutrophils ± chronic inflammation)
  - Canalicular cholestasis, cholate stasis, bile lakes, bile infarcts
- Venocentric-type cirrhosis
  - Venous outflow obstruction: Centrilobular congestion, sinusoidal dilatation and congestion, centrilobular hepatocyte atrophy/necrosis, ± peliosis, perivenular/perisinusoidal fibrosis

- Other organ findings
  - Portal hypertensive gastropathy (dilated, tortuous submucosal vessels in gastric body), erosive/hemorrhagic gastritis (alcohol use), chronic active colitis/inflammatory bowel disease (PSC)
  - Chronic pancreatitis with interstitial fibrosis, loss of acini and ducts, islet aggregation, dilated ducts ± concretions
  - Iron deposition in pancreas, adrenal glands, myocardium (hemochromatosis)
  - Panlobular emphysema (AAT deficiency), pneumonia, ↑ wall thickness of pulmonary veins and capillaries (hepatopulmonary syndrome)
  - Copper accumulation in brain, kidneys, cornea (Wilson disease)
  - Type 2 astrocytosis in cerebral cortex and basal ganglia (hepatic encephalopathy), cerebellar atrophy with loss or Purkinje cells in vermis (chronic alcoholism), peripheral neuropathy
  - Wernicke encephalopathy (areas of hemorrhage and necrosis in mamillary bodies and walls of 3rd and 4th ventricles)
  - Korsakoff syndrome (healed Wernicke lesions with macrophage infiltration and cyst formation [thiamine deficiency in chronic alcoholism])
  - Pigmented yellow green casts in distal tubules and collecting ducts and acute tubular injury (hepatorenal syndrome)

ANCILLARY TESTS

Histochemistry

- Trichrome to evaluate fibrosis
- Rhodanine (copper) and Victoria blue/orcein (copper-binding protein) in Wilson disease, also present in chronic cholestatic diseases
- Iron stain, PAS-D (A1AT)

Immunohistochemistry

- Hepatitis B surface and core antigens, A1AT
- CK7 highlights bile duct epithelium and hepatocytes with chronic cholestasis

Microbiology

- Postmortem blood, urine, ascites fluid, pleural/pericardial fluid, tissue cultures

DIFFERENTIAL DIAGNOSIS

Acute Liver Failure

- Similar clinical presentation but for < 26 weeks duration **without** history or signs of underlying chronic liver disease
- Some similar etiologies (hepatitis B ± D, autoimmune hepatitis, Wilson disease, drug induced)
- Radiographic findings: Hepatic atrophy or hepatomegaly, surface nodularity due to alternating necrosis and regeneration, evidence of portal hypertension
- Macroscopic findings: Necrosis and regenerative nodules **without** fibrosis/cirrhosis
- Microscopic findings: Varying degrees of necrosis, parenchymal collapse, ductular reaction, regeneration, **no** bridging fibrosis

REPORTING CRITERIA

Final Report Should Include

- Etiology of CLF, presence of complications, effects on other organs
- Whether it was cause of death or contributing factor
- Implications for living family members (hereditary diseases)

SELECTED REFERENCES

1. Tsochatzis EA et al: Liver cirrhosis. Lancet. 383(9930):1749-61, 2014
2. Liberal R et al: Autoimmune hepatitis: a comprehensive review. J Autoimmun. 41:126-39, 2013
3. Panella M et al: Unsuspected hereditary hemochromatosis at forensic autopsy: its presentation, confirmation, and implications. Am J Forensic Med Pathol. 32(1):20-4, 2011

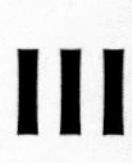

CHRONIC LIVER FAILURE

Causes of Chronic Liver Failure

(Left) *This liver shows the characteristic features of alcoholic steatohepatitis: Steatosis ➔, ballooning degeneration of hepatocytes with abundant Mallory-Denk bodies ➔, and pericellular neutrophilic inflammation ➔.* ***(Right)*** *Chronic autoimmune hepatitis is characterized by lymphoplasmacytic infiltrates involving the portal tracts ➔ and periportal regions. Lymphocytes and plasma cells surround individual hepatocytes at the interface ➔.*

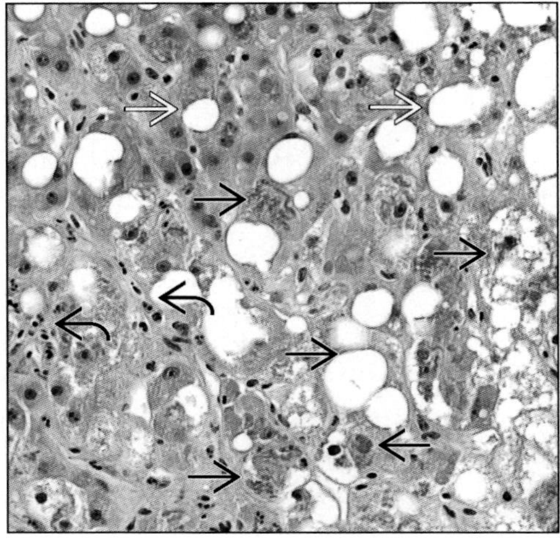

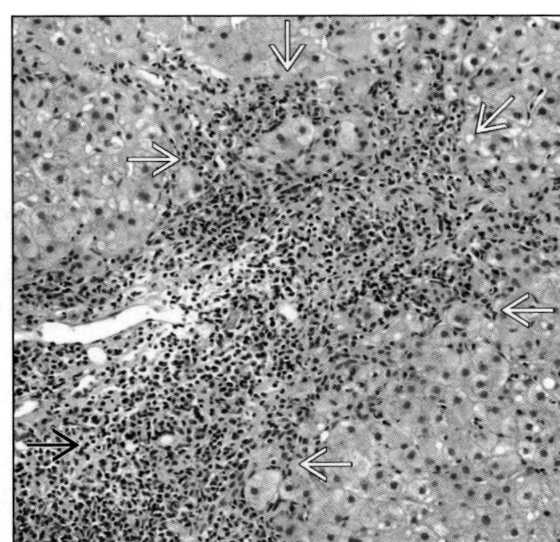

(Left) *Periodic acid-Schiff stain with diastase digestion (PAS-D) highlights numerous α-1-antitrypsin globules (bright pink) ➔ in the cytoplasm of periportal hepatocytes in this case of chronic liver failure due to α-1-antitrypsin deficiency.* ***(Right)*** *This iron stain shows diffuse hepatocellular siderosis (blue granules) ➔ without significant Kupffer cell siderosis in this patient with hereditary hemochromatosis.*

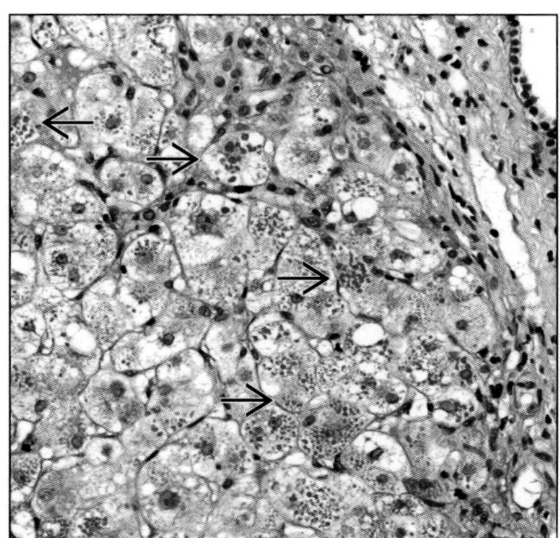

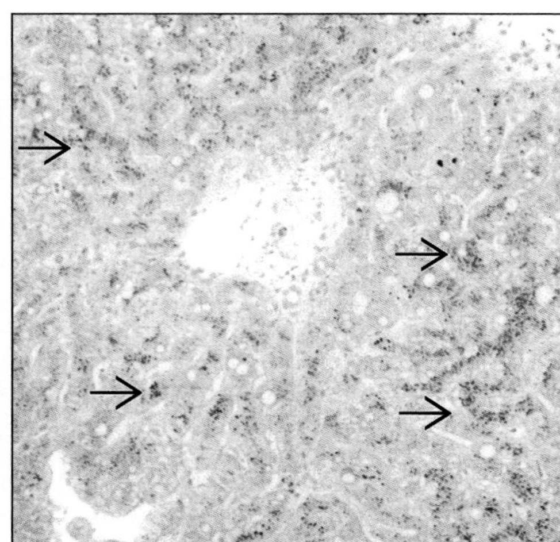

(Left) *The "florid duct lesion" is characteristic of primary biliary cirrhosis. This portal tract contains a poorly formed periductal granuloma ➔ with associated chronic inflammation including eosinophils ➔ and lymphocytes infiltrating the residual, nearly destroyed bile duct ➔.* ***(Right)*** *The fibro-obliterative lesion is a characteristic finding in primary sclerosing cholangitis. The bile duct in this portal tract has been replaced by a round, fibrous scar ➔.*

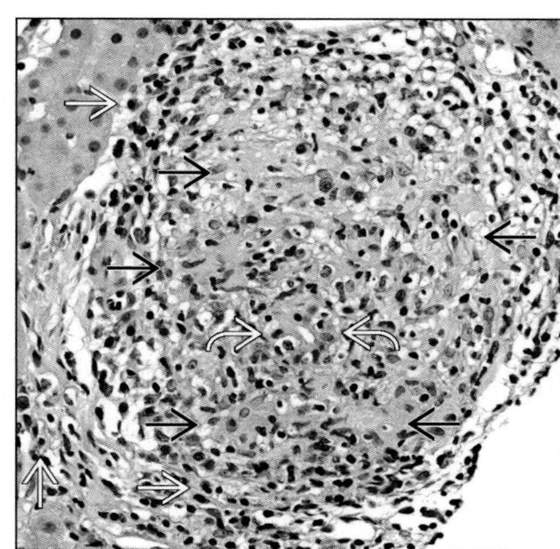

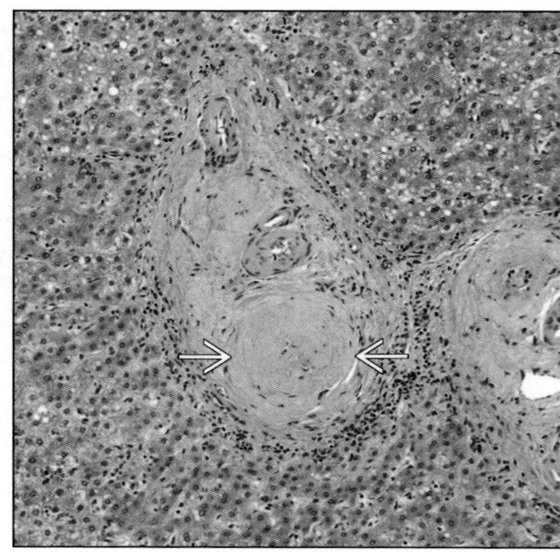

Complications of Chronic Liver Failure

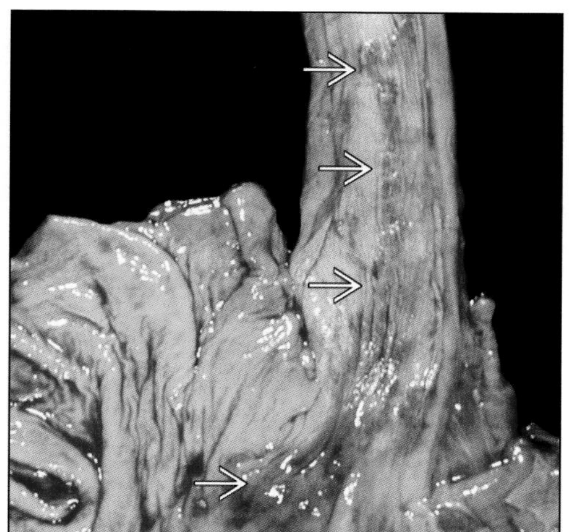

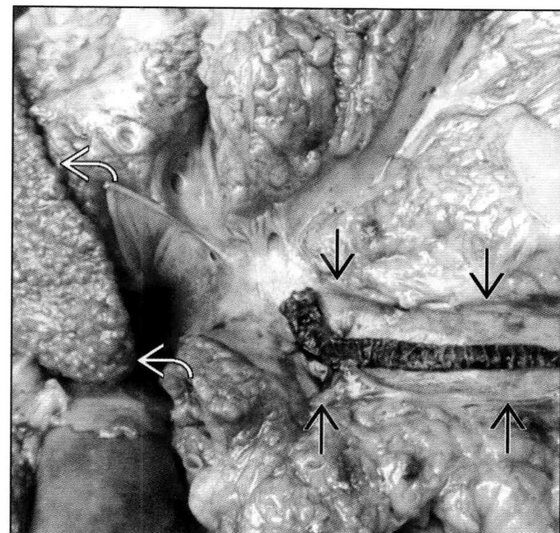

(Left) *Esophageal and gastric varices ➡ are a common complication of portal hypertension due to cirrhosis and may cause massive gastrointestinal bleeding. (Courtesy D. Rubin, MD.)* ***(Right)*** *Portal vein thrombosis ➡ occurred in a patient with cirrhosis ➦ due to chronic hepatitis B infection.*

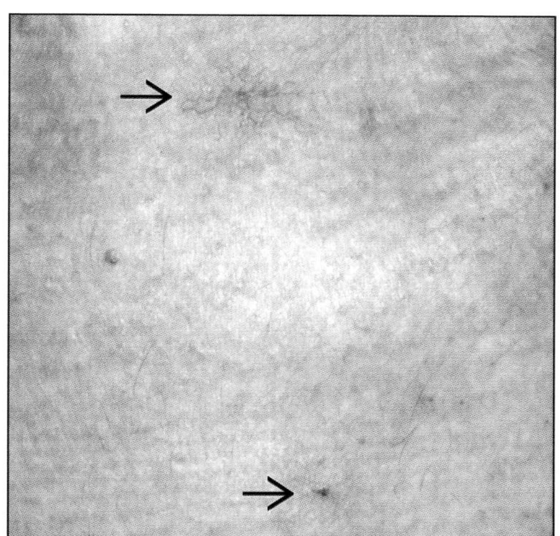

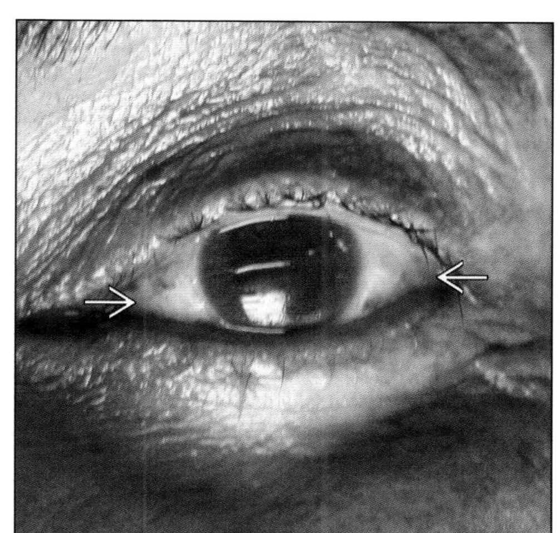

(Left) *Spider angiomas occur in hyperestrogenemic states such as cirrhosis. They appear as a red papule (dilated arteriole) with thin veins radiating outward from the center ➡. These occurred in a patient with cirrhosis due to chronic hepatitis C infection.* ***(Right)*** *Scleral icterus ➡ is caused by hyperbilirubinemia in this patient with cirrhosis due to chronic viral hepatitis C infection.*

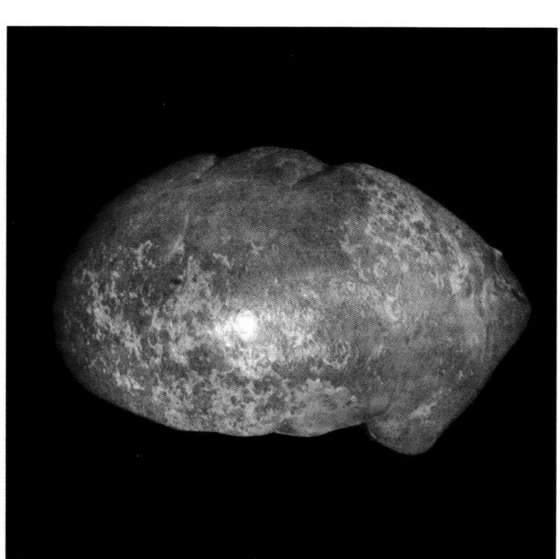

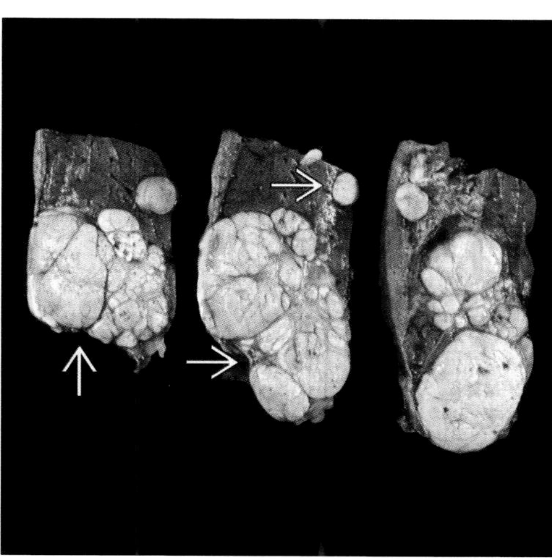

(Left) *Splenomegaly is a common complication of portal hypertension. This spleen from a patient with alcoholic cirrhosis weighed 460 g (normal weight: 150-200 g).* ***(Right)*** *Hepatocellular carcinoma in a patient with chronic hepatitis B infection appears as multinodular pale tan masses ➡. The background hepatic parenchyma is not cirrhotic. (Courtesy D. Rubin, MD.)*

CHRONIC RENAL FAILURE

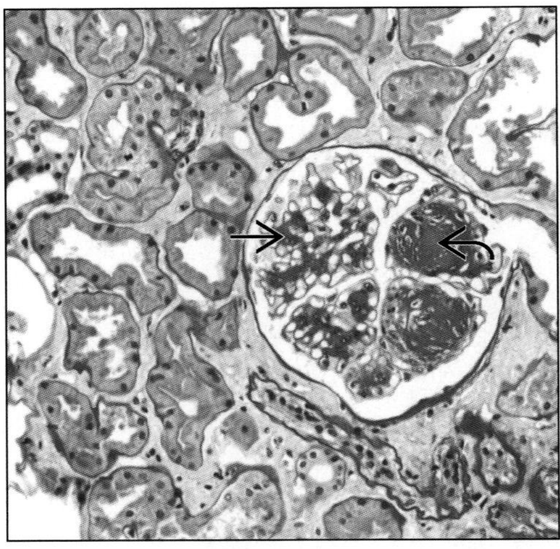

PAS stain highlights mesangial matrix ➡ and the nodules ↪ in diabetic nephropathy are strongly positive. The nodules are composed mainly of matrix with minimal or no cellular proliferation.

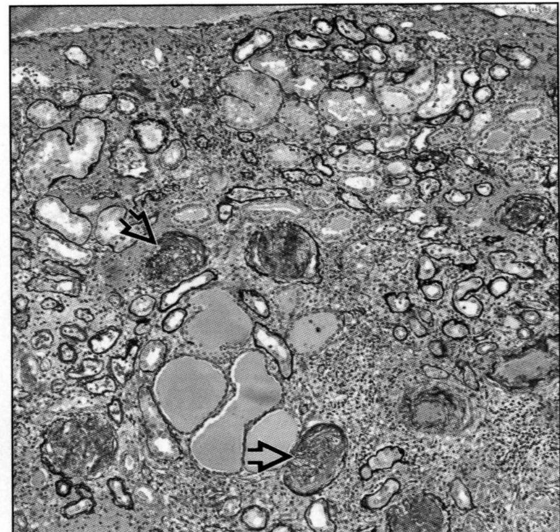

In arterionephrosclerosis, solidified-type global sclerosis is characterized by corrugation of the glomerular basement membranes ➡ involving the entire glomerular tuft.

TERMINOLOGY

Abbreviations

- Chronic renal failure (CRF)

Synonyms

- Chronic kidney disease (CKD)

Definitions

- Renal function deterioration with glomerular filtration rate (GFR) < 60 mL/minute per 1.73 m^2 &/or kidney damage for ≥ 3 months due to diseases causing destruction of parenchyma leading to fibrosis, glomerulosclerosis, and vascular damage

ETIOLOGY/PATHOGENESIS

Glomerular Diseases

- Most types of glomerulonephritis can progress and cause CRF in variable time interval
  - Membranous glomerulopathy: ~ 33% progress to end-stage renal disease (ESRD)
  - Primary focal segmental glomerulosclerosis: Significant fraction of cases progress to ESRD
  - IgA nephropathy: Progresses to ESRD in ~ 30% of cases
  - Membranoproliferative glomerulonephritis: Slow progress to ESRD in ~ 10 years
  - Lupus nephritis: Median progression to ESRD is 10 years in ~ 25% of cases
  - Fibrillary glomerulopathy: 40-50% progress to ESRD in 2-4 years
  - Anti-GBM crescentic glomerulonephritis: Most cases progress to ESRD

Tubular/Interstitial Diseases

- Chronic pyelonephritis
- Chronic interstitial nephritis (e.g., urate nephropathy, lithium toxicity, oxalate nephropathy, 2,8 dihydroxyadenuria)
- Chronic infections
  - Tuberculosis
  - Xanthogranulomatous pyelonephritis
  - Malakoplakia
- Autosomal dominant adult polycystic kidney disease (ADPKD)
  - Mutations in polycystin 1 (*PKD1*) 16p13.3 and polycystin 2 (*PKD2*) 4q21

Vascular Diseases

- Hypertensive nephrosclerosis: Vascular and parenchymal damage associated with high blood pressure
- Renal artery stenosis secondary to atherosclerosis, fibromuscular dysplasia, dissecting aneurysm, vasculitis, retroperitoneal fibrosis, and neurofibromatosis

Metabolic

- Diabetic nephropathy

Paraprotein-Associated

- Amyloidosis (e.g., light chain [AL], secondary amyloidosis [AA], transthyretin, and others)
- Light/heavy chain immunoglobulin deposition disease

CLINICAL ISSUES

Epidemiology

- Incidence
  - Glomerular diseases affect 12-16% of patients with CRF
  - ADPKD is ~ 3% of patients with CRF
  - Hypertensive nephrosclerosis is 29-38% of patients with CRF

CHRONIC RENAL FAILURE

Key Facts

Terminology

- Renal function deterioration with glomerular filtration rate (GFR) < 60 mL/min per 1.73 m^2 &/ or kidney damage for ≥ 3 months due to diseases causing destruction of parenchyma leading to fibrosis, glomerulosclerosis, and vascular damage

Clinical Issues

- Glomerular diseases affect 12-16% of patients with CRF
- ADPKD is ~ 3% of patients with CRF
- Hypertensive nephrosclerosis is 29-38% of patients with CRF
- Diabetes nephropathy is ~ 50% of patients with CRF and ≥ 1/3 of patients in dialysis
- Progression to ESRD is variable depending upon etiology of renal disease

Microscopic Pathology

- Varies depending on etiology of renal failure
- When process is advanced, it may not be possible to determine etiology

Ancillary Tests

- Special stains (AFB, GMS) are contributory for specific diagnosis of infections
- Panel including IgG, IgA, IgM, C3, C1, light chains, albumin, and fibrinogen is necessary in cases of glomerular diseases
- Electron microscopy should be performed in cases of glomerular diseases

---

  - Diabetes nephropathy in ~ 50% of patients with CRF and ≥ 1/3 of patients in dialysis
- Age
  - Glomerular diseases present in children and young adults
  - ADPKD become symptomatic at 40-50 years
  - Hypertensive nephrosclerosis presents in adults and older patients
  - Diabetic nephropathy may present in young adults in type 1 and in older adults in type 2

Presentation

- Glomerular diseases
  - Hematuria
  - Proteinuria
  - Hypertension
  - Progressive increase of creatinine
  - Metabolic abnormalities
- Tubular/interstitial diseases
  - Chronic pyelonephritis/other infections
    - History of recurrent infections
    - Urinary anomalies: Obstruction, nephrolithiasis, posterior urethral valves
    - Back pain
    - Fever
    - Pyuria/bacteriuria
    - Hypertension
    - Increased creatinine
    - Proteinuria usually nonnephrotic range
  - Chronic interstitial nephritis
    - Nonspecific urinary sediment abnormalities
    - Proteinuria, nonnephrotic range
    - Gradually progressive renal failure
  - ADPKD
    - Hypertension
    - Hematuria
    - Flank pain
    - Infections
    - Nephrolithiasis
    - Cysts involving liver, pancreas, and spleen, and aneurysms in circle of Willis
- Hypertensive kidney disease
  - Longstanding elevated blood pressure
  - Proteinuria variable degree may be nephrotic
  - Progressive renal failure
- Renal artery stenosis
  - Renovascular hypertension
  - Progressive renal failure
- Diabetic nephropathy
  - Proteinuria initially in nonnephrotic range with progression to nephrotic proteinuria
  - Progressive renal failure
  - Hypertension
  - Neuropathy
  - Retinopathy

Laboratory Tests

- Serum creatinine
- Blood urea nitrogen (BUN)
- Cystatin C (CysC)
- β-2-microglobulin
- Urinalysis: Albuminuria
- Urine cultures
- Antinuclear antibodies (ANA), antineutrophil cytoplasmic antibodies (ANCA), anti-GBM antibodies
- Hepatitis C and B serologies
- Serum/urine protein electrophoresis

Treatment

- Drugs
  - Angiotensin converting enzyme (ACE) inhibitors
  - Angiotensin receptor blockers (ARBs)
  - Antihypertensive medication
  - Antidiabetic medication
  - Antibiotics
  - Statins
- Renal replacement therapy
  - Hemodialysis
  - Peritoneal dialysis
  - Transplantation

Prognosis

- Glomerulonephritis progress to ESRD in variable interval time

CHRONIC RENAL FAILURE

- Hypertension progression to ESRD is slow
- Diabetic nephropathy progress to ESRD in 5-10 years after proteinuria is present
- ADPKD progresses to ESRD faster in type 1

IMAGE FINDINGS

CT Findings

- Asymmetrically or symmetrical contracted kidneys
- Coarse patchy cortical scars
- Blunting/deformity pyelocaliceal system
- In ADPKD, bilateral enlarged cystic kidneys

Angiography

- Renal artery stenosis can be identified

MACROSCOPIC FEATURES

External Examination

- Sallow/yellow appearance of skin
- Muscle atrophy

Organ Examination

- Kidney
  - Glomerular diseases
    - Marked reduction of kidney size
    - External surface with granular appearance
- Tubular interstitial diseases
  - Chronic pyelonephritis
    - Kidney size may be reduced
    - Irregular cortical scars with U-shaped broad base appearance overlying blunted/deformed calyces
    - Renal poles are more involved
    - Scars are demarcated from adjacent parenchyma
    - Thinned cortex
  - Chronic interstitial nephritis
    - Kidney usually reduced in size and shrunken
  - Chronic infections
    - Renal tuberculosis: Initial lesions involve renal pelvis, calyces, and papillae; ulceration and caseous material can obstruct ureteropelvic junction causing hydronephrosis; cortical multiple small yellow nodules
    - Xanthogranulomatous pyelonephritis: Kidney may be enlarged with yellow mass lesions that are usually unilateral involving pyelocalyceal regions
    - Malakoplakia: Enlarged kidney with raised multiple yellow nodules distributed through parenchyma and pelvic lining
  - ADPKD
    - Markedly enlarged kidneys, bilateral
    - Weight range from 4.5-10 lb
    - Cobbled appearance of external surface
  - Hypertensive nephropathy
    - Reduction of kidney size
    - Finely granular appearance of external surface
    - Thinned cortex
  - Renal artery stenosis
    - Narrowing of renal artery
    - Friable lipid debris, calcification, and dense fibrosis in atherosclerosis
    - Multiple ridges of hyperplastic muscle alternating with dilated segments with thin wall, in muscular dysplasia involving distal 2/3 of main renal artery
  - Diabetic nephropathy
    - Enlarged kidney in early stage
    - Normal size or reduced size in advanced stage
    - Irregular external surface
    - Papillary necrosis with pyramid loss may be present
- Other organs
  - Heart
    - Congestive heart failure
    - Atherosclerotic coronary artery disease with significant wall calcification
    - Mitral valve annulus and aortic cusps calcification
    - Uremic cardiomyopathy
    - Pericarditis
    - Sudden cardiac death (especially with dialysis)
  - Lung
    - Edema
    - Uremic pneumonitis
  - Gastrointestinal tract
    - Mucosa inflammation, erosion, ulceration
    - Angiodysplasia
    - Ischemic changes
    - Acute/chronic pancreatitis
  - Central nervous system
    - Ischemic/hemorrhagic infarcts
    - Uremic encephalopathy
    - Atherosclerosis
  - Bones and joints
    - Amyloid β-2 microglobulin deposition
    - Destructive arthropathy
    - Bone cysts/fractures
    - Osteitis fibrosa/osteomalacia

MICROSCOPIC PATHOLOGY

Histologic Features

- Glomerular diseases
  - Variable mesangial/endocapillary proliferation seen in nonsclerotic glomeruli
  - In advanced stage, global glomerulosclerosis is seen in all types of glomerular diseases
- Chronic pyelonephritis
  - Tubular atrophy
  - Dilated tubules with hyaline casts (thyroidization)
  - Variable degree of interstitial mononuclear inflammation
  - Interstitial and periglomerular fibrosis
  - Glomeruli are not significantly involved except for late development of focal segmental sclerosis
  - Calyceal system shows chronic inflammation
- Chronic interstitial nephritis
  - Morphology varies depending upon etiologic agent
  - Interstitial fibrosis and tubular atrophy are common
  - Interstitial inflammatory infiltrates of variable degree composed of lymphocytes, plasma cells
  - Lithium nephropathy: Tubular dilatation is characteristic with single cell lining and segmental glomerulosclerosis

- Urate nephropathy: Urate crystals with birefringent needle-shaped appearance in tubular lumen &/or interstitium surrounded by foreign body giant cell reaction

- Chronic infections
  - Renal tuberculosis
    - Granulomatous inflammation with caseous necrosis
    - Interstitial fibrosis and tubular atrophy
    - Large coalescent granulomas may form large masses
  - Xanthogranulomatous pyelonephritis
    - Diffuse granulomatous inflammatory tubulointerstitial infiltrate with numerous foamy cells, lipid-laden macrophages, and occasional multinucleated giant cells
    - Additional inflammatory cells include lymphocytes, plasma cells, and neutrophils
  - Malakoplakia
    - Nodules composed of clusters of macrophages with foamy eosinophilic cytoplasm (von Hanseman cells)
    - Additional inflammatory infiltrate composed of lymphocytes and plasma cells
    - Michaelis-Gutmann bodies inclusion (4-10 μm) in macrophages or interstitium
- ADPKD
  - Early stage cysts of variable size (0.5-5 cm) with normal intervening kidney parenchyma
  - Late-stage cysts with fibrotic and atrophic intervening kidney parenchyma, global glomerulosclerosis, and glomerular cysts
  - Cyst lining is usually single layer with flattened-appearing tubular cells
- Hypertensive nephropathy
  - Arteries: Intimal fibrosis, elastic lamina reduplication, media hyperplasia
  - Afferent arterioles show hyalinosis
  - Glomerular ischemic changes
    - Glomerular basement membrane (GBM) thickening and wrinkling
    - Global glomerulosclerosis with solidified obsolescent glomeruli
    - Segmental glomerulosclerosis
    - Tubular atrophy
    - Interstitial fibrosis
- Renal artery stenosis
  - Proximal tubules with marked reduction in size, resulting in significant glomerular crowding
  - Glomeruli are reduced in size with mild Bowman space dilatation
  - Mild to moderate hyperplasia of juxtaglomerular apparatuses
  - Fibromuscular dysplasia shows 3 patterns: Intimal fibroplasia, medial muscular dysplasia, and periarterial dysplasia
- Diabetic nephropathy
  - Mesangial expansion, nodular in advanced stage
  - GBM thickening
  - Hyaline caps and capsular drop
  - Hyaline insudation/accumulation in arterioles (afferent and efferent)

ANCILLARY TESTS

Histochemistry

- Acid-fast bacilli useful for confirmation of renal tuberculosis
- von Kossa stain useful to identify Michaelis-Gutmann bodies in malakoplakia
- Elastic stain to evaluate renal artery stenosis caused by fibromuscular dysplasia

Immunofluorescence

- Panel including IgG, IgA, IgM, C3, C1, light chains, albumin and fibrinogen is necessary in cases of glomerular diseases

Electron Microscopy

- Transmission
  - Necessary in cases of glomerular diseases for identification of electron-dense deposits and GBM abnormalities

REPORTING CRITERIA

Final Report

- Should include
  - Etiology of CRF
  - Whether CRF was cause of death or contributory factor
  - Effects/complications in other organs of CRF

SELECTED REFERENCES

1. Lopez-Giacoman S et al: Biomarkers in chronic kidney disease, from kidney function to kidney damage. World J Nephrol. 4(1):57-73, 2015
2. Buettner M et al: Nephropathy in illicit drug abusers: a postmortem analysis. Am J Kidney Dis. 63(6):945-53, 2014
3. Díez R et al: Renal AA amyloidosis in patients with type 2 diabetes mellitus. Nephron Extra. 4(2):119-26, 2014
4. Iwakiri T et al: Association between renal vasculature changes and generalized atherosclerosis: an autopsy survey. J Atheroscler Thromb. 21(2):99-107, 2014
5. Santoro A et al: Chronic renal disease and risk of cardiovascular morbidity-mortality. Kidney Blood Press Res. 39(2-3):142-6, 2014
6. Tomino Y: Pathogenesis and treatment of chronic kidney disease: a review of our recent basic and clinical data. Kidney Blood Press Res. 39(5):450-89, 2014
7. Tuttle KR et al: Diabetic kidney disease: a report from an ADA Consensus Conference. Am J Kidney Dis. 64(4):510-33, 2014
8. Zachariah D et al: Sudden cardiac death in end stage renal disease: unlocking the mystery. J Nephrol. Epub ahead of print, 2014
9. Zhao J et al: Assessment of renal fibrosis in chronic kidney disease using diffusion-weighted MRI. Clin Radiol. 69(11):1117-22, 2014
10. Roberts WC et al: Cardiac findings at necropsy in patients with chronic kidney disease maintained on chronic hemodialysis. Medicine (Baltimore). 91(3):165-78, 2012

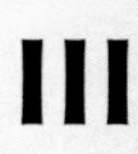

CHRONIC RENAL FAILURE

Gross and Microscopic Features

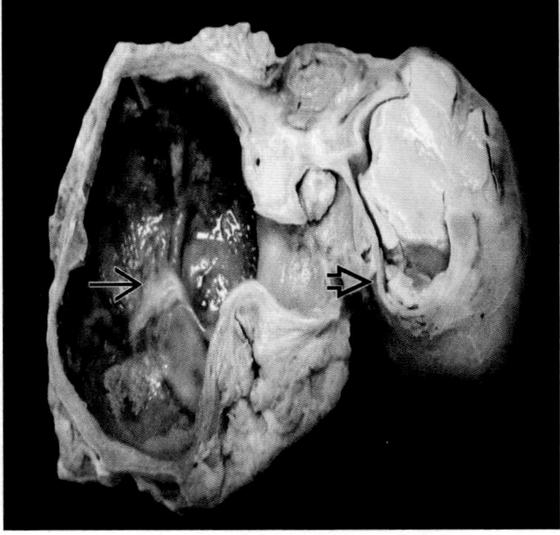
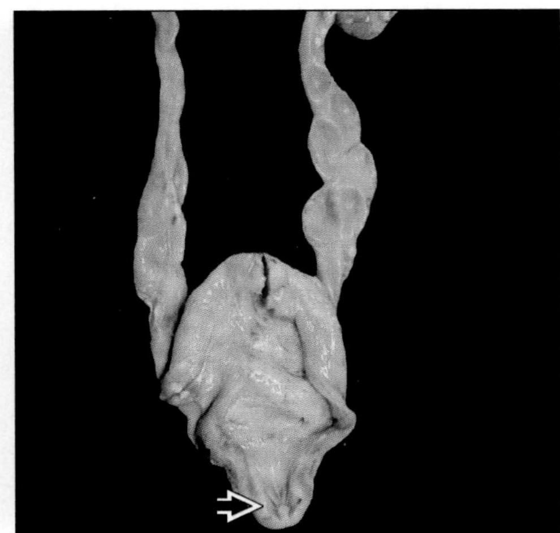

(Left) *In chronic pyelonephritis, kidney is reduced in size, with marked destruction of renal parenchyma & dilatation of calyces, forming cyst ➙. Note abscess filled with necrotic debris ➙.* ***(Right)*** *Posterior urethral valve ➙ is an obstructing membrane in the posterior male urethra as a result of abnormal in utero development. It is the most common cause of bladder outlet obstruction in male newborns, can cause hydroureter & hydronephrosis, and is a risk factor for chronic pyelonephritis.*

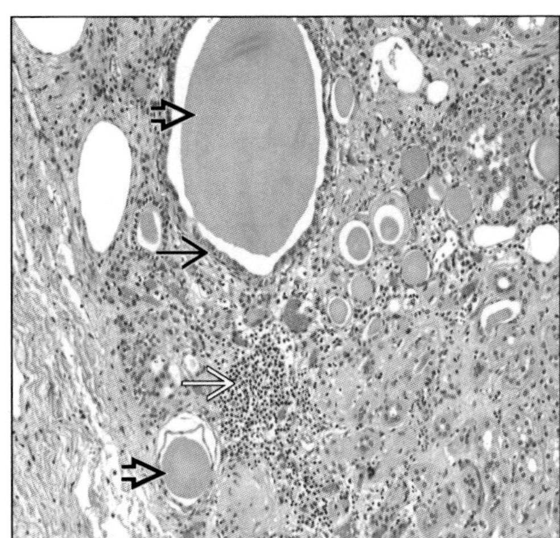
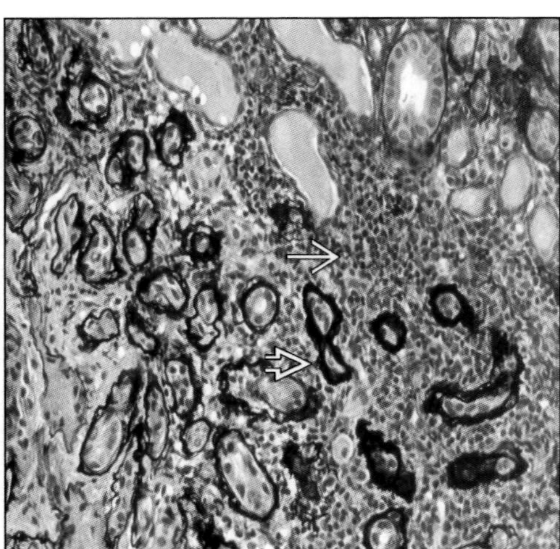

(Left) *This section of a case of chronic pyelonephritis shows tubular thyroidization, which is characterized by atrophic tubules ➙ with attenuated epithelium and luminal colloid-like hyaline casts ➙. Patchy chronic inflammation is seen in the interstitium ➙.* ***(Right)*** *In chronic pyelonephritis, tubulointerstitial inflammation ➙ containing lymphocytes, plasma cells, and mononuclear cells with associated geographic/jigsaw pattern of interstitial fibrosis and tubular atrophy ➙ are characteristic.*

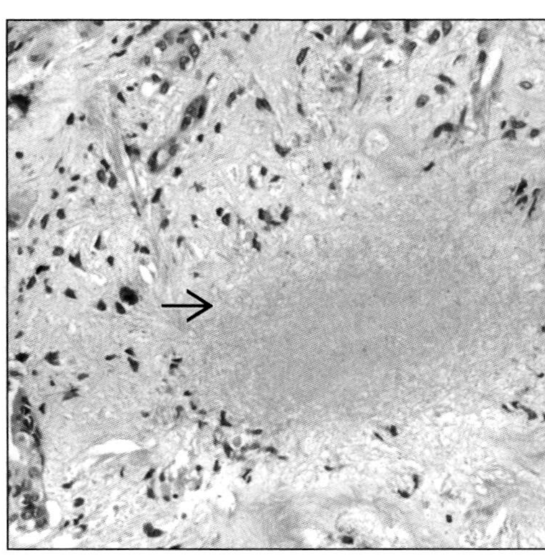
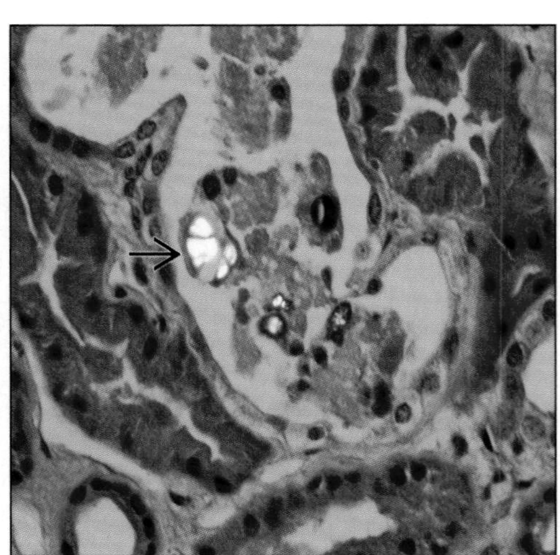

(Left) *In urate nephropathy, there is accumulation of needle-like crystals ➙, associated with an inflammatory infiltrate in the interstitium, characteristic of a gouty tophus.* ***(Right)*** *2,8 dihydroxyadeninuria crystalline nephropathy, a rare autosomal recessive inherited disorder of purine metabolism, clinically varies from an asymptomatic state to recurrent nephrolithiasis, recurrent urinary tract infection, and CRF. Crystals are present in tubular lumina and are polarizable ➙.*

Gross and Microscopic Features

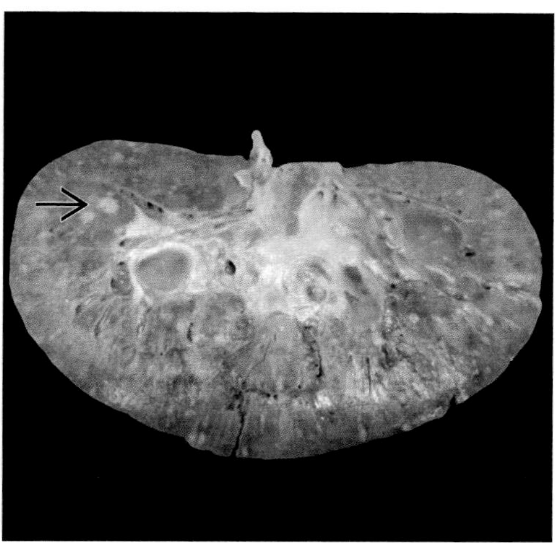

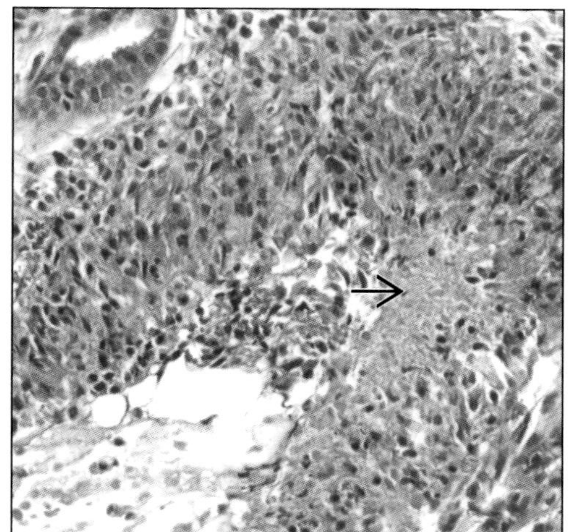

(Left) *Gross specimen from a case of miliary tuberculosis shows numerous small foci of caseous necrosis ⇒ in the cortex and medulla.* ***(Right)*** *Granulomas with caseous necrosis are characteristic microscopic features of tuberculosis ⇒. Tuberculosis involving the kidney is most commonly seen in immunosuppressed patients with HIV infection or transplants. Fungal infections may also manifest with necrotizing granulomas. Special stains are necessary for identification of microorganisms.*

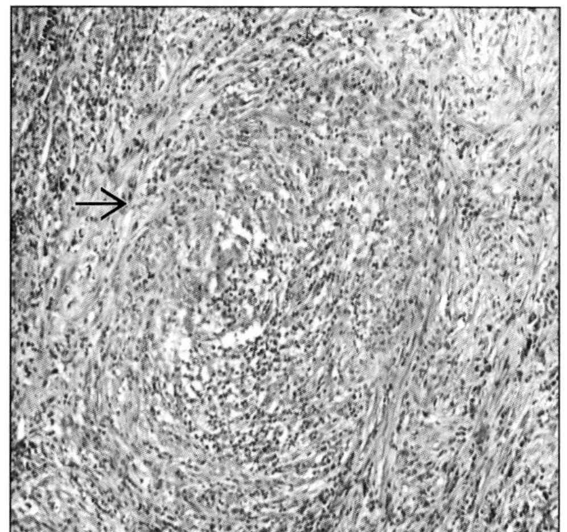

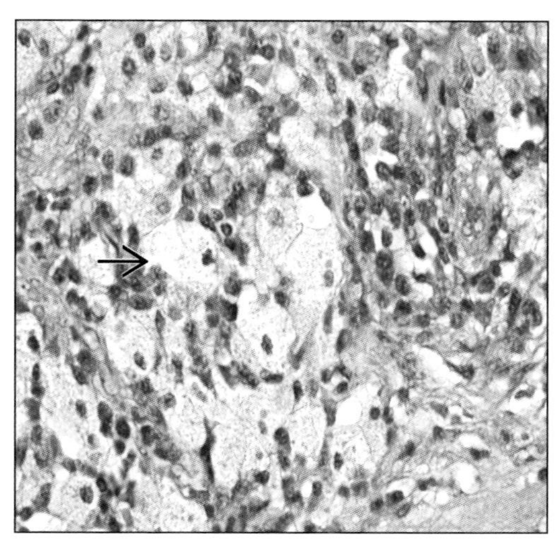

(Left) *Xanthogranulomatous pyelonephritis is a variant of chronic pyelonephritis, characterized by mass lesions with many foamy macrophages forming granulomas ⇒. Proteus mirabilis is the most common causative agent.* ***(Right)*** *At higher magnification in a case of xanthogranulomatous pyelonephritis, there is prominent foamy macrophage infiltration ⇒ with scattered lymphocytes and plasma cells.*

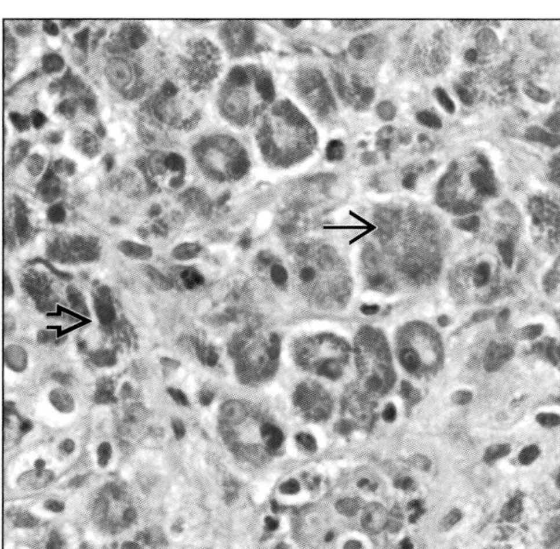

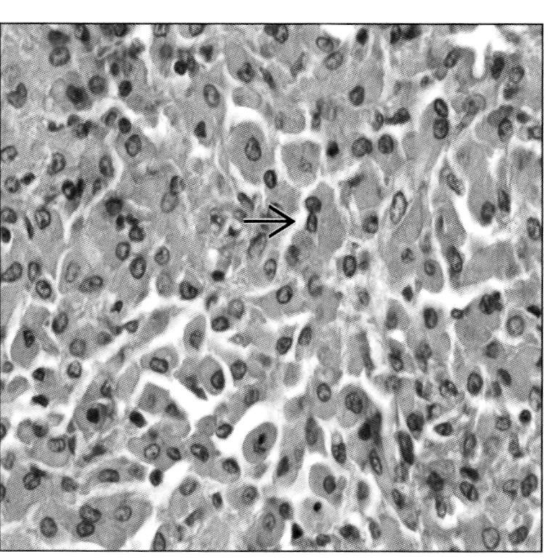

(Left) *Malakoplakia is caused by chronic bacterial infection. Histologically, macrophages with foamy cytoplasm ⇒ containing PAS-positive Michaelis-Gutmann bodies ⇨ are seen.* ***(Right)*** *Megalocytic interstitial nephritis is closely related to malakoplakia and it is caused by chronic gram-negative bacterial infection. The lesion is characterized by interstitial infiltration of histiocytes with eosinophilic granular cytoplasm ⇒. In contrast to malakoplakia, there are no Michaelis-Gutmann bodies.*

CHRONIC RENAL FAILURE

Gross and Microscopic Features

(Left) Autosomal dominant polycystic kidney disease on gross examination shows replacement of the kidney parenchyma by multiple cysts ➡ with variable size, thin walls, and containing clear or hemorrhagic fluid. *(Right)* Autosomal dominant polycystic kidney disease on gross examination shows multiple cysts ➡ of variable size with thin walls and smooth-appearing internal surfaces. The pyelocalyceal system is distorted and dilated ➡.

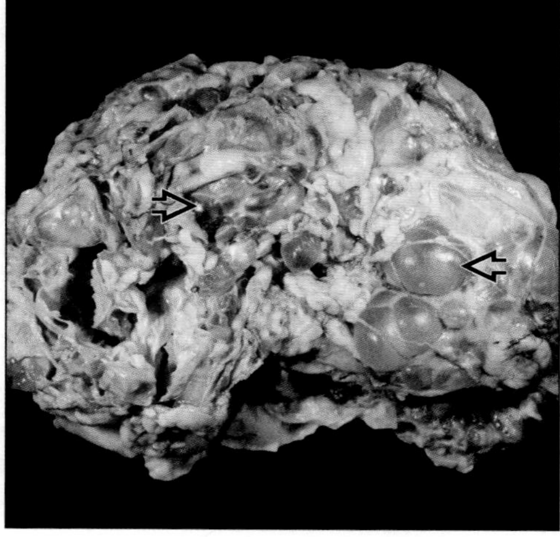

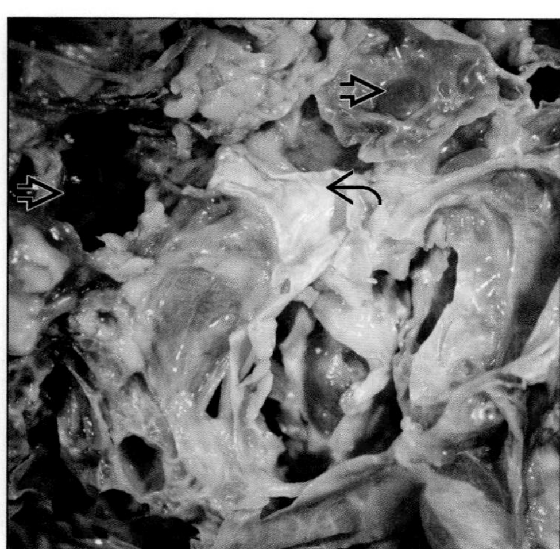

(Left) H&E section of a case of ADPKD demonstrates cysts walls ➡ lined by an attenuated layer of epithelial cells with scant parenchyma containing atrophic tubules and interstitial fibrosis ➡. *(Right)* In ADPKD, other organs are frequently involved. In 15% of cases, aneurysms ➡ in the circle of Willis can be identified. They may rupture and be the cause of death with extensive subarachnoid hemorrhage ➡.

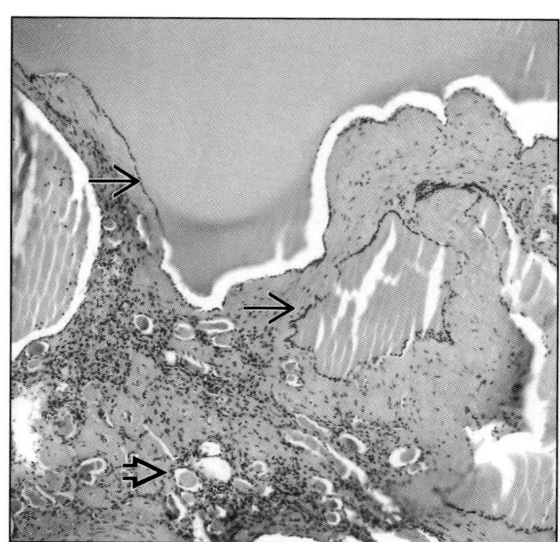

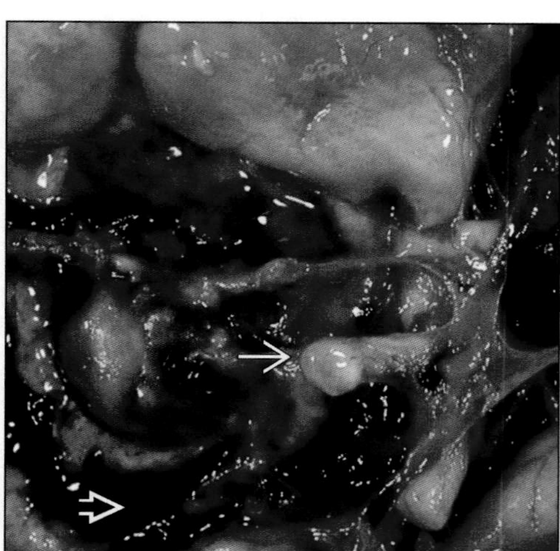

(Left) Hypertensive nephrosclerosis initially affects arterioles and arteries, but with progression of the disease, the glomeruli are involved and develop global glomerulosclerosis ➡. The arteriole appears thickened and with reduplication of elastic lamina ➡. *(Right)* In hypertensive nephrosclerosis, the arterioles show thickening of the wall with deposits of hyaline material in subendothelial distribution that eventually becomes circumferential ➡.

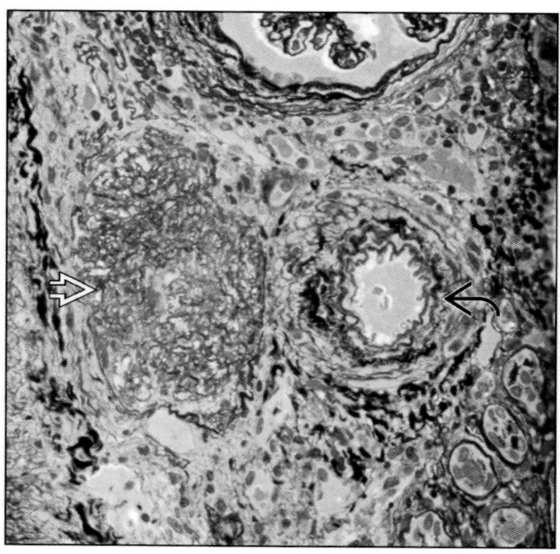

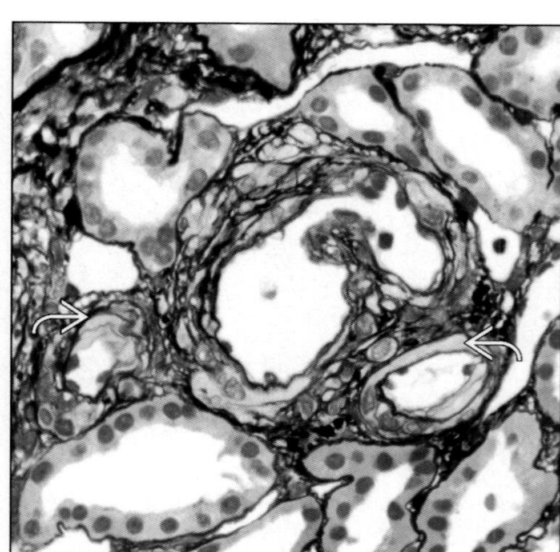

Microscopic Features

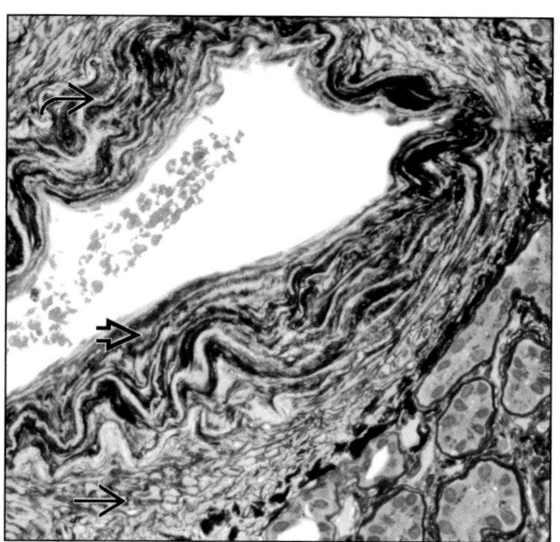

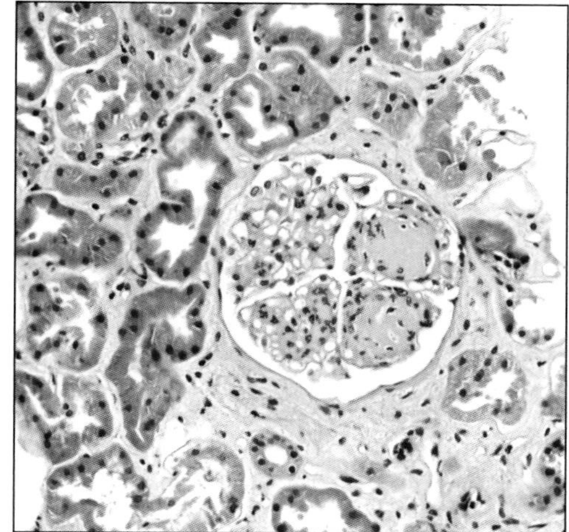

(Left) The large arteries in hypertensive nephrosclerosis show varying degrees of tunica media thickening ⇨ and intimal fibrosis ⇨ with reduplication of internal elastic lamina ↪. **(Right)** Diabetic nephropathy is characterized by expansion of the mesangial matrix ± nodular formation. The nodules are of different size and involve the glomerular tuft irregularly. The nodules are composed mainly of matrix.

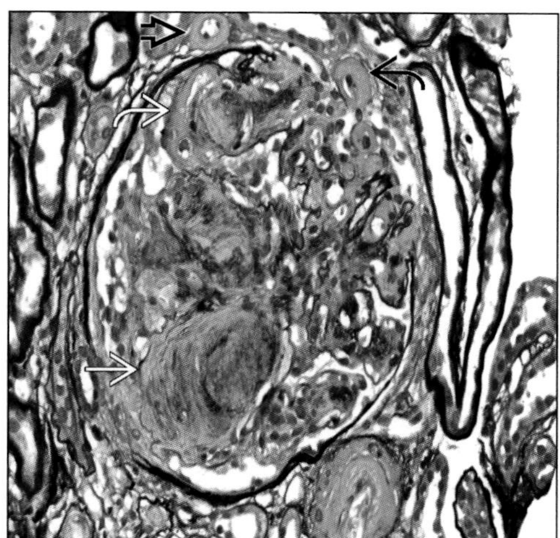

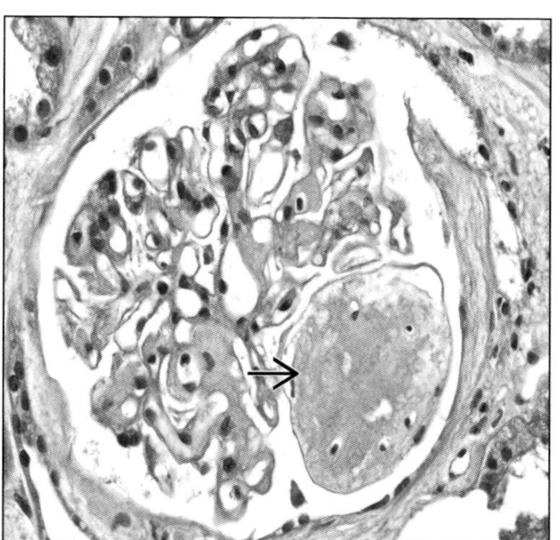

(Left) In the advanced phase of diabetic nephropathy, the mesangial matrix expansion often forms nodules known as Kimmelstiel-Wilson nodules. On silver stain, the matrix shows a lamellated appearance ➡. There is hyaline deposition (insudation of plasma proteins) in afferent ⇨ and efferent arterioles ↪, and hyaline caps are also present ↪. **(Right)** In amyloidosis, there is mesangial expansion with acellular amorphous eosinophilic material ⇨ that is paler than the normal mesangial matrix.

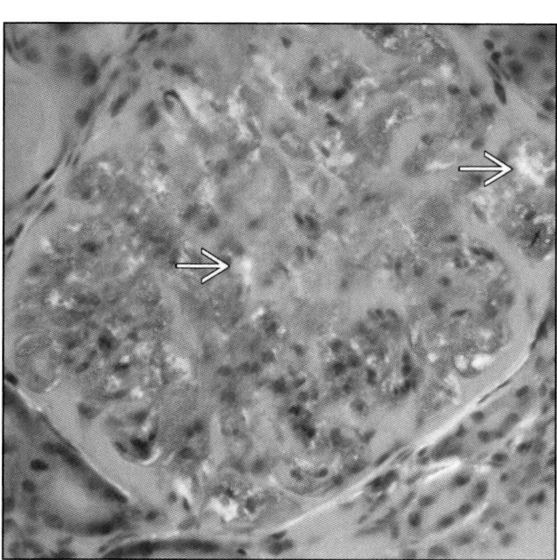

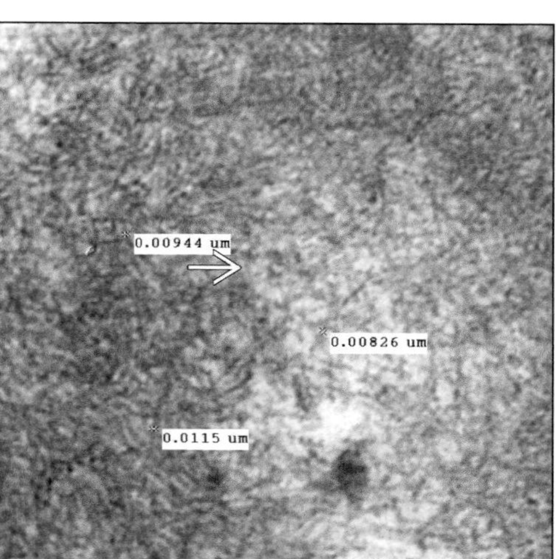

(Left) The amyloid deposits in the mesangium show birefringent apple-green color ➡ under polarized light. This characteristic feature is useful for diagnosis. **(Right)** On ultrastructural examination, amyloid deposits show randomly arranged nonbranching fibrils ➡ with diameters varying from 0.8-1.2 μm. These features are characteristic and allow differentiation from fibrillary or immunotactoid glomerulopathies where the deposits are larger.

DEMENTIA AND NEURODEGENERATIVE DISEASE

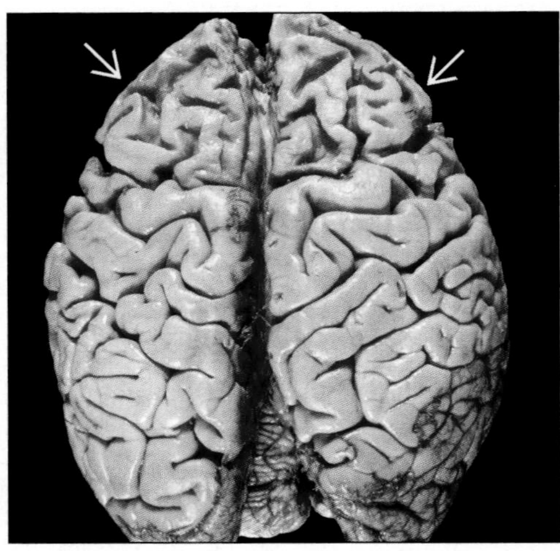

Autopsy specimen of frontotemporal dementia shows striking atrophy of the frontal gyri ➔ with normal-appearing parietal and occipital lobes. (From Osborn's Brain.)

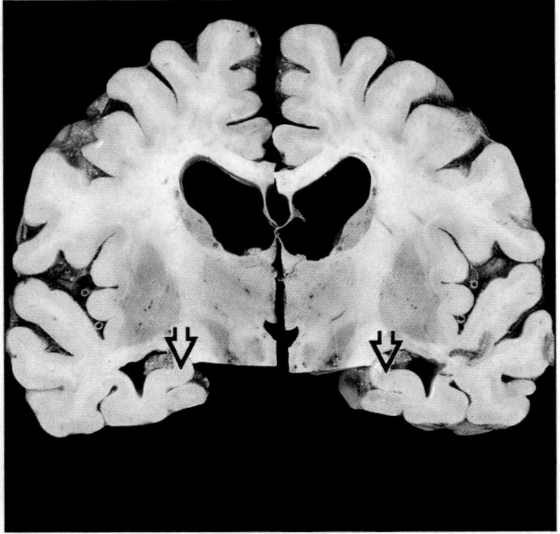

Coronal autopsy section from a patient with early Alzheimer disease shows enlarged lateral ventricles. The hippocampi ⇨ appear mildly atrophic. (From Osborn's Brain.)

ETIOLOGY/PATHOGENESIS

Alzheimer Disease (AD)

- Most common neurodegenerative disease, incidence ↑ with age

Tauopathies

- AD, Pick disease, corticobasal degeneration (CBD), progressive supranuclear palsy (PSP), argyrophilic grain disease

Multi-Infarct Dementia

- Shared risk factors for atherosclerosis

Frontotemporal Dementias (FTD)

- Pick disease, FTD with inclusions (positive for tdp-43, neurofilament, fused in sarcoma protein [FUS], p62, ubiquitin)

Amyotrophic Lateral Sclerosis (ALS) With Dementia

- Spectrum from ALS only to ALS with frontotemporal dementia to pure frontotemporal dementia with ubiquitin positive inclusions

Synucleinopathies

- Parkinson disease (PD), Lewy body dementia (LBD), multisystem atrophy (MSA)

Other Heritable Conditions

- Huntington disease (HD), spinocerebellar ataxias, Friedrich ataxia, inherited amyloidoses

Other Acquired Conditions

- Acquired-B12 deficiency, chronic traumatic encephalopathy, Wernicke-Korsakoff

CLINICAL ISSUES

Epidemiology

- Incidence
  - AD is most common neurodegenerative disease
    - Not a normal part of aging but incidence ↑ with advancing age: Incidence 1/100 in 65-59 year olds
    - Prevalence doubles with 5-year increments after age 70
    - Younger onset with inherited AD (mutations in amyloid precursor protein [APP], pre-senilin 1, pre-senilin 2; all autosomal dominant)
    - Down syndrome (APP gene on chromosome 21)
  - Multi-infarct dementia occurs with other risk factors for and manifestations of cardiovascular disease
  - Note that patients with autosomal dominant inherited diseases with trinucleotide repeats (e.g., HD) may show earlier onset in successive generation
  - PD also increases with increasing age but has early-onset heritable forms in 10% of cases
    - Heritable forms may be autosomal dominant or recessive

Presentation

- AD: Insidious onset, disturbances in recent memory function, visuospatial disorders, behavioral change
- Multi-infarct dementia: Stepwise deterioration
- FTD: Progressive aphasia, behavioral change, semantic dementia (language difficulties)
- Movement disorders
  - PD: Tremor, rigidity, responsive to L-dopa
  - LBD: Tremor, rigidity, not responsive to L-dopa, with visual hallucination
  - HD: Chorea
  - Corticobasilar degeneration: "Alien limb"
- Prion diseases: Rapidly progressive dementia (< 1 year), ataxia, myoclonus, sleep disturbances

DEMENTIA AND NEURODEGENERATIVE DISEASE

Key Facts

Clinical Issues

- Common causes of death
  - Aspiration pneumonia, other infections, choking, or respiratory failure
  - Other infections
  - Pulmonary thromboembolism
  - Falls due to extrapyramidal symptoms, weakness, orthostatic hypotension, and deconditioning from immobility
  - Decreased nutritional intake, generalized deconditioning contribute to comorbidity

Macroscopic Pathology

- Routine sampling
  - Frontal, temporal, anterior cingulate, parietal (ink the precentral gyrus before sectioning), occipital cortex
  - Hippocampus, amygdala
  - Caudate, putamen, globus pallidus, subthalamic nucleus
  - Midbrain (with substantia nigra), pons (with locus ceruleus), medulla
  - Cerebellar vermis, dentate
  - Target to suspected disorder based on clinical signs and symptoms

Diagnostic Checklist

- Alzheimer: Plaque frequency does not correlate well with clinical dementia, but tangle frequency and distribution does
- Parkinson: Most of the loss of pigmented neurons in pars compacta of substantia nigra occurs laterally and ventrally, whereas in normal aging, what loss there is occurs medially and dorsally

Laboratory Tests

- Genetic testing: *SNCA* (synucleinopathies), *PSEN1* (AD), huntingtin (HD)
- Autonomic testing: Impaired in PD, MSA
- Cerebrospinal fluid testing for prion disease (14-3-3 protein and tau)

Prognosis

- Aspiration pneumonia, infections, respiratory failure are common causes of death
- Decreased nutritional intake, general deconditioning contribute to comorbidity
- Falls due to extrapyramidal symptoms, weakness, orthostatic hypotension, and deconditioning from immobility

IMAGE FINDINGS

CT Findings

- AD
  - Enlarged ventricles
  - May be lobar hemorrhage if associated amyloid angiopathy
- Cerebellar, pontine atrophy in MSA

MR Findings

- AD: Hippocampal atrophy; frontal, temporal, and parietal atrophy
- MSA: Atrophy of putamen, pons, ("hot cross bun" hyperintensity of pons), cerebellum
- FTD: Severe focal frontal and temporal atrophy
- Creutzfeldt-Jakob disease (CJD): Hyperintensity of cortical ribbon, caudate, putamen

MACROSCOPIC FEATURES

External Examination

- Cachexia, features of Down syndrome, muscle atrophy indicating denervation, contractures
- Evidence of deep vein thrombosis (asymmetrical calf swelling), decubitus ulcers, fractures from recent falls, tongue biting from seizures

Internal Examination

- Aspiration pneumonia
- Atherosclerotic disease (multi-infarct dementia)

Brain Examination

- Pattern of atrophy
  - AD: May be thinning of cortical ribbon, ventricular enlargement, diffuse atrophy
  - HD: Flattening or concavity of caudate nucleus
  - FTD: "Knife edge" atrophy of temporal lobes, frontal atrophy
  - MSA: Atrophy of putamen, inferior olivary nuclei, pons, and cerebellum
  - SCA: Pontine, olivary, or cerebellar atrophy
  - CBD: Asymmetrical frontal and parietal atrophy, sometimes caudate and thalamus
  - PSP: Atrophy of subthalamic nucleus, superior cerebellar peduncle
  - ALS: May be atrophy of motor cortex (precentral gyrus); may be frontal and temporal atrophy if coexisting FTD
- Pigmentation
  - Discoloration of putamen in MSA, globus pallidus in PSP and CBD
  - Loss of pigment in substantia nigra in PD, LBD, MSA, PSP, CBD
  - Pallor of locus ceruleus in PD, LBD, MSA, and AD
- Sampling
  - Target to suspected disorder based on clinical signs and symptoms
  - Cortex: Frontal, temporal, anterior cingulate, parietal, occipital
    - Ink precentral gyrus (motor cortex) before serially sectioning
  - Hippocampus, amygdala
  - Basal ganglia and thalamus: Caudate, putamen, globus pallidus, subthalamic nucleus, mamillary bodies

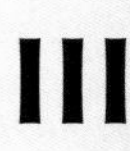

- Brainstem: Midbrain (with substantia nigra), pons (with locus ceruleus), medulla
- Cerebellum: Vermis, dentate
- Cervical, thoracic, and lumbar cord (esp. in ALS, spinocerebellar ataxias, Friedrich ataxia, B12 deficiency)

MICROSCOPIC PATHOLOGY

Histologic Features

- Amyloid plaques, neurofibrillary tangles (AD)
- Neuronal inclusions
  - PD, LBD: Lewy bodies (alpha synuclein [+])
  - PSP, CBD: Balloon neurons
  - ALS: Skein-like inclusions
- Glial inclusions
  - MSA: Cytoplasmic in oligodendrocytes
  - PSP: Tufted/"thorny" astrocytes
  - CBD: Astrocytic plaques
- Spongiotic degeneration
  - Prion disease: Throughout cortex, thalamus, &/or cerebellum
  - AD, LBD: Superficial cortex only (in severe forms)
- Neuronal loss
  - PD: Atrophy and loss in substantia nigra (midbrain)

ANCILLARY TESTS

Histochemistry

- Congo red (or beta amyloid IHC)
  - Staining pattern
    - Extracellular amyloid plaques of AD and prion disease
    - Amyloid in media of vessels in amyloid angiopathies
- Silver stains: Bielschowsky, Gallyas, or Bodian
  - Stain plaques and wide variety of inclusions with varying sensitivities

Immunohistochemistry

- Ubiquitin: Highlights intraneuronal inclusions (e.g., SCA, Huntington, and ALS)
- A-synuclein: Lewy bodies and Lewy neurits in neuronal processes, glial cytoplasmic inclusions in MSA
- Tau: Hyperphosphorylated tau seen in neurofibrillary tangles of AD, Pick bodies in Pick disease, inclusions of CBD, PSP

DIAGNOSTIC CHECKLIST

Pathologic Interpretation Pearls

- Normal aging
  - Both diffuse plaques and varying number of neuritic plaques (amyloid plaques with a core of dystrophic neurites)
  - Hippocampal neurofibrillary tangles found in normal aging (but cortical tangles specific for dementia)
- AD
  - Only neuritic plaques relevant to a diagnosis of AD; must be interpreted in context (patient age, signs and symptoms)
  - Plaque frequency does not correlate well with clinical dementia severity, but tangle frequency and distribution does
  - β-amyloid plaques are extracellular; neurofibrillary tangles are intracellular
- PD
  - Lewy bodies are never a normal finding in aging
  - Loss of pigmented neurons in pars compacta of substantia nigra (lateral and ventral), whereas in normal aging, loss is medial and dorsal

REPORTING CRITERIA

Cause of Death

- Generally secondary effect of dementia rather than neurodegeneration alone
  - Aspiration, sepsis, or other systemic findings

Clinicopathologic Correlation

- AD diagnosis requires clinical history of dementia, and absence of another cause of dementia
- Findings of AD frequently coexist with LBD
- Multiple vascular subcortical lesions are more suggestive of multiinfarct dementia than lacunar infarcts

SELECTED REFERENCES

1. Cure S et al: Systematic literature review and meta-analysis of diagnostic test accuracy in Alzheimer's disease and other dementia using autopsy as standard of truth. J Alzheimers Dis. 42(1):169-82, 2014
2. Bigio EH: Making the diagnosis of frontotemporal lobar degeneration. Arch Pathol Lab Med. 137(3):314-25, 2013
3. Jordan BD: The clinical spectrum of sport-related traumatic brain injury. Nat Rev Neurol. 9(4):222-30, 2013
4. Kojima G et al: Creutzfeldt-Jakob disease: a case report and differential diagnoses. Hawaii J Med Public Health. 72(4):136-9, 2013
5. Nelson PT et al: Correlation of Alzheimer disease neuropathologic changes with cognitive status: a review of the literature. J Neuropathol Exp Neurol. 71(5):362-81, 2012
6. Thompson PM et al: Pathologic lesions in neurodegenerative diseases. Prog Mol Biol Transl Sci. 107:1-40, 2012
7. Dickson D et al: Neurodegeneration: The Molecular Pathology of Dementia and Movement Disorders. 2nd ed. New Jersey: Wiley-Blackwell, 2011
8. Fearnley JM et al: Ageing and Parkinson's disease: substantia nigra regional selectivity. Brain. 114 (Pt 5):2283-301, 1991

Gross and Microscopic Features

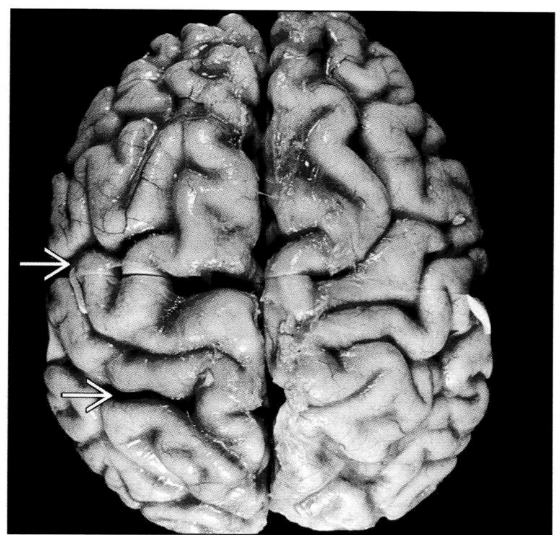
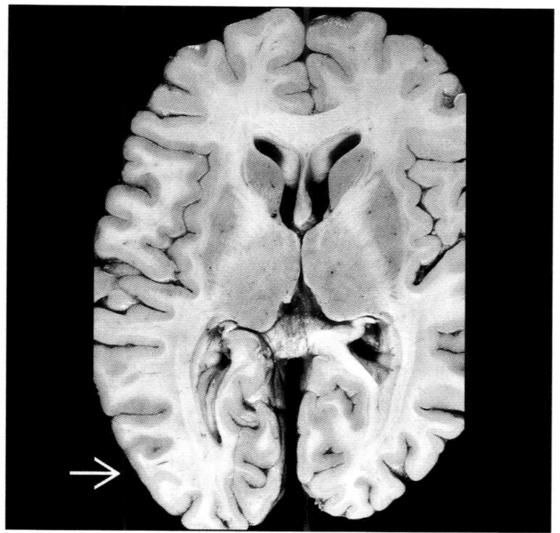

(Left) *Autopsy case of dementia with diffuse Lewy bodies shows mild, generalized volume loss without specific lobar predominance. Atrophy is manifest in part as widening of the sulci ➔. (From Osborn's Brain.)* ***(Right)*** *Axial section in the same case shows mildly enlarged ventricles with no other definite abnormalities identified. The occipital lobes ➔ appear normal. (From Osborn's Brain.)*

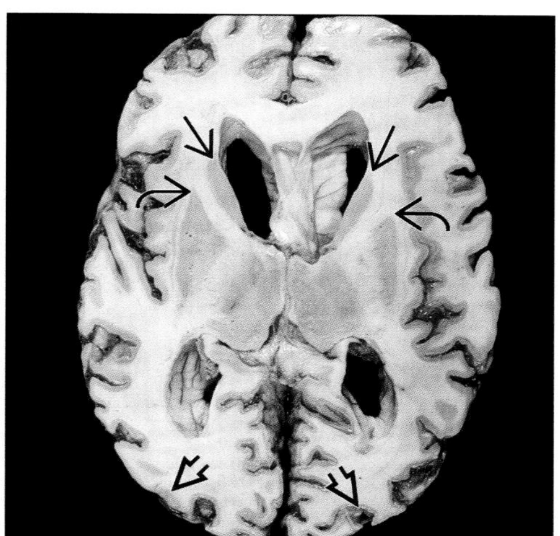
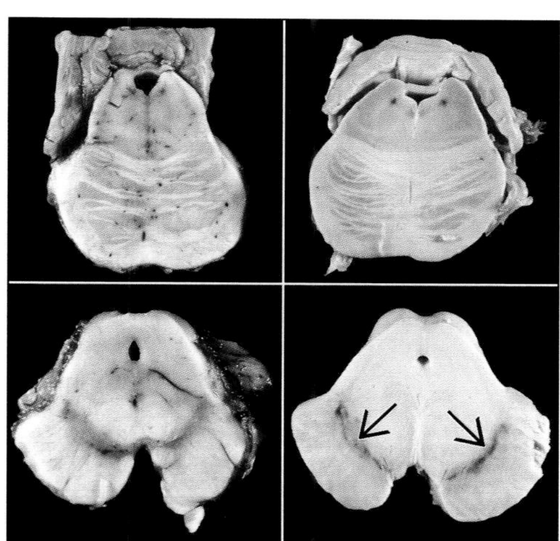

(Left) *Autopsy of sporadic Creutzfeldt-Jakob disease shows marked atrophy of the caudate nuclei ➔ and anterior basal ganglia ➔. The cerebral cortex is severely thinned, especially in the occipital lobes ➔, where it is almost inapparent. (From Osborn's Brain.)* ***(Right)*** *Autopsied sections compare normal midbrain (left) to one affected by Parkinson disease (right). Note midbrain volume loss in Parkinson disease and abnormal pallor of the substantia nigra ➔. (From Osborn's Brain.)*

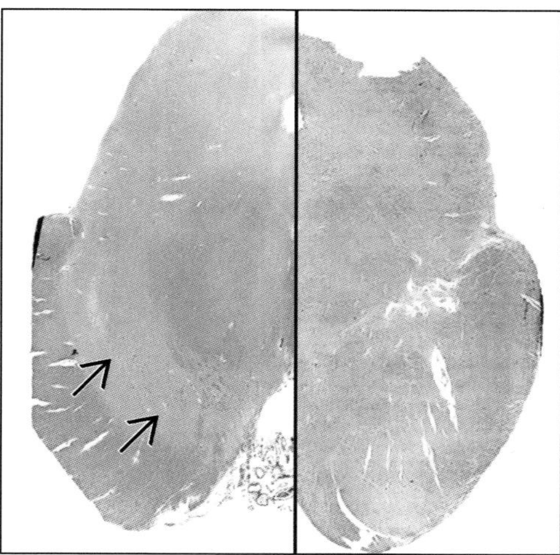
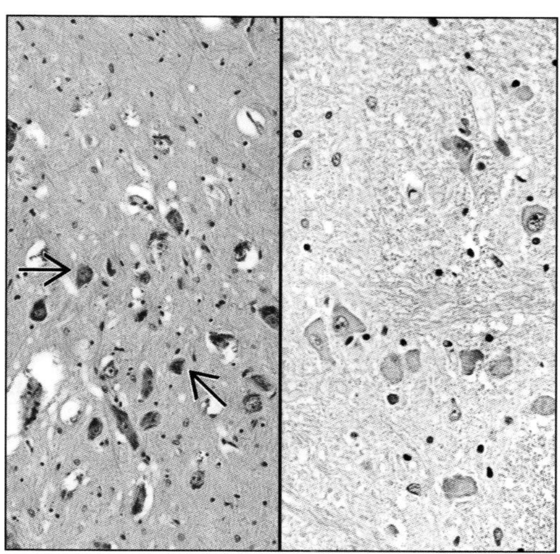

(Left) *These side-by-side photomicrographs are from patients with (right) and without (left) Parkinson disease. Pigmented cells can be seen in the substantia nigra area of the normal brain ➔.* ***(Right)*** *These side-by-side photomicrographs at higher magnification show the substantia nigra neurons. The normal comparison shows retention of pigment ➔, and the Parkinson patient shows pigmentary "incontinence."*

INDEX

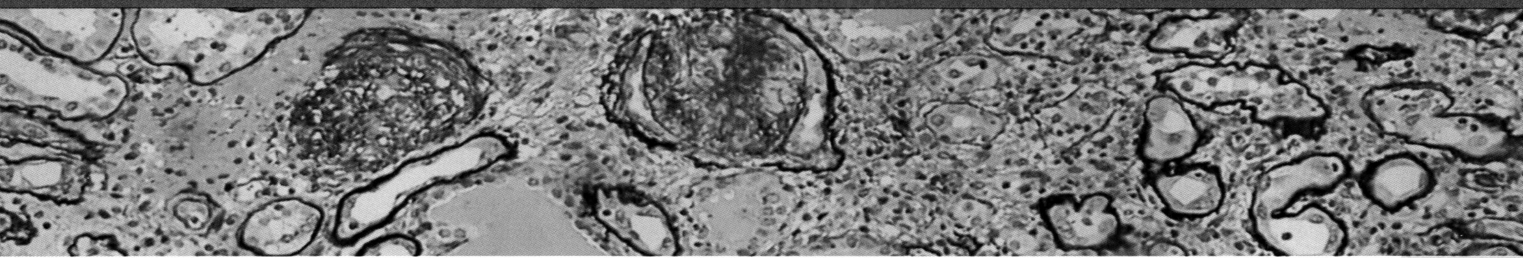

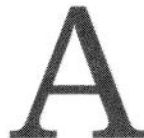

INDEX

B

INDEX

D

E

F

G

INDEX

H

I

J

K

L

M

INDEX

N

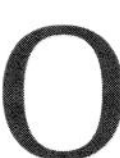

O

P

Q

R

S

T

U

MW01225459

Dreamers
Skeptics
and Healers

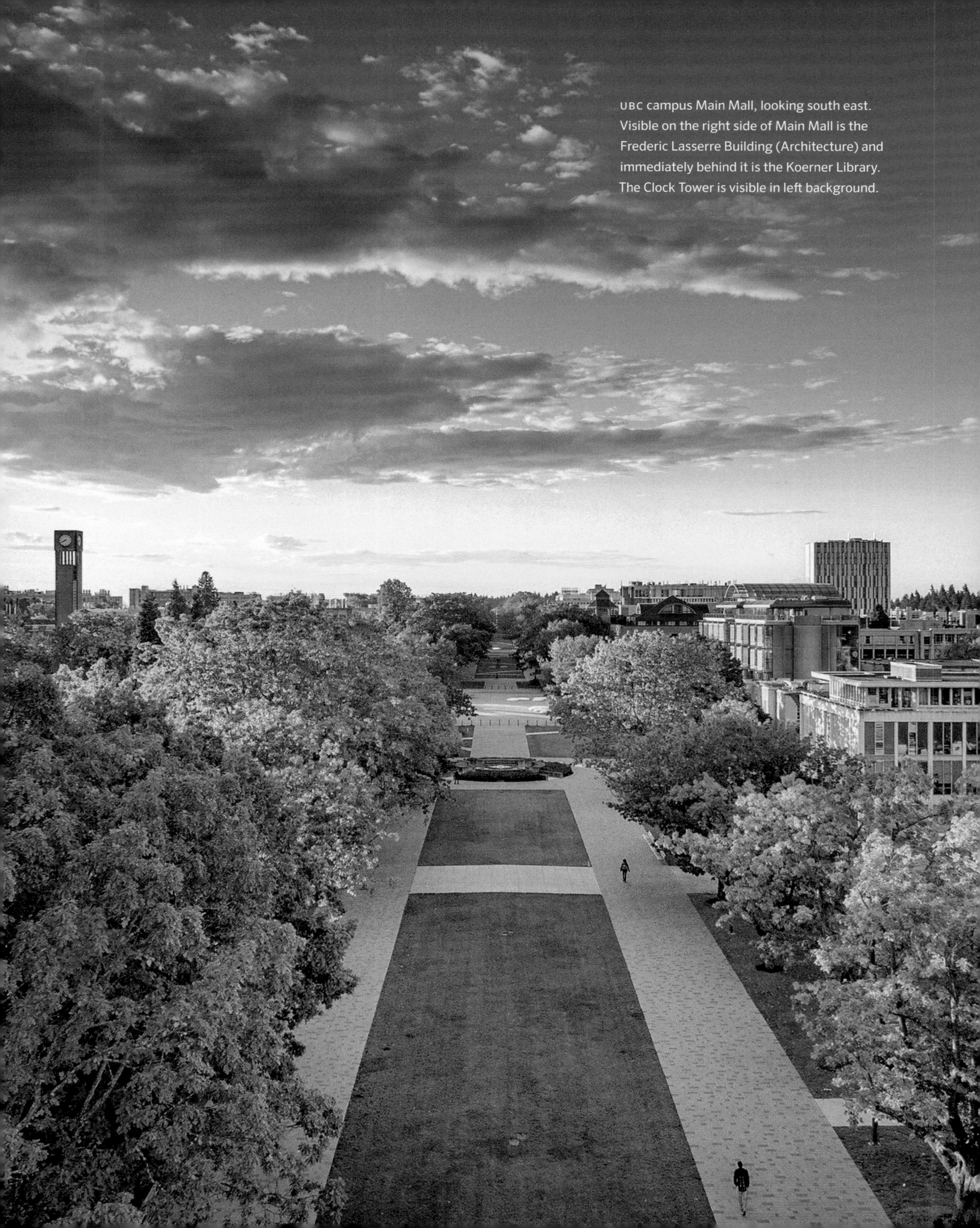

UBC campus Main Mall, looking south east. Visible on the right side of Main Mall is the Frederic Lasserre Building (Architecture) and immediately behind it is the Koerner Library. The Clock Tower is visible in left background.

THE UBC FACULTY OF MEDICINE AT 70 YEARS

Dreamers Skeptics and Healers

THE STORY OF BC'S MEDICAL SCHOOL

Wendy Cairns · John Cairns · David Ostrow · Gavin Stuart

PAGE TWO
BOOKS

Cataloguing in publication information is
available from Library and Archives Canada.
ISBN 978-1-989603-89-5 (hardcover)

Page Two
pagetwo.com

Edited by Lesley Erickson
Copyedited by Rachel Ironstone
Jacket and interior design by Fiona Lee
Front cover photo © Paul H. Joseph, Photographer
Back cover photo University of British Columbia
Archives [UBC 1.1/2673]
Printed and bound in Canada by Friesens
Distributed in Canada by Raincoast Books
Distributed in the US and internationally by
Publishers Group West, a division of Ingram

21 22 23 24 25 5 4 3 2 1

WE ACKNOWLEDGE the Indigenous Peoples of all the lands on which BC's medical school is situated. UBC was founded on the Point Grey campus which is located on the traditional, ancestral, and unceded territory of the xʷməθkʷəy̓əm (Musqueam) people. We recognize that the medical school is now spread across the province on the territories of many Indigenous Peoples. We acknowledge the importance of these lands, which we each call home. We do this to reaffirm our commitment and responsibility to improve relationships between nations and to enhance our own understanding of local Indigenous Peoples and their cultures. We acknowledge the traditional, ancestral, and unceded territory of all the Inuit, Métis, and First Nations Peoples that call this place home. Please take a moment of reflection to acknowledge the harms and mistakes of the past and to consider how we can each, in our own way, try to move forward in a spirit of reconciliation and collaboration.

Contents

Foreword

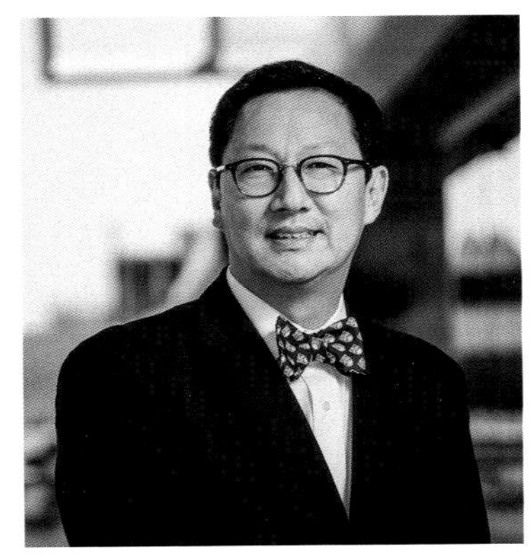

SINCE UBC'S FACULTY of Medicine opened its doors in 1950 with sixty students, it has grown to become one of the world's best medical schools—a global leader in both the science and the practice of medicine.

Building on initial work by the late Wendy Cairns, John Cairns, David Ostrow, and Gavin Stuart have done a tremendous job bringing the Faculty of Medicine's history to life in *Dreamers, Skeptics, and Healers*.

The book tells the fascinating story of the Faculty of Medicine's first seventy years—from its rocky launch, through its coming of age and the years of growth to the present. In these pages, you'll meet many of the students, professors, researchers, alumni, and administrators who have been part of the Faculty's story over the years.

When I joined UBC as president and vice-chancellor, I also became a faculty member in the Faculty of Medicine. Reading this book reinforces my pride in being part of the Faculty of Medicine family. I hope that you find *Dreamers, Skeptics, and Healers: The Story of BC's Medical School* as inspiring and fascinating as I did.

SANTA J. ONO
President and Vice-Chancellor
University of British Columbia

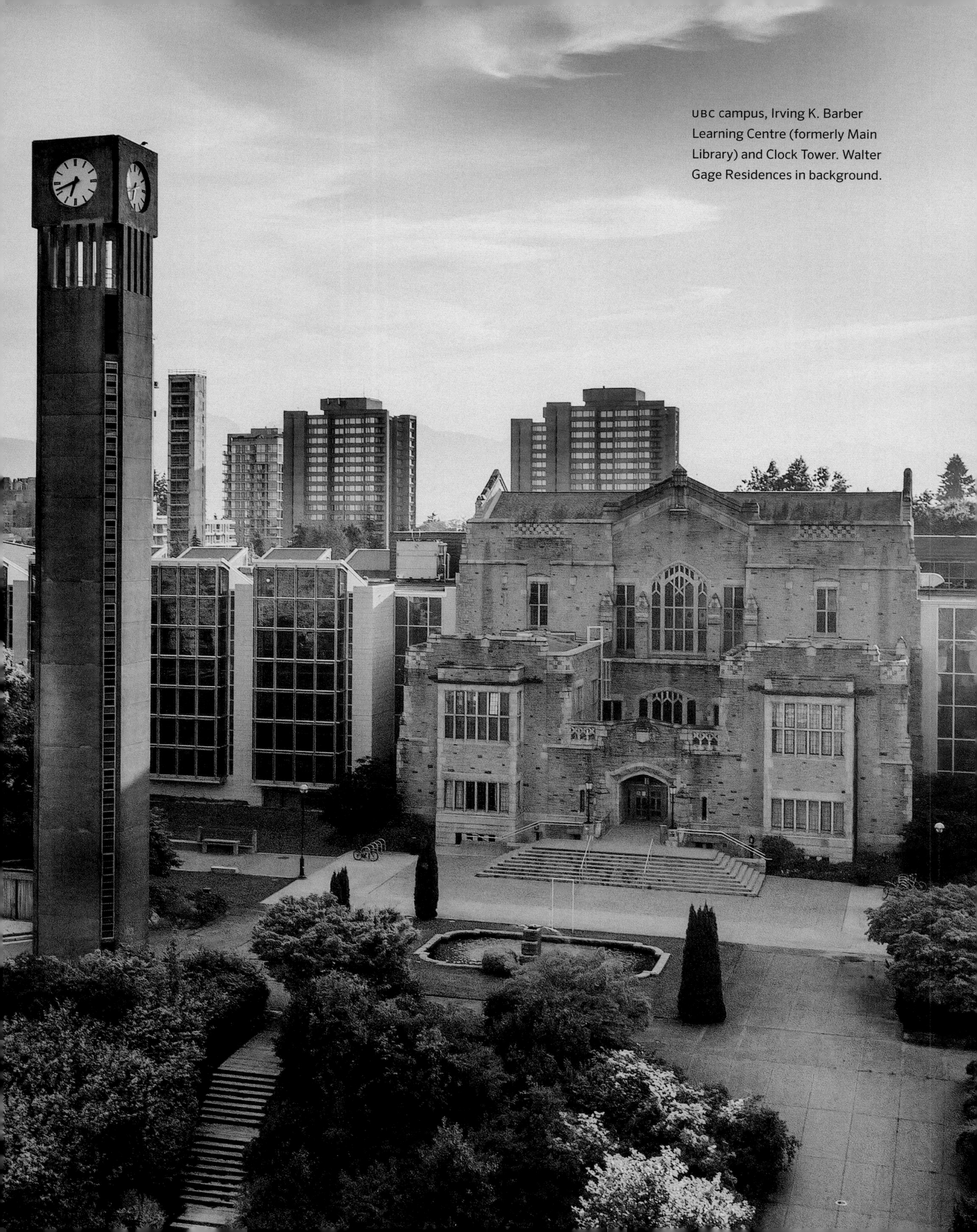

UBC campus, Irving K. Barber Learning Centre (formerly Main Library) and Clock Tower. Walter Gage Residences in background.

Preface

THE IDEA OF writing the Faculty of Medicine's story of adversity and ultimate success first came to Wendy Cairns back in 1998, shortly after her husband, John, became Dean of Medicine at the University of British Columbia. She worked on the project through to 2003, drawing on data from an array of previous works and UBC's rich archival sources. She interviewed many individuals who had played key roles during the Faculty's first fifty years. Wendy wrote extensively on the period from 1870 through 1996 but eventually abandoned the task, feeling somewhat overwhelmed by the scope of the story and its complexity. She and John saved her written work and voluminous reference materials. Wendy died tragically in 2018, a few months after having a massive stroke. Gavin Stuart, John's successor as dean, had already proposed that the exciting expansion and distribution of the medical program across the province since 2003 be formally recorded, and soon, he, John Cairns, and David Ostrow, former CEO of Vancouver Coastal Health Authority, agreed to collaborate to bring the story to fruition.

We have taken Wendy's writings as foundational and edited and integrated them with our own narratives from 1996, where she left off, to the present. Our references are listed in "Further Reading" and we have called upon many colleagues and the UBC archives for fact-checking.

The story is a long one, and we have had to be selective with the riches of material available from the first seventy years of the Faculty. It has a broad provincial reach, includes hundreds of academic faculty members and thousands of clinical faculty members, and has graduated several thousand MDs. In the context of a complex intersect with numerous hospitals and medical practices, it has been a challenge to define and adhere to a coherent narrative of manageable length and general interest. We have chosen to proceed as much as possible in chronological order in an effort to minimize diversions and repetition.

The Faculty of Medicine (FoM) is one of twenty-six faculties and schools at UBC. The mission of the Faculty is "Health through knowledge and innovation." The FoM is home to 4,500 students, 600 academic and 9,000 clinical faculty members, and 2,000 staff. The broad entity of the FoM comprises a matrix of educational and research programs delivered by nineteen departments and three schools housed on the Point Grey Campus of UBC and within the Clinical Academic Campuses of the Vancouver teaching hospitals. Equally important elements of the Faculty are located on the university-affiliated campuses as well as the major Clinical Academic Campuses and Affiliated Regional Centres in Surrey, Prince George, Victoria, and Kelowna. Programs are augmented by other hospitals and clinical settings across the province. The Doctor of Medicine (MD degree) undergraduate program, the Postgraduate Medical Education program (speciality and/or subspeciality training programs recognized by the Royal College of Physicians and Surgeons of Canada and the College of Family Physicians of Canada), and the Continuing Professional Development (CPD) programs constitute the largest components of the FoM's educational activities. These may be conceptualized as programs of the "medical school," although there is no such formal designation employed at UBC (in contrast to several other Canadian Faculties of Medicine or Health Sciences). The FoM also provides outstanding health professional education programs within its School of Audiology and Speech Sciences, its Department of Occupational Science and Occupational Therapy, its Department of Physical Therapy, its undergraduate science programs in physiology and biochemistry/molecular biology, and its medical laboratory technology and graduate education programs within a wide range of Faculty departments. Other excellent professional graduate programs in genetic counselling, population and public health, reproductive and developmental sciences, and global surgical care are offered within the Faculty. Health research is conducted not only within fields of priority (precision health, heart and lung health, cancer, brain and mental health, population health, and chronic diseases) but also across the breadth of health and life sciences disciplines within the FoM.

When we use the terms "Faculty of Medicine," "FoM," or simply "Faculty" (with a capital "F"), we are referring to the broad entity described above. When we refer to the "medical school," we are referring to the FoM's enterprises of physician education and related medical research, while acknowledging that there is no formally designated medical school at UBC. We celebrate the rich history and success of many of the other "non-physician" programs within the Faculty. While their full history is not covered in this book, it is a critical part of the history of the Faculty that one hopes will be captured in a subsequent book. The teachers and researchers formally appointed to the FoM as either academic or clinical faculty members are collectively referred to as "faculty members" or simply "faculty" (with a small "f").

The names of many facilities in which the FoM fulfills its mission have changed over time. For example, the Vancouver General Hospital (VGH) began as the City Hospital, then became Vancouver City Hospital, then Vancouver General Hospital beginning in 1902. The name of the hospital complex changed several times in the 1990s and early 2000s, and today the designation Vancouver General Hospital is applied to the complex of buildings located at the 12th Avenue and Oak Street site and operated by Vancouver Coastal Health. Faculty academic building and department names have also changed over the years. In general, we have tried to use the designation of a given facility, building, or department that was in use at the time we are referring to it, acknowledging that the name might have changed when the entity is next referred to.

While modern health care is undoubtedly a multidisciplinary team process, the focus of this history is on the development of the missions in education and research of the *medical* portion of the FoM. The visions and achievements of key leaders are described, acknowledging that they are embodiments of the visions and aspirations of countless colleagues who may not be named in this broad narrative. Stories of some of the leaders and the entities that make up the FoM have already been told in prior publications and will no doubt be covered in others to come.

This volume is the first comprehensive documentation of the history of the entire medical school. We hope the reader will enjoy reading this story as much as we have enjoyed researching and writing it.

The Great Trek,
October 1922.

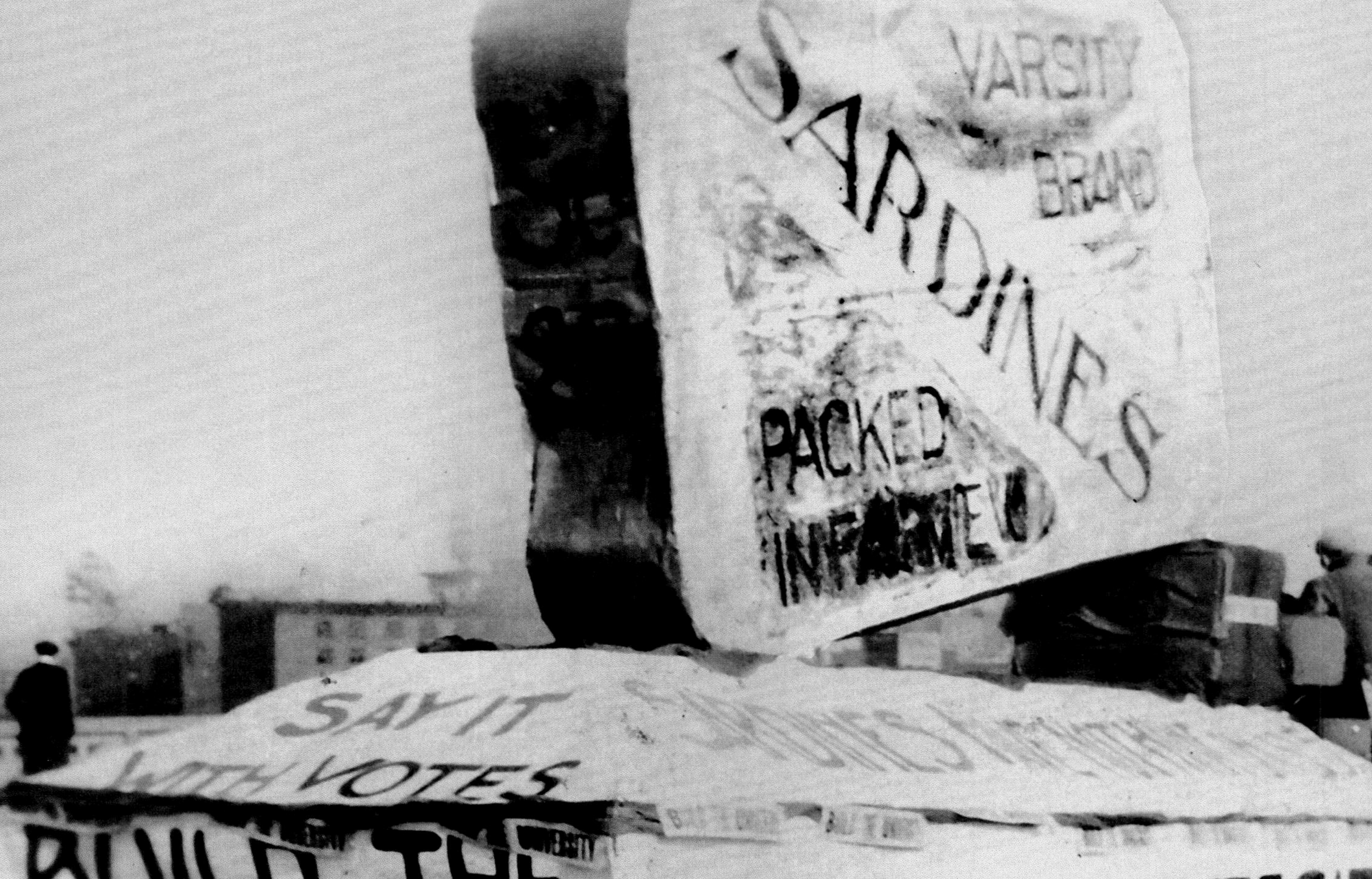

Introduction

THIS STORY OF UBC's Faculty of Medicine is being published during our seventieth anniversary year, 2020–21. The complete complex tale, however, goes back 150 years to 1870, even before British Columbia joined Confederation. The aspirations for a medical school were held by BC physicians with key roles in the Confederation negotiations, in provincial cabinets, and in leadership roles at the University of British Columbia in its earliest days. Resource rich and growing rapidly, the province was served by 554 physicians by 1920, most of them graduates either of McGill's medical school, which had been founded as the Montreal Medical Institution in 1823 by Edinburgh-trained physicians, or of the University of Toronto's program, established in 1843 as part of King's College. Other Canadian medical faculties were at Queen's University (1854), Laval University (1854), University of Montreal (1889), Dalhousie University (1868), the University of Western Ontario (1881), and the Manitoba Medical College (1883). During the first half of the twentieth century, medical faculties were established at the University of Alberta in Edmonton (1913), the University of Saskatchewan (1926), and the University of Ottawa (1945). And yet it was 1950 before UBC enrolled its first class of medical students.

We have identified several themes characterizing the development of our uniquely British Columbian medical school. For over a hundred years, BC had a succession of provincial governments willing to rely on other provinces and countries to educate and train the physicians required to care for British Columbians. Confronted by two world wars and recurrent economic adversity, governments of all parties were resistant to committing the funds necessary to create and operate a medical school. Accordingly, BC was very late in establishing a medical school, and even many years after it opened in 1950, the ratio of medical students to population continued to be the smallest of any province in Canada. Funding was a chronic problem from its inception, and the provincial Ministry of Health was, for many years, relatively unengaged.

The rugged individualism and entrepreneurial spirit which drove miners, ranchers, fishers, and loggers from more settled regions of the country to seek their fortunes in the harsh splendour of the west found a parallel in the medical profession. The forceful and often contentious personalities of these practitioners led them to either challenge or ignore the more conventional foundations of traditional institutions established in older North American centres. These characteristics ultimately played a role in the genesis of an innovative Faculty of Medicine with a strong commitment to a province-wide mission, but also gave rise to controversy as to the location and the nature of a new medical school, further delaying its founding. The establishment of UBC on the Point Grey peninsula, ten kilometres from the downtown hospitals, was a unique hurdle, challenging the early planners and ultimately precluding the establishment of a large, full-service university campus hospital. Rivalries between Vancouver's two major adult hospitals (Vancouver General and St. Paul's) have been a part of our history, as have been clashes between the visions and aspirations of academic leaders and practicing specialists and generalists.

The motto of UBC is "Tuum Est," which can be roughly translated as "It's up to you." This emphasis on the individual setting their own pace, as it were, is wonderful for encouraging self-starters and innovators. However, it risks giving rise to conflicts between strong-willed individuals. This seemed to characterize the early years of the Faculty. But by the time the medical school had reached its fortieth year, in 1990, a level of maturity had developed, and cooperation between individuals, departments, and even sites had become the norm, albeit still with an element of edginess.

Although the Faculty of Medicine was characterized early on by many innovations in the teaching of anatomy, student experiences with family practice settings, and institutional responsibility for continuing medical education, the curriculum was in most ways traditional and based on Eastern Canadian models. In response to criticism from accrediting bodies in the mid-1990s, a new problem-oriented curriculum was created, launching an era of innovations in medical education. These include the development of a distributed model of medical education, employing cutting-edge audio-visual technologies for teaching and administration of a program that spans four major geographic sites and over eighty individual teaching sites.

From its earliest days, the medical school has had a province-wide vision, a natural perspective for the only medical school in BC. This vision was nurtured to full flower with the conceptualization of a dramatically expanded but single BC medical school, with distributed sites and a common curriculum and leadership. The innovative model captured the support of provincial governments and the allocation of dramatically increased operating and capital budgets. These concepts have been enhanced by recruitment of Indigenous students, students from rural areas, and students from less-served populations and by a renewed focus on primary care. The distributed programs for medical students and postgraduate trainees have been eagerly embraced by physicians and communities throughout the province, and early indications are that UBC medical school graduates are returning to local communities and contributing to addressing chronic problems of physician supply. The UBC approach has garnered international attention.

In British Columbia, the provincial government has a unique relationship with Indigenous Peoples. BC entered Confederation with only one historical treaty between the Crown and First Nations on Vancouver Island (the Douglas Treaties of 1854) followed by a second (Treaty 8, signed in 1899), which had effect over North-Eastern BC, Alberta, and part of the Northwest Territories. Recent recognitions of First Nations autonomy include the Nisga'a Treaty, which came into effect in 2000. The creation of a First Nations Health Authority in 2013, to which Health Canada transferred authority over First Nations' health, was unique in Canada and has provided an impetus for strengthening relations with First Nations communities. By the late 1990s, it was recognized that more effort was required to increase the enrollment of Indigenous students in the Faculty of Medicine and to support them to succeed. The resulting Indigenous program with its strong infrastructure has led to the enrollment and graduation of substantial numbers of Indigenous students, and the woefully low proportion of Indigenous physicians to population in the province is improving.

Alongside the development of innovative pedagogy, the Faculty of Medicine's research enterprise, once lagging far behind those of the long-established competing Canadian medical schools, has grown enormously, and UBC is now ranked among Canada's foremost research-intensive medical schools. The Faculty of Medicine has become the largest research enterprise of the University of British Columbia. Over the past thirty years, the administrations and boards of Vancouver teaching hospitals have become strongly committed to health research, have facilitated its conduct, and have steered philanthropic resources to the building and operation of extensive research infrastructure.

Dreamers, Skeptics, and Healers opens by outlining the eighty years of adversity prior to enrollment of the first students in 1950. The long-held aspirations for a BC medical school persevered over struggles against great odds and clashing local visions as to its nature and location. Medical and academic visionaries were ultimately pragmatic and accepting of awkward geography, initially primitive facilities, and the vagaries of government support in the inevitable cycles of boom and bust in a frontier economy. Challenges of minimal funding, physical facilities, and hospital teaching beds characterized the initial years of the young school.

Currently, seventy years after its founding, the Faculty of Medicine is experiencing great success with a distributed model of medical education that is addressing provincial needs and gaining international recognition for its innovation and achievements. Exceptional health and life sciences research is thriving in the environment of a research-intensive university. The future looks bright.

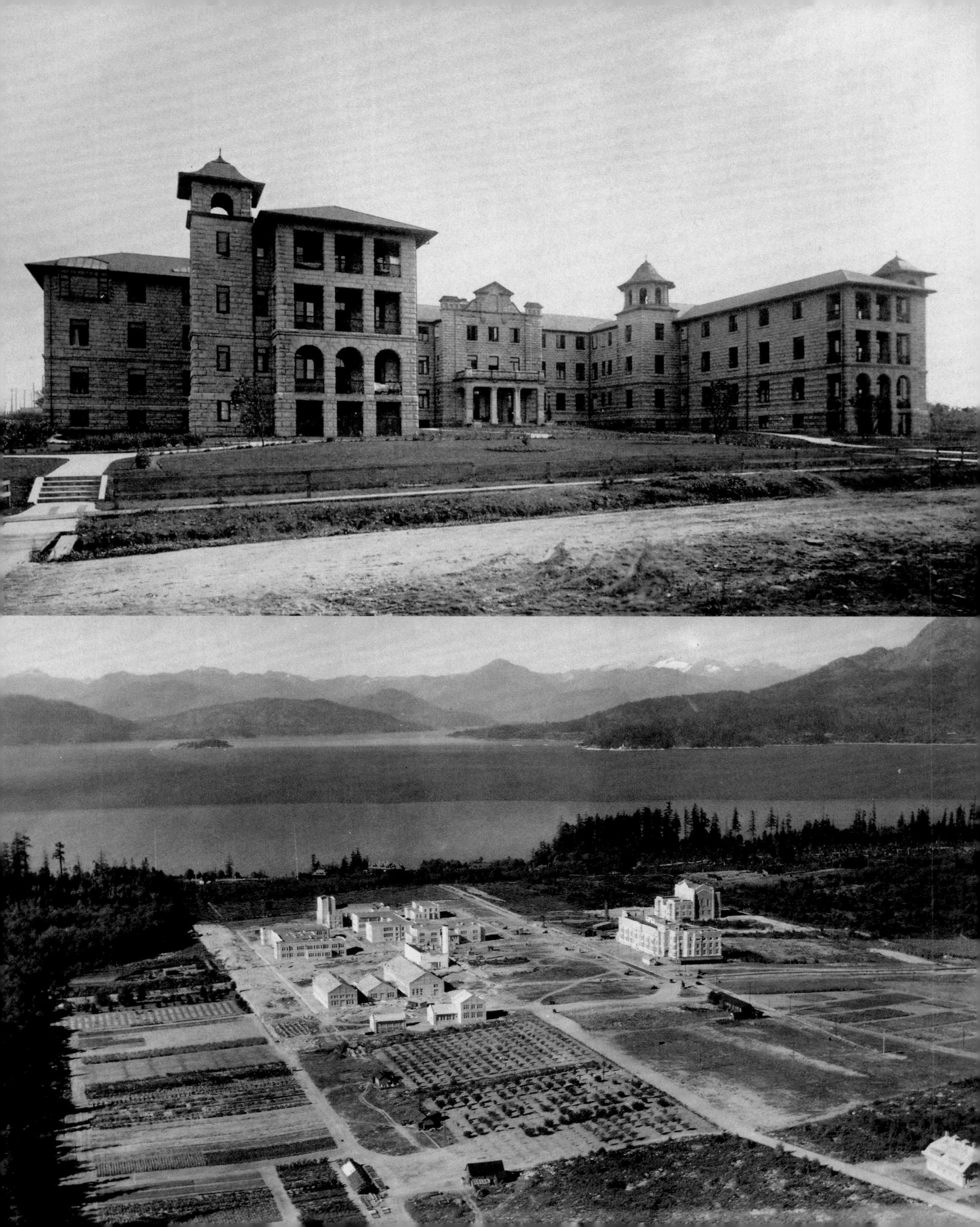

1

Setting the Scene

1870–1949

TOP FACING Heather Pavilion, Vancouver General Hospital, c. 1906

BOTTOM FACING UBC Campus. Looking due north. To the right of the Main Mall (running from south east to north west) is the Science Building (later to become the Chemistry Building) and immediately behind it is the Main Library. To the left of the Main Mall are several agricultural, arts and sciences buildings. The Faculty of Medicine temporary buildings were eventually located just to the right of the three large Agriculture barns and opposite the Chemistry Building. 1927

FACING Hon. John Sebastian Helmcken, Vancouver Island physician, member of BC delegation charged with negotiating terms of union with Dominion of Canada, c. 1854.

Helmcken's vision initiated a long and turbulent course of events leading to the establishment of BC's medical school and its eventual rise to national and international recognition.

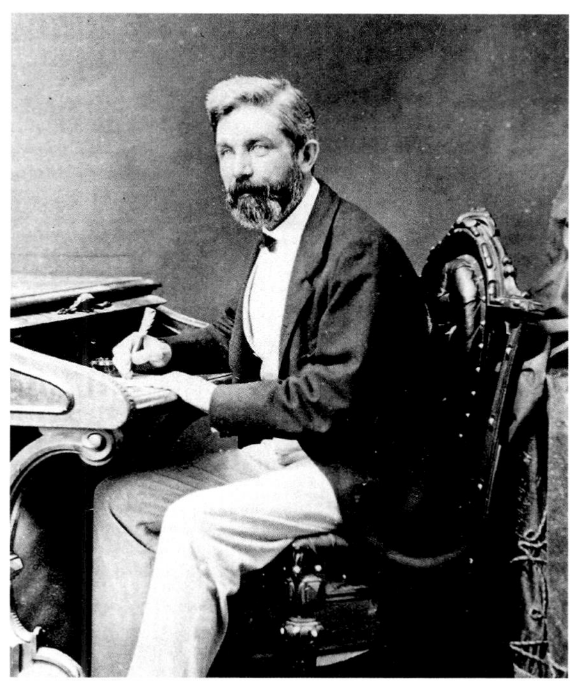

JOHN SEBASTIAN HELMCKEN, a Hudson's Bay physician and later president of the British Columbia Medical Association, was convinced that BC must join the newly formed Dominion of Canada. In 1870, he was chosen as a delegate to the Confederation negotiations in Ottawa to draft BC's terms of union. He was determined that the creation of a marine hospital and associated medical school at the Royal Navy base of Esquimalt on Vancouver Island must be an essential condition for BC's participation in the federation. BC joined Confederation in 1871, and the promise of completion of the Canadian Pacific Railway linking BC to the rest of Canada was duly fulfilled in 1885, opening up the port of Vancouver and stimulating a growth in population which soon outstripped that of Victoria, the provincial capital. The resource-rich province attracted entrepreneurs to exploit its fishing, logging, mining, and, later, hydroelectric assets. However, it would be eighty years before Helmcken's dream of a medical school for BC began to be realized, and a further sixty years until the Island Medical Program was established in Victoria as an integral component of University of British Columbia's newly distributed Faculty of Medicine. His vision initiated a long and turbulent course of events leading to the establishment of BC's medical school and its eventual rise to national and international recognition.

Early Health Services

In the nineteenth century, health services for settlers in the rapidly growing province were of the most rudimentary sort. The first hospital was the Royal Jubilee, opened in Victoria in 1858. In 1862, the Royal Columbian Hospital opened in New Westminster originally to care for men only. The first formal care facility in the city of Vancouver, at that time smaller than Victoria, was an infirmary tent established for the care of injured railway workers in 1886 by the Canadian Pacific Railway on property near the original centre of the young city. The infirmary was incinerated during the great city fire of 1886 and was replaced by a nine-bed, single storey wooden structure which was taken over by the city's Health Committee in 1887, becoming known as the "City Hospital." When smallpox struck from 1888-92, afflicted patients were cared for in the "Pest House," erected on Deadman Island in Vancouver's Coal Harbour. With the general populace

Nursing Education in Vancouver

The hospital-based schools of nursing established at Vancouver City Hospital and St. Paul's Hospital were consistent with practices across North America, but UBC was a pioneer in the creation of a university-based nursing school. UBC's School of Nursing opened in 1919 as part of the Faculty of Applied Science, shortly after UBC itself was founded and thirty years before the Faculty of Medicine was created. Nursing has sustained its academic missions independent of the Faculty of Medicine; although, since 2015, both nursing and undergraduate medical education interact officially within UBC Health, a partnership of all health professional programs at UBC.

TOP FACING Deadman Island, Coal Harbour, Vancouver, site of the "Pest House" erected to care for smallpox victims during the epidemic of 1888–92.

BOTTOM FACING Vancouver City Hospital, opened on corner of Pender and Cambie in 1888.

experiencing a shortage of beds, despite excluding all cases of venereal disease and drunkenness from the hospital, City Council soon allotted $2,000 for the building of a new thirty-five-bed Vancouver City Hospital on the southeast corner of Pender and Cambie Streets near the current Victory Square. It opened with a staff of five in 1888 and established a Training School for Nurses in 1899. The rapid growth of Vancouver would soon necessitate larger, more modern hospital facilities. By 1902, the provincial government was persuaded to incorporate the hospital under the Vancouver General Hospital Act with a special clause providing for a municipal contribution of $50,000. In 1906, the hospital moved to occupy the newly built Heather Pavilion at the corner of Heather Street and 10th Avenue. The new hospital, the largest in Western Canada, had 150 beds and 72 staff. The structure is now a heritage building at the core of the VGH.

The overcrowding at the Vancouver City Hospital was the impetus for the Bishop of New Westminster Diocese to approach the Sisters of Providence in Montreal in 1892 to initiate plans for a new Catholic hospital. Mother Therese and Sister Rodrigue came up from a Sisters of Providence mission in Portland, Oregon, purchased land on Burrard Street, and in 1894 St. Paul's Hospital was opened as a four-storey, twenty-five-bed hospital at a total cost of $28,000. It was active by 1907 as a training school for nurses, and physicians were consulted only in a supporting role to the nurses when necessary. By 1911, the hospital held 115 beds. The Sisters canvassed logging and mining camps in the BC Interior and up the coast of the province, selling $10 tickets which guaranteed hospital care at St. Paul's for illness or injury for a year. In 1912, the initial structure was replaced by a permanent brick building, which remains on the original site.

Until the nineteenth century, most physicians and surgeons in North America learned their profession through a traditional apprenticeship model. Medical education was accomplished in a haphazard fashion; students learned through observation and paid for the opportunity. By the start of the twentieth century in North America, there were more than 250 proprietary medical schools, many of dubious quality. The idea that medical schools should be affiliated with universities hadn't taken hold.

In 1912, however, the Flexner Report, commissioned by the Carnegie Foundation, recommended

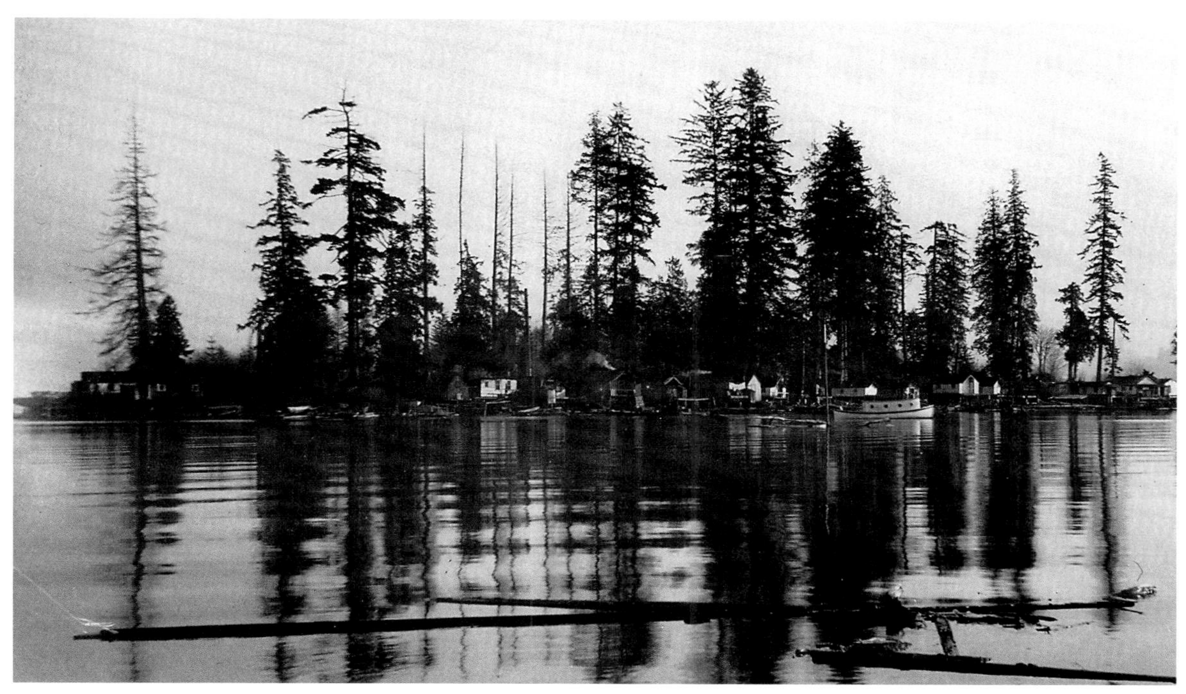

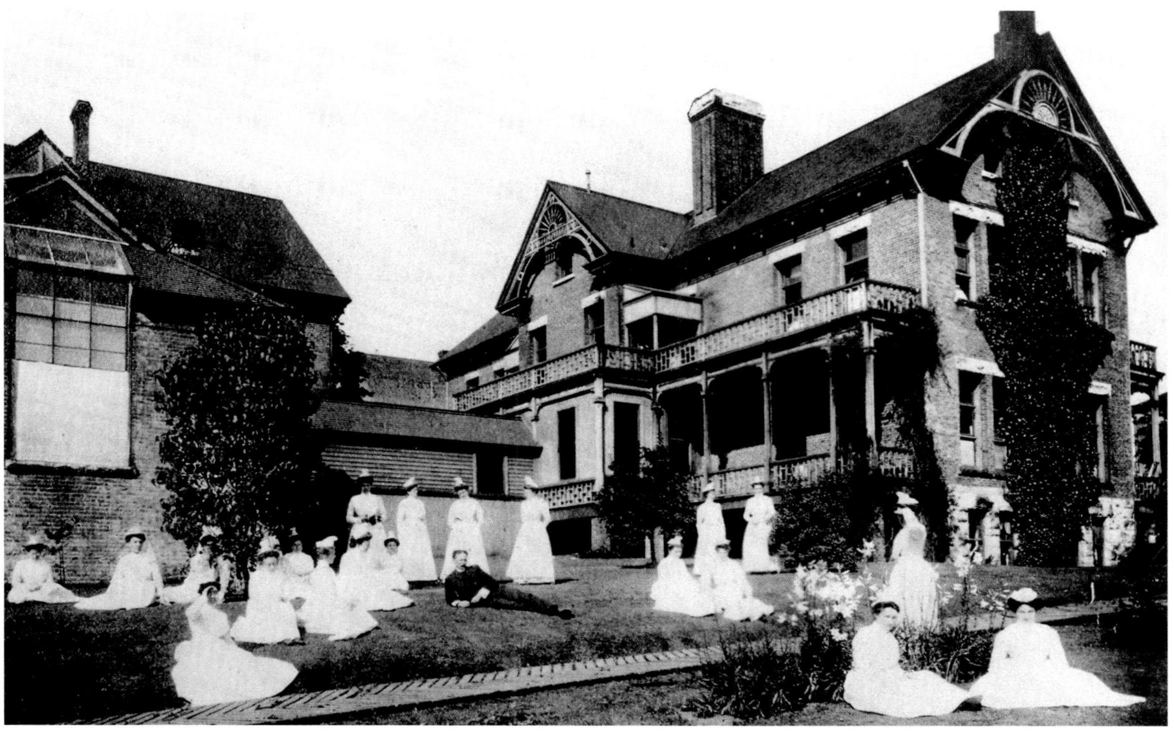

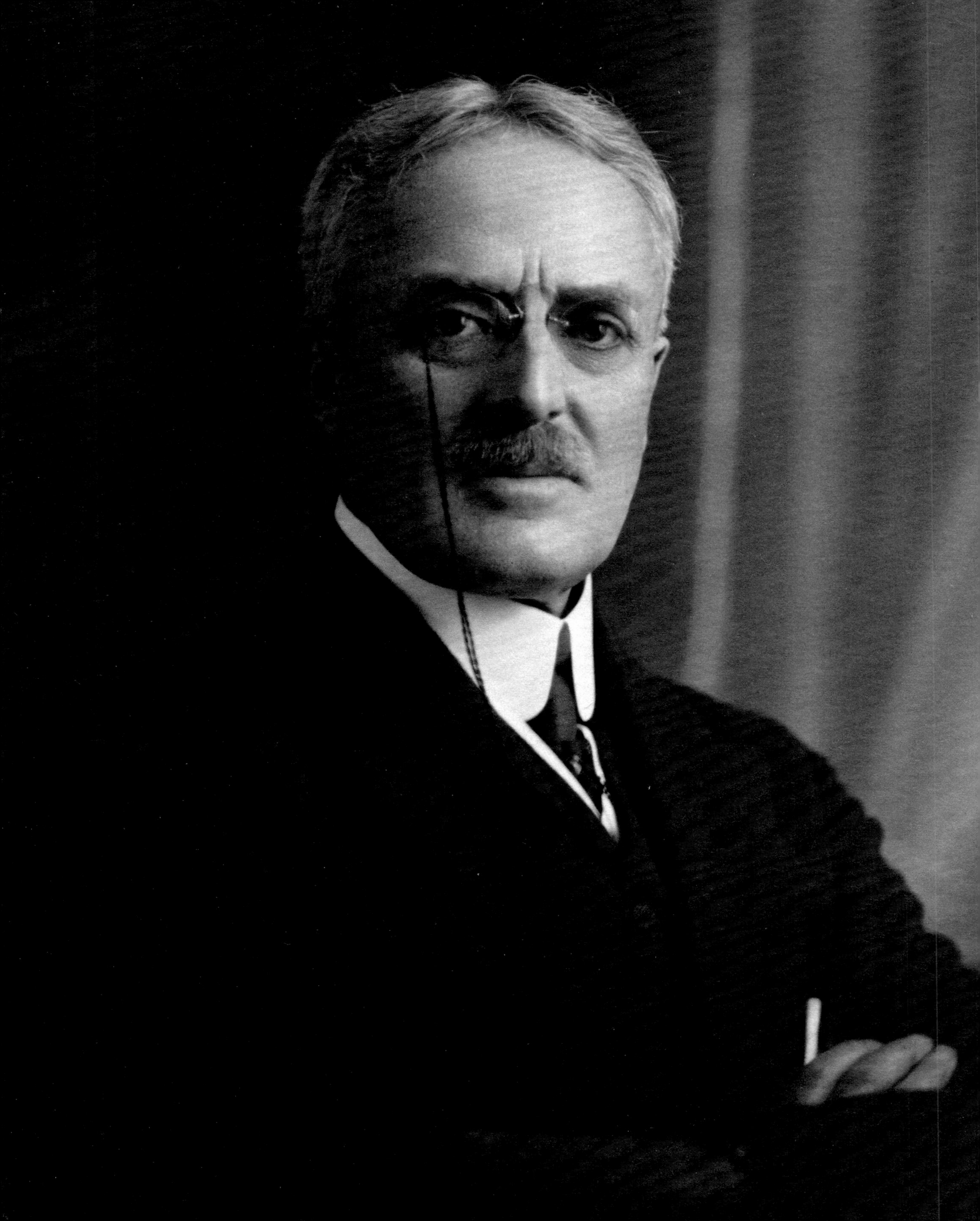

St. Paul's Hospital, facing Burrard St., c. 1904.

FACING Frank Fairchild Wesbrook, physician, inaugural President of UBC (1913–18).

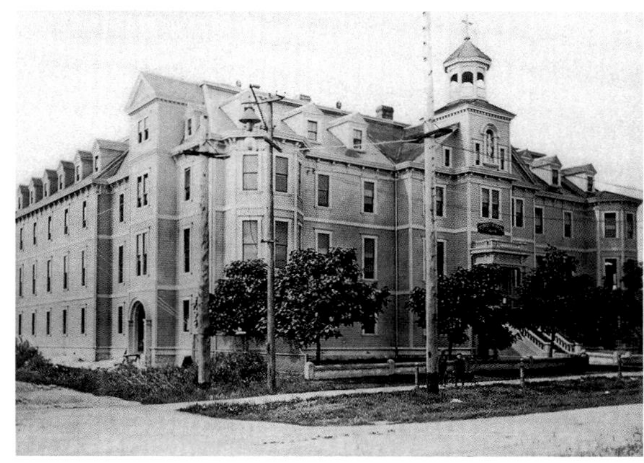

sustaining only those medical schools attached to universities, which offered basic science instruction, were aligned with a teaching hospital, and had paid staff physicians to teach. Within five years of this report, the number of medical schools operating in North America had dropped to under ninety. At the time, doctors-in-training were required to receive a scientific, theoretical underpinning from universities before their later clinical experience with hospital patients. Students spent their initial years immersed in basic sciences and their later years learning at the bedside. The proximity of university and hospital posed no particular problem for most of Canada's medical schools in Halifax, Quebec City, Montreal, Toronto, and Winnipeg, where institutions of health care (hospitals) were generally in the vicinity of institutions of higher learning. However, this was to become an issue of major importance in the eventual struggle to establish a medical school in British Columbia.

It is ironic, given the delay in establishing a Faculty of Medicine, that some of the principal movers in the founding of the University of British Columbia were themselves physicians. Dr. Henry Esson Young, a McGill graduate, played an important role as BC's minister of education in the establishment of UBC. In 1908, he introduced an act to establish a provincial university, to provide "such instruction in all branches of a liberal education as may enable students to become proficient, and qualify for degrees, diplomas, and certificates, in Science, Commerce, Arts, Literature, Law, Medicine, and all other branches of knowledge." Land in heavily forested Point Grey peninsula was granted in 1911 (University Endowment Lands), but it was to be another fourteen years before a university campus finally opened on the site.

Frank Fairchild Wesbrook, a graduate of Manitoba Medical College and then Dean of Medicine at the University of Minnesota, was appointed UBC's first president in 1913. Within a few months of his arrival in Vancouver, the outbreak of war delayed construction on the new campus, and in 1915, the university began its operations in temporary quarters on the Fairview campus adjacent to the Vancouver General Hospital. Wesbrook's advice and assistance were instrumental in establishing the "Fairview shacks," a bacteriology and pathology laboratory, which became the foundation for the science departments of the university. His dream of a medical school, however, had to be put on hold as the war persisted. Sadly, President Wesbrook died at the age of fifty in October 1918.

Wesbrook's successor as president, agronomist Leonard S. Klinck, learned that the Rockefeller Foundation had set aside $5 million to advance

TOP FACING UBC's Fairview Campus and "shacks," looking eastward, Oak St. running left to right in the foreground and 12th Ave. to the right running west to east. The Heather Pavilion is visible beyond the tennis courts.

BOTTOM LEFT FACING Leonard S. Klinck, agronomist, second President of UBC (1919–44).

BOTTOM RIGHT FACING Robert E. McKechnie, physician, inaugural President BCMA (1899), Chancellor of UBC (1918–44).

Canadian medical education. In response to his request for funds, the foundation sent Robin Pearce to review the state of medical education in Vancouver. In 1921, Pearce met three prominent doctors who were keen to establish a medical school in the city: J.M. Pearson, a senior internist and founder of the Vancouver Medical Library; R.H. Mullin, Director of Laboratories at VGH and Professor of Bacteriology at UBC; and M.T. McEachern, superintendent at VGH. The trio pressed enthusiastically for a medical school to be centred at VGH. The lack of dedicated teaching beds at VGH and the absence of support from the Victoria Medical Society for a medical school in Vancouver were obstacles to be overcome. However, the most troublesome difficulty, reported by Pearce, concerned "the present [Liberal] government, which is opposed to the University generally, will not vote funds for buildings or development, and provides only the meagre maintenance budget necessary for the present work." The attitude of that government was epitomized in a statement made in the legislature by Alberni's member of the Legislative Assembly, Richard J. Burde, who declared "the University... is bunk."

It was anticipated that a Conservative government, which had started UBC, would be elected and then move UBC to its new Point Grey site, making available the vacated Fairview shacks beside VGH to house a medical school. Simultaneous with the Rockefeller Foundation visit, there were discussions between Chancellor Robert E. McKechnie (unbeknownst to President Klinck) and the University of Alberta, regarding a shared medical program. Unfortunately for the University of BC, this did not gain traction, and the foundation committed its entire Western Canada allocation to Alberta.

The Great Trek of 1922, a student-led demonstration and fundraiser marching from Vancouver Fairview to Point Grey, finally provoked the resumption of construction on the Point Grey Campus which opened to students in 1925. Chancellor McKechnie was another dedicated champion of the need for a medical school. He was a Nanaimo-based surgeon and the first president of the BC Medical Association (1899-1900). He helped establish the American College of Surgeons and served as one of its first regents, thus ensuring a unique Canadian professional link to American colleagues that continues to this day. Throughout his twenty-six years (1918-44) as chancellor, he applied his considerable diplomatic and administrative talents to the promotion of a new medical school, but to no avail as the province struggled to recover from World War I and the subsequent depression.

Over several decades, there was increasing anxiety among potential medical students that medical schools in other provinces, supported by their legislatures, might no longer reserve slots for BC applicants. Unfortunately, in the face of annual budget cuts from an uncomprehending provincial

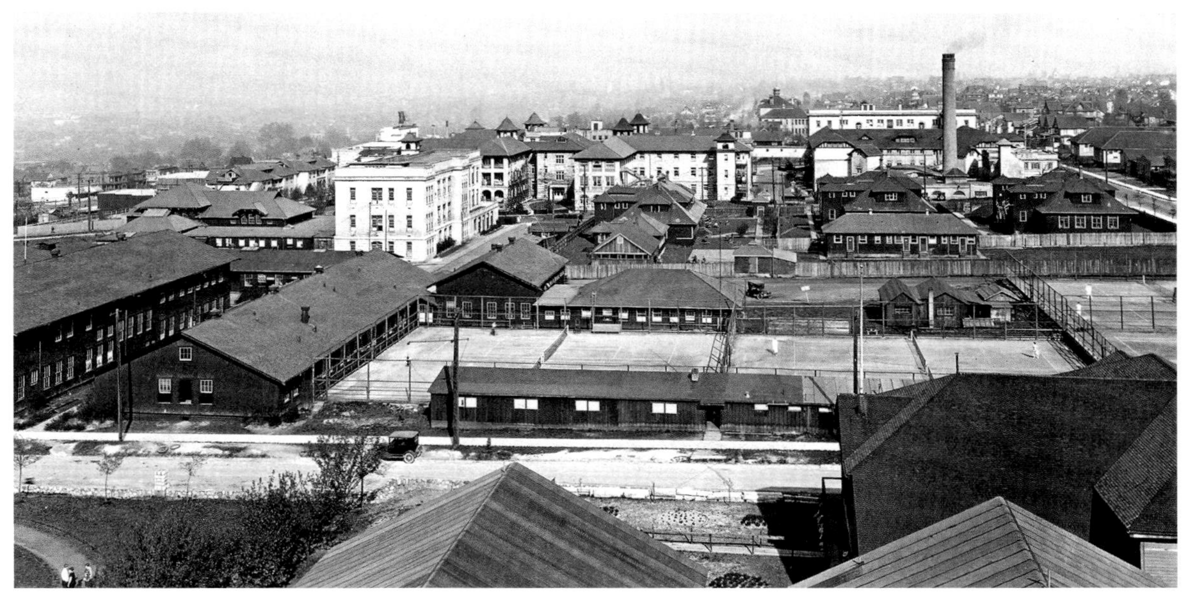

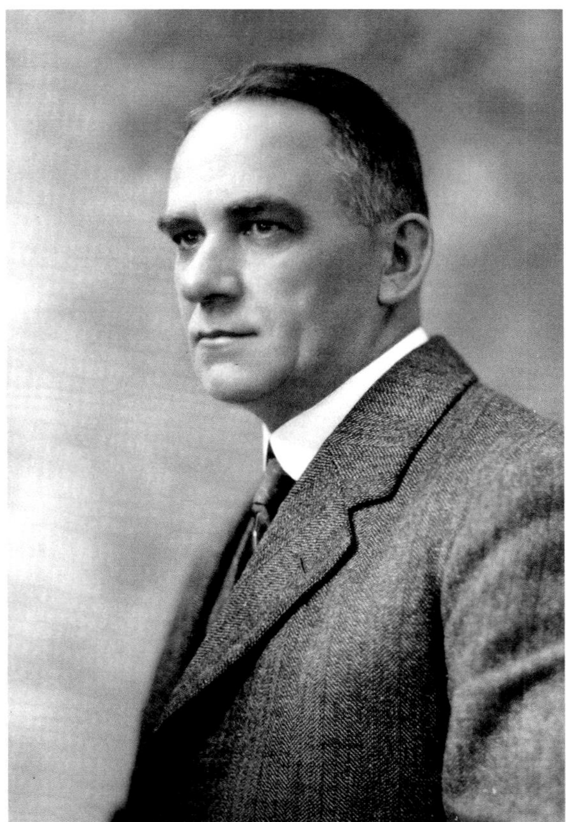

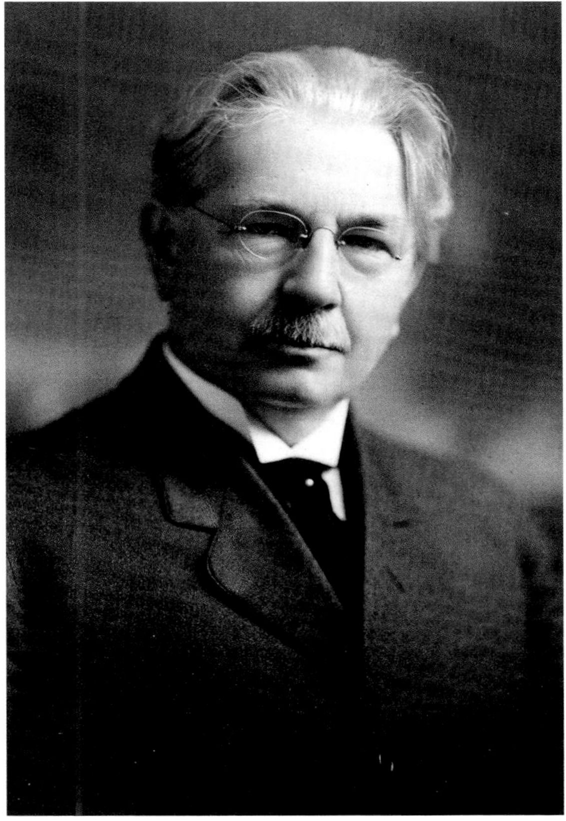

The Great Trek culminated at the Science Building (later to become the Chemistry Building), UBC Point Grey campus. This photo was taken the following year depicting the laying of the cornerstone.

FACING Claude E. Dolman, microbiologist, Head of UBC Department of Bacteriology and Preventive Medicine (1935–51) and then of Bacteriology and Immunology (1951–61).

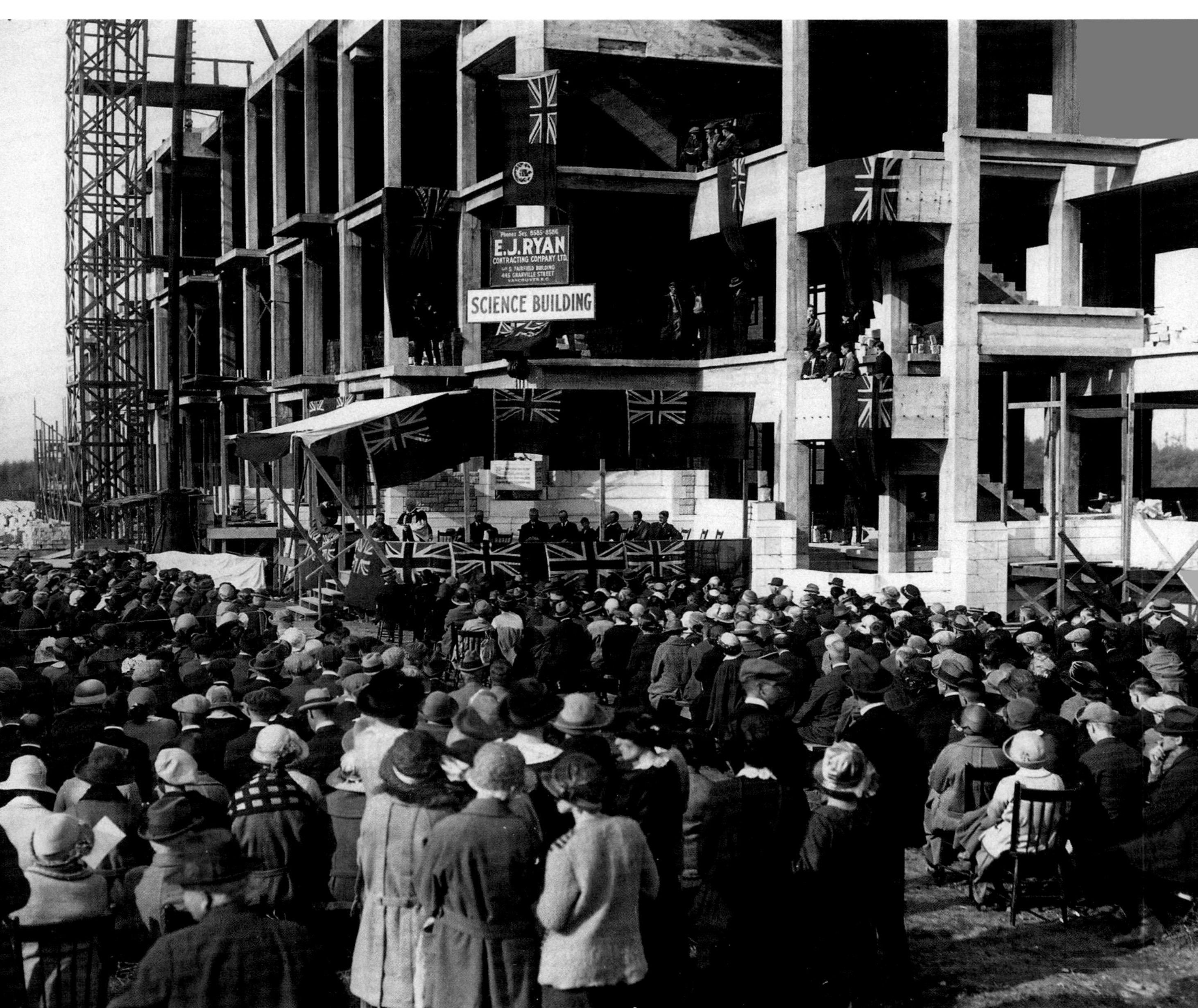

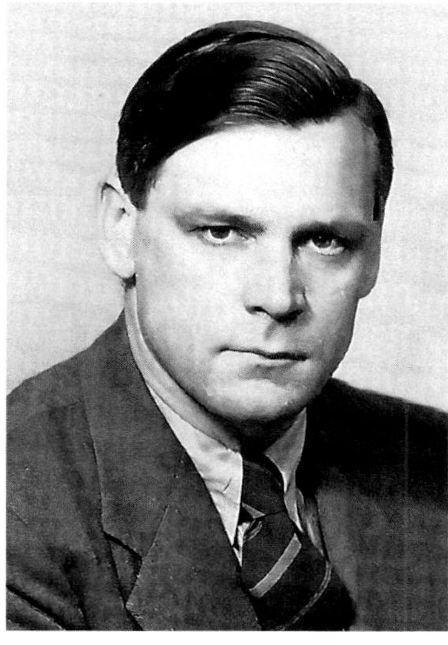

government, UBC could do nothing to address the entreaties of students and their families. It would not be until the return of veterans from World War II that definitive action would be taken.

The Arrival of Claude Dolman

When Claude E. Dolman arrived in Vancouver in September 1935 to take up his new roles as Director of the Provincial Laboratories and Head of the Department of Bacteriology and Preventive Medicine at UBC, he discovered a university in chaos–its budget slashed from $600,000 to $200,000 by the provincial government; its long-serving President Klinck (1919-44) lacking the confidence of his faculty members; and its infrastructure almost non-existent. He also observed that medical services in Vancouver and British Columbia were still in a relatively primitive state having developed in fits and starts.

A bright young microbiologist, Dolman had been an assistant in Alexander Fleming's laboratory at St. Mary's Hospital Medical School, London, when the discovery of penicillin was made. His success at St. Mary's prompted him to apply for an opportunity in Canada as a research assistant at Connaught Laboratories with John G. FitzGerald, who was also Dean of Medicine at the University of Toronto. Dolman immigrated to Canada in 1932 and by the next summer had established a reputation sufficient to be invited to Vancouver to give a series of lectures. The following year, when he was offered the provincial and UBC positions, he eagerly took them up.

A tenacious, uncompromising perfectionist, Dolman did not generally endear himself to his colleagues. However, working with a sympathetic Dr. George M. Weir, Minister of Education and Provincial Secretary, he was able to acquire sufficient funding for construction of the Institute for Preventive Medicine on the UBC campus. Using this as a nidus, he began to draft plans for the initial years of a new medical school, an initiative that would lead him to become a central player in the controversial beginnings of UBC's Faculty of Medicine.

Sowing the Seeds of the Town versus Gown Conflict

In 1943, Dolman forwarded Weir, who was now acting director of training for the Department of Veterans Affairs in Ottawa, the "Memorandum on the Establishment of an Institute of Preventive Medicine and a Faculty of Medicine at the University of British Columbia," which would ultimately spark conflict with clinical physicians in town. He suggested a budget of $2 million for a student enrollment of forty,

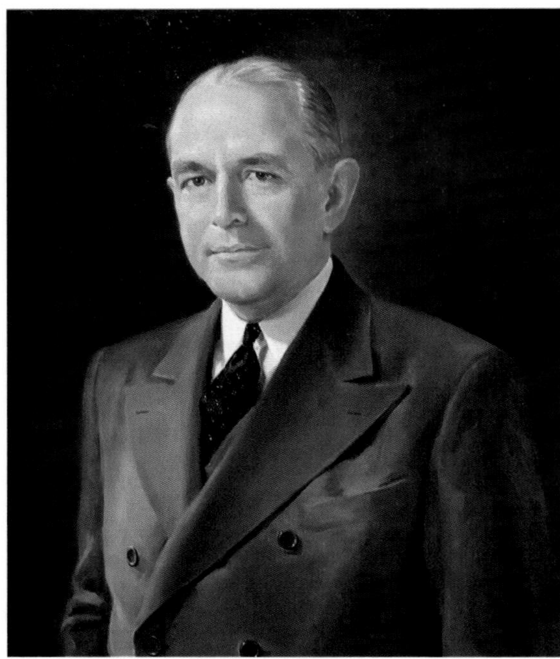

George F. "Fritz" Strong, internist, President of Vancouver Medical Association (1929–30), President of BCMA (1935–36).

with an annual operating grant of $150,000. These projections assumed that students would use the clinical facilities of Vancouver General Hospital and the UBC Institute and other campus buildings for their basic science studies.

Meanwhile, the British Columbia Medical Association (BCMA) reflected the views of the "downtown doctors" who recognized the need to establish a medical school in the province, while fearing that the development of a hospital on the UBC campus would be detrimental to current practitioners by bringing in competitors for the local physicians. They enlarged and reactivated their Committee on Medical Education, intending to promote the creation of a medical school and to exert local professional influence on its development. Dolman was asked to represent the Vancouver Medical Association on this committee, which was chaired by the city police surgeon, K.D. Panton. Using Dolman's "Memorandum" as its foundation, the committee produced a brief that was sent to UBC President Klinck in January of 1944, with a copy to the minister of education. Dean J.N. Finlayson of the Faculty of Applied Science was soon appointed chair of a UBC committee to begin planning for a medical school, and at Dolman's urging, a joint UBC-BCMA committee was formed. Two subcommittees were then established, with Dolman as chair of one that was to detail the exact costs of facilities and operations and George Frederick "Fritz" Strong as chair of the other, which was to serve as a citizens committee, ensuring appropriate community input. Strong had graduated from the University of Minnesota, interned at VGH, and then practiced internal medicine and cardiology in Vancouver. A formidable figure, he would eventually become president of the Royal College of Physicians and Surgeons of Canada. He was the driving force behind the Western Society for Rehabilitation, and the GF Strong Rehabilitation Centre in Vancouver (opened 1949) was named after him.

Dolman's unwavering commitment to his principles, particularly the importance of high academic standards, contrasted strikingly with Strong's more pragmatic approaches and his desire to maintain the solid power base he and his clinical colleagues had established in the local medical community. With his sense of the importance of local influence, the forceful Strong gathered around him colleagues with compatible viewpoints. Dolman and Strong were both passionate advocates for a BC medical school, and although they shared many

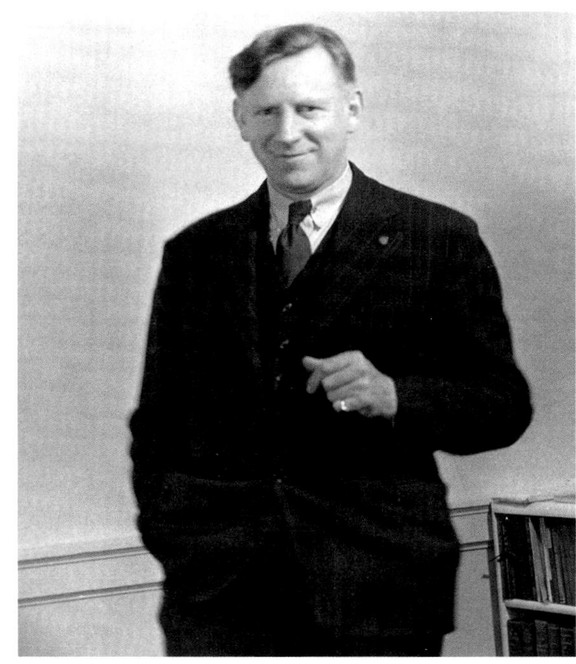

Norman A.M. "Larry" MacKenzie, authority on international law, third President of UBC (1944–62).

philosophical viewpoints and their relationship was initially cordial, their forceful personalities led to repeated clashes and public conflict. The BCMA group leaned toward Strong's views and heartily endorsed a model based on acquiring clinical skills in the community. They saw the role of the dean as part-time in nature, to be filled by a senior clinician in practice. Dolman's view, hardening over time, would have had medical students learning strictly at a university-controlled hospital and a medical school established only when this approach could be assured. The seed of the town versus gown conflict had been planted.

The Idealist versus the Pragmatist

Claude Dolman's strong views would also cause him to clash with another pragmatist, Norman "Larry" MacKenzie, UBC's third president. When MacKenzie arrived on campus in 1944, he identified two major challenges ahead: 1) increasing enrollment to accommodate the large number of returning veterans, and 2) establishing a Faculty of Medicine. Although MacKenzie had initially studied medicine, his passion was law. He used all of this knowledge in taking on the running of the young university. He held lofty goals for UBC, and during his eighteen years as president, he oversaw the addition of numerous faculties and schools to meet the needs of the province. Although an accomplished academic, he was a man of great common sense and would compromise his principles in order to achieve consensus. MacKenzie was flexible, conciliatory, and gifted in the art of friendship. This provided a sharp contrast with Claude Dolman. While Dolman insisted obstinately on holding out for "the best," MacKenzie demanded only "the possible," as long as it was practicable and acceptable to the majority of those involved.

The joint UBC-BCMA committee gathered data from the deans of five Canadian medical schools. Their report was delivered to the office of the premier in September 1944, making the following recommendations for the proposed UBC Faculty of Medicine:

- That preclinical studies be pursued at the university with the clinical years downtown.
- That two buildings would be needed on the campus (the Institute for Preventive Medicine and a Medical Science Building, plus a smaller building to house laboratory animals), as well as a third clinical building to be located adjacent to the

Vancouver General Hospital (to house Departments of Pathology and Pathological Chemistry plus lecture theatres, library, and clinical offices).

- That the proposed budget be $1.5 million for buildings with an annual operating budget of $200,000.

The committee was convinced that all preclinical activities and the headquarters of the medical school should be on the campus, allowing strong linkages with other academic elements of the university functionally, administratively, and geographically. At this point in the planning, a new hospital on campus was not regarded as essential to the establishment of the school; instead it was felt that clinical facilities could be housed at the VGH site. It was also agreed that UBC's Board of Governors would hold the power of appointment to the Faculty and that the dean would (through the Senate) control all matters related to curriculum, academic discipline, and requirements for graduation of the medical students.

By this time, it was expected that the economic environment in BC might improve. After further refinements of their cost estimates, Dolman and a small group of others met with Premier John Hart, Liberal leader of the Liberal-Conservative coalition government, in January 1945. Subsequently, in the Speech from the Throne, a government proposal for $5 million for new buildings on campus was tabled. However, Dolman saw these funds as targeted only for his institute and the Provincial Laboratories. He was dismayed to learn that this amount was to be distributed broadly for the wider university and that G. Amyot, the provincial health officer, favoured a downtown location for the laboratories. Dolman's unwavering conviction as an immunologist was that prevention was fundamental to health policy and education; he believed the new institute on campus should be the cornerstone of a modern progressive medical school.

Gravely concerned about the well-being of large numbers of returning veterans, President MacKenzie led UBC in the bold gesture of accepting into its ranks any qualified veteran who wished a university education. There was also ongoing pressure to establish the medical school without further delay. The UBC Pre-Medical Undergraduate Society, many of whom were World War II veterans, in conjunction with the University Branch of the Canadian Legion, prepared a brief for the provincial government, advocating the establishment of a medical school at UBC by autumn 1946. It included a letter from K.D. Panton, stating that the Committee on Medical Education of the BC Medical Association "strongly endorses their plans." The brief summarized the case for establishing a medical school, outlined the building and operating budget requirements, and summarized the progress to date. The motif of the Pre-Medical Nursing Ball held at Brock Hall in November 1945 was "Faculty of Medicine in 1946." Soon thereafter, MacKenzie asked Dolman, "What could you do with sixty thousand dollars?" Wishing to allow "some sort of start to be made," he requested that Dolman outline a first-year course in medicine, thereby allowing the inclusion of a $60,000 amount in the UBC estimates for the following academic year (1946-47). Although opposed to a premature launch of the medical school, Dolman reluctantly provided recommendations for faculty members and curricula for the basic sciences.

Duelling Visions

The desirability of a survey of representative North American medical schools to ascertain the features of a good school had been extensively discussed since late 1944, and eventually MacKenzie and the UBC Board of Governors asked Dolman to conduct the survey. In 1946, Dolman travelled to twenty-two American and eleven Canadian medical schools, interviewing 272 deans, professors, and presidents. Despite a brutal schedule, he kept up a running correspondence with President MacKenzie to keep him apprised of his findings. During his travels, he received word that the BC legislature had passed the $60,000 request from UBC for a first-year medical course to begin in autumn 1946, but he continued to advocate for a delay.

Dolman's "Report on a Survey of Medical Education," delivered to the president and Board of Governors on May 3, 1946, was to become a model of exhaustive and well-documented research in the area of medical school planning. It consisted of forty-five typed pages of detailed data on the schools he had visited and the viewpoints of the academic and administrative leaders he had interviewed. Requests for the report later came from all over the world, so that the first printing of two thousand copies was depleted and a second printing had to be made in February 1947.

His vision for a medical school and clinical training facilities on the UBC campus had crystallized, and his conclusions were emphatic and resolute. Among his ten prerequisites for a first-class medical school at UBC were the following:

- "That quite apart from such teaching affiliations with local hospitals as may be feasible on terms satisfactory to the University, there should be a University Hospital staffed entirely by the Faculty of Medicine," and
- "That the whole school be located on the campus as the only satisfactory means of securing the desired physical contiguity and spiritual affinity between the medical science and clinical departments within the Faculty of Medicine and other Faculties at the University."

His cost estimate for this campus hospital was $3.5 million. He declared that the Faculty must have complete control over a minimum of six hundred hospital beds, and he bluntly dismissed

Please Return to: With compliments & kind regards

Wm C Gibson Claude Dolman.

1690 Wesbrook Crescent.
Vancouver, B.C.

REPORT

ON A SURVEY OF

MEDICAL EDUCATION

IN CANADA AND THE UNITED STATES

C. E. DOLMAN

M.R.C.S. (Eng.), L.R.C.P.; M.B., B.S.;
M.R.C.P.; D.P.H.; Ph.D. (Lond.); F.A.P.H.A.

Professor and Head of the Department of Bacteriology and Preventive Medicine;
Professor and Head of the Department of Nursing and Health;
Director, Division of Laboratories, Provincial Board of Health;
and
Research Member, Connaught Medical Research Laboratories, University of Toronto

1946

FACING Front cover of Dolman's report to the UBC President and Board of Governors, 1946. Dolman's signature is seen in the upper right corner.

offering faculty appointments to any disgruntled "middle-aged failures or mediocrities," "exiles or transients of all ages." The clinical staff had to be full-time, that is, have no private patients compensating them directly for their medical care. His report was received warmly by the UBC board and some of the BCMA leaders.

Knowing that Dolman's intransigence and single-mindedness had begun to exasperate those who just wanted to get on with starting the medical school, Strong was concerned that Dolman's UBC survey report could be biased and therefore determined to conduct his own survey on behalf of the BCMA. Strong visited a few of the same schools of medicine as Dolman, in addition to several others, and interviewed a much smaller number of academics and administrators. Strong's report was considerably shorter, less scholarly, and more pragmatic than Dolman's. Although it stressed the need for a high-quality medical school, it concluded that the major costs of building and maintaining a new facility on the campus away from the already available facilities pointed to the need for further study. Its conclusions were in many respects similar to Dolman's, but the body of the report contained a number of statements with which Dolman strongly disagreed, namely that it was not only impossible but undesirable to establish "another Johns Hopkins," that a university hospital could only be attained at tremendous cost, and that the heads of major clinical departments need not be full-time members of the departments. It opposed the idea of a "split" school and presented points in favour of locating the entire school near one of the community hospitals. The location of the teaching hospital was the major issue. With forceful and divergent views documented, a decision was made to seek external consultants. As expected, the choice of consultants was disputed, but there was eventual agreement between the BCMA and UBC upon eight leaders in medical education to review the reports and to provide advice.

Panton sent a letter to President MacKenzie claiming a general failure of UBC to consult with the BCMA education committee and in particular regarding the appointment of Dolman to conduct the survey. The president replied, generally refuting Panton's claims and concluding by saying, "if a Medical School does become an integral part of the University of British Columbia, all of the final decisions that are made in connection with it will have to be made by the Senate and Board of Governors of the University of British Columbia and by no one else." No longer confident in Panton's leadership of the committee, Dolman resigned.

The external consultants were unable to come to Vancouver as a group. One group came down clearly in favour of Dolman's recommendations. Another group advocated a point of view more favourable to the Strong camp in that it did not regard the campus location of the proposed teaching hospital as essential, but it did oppose an adapted VGH as the venue. All of the visiting experts had met with the Senate-Faculty committee, chaired by Dean Finlayson. It was agreed to form yet another subcommittee to draw up a short report to present to the Senate. Even though the visiting experts had not considered a campus location essential for the school, the December 1946 "Report to the Senate-Faculty Committee on Faculty of Medicine" came to the following four conclusions:

1. A University hospital is an essential part of a modern medical school. No existing hospital in Vancouver could be satisfactorily adapted to function as a University hospital.
2. In view of the importance of the integration of the so-called preclinical and clinical parts of the curriculum, all departments of the Faculty of Medicine should be housed in proximity.
3. There should be a nucleus of full-time appointees in each of the major clinical departments.
4. A good medical school is costly, but to create a Faculty of Medicine of less than excellence would be an unjustifiable expense.

The report went on to outline the objectives of a modern medical school and to revise the capital cost estimate of a university-based school to $6 million with an annual operating budget of $400,000. To Dolman's disappointment, the Senate agreed only to receive the report. It was now time for the university to approach and seek a choice by the government between the options of proceeding with the medical faculty at the university, including a new hospital of five hundred beds and a permanent subsidy of $400,000 a year, or postponing action. This latter choice would have denied the opportunity for BC students to take up medicine as a career, as there were few openings for them in already overcrowded schools throughout Canada and the US.

The Death of Dolman's Dream

In mid-January 1947, President MacKenzie went with Chancellor Eric Hamber to visit Premier Hart and Minister Weir. Two days later, he told Dolman that although they had made no formal request, they had learned that the provincial government did not favour building a campus hospital, wanting to avoid the heavy financial burden of constructing and operating such a facility. UBC's location at the far end of the Point Grey peninsula, no doubt favouring academic contemplation, was not a practical site for a major hospital. It is likely that the dissension and discord within the academic and clinical medical communities provided a cash-strapped government with additional valid rationalization for denying the approval of a campus-based hospital.

The outcome of this meeting was a bitter disappointment to Dolman who felt that MacKenzie had essentially abandoned his advice, leaving the decisions to the local doctors. Dolman had little

It was now time for the university to approach and seek a choice by the government between the options of proceeding with the medical faculty at the university or postponing action.

insight into MacKenzie's challenges from trying to balance the pressing needs of eleven other faculties. Fritz Strong asked, "Is the university going into the hospital business?" Many local physicians felt that VGH would always be the "mother house" of medicine in the province, with or without an associated medical school.

Shortly thereafter, Panton resigned as chairman of the BCMA's Committee on Medical Education when members of the committee would not endorse a letter he had written to Premier Hart, urging establishment of a medical school as soon as possible and claiming the province could not afford the luxury of a medical school on the campus. Panton's resignation and his subsequent letter to the premier and the *Vancouver News-Herald* started another heated debate in the press with comments from various parties, including the pre-med students, the VGH clinicians, the politicians in Victoria, and the press in Vancouver. Panton accused the government of "effacement and deference to university plans." Dolman retorted, "Admittedly, perfectionism is scorned as outmoded by the cruder forms of contemporary realism. But in this vital question of a medical school, surely it is not too much to hope that we might have the sagacity to follow the best advice obtainable, whose gist was that the more idealistic plan would prove the more fruitful, and that true realism lay in a far-sighted vision rather than in opportunism and improvisation."

On February 17, 1947, a significant reference was incorporated in Premier Hart's policy speech to the provincial legislature. This included a grant of $1.5 million for capital expenditure on buildings and $100,000 for operating costs of a medical faculty. It was suggested that the Normal School facilities beside the VGH where teachers were being trained could be an adequate site for the medical school. After all of the planning and dialogue, this appeared to be a retrenchment of the government's position, leaving the university to decide on next steps.

The W.K. Kellogg Foundation had recommended an optimal size of 450 to 700 beds for a teaching hospital, whereas the other consultants had recommended a large increase in beds and expansion in keeping with the profile of a major teaching hospital. Strong's vision was to have VGH become one of the largest hospitals in the country. MacKenzie arranged a meeting of the full Board of Governors of UBC and the Board of Directors of the VGH to consider the feasibility of starting a medical school in cooperation with VGH, planning to keep as much of the school as possible on the campus.

Against a background of increasing criticism from the press and others, the legislature unanimously voted on March 26, 1947, for immediate organization of a Faculty of Medicine. The Senate of UBC, however, had again determined to refer the matter back to a subcommittee. The UBC board met on March 31 and resolved unanimously "that it will

Hon. John Hart, Liberal, Premier of BC (1941–47).

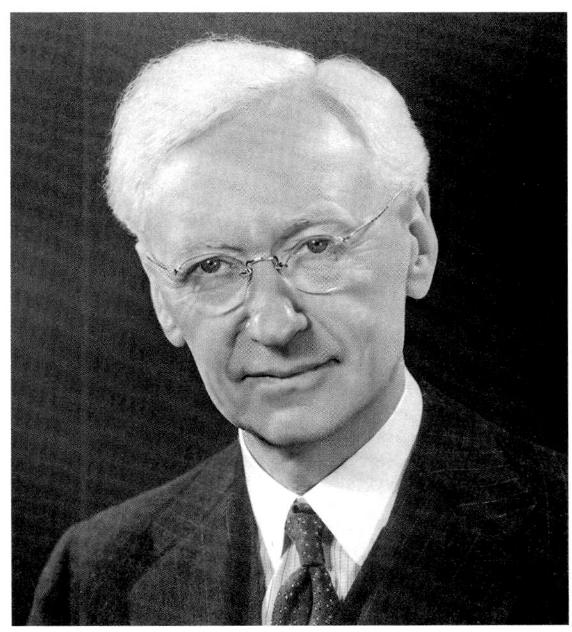

be impossible to give the first year of the medical course in 1947," stating that its establishment could only be done on the following conditions:

1. That it shall be a medical faculty of high standing.
2. That sufficient money shall be guaranteed to ensure that, if the faculty is started, the students who register in it can finish the clinical as well as the preclinical years.
3. That a minimum of four hundred teaching beds must be available at the end of the second year of this course for the students entering the clinical work.

This relatively modest stance constituted the final negotiating position for the UBC Board of Governors and President MacKenzie.

In November 1947, Dean of Law George Curtis put forward to the Senate a resolution that passed unanimously. It endorsed the development of the Faculty of Medicine, and at last, in April 1948, the government announced that the FoM would be established by the fall of 1949. Shortly afterwards, the government declared that it would improve the ward facilities of the VGH, establishing a seven-hundred-bed acute care unit and thereby freeing up four hundred beds, which would be available for teaching purposes. The Faculty of Medicine was established in 1949 and under the leadership of a new dean, Myron Weaver, sixty students were admitted to the first year of the UBC medical school in the fall of 1950.

After decades of discussion and debate, the vision of excellence promulgated by Dolman was superseded by the pragmatic and feasible plan of President MacKenzie and the doctors at VGH. Although Dolman withdrew from the Faculty of Medicine and refused repeated requests to bring the Department of Bacteriology into the Faculty, he continued as a professor of bacteriology at UBC and a member of the Royal Society of Canada until his death in 1994. Claude Dolman married Clarisse Leonore Aszkanazy (UBC '43, Bacteriology) in 1955. Clarisse received her MD at the University of Toronto ('47) and eventually returned to Vancouver, becoming the first qualified neuropathologist at VGH. Affectionately known as "Lore," she and Claude had three children, each of whom received an MD degree from UBC and practice in Vancouver: John ('80, anesthesiologist), Peter ('84, ophthalmologist), and Jennifer ('84, family physician and pastoral care provider).

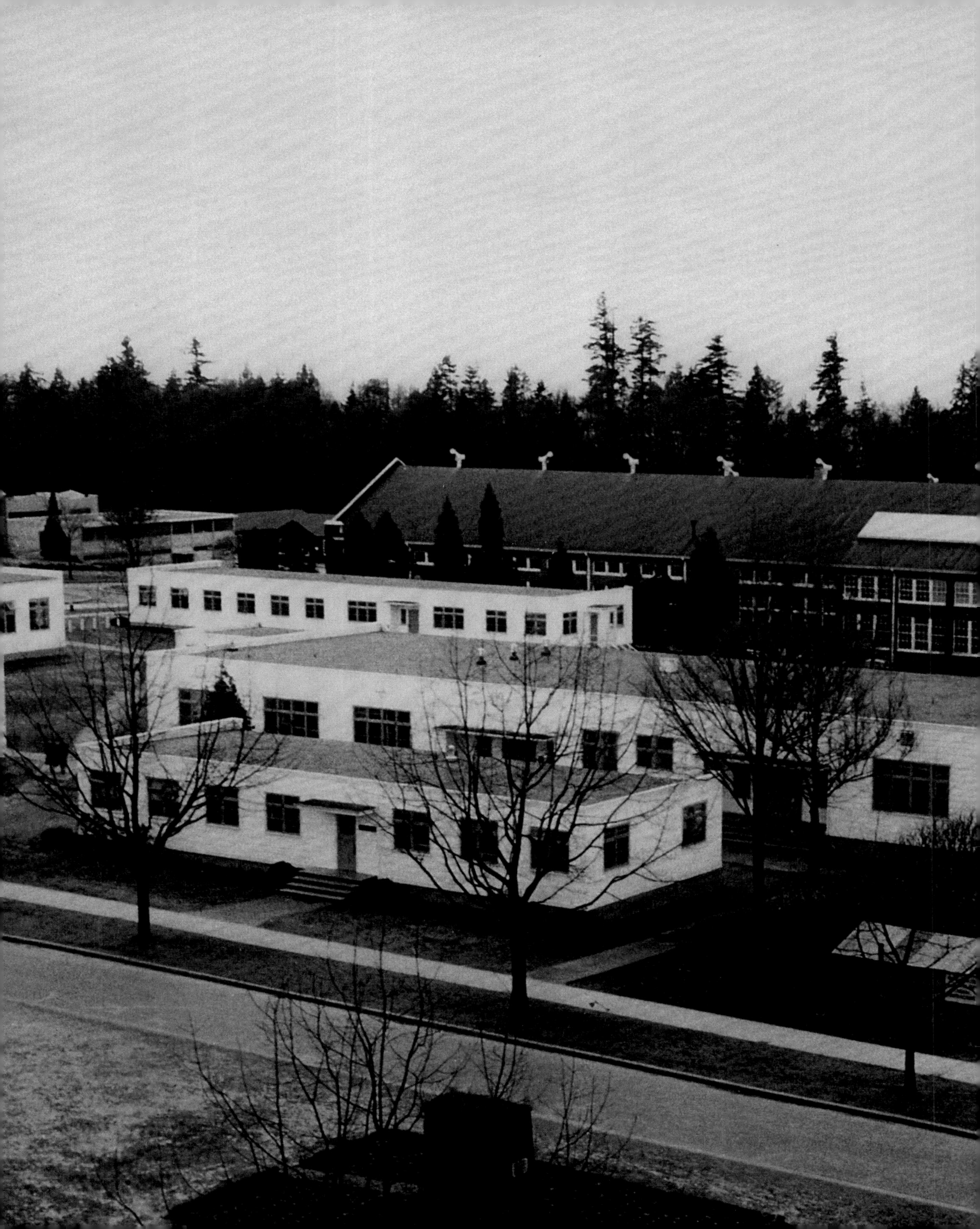

2

The Fledgling School

1950–56

FACING Original quadrangle of Faculty of Medicine with temporary buildings on the UBC Main Mall opposite the Great Trek Cairn, Agriculture Barn immediately behind, c. 1950.

FACING Myron M. Weaver, internist, inaugural Dean of Medicine (1949–55).

During the Faculty of Medicine's first decade, neither the economy nor public opinion provided much support. This impecunious start was to become a longstanding legacy of the medical school.

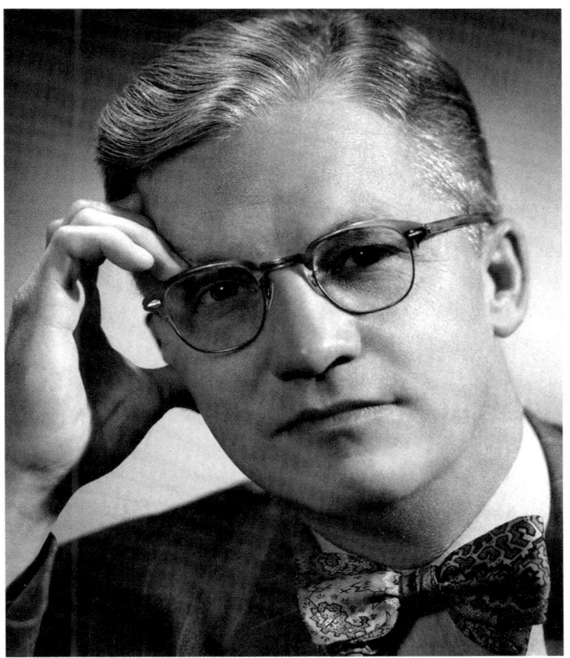

LIKE THE ESTABLISHMENT of the Faculty itself, the matter of who would be the founding dean sparked fierce debate. In August 1948, President MacKenzie suggested that a basic scientist would be better able to know the students, a view perhaps to be expected from a traditional university academic. Some UBC leaders believed that a clinician would be too expensive. Most understood that the dean would have to be acceptable to the medical profession and the British Columbia Medical Association.

In surveying outstanding schools in the United States, Fritz Strong and Claude Dolman had both met Myron M. Weaver, who had received his MS, PhD, and MD degrees at the University of Chicago. By 1944, he was an assistant dean of the University of Minnesota Medical School, the president of which was a good friend of President MacKenzie. In addition to his laboratory background, Weaver had considerable clinical experience as a physician with interests in diabetes and nutrition, as well as a non-clinical specialty in medical economics. Ultimately, he appeared to have the requisite characteristics and was appointed as the Dean of Medicine at University of British Columbia as of July 1, 1949. He and his wife moved into a duplex on Fourth Avenue near the university. He was an affable, pleasant person, skilled at persuading people to work together and exuding a spirit of dedication and commitment. His personable nature endeared him to those with whom he worked, and the adverse conditions which prevailed at UBC were to some extent mitigated by the hospitable and personal welcome he extended to his new recruits.

When Weaver first arrived, the formidable Gordon Shrum, head of physics, provided him with inauspicious quarters in a narrow corridor in the physics building for a year while accommodations were being prepared for the Faculty. Along with his secretary, Marguerite Service, Weaver worked at an unrelenting pace, including during evenings and weekends, to organize the Faculty in time for the arrival of its first students in the fall of 1950. During the Faculty of Medicine's first decade, neither the economy nor public opinion provided much support. Meagre funding was available to UBC overall, and hiring outstanding faculty members was a continuous struggle. This impecunious start, with funding barely sufficient for buildings and desks, was to become a long-standing legacy of the medical school.

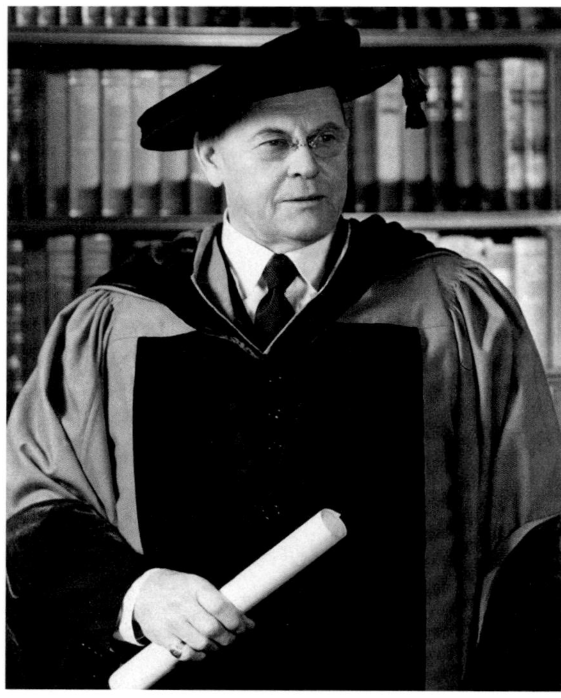

Hon. Eric W. Hamber, banker, businessman, Lieutenant Governor of BC (1936–41), Chancellor of UBC (1944–51).

Originally the Faculty of Medicine budget was separate from the remainder of the university budget to avoid the implication that medicine was taking money away from other areas. The academic community in general recognized that the new faculty was an important part of the university, and with few exceptions it was tolerated and welcomed. On the other hand, the Ministry of Health had no understanding of the educational mission of the Faculty of Medicine, and the Ministry of Education saw no reason why they should fund what they saw as hospital work. The failure to resolve this lack of agreement as to funding responsibilities would have significant implications for the Faculty in the years ahead.

Weaver's Appointments

Weaver saw the appointment of a nucleus of good faculty as a priority. In describing his ideal faculty members, he was quoted as saying, "They stimulate the imaginations, and stir the ambitions of their students, and an esprit de corps results which is the mark of a really first-class medical school."

Although there had been considerable friction among members of the academic and medical communities, once the Faculty of Medicine was established, faculty members were treated with cordiality and generosity by members of both communities. Chancellor Eric Hamber and his wife took an especially active role in the recruitment of new faculty, asking the mostly young candidates for academic positions to give a small speech in front of various committees and then informally interviewing them at dinners and cocktail parties. Early faculty spoke with appreciation of the fine parties hosted by prominent Vancouverites, with the Hambers frequently playing a leading role.

Academic and Clinical Faculty

From the beginning and continuing to the present, faculty members were either in full-time employment with UBC (mostly scientists and a few physicians, collectively referred to as "academic faculty") or were practicing physicians teaching for modest or no stipends (referred to as "clinical faculty"). An *academic faculty member* receives at least a portion of their salary through UBC and has a high level of accountability to their UBC department head. If the member is a non-clinician, their income is likely to flow almost entirely through UBC's financial system, although the funds may originate from either UBC's annual BC government grant or from a variety of other sources. If the member is a clinician (most of whom are physicians), a portion of their income flows through UBC under arrangements analogous to those for a non-clinician. However, a major difference is that academic faculty members who are clinicians are likely to be providing patient care and receiving income from the provincial health care budget (via direct billings to the Medical Services Plan [MSP] or clinical care stipends) which may constitute the majority of their total income.

A *clinical faculty member* (most of whom are health professionals–mainly MDs–but some of whom are non-clinicians and classified as clinical faculty in reference only to their accountability and financial arrangements vis-à-vis UBC) receives their income from some source external to UBC and has only limited accountability to their UBC department head. A clinical faculty member who is a clinician is primarily engaged in patient care and derives their income from MSP billings or clinical care stipends. Clinical faculty members far outnumber academic faculty members and are vital to the teaching missions of the FoM, and yet in earlier years they received little or no financial compensation or recognition for teaching. Modest financial compensation for teaching and administrative roles became more common during the 1990s, but most such duties remained largely uncompensated.

The development of the Faculty initially focused on the core basic science departments–anatomy, physiology, biochemistry, and pharmacology–and that of pathology. The first four clinical departments in the 1950s were those of medicine, surgery, obstetrics and gynecology, and the developing area of pediatrics. Psychiatry started as a division within medicine, eventually becoming an independent department in 1953, a course followed by several disciplines. Other clinical departments, largely centred at Vancouver General Hospital, were added over the next several years.

The new department heads were, generally speaking, the youngest of any medical school in Canada, with an average age of about thirty-five. They were all recruited from other universities in Canada and the US, with the exceptions of the Departments of Obstetrics/Gynecology and Psychiatry, for which a senior local clinician was appointed. A new and innovative approach to studies resulted because no one was concerned about tradition. A common observation of all the early faculty recruits was the sense of excitement and esprit de corps they encountered. This leadership group generally believed that a united school on the UBC campus had been agreed upon during negotiations over the founding of the medical school and that funds would be forthcoming to build a university hospital on campus. This dream was not to be realized until 1980, and then only in a limited fashion.

FACING Husband and wife team Sydney Friedman, inaugural Head of Department of Anatomy (1950–81), and Constance Friedman.

The Basic Science Departments

The department heads that Weaver recruited for the basic sciences made key hires and introduced numerous innovations to bridge the gap with clinicians and engage first year students. However, it was clear that not all the faculty shared the same vision. Although relationships with clinicians at VGH were cordial and socially smooth in the early days of the school, Sydney Friedman, the first head of the Department of Anatomy, observed that academics were not close with clinicians, as they lived in separate worlds. He felt that the clinicians did not have much interest in the basic medical sciences, and the academics on the campus found few reasons to make the trip to the hospital, feeling, if not exactly unwelcome, at least unrecognized. Even parking, which was at a premium, made movement between sites awkward.

The Department of Anatomy

Friedman's appointment as head of the Department of Anatomy would have a lasting impact on the new school. Friedman had received his MD and his PhD at McGill. In 1950, he was eager to move on to a greater challenge but wanted particularly to stay in Canada. He originally chose an academic appointment over clinical practice to focus on his research on hypertension. His wife, Constance, who had a PhD in anatomy, had worked with him at McGill. She was hired by UBC on a yearly contract as a research associate professor, helping to circumvent the strict nepotism rule, which forbade the hiring of faculty relatives. Under their guidance, the Department of Anatomy eventually became one of the outstanding centres of its kind in North America and spawned a series of leaders both within the Faculty and beyond.

Funding for the anatomy department was never a problem; Friedman was able to offer salaries to his faculty members that were competitive with those offered in the United States. A strong emphasis on research was a feature of the department. From Hans Selye's lab at the University of Montreal, Friedman recruited Associate Professor Paris Constantinides, who would become an acclaimed researcher in cardiovascular disease. He also developed his own medical scientists, identifying promising students from the UBC medical school and training them in the hopes that they would pursue academic careers. With the help of the Simmons & McBride funeral home, Friedman established a fund which brought in such eminent speakers as the distinguished Selye from Montreal. Having prestigious guest speakers was important for the credibility of the young school, both internally and externally.

Attempting to mitigate the clinical-basic science split, Friedman started off by attending VGH grand rounds, believing that this would give the clinicians

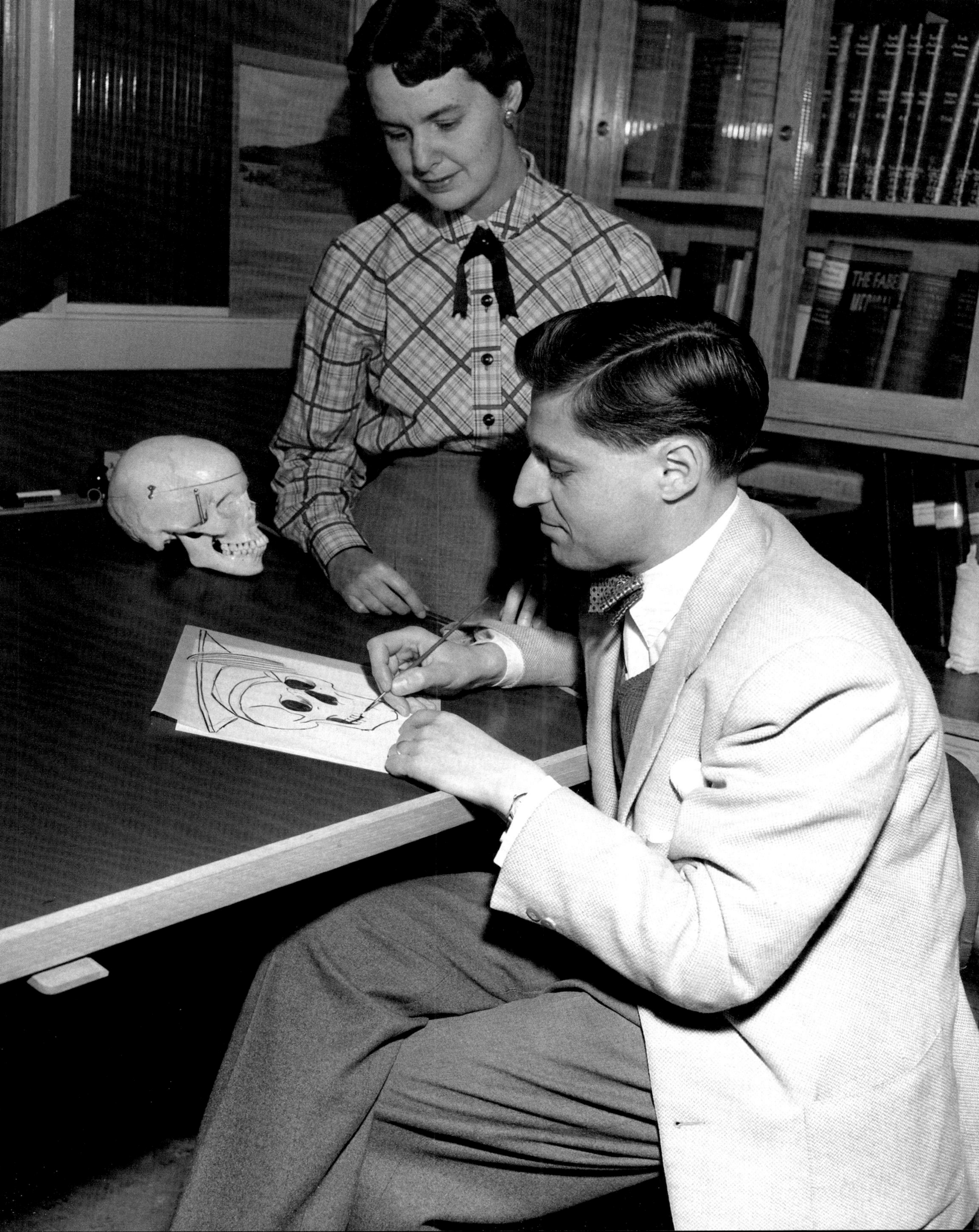

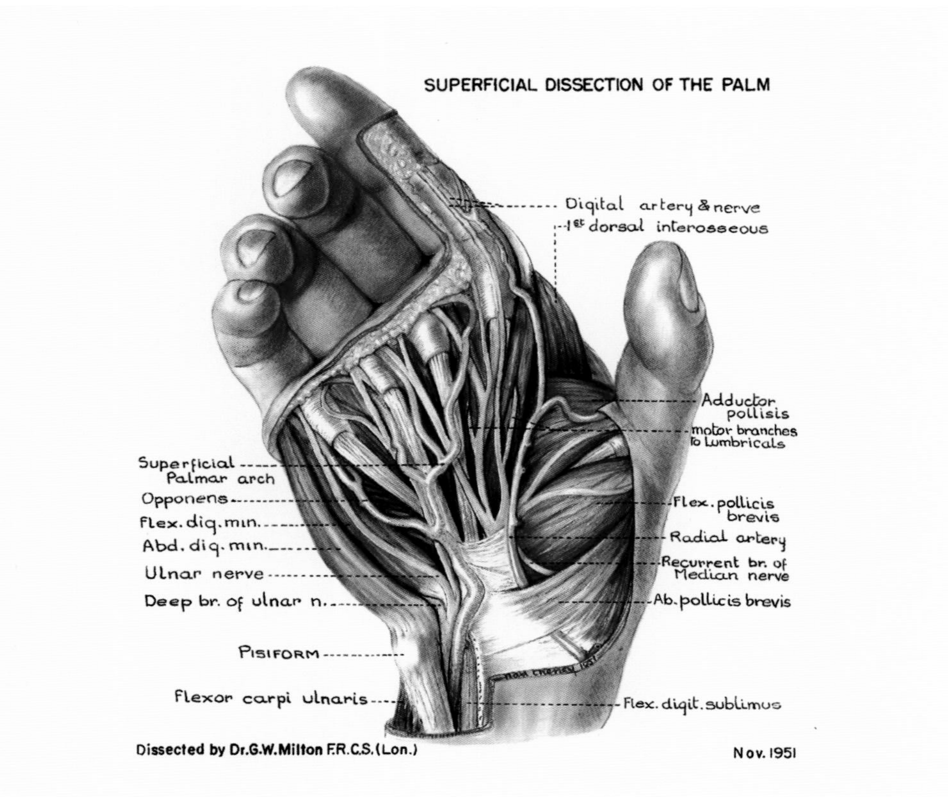

the sense that the basic scientists were interested in what their clinical colleagues were doing. He then started a course in anatomy for surgical trainees. However, he felt that the UBC faculty and the clinicians at VGH did not share a vision for medical education and academic medicine. He still thought that, ideally, delaying the start of the medical school until there was a commitment from the government to fund construction on campus would have been preferable. Also, he felt that Dean Weaver and President MacKenzie were not strident enough in their support of the school on the UBC campus.

The teaching of anatomy at UBC introduced some innovations, relating the course to clinically relevant aspects and integrating histology, gross anatomy, radiology, and neuroanatomy. It was among the first programs in North America to incorporate the use of television for gross anatomy, even as the dissecting rooms continued to be housed in antiquated huts. The immediacy of the display allowed the students to ask questions and hear the response as everyone witnessed common images.

Anatomical illustration was a highlight of any course offered by Friedman. He felt that anatomy was above all a visual science, not abstract or theoretical. He wanted his students to achieve a three-dimensional sense of what they were viewing. His two-handed blackboard drawings became legendary. Students would look forward with anticipation to his fabled session in which, as he spoke, he would pick up a piece of chalk in each hand and, using them simultaneously, proceed with rare and awe-inspiring skill to delineate the symmetry of the human body and its internal features.

D. Harold Copp, inaugural Head of Department of Physiology (1950–80).

FACING Anatomical drawing by Nan Cheney, 1951, Nan Cheney Anatomical Illustrations.

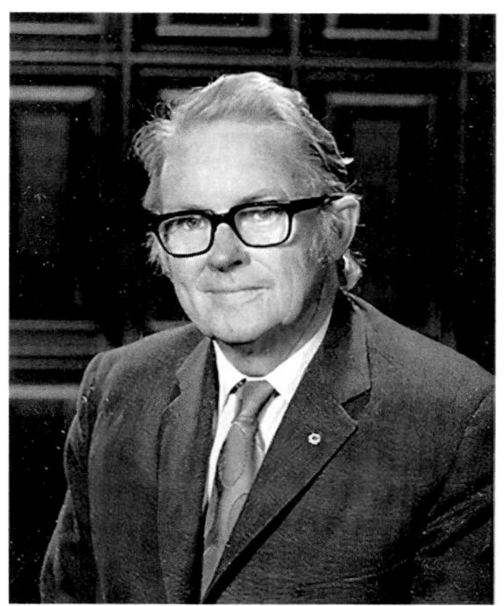

Soon after his arrival at UBC, Friedman was introduced to medical artist Nan Cheney, who came to have a significant influence on his career. She had moved with her radiologist husband from Montreal to Vancouver. Her works eventually illuminated a number of popular anatomical and clinical texts and, to the present day, many of her illustrations hang in the lobby of the Life Sciences Centre on the UBC campus.

The Department of Physiology

For the Department of Physiology, Weaver recruited Douglas Harold Copp, who, like Friedman, was eager to live in Vancouver and to participate in the development of a new medical school. Copp had obtained his medical degree at the University of Toronto. With the outbreak of war in 1939, he went to the University of California, where he worked on radioactive isotopes and received a PhD in biochemistry. In connection with the top-secret Manhattan Project to develop the atomic bomb, he was given the responsibility of studying particularly plutonium and strontium-90 and the effects of radiation on human bone marrow. This work stimulated his interest in bone and in calcium metabolism. Following the war, he returned to teach at Berkeley. A manifestation of the prevailing McCarthyism in America was a demand that he sign a loyalty oath. He found this offensive to his Canadian academic sensibilities, and he resigned from his position and called Weaver to accept a position at UBC.

Copp's research on calcium regulation required that he develop an accurate technique for measuring blood calcium. Early in his work at UBC, he devised a titration technique, using a colorimeter, burette, pipette, plus graph paper, and "the most important thing, an eraser so you can use the same piece of graph paper over and over again." This technique eventually helped lead him to his major scientific achievement, the discovery in 1961 of calcitonin, a hormone which regulates the level of calcium in the blood. His work would eventually earn him numerous prestigious awards, including the Gairdner Award, the Flavelle Medal, and the Jacob Biely Faculty Research Prize.

The Department of Biochemistry

The founding Head of Biochemistry was Marvin Darrach, who was recruited from Merck, where he had been very involved in the research, development, and marketing of cortisone and related agents. Prior to the establishment of the Faculty of Medicine, biochemistry teaching and research had been the purview of the Faculty of Arts and Sciences.

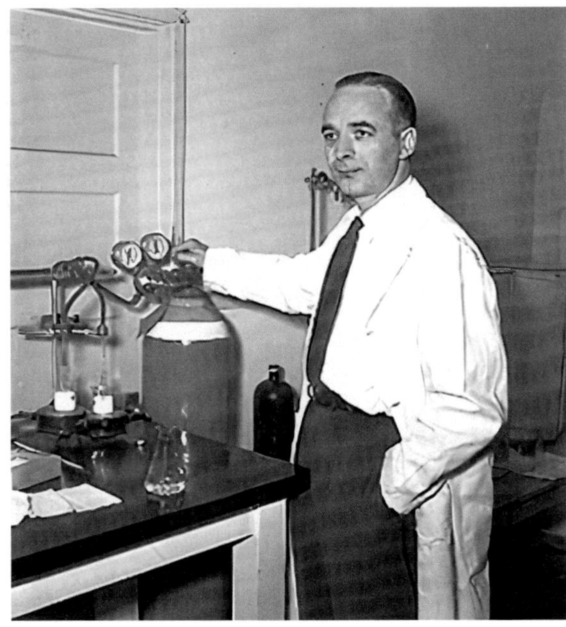

Marvin Darrach, inaugural Head of Department of Biochemistry (1950–72).

However, in 1950, the Department of Biochemistry was created as a separate department within the new Faculty of Medicine. The department was to be responsible for the teaching of biochemistry to medical students but was also assigned the much larger responsibility for the teaching of biochemistry to undergraduate students in other faculties and for a burgeoning program of graduate education in biochemistry. Nevertheless, the department's budget came entirely from the Faculty of Medicine. The department members often felt that they lost out on Faculty budget decisions because, compared to the Department of Anatomy, their teaching of medical students was relatively modest.

While he was still at the University of Minnesota, Myron Weaver had met a University of Toronto graduate, Sidney Zbarsky, who was teaching physiological chemistry in Minneapolis. In 1949, Zbarsky accepted a position to teach biochemistry in UBC's Department of Chemistry, eventually moving to the new Department of Biochemistry once the medical school was established. He always felt Darrach was lacking in imagination and failed to advance the department. He observed ruefully that Darrach "was happy to return unspent budget funds to the Faculty at year end," funds that were eagerly received by more aggressive departments such as anatomy. Despite Zbarsky's criticisms, Darrach remained as department head from 1950 to 1972.

The Department of Pharmacology

The new Head of Pharmacology, James Foulks, was recruited from New York to UBC in 1951. Arriving with his wife and baby in a new city and new country to build a department from the ground up in a new medical school, Foulks had no time to second-guess his decision. In the first year, he gave some sixty to seventy lectures, operated a laboratory twice a week with the assistance of a single teaching fellow from the Department of Anesthesiology, and gave weekly basic science refresher lectures to anesthesiology residents at the Vancouver General Hospital.

Foulks observed there was not a great deal of interest among clinical appointees at the hospitals in the activities of the basic scientists on campus, probably because of geographical separation and time constraints. Like Friedman and Dolman, Foulks envisioned UBC as having the potential to develop a large, outstanding medical school of the same rank as the best in the US. The prevailing thinking in the 1950s was that a medical school could be either a research-intensive institution or a centre of clinical excellence, but not both.

LEFT Student in William Boyd Pathology Museum, VGH.

RIGHT John William Boyd, inaugural Head of Department of Pathology (1951–54).

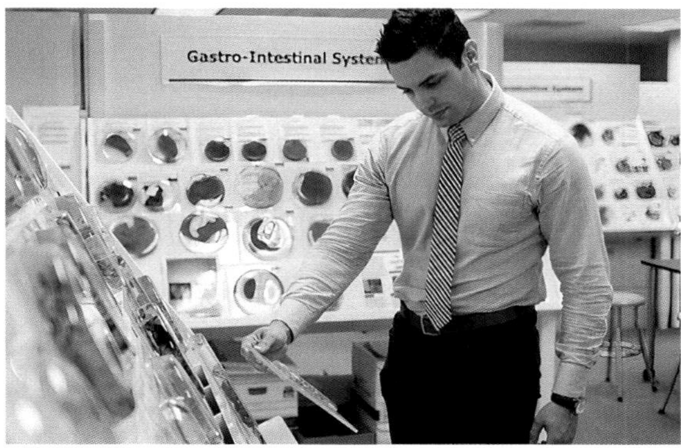

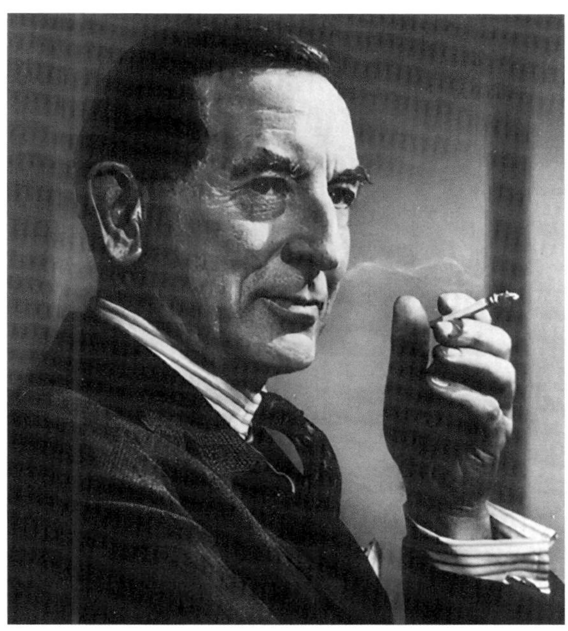

The Department of Pathology

The Head of the Department of Pathology, John William Boyd, was one of the world's leading pathologists, in demand everywhere for his impressive lectures and famous for the lucid, humorous, and effective manner in which he illuminated his subject. He was a prolific author of textbooks and was one of the few textbook writers of the time to become a millionaire from his work. After attaining prominence at the University of Manitoba, he moved to Toronto to continue his academic pursuits. During a guest lectureship at UBC, he observed, "I'd just like to come out here and live for the rest of my life." Robert "Bob" Kerr, the founding Head of the Department of Medicine, overheard him and persuaded Weaver to offer him a position as Head of Pathology. Willing to defer his retirement for several years, Boyd accepted the offer and moved to Vancouver in 1951.

Remembered as an immensely capable teacher by his students, Boyd instituted a weekly Friday afternoon tea party-cum-quiz session, where he would present slides of pathological histology and invite various attendees at the gathering to stand up in front, describe their observations, and identify the mysterious picture on display. His fellow department head, Harold "Rocke" Robertson of Surgery, recalled his hosting a cocktail party one night and announcing in the course of the evening that he was celebrating the news from his publisher that sales of his textbooks had just reached one million. The Professor William Boyd Pathology Museum is now housed in the Gordon and Leslie Diamond Health Care Centre at Vancouver General Hospital.

The Clinical Departments

Until early in the twentieth century, clinical medicine was divided into essentially the three specialties of surgery, internal medicine, and obstetrics and gynecology. Along with the newly developing field of pediatrics, these were the clinical departments in the new medical school. The principal clinical appointees at the beginning were Rocke Robertson,

A "Little Explosion"

Foulks was remembered by his students as a very talented teacher; they listened intently to his words of wisdom delivered in a strong Texan accent. One of the members of the class of 1956, Gerry Philippson recalled an occasion when Foulks had arranged for Eric Webb, an anesthetist, to demonstrate the explosive nature of certain anesthetic gases by pumping several of them into clear plastic bags into which he would then introduce an electric spark. After first using cyclopropane, which made an "impressive little explosion," he explained that the next, nitrous oxide, would not explode. A split second later, an enormous blast nearly blew the windows out of the temporary wood-frame building. The metal connector for the apparatus flew past Philippson, crashing against the back wall. Stunned, Webb stood in front of his apparatus with blood dripping from his forehead, which the connector had glanced on its trajectory. Webb had forgotten to close the cyclopropane valve.

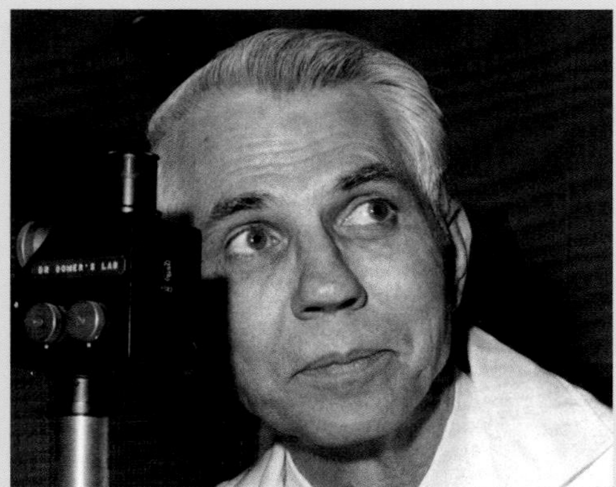

James Foulks, inaugural Head of Department of Pharmacology (1950–71).

Professor of Surgery; Bob Kerr, Professor of Medicine; Alec M. Agnew, Professor of Obstetrics and Gynecology; and John F. McCreary, Professor of Pediatrics and later Dean.

The appointees within the university clinical departments were drawn from the city's practitioners. They held mixed views on the new medical school. Some were antagonistic toward giving the university control of their practices with little compensation, while others recognized the value of the university to the community and the prestige of working in a large academic centre. It was, however, only with the enthusiastic participation of these clinicians in the educational mission that the school could provide the students with the requisite foundation in clinical skills.

Weaver obtained agreement from the VGH's Board of Trustees that any clinician appointed to the Faculty of Medicine would also be appointed to the respective hospital department and that the head of each department would also be department head at the hospital. Lawrence E. Ranta, Associate Professor of Bacteriology, was appointed Assistant to the Dean. Having been the man in the middle of the bitter battle of personalities between Strong and Dolman, he was familiar with the political background to the Faculty's beginnings and brought substantial strengths to the administrative team. A diplomatic, kind man, he eventually became medical director of the VGH (1952–75). He was very supportive

Lawrence Edward Ranta, Associate Professor of Bacteriology, Assistant to Dean Weaver, Medical Director, VGH (1952–75).

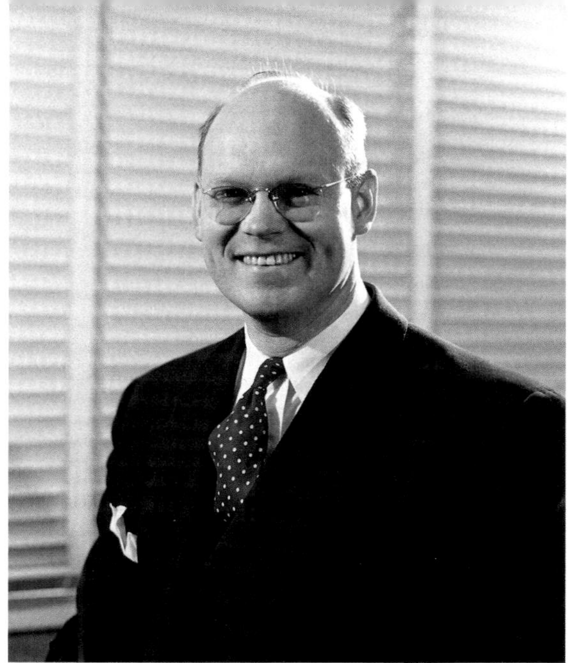

of the new medical school and was quietly effective in implementing necessary changes within the hospital.

Although the clinical faculty members felt welcome at the VGH, they were concerned that they would not be given enough teaching beds. As a general hospital, the VGH held many beds over which the university had no control, and there were recurrent arguments about how many beds would come under university control. Eventually, in his negotiations with the VGH board to appoint UBC appointees to their respective hospital departments and to establish department headships jointly at UBC and VGH, Weaver agreed to withdraw the UBC claim for a campus-based hospital in favour of a major new hospital facility to be constructed at the VGH site. It would open as the Centennial Pavilion in 1959.

The Department of Surgery

The founding Head of Surgery, Rocke Robertson, born in Victoria, BC, obtained his MD from McGill in 1929. After serving with distinction in the Canadian Army in Europe, he returned to Canada to work at Vancouver's Shaughnessy Veterans Hospital. For five years, he was chief of surgery there, all the time considering a return to a staff position at McGill but holding off in the expectation that the much-needed medical school would eventually get off the ground at UBC.

He took on the headship at a time when many general surgeons operated on a wide variety of problems, but increasingly, surgical specialization was developing. Following World War I, orthopaedics had been led by Frank P. Patterson Sr., a highly respected, hard-working practitioner but a rather forbidding teacher who was one of the two earliest surgeons in English-speaking Canada to confine his work to orthopaedics. He was succeeded in 1936 by John R. "Jack" Naden who was later succeeded by Frank Patterson Jr. as Head of the Division of Orthopaedics. Leadership of other specialities included J.A. "Oakey" Smith (eye, ear, nose, and throat), Archibald Hunter (urology), and Frank Turnbull (neurosurgery). Turnbull was much admired for his thorough and meticulous technique as a neurosurgeon and was also active in many university, civic, and national medical and academic organizations. Specialist trainees, until about 1944, were not certified as having undergone complete training in their area but would call themselves specialists depending upon their experience and practice. While at Shaughnessy, Robertson had formalized some postgraduate training activities for interns and residents.

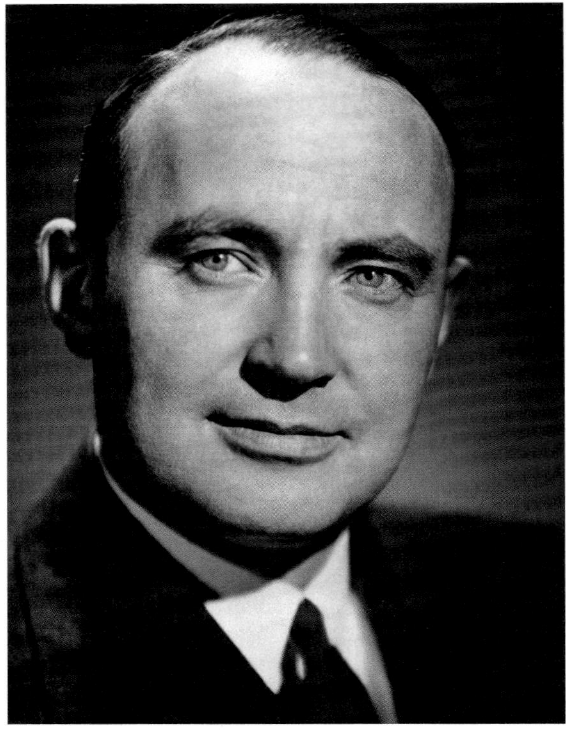

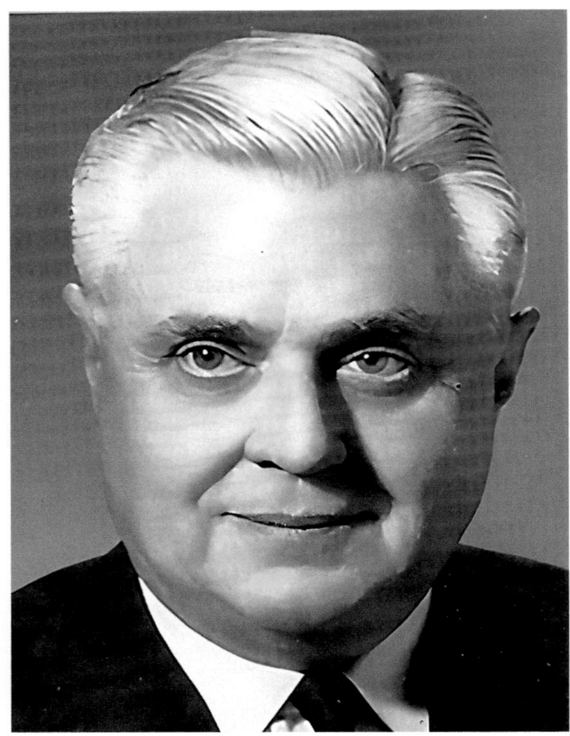

Robertson and his surgical associates at the VGH, along with their wives, entertained the medical students and interns on their services. Every week, Mrs. Robertson, Mrs. Alan McKenzie, or Mrs. Murray Johnson would produce a supper at the lab for students, trainees, and staff. Occasionally they would rent the Kerrisdale Arena; make up teams of students, trainees, and faculty; and face off against each other in friendly, highly unskilled hockey matches.

Robertson was a strong advocate for centring the medical school's clinical activities on the downtown city hospitals, recognizing the many benefits to quality of care. Any patient neglect or improper care was likely to come to attention in a learning environment, where a larger number of people would have access to a patient. Surgical errors would be much more apparent. Pathology conferences, surgical theatre clinics, and other teaching activities were a good influence on the staff physicians and surgeons who in the past would have had little opportunity to attend such sessions. Smaller outlying towns benefitted from the touring groups who held clinical days around the province. Robertson favoured the model of teaching in a large clinical municipal facility rather than in an "ivory tower" on an isolated academic campus. He was of the strong opinion that the school was underfunded.

The Department of Medicine

The Head of Medicine, Bob Kerr, following his recruitment by Dean Weaver from Toronto in 1950, quickly teamed up with Murray Baird, Head of Medicine at the Shaughnessy Veterans Hospital. They presented clinical situations and actual patients to the medical students, discussing the physiological basis for each medical condition. Accommodated in the TB Auditorium at Vancouver General, this program correlated basic science with clinical

LEFT FACING Harold "Rocke" Robertson, inaugural Head of Department of Surgery (1950–59), Acting Dean (1955–56).

RIGHT FACING Robert Kerr, inaugural Head of Department of Medicine (1950–74).

findings, not common practice in other schools at the time, and served, in Kerr's view, to stimulate the students and enhance their appreciation of the basic sciences.

Kerr's first undertaking as department head was to meet with all the physicians who might potentially become members of the Faculty or who were interested in teaching. About twenty internists were recruited and were each paid as much as $150 per year to conduct a series of bedside clinics with four to five students present. The students would change teachers halfway through the term in order to broaden their exposure to clinical techniques and approaches.

By the time the students were in their third year, Kerr had funded a teaching fellow who was a junior member of the Faculty. Among the early appointees were Hal Robinson, who later became Director of the Canadian Arthritis and Rheumatism Society, and Orm Murphy, who practiced internal medicine and became Medical Director of Shaughnessy Hospital. There were also lectures in therapeutics conducted by Arthur W. Bagnall. Donald "Mac" Whitelaw, a downtown practitioner whom Kerr recruited from his busy practice to become an associate professor, led the outpatient clinic at VGH. With as many as ten thousand patients per year, it was another teaching opportunity and patients were generally pleased with the thorough attention provided. Working with Kerr, Murray Baird developed student teaching at the Shaughnessy site where the large numbers of veterans provided a great patient resource.

William B. "Bill" Hurlburt, Head of the Department of Medicine at St. Paul's Hospital (1954–77), organized teaching clinics in 1954. He led efforts to develop the Clinical Investigation Unit (led by Howard Rice, builder of St. Paul's Hospital's heart-lung bypass machine) and in 1959 hired Doris Kavanagh-Gray as St. Paul's Hospital's first full-time specialist to develop the cardiac catheterization

Donald S. Munro, Consummate Clinician

The majority of lectures on physical examination and diagnosis were presented by Donald S. Munro. He was known to students and colleagues as a consummate clinician. Donald Ricci (UBC MD '70) recalls that once, as Munro and the students were finishing a clinical session over coffee, he told them they should walk him to the emergency room as he was experiencing a dissecting aortic aneurysm. He was correct! He was treated by the very colourful surgeon Peter Allen, who insisted that the mean blood pressure be controlled within a very tight limit. Robert Meek (UBC MD '68) recalls being an intensive care unit resident at the time, responsible for titrating the BP. One day it was a bit high, so he said to the nurse, "His pressure is ninety-six, give him some verapamil." Munro, who apparently had never been awake and never spoken during his two-week stay in the ICU, said, "Young man, don't you know you don't give verapamil to a patient with a mean pressure of only ninety-six?"

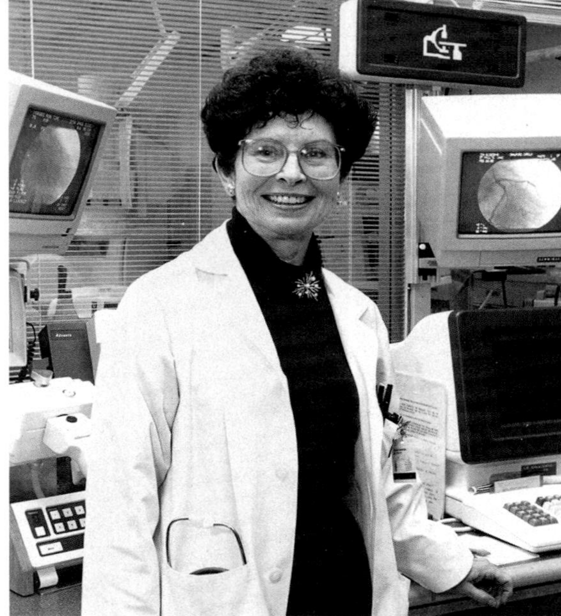

Doris Kavanagh-Gray, pediatric and adult cardiologist, founding Head of Cardiology at St. Paul's Hospital (1959).

laboratory and cardiac investigation service. She was a pioneer, establishing cardiac catheterization at St. Paul's, working closely with the hospital's innovative team of cardiac surgeons led by Robert Gourlay, chief of surgery (1958–72). In 1965, Hurlburt recruited Dwight Peretz from McGill to establish a state-of-the-art combined Intensive Care and Coronary Care Unit. Kavanagh-Gray was head of the Division of Cardiology for about thirty years, recruiting John Boone and Arthur Dodek and serving as a role model and mentor for many young female specialists.

Despite the earlier uneasy relationship between the BC Medical Association and the university, Kerr found that the professional group was tremendously cooperative. Holding their annual meeting in the Hotel Vancouver that first autumn, of 1950, the BCMA invited the whole first class and many members of the faculty to join them for lunch, where they had them stand and be recognized.

Kerr remained Head of the Department of Medicine until 1974. He established this key department in the setting of a VGH in which many practicing physicians held reservations about the advent of formal teaching in their midst. He formed excellent working relationships with them, establishing active teaching of internal medicine within VGH and eventually Shaughnessy Veterans Hospital and St. Paul's. It gave him great satisfaction later to know that after the introduction of standardized multiple-choice exams in 1967–68 by the Medical Council of Canada, the UBC medical graduates consistently ranked first in Canada. He was similarly gratified that hospital superintendents and medical associates across the country frequently told him that they were pleased with the quality of interns who had received their education in Vancouver.

Although his term was long by today's standards, the era of defined terms and reappointments had not yet become common among Canadian medical schools. He was later criticized for insufficient development of clinical research, but his intent was clear in a 1985 interview, when he stated, "Research accomplishments were not as great as might have been; however, I felt that our main purpose in the early years was to develop a sound clinical teaching program and I think we accomplished that." Under Kerr's leadership, several divisions emerged: psychiatry, neurosciences, dermatology, respirology, and nephrology. They, too, worked in primitive conditions.

PSYCHIATRY. Psychiatry began as a division within the Department of Medicine under the leadership of George A. Davidson. He recruited several practicing psychiatrists as teachers to present lectures and

James Tyhurst, Head of Department of Psychiatry (1959–70), with Detwiller Pavilion in background.

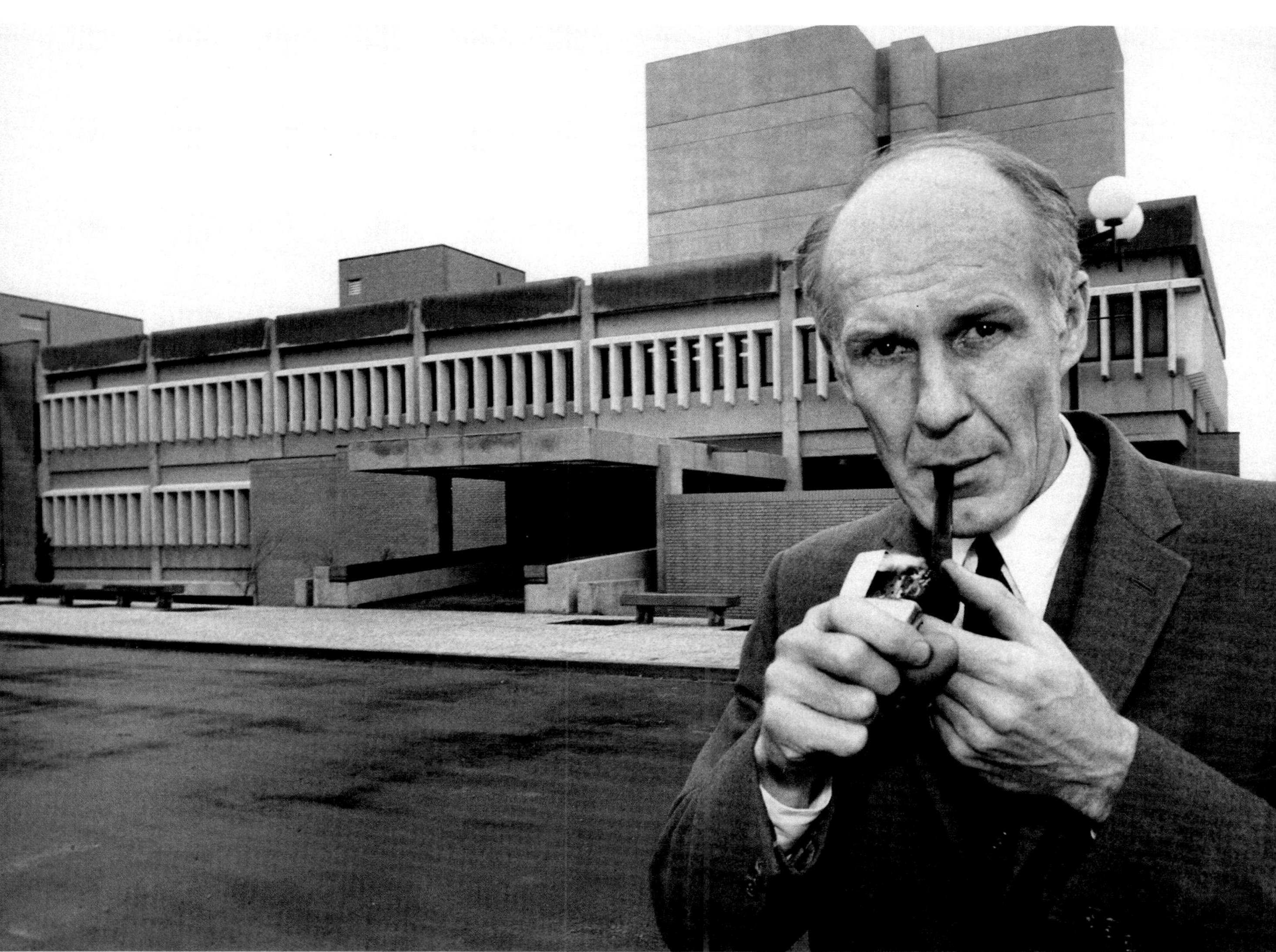

Fred Bryans, Head of Department of Obstetrics and Gynecology (1959–78).

FACING William C. Gibson, neurologist, inaugural Director of the Crease Clinic for Neuropsychiatric Research (later Division of Neurological Research, Department of Psychiatry) (1949–58), Professor of the History of Science and Medicine (1959–78).

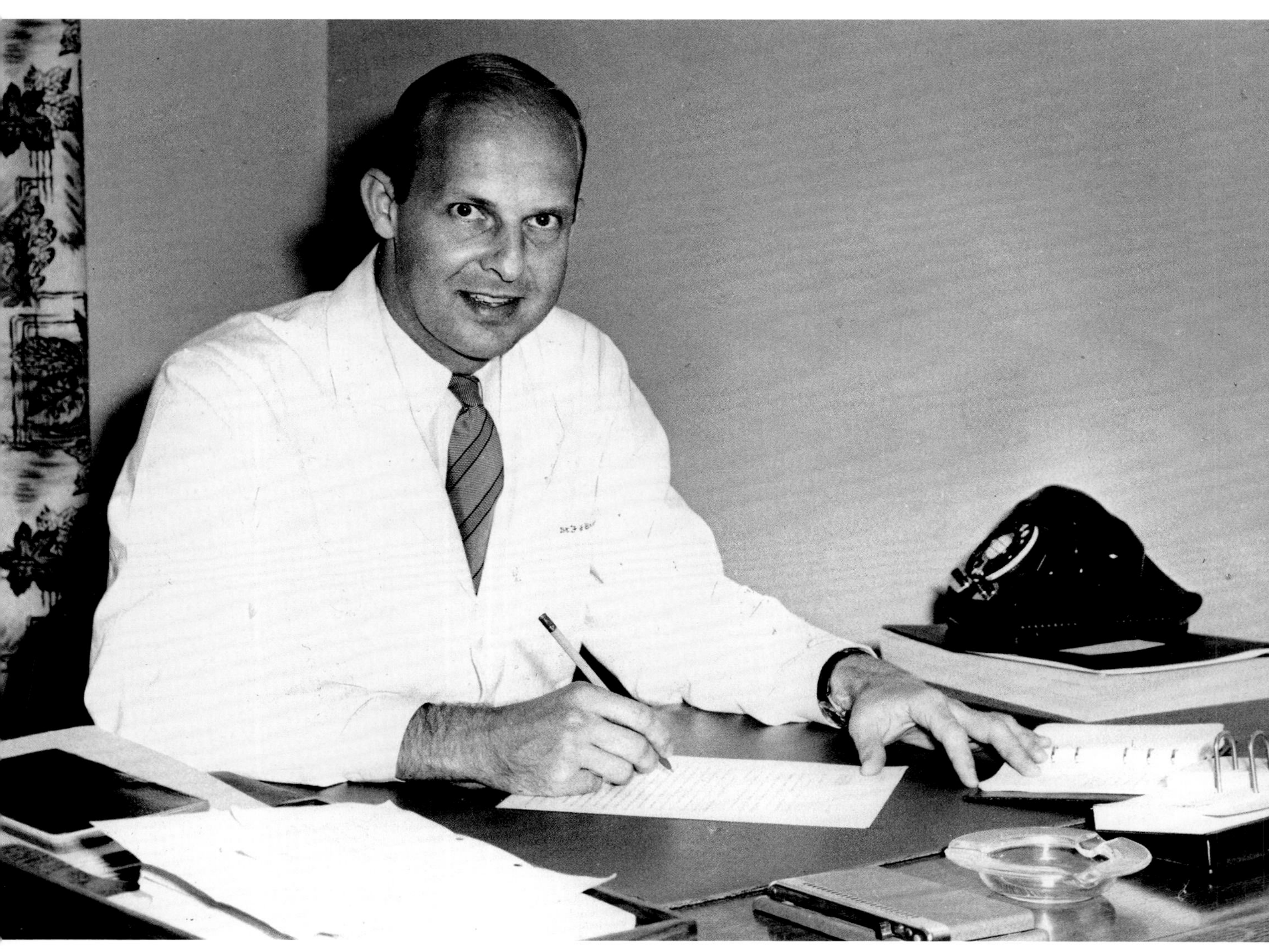

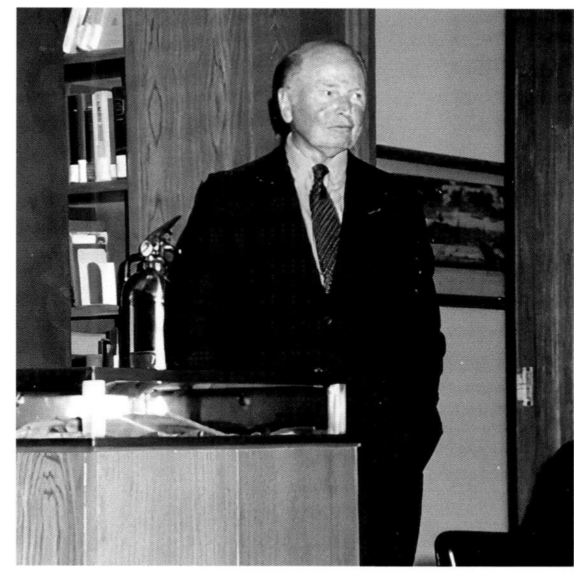

conduct clinics on the basics of human behaviour. A separate psychiatric unit was established at VGH with designated teaching beds and outpatient facilities. By 1953, Donald Ross from the University of Manitoba was appointed the first head of a separate department, to be followed in 1959 by McGill-trained James Tyhurst.

NEUROSCIENCES. In the field of mental health and investigations into disorders of the brain, Arthur Crease operated a facility outside of Vancouver on the lands of what would become the Riverview Hospital, handling the treatment of a wide range of neurological and psychiatric conditions. Just before his retirement in 1949, as the medical school was being founded, he recruited the young William C. Gibson, a Victoria-born McGill graduate who had completed his residency in neurology and psychiatry to head the Crease Clinic Unit for Neuropsychiatric Research on the UBC campus. A tiny corridor of a twenty-by-four-foot former radio shack used for RCAF training during the war served as the initial facility.

DERMATOLOGY. Donald Cleveland, an able dermatologist, speaker, and administrator, was appointed Head of Dermatology, a division of Medicine which included four or five practitioners at the VGH. Cleveland suffered a debilitating stroke and was succeeded in 1950 by Donald Williams, who had done his postgraduate work at the Mayo Clinic. Williams remarked that the shocking contrast between one of the most sophisticated clinical settings in the world and the primitive working environment found in Vancouver was offset by the deep satisfaction he derived from teaching students in the context of caring for patients.

RESPIROLOGY. The respiratory disease division, headed by Stefan Grzybowski, an expert in TB management, was housed in a frame building on the north side of 10th Avenue between Heather and Willow in what had been the Nurses' Annex. Tuberculosis was prevalent in the 1950s until the discovery of chemotherapeutic agents all but eliminated the need for isolated hospital beds and sanatoria for TB patients.

The other very serious infectious illness of the 1950s, of course, was polio. A special polio unit was established under the supervision of C.G. "Chargo" Campbell. Prior to modern developments in the control of respiratory function, some patients were placed in iron lungs, the body-encasing tank respirators which produced positive and negative external pressure to breathe for the person.

NEPHROLOGY. Russell Palmer and W.W. Simpson, with the aid of maintenance personnel at the VGH, built a dialysis machine which was used at Shaughnessy and the VGH for patients with acute renal failure. An excellent program of dialysis, which brought in patients two or three times a week, was developed for adults by John Price, and for children by David Lirenman. The program also flourished at St. Paul's under Angus Rae. Dialysis therapy demonstrated conclusively that patients in renal failure could continue to live productive lives for many years. A division of nephrology was established in 1979.

The Department of Obstetrics and Gynecology

Alec M. Agnew, the first head of the Department of Obstetrics and Gynecology, was a respected and capable surgeon who had been head of the VGH department since 1948. Fred Bryans joined him, and together with other clinicians they set up a teaching program, using one wing of the first floor of the Laurel Pavilion at VGH. In their third year, students attended the Women's Clinic there, and in fourth year observed deliveries, although there were never as many patients as the teachers would have liked. Agnew's clash with the chief at St. Paul's Hospital precluded cooperation with that facility. To address the patient shortage, the Grace Hospital, located on the corner of Heather Street and 26th Avenue, was brought into the fold. The popular hospital was run with devotion by the Salvation Army in compact facilities and handled a large volume of primary obstetrics, including staff patients and those without health insurance. It and the United Church Home for Unwed Mothers provided a useful teaching resource for the nascent and clinically oriented department.

The Department of Pediatrics

In the fall of 1950, Dean Weaver recruited John F. "Jack" McCreary as the head of pediatrics. McCreary was ultimately to leave an indelible stamp on the character of UBC's Faculty of Medicine.

His first job as the head was to negotiate with the minister of health in the coalition government as to where they would set up the pediatric department. After a great deal of soul searching, a semi-private building at 715 West 12th Avenue on the VGH site would become a new home for the Health Centre for Children. With approximately two hundred beds, facilities for outpatients, academic offices, and some research space, the unit was officially opened by Prince Philip, Duke of Edinburgh, on August 7, 1954.

The topic of normal growth and development of children was introduced to the medical students in 1951. Using a public health clinic established on the UBC campus in the Wesbrook Building under the directorship of John Read, with social worker Eleanor Bradley and public health nurse Joan Morrison, the Child Health Program provided well-baby care, immunization, counselling, and periodic health maintenance of local families. It allowed medical students, interns, and residents the experience of working directly with the families to which they were assigned and an opportunity to observe the normal development of healthy children. In 1956, McCreary and Donald Paterson co-edited a formal textbook entitled *Paediatrics* with thirty-six contributing authors, mostly from the Vancouver department.

Rustic Huts and Makeshift Libraries

New faculty and students who arrived on campus in 1950 would have found only a few scattered, low, temporary buildings, including some army huts and, still under construction, a permanent building (eventually named the Wesbrook Building) to house the Institute for Preventive Medicine, a concession to Claude Dolman, who had struggled so valiantly for a campus hospital. There was apprehension among the new faculty members that the institute was being built to placate Dolman and that it would subsume all new funding intended for the medical school. There was some resentment at this use of what they felt was "their" money, especially since the new building was not to be occupied by any part of the Faculty of Medicine. In fact, Minister of Education William T. Straith was so confused by the turn of events that at the opening ceremonies in 1951, he presented the keys of the building to Dean Weaver, whose Faculty would not be using it at all. Dolman's plans for a world-class public health centre which would have been the envy of all university medical schools finally ended up housing, in addition to Bacteriology, the Pacific Salmon Fisheries Commission, the Student Health Service, the School of Nursing, and a number of miscellaneous organizations with no other home.

All accommodations for the new medical school, like much of the rest of the university, were primitive. Through the entrepreneurial skills of physics professor Gordon Shrum and the influence of Chancellor Eric Hamber, several hundred huts, formerly armed forces barracks on Little Mountain and slated to be dismantled by the CPR, were commandeered and moved to the Point Grey Campus, to help accommodate the nearly six-fold increase in students following World War II. It had been originally planned that the Faculty of Medicine would be accommodated in several renovated huts. However, as recalled by Marguerite Service, secretary to Marvin Weaver, the new dean's eye fell on four white, single-storey temporary buildings located on the Main Mall, adjacent to the Bus Stop Cafeteria and immediately opposite the Great Trek cairn. These buildings had been allocated to the Department of Psychology, but Weaver was able to argue successfully that they would be much more suitable than

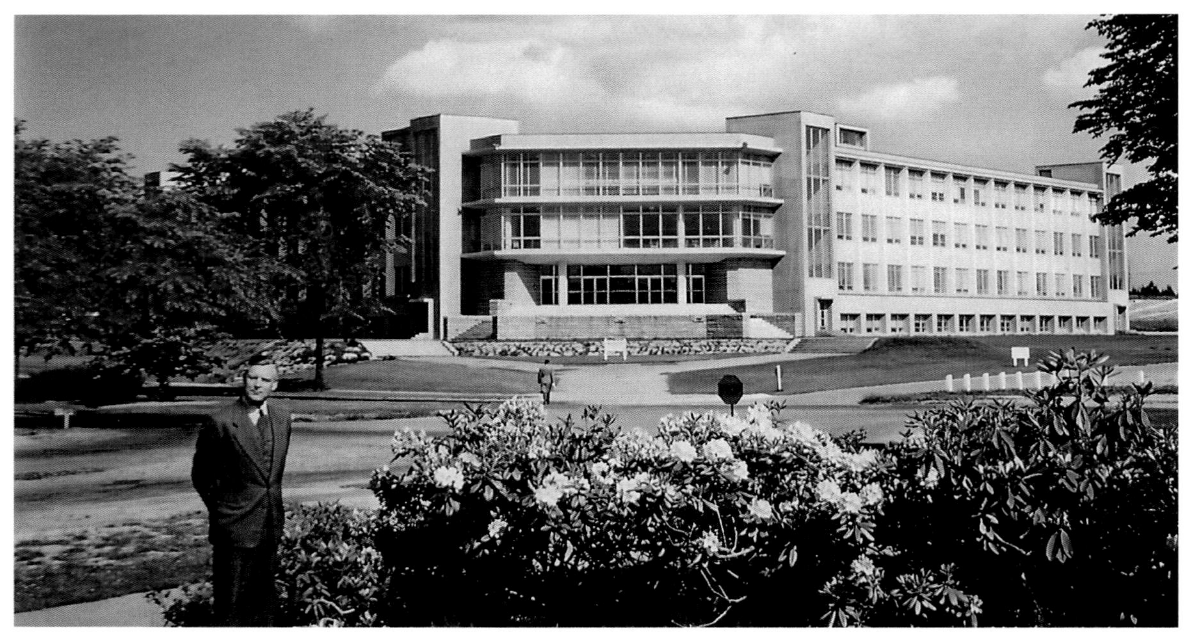

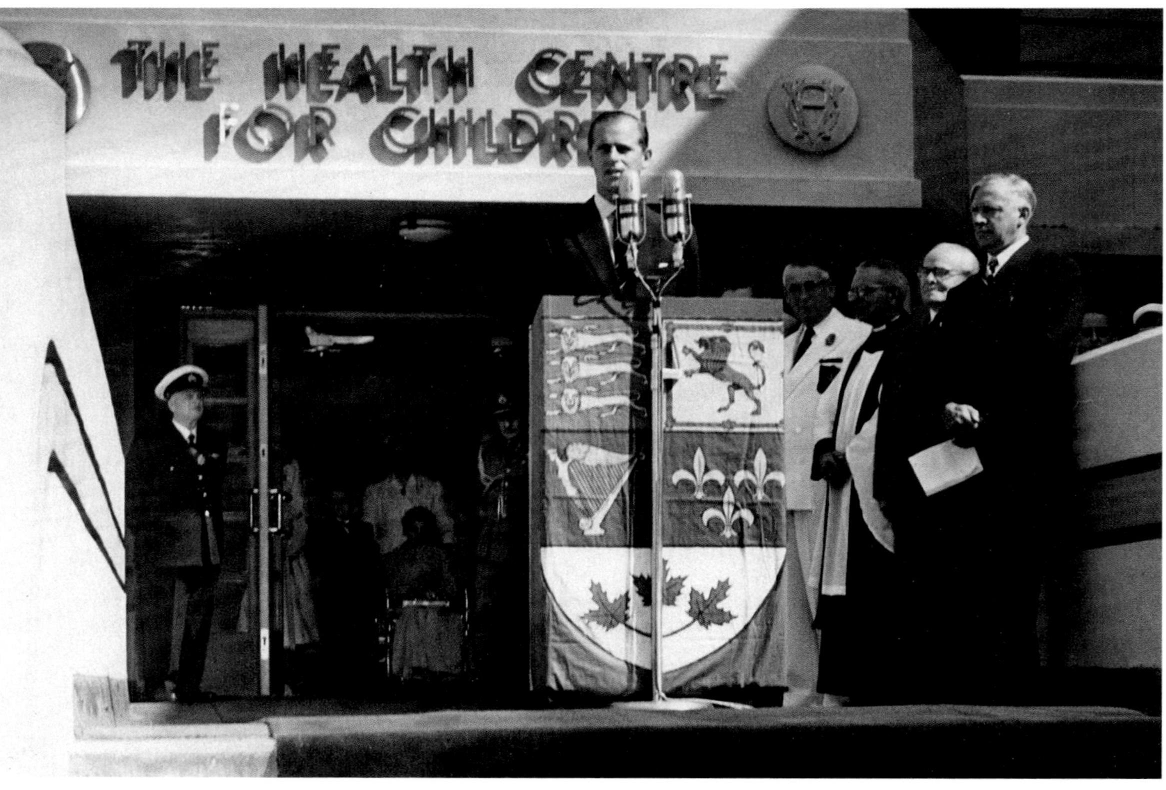
THE HEALTH CENTRE
FOR CHILDR

TOP FACING Claude Dolman in front of what was to be named the Wesbrook building, 1951.

BOTTOM FACING HRH Prince Phillip opening the Health Center for Children at VGH site, August 7, 1954.

renovated army huts as a home for the new Faculty of Medicine. The Faculty provided $5,000 to renovate army huts for the psychology department, and preparations to house the nascent Faculty were launched. To ensure timely completion of the renovations by September 1950, Weaver contracted his own journeymen to have the work done. Arranged in a quadrangle, there were four huts: one was the dean's office, one a 2,500-square-foot building for the anatomy and physiology laboratories, another for lectures, and the fourth for lectures and offices. Students in the early years recall walking over to the Bus Stop Cafeteria for coffee and a UBC cinnamon bun during breaks from anatomy and physiology labs.

In addition to space for dissections, there was a basic requirement for a suitable place to appropriately house cadavers. Eventually, Alex Wood, Head of the university's Department of Animal Nutrition, arranged for a room in Agriculture's dairy barn to be set aside for the storage of cadavers. Thanks to the intervention of William Gibson, Director of Neurological Research, who had contacts in a long-established histology laboratory in the UK, sixty sets of all the tissues of the body arrived from Oxford via an eleventh-hour shipment through the Panama Canal, just one week before the students began their studies of histology. This key contribution from Gibson was to be followed by many others of increasing magnitude over subsequent years. A year later, Friedman was able to have a small morgue added to the end of the anatomy and physiology hut, ending the necessity for clandestine, late-night transfers of cadavers between the dairy barn and the anatomy laboratory. He also ensured that an Anatomy Act was in place in BC, giving the university's anatomy department head total control of cadaver procurement and dissection. UBC became one of the first medical schools in North America to start a voluntary donation program, encouraging people through newspaper ads to leave their bodies for scientific purposes.

Resources were very limited in the 1950s, and government was not investing in universities. According to Friedman, this lack of resources was an impediment to the school's ability to attract some distinguished faculty members. In 1951, he was granted approval from Weaver to review some of the developments that were occurring in buildings in new medical schools all over post-war Europe. Following a six-week visit to Edinburgh, Oslo, Holland, Belgium, and Italy, he wrote a report extolling the virtues of the Karolinska Institute in Stockholm, which had impressed him greatly and on which the UBC school later modelled the planned basic sciences buildings. But despite frequent reassurances from President MacKenzie that construction would begin within a year or two, it took ten years for these buildings to materialize.

In the early years, library services were almost non-existent. Medical students borrowed their professors' journals and were expected to purchase

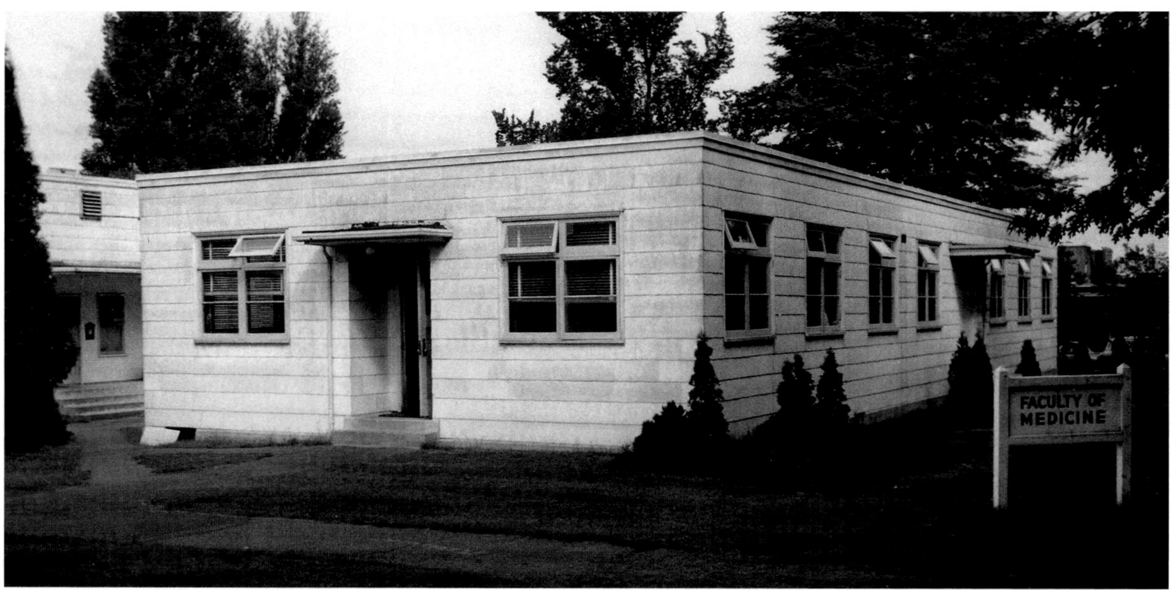

their own standard texts, such as *Gray's Anatomy*. By the time the first students were approaching their second year, however, it was essential to have access to a library. A small balconied, windowless space of the Main Library on the campus housed whatever medical books could be acquired. As the first chair of the library committee, Sydney Friedman asked the newly arrived Bill Gibson for assistance in setting up a good medical library for the new Faculty. The first dedicated medical library space was in a wood-frame building on the north side of 10th Avenue on the site where the Eye Care Centre would eventually be constructed. More permanent clinical library space would be established in the UBC clinical building along Heather Street and 10th Avenue in 1957. There would be no dedicated medical library on the UBC campus until 1964.

In the beginning, the Department of Biochemistry's laboratories and offices were housed in two of the renovated army huts located behind the chemistry (then science) building and the physics building. About 1959, at a cost of approximately $80,000, the Faculty of Medicine's temporary buildings and huts were to move to what was to become the health sciences sector of the campus where the Woodward Library and Instructional Resources Centre were eventually to be built. The basic sciences would move into permanent facilities in 1961. In their new geographic location, the temporary buildings and huts would live on as classroom space and a home for continuing education while the dean's office remained in its humble quarters until 1973.

Creating Facilities for Clinical Education

In the 1930s and '40s, doctors with admitting privileges had treated non-paying (staff) patients, who comprised more than seventy-five percent of VGH's patient population, in long, open wards in the Heather Pavilion for no remuneration. When the medical school opened in 1950, construction of a new wing of VGH was nearing completion, pursuant to agreements with the provincial government to make new beds available to accommodate clinical teaching of medical students. The new wing

FACING Faculty of Medicine Administrative Offices (the "Dean's Hut"), originally located on the Main Mall (1950) and later moved to the site of the Health Sciences complex.

LEFT UBC Wing (Offices, Laboratories, and Library) on corner of Heather St. and 10th Ave. at VGH (opened 1957), adjacent to Heather Pavilion extension along 10th Ave. (opened 1951).

RIGHT Students in clinical lecture theatre in UBC Wing at VGH, c. 1957.

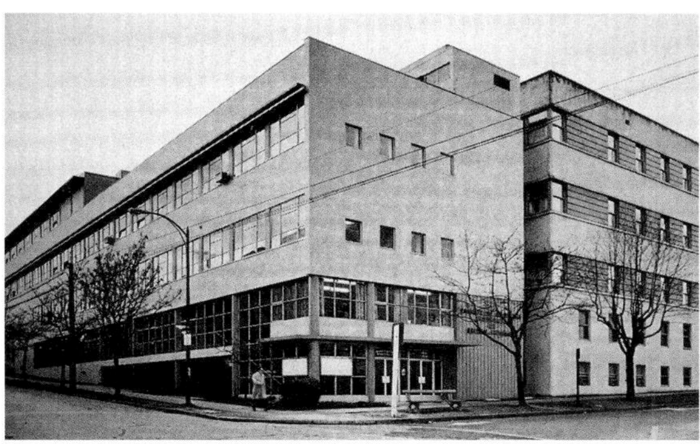

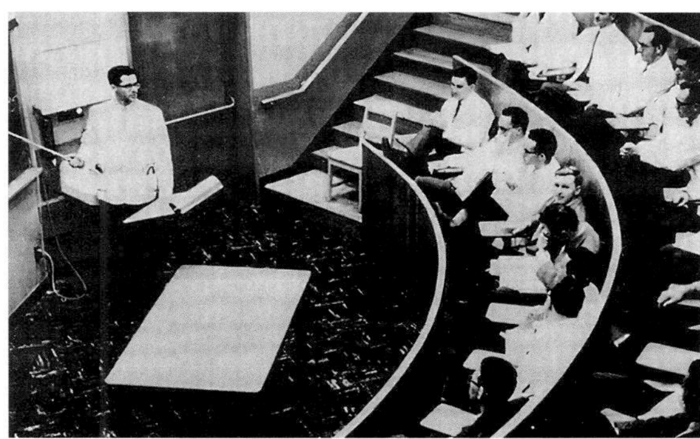

opened in 1951 on the corner of 10th Avenue and Heather Street, comprising A floor (psychiatry), B floor (medicine, wards B3 and B4), and C floor (surgery, wards C3 and C4), with direct connections to the open wards of the old Heather Pavilion on the B and C floors. Department heads could now have their own offices, as well as space for a secretary and an examining room, with a seminar room down the hall. Since all their teaching took place in the hospital, it was a very convenient arrangement for the professorial staff to have their offices only steps away from the beds where the students were caring for their patients. Patients would not necessarily know beforehand that they would be participating in the education of medical students; the concept of patient consent was not yet established. Head of surgery Robertson found the new quarters at the Vancouver General in 1951 very agreeable compared to those he and his academic colleagues had known earlier.

Beginning in 1952, with the start of their clinical education, students received most of their lectures in the TB Auditorium in the Willow Chest Centre building at the VGH. Although the new VGH wing provided access to patients for teaching purposes and modest academic clinical space, Dean Weaver, along with Kerr from medicine and Robertson from surgery, pressed the new medical school's need for clinical teaching and administrative space. They approached the coalition government under Premier Byron Johnson and were able to obtain $500,000 from each of the Ministries of Health and Education for a new extension along Heather Street on the east end of the VGH. Opened in 1957, this building provided them with a plethora of new space: in addition to facilities for Surgery and Medicine, there was room for the Department of Pathology, autopsy rooms, research facilities, two new lecture theatres–one seating over 150, the other a steeply sloped amphitheatre seating about 100–as well as seminar rooms and more offices. Eventually, clinical research facilities were developed on the fourth floor. Meanwhile, planning for expanded patient care facilities at VGH proceeded, and in 1959, the 504-bed Centennial Pavilion (commemorating the 1858 founding of the Crown Colony

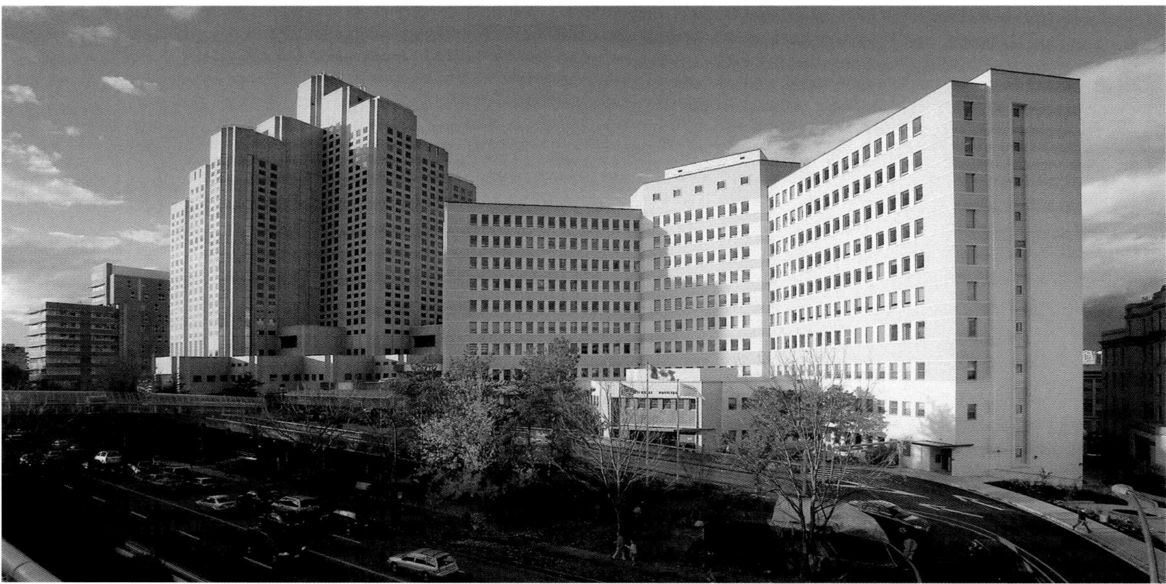

of British Columbia) was opened for the care of private patients, while public patient accommodations in the new Heather Pavilion (opened in 1951) became UBC "teaching beds." Although the new facilities were a marked improvement and placated most clinical faculty members, many continued to dream of a unified school on campus.

The First Students

There were 250 applicants for the sixty positions available for the first class in 1950. The selection process was based primarily upon the presentation of excellent marks from pre-med or arts years. Much importance was placed on letters of reference, of which three were required. A committee of eight, including the dean and several of the full-time department heads, would sift through the applications, transcripts, and references, and meet to assign rankings from A to D. The ranking, however, was based entirely upon the documents provided by the applicant, and not upon interviews conducted in person. Professor Geoffrey Andrew, deputy to the president and a member of the Faculty Admissions Committee, recalled that it was one of his mandates to resist any attempt to impose quotas on women, Jews, or foreign students in the medical class.

In the reminiscences of early faculty members, there is frequent mention of the high quality of the first cohort of students in the UBC medical school. One third of the inaugural class were veterans of World War II and were older on average than subsequent students. The war experience of a large segment of the first class gave them the added benefit of a veteran's pension; medical school fees, always a matter of contention, were $440 per year. Many students were married and had children; three were women. A sense of pioneering and adventure led to a strong group identity, and the friendships begun then became lifelong. The first graduating class celebrated their sixty-fifth reunion in December of 2019 with five attendees!

The first students were wined and dined by the medical and university community. They instigated a Medical Ball in 1951 at the Hotel Vancouver.

FACING Centennial Pavilion, VGH (right foreground), opened in 1959 and renamed the Leon Judah Blackmore Pavilion in 2017. Jim Pattison Pavilion is to the left, and Gordon and Leslie Diamond Health Care Centre in left background.

Margaret Cox (UBC MD '55) recalled it as a formal affair with the women attired in long dresses and corsages, the men in tuxedos (if they could afford to rent one). The evening began with a banquet, but with BC liquor laws, it was not possible to order wine or other alcoholic drinks with dinner, and attendees brought their own in paper bags concealed under the table, ordering mixers as required. The Irish regiment was dining in an adjacent banquet room and their pipe band marched in and played at one point. The evening concluded with dancing to the music of bandleader Dal Richards. For many years the Medical Ball was held at the Commodore, but it eventually moved to the Pan Pacific Hotel. Dal Richards returned to perform at the Fiftieth Anniversary Medical Ball in 2000.

The MD Curriculum

The curriculum in the Faculty's early years was traditional and conservative, despite the fact that several early leaders including Weaver, McCreary, and Friedman had travelled extensively and seen educational innovations in the US that they wanted to bring to BC. In their first and second years, students received lectures in each of the basic science courses—physiology, anatomy, biochemistry, and pharmacology—along with extensive and comprehensive laboratory experiences. There was considerable emphasis on acquiring facts, as opposed to solving problems, but the ability to integrate material and apply it to clinical situations was also stressed. Students were examined using questions requiring written essay-style answers, and in anatomy, there were harrowing oral examinations based upon cadaveric and skeletal specimens. There was very little direct contact with patients in the first two years.

Professors Copp, Friedman, and Foulks introduced a program of taking into their labs first-year students who wanted to work with them during the summer, paying them from their research grants, introducing them to the necessary discipline and techniques of scientific investigation, and stimulating the pursuit of careers in research. Some of these students were supported by summer studentships from the Medical Research Council (MRC).

For a number of years at the beginning, Friedman and Copp worked with determination, but little success, to achieve an integrated Faculty of Medicine and a university hospital. Donald Williams (eventually to be appointed in 1961 as the first associate dean of continuing medical education) deplored the fact that faculty members were too busy in their own areas to devise ways of integrating and coordinating the two facets of medical knowledge and that no committee was struck to transfer ward rounds, special meetings, or designated resources from the VGH to the campus and vice versa in order to allow the first- and second-year

Exam Results

It was the practice in the early years that, following exams in the basic sciences, the results would be posted on a designated bulletin board in the relevant building. Word spread quickly on the day of the posting, and students would crowd around the board to learn how they (and their classmates) had fared. The practice in Anatomy was more theatrical. Students would return to the lab after coffee break, and Dr. Friedman would take up his position seated in the centre of the room with the closed-circuit TV camera focused on him. He would review the focus and intent of the exam, the number of candidates, the mean and standard deviation of the marks, the number of passes and failures, and then, one by one, he would read off in alphabetical order each name followed by their percentage. Most would pass, but the few failures were public and traumatic.

students to see the relevance to patient care of all their basic science learning. In contrast to current pedagogy, the thinking was that clinical medicine should be brought to the campus, rather than the other way around.

The friends and social contacts of the Friedmans and of Copp tended to be on the campus and from a wide variety of academic endeavours, rather than in the practicing medical community. Research efforts involved collaboration with other scientists. There was camaraderie among the university people, and no sign of jealousy over government funding. Although relationships with clinicians at VGH were cordial and socially smooth, Friedman observed that they were not close.

FACING Alexander "Al" Boggie's acceptance letter, 1950.

The students' education was characterized by a marked change in the second half of their second year when they moved from the basic sciences to their clinical training at the various city hospitals, mainly the Vancouver General, Shaughnessy, and, to some degree, St. Paul's.

In years three and four (the clinical years), when increasingly more time was spent on the "public" hospital wards, much attention was paid to the presentation of cases. Clinical reasoning and the diagnostic process were illuminated through observing clinicians in action at medical and surgical rounds, clinical pathological conferences, and grand rounds. Didactic lectures covering all of the common disease entities, system by system, were accompanied by two bedside clinics a week with a clinician. One afternoon a week, each student would be assigned a patient on whom they would write up the history and physical examination, which would be evaluated by a departmental teaching fellow. They would see about thirty-six patients over the course of the year, thereby covering a great many of the common medical conditions.

The students would finally be tested by being assigned a patient to examine and record their findings. Then, with two or three clinicians accompanying them to the bedside, they would spend one or two hours presenting the history, physical findings, and diagnosis, and being quizzed by their teachers. An important feature of the early program in the Department of Medicine was the oral

IMPORTANT: PLEASE READ ENTIRE LETTER CAREFULLY

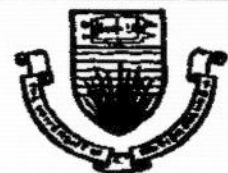

THE UNIVERSITY OF BRITISH COLUMBIA
VANCOUVER, CANADA

FACULTY OF MEDICINE
OFFICE OF THE DEAN

March 15, 1950

APR 11 1950
D. V. A.
REHAB.

Mr. Alexander Boggie,
2954 West 33rd Avenue,
Vancouver, B. C.

Dear Mr. Boggie,

You have been accepted tentatively as a member of the First Year Class in Medicine which will begin instruction on September 7, 1950.

REGISTRATION WILL BE ON TUESDAY AND WEDNESDAY, SEPTEMBER 5 and 6, 1950.

YOUR ACTUAL ADMISSION TO THE FACULTY OF MEDICINE IS CONTINGENT UPON YOUR COMPLETION OF PRE-MEDICAL COURSES IN WHICH YOU ARE DEFICIENT, IF ANY, AND UPON YOUR MAINTENANCE IN THE REMAINDER OF YOUR COLLEGE WORK OF AN AVERAGE WHICH IS ACCEPTABLE TO THE SCREENING COMMITTEE.

You will find enclosed a statement of account from the Bursar for $50.00 (fifty dollars), which is a deposit toward the fees of the first term. This preliminary fee is to be paid by March 29th, 1950, and it is not refundable if you subsequently enter another medical school, or if, without adequate reason, you should fail to register in this Faculty of Medicine in 1950.

Your attention is directed to the requirement that you provide yourself with a microscope of approved design. This should be of a substantial construction and equipped with the following accessories: objectives - 16 mm., 4 mm. and 1.8 mm. oil immersion; oculars 5 X and 10 X; triple nose piece; and substage condenser with an iris diaphragm. You may obtain such an instrument from any source which is available to you.

You will enjoy reading "Doctors in the Making" before registration. It gives specific suggestions as to how you may study medicine most effectively.

If you are attending the University of British Columbia at this time, or are living in Vancouver or its vicinity, you are invited to stop in at my office. Any details regarding the completion of your entrance requirements, or any question which you may have in mind regarding points raised in this letter or the medical course at the University of British Columbia can be discussed at that time.

Yours very truly,

M. M. Weaver

M. M. WEAVER, M.D.,
Dean of Medicine.

MMW:MAE.
Enc.

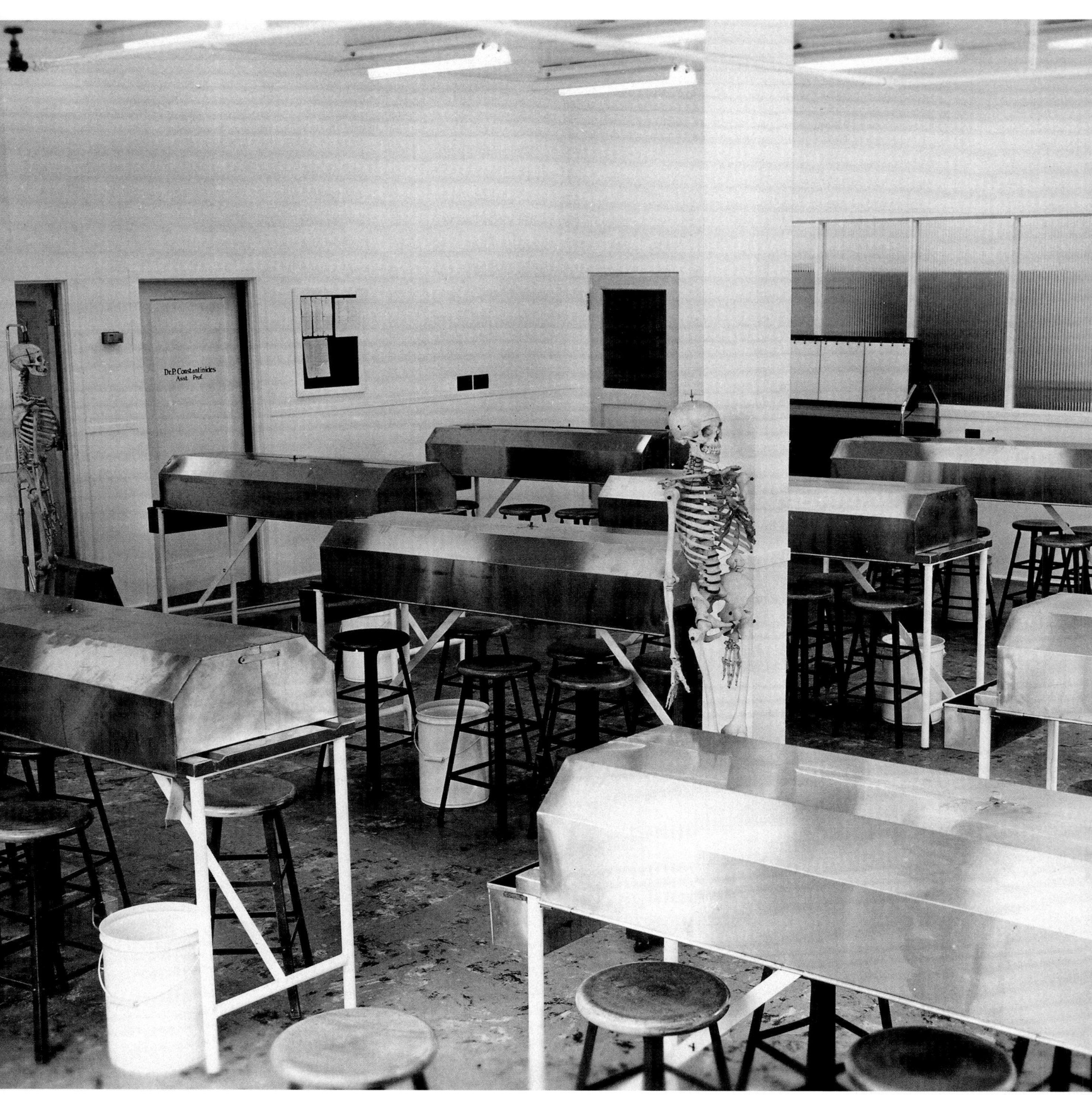
Dr. P. Constantinides
Asst. Prof.

FACING Anatomy Dissection Laboratory, 1950.

examination, a strenuous and challenging ordeal conducted by Professors Kerr and Whitelaw. During their surgical training, the students were exposed to a wide mix of patients on the two general surgery wards at the VGH. Most of their time was spent with general surgical cases, but they would also have short exposures to neurosurgical, orthopaedic, plastic, and eye, ear, nose, and throat patients.

In the early years, although students were given patient assignments on the wards and made rounds with the residents, there were no clinical clerkship experiences or direct patient care responsibilities as a formal part of their education. The only practical training the students had, apart from assisting in delivering babies, was in history taking and physical examination. By the end of their four years, some of them had never set up an intravenous line or tied a surgical knot unless they engaged in extracurricular activities. Experience with such techniques was considered to be part of the routine of internship following year four.

Some students were very keen to gain clinical experiences and many, even in their first and second years, would work evenings and weekends in the emergency departments of VGH, Shaughnessy, and St. Paul's, taking histories, performing venipunctures, starting IVs, and suturing—essentially acting as early physician assistants. Prior to the advent of Medicare in 1964, all "public patients" were potential subjects of the students' endeavours, and most of the clinical faculty provided access to their "private" patients as well. Following year three, many had the chance to work with practitioners in both Vancouver and in smaller communities around BC, gaining valuable clinical experience with deliveries, minor surgery, first-aid procedures, the management of patients, and the art of medical practice. This externship program ran for many years and was popular with students as well as the supervising doctors who gave generously of their time to support it.

Dean Weaver and his department heads felt that a thesis should be one of the requirements for a medical degree. They believed that it would be a useful academic enterprise, giving the students some focus of creativity on a scholarly undertaking that required a certain amount of independent exploration, perusal of medical literature, and formulation of an argument. The topic was usually selected by the student in consultation with a faculty member sponsor, who would criticize and evaluate the work. The thesis became a feature of UBC's medical training for the first few years, but eventually the requirement was discontinued.

Prior to the creation of the Faculty of Medicine, postgraduate training in BC was conducted primarily in Vancouver and followed an apprenticeship model. When the Faculty was established in 1950, post-MD education was focused on highly individualized rotating internship positions funded by hospitals

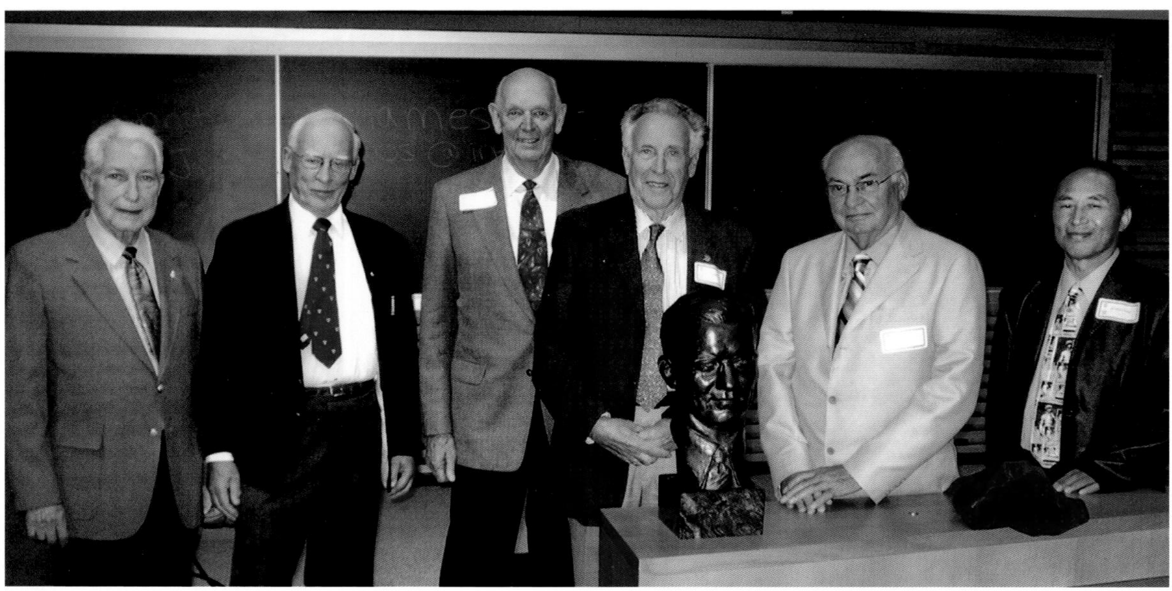

in Vancouver, New Westminster, and Victoria. Organized postgraduate specialty training programs gradually developed in many disciplines beyond the traditional one year of "rotating internship" to several years of training in the given specialties, including obstetrics and gynecology, surgery, medicine, and pediatrics.

Weaver's Legacy

As the first Dean of the medical school, Myron Weaver was exceptionally hard-working, and the stress of medical and university politics took a toll on his mental and physical health. After a myocardial infarction in 1955, he stepped down as Dean and moved to Albany, New York, where he worked for a few years in Student Health Services. He died there of a recurrent infarction in 1963.

Assessments of Weaver's legacy as the first dean were mixed. There was consistent agreement among his early department heads that he was a hard-working, conscientious, pragmatic administrator, but was possessed of neither great intellectual strength nor exceptional vision. He was a kindly, likable person who lacked the authority to challenge the opposition he encountered from stronger leaders around him. He had the insight to recruit some able leaders and excellent teachers and on occasion was imaginative, as when he attracted William Boyd to extend his career in academic pathology. He was revered by the medical students. Members of the first class presented the Faculty with a bronze bust of Weaver on the occasion of their sixtieth reunion in 2014. Although his achievements were constrained by the increasing tensions between the hospital clinicians and the campus-based scientists, as well as the continued debate about a university hospital and its location, he was able to overcome a myriad of challenges to launch the Faculty. From the perspective of over seventy years since his initial appointment, the accomplishments appear enormous.

Physiology Teaching Laboratory, 1951. Note kymograph drums right foreground and freshly varnished records drying in background.

FACING Members Class of 1954 present bust of Myron Weaver to UBC on their 60th reunion, 2014. From left: Gordon Heydon, Albert Cox, Bill Bell, Al Boggie, Alfred Gerein, and sculptor Arthur Cheung.

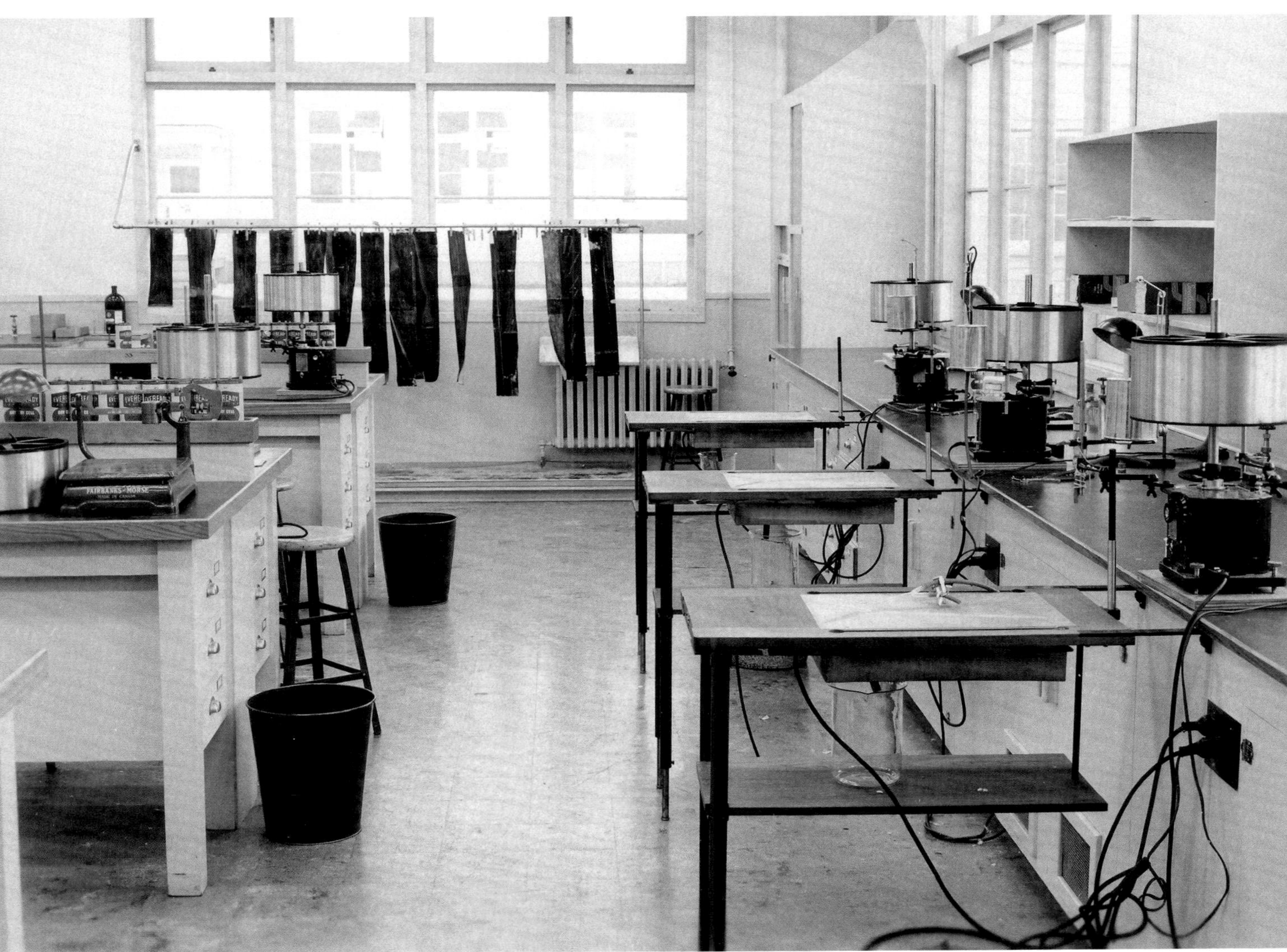

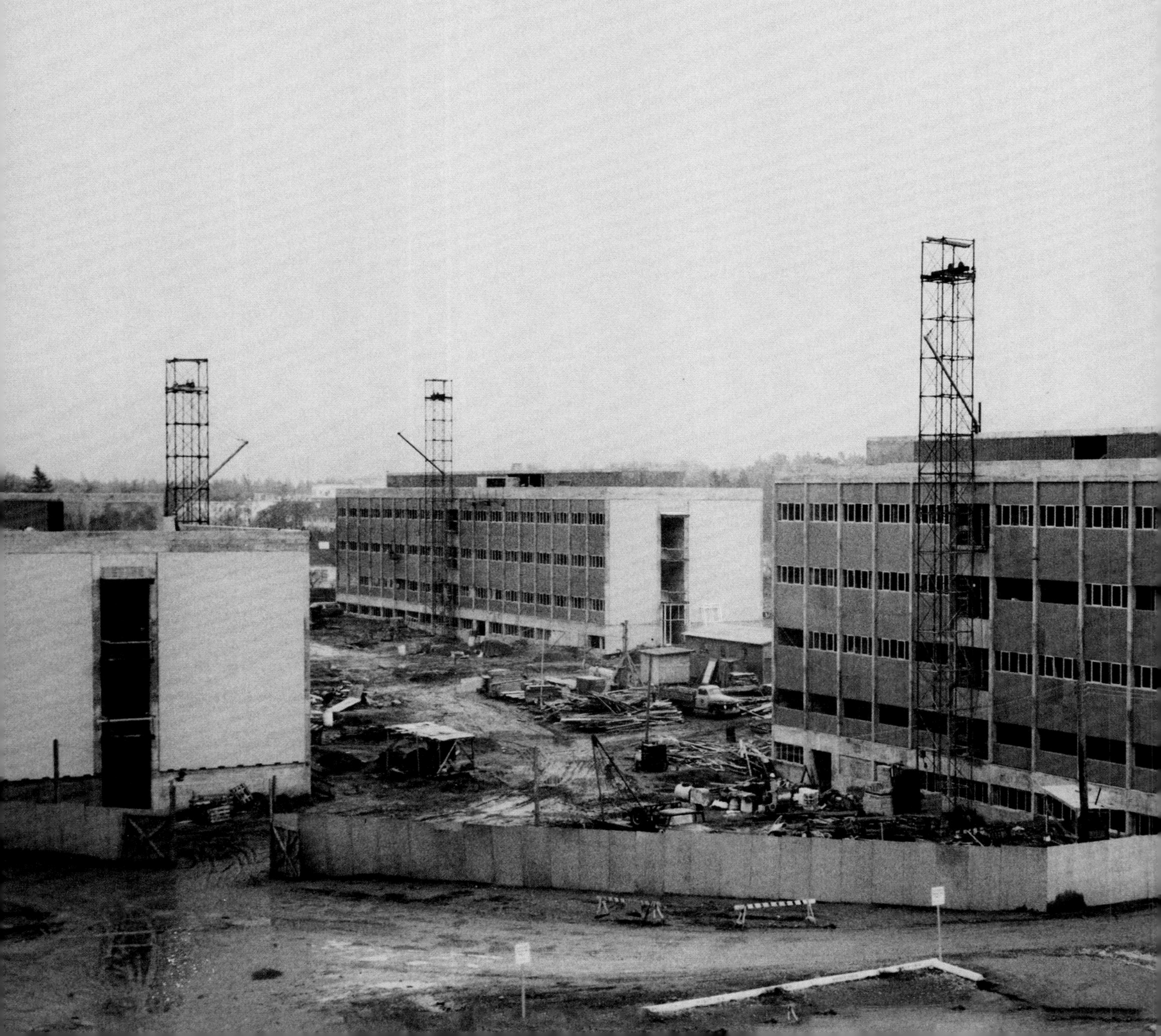

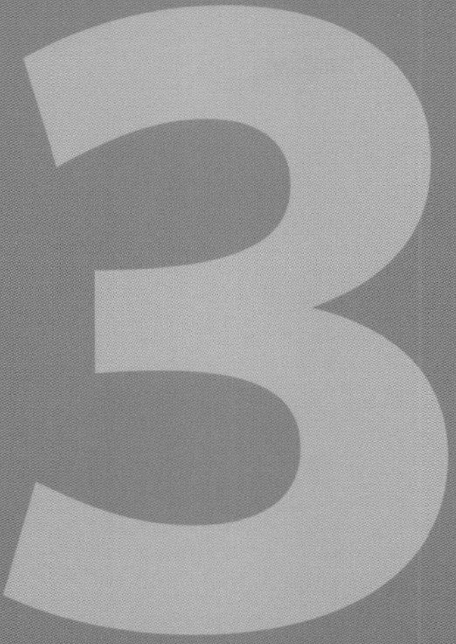

3 Growing Pains

1956–72

FACING Basic sciences buildings under construction: Block A (Biochemistry and Physiology) in the left foreground, Block B (Anatomy and Cancer Research) in the left background, and Block C (Pharmacology and Kinsmen Laboratory) in the right foreground.

FACING John Patterson, ophthalmic pathologist, second Dean of Medicine (1956–58).

McCreary's dynamic personality and strong vision were to help the fledgling school come of age and to boost it into contention with leading Canadian faculties of medicine.

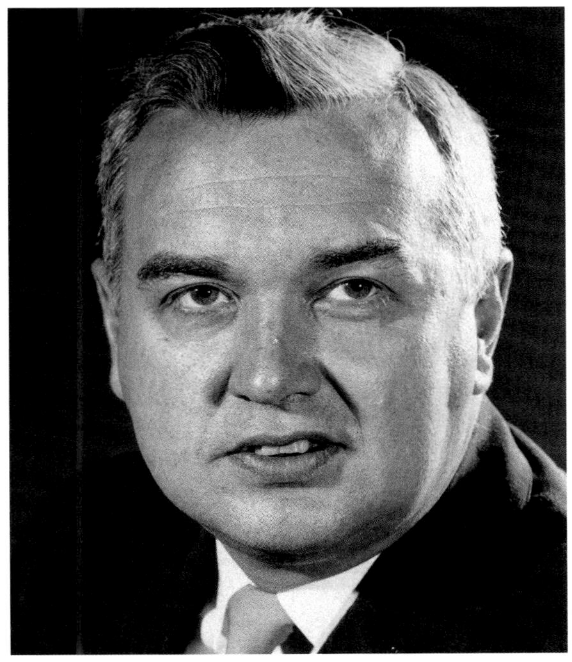

AFTER WEAVER STEPPED down in 1955, Rocke Robertson, who did not wish to be dean himself, agreed to serve as acting dean until a replacement could be found. His commitment at this time was continuing to lead the Department of Surgery. Nonetheless, he did his utmost to fulfill his responsibilities, handling with dispatch the inevitable crises, such as a fierce competition for research space between Pharmacology and Biochemistry. He proved to be a consummate administrator and later went on to become principal of McGill University.

University of British Columbia recruited its second Dean of the Faculty in 1956. John Patterson was an outgoing, affable eye pathologist and Associate Dean at Case Western Reserve University in Cleveland. His university had initiated what many considered the most advanced medical curriculum in the US, integrating the basic and clinical sciences, focusing on organ systems, and featuring an introduction to patients in the first year. Despite the interest of Robertson and Sydney Friedman in a systems approach, Patterson's time in BC was not to be long. He quickly committed himself to building a new hospital on the campus. His systems approach alienated the basic scientists who were more focused on preserving their departmental teaching, and he further alienated Friedman, Harold Copp, and Marvin Darrach by advocating that their respective departments of Anatomy, Physiology, and Biochemistry pool their resources. President MacKenzie supported the department heads, and Patterson found himself pilloried at a Senate meeting when he was publicly rebuked by the president. He said, "I suddenly find they've cut my throat when I didn't anticipate it." Bob Kerr and Copp recalled that although there were disagreements with Patterson's ideas about medical education, his main difficulty was his problematic interpersonal approaches. When an offer arose for the position of Dean of Medicine at Vanderbilt University in Nashville, Tennessee, Patterson found it was not difficult to leave the UBC situation, with all its political strife. His brief stint as dean was over after two years, and according to Copp, there was much celebration when he departed in 1958.

McCreary's Vision

When John Patterson resigned, a search for a new dean was launched for the third time. Deputy

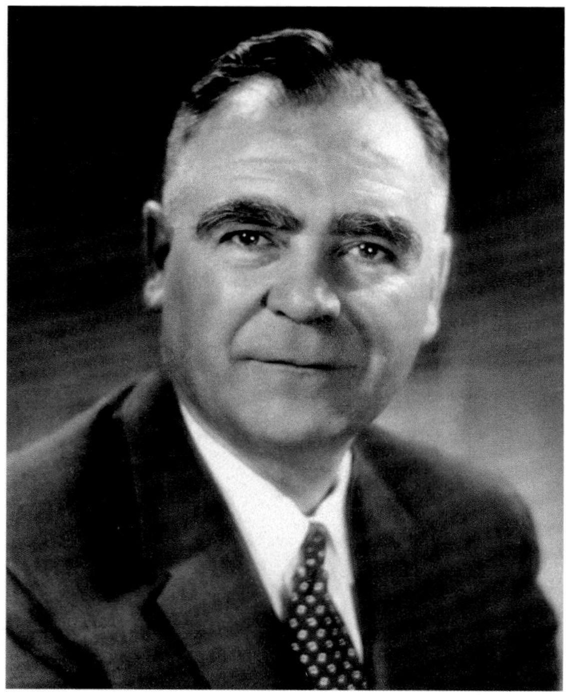

John F. "Jack" McCreary, inaugural Head of Department of Pediatrics (1951–59), third Dean of Medicine (1959–72).

President Geoffrey Andrew chaired the committee and quickly the Faculty recognized that the charismatic Jack McCreary, Head of Pediatrics, seemed to be the logical successor. In addition to his well-known clinical abilities, McCreary was held in high regard for his organizational and administrative skills. His dynamic personality and strong vision were to help the fledgling school come of age and to boost it into contention with leading Canadian faculties of medicine.

The new dean was confronted by substantial hurdles. Weaver's illnesses, an interim deanship by Robertson, and the brief tenure of Patterson had led to a loss of cohesion within the school. The basic sciences were well established with strong leadership, but the clinical departments were less so and focused primarily on their own visions, rather than on a unified set of Faculty priorities. The school was still significantly underfunded compared with other Canadian medical schools. The funding deficit led to conflict between clinical faculty, who were particularly affected, and the academic faculty. There remained lack of consensus in the community as to the optimal location for a major teaching hospital. McCreary was a popular lecturer and a gifted teacher, but he never lost sight of his clinical roots and held the care of patients to be the loftiest and most rewarding goal of a medical education. It was clear that his understanding of clinical practice would bring insight to the challenges and exigencies of the clinicians and would encourage their participation in academic affairs. His clinical perspectives strengthened his belief in the need for a campus hospital.

McCreary perceived that his first duty was to unify the medical school and try to steer it on a clear and consolidated course. Accordingly, he set up a long-range planning group of department heads. With financial support from both the Rockefeller Foundation and the John and Mary R. Markle Foundation, he and his team spent almost a year examining new medical schools, construction of new university hospitals, and health care delivery in North America and Europe.

The planning group highlighted three issues. The first was a purely Canadian phenomenon. In 1957, the federal government had agreed with the provinces to partially fund the cost of acute hospitalization. This was the first tentative step toward what was to become Medicare. McCreary felt that this arrangement placed an undue emphasis on in-patient care and left the patient responsible for the cost of community-based care. Furthermore, this model focused medical teaching on acute care rather than comprehensive care. Subsequently, McCreary's planning group initiated community-based medical student teaching with family practice units in two locations (one opposite the VGH on Heather Street and one on the university campus). A third community teaching site, the REACH (Research, Education, and Action for Community Health) Centre, was established at a pediatric care centre in the city's east end, founded by pediatrician Roger Tonkin and staffed mainly by family practitioners. All three projects were initiated with philanthropic funding.

Second, McCreary realized that there was no formal process for continuing medical education in an era of rapid scientific advancements. The BC Medical Association was more interested in public policy issues, and in fact this wasn't really their responsibility. McCreary felt that as BC's only medical school, the UBC Faculty should take on the role of maintaining the currency of its graduates and of others practicing in the province.

The third issue considered by McCreary was that primary health care–provided in the patient's home or physician's office–was being handled almost exclusively by physicians. This was in sharp contrast to what happened in hospitals, where nurses, pharmacists, physiotherapists, and other health professionals provided a considerable portion of the care. He believed that the physician monopoly on primary care seriously limited the scope of practice of all health professionals and could be exacerbated with the advent of Medicare. His prescient view was that if, in this young medical school where various professional faculties had not been too long entrenched, health professional students could be brought together to work in teams, then a new concept could be developed that would mold the health science professionals together at the beginning of their training. Each of the professional groups would become aware in the formative years of their education of the strengths and limitations of their own and other health professions.

In 1960, the concept of a health sciences team approach was a radical departure from the norm. Although the School of Nursing did not have any serious objections to McCreary's plan, leaders of the other professional schools were defensive, with each group anxious to protect its own domain, fearful of reducing the power or influence or set of responsibilities already accrued. McCreary's vision was that of a new UBC-based health science centre and teaching hospital where integrated care could be delivered. Although his vision came to fruition in the form of new buildings and a library on campus, it would take other forces to move closer to a successful model of integrated patient care.

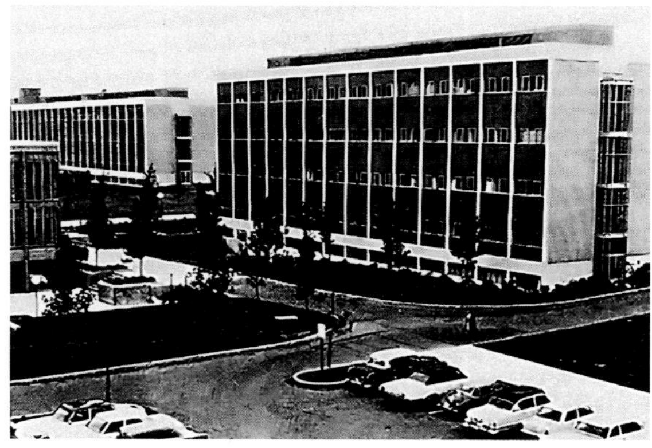

Basic science buildings shortly after completion in 1961 (Block A in left foreground, Block B in left background, and Block C in right foreground).

FACING The Charles Woodward Memorial Room of the Woodward Library (opened 1964). Students perusing some of the priceless volumes, Gobelin tapestries hanging behind them (top: Masters of the Spirit, bottom: Masters of Science).

A New Health Sciences Centre

McCreary's vision of a health sciences centre included the construction of appropriate space for the basic sciences, a medical library, and a full-service teaching hospital. Delays with new construction on campus had long preceded Jack McCreary and were limiting any further recruitment and development of the Faculty. The premier finally agreed to fund a building plan, but only on condition that the university come up with fifty percent of the necessary monies–the first time that this tactic had been employed for a public university in Canada. By 1961, a fundraising campaign had yielded a total of $10 million from private sources, including two very substantial gifts from Walter and Leon Koerner who had immigrated to Canada from their native Czechoslovakia during the Nazi era. They had become prominent philanthropists, eventually bestowing their generosity through the Leon and Thea Koerner Foundation on not just UBC but a wide range of educational, social service, and cultural activities throughout the province. Accessing these new resources, and at a remarkably low cost of just over $2 million, buildings A, B, and C, as they were first called, were constructed to the specifications of their occupant department heads. Having functioned up until this point in meagre, sometimes shared huts, the departments wanted their own space. Former Dean Patterson had attempted to integrate the various medical disciplines with interdisciplinary laboratories in a single tower. However, this vision was replaced with a more independent one based upon Sydney Friedman's recommendations after his visit to Europe and the Karolinska Institute. In the new UBC structures, the Biochemistry and Physiology departments shared Block A, Anatomy and cancer research Block B, while Pharmacology, Pathology, and the Kinsmen Laboratory of Neurological Research occupied Block C. Although this may have enhanced their sense of identity, it ultimately stifled collaboration across departments.

The temporary buildings and huts, now located on what was becoming the health sciences region of the campus in proximity to the Wesbrook Building, had been condemned as uninhabitable, yet after eleven years they were still, in 1961, serving as administrative space, offices, laboratories, and classrooms for the medical school. BC was lagging far behind the other provinces in government support of higher education. Faculty members deplored Premier Bennett's policy of building roads while forgoing the investment they thought it should have been making in education.

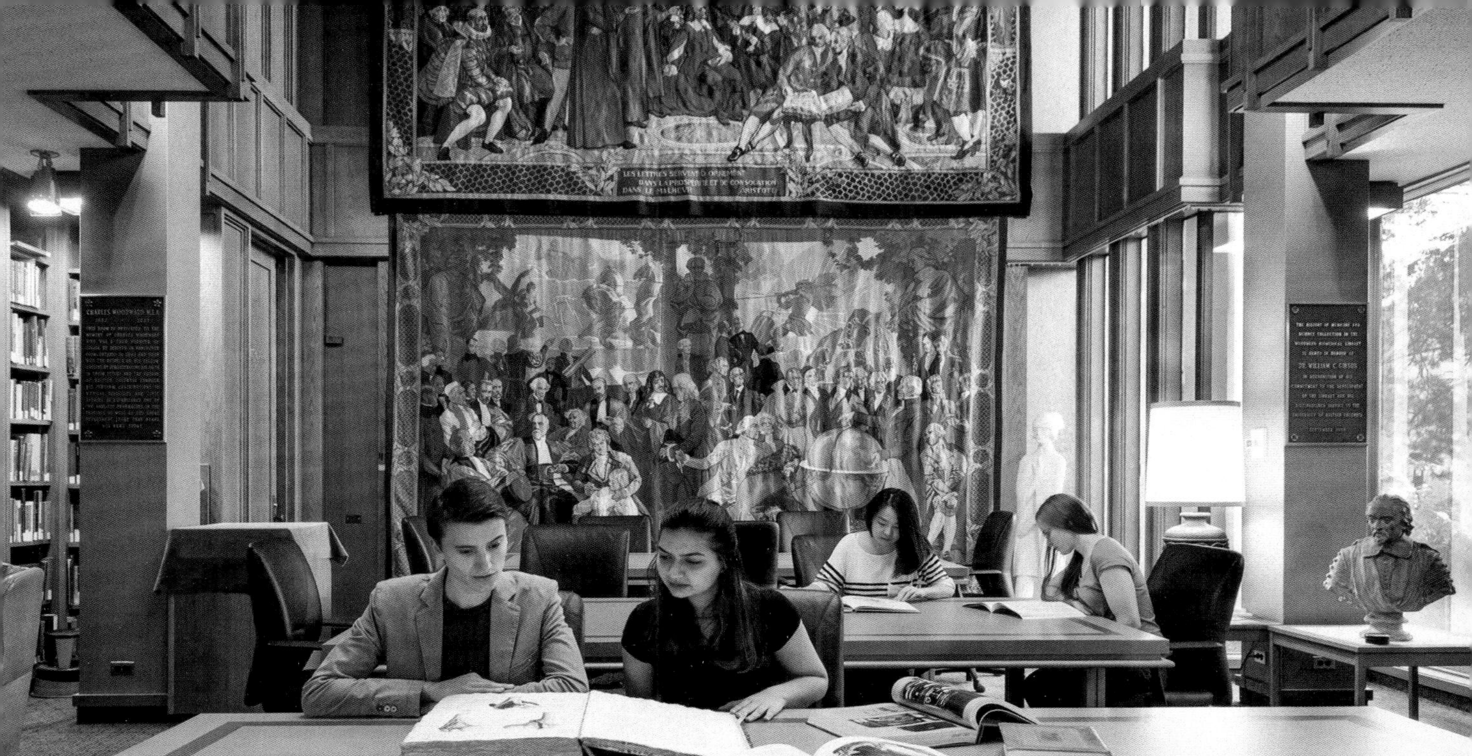

Bill Gibson, founding Director of Neurological Research, and his successor, Patrick McGeer, were becoming frustrated with the ongoing delay of any substantial action in building facilities for the medical school and the contest between the VGH and UBC for provincial government funding. Gibson, newly elected president of the UBC Alumni Association, publicly decried the lack of support for UBC from the province. In a statement to the press, he denounced W.A.C. Bennett's Social Credit government, which was leading one of Canada's wealthiest provinces and yet contributing the lowest per-student grant and lowest overall subsidy to its university of any of the western provinces. McGeer, a UBC graduate and now neuroscientist faculty member, publicly described the inadequate funding situation as a crisis.

The Woodward Biomedical Library

A medical library was a major achievement during McCreary's tenure. Bill Gibson and fellow neurologist S.E.C. "Ward" Turvey, impressed by the Wellcome Library in London, led initiatives toward its establishment. Turvey, who shared an office with Robert E. McKechnie, introduced Gibson to Percival Archibald "Puggy" Woodward, the entrepreneurial and feisty son of grocery store magnate Charles Woodward. It was the younger Woodward who had pioneered the concept of the modern supermarket in Western Canada. During one of his periodic bursts of enthusiastic philanthropy, Woodward learned from Turvey, McKechnie, and Gibson of the dire need for a proper medical sciences library at UBC. He made a generous gift, and the outstanding Woodward Biomedical Library opened its doors on the UBC campus in 1964.

The library is a UBC gem, a striking contrast to most of the neighbouring structures, which were built with a frugal eye on limited budgets. The splendid Memorial Room is dedicated to Charles Woodward and houses an impressive collection of significant works on the history of biomedical sciences. The beautiful gallery around the reading

Dean and Department Heads about 1960. Left to right, front row: Marvin Darrach, Robert Kerr, William Gibson, John McCreary, Harold Taylor, unknown, Donald Williams, Brock Fahrni. Back row: James Foulks, Fred Bryans, unknown, unknown, James Mather, Alan MacKenzie, James Tyhurst.

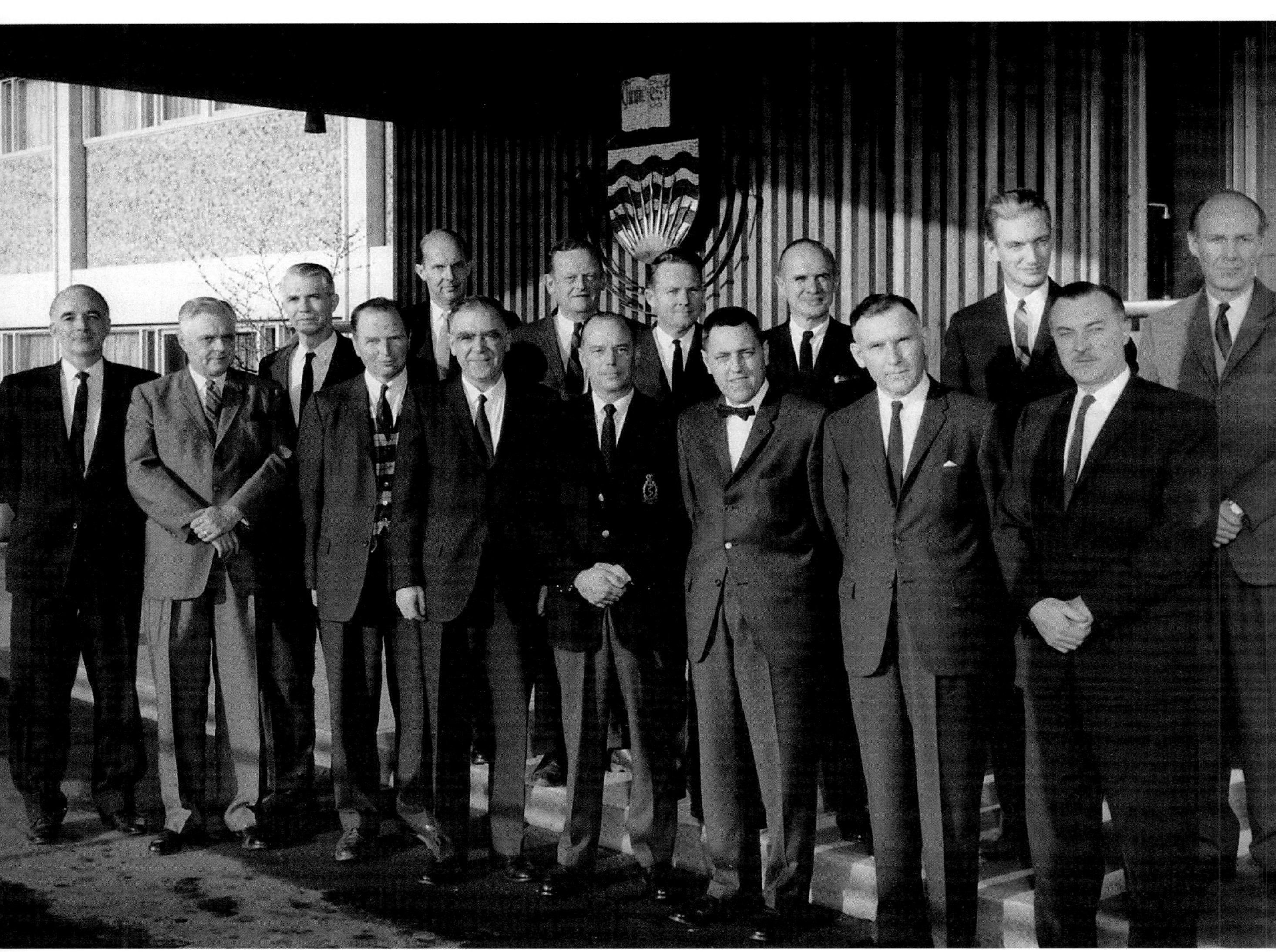

room holds some of the rarest scientific books, and a special case encloses a first edition (1543) of Vesalius's *The Fabric of the Human Body*. The adjacent seminar room is named after the illustrious Oxford scientist Sir Charles Sherrington, with many memorable items donated from his estate. Gibson's tireless efforts and numerous contacts with generous patrons around the world brought in whole collections of rare books, biological drawings by Leonardo da Vinci, special facilities for blind students, a striking Francis Loring bust of Frederick Banting, and, following extensive sleuthing and determination, William Harvey's seventy-two-page 1628 first edition of *De Motu Cordis* in which the author describes the circulation of the blood in the human body. Two exquisite Gobelin tapestries grace the walls of the Memorial Room: the *Masters of Science* (1948), depicting Edward Jenner, Louis Pasteur, and others; and the *Masters of the Spirit* (1954), featuring philosophers and writers dating back to ancient Greece.

Student-Faculty Retreats

The class of '68 organized a very successful retreat, held at Whistler in the autumn of 1966. Attended by about seventy students from years two, three, and four and at least twenty faculty members, the two-day event had a formal program of talks, primarily by students, evening receptions, and skits, as well as free time for hikes and other outdoor activities, all designed to improve student-faculty communication and relationships. It was repeated at Whistler the next year and later moved to Manning Park Lodge. Unfortunately, the party aspects came to dominate, and following some damage to furniture at Manning Park, the event ended somewhat unceremoniously after 1971.

Another Failure to Launch a Campus Hospital

In 1959, the UBC Board of Governors had approved the start of a planning process for a modern campus hospital. McCreary and his long-range planning group appointed a coordinating committee, funded by the Leverhulme Trust, to focus on the campus hospital concept and to ensure coherence with the long-range planning for all aspects of the Faculty.

As a member of the Royal Commission on Health Services (also known as the Hall Commission) set up by the Diefenbaker government in 1961, McCreary was able to influence the development of national health policy but would meet difficulties with implementation in BC. In 1964, the Hall Commission recommended that a Health Resources Fund be established to assist financially in the construction of health training and research facilities in Canada. In July 1966, an act of Parliament created a $500 million fund from which $300 million was to be allocated to the provinces on a per capita basis over five years for the development of health training facilities, with contributions payable to the provinces in amounts of up to fifty percent of the costs of the projects approved by the Minister's Advisory Committee.

In 1963, the provincial legislature had passed the University of British Columbia Health Sciences Act, and in 1967 President John B. Macdonald established the temporary Curtis Committee to plan the administrative structure of a health sciences centre. In anticipation of the creation of the health sciences centre, in 1962 McCreary had orchestrated the appointment of the respected health economist Lloyd Detwiller to manage the planning. There were to be six administrative divisions within the centre: continuing education, health services research and development, interprofessional education, hospital administration, business administration, and health systems.

At last, McCreary thought he had provincial approval to go ahead with planning a campus hospital using resources from the Health Resources Fund. Linked with the idea of the health sciences centre, the ambitious plan called for a $36-million, fourteen-building complex which would serve three functions. It would be a provincial referral centre for difficult medical cases, a major research facility, and a pioneering centre for the integrated teaching concept being developed by McCreary and his team. It was expected that, when complete, it would accommodate 1,400 students in the fields of medicine, dentistry, pharmacy, nursing, social work, and rehabilitation medicine.

But once again there was a serious lack of agreement among the various parties about the vision, and about what could or should be built on campus. Echoes of earlier discord could be heard in the differing viewpoints regarding campus facilities. As the new head of the Department of Psychiatry, James Tyhurst was a strong advocate for a new psychiatric unit on campus. A phase-one, three-storey building opened in 1967, followed in 1968 by a five-storey extension, eventually designated as the Detwiller Pavilion and housing the Kinsmen Laboratory of Neurological Research on its top two floors. It was expected to be the first wing of the long-awaited campus-based 410-bed teaching and referral hospital that McCreary envisioned as his hub for the centre. Tyhurst felt that a psychiatric hospital should be a warm, human place where patients would not feel they were entering a "sterile sort of whitewashed bedlam." However, when members of the government came from Victoria to open the new facility, they were shocked at its seeming extravagance and sent plans for the remaining buildings back to the drawing board for redesign and cost revisions. Irreverent references to the "Psycho-Hilton" were often heard. Tyhurst's positive inputs were later eclipsed by sexual assault allegations against him by former patients, for which he was eventually acquitted on appeal but then successfully sued in civil court.

Differences among the visions of McCreary, academic faculty, and clinicians at VGH led to interminable battles over the concept of a health sciences centre, and when the Social Credit government fell to the New Democratic Party in 1972, the entire

Husband and wife team Patrick McGeer (UBC MD '58), neuroscientist, MLA and Cabinet Minister, and Edith McGeer, neuroscientist.

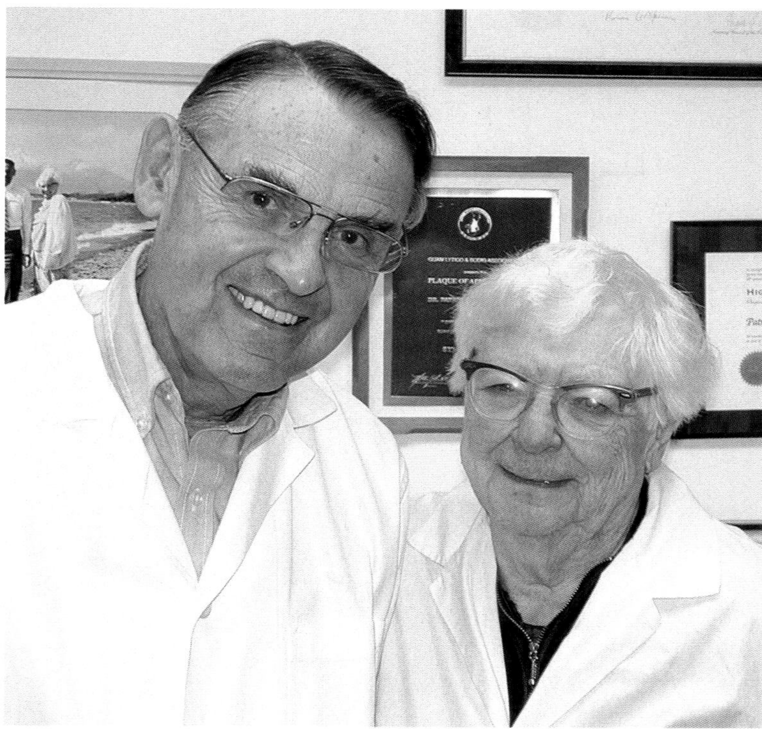

project was stopped completely. To the dismay of many, the beautifully planned campus hospital was never constructed as originally planned. The plans later materialized as the acclaimed University Hospital in London, Ontario. As a compromise, McCreary accepted the building of an extended care hospital (the Purdy Pavilion, opened in 1977) to become part of the new complex. It is ironic that McCreary, who had been so instrumental in bringing the Health Resources Fund into being on a national level, led the institution which benefitted from it so little and so late.

Departmental Innovations

Complementing the major capital developments and evolving focus of health sciences education during McCreary's era were several important innovations at the department and program level.

The Department of Continuing Medical Education

In 1960, Dean McCreary asked Donald Williams, Head of Dermatology at VGH, to start a Department of Continuing Medical Education. He accepted immediately, closed his busy consulting practice, and developed a five-year plan for his new department. Williams defined continuing medical education in a number of lectures. While delivering the Sir Thomas and Lady Edith Dixon Lecture in May 1969 at the Royal Victoria Hospital in Belfast, he stated that "continuing medical education is first the scholarly habit of planned daily reading and study in a home library sanctuary as an integral part of a doctor's workday; secondly, the periodic return every three to five years for three months or more of intensive study; third, the day-to-day informal and formal colleague association and patient care in the community hospital, teaching hospital, group

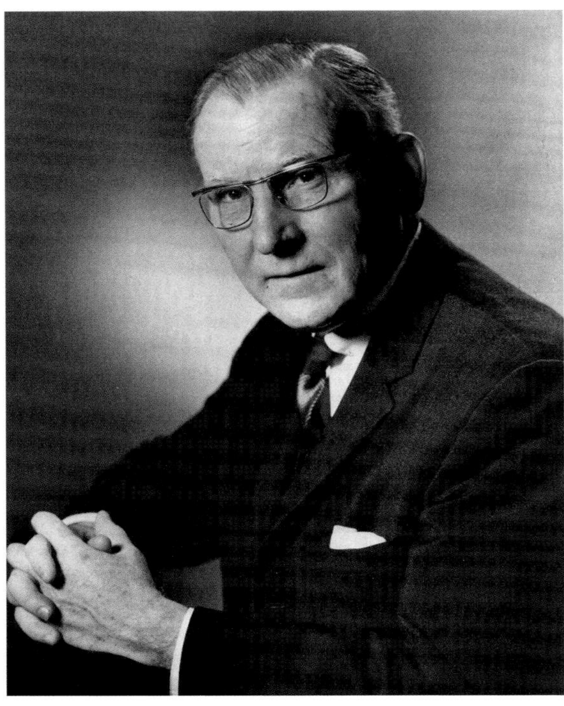

Donald Williams, Head of Division of Dermatology until 1960, then appointed inaugural Associate Dean of Continuing Medical Education.

practice, and by consultation; fourth, attendance at scientific sessions of learned societies; and fifth, attendance at short courses."

Unique amongst his peers, he produced an annual report every year. At the beginning of each year, Williams would determine what the continuing medical education needs were for each region and then invite the department heads to identify their best teachers and ask them to go to the outlying centres for these sessions. The system had the added advantages of encouraging referrals to Vancouver from the areas visited and strengthening the regional centres. The twenty-four community hospitals throughout the province each hosted two or three faculty members per month during the academic year to present updates on topics of the local doctors' choosing. The result was that ninety-six percent of the physicians in British Columbia were provided with courses within twenty-five miles of their communities. The program became so successful that observers from other medical schools around the world came to spend time and learn about its methodology. Williams was later to put the same principles into use when his mandate was expanded to include the other health professional programs. In subsequent years, the Department of Continuing Medical Education evolved to become a large program, continuing to be led by an associate dean but no longer with the designation of "Department."

The Department of Public Health

After World War II, physicians in public health focused on issues of sanitation, engineering, and nutrition. Governments opened public health services and established programs to diminish the spread of contagious diseases and improve the health of the general population. James Mather was the first head of UBC's Department of Public Health. Like former dean Weaver, he achieved his ends by steering people in the general direction he wanted them to go without antagonizing anyone along the way. He recruited people like Stuart Murray, the city health officer, and George Elliot, another friend from wartime military service, who had become Deputy Minister of Health.

At an early stage, a training program was developed within the provincial public health system whereby practicing physicians could return to pursue a formal course of studies to earn a master of science degree in public health. The Faculty

Department of Public Health became the Department of Health Care and Epidemiology in 1968 and in 2008 evolved to become the School of Population and Public Health which includes teaching and research in global health, biostatistics, health services policy, and occupational and environmental health.

The Department of Neuroscience Research

By the late 1950s, William Gibson had moved the Department of Neuroscience Research into one of the temporary buildings occupied by biochemistry on the health sciences site. The Kinsmen Clubs of BC raised the necessary capital to equip new facilities that were established in Block C of the new basic sciences building complex opened in 1961. For administrative purposes, the department lost its separate identity and was made a division within the Department of Psychiatry and clinical neurology became a division within the Department of Medicine.

Patrick and Edith McGeer, both PhD chemists who had met and married at the DuPont Experimental Station in Wilmington, Delaware, arrived in Vancouver from the United States in order that Patrick could enroll in the medical school class entering in 1954. Following his internship at the VGH, the couple were recruited to the young Faculty, joining the Department of Neuroscience Research.

In 1961, Patrick McGeer and Gibson conducted the first clinical trials using large oral doses of dl-DOPA in patients with mental disorders and later Parkinson's disease. Gibson eventually turned over the leadership of the Department of Neuroscience Research to McGeer in order to pursue another of his major interests as Professor of the History of Medicine and Science. The McGeers went on to make many contributions to neuroscience. Based on his own convictions and awareness of the frustrations of those in the medical school with the provincial government, McGeer also entered the political fray himself. Following a brief stint in municipal affairs, he was elected to the BC provincial legislature in 1962. He remained a member of the legislative assembly and then a cabinet minister until 1986, holding a series of portfolios of direct relevance to the development of the Faculty of Medicine.

Don Williams versus the Pharmaceutical Industry

As associate dean of continuing medical education, Don Williams was well known for his strong views on the nefarious influences of the pharmaceutical industry on physicians' prescribing habits. For many years, through the 1960s and '70s, he graphically illustrated the magnitude of pharmaceutical detailing by arriving at one of his lectures bearing a huge box. Partway through the session, he would pause for dramatic effect, then open the box and splay its contents (hundreds of samples received by him so far that year) onto the floor in front of the suitably impressed third-year students. His message about the importance of independent continuing medical education in contrast to "education" by the pharmaceutical industry could not have been clearer.

In September 1966, it was announced with great fanfare that Juda H. Quastel, an eminent biochemist and pioneer of modern neurochemistry, accompanied by eight of his research associates and graduate students, would leave McGill University to establish a new research unit in the Kinsmen Laboratory of Neurological Research. Amongst other achievements, he had published some of the earliest metabolic studies among patients with phenylketonuria, caused by an inherited enzyme deficiency resulting in severe neurological disorders. Juhn Wada, who had come from Wilder Penfield's Montreal Neurological Institute, established a seizure investigation unit and the epilepsy surgery program. The Wada test for cerebral hemispheric dominance of language function became the gold standard and is widely conducted prior to epilepsy surgery. Soon the group was expanded to include S.C. Sung, who did some original work on enzymes involved in muscular dystrophy; Louis Woolf from Oxford, who had helped develop a safe diet for phenylketonurics; and Toshiaki Hattori, who contributed a great deal to the understanding of the biochemical neuroanatomy of the basal ganglia. H.C. "Chris" Fibiger made numerous contributions to neuroscience research and served as Head of the Division of Neurological Sciences (Department of Psychiatry) and chair of the university's graduate program in neuroscience prior to leaving for industry in 1998.

The Department of Biochemistry

It was almost by accident that in September of 1956, a graduate chemist named Michael Smith, fresh from receiving his PhD at the University of Manchester, arrived in Vancouver to do some postdoctoral work. It happened that a brilliant young Punjabi immigrant and eventual Nobel Prize winner, Gobind Khorana, was working at UBC in a field that interested Smith. Just a month before Smith's arrival, Khorana had stumbled upon a way in which chemists could isolate pieces of DNA. This historic development was one of the underpinnings of the biological revolution which brought molecular biology and modern genetics to the scientific forefront. It had the further pivotal effect of steering Smith away from organic chemistry and into biochemistry, the field in which he was to make a profound difference later in his career.

After marrying a Vancouver native, he followed Khorana to the University of Wisconsin as a postdoctoral fellow, and then returned to Vancouver in 1961. Although not appointed to the university at this point, but conducting research and running the chemistry division of the Fisheries Research Board of Canada's laboratory located on the UBC campus, he was involved informally with the university because of collaborations he undertook with biochemist Gordon Dixon and his graduate and postdoctoral students. Biochemistry head Marvin

Michael Smith, biochemist, Nobel laureate (1993), and leader of the genetic/genomic revolution at UBC in the late 1990s.

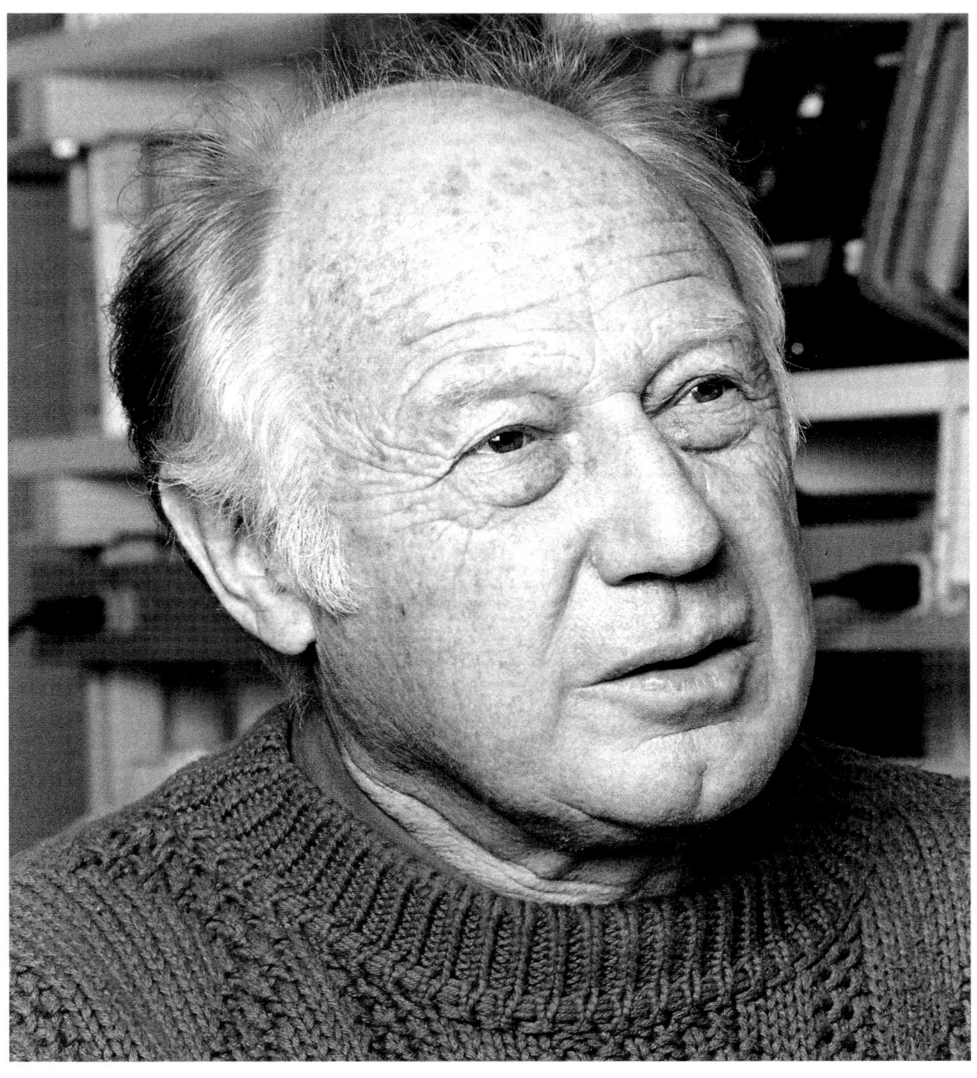

TOP Sydney Israels, neonatologist, Head of Department of Pediatrics (1965–77).

BOTTOM Stephen Drance, glaucoma ophthalmologist, Head of Department of Ophthalmology (1973–90).

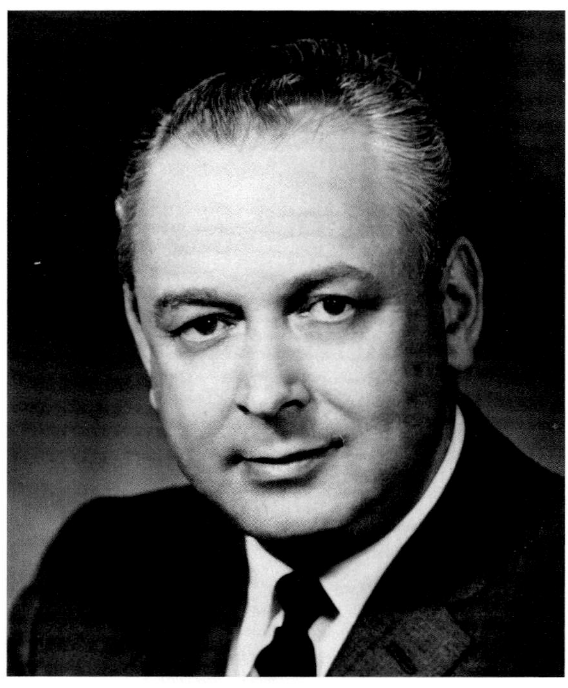

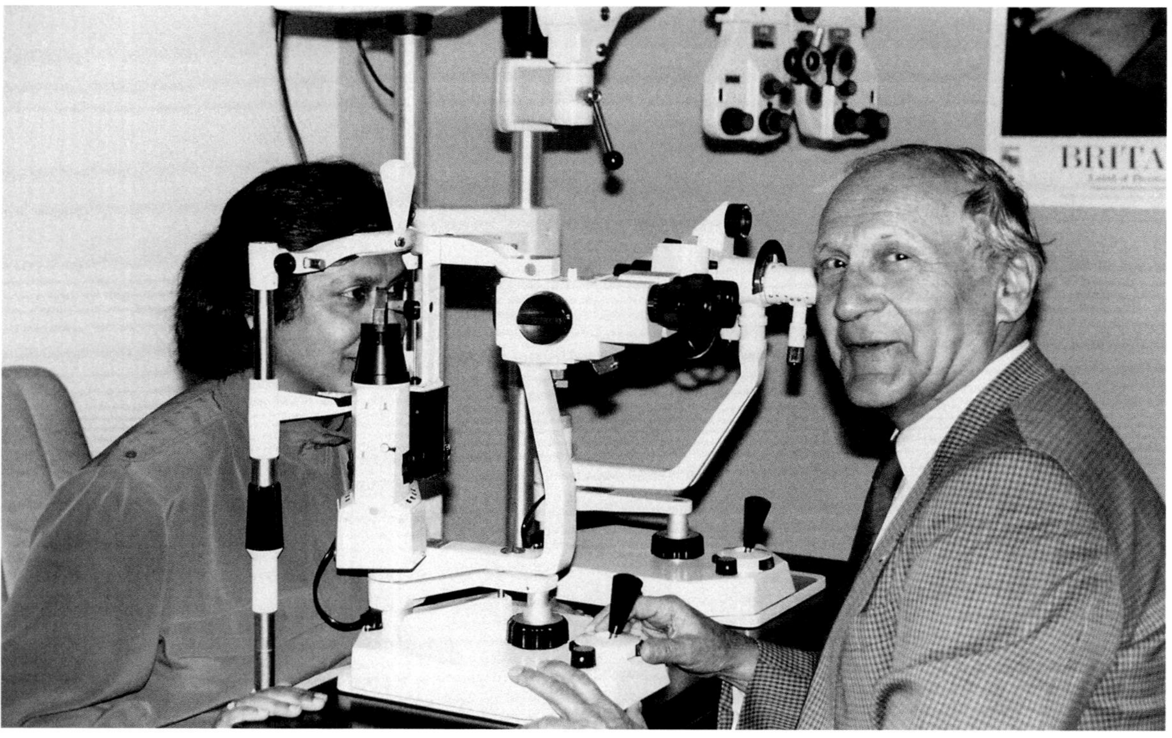

Darrach enabled a successful application for a Medical Research Council associateship that provided Smith with the means to relocate to the university department in 1966. Smith's research there eventually led to receipt of the 1993 Nobel Prize in Chemistry (shared with Kary Mullis, inventor of the polymerase chain reaction) for his work in developing site-directed mutagenesis, which has led to fundamental new diagnostic strategies and potential treatments for genetic diseases.

The School of Rehabilitation Medicine

Brock Fahrni was appointed the first Director of the School of Rehabilitation Medicine when it was founded in 1961. A clinical instructor in the Department of Medicine, he had a particularly strong interest in the care of the elderly and chronically disabled and some revolutionary ideas about their treatment. The school offered a combined course in physiotherapy and occupational therapy, initially as a certificate course in physical medicine therapy. A year later, it became a degree program, and eventually, in 1983, it evolved to offer separate BSc degrees in occupational therapy and physical therapy.

The Department of Ophthalmology

In 1963, Stephen Drance was recruited to pursue a practice focused on glaucoma and to establish departmental research. In 1965, under the leadership of Alfred Elliot (Head of Ophthalmology, 1961–73) and with support from the Canadian National Institute for the Blind and Leon J. Koerner, the Ophthalmology Research Unit was established in space leased from VGH, with Drance as director. Educated and trained in England, Drance had been appointed at the University of Saskatchewan from 1957 to 1963 under renowned medical dean J. Wendell MacLeod. He had implemented geographical full-time faculty appointments whereby the university collected the clinical billings of faculty members who, in return, were paid a reasonable salary to fulfill clinical, research, and teaching duties. Dean McCreary enthusiastically appointed Drance in Vancouver using this model. However, six years later, Drance discovered that he was the only faculty member subject to this system and insisted on changes to his compensation package. The failure of this early practice plan experiment presaged future faculty member resistance to practice plans within the UBC FoM, despite widespread adoption of such plans in other Canadian medical schools.

The Department of Pediatrics

Shortly after his appointment as Dean, McCreary recruited Sydney Israels, a Saskatchewan native and high achieving graduate of the University of Manitoba to be the head of pediatrics. Israels tackled the job with characteristic vigour and dedication, and in the course of his career made a lasting mark upon the institution he served so

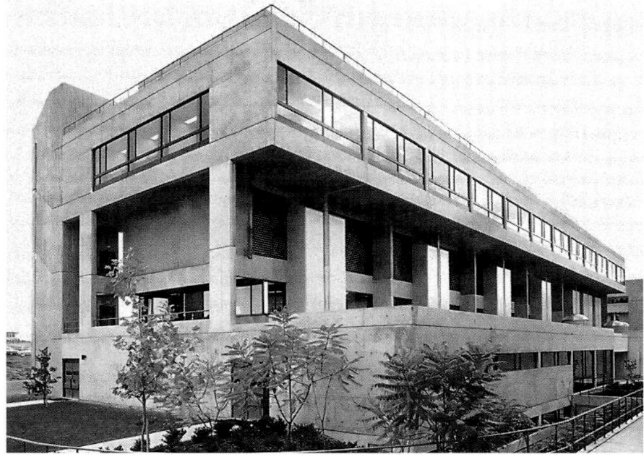

The Instructional Resources Centre, its architecture characteristic of the New Brutalism movement (opened 1972).

tirelessly. He made it his business to expand and strengthen the department, fortifying existing subspecialties and introducing many new ones. He also strongly encouraged research and fostered good relations with the community practitioners whom he involved in education as actively as he could. A number of patient care programs were instituted under his leadership, including parent participation in the care of sick children, interdisciplinary approaches to care of the chronically ill child, a fibrocystic clinic, an oncology program, and a program for identifying and preventing child abuse.

The Department of Obstetrics and Gynecology

Dr. Fred Bryans graduated from the University of Toronto and did postgraduate training at Toronto and Harvard and held a travelling fellowship in Europe for one year. After arriving in Vancouver in 1954, he became Head of the UBC department from 1959 to 1978. As Head, Bryans utilized his training in both basic sciences and clinical care to establish a strong department during the McCreary era by making strategic linkages to other academic units. This included Sidney Segal, a leading neonatologist; Betty Poland, who was a bridge to genetics and worked on the morphological causes of abortion; and Molly Towell, who was a hard-working researcher on the cardiovascular and respiratory effects of intrauterine hypoxia. Towell was a strong clinician as well, bringing the department into the emerging field of high-risk pregnancy and antenatal supervision and testing.

McCreary's Legacy

The McCreary years were marked by substantial growth in the young school. By 1972, the Faculty had moved from its primitive on-campus huts into modern basic sciences buildings, a state-of-the-art Woodward Medical Library, and a large although spartan Instructional Resources Centre, which was a part of McCreary's vision for comprehensive health sciences education and leadership. Opened in 1972, the IRC was built in juxtaposition to the Woodward Library and linked to it by a common atrium. The FoM had established its clinical teaching presence in VGH, the Children's Health Centre at VGH, St. Paul's Hospital, and in several family

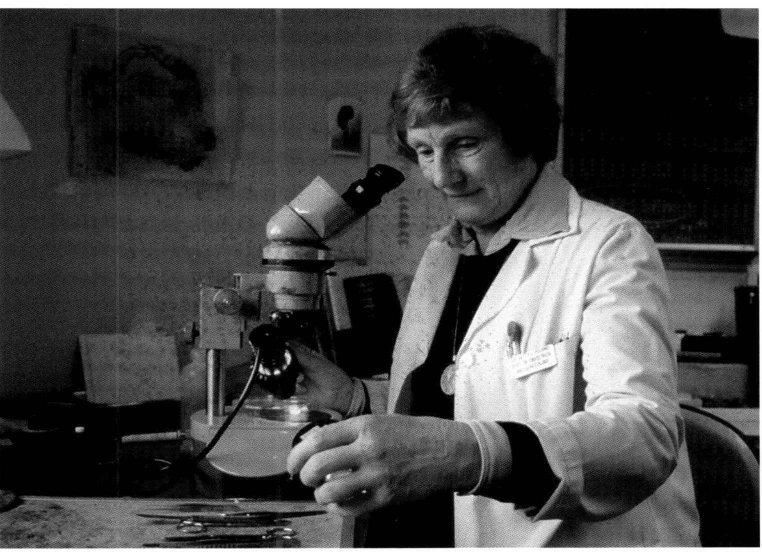

Betty Poland, obstetrician/gynecologist, embryologist, and geneticist.

practice clinical settings, but apart from the Heather Street academic wing at VGH, there was little additional formal space for faculty and students within the Vancouver teaching hospitals. Despite McCreary's sustained efforts to convince provincial and federal governments to fully pursue his concept of a major university teaching hospital and health sciences complex on the UBC campus, there had been little progress toward this goal. Only the Detwiller Pavilion (psychiatric care and neurosciences research) and the Purdy Pavilion (chronic care) had been built on campus. By 1972, the provincial government had only grudgingly agreed to a modest expansion of enrollment from sixty to eighty students in the first-year class and was only inching toward the funding of expanded facilities. Some of the major obstacles to the school's advancement remained to be dealt with. Nevertheless, fulfillment of many aspects of McCreary's vision would come with the dawn of the new millennium.

McCreary stepped down as Dean in 1972 but continued to serve as Coordinator of Health Sciences (having been appointed interim Director of Health Sciences in 1967 and then Coordinator of Health Sciences in 1970). Bill Webber, an associate dean, became acting dean for the next four months. Until his retirement in 1975, McCreary worked energetically to realize his vision for the integrated education of health professional students. Harold Copp succeeded McCreary as Coordinator of Health Sciences and was in turn succeeded by John Gilbert, who served until 2001 when the position evolved to that of Principal of the newly established College of Health Disciplines. McCreary's early death on October 14, 1979, occasioned an outpouring of grief, tributes, and affection. On May 16, 1980, the Honourable Patrick L. McGeer, by now provincial Minister of Universities, Science, and Communications together with the Honourable Monique Begin, federal Minister of Health, officiated at the naming of the John F. McCreary Health Sciences Centre on the UBC campus. The commemorative plaque remains in the IRC building.

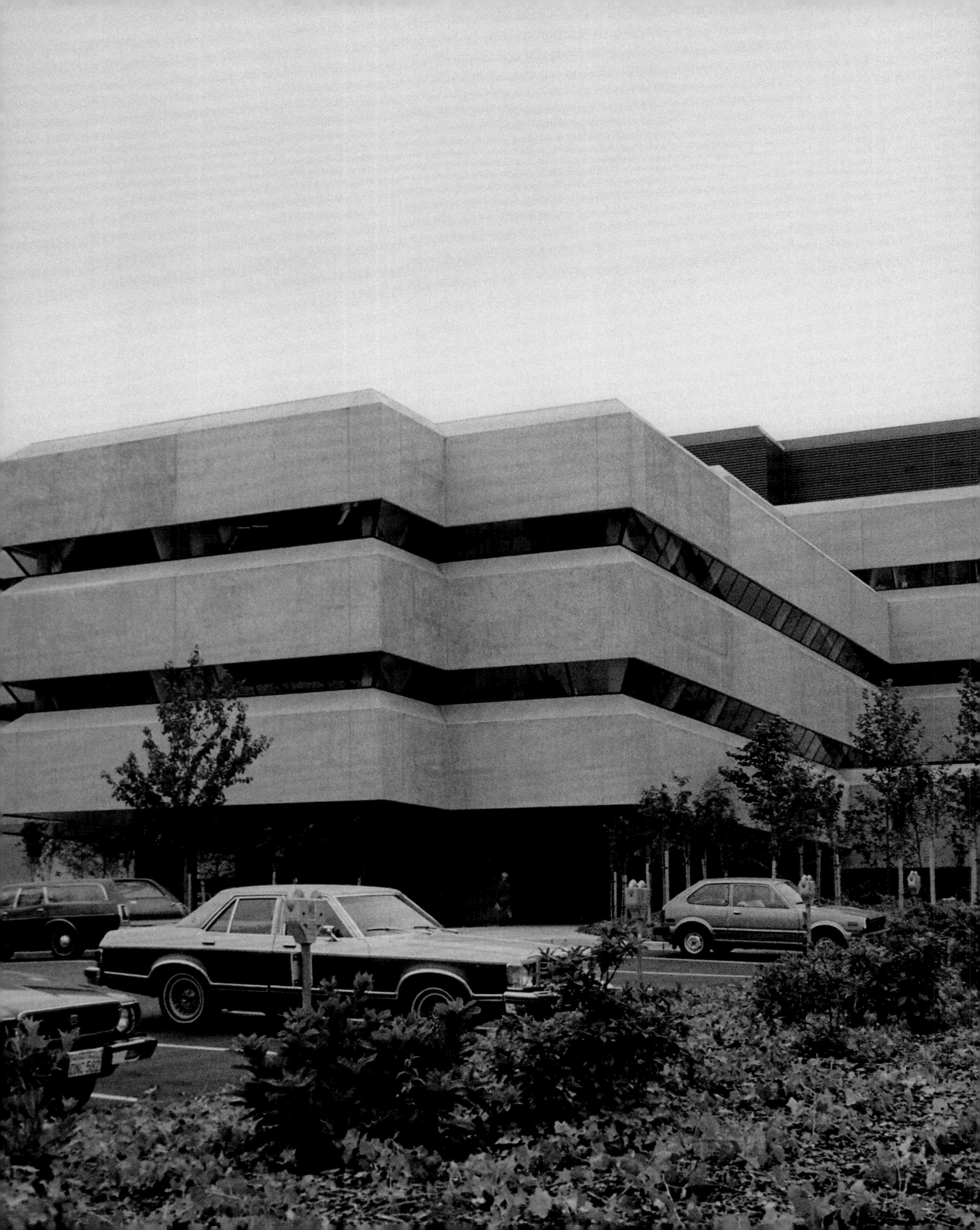

4

Coming into Its Own

1972–90

FACING Koerner Pavilion, UBC Hospital (opened 1980).

FACING Walter Gage, mathematician, sixth President of UBC (1969–75).

There was a sense among the UBC leadership that it was time for its young medical school to move beyond its humble beginnings to increased student enrollment, greater research stature, and wider national prominence.

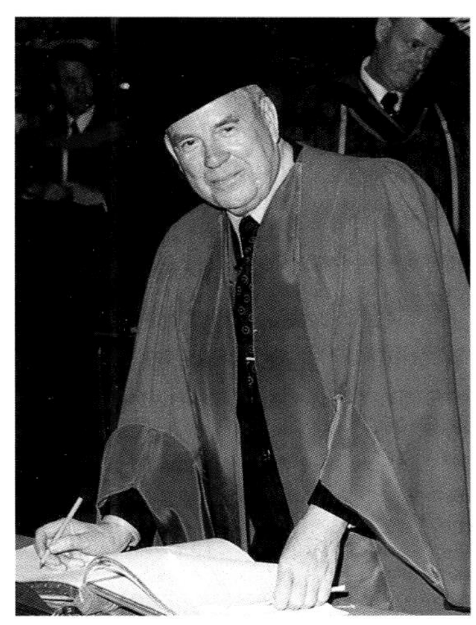

DAVID V. BATES became UBC's fourth Dean of Medicine in July 1972. Having attended Cambridge University and later worked at St. Bartholomew's Hospital in London, he joined McGill University's Faculty of Medicine in 1956. He had become Head of the Department of Physiology in 1967 and later director of the respiratory division of the Royal Victoria and Montreal Children's hospitals. He was one of Canada's leading respirologists and had established a reputation as a highly accomplished clinician-scientist. There was a sense among the UBC leadership that it was time for its young medical school to move beyond its humble beginnings to increased student enrollment, greater research stature, and wider national prominence. Bates appeared to be the ideal individual to lead the FoM toward this loftier vision.

During his recruitment, Bates laid out for UBC president Walter Gage his broad objectives: 1) receipt from Ottawa of BC's share of the Health Resources Fund (established by the Pearson government in 1966 for the support of developing medical schools); 2) expansion of the first-year class to around one hundred; and 3) growth and academic development of the full-time faculty.

To assist him in the Faculty's missions while he focused on these strategic undertakings, Bates retained McCreary appointees Associate Dean of Continuing Medical Education Donald Williams, Associate Dean of Admissions Donald Graham, and Associate Dean Bill Webber (associate dean of everything else, or "odds and ends" as Webber described it). He soon created additional portfolios, appointing popular clinician and teacher Roland Lauener, based at the VGH, as Associate Dean of the Undergraduate Medical Curriculum and David Lirenman as Associate Dean of Residency Education and assigning research responsibilities to Bill Webber.

A New Plan for Hospital Development

Bates believed that McCreary's vision of a university hospital on the UBC campus, discussed for many years with the Social Credit government, would come to fruition under his own deanship. Mere months after his arrival, and to the amazement of local pundits and most UBC faculty members, after almost twenty years in power, the Social Credit party was defeated by the New Democratic Party in September 1972. McCreary's vision for medical developments on the UBC campus was immediately put on hold.

The contrasting NDP vision was eventually revealed by Minister of Health Dennis Cocke in the spring of 1974 during a lunch with Bates and President Walter Gage. Cocke declared that at a

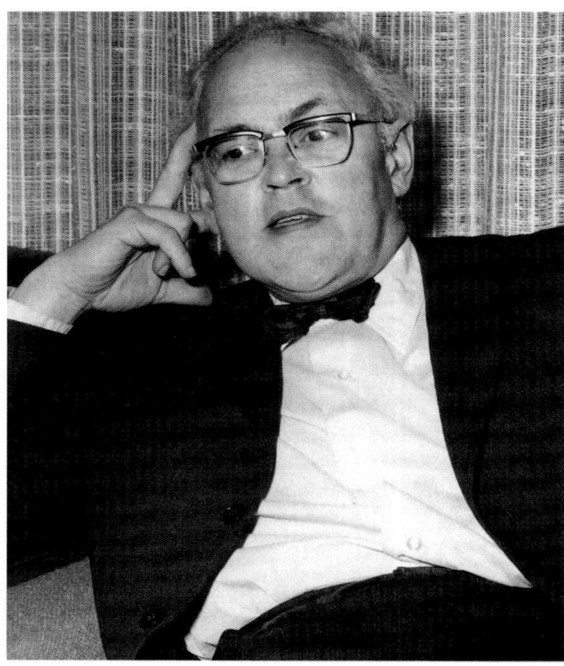

David Bates, respirologist, fourth Dean of Medicine (1972–77).

press conference later that afternoon he planned to announce the establishment of a huge new British Columbia Medical Centre (BCMC), under the chairmanship of logging executive and NDP friend Jack Christensen. It was to be built not on the UBC campus but at the site of the Shaughnessy Veterans Hospital, about three kilometres south of VGH and ten kilometres from the campus. Not only that, but the government was planning to fund an increase in the number of first-year medical class places to 260, up from the current 80 (he modified this to 160 when Bates convinced him that 260 was not feasible). Although McCreary's concept of a campus-based major teaching hospital appeared to have been cast aside, Bates saw enormous opportunity in the provincial government's vision.

Renowned West Coast architect Arthur Erickson drew up a revolutionary design for a splendid complex of four hospitals joined at the centre with a gallery of glass, boutiques, and coffee shops. There were to be seven hundred general beds, a new children's hospital, and a new women's facility. Bates remained enthusiastic, but a majority of the academic and clinical faculty had strong misgivings about the unrealistic nature of the grand design, mistrusting the large and growing bureaucracy. As projected capital and operating costs soared, local politicians had begun to question the wisdom of the ambitious plan. By January of 1975, the pace of planning for the centre was already slowing down, and in July the Greater Vancouver Regional Health District voted to oppose immediate construction on the site. In the autumn 1975 election, the NDP was resoundingly defeated. In December, the renewed Social Credit party, now led by Bill Bennett, son of the fabled W.A.C. Bennett, took the reins of government. BCMC office staff and over three hundred volunteers in the midst of the three-year development program were stunned when the new health minister, Bob McClelland, announced at a press conference in March 1976 that the project was to be abolished.

On June 4 to 6, 1975, the twenty-fifth anniversary of the entry of UBC's first students into the Faculty of Medicine had been marked by a three-day symposium on future patterns of health care, the future of medical education, and science policy and medical research. At the symposium, William Gibson noted that the entire research budget of the school amounted to $5 million per year. A panel of distinguished scientists encouraged the UBC Faculty of Medicine to embrace a bold vision of focused research. One speaker, Sir Richard Doll, applauded the appointment in the UK of a chief scientist in order to ensure that the "right questions" were being asked in the health system and that the academy could work to provide the answers for the system. This was a prescient comment in the Canadian context, as it would be several more decades before Prime Minister Justin Trudeau established the office of a chief science advisor.

In his address at the symposium, Dean Bates lauded the considerable progress that had been made since the Faculty's shaky beginnings, but had to lament the ongoing physical separation of clinical and basic science departments, the dearth of resources to support geographic full-time faculty and research, and the short-staffed teaching hospitals. This lamentation appeared to be even more relevant by the spring of 1976.

How to proceed after these developments? At this critical juncture, the Faculty of Medicine now had a key ally in government: Pat McGeer, a graduate of UBC's medical school and an accomplished neuroscientist and UBC faculty member. He had been elected as a Liberal, but perceiving that he would have more influence as a cabinet minister for the Social Credit government, he switched parties to become BC's Minister of Education. He realized that British Columbia's sizeable portion of the Health Resources Fund remained unclaimed after ten years. Ottawa now had decided to close out the fund and required the province to claim it within three months or see it disappear altogether. McGeer issued an ultimatum to the university: come up with a plan for the campus hospital in sixty days, or lose the funding.

In March of 1976, UBC President Douglas Kenny appointed a troika of prominent faculty members (Stephen Drance, Head of Ophthalmology; Bill Webber, Associate Dean; and Morton Low, an acting associate dean) to create a new plan, in effect to become informal designers of the long overdue facilities. Their eventual proposal, including an increase in the size of the medical class, went forward with the agreement of all the organizations they had consulted, if not some of the individuals. The FoM and the Senate approved the proposal, and the VGH, as the primary teaching hospital, and the Vancouver Medical Association, representing the practicing medical profession, jointly lent their support.

The Appointment of John Dirks as Head of Medicine

Bates had recognized early on that an issue requiring immediate attention was leadership of the Department of Medicine, usually the largest and most academically accomplished of departments in a faculty of medicine. The most recent Royal College-Medical Research Council review had concluded that the department had not kept pace with advances in modern medical education, noting that some long-standing members of the department had

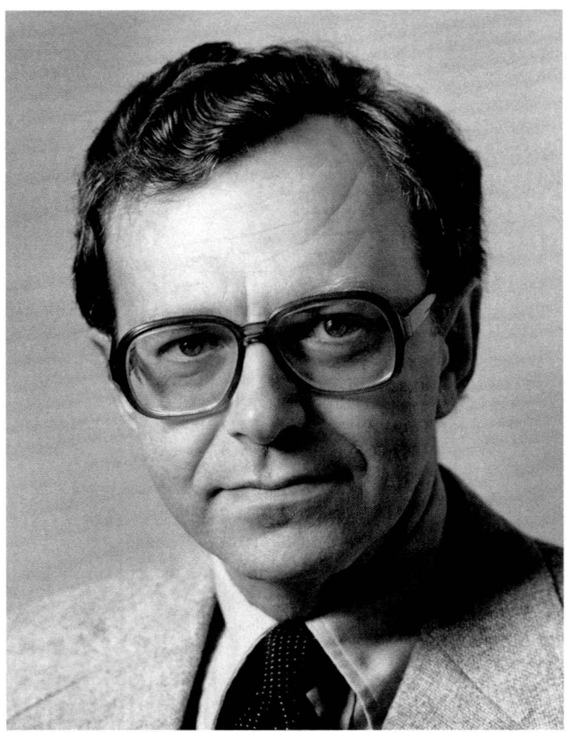

John Dirks, nephrologist, Head of Department of Medicine (1976–87).

not been put on tenure track and that there was very little meaningful research being done. Still under its original head, Bob Kerr, more than two decades since the founding of the FoM, the Department of Medicine was in urgent need of leadership renewal.

The search proved to be long and challenging, but eventually the search committee recommended well-known Toronto cardiologist Douglas Wigle, boosting the morale of academic clinicians hoping for a new dynamism in this key department. Wigle took up his new position in 1974, but the aspirations of local faculty and potential returnees to Vancouver were dashed when he abruptly reneged within weeks of his arrival. He returned to Toronto, claiming anxiety about the real estate situation and other financial matters. There were many who believed that an important determinant of the failed appointment was the magnitude of the challenge of bringing the department to national stature.

Planning for expansion of capital facilities and enrollment were important foci throughout Bates's term, but he also worked hard to raise the academic stature of the FoM. Although finding a new head of medicine was a top priority, the appointment was not made until almost four years after Bates had highlighted the need and almost two years since the abortive Wigle appointment. The academic issues had become even more evident. In 1976, the department had few formal divisions, with most subspecialties subsumed by the Division of General Internal Medicine. It commanded very limited space, conducted minimal research, and had only twenty-three full-time faculty members and about six percent of the total Faculty budget, unusually low for a department commonly the largest in any medical school. Attending physicians and clinical instructors were, for the most part, inclined to regard the university as peripheral to their activities.

In April 1976, John Dirks became the Head of Medicine. A native of Winnipeg and a graduate of the University of Manitoba, he had developed his Division of Nephrology at McGill's Royal Victoria Hospital into one of the strongest in North America. Known to be exacting and uncompromising, Dirks had the requisite thick skin for success as an outsider thrust into an onerous job. As UBC's Head of Medicine, Dirks was also to be Head of the Department of Medicine of VGH, despite some objection among the hospital's clinicians to the idea of bringing in an outsider. Dirks had also been alerted by Bates

McGeer issued an ultimatum to the University: come up with a plan for the campus hospital in sixty days or lose the funding.

William "Bill" Webber, anatomist (UBC MD '58), fifth Dean of Medicine (1977–90).

LEFT FACING William "Bill" Hurlburt, internist, Head, SPH Department of Medicine (1952–77).

RIGHT FACING James Hogg, Pulmonary Pathology Researcher.

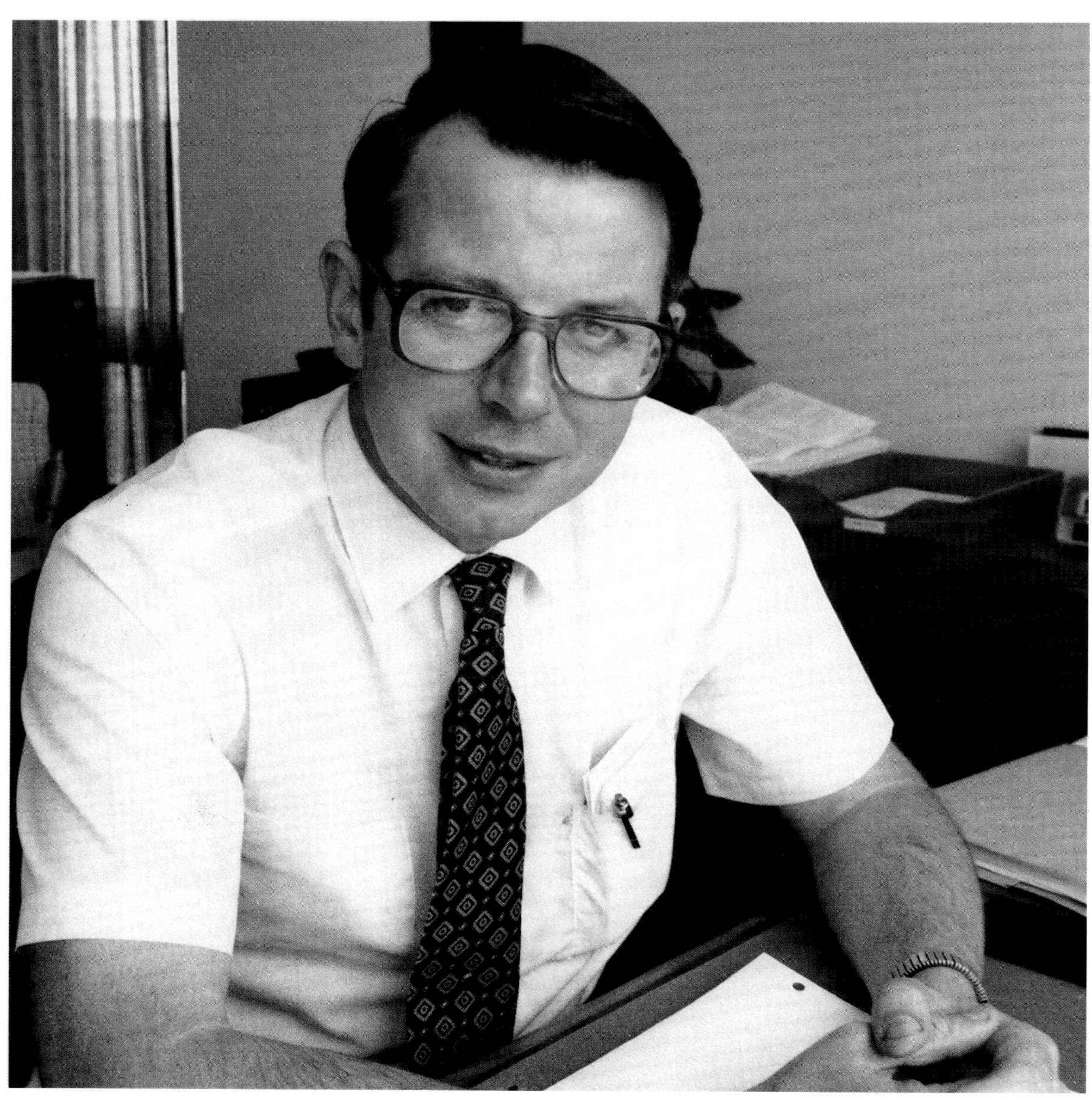

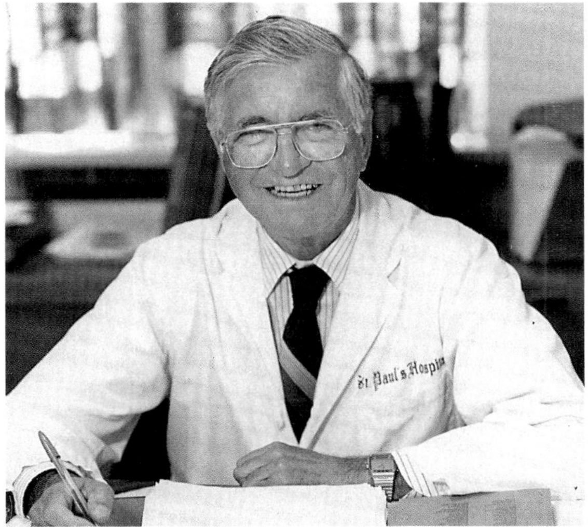

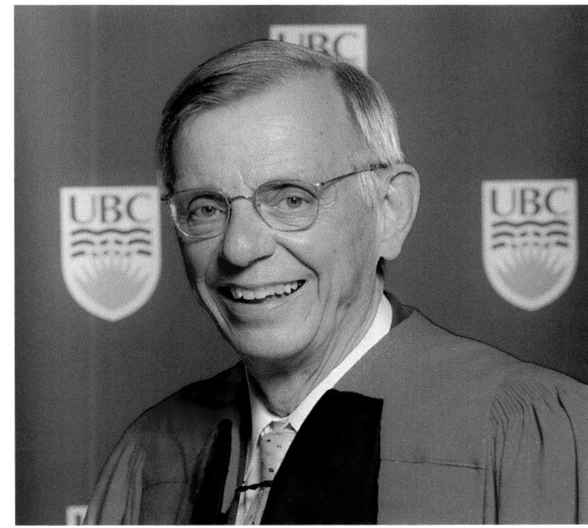

of the long and persisting hostilities between the VGH and the medical school and the absence of an affiliation agreement between the two institutions.

One of his first acts was to appoint Max Walters as chief of cardiology in the hopes of bringing the VGH cardiology service into the UBC Department of Medicine. An exemplary physician who inspired his students, Walters had built a strong clinical division with all the facilities necessary to handle angiography and various other diagnostic and therapeutic procedures. Donald Ricci (UBC MD '70) remembers Walters for his elegant three-piece suit, white shirt, and cuff links; his total command of clinical cardiology; and his warm bedside manner. The Walters appointment was well received, but unfortunately Dirks's single-minded pursuit of academic goals and his idealistic vision were perceived as impractical and high-handed, and progress was turbulent and slow.

At St. Paul's Hospital, Head of Medicine Bill Hurlburt, very supportive of Dirks, had struggled to establish a strong clinical education program which had become popular with students, but the hospital department conducted virtually no research. Hurlburt had strengthened clinical respirology in the early 1970s with the recruitment of Richard "Dick" Donovan from McGill and Graham Copeland from Toronto. In 1977, James Hogg, one of the country's leading pulmonary pathologists and a former colleague of Bates and Dirks at McGill, along with his younger respirologist colleague, Peter Paré, were recruited, marking a turning point in the academic affairs of St. Paul's Hospital. Although these developments initially caused tensions with the VGH respirology group under Stefan Grzybowski, it became apparent that the two groups would be complementary, and research thrived in both.

Bill Webber Becomes Dean

The government commitments to extensive new clinical and academic facilities and further expansion of medical school enrollment were secured during Bates's tenure as dean but would be realized only during the term of his successor. In 1977, Bates stepped down early from his deanship after only five years. There were those who felt that he had failed to gain the trust of many of the clinical faculty who accused him of being naive and inconsistent in his dealings with them. Stephen Drance felt Bates would have made a wonderful dean in a university where there was already a tradition of excellence and quality, in contrast to circumstances in UBC's still young medical school. Having sustained his expertise in respiratory research during his deanship, Bates took on the headship of the Division of Respiratory Medicine, his studies on air pollution gained momentum, he served on a variety of expert environmental panels, and in 2002 he received the Order of Canada. He continued to live in Vancouver as an emeritus professor until his death in 2006. The David Bates Memorial Lecture in occupational and environmental health has continued annually since that time in the UBC School of Population and Public Health.

By the time Bates stepped down, the Vancouver medical community and the Faculty of Medicine were in turmoil. The changing roles of various city hospitals and lingering questions about the appropriate degree of influence a medical school should exert on the activities within them posed problems for administrators of all the institutions involved. Tensions between hospital staff and university faculty were evident, as were significant ill feelings toward the dean's office on the part of some clinical faculty who did not respect Bates and resisted the relentless and sometimes insensitive efforts of Dirks to bring the Department of Medicine into the Canadian academic mainstream. It was essential that the next dean be a conciliator and communicator of the first order, someone who could look at problems with a calm and objective view and work out compromises which would allow development to move ahead without alienating any of the important players in the increasingly complex enterprise of medical education in the province. Such a mediator was already present in the person of William A. Webber.

Having graduated in 1958 with the Hamber Medal at the top of his medical class—UBC's fifth—and following his internship at VGH and research training at Cornell University, Webber had returned to UBC as an assistant professor of anatomy in 1961. An outstanding and much-loved teacher, he had demonstrated his administrative acumen early in his academic career, steadfastly serving the Faculty in a number of capacities over the following two decades, most recently as acting dean prior to Bates's arrival and then as associate dean. Although little known on the national and international stage, Webber was respected at UBC for his deep understanding of its workings, personalities, and bureaucracy. An articulate spokesperson for the academic mission, he was noted for his open-minded and statesmanlike approach to controversial issues.

As a basic scientist rather than a practicing physician, Webber was not regarded as the most appropriate appointee to the deanship by some members of the BC Medical Association and a minor town-versus-gown brouhaha erupted at the news of his appointment. With characteristic goodwill and

David Hardwick, pediatric pathologist (UBC MD '57), Head of Department of Pathology (1976–90), Associate Dean of Research and Institutional Planning (1990–96).

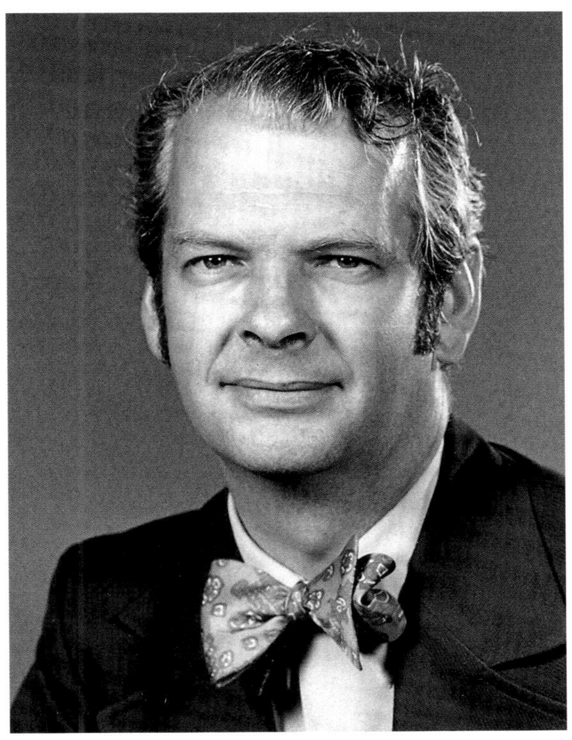

deft political skills, Webber made it his business to introduce himself early and often to the BCMA's executive, maintaining as direct a link with the organization as he could, attending their annual meetings and discussing common concerns. He came to feel familiar with the issues of clinical, or "town," medicine.

Webber identified three important aspects of his mandate. First, the continuing low number of BC graduates from the Faculty of Medicine relative to the population meant that it was important to expand the undergraduate enrollment, which had risen to eighty under Bates and was due to increase to 160. Second, the dearth of space and facilities for medical education, especially in the clinical departments, pointed to the need for development of the acute care component of the campus hospital, now in the early stages of construction but still in need of considerable organizational planning. And third, new academic space at the teaching hospitals and in the basic science buildings was warranted by the expanded enrollment and essential for enlarging the Faculty base and enhancing research capability. After discussions with new university president Douglas Kenny, Webber felt that he had the support of the administration to follow through on his ideas about expansion and development.

The inimitable bow-tied David Hardwick, a graduate of UBC's fourth medical class (1957), was a close friend of Bill Webber and a key strategic colleague throughout his deanship. His counsel proved to be a resource to all subsequent deans. He had been appointed to the Department of Pathology in 1965, and on the departure of Harold "Hal" Taylor in 1966, he took over the MD undergraduate pathology course, restructuring and codifying it into an educational program which ran for over thirty years. He became Head of Pathology in 1976 (to 1990), but his influence came to be felt far beyond his discipline. Seeing himself as a teacher, a social activist, and a researcher, he was elected to the UBC Senate and was appointed as faculty advisor to UBC presidents, for many years furthering FoM interests and working with legal advisors in the president's office. Hardwick's ongoing mission within the Faculty was to ensure that people understood the dynamic of the social system in which they worked and to create administrative structures that are coherent with the social culture and offer cooperative relationships amongst institutions.

St. Paul's Hospital, Vancouver. View from Burrard St., with the foreground showing all permanent structures and additions up to 1960. Phase I Providence Wing (left background) (opened 1983) and Phase II Providence Tower (centre background) (opened 1991).

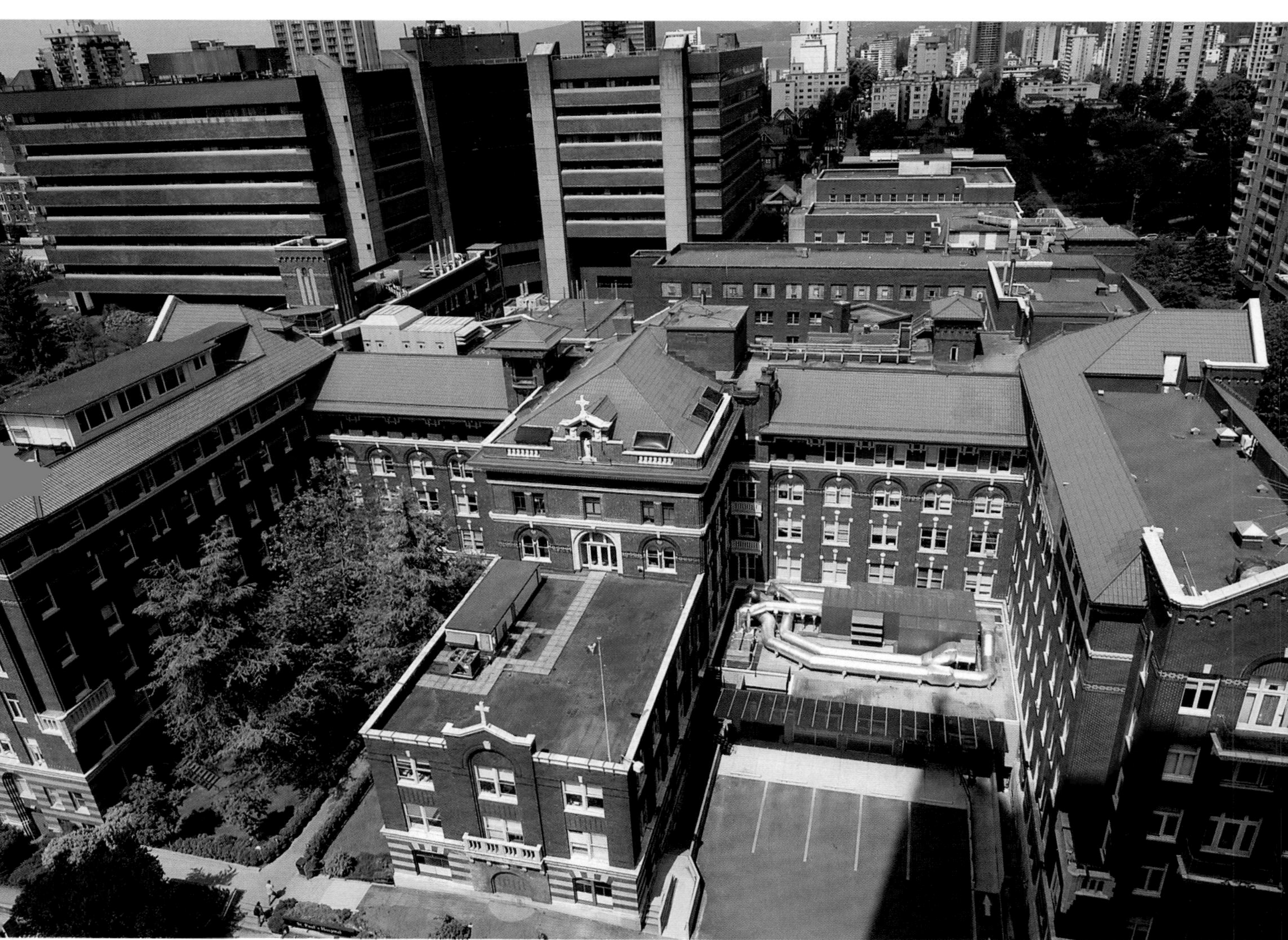

Despite an increase in the first-year class size to eighty in 1972, BC continued to have by far the lowest number of medical students per capita of any province, as short-sighted provincial governments had been able to opt out of the responsibility for educating their own doctors. The pre-emptory announcement of expansion to 160 by Minister Cocke in 1974 was recognized as unrealistic, but the class size did reach 120 by 1980. Still, British Columbia did not train physicians in proportion to its needs. Although the province's natural attractions drew large numbers of physicians from outside, many from foreign shores, to practice for varying lengths of time in communities throughout the province, there were serious shortages in rural areas. There was ongoing disagreement among politicians, journalists, and citizens about the need for increasing the class size. Incredibly, enrollment did not increase again for a further twenty years.

New Facilities and Buildings

BC's share of the federal Health Resources Fund became available as the provincial government began to act on the recommendations of UBC president Kenny's advisory committee in 1976. The final package from the provincial government comprised a new two-hundred-bed, $30-million children's hospital, new facilities on the Shaughnessy site for a women's hospital near the Grace Obstetrical Hospital, more money for academic facilities at the VGH, expansion of academic facilities in a new clinical building at St. Paul's Hospital (henceforth to have a more important role in the FoM), and, at long last, money to build a 280-bed acute care hospital on the UBC campus. The agreement to increase the class size went hand in hand with the long-sought but hitherto elusive growth in clinical and teaching space.

Hardwick had been influential in persuading Deputy Minister Walter Hardwick (his older brother) and Minister McGeer not to channel all of the Health Resources Fund money to the campus hospital, but to allocate significant amounts to the Laurel Street development at the VGH, the BC Children's Hospital, the Grace Maternity Hospital, and St. Paul's. Following the release of the health resources funds, planning and action resumed in earnest. In 1982, academic space became available at the new BC Children's Hospital and the Grace Maternity Hospital. New clinical areas were developed at St. Paul's and the new BC Cancer Control Agency (now known as BC Cancer). As the population of veterans declined, some space in the Shaughnessy Hospital was designated for research, and a family practice teaching unit was started there.

Philanthropy allowed the construction of the first phase of the Jack Bell Research Centre at the

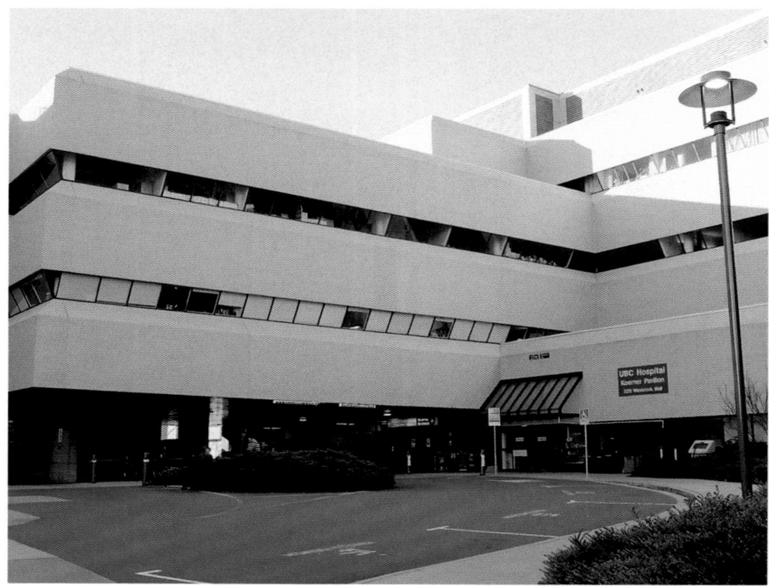

Koerner Pavilion (opened 1980).

VGH site and in 1983 the Eye Care Centre. The three basic sciences buildings on the Point Grey Campus were substantially enlarged, and a 250-seat lecture theatre was added to the existing five lecture halls in the Instructional Resources Centre, which had first opened in 1972 as part of McCreary's vision for comprehensive health sciences education and leadership.

The Koerner Pavilion

The long-awaited campus-based hospital which opened in 1980 was a far cry from McCreary's vision of a seven-hundred-bed university teaching hospital, but the government and many practicing physicians felt that a community hospital of modest size best fit provincial needs. Key philanthropic support from the Leon and Thea Koerner Foundation and Walter Koerner's particular interest in the medical school were appropriately acknowledged when the acute care unit was named for him when it opened in 1980. The opening was marked by an international symposium, which embodied the growing optimism within the medical school. The acute care unit and research facility, so long the dream of those who wished for a truly academic centre for teaching medical practice, was now a reality, awaiting only the bustle of some first-rate investigators within its walls to fulfill its promise.

Laboratory and teaching spaces in the new hospital were adjacent to clinical areas; it was designed to incorporate educational and research roles within its primary function of providing patient care. Pursuing McCreary's vision of training health professionals together, Medical Director George Price and Hospital Director Lloyd Detwiller were enthusiastic that the design would allow all health sciences students the opportunity to see patients not only in hospital beds but also in nearby outpatient offices. Doctors with admitting privileges understood that their patients were to be available for teaching purposes.

To avoid duplication of services offered at other city hospitals, the plan was to emphasize general medicine and surgery. It would become the major treatment and research centre in gastroenterology,

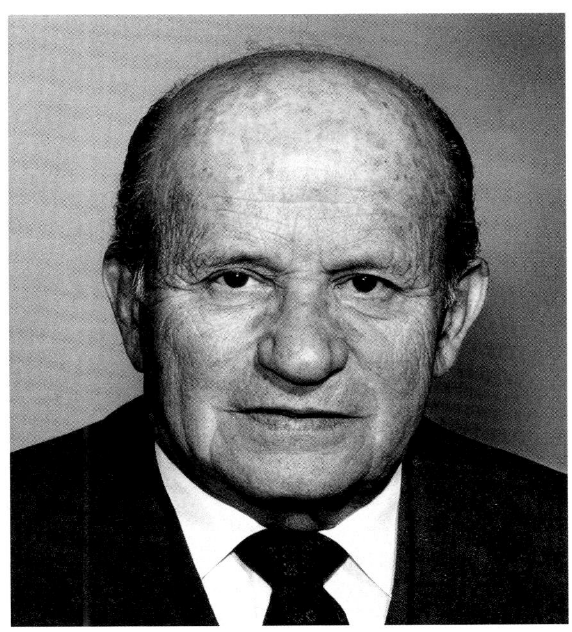

Walter Koerner, philanthropist.

metabolism/endocrinology, neurology, drug metabolism, sports medicine, hospital dentistry, and some vascular surgery. Cardiac surgery; eye, ear, nose, and throat surgery; neurosurgery; and obstetrics would not be provided.

Uniquely, the discipline of sports medicine flourished on the Point Grey Campus during this time. In 1979, doctors Jack Taunton, Don McKenzie, and Doug Clement established the Allan McGavin Sports Medicine Clinic in close collaboration with the new acute care hospital. The sports medicine program would eventually offer graduate and postgraduate educational programs under the auspices of Family Medicine, Orthopaedics, Medicine, Physical Therapy, and others. In 1985, as part of community engagement, Doug Clement and his wife, Dianne (both Canadian Olympians), together with Jack Taunton and his wife, Cheryl, started the Vancouver Sun Run, which is now Canada's largest and most influential 10K run annually. Several decades later, in 2018, the sports clinic, together with the Centre for Physical Activity and Exercise Medicine, would move into the new Chan Gunn Pavilion on the Point Grey Campus.

The faculty members based on the UBC campus were for the most part young, energetic, enthusiastic, and happy to have the opportunity to start something fresh in the early phases of their careers. John Fleetham, at the time a thirty-year-old new recruit from Manitoba to the Division of Respiratory Medicine, recalls the opening days when the hospital contained only four patients and four residents. There were huge demands on faculty time to set up wards, labs, and offices–an opportunity unlikely to occur more than once in a lifetime. In an inspired move, Dirks promoted Max Walters from Head of Cardiology at VGH to Head of Medicine at the Koerner. Walters's community stature and clear commitment to the success of the new facility were critical to its development.

The establishment of the campus hospital initially increased the tensions among the teaching hospitals; this new player in the mix meant a greater threat to perceived territorial imperatives. The Council of University Teaching Hospitals (COUTH) was created in the early 1980s; the leadership comprised six hospital CEOs and the Dean. Webber saw it as a forum in which to work out compromises, to find courses of action which would be equally beneficial, and to appoint Faculty department heads from hospitals other than the VGH exclusively, thereby fostering a greater institutional sense of involvement with UBC.

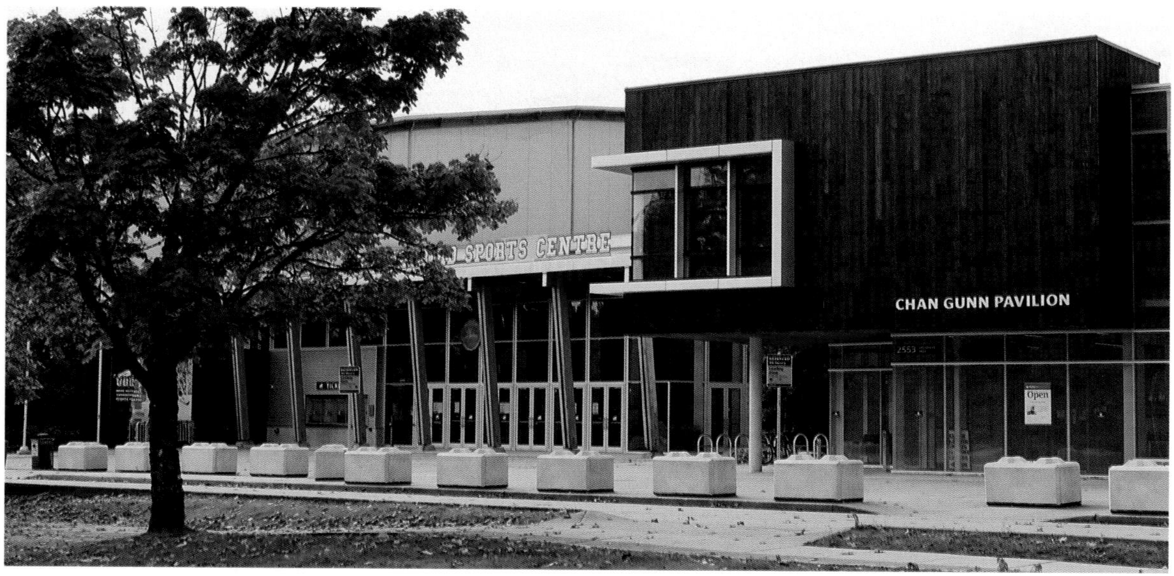

The BC Children's Hospital and Variety Research Centre

The BC Children's Hospital opened on the Shaughnessy site in 1982, after decades of gradual, disjointed expansion: the Children's Hospital on 59th Avenue (1933; later to become the centre for chronic care and developmental pediatrics), the Health Centre for Children at the VGH site (1954), and small services at St. Paul's and Mount Saint Joseph hospitals. All pediatric services moved from the VGH to the new site, designated as the provincial centre for tertiary pediatric care.

Rob Hill, head of pediatrics at this critical transitional time (1977-87), recalled that during the planning the government bureaucrats had no understanding of the needs of an advanced tertiary care pediatric teaching institution. They could not comprehend why the kind of facility envisioned by professionals required anything other than the standard hospital equipment used elsewhere in the province. An adequately sized, separate pediatric emergency department seemed an unnecessary frill to the government planners. Future needs for ambulatory space and pediatric services seemed beyond their vision.

The only funding for education infrastructure was approximately $2 million diverted from the Health Resources Fund allocations for the campus hospital and amounting to about four percent of the total projected cost—far less than what was needed. Ministry of Health officials refused to consider funding anything that might be deemed "academic" space, such as seminar rooms or libraries, despite the fact that in order to be accredited, all provincial hospitals needed conference rooms and libraries. The final design was fraught with concessions and inefficiencies. Nearby residents demanded a long, low profile resulting in lengthy corridors and widely distant service areas; two distinct government ministries would not fund the academic and service missions in a coordinated manner, leading to confusion as to the source of funding for furniture and equipment; the emergency room and academic space were less than adequate; and there was no room for the needs of residents and medical students.

FACING Chan Gunn Pavilion, UBC Point Grey campus (opened 2018).

TOP BC Women's Hospital, originally opened in 1982 as the new Grace Hospital.

BOTTOM BC Children's Hospital (opened 1982).

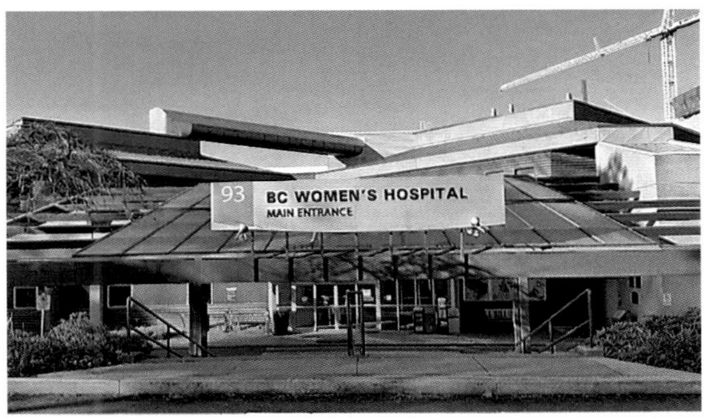

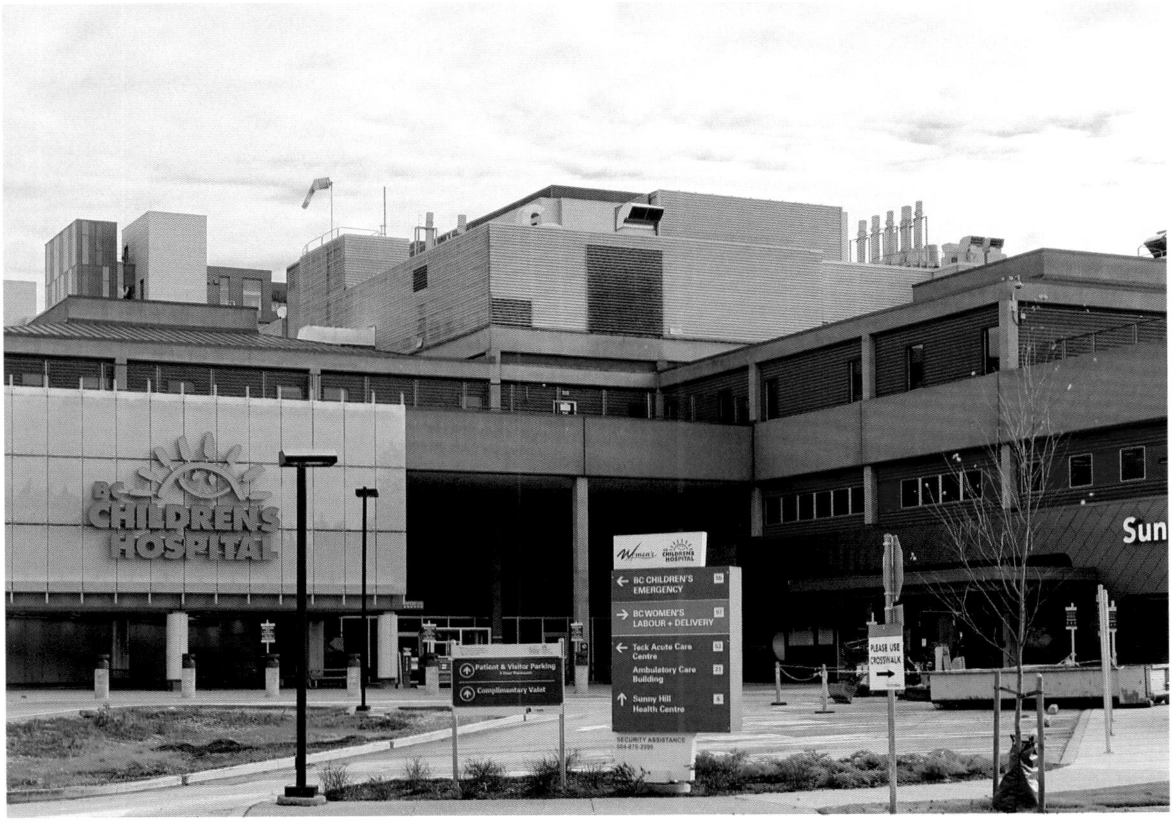

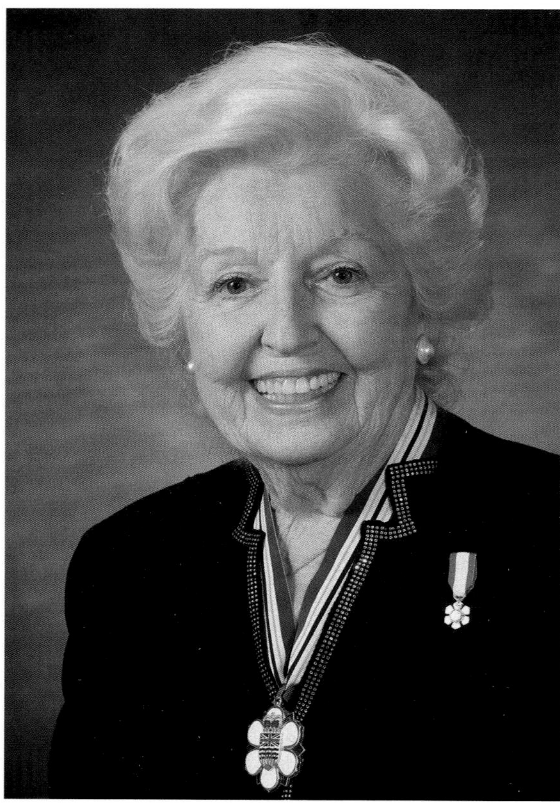

Grace McCarthy, MLA (1966–72, 1975–91), Cabinet Minister of BC Legislature, and supporter of BC Children's Hospital.

LEFT FACING Clyde Slade, internist and psychiatrist, inaugural Head of Division of Primary Care of Department of Health Care and Epidemiology (1967–78).

RIGHT FACING Peter Grantham, family physician (UBC MD '58), inaugural Head of Department of Family Practice (1978–88).

The previously established Health Centre Society became the new BC Children's Hospital Foundation to raise funds and public support for the important research component of the pediatric health centre. When the Variety Club organizations became convinced of the benefits of supporting a pediatric research facility, the new foundation and the faculty were happy to join forces. After local MLA Grace McCarthy, a strong supporter, used her influence to overcome Shaughnessy Hospital's jurisdictional claims over buildings on the site, the government approved construction of a research building. The Children's Variety Research Centre opened in 1985, a superb facility and a striking contrast to the neighbouring hospital, not only in the story of its relatively painless development but also in the exemplary and functional structure it became.

Department Developments, New Stars, and Research Breakthroughs

By the early 1980s, the facilities were less primitive and more in keeping with health and research centres in other major Canadian cities. With money available from the class expansion, it became feasible to recruit strong personnel and to develop the academic strengths not only of the key Department of Medicine, but in many other disciplines.

The Department of Family Practice

Whereas primary care in many other Canadian provinces was often provided by specialists chosen directly by their patients, in BC a more appropriate model had developed in which a general practitioner is a patient's first contact when health issues arise and may refer the patient to a specialist as required. Yet, somewhat surprisingly, for many years family practice had no formal departmental status in the FoM.

In 1967, Clyde Slade, a certified internist and psychiatrist, had been appointed in the Department of Health Care and Epidemiology to head the new Division of Primary Care. In 1969, he and McCreary had recruited Al Boggie, a member of the first UBC medical class, to move from Vernon to Vancouver to establish a family practice residency program centred at the VGH. In 1973, the Department of Health

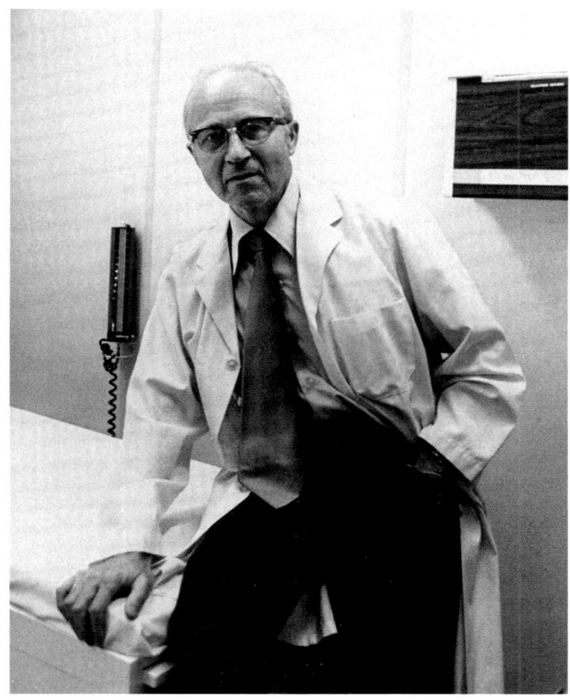

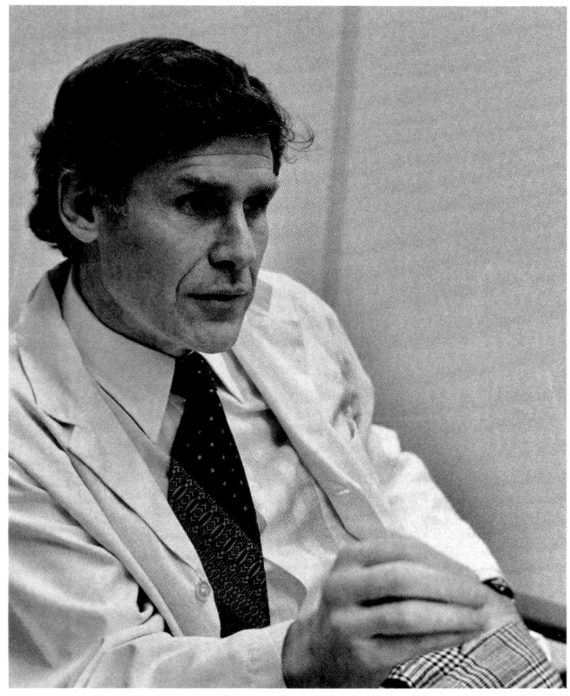

Care and Epidemiology and its Division of Primary Care moved into the new James Mather Building on the UBC campus.

Over considerable opposition in the UBC Senate, Dean Bates had advocated for the creation of a Department of Family Practice. Slade was able to persuade the Royal Canadian Legion to endow a chair of family practice, and the new department was launched in 1978 with Peter Grantham as the inaugural Head. Grantham was somewhat uneasy about his lack of an academic background, but remembering with consternation his years as a medical undergraduate at UBC having not a single encounter with a general practitioner, he was motivated to tackle the challenge. The establishment of the department recognized the body of knowledge unique to those who were generalists, who took care of people in the context of families and communities, and whose focus was broader than that of the specialist.

Grantham and Boggie sought to expose the residents to a much wider variety of conditions by placing them not only in the VGH and UBC campus family practice facilities, but also in the innovative REACH Centre, a university-based outreach clinic which provided pediatric, adolescent, and family health care in a setting with a combination of medical, dental, social, and educational services for its multiethnic patient community. The REACH Centre is still active on Commercial Drive, and the UBC campus unit is now located on University Boulevard. In 1981, Mark Longhurst, a practitioner in Revelstoke who had obtained his master's degree in education, began to transform the family practice residency program. Boggie had initiated obstetrical and pediatric experiences for family practice residents in Vernon and Kelowna, and Longhurst now established a formal rural practice program.

In 1982, Carol Herbert, a 1969 graduate of UBC's medical school, joined the department. She had

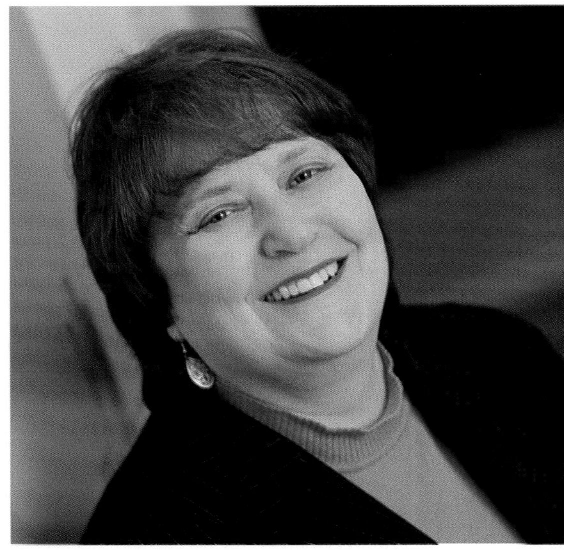

Carol Herbert, family physician (UBC MD '69), Head of Department of Family Practice (1988–98).

been tempted to pursue a career in biochemistry and later to specialize in pediatrics but had found her true calling in the people-oriented discipline of family medicine. As a busy physician and clinical instructor at REACH, she became a passionate voice for the view of medicine as patient-centred. She initiated the department's research program and developed the Division of Behavioural Medicine and the Sexual Assault Service, initially at Shaughnessy and then at VGH. Based on the experiences of Herbert and others who had worked in the trenches, a variety of changes in the medical school curriculum were introduced to enhance the psycho-social perspectives of the program, with a stronger emphasis on communication skills and the doctor-patient relationship.

Since 1982, the Department of Family Practice has also trained doctors for rural practice through its community-based residency training program. The family practice postgraduate residency program has developed to include nineteen regional, rural, and decentralized training sites throughout British Columbia. Rooted in principles of social accountability and the delivery of high-quality primary care, the department has become the largest in the Faculty of Medicine with more than three thousand UBC clinical faculty members across the province. The department's successes in advancing primary care have been internationally recognized and have directly influenced the FoM's educational programs.

The Department of Medical Genetics

The Division of Medical Genetics in Paediatrics at the Health Centre for Children, established in 1967, became the Department of Medical Genetics in 1972. Under the leadership of James Miller, strong collaborations with the Department of Pathology were established. In 1978, an energetic young geneticist, Patricia Baird, was appointed acting head, becoming Head the following year. The department was at a low ebb. There were doubts about the viability of the graduate program, inadequate space for clinical activities in a decrepit rented apartment building on West 10th Avenue, minimal lab space on campus in the James Mather Building, and a scarcity of clinical faculty.

During the following decade, however, the department underwent a busy recruiting phase. Persuading bright young graduates to work at UBC using their own award money initially, Baird was able to build the department out of "chewing gum and string." Within ten years, she and her colleagues managed to quadruple the department's space, increase the faculty from five to eighteen,

Patricia Baird, medical geneticist, Head of Department of Medical Genetics (1979–89), Chair, Royal Commission on Reproductive Technologies.

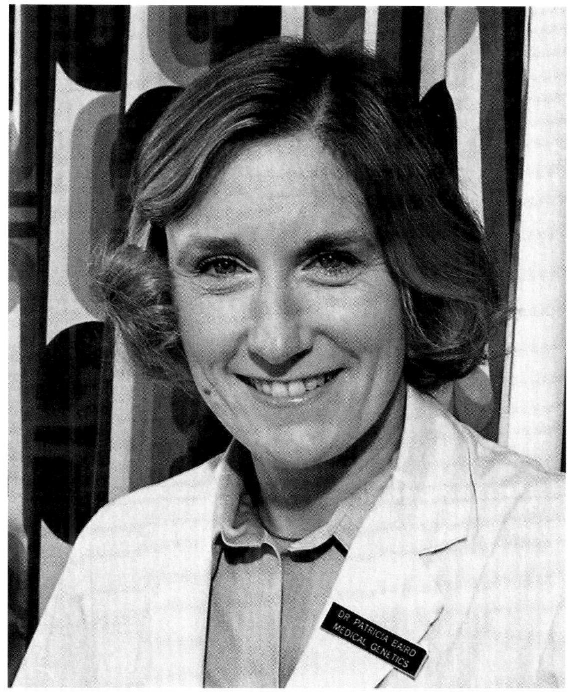

increase the support staff twenty-four-fold, and, most significantly, vastly expand the department's research and clinical activities. The department's innovative spirit gave rise to the genetic counselling master's degree program, graduates of which have come to support medical genetics services across North America.

The research funding attracted by the Department of Medical Genetics climbed dramatically. Baird's work on the distribution of birth defects and genetic disease in the population led to her later appointment as chair of the Royal Commission on New Reproductive Technologies. Several members of the young department made research contributions which became recognized internationally.

Michael Hayden's focus on Huntington disease and lipoprotein disorders broke new ground in both. Hayden went on to spectacular research achievements and in 1992 founded the Centre for Molecular Medicine and Therapeutics on the Shaughnessy site. Additional outstanding achievements included Paul Goodfellow's work in multiple endocrine neoplasia, Rob McMaster's use of molecular genetic approaches in genetics and the immune response, Diana Juriloff's unravelling of the genetic background to birth defects, Ann Rose's molecular research using nematodes, Judith Hall's clinical research with families deriving insights into the natural history and causes of genetic diseases and birth defects, and Connie Eaves's efforts in understanding the control of hematopoiesis.

The Department of Anatomy

Within the Department of Anatomy, a key appointment was that of Charles "Chuck" Slonecker in 1981, who succeeded Sydney Friedman after his thirty-one years as Head of Anatomy. Slonecker had joined the Faculty in 1968 after completing his degree in dentistry and a PhD in cellular immunology at the University of Washington in Seattle. Teaching neuroanatomy provided the affable Slonecker with an opportunity to interact with clinical teachers in the hospitals. During a successful ten-year term, he established a graduate program and recruited junior faculty, including several women. His approaches endeared him to students who benefitted from his support as they passed through UBC, and led to significant international recognition. In his later years at UBC, Slonecker and his wife, Jan, served presidents David Strangway and Martha Piper as enthusiastic UBC representatives and hosts on countless occasions.

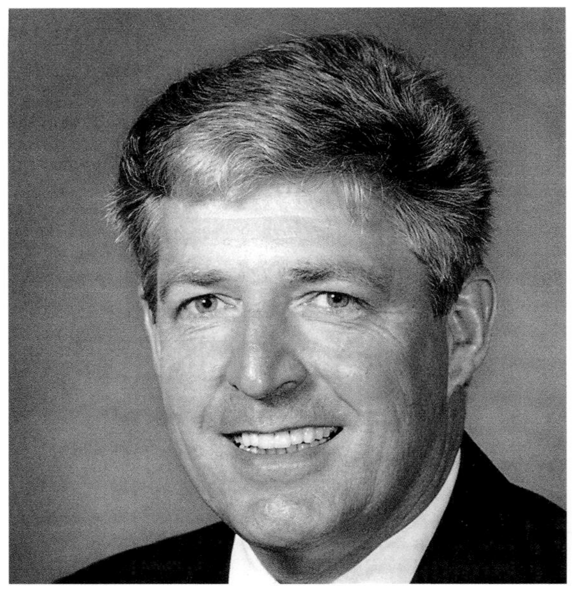

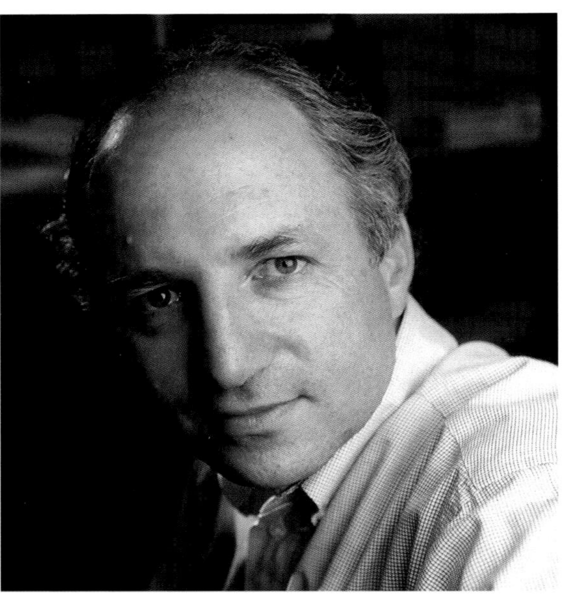

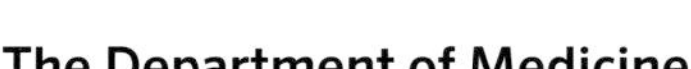

The Department of Medicine

Although the Head of the Department of Medicine, John Dirks, had been recruited by Dean Bates, he served most of his turbulent tenure (1976–87) under Webber. With the expansion of the medical school and the new campus hospital came new resources and academic space. Appreciating the importance of the Department of Medicine, Webber gave Dirks the opportunity to recruit several stars. Dirks appointed Roger Sutton, an expert in calcium metabolism, in nephrology. The BC Cancer Agency's development under Tom Hall and David Boyes, a leader in the epidemiology of cancer, permitted the reorganization of the Division of Hematology into an academic division that initiated a leading-edge bone marrow transplant program under Alan Eaves.

In the Division of Neurology, Dirks appointed Donald Paty, an alumnus of Emory and Duke Universities, as Head. Coming from London, Ontario, in 1980, Paty established the multiple sclerosis program at UBC, comprising one of the best clinics in the world, a renowned genetics program and a clinical trials program that became a model in the field. He collaborated with radiologist David Li in the use of magnetic resonance imaging (MRI) in the evaluation of the natural history of MS and in clinical trials. The following year, neurology gained British emigre Donald Calne, a world leader in Parkinson's disease and movement disorders, from the National Institutes of Health in the US. He had been invited to participate in a grant application being proposed by neurologists to build the positron emission tomography (PET) scanner on the UBC campus as part of TRIUMF, Canada's national particle accelerator centre. Calne went on to make the Neurodegenerative Disorders Centre at Vancouver Hospital and Health Sciences Centre and UBC one of the top resources of its kind.

An affiliation agreement signed by UBC and St. Paul's Hospital paved the way for Dirks's appointment of John Ruedy as Head of Medicine in 1977. At McGill, Ruedy had led the first division of clinical pharmacology in Canada, and then a newly formed Department of Clinical Pharmacology. However, his primary interest was teaching and practicing general

Donald Paty, neurologist, Head of Division of Neurology (1980–96).

LEFT FACING Charles Slonecker, anatomist, Head of Department of Anatomy (1984–95).

RIGHT FACING Michael R. Hayden, medical geneticist, founding Director of Center for Molecular Medicine and Therapeutics (1992–2007).

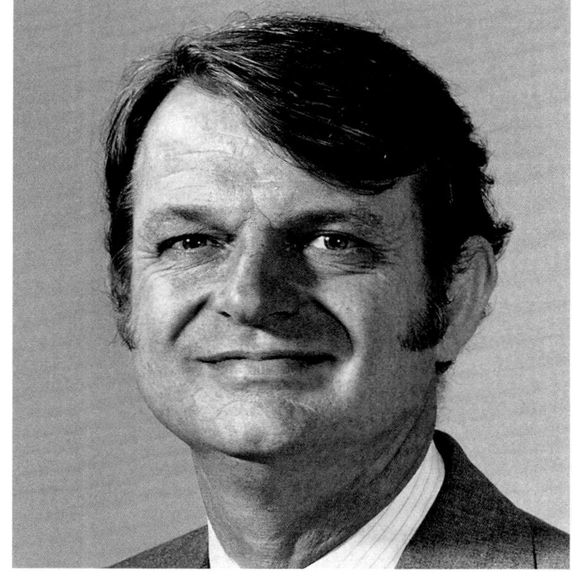

internal medicine, and in the St. Paul's department he found a cohesive group with a strong commitment to general medicine, pride in their record of teaching and clinical care, and limited development of subspecialties. Whereas Dirks encountered difficulties in getting clinical faculty at the VGH to teach, Ruedy found the opposite at St. Paul's, where Hurlburt's philosophy of assuming voluntary teaching from his staff had worked well. Deeply interested in postgraduate (residency) training, Ruedy took on the additional role of Associate Dean of Postgraduate Education in 1982. Ruedy was recruited to be Dean of Medicine at Dalhousie in 1993.

Around 1983, the first few cases of a mysterious, rapidly fatal, apparently infectious disease began to appear among the homosexual white population from the city's West End who were being served by a group of family practitioners at St. Paul's. A similar phenomenon began to show up in hemophiliacs, and soon it became evident that this was a bloodborne illness: HIV-AIDS. Care of these patients became a focus of St. Paul's. Advocacy by the board, strongly supported by the Sisters of Providence, led to St. Paul's becoming the provincial centre for HIV-AIDS care. Volunteer organizations working with the hospital raised the funds for a chair in AIDS. The organization of clinical services and the clinical studies conducted by Ruedy, respirologist Julio Montaner, and epidemiologist Martin Schechter laid the groundwork for the selection of St. Paul's by Health and Welfare Canada as the base for the Canadian HIV Trials Network. As expensive new drugs became available, they were able to convince the provincial government to fund the BC Centre of Excellence in HIV/AIDS and to recruit Dr. Michael O'Shaughnessy from Ottawa. Schechter, Montaner, and O'Shaughnessy co-chaired the XIth International AIDS Conference, held in Vancouver in 1996, thereby acknowledging BC's global leadership in the field.

As Dirks pursued his efforts to recruit researchers and to build the academic profile of the Department of Medicine, he tried to impose ceilings on faculty members' incomes, and he advocated practice plans. Under these plans, fees for medical services within a group, such as a division within medicine,

Donald Calne, neurologist, Director of the Neurodegenerative Disorders Centre at Vancouver Hospital Health Sciences Centre and UBC (1981–2001).

LEFT FACING Hematologists Gordon Phillips (l) and Alan Eaves (r), pioneers in bone marrow transplantation for hematologic malignancies.

RIGHT FACING Julio Montaner, respirologist (l); John Reudy, clinical pharmacologist (c); and Martin Schechter, epidemiologist (r) – all pioneers and world leaders in HIV/AIDS diagnosis and treatment.

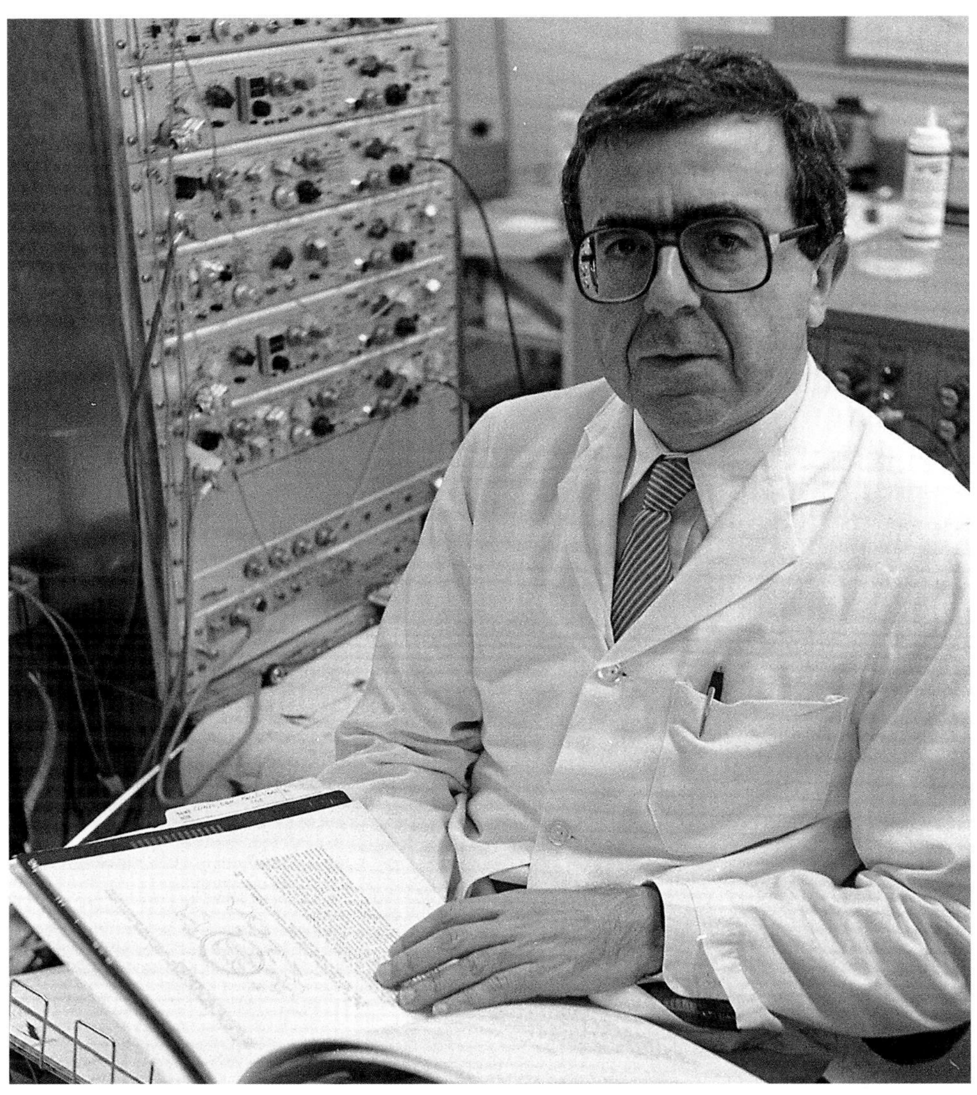

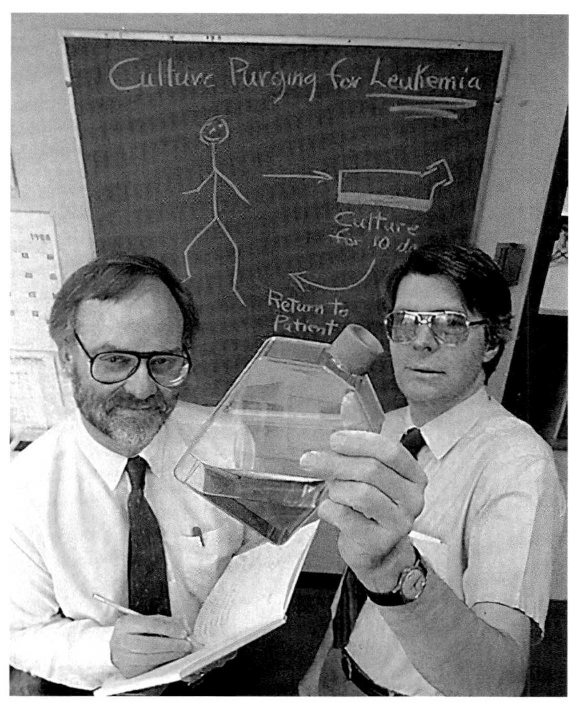

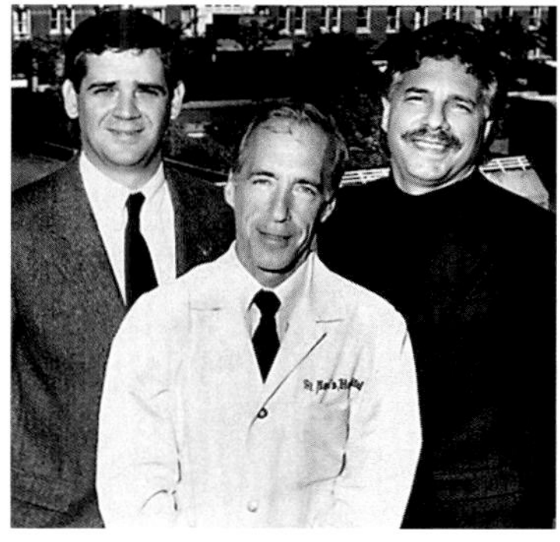

would be pooled into a fund from which its members would pay each other a negotiated salary and use the remainder to cover costs of such services as secretarial or laboratory support or to further the academic mission of their discipline. These attempts were met with resentment and antipathy by clinical faculty. According to some of his colleagues at the time, Dirks was not sufficiently sensitive to others' opinions. There were rumblings of discontent, vague threats of legal action, and attempts to circumvent the authority of the department head by going behind his back to the Dean. The conflict between Dirks and the established clinical community had substantial impacts. Many of the new recruits to the VGH in the late 1970s and early '80s felt they were treated with suspicion by the establishment, as one of "Dirks's boys," even if they brought new clinical skills to the organization.

Dissatisfactions with Dirks and opposition to what was seen as diversion of resources to the new campus hospital led to controversy over his first reappointment in 1981. Could he be reappointed as head of the academic department if the VGH was not willing to reappoint him as head of the hospital department? A compromise was eventually negotiated, whereby Dirks was replaced as chair of a committee designed to consider questions of bed allocations and hospital appointments by a deputy head in matters pertaining to the clinical faculty. The manoeuvre was sufficient to cool the heated atmosphere and allow the department to focus on its educational and research mandates. However, when his second reappointment came up in 1986, Dirks was asked to step down as Head of Medicine at VGH while carrying on as UBC Head.

By the time John Dirks left Vancouver to become the Dean of Medicine at the University of Toronto in 1987, the department he had led for eleven years had undergone enormous changes. There had been extensive expansion of the subspecialties, several of

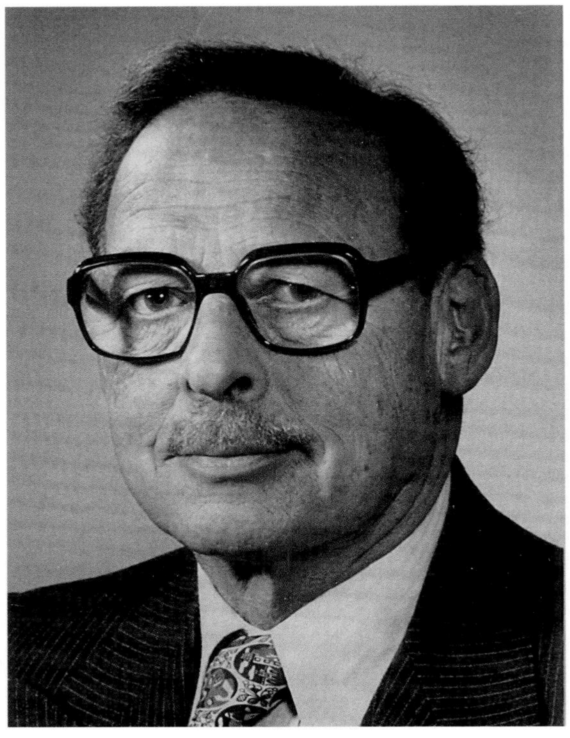

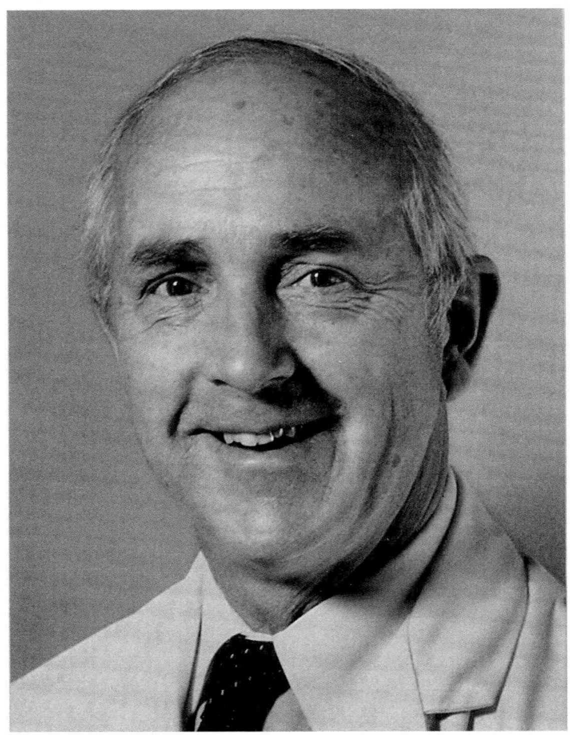

them achieving national stature. Research funding had increased thirty-fold. The lingering town-versus-gown struggle characteristic of the university's relationship with its physician-teachers was not only unresolved, it had intensified. Nevertheless, over time the value of the talented new physicians he had recruited was recognized locally as they contributed to the clinical expertise, academic stature, and national reputation of the organization.

The Department of Surgery

The Department of Surgery had been headed by Cam Harrison since 1966. Although he was well recognized in surgical research and gastrointestinal physiology and had strengthened research, the department required fresh leadership. In 1976, Bates appointed the dynamic Frank P. Patterson Jr., former Head of the Division of Orthopaedics. When Patterson stepped down in 1981, Webber appointed A.D. "Herb" Forward who built up the department, strengthening its postgraduate and undergraduate education programs and identifying some young surgeons who were sent away to train in basic science research. In 1987, Forward stepped down, and Doug Courtemanche, the Head of Plastic Surgery, was acting head for a year. During this time, a lung transplant program was founded at VGH by thoracic surgeon Bill Nelems and respirologist David Ostrow. Wallace B. "Wally" Chung, head of the Division of General Surgery, inaugural Head of the Division of Vascular Surgery, and Head of Surgery at UBC Hospital (1981–91) was known for his development of innovative vascular surgery techniques. Together with his wife, Madeline Chung, an obstetrician and gynecologist, he donated his collection of over 25,000 artifacts to UBC in 1999, creating the library's Wallace B. Chung and Madeline H. Chung Collection.

LEFT FACING Frank P. Patterson, orthopedic surgeon, Head of Division of Orthopedics (1951–73), Head of Department of Surgery (1976–81).

RIGHT FACING Herb Forward, general surgeon, Head of Department of Surgery (1981–87).

Over time the value of the talented new physicians was recognized locally as they contributed to the clinical expertise, academic stature, and national reputation of the organization.

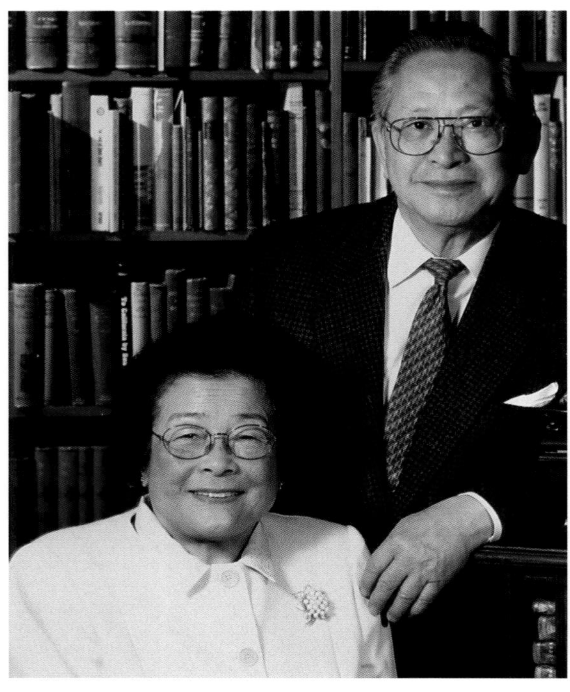

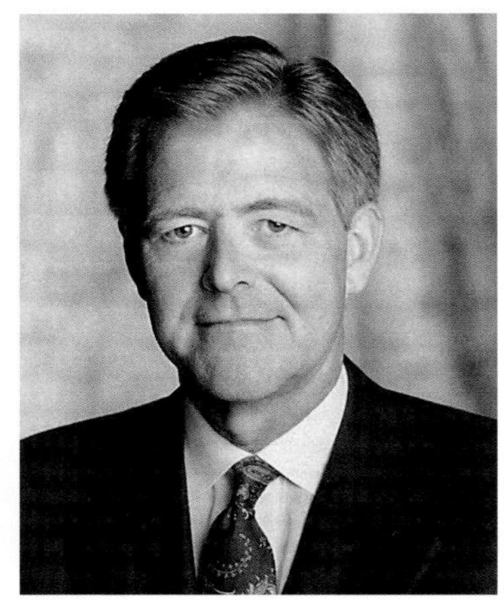

The Department of Orthopaedics

Ken Morton took on the headship of the orthopaedics division from Patterson in 1973. By 1982, he, along with Brian Day and Robert McGraw, had established a movement to break away from Surgery. They summarized their rationales in a publication which became a kind of how-to manual on separating orthopaedics from an academic department of surgery. In 1984, they achieved Senate approval for a freestanding Department of Orthopaedics, and Robert McGraw became its first Head. He emphasized growth and subspecialization, engendering a high level of research accomplishment, patient care, and educational dynamism within orthopaedics, to the point where the new department became recognized across the country. Today there are eight orthopaedics divisions—pediatrics, spine, reconstructive orthopaedics, athletic injuries, upper extremity, comprehensive, oncology, and trauma—as well as a strong research division.

The Department of Obstetrics and Gynecology

By 1978, with the advent of new funding from the expansion budget, small departments like Obstetrics and Gynecology, long constrained by paltry resources, were able to recruit new full-time members. Victor Gomel, a local specialist who brought the department into the modern era of minimally invasive surgery, took the reins from Fred Bryans in 1978 and had the entrepreneurial and managerial skills to extract the optimal amount of space from hospitals and budgetary increases from the dean. Gomel would later become a world leader in gynecologic laparoscopy.

From its early days, the department had had a liberal policy toward termination of pregnancy. David Claman, a crusader for the right of women to choose to end pregnancy, was later joined by Garson Romalis. Following the change of the Criminal Code Canada in 1969 to allow abortion under specified

Victor Gomel, obstetrician/gynecologist, Head of Department of Obstetrics and Gynecology (1978–93).

LEFT FACING Wallace B. Chung, vascular surgeon, Head of Division of General Surgery, inaugural Head of Division of Vascular Surgery and Head of Surgery at UBC Hospital (1981–91), and Madeline Chung, obstetrician/gynecologist.

RIGHT FACING Robert McGraw, orthopedic surgeon, inaugural Head of Department of Orthopedics (1984–96).

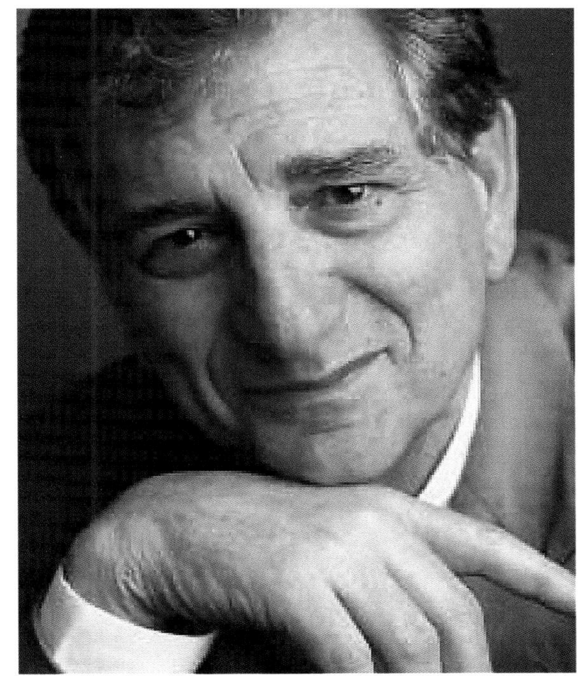

terms, the rate of abortions at VGH rose from 50 per year to 3,800 by 1975. Termination cases were being squeezed into crowded wards and operating room schedules. A highly skilled group of OB/GYN practitioners in this domain pushed for the creation of a day care surgery unit at VGH. Their willingness to take on the controversial procedure allowed other hospitals, like St. Paul's, St. Vincent's, and Grace Hospitals, to avoid the issue and send cases to VGH. In addition to the scheduling challenges, the inherent risks were all too clearly evident when Romalis narrowly escaped death in 1994 from a fanatic's bullet while sitting in his home and in 2000 survived a stabbing attack near his office.

When it became clear in the early 1970s that obstetrical ultrasound had merit in measuring the fetus to judge its maturity, the department's wish to develop an ultrasound unit ran into conflict with the VGH policy that all imaging would be centralized under the radiology department. The policy became irrelevant when the OB/GYN department was relocated to its new facility at the Women's and Children's. With the more recent work of Duncan Farquharson, obstetrical imaging developed into a first-class department service. Peter McComb developed an excellent residency program, and Sidney Effer performed epidemiological studies in relationship to low birth weight babies, an aspect of the clinical excellence that has become a hallmark of the department and the hospital.

The Department of Ophthalmology

After being appointed by Bates as Head of the Department of Ophthalmology in 1973, Stephen Drance came to the realization that to make the sorts of changes he desired, he could not rely on either the university or the VGH for the necessary financial support. He had learned from the successful efforts of his predecessor, Alfred Elliot, that raising money was part of the job, and that if he

A Student-Led Strike for Better Education

In 1980, fourth-year students John Wade and Dianne Miller led a day-long strike by UBC medical students regarding teaching in their senior year and extending into the postgraduate years. Students had found themselves on 1:3 call, often doing difficult scut work, clinical tasks that others couldn't do—starting IVs in bone marrow transplant patients, starting scalp IVs in infants in the ICU—and without any formal teaching inserted into their weekly academic lives. The day-long strike was almost one hundred percent successful and led in part to the establishment in the academic half-day for fourth-year students.

wanted to develop anything, he would have to go after the funding himself. He led a highly successful fundraising campaign that culminated in the opening in 1983 of the Eye Care Centre on 10th Avenue, a splendid, state-of-the-art clinical and academic research facility. Even today, UBC President and Vice-chancellor Santa Ono has his vision laboratory and graduate students located there. Drance ensured that the fundraising efforts put an amount in trust for research space, allowing him to search for a top-notch director of research who would be able to develop the space to their own specifications.

Having met Max Cynader, Professor of Physiology and of Psychology at Dalhousie, during a UBC visit in 1981, Drance set out to recruit him to direct the basic and applied research arm of the Department of Ophthalmology and to bring with him Dalhousie colleagues, including Robert Douglas, Joanne Matsubara, Christopher Shaw, and Nicholas

LEFT FACING Jack Rootman, orbital ophthalmologist, artist, and Head of Department of Ophthalmology (1990–2002).

RIGHT FACING Max Cynader, neuroscientist, founding Director, UBC Brain Research Center, 1998.

Swindale. Cynader and colleagues arrived in 1988, beginning an era of fruitful research for ophthalmology and neurosciences. Cynader's personal research achievements and his entrepreneurial skills led to his appointment as founding director of the UBC Brain Research Centre in 1998.

In 1988, Jack Rootman succeeded Drance as Head of Ophthalmology. A world-renowned expert in orbital surgery, he has written three books on this specialty. Rootman is also a celebrated artist who saw a direct connection between the skills of the surgeon and the artist, and the degrees of concentration required of each.

Students and Residents

In this era of expansion, both students and faculty recognized the need for a facility that provided dedicated space for students and alumni, especially for the students' social and recreational lives. There had been library and study space for faculty and students in an old army hut on 10th Avenue. When the library moved to the new Heather Street building, the hut became a student lounge, but although it was renovated in 1966 as an outcome of student activism, the facilities were considered by many to be inadequate. A Medical Alumni Association was formed in 1984, and subsequently David Hardwick and a group of very keen students proposed the creation of a Medical Student and Alumni Centre

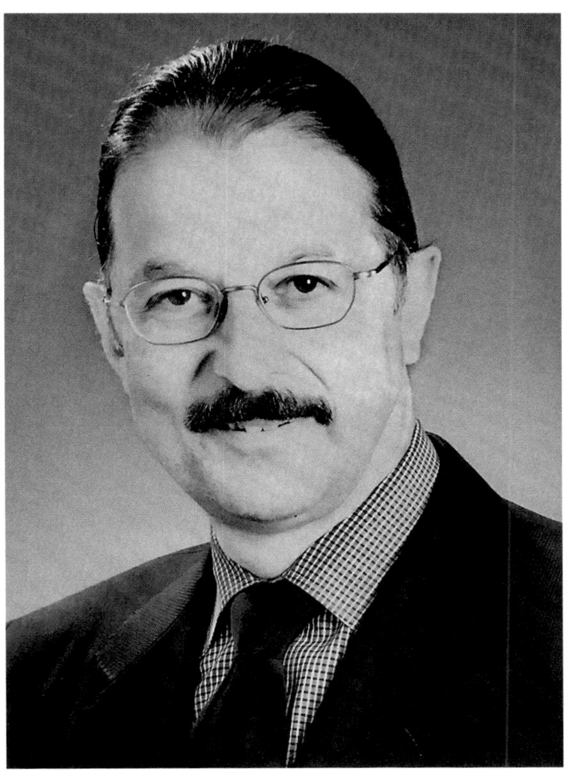

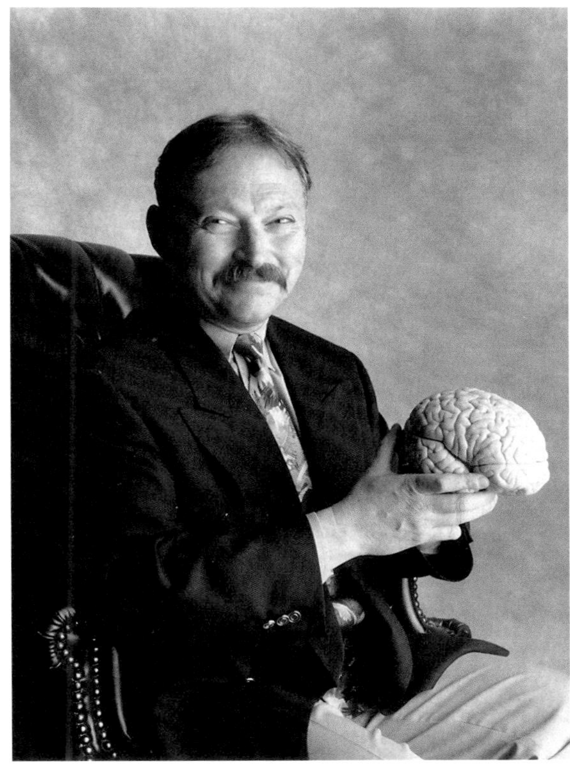

(MSAC). A site on the corner of Heather Street and 12th Avenue was leased from the VGH, fundraising began, and by 1989, there was a groundbreaking ceremony at the site. Key individuals in the fundraising included Hardwick, Webber, Richard Beauchamp, and Curt Latham with a total of $960,000 raised. Upon completion of phase one of the MSAC, medical students conducted a "reverse trek" from Point Grey to the site at VGH followed by the Centre's grand opening including a ribbon cutting ceremony led by the new dean, Martin Hollenberg, in 1990.

There was to be a further expansion supported by students and alumni, and at its opening in 1996 it was announced that more than $1.25 million had been raised. The expanded centre was dedicated as the William A. Webber Medical Student & Alumni Centre in 2007 and now contains rooms for remote video conferencing as well as recreational space for students. In recognition of its success, and the distributed curriculum, an MSAC space was constructed in 2014 at the Royal Jubilee Hospital in Victoria and in 2017 at the University Hospital of the North. A sophisticated provincial audio-visual network supports regular interaction amongst students at all the MSAC sites.

The Faculty of Medicine also had to untangle the funding of residents (postgraduate trainees). By the early 1980s, there were over five hundred residents training in BC, and they were still enrolled in individual hospital programs with their salaries paid by the hospitals. They formed what was essentially a trade union and negotiated for significant increases in remuneration and benefits.

Prior to the creation of the Faculty of Medicine, postgraduate training in BC had been focused

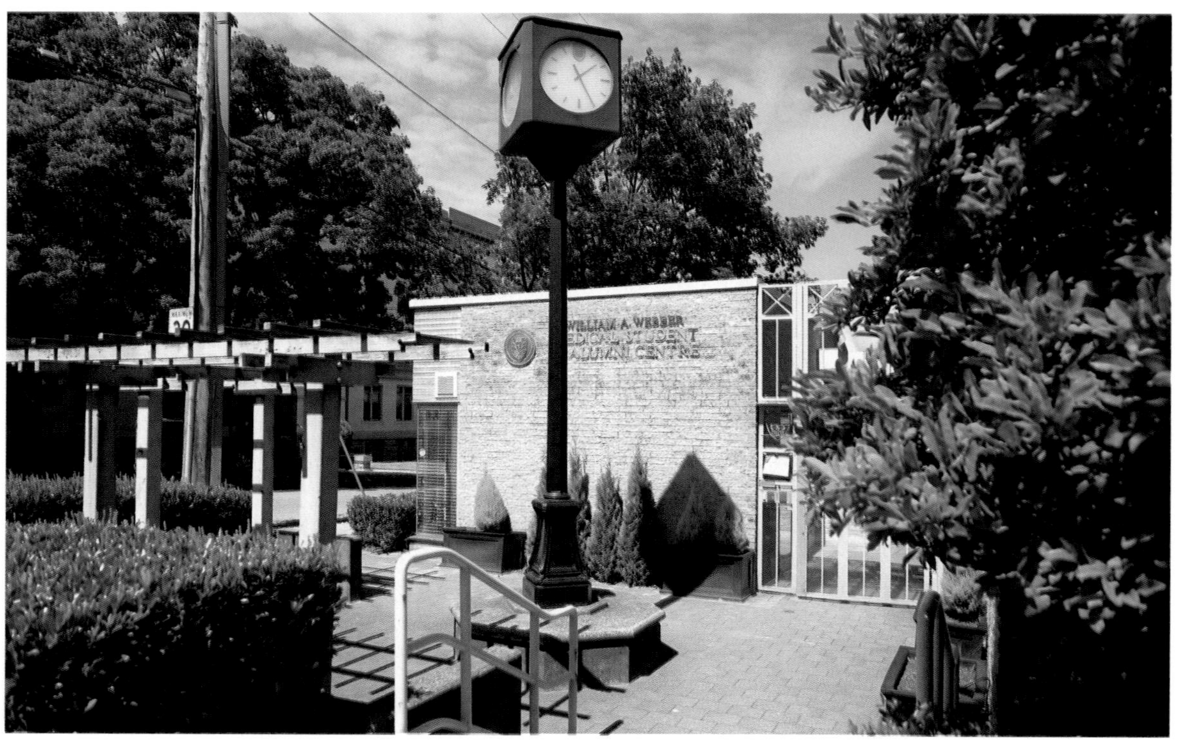
WILLIAM A. WEBBER
EDICAL STUDENT
ALUMNI CENTRE

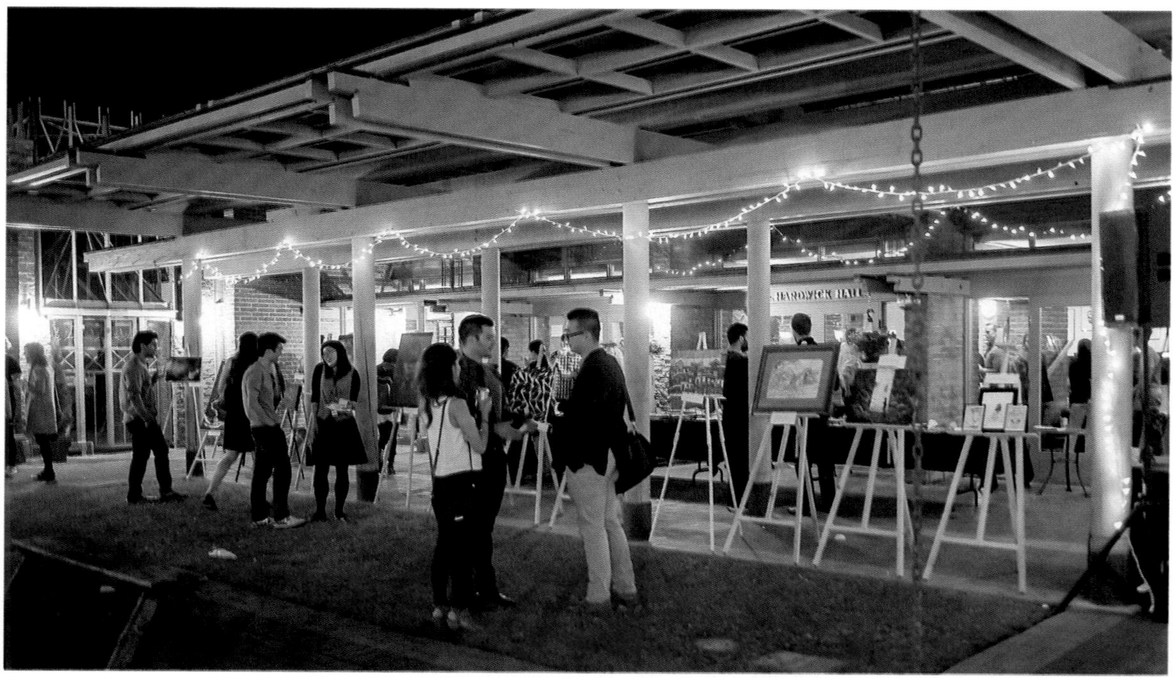
HARDWICK HALL

TOP FACING Medical Student and Alumni Center (MSAC) (opened 1990), 12th Ave. entrance.

BOTTOM FACING MSAC Courtyard, MSAC resident Talent Night.

Weepers

Both Don Ricci (UBC MD '70) and John Wade (UBC MD '80) recalled the Friday evening parties that regularly took place in a medical student lounge on the north side of 10th Avenue opposite the Heather Pavilion. After classes, many students would go to the emergency room at VGH, where they would learn to put in IVs, perform arterial punctures, take histories, and perform physicals, and then later in the day move to the student lounge where, fortified by one-hundred-proof alcohol from the clinical chemistry lab, the festivities lasted into the night. Later on, the event became more formalized as "Weepers" and took place in the basement of the doctors' residence on Heather and 12th. This Friday party was frequented by the many British and other foreign interns and residents who came to Vancouver in those days. Social interactions were facilitated by the existence of a tunnel from the doctors' residence to the VGH student nurses' residence across 12th Avenue, allowing for discreet travel back and forth.

primarily in Vancouver and followed an apprenticeship model. When the Faculty was established in 1950, post-MD education focused on highly individualized rotating internship positions funded by hospitals in Vancouver, New Westminster, and Victoria. During his tenure as Dean in the 1950s and '60s, McCreary had seen the need to shift intern and residency training from the hospital-based apprentice model to a university education status and had charged David Hardwick with developing a description of the programs that allowed university recognition of a variety of advanced courses. Organized postgraduate specialty training programs gradually developed in many disciplines beyond the traditional one year of internship to several years of focused training in the given specialties including OB/GYN, surgery, medicine, and pediatrics.

In the 1970s, universities, rather than hospitals, were assigned the responsibility and authority for postgraduate education, and the rotating internship, which had once qualified the trainee to be licensed as a family physician, was phased out. The Royal College of Physicians and Surgeons and the College of Family Physicians formally took on the role of accrediting university-based training programs, conducting the certification examinations and granting fellowships in the colleges.

When the issue of funding emerged in the 1980s, a provincial residency advisory committee was struck. It was chaired by Webber and comprised representatives from government, the BCMA, the College of Physicians and Surgeons, and the FoM. Through discussions with the teaching hospitals, the Ministry of Health agreed to take over the hospital budgets for remuneration, make up shortfalls, and provide standard allocations to the various hospitals through a central paying agency. Although the Ministry of Education refused to fund the educational components of internships and residencies, the Faculty of Medicine could now include

The Webber Boot

In the accompanying photograph, Dean Webber presents the "Webber Boot" to Jamie Appelby (UBC MD '82). Dean Webber was a great soccer fan who, along with his sons Eric (a Vancouver pediatric surgeon) and Geordie, used to play pick-up games on Sunday mornings with Jamie and some of his classmates. It was his class that came up with the idea of the Webber Boot. That class team toured England and played some games against other medical school teams there during their break between third and fourth year.

The boot actually belonged to Jim Hunter (UBC MD '85). There also used to be a "Lauener Sock," the women's soccer trophy named for Roland Lauener, then undergrad dean. The Webber Boot tournament is still played, now as a co-ed event.

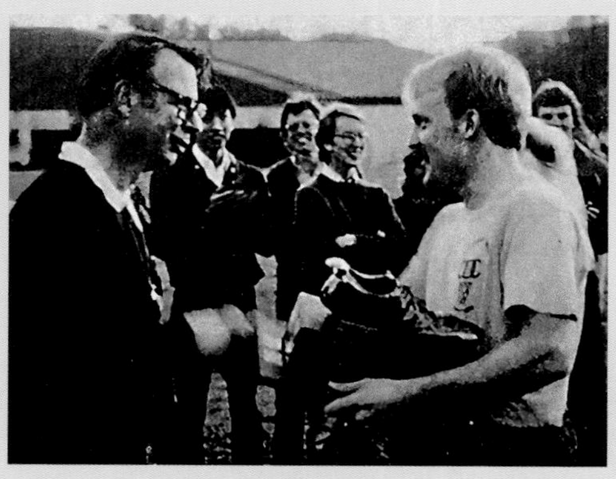

interns and residents as students in their annual budget submissions to UBC. This model continues today wherein the Resident Doctors of BC negotiates wages and benefits with the Health Employers Association of BC (HEABC), which works on behalf of the Ministry of Health. There are now some 1,360 postgraduate learners in seventy-five distinct UBC training programs across the province.

Webber's Legacy

In the latter part of Webber's deanship, the need for more good people was the rationale for directing the Faculty of Medicine's component of President David Strangway's immensely successful World of Opportunity campaign into recruitment. With endowments, matching government money, and interest rates as high as eighteen percent, it was possible to create over a dozen new chairs. The increased research capacity led to the FoM's involvement in ten of the fourteen Networks of Centres of Excellence established jointly by Canada's research funding councils in 1989. Webber recalled that when he became Dean, the Faculty had about $8 million a year in research funding, and when he stepped down, that figure had increased to about $40 million.

Webber served as Dean at a time when the feminist movement was gaining momentum, and he oversaw the transformation of the Faculty into a more woman-friendly environment. By the end of his second term, about one-quarter of the senior women academics at UBC were in the Faculty of Medicine, and one-quarter of the full or associate professors in the FoM were women. No other faculty had as many. Some outstanding scholars and leaders arose from their ranks: Patricia Baird, Head of Medical Genetics; Judith Hall, Head of Pediatrics; Judith Johnston, Director of the School of Audiology and Speech Sciences; Carol Herbert, Head of Family Practice and then Canada's second female Dean of Medicine at the University of Western Ontario; and Joanne Emmerman and Joanne Weinberg, who held senior positions within the Faculty and the research community. Hall fondly recalls several gatherings of senior female faculty members, sometimes at her Mayne Island cottage, to discuss the many career development and academic issues they were facing.

Another source of pride to Webber was the network of medical libraries across the city's teaching hospitals. Partly because it was necessary, and partly to keep groups happy at the various hospitals, UBC agreed to upgrade the old facility at the VGH and to establish a branch library at St. Paul's and, with a donation from the Hamber Foundation, another at the Shaughnessy-Children's-Grace site.

Webber will long be remembered by the thousands of students who passed through the Faculty before, during, and after his tenure as Dean, as a warm, caring, and committed mentor whose overriding interest was the welfare of the students. The only person who might have remembered more names of UBC medical graduates was his trusty wife and partner, Marilyn. Together, through over forty years, they welcomed countless students as guests in their home near the campus. Sadly, Bill Webber died with colonic cancer in 2006.

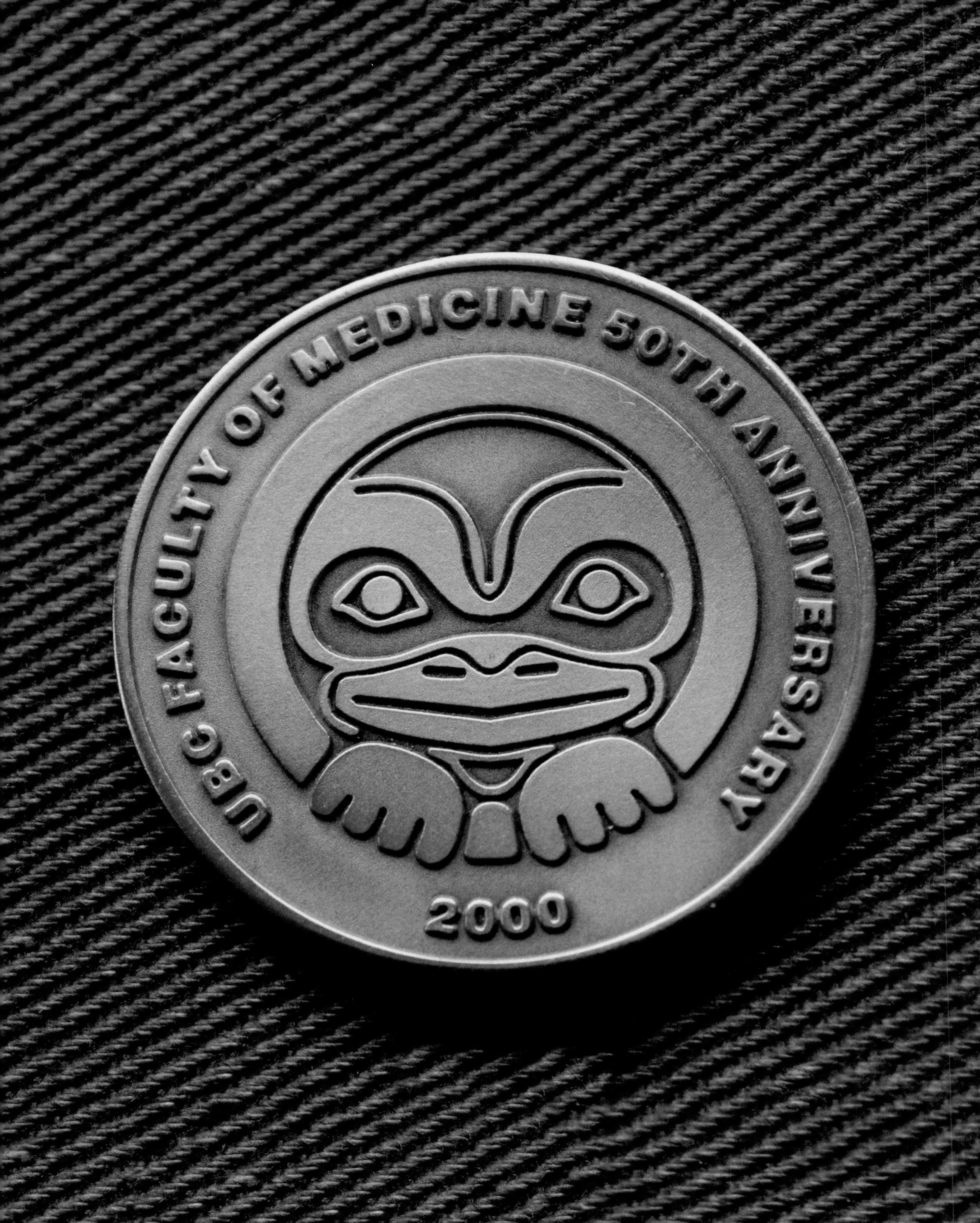
UBC FACULTY OF MEDICINE 50TH ANNIVERSARY
2000

5

The Great Turnaround

1990–2003

FACING Logo of the Golden Jubilee (2000) and subsequently adopted as Faculty of Medicine logo, created by Lyle Wilson, a Haisla artist.

FACING Martin J. "Marty" Hollenberg, anatomist, sixth Dean of Medicine (1990–96).

Despite great strides forward in the 1970s and '80s, the Faculty still had inadequate infrastructure and a paucity of clinician-scientists, only a third to a half of that in leading Canadian medical schools.

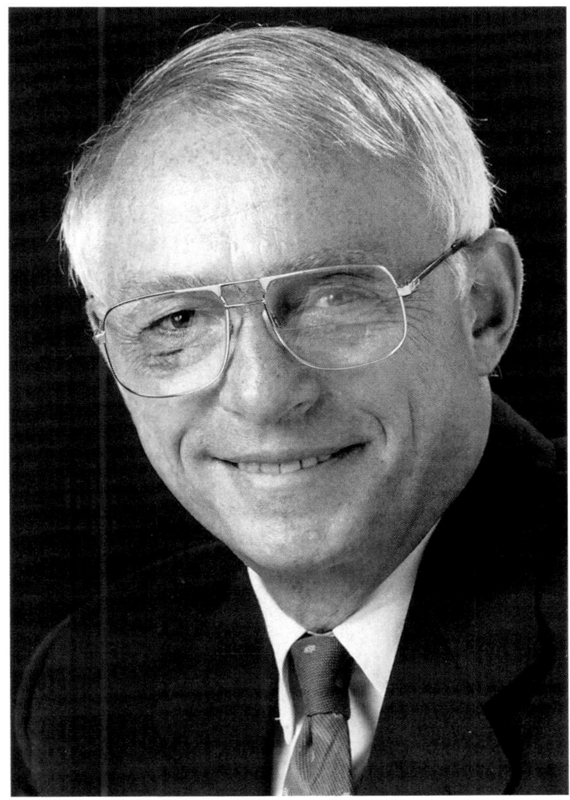

MARTIN HOLLENBERG became the University of British Columbia's sixth Dean of Medicine in 1990. A graduate of the University of Manitoba, he obtained his PhD at Wayne State University, served in the Department of Anatomy at UBC (1971–75), and then in the new University of Calgary Faculty of Medicine (1975–78). He had been a successful dean of medicine at the University of Western Ontario (1978–85) and was happily returning to his research in 1990 when the call came to explore his interest in the deanship at UBC. He was attracted to the idea of leading the only medical school in the province in contrast to the Ontario scenario of five competing schools, and he felt that as a previous dean of medicine, he would not have to face a steep learning curve in the position. There was also the unfailing appeal of living in beautiful Vancouver, where he and his young family had spent four happy years in the early 1970s.

Hollenberg arrived at UBC aware that a succession of problematic and short-term presidencies had ended in 1988 with the appointment of President David Strangway (1988–97), a brilliant physicist and visionary leader who soon revealed his talent for working effectively with governments and for raising funds from Vancouver's wealthy but heretofore tight-fisted philanthropic community. Somewhat surprisingly for a relatively new and publicly funded university, UBC was increasingly achieving international recognition, particularly for its faculties of science, applied science, and forestry and for its library. *Maclean's* magazine had also begun to recognize some of UBC's attributes in its rating of Canadian universities. UBC's reputation in medical research was to be boosted still further by Michael Smith's Nobel Prize, awarded in 1993.

Hollenberg had wondered why UBC was not one of the top-ranked medical schools in the country, with its splendid setting in a vibrant city with large urban hospitals nearby. He soon became aware that despite great strides forward in the 1970s and '80s, the FoM still had inadequate infrastructure and a paucity of adequately funded geographic full-time clinician-scientists, only a third to a half of that in leading Canadian medical schools. Although clinical research had grown in the prior decade, it was

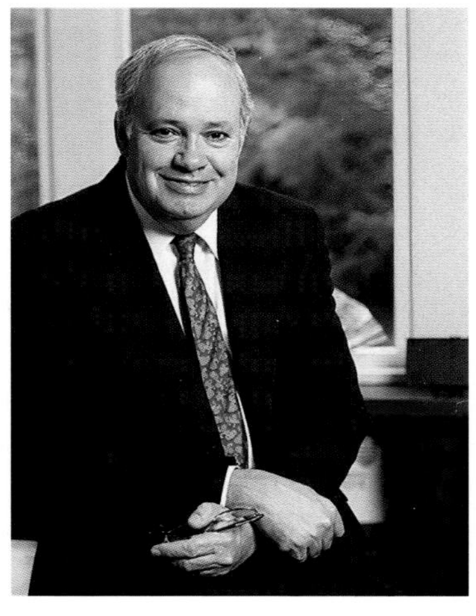

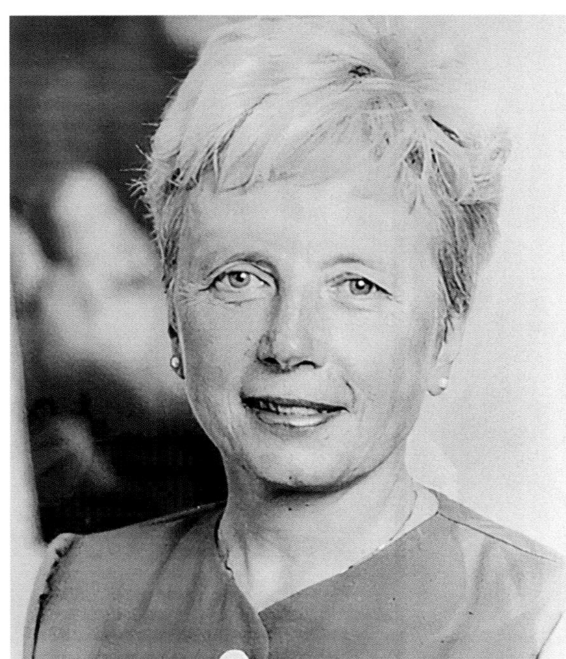

still modest in scope and impact by comparison to more established schools. Inadequate government funding meant that UBC's medical leaders had to rely on clinical faculty to a greater extent than in many better-funded faculties of medicine. Hollenberg recognized the discontent simmering among the members of clinical faculty, but with recurrent budget cuts there was little he could do to address their needs.

Academic Excellence in an Era of Decreased Funding

Early in his term, Hollenberg appointed David Hardwick as Associate Dean of Research and Institutional Planning: in effect, vice-dean. Together they developed a grand plan (Medicine 2000) modelled on the faculties of medicine in Calgary and Hamilton, incorporating research themes, each identified with the hospital where existing and evolving clinical programs and people offered the attraction of critical mass and the potential for growth. The themes were made attractive for funding from a variety of sources, not only government and individuals but also industry, charitable organizations, and service groups. The plan was enthusiastically received by both hospital administrators and researchers.

Hollenberg was asked to chair the Planning and Steering Committee of the Council of University Teaching Hospitals (COUTH), which allocated areas of major clinical focus among the teaching hospitals. Some of them were obvious: cancer and the health of women and children. Others were less so and subject to ongoing controversy: neuroscience was assigned to VGH, cardiovascular medicine and surgery to St. Paul's, and pulmonary to both major hospitals. The research themes of Medicine 2000 were aligned as much as possible with the areas of clinical focus. Existing hospital-based research institutes were encouraged, and new ones sprang up. Substantial additional academic space was opened

LEFT FACING David W. Strangway, physicist, tenth President of UBC (1985–97).

RIGHT FACING Peggy Ross, anesthesiologist (UBC MD '58), inaugural Associate Dean of Equity (1993–99).

in the Laurel Pavilion of VGH in 1996. The Vancouver teaching hospitals doubled or tripled their research space throughout the 1990s, although UBC investment was conspicuously minimal until a series of major federal health research initiatives were to begin late in the decade.

As Dean, Hollenberg became the CEO of an enormous and diverse organization. In 1993, he created the post of associate dean of equity to "foster an atmosphere of sensitivity and accountability to gender and equity issues and to develop policies and guidelines for dealing with complaints regarding these issues in a fair and equitable manner." Its first occupant, anesthetist Peggy Ross (UBC MD '58), had her hands full dealing with allegations of harassment and discrimination. Awareness of the importance of appropriate treatment of support staff, patients, trainees, and colleagues gradually spread though faculty members. Dorothy Shaw would be appointed to succeed Ross in 1999.

The dean's office also had to contend with having little infrastructure to support the enterprise. There was no human resources department to handle personnel matters, no procedures in place to track commitments made in the course of recruitments, and no finance department to prepare budgets, monitor expenditures, and provide timely data on the Faculty's finances. Hollenberg found the details of UBC budgeting and the Faculty's finances obscure and was uncertain of resources to fund development and recruitment. Planning and recruitment were hampered by the provost's policy whereby on retirement of a faculty member, the salary was immediately absorbed into an "academic reserve fund" controlled by the provost and returned to the Faculty only in part, when funds were available and a satisfactory case had been made. Commissioning an Ernst and Young analysis of FoM finances, Hollenberg attempted to make the case for returning the academic reserve funds to the FoM on a regular basis, but he was not successful.

Hollenberg continued to recruit and to sustain vital educational programs. He had concluded that without critical faculty appointments and program supports, accreditations of the MD undergraduate and residency programs were at risk, and the research enterprise would continue its ongoing decline. In university budget submissions, he maintained the practice of listing as assets funds primarily controlled by the clinical departments and divisions. They derived from clinical earnings, were committed to the departments where they originated, and could not be used for anything other than compensation of the clinicians who had earned the income. A lack of financial sophistication at the centre and a failure to understand the components of the FoM budget meant that as far as the university was concerned, the FoM had a balanced budget. The financial obligations incurred as new appointments were arranged often did not have designated

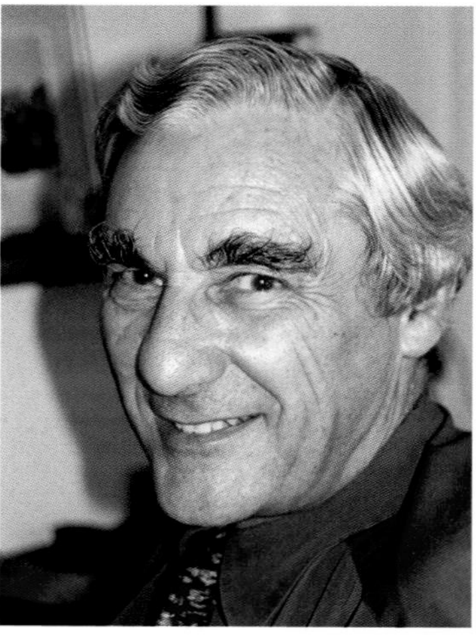

Andrew Eisen, neurologist, Interim Head of Department of Medicine (1987–92).

university funds to back them up. Hollenberg knew that debt was accumulating but was certain that "without that debt, the house of cards which was the Faculty of Medicine might well have collapsed." He regarded it as an interest-free loan, without which, he was convinced, the Faculty would never have been able to recruit the heads they did and would have been in danger of disintegration.

The Department of Medicine

In the Department of Medicine, neurologist Andrew Eisen had become acting head when John Dirks stepped down in 1987. With an echo of the challenge faced by Dean Bates in the early 1970s, searching for a new permanent head became Hollenberg's first major recruitment task, and it was a formidable one. Some of the delay was attributable to a plan to have the department head sited at the UBC hospital, which as of 1991 had been organizationally merged with the Shaughnessy Hospital, the whole amalgam known as the University Hospital (now UBC Hospital). It seemed important to the Faculty and to administrators of the campus hospital that the next leader of the largest department be firmly rooted in the university camp, and Hollenberg agreed. Eisen's interim leadership continued for four and a half years.

In spring 1992, Hollenberg appointed cardiologist John Mancini as Head. He had served as Chief of Cardiology in the Veterans Administration Medical Centre, University of Michigan in Ann Arbor. He was attracted by the COUTH vision of a coordinated rather than competitive system among the several teaching hospitals of the city. He looked forward to working with the new CEO of the University Hospital, Lionel MacLeod, a well-liked and effective former Dean of Medicine at University of Calgary.

Heavily involved in planning the administrative and service structure of the University Hospital, Mancini was soon aware of rumours of the closure of the Shaughnessy site and a merger of the UBC Hospital with VGH. Indeed, the Minister of Health announced in March 1993 that Shaughnessy Hospital would be closed. Careers were disrupted, research programs lost their headquarters, and lives were turned upside down as faculty clinicians suddenly found themselves without admitting privileges and infrastructure. At a board meeting of the University Hospital, Minister of Health Elizabeth Cull summarily informed its members that the board they had generously served would now be

G.B. John Mancini, cardiologist, Head of Department of Medicine (1992–2002).

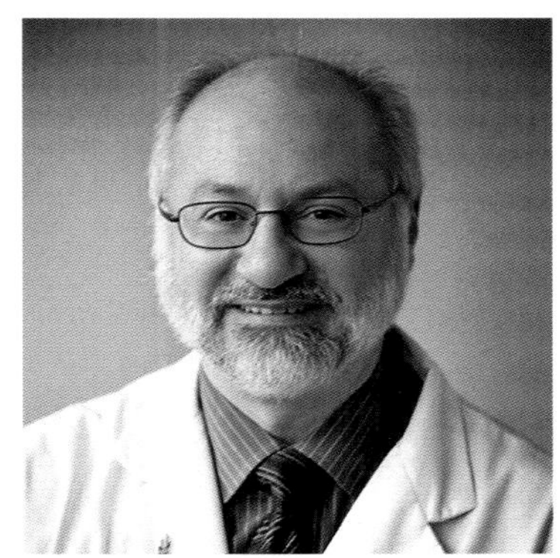

disbanded and UBC Hospital was to be merged with Vancouver General to form the Vancouver Hospital and Health Sciences Centre (VHHSC).

As head of the university Department of Medicine, Mancini was now asked to move to the VGH. Roger Sutton, the incumbent hospital head of medicine, disagreed with the plan, and many clinical faculty members expressed grave concerns about being "taken over" by UBC if Mancini were to be appointed hospital head. Mancini met severe resistance to his ideas about a departmental practice plan. He thought that at the very minimum he could encourage divisional practice plans, but the hospital administration did not cooperate. Mancini maintained that the distribution of clinical resources to his department was dramatically out of line with its patient load and the pressures on Medicine in the emergency room. He was forced to make massive cuts and to shut down entire wards at the UBC site, generating not just unfavourable press coverage but internal conflict. Cutbacks to the UBC-derived academic budget exacerbated the resource deficiencies. Eventually an extraordinary review of the Head of Medicine was ordered by the Vancouver General Hospital. Mancini offered his resignation to CEO Murray Martin, who refused it, and Mancini continued as university and hospital head of medicine, although his relationship with Martin remained testy.

Hollenberg suggested to his successor, John Cairns, that he not reappoint Mancini as head of the Department of Medicine, a view also expressed by Murray Martin, CEO of the VHHSC. Recognizing Mancini's strengths in a time of Faculty turbulence, the new dean reappointed him for a further five years, a decision he never regretted. Mancini was ultimately credited with organizational restructuring, mission-based budgeting, the establishment of divisional business plans, the creation of an Academic Enhancement Endowment fund (providing grants-in-aid to foster excellence in teaching and/or research) and a departmental Resident Research Day, and the promotion of the experimental medicine (graduate medicine) and the clinician investigator programs. New divisions of general internal medicine, allergy and immunology, and critical care medicine were established. He increased the numbers of women and of clinical faculty on the department promotions committee and implemented policies for promotion of clinical faculty. Research grants increased substantially.

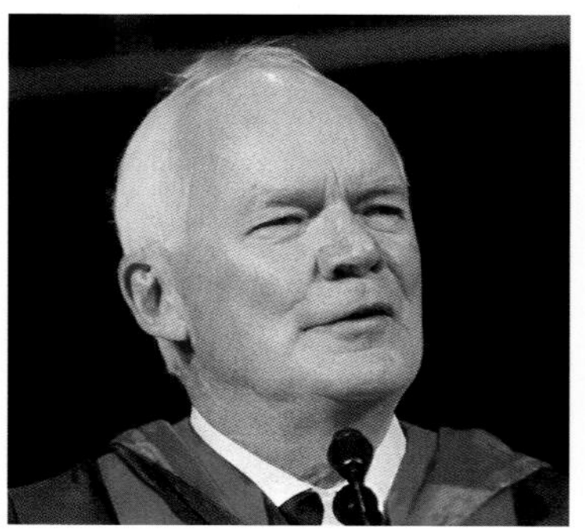

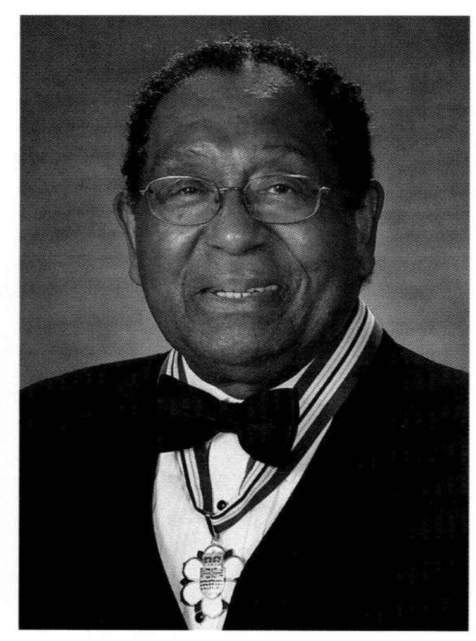

The Department of Surgery

Throughout Hollenberg's time as Dean (and during the first several years of that of his successor), the Head of Surgery was Richard Finley, a University of Western Ontario graduate and former Head of Surgery at Victoria Hospital in London, Ontario, who had been appointed by Webber in 1988. With the assistance of David Hardwick, Finley immediately established a strategic planning process, assembling the leaders of each division of surgery in the city's teaching hospitals, representatives of the young surgeons and of those from outside the city, to devise a mission statement based on some fundamental and agreed-upon principles. The department set out to provide the best clinical care for their patients while fulfilling and augmenting its educational responsibilities.

They began to focus on the entire undergraduate curriculum, as opposed to the clerkship only. Andrew Seal, a favourite of the students, established the Surgical Club where first- and second-year medical students could come to sessions at least once a month to hear seasoned surgeons discuss their practices and then accompany them into the operating rooms and their offices. Along with the dedicated participation of Director of Undergraduate Education Ian Turnbull, and similarly devoted educators Judy Vestrup and David Fairholm, the bedside teaching program was strengthened enormously. The heads of surgery at St. Paul's (John MacFarlane), Shaughnessy (Howard Fenster), Children's (Phil Ashmore), and UBC (Andrew Seal) were all keenly supportive of a strong education program. The department was proud that the Licentiate of the Medical Council of Canada (LMCC) results for undergraduates in surgery consistently put UBC in the top three or four in the national rankings. Former department head Herb Forward became director of residency education, initiating a residency training program in Prince George in 1990 and adding six-month rotations in several BC communities, among the first such rural programs in Canada.

In the 1990s it became a condition of employment that any new Vancouver surgical appointee, in addition to needing to be a good clinical surgeon, must have had at least two years of post-residency training in an area of expertise and must go into the full-time university stream. The academic quality of surgery was maintained by insisting on the

Robert Woollard, family physician, Head of Department of Family Practice (1998–2008).

LEFT FACING Richard Finley, thoracic surgeon, Head of Department of Surgery (1989–2001).

RIGHT FACING Felix Durity, neurosurgeon (UBC MD '63), Head of Division of Neurosurgery (1991–97).

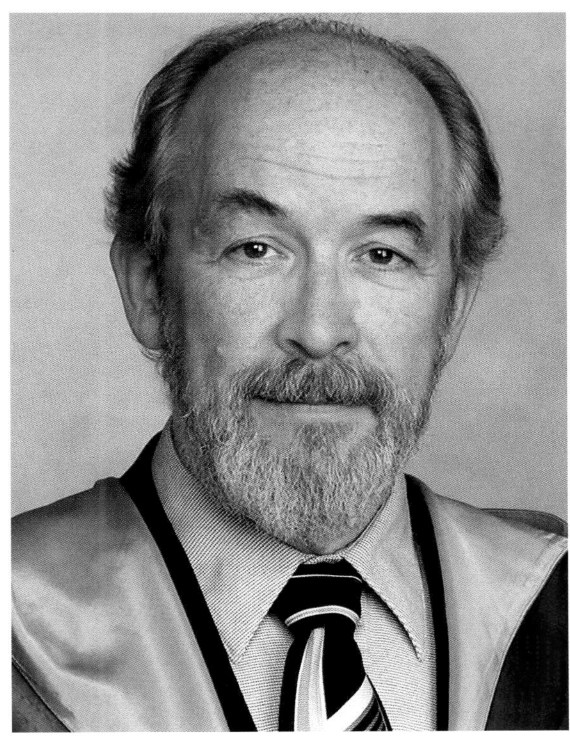

standards of training they had earlier identified, by linking each new faculty member with a basic science group and by having their divisions protect their clinical time. Particularly strong areas of basic science research were developed within the prostate cancer group (under Larry Goldenberg and Lorne Sullivan), the Solid Organ Transplant Program (under Stephen Chung and greatly enabled by Finley's successor, Garth Warnock), the neurosurgery program (under Felix Durity, noted for his innovations in skull-base surgery and his humanitarian work in Africa), and the vascular biology group. Finley exerted a degree of control over the distribution of funding and operating room time, rewarding those divisions that most vigorously pursued educational and research endeavours. The COUTH process of concentrating large surgical services in selected teaching hospitals was a significant factor in the effort to enhance the academic endeavour.

In 2000, late in his second term and under a new dean, Finley determined that the Department of Surgery's new evidence-based benchmarks for surgical waiting times were being met in only about fifty percent of cases. The situation was taken public to the Vancouver newspapers, radio, and television. Substantial additional government funding followed meetings with Minister of Health Mike Farnworth, and a major reorganization of the Vancouver hospital framework resulted. Although there were challenges posed by persisting inadequacies of infrastructure and personnel, the new resources would have a positive impact on reducing wait times and on encouraging existing subspecialty surgeons to resist offers from neighbouring Alberta and new recruits to pursue opportunities in BC. By the time he completed an extended second term in 2002, Finley would be recognized for having successfully navigated the challenges of turmoil in the health care system and limited academic funding to strengthen the clinical and academic missions of the department.

The Department of Family Practice

Carol Herbert led the relatively new Department of Family Practice from 1988 to 1998, a decade of enormous growth. Research and scholarly activity took root as faculty and staff were recruited,

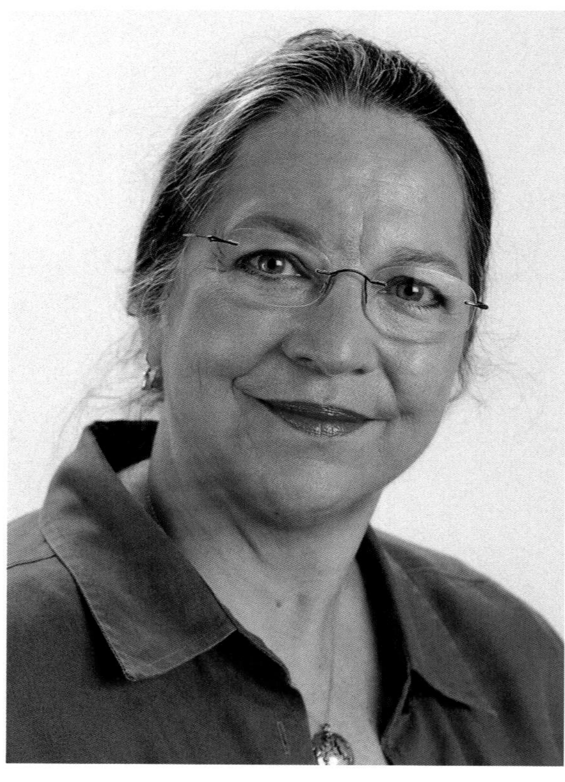

Judith Hall, pediatrician and geneticist, Head of Department of Pediatrics (1990–2000).

programs developed, and learning opportunities for students and residents expanded. Emphasizing its community-based philosophy, the department placed residents in St. Paul's Hospital, Victoria, Chilliwack, and Prince George, as well as in an increasing number of rural and remote settings. It expanded to over a hundred residents in seven programs, even though the required new funding was not guaranteed by the provincial government. Partnerships in the community gave rise to additional services and the divisions of palliative care and maternal-newborn care were added to the previously established divisions of sports medicine, emergency medicine, community geriatrics, and behavioural medicine.

In 1998, Herbert would leave to become Dean of Medicine at the University of Western Ontario. Hollenberg's successor, Cairns, appointed Robert "Bob" Woollard as the Head of Family Practice. Woollard had chaired senior committees, councils, and task forces for the BCMA, Canadian Medical Association, and College of Family Practice of Canada in the areas of medical education, environmental health, and ethical relations with industry. He continued to place departmental emphasis on serving the community and responding to provincial needs. He was soon to be assigned a major role in the implementation of the new MD undergraduate program and eventually in the implementation of additional resources that would come to the FoM for the expansion of educational activities within the BC health care system.

The Department of Pediatrics

Following the accidental death of pediatrics Head Donald Hill in 1989, Judith Hall was appointed as the new head, having run the clinical genetics program for the previous ten years. She was immediately confronted by issues of shortages of pediatric subspecialists to staff BC's only tertiary care hospital for children, overwhelmed clinicians with little time or energy for research, and a pediatric residency program "on notice to close." Recurrent budget cuts by UBC and the hospital, themselves experiencing government cuts, were discouraging for Hall and others trying to build up academic programs. From 1989 to '98, five different CEOs directed the BC Children's Hospital and Sunny Hill Health Centre and

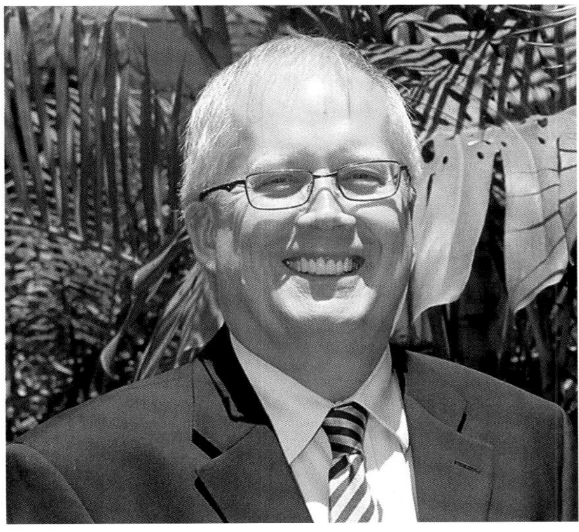

Robert Armstrong, developmental pediatrician, Head of Department of Pediatrics (2000–10).

the Women's Hospital and Health Centre, each of them facing serious financial constraints. Explaining the importance of the academic mission became a vital and recurrent task for Hall as new administrative leaders grappled with the complexities of the needs of physicians, residents, and students. Despite adversity, academic and service pediatrics grew stronger during the 1990s.

Strong subspecialty divisions developed in infectious disease and immunology, neonatology, adolescent health, rheumatology, oncology, neurology, and developmental pediatrics. Under its new director, Barrie MacLean, the residency program was rejuvenated and fully accredited, and later strengthened academically under its next director, Andrew McNabb. The BC Pediatric Society was established, improving communications among pediatricians and leading to travelling specialty clinics and a continuing medical education program. The administrative staff compiled a time-based survey of department member activities and responsibilities, at first locally and then nationally. The survey recommendations were used by other academic pediatrics departments across Canada but led to only modest funding adjustments in BC.

With expert guidance from Aubrey Tingle, the BC Children's Hospital Foundation provided substantial resources for support of investigators and the development of research infrastructure, fostering increasing success with external grant funding and publications.

Hall completed her second term in 2000. Sensitized to the need for the department head to have experience with and insight into the complexities of hospital administration, Dean Cairns appointed Robert "Bob" Armstrong as her successor. He had been Medical Director at Sunny Hill Health Centre and Vice-president, Medical Services and Quality at BC Children's Hospital (a name which has undergone frequent revisions and, as of 2020, is BC Children's Hospital and Women's Hospital and Health Centre). His direct experience with hospital administration would prove to facilitate his management of hospital relations as the department head.

The New MD Curriculum

By the time of Hollenberg's deanship, the school had been using the same curriculum for much of its first forty years; its characteristics were similar to medical curricula that had been in effect throughout the middle decades of the century in the majority of North American medical faculties. Although the Faculty was justifiably proud that its graduates regularly placed near the top in the LMCC's annual qualifying examinations and had gone on to obtain

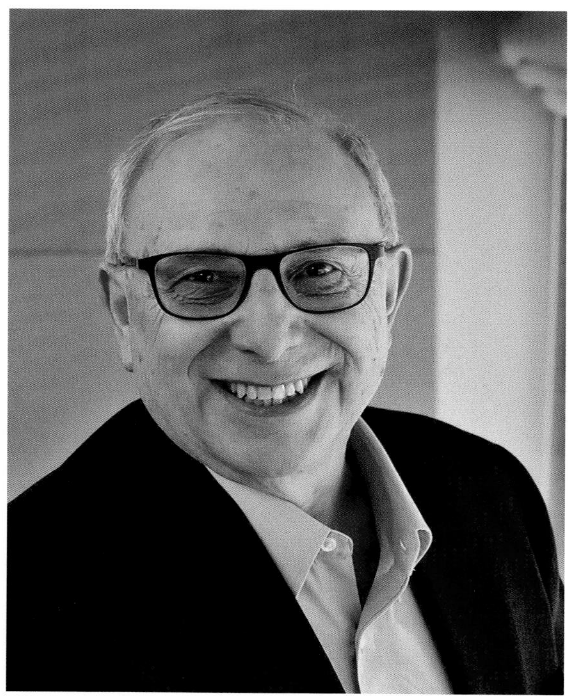

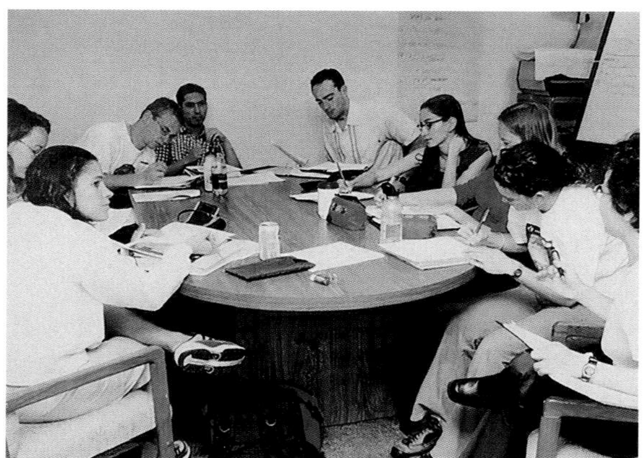

desirable residencies around the continent, the program had nevertheless come in for substantial criticism over the preceding decade. The joint Liaison Committee on Medical Education (LCME) and Committee on Accreditation of Canadian Medical Schools (CACMS) accreditation survey of UBC (April 19–22, 1993) characterized the medical undergraduate curriculum as being outdated and in need of major changes. The report was clear: reform was necessary if UBC was to retain its accreditation as one of Canada's sixteen medical schools.

The Faculty Executive Committee acted quickly to address this present threat to its accreditation. In November 1993, it established a Strategic Planning Committee that was "to make recommendations on any and all aspects of the undergraduate medical education program at the University of British Columbia, with a view to maintaining and enhancing the quality of the program." The committee was asked to address the entire curriculum and its administration and was given one year to make its recommendations. The committee, chaired by respirologist David Ostrow, comprised Joanna Bates, Mark Broudo, Andrew Chalmers, David Fairholm, Lili Kopala, Christine Loock, William Ovalle, Gordon Page, William "Wes" Schreiber, Andrew Seal, Laurie Summers, and Bruce Tiberiis. A goal was identified: to enable the MD graduate to develop defined knowledge, attitudes, and skills necessary to enter postgraduate training in any discipline. The prescribed competencies were to reflect the mission statement of the Faculty: "to advance the knowledge, understanding, and health of our society through education, scholarship, and health care with excellence as the most important criterion."

The committee recommended problem-based learning in small group tutorials as the basis for directed self-learning, supplemented by a few lectures and laboratories all based around physiological systems. Students were to be assigned to attend the offices of family physicians early on in the first year, and clinical skills were to be taught from the beginning of the course in conjunction with each of the problem-based-learning physiological systems. There would also be a course on the physician and society (Doctor, Patient, and Society), and some innovative approaches to student assessment were to be initiated. The specific

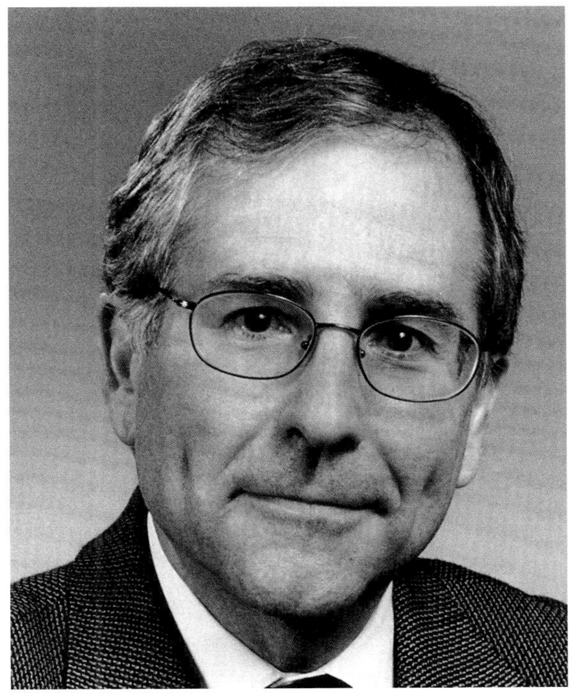

John A. Cairns (UBC MD '68), cardiologist, seventh Dean of Medicine (1996–2003).

LEFT FACING David Ostrow, respirologist, Professor Emeritus, Department of Medicine, President and CEO Vancouver Coastal Health (2009–14).

RIGHT FACING MD student tutorial group with faculty leader early in the era of the "new curriculum."

recommendations mirrored educational innovations that had occurred at the medical schools of McMaster and Harvard. The clerkship was to be greatly expanded from fourth year to include the third-year students in order to provide more in-depth clinical experiences.

The planning process brought together clinicians and laboratory scientists and required faculty to think about MD undergraduate education with a new intensity. The exercise was rejuvenating and stimulated a much greater commitment to and involvement in medical education within the Faculty. The committee report was delivered within six months, and a new curriculum was approved in principle by the Faculty Executive in November 1994. The initial implementation target was autumn 1996, but in late 1995 it was decided to postpone it until 1997 because of unresolved issues about the adequacy of resources, persisting reservations among many academic faculty members, and significant resistance from clinical faculty who carried responsibility for most of the teaching after years one and two and yet received only token or no financial compensation for their services. They believed their teaching loads would increase with negative impacts on their clinical responsibilities, and they shared reservations as to the soundness of the new pedagogy. It would take the considerable negotiating skills and goodwill generated by the next dean to finally overcome these obstacles and implement the new curriculum.

The Appointment of John Cairns

John Cairns became UBC's seventh Dean of Medicine when Hollenberg stepped down in 1996. Although Hollenberg retired, he kept busy tutoring in the Faculty, pursuing his research on the development and regeneration of the vertebrate retina and exploring possibilities for UBC's medical school in certain international forums, particularly with regard to cooperative projects and exchanges in medical education.

Cairns was drawn to the position by the prospect of a return to his alma mater (he had been the gold medallist in the class of '68) and by the dramatic growth in the stature of UBC. Following clinical and research training in cardiology at McGill's affiliated

FACING Andrew Chalmers (UBC MD '71), rheumatologist, Associate Dean of MD Undergraduate Curriculum (1993–99).

teaching hospitals, Cairns had been recruited to McMaster University in Hamilton, Ontario, world-renowned for its problem-based curriculum of medical education. He had been Coordinator of the Regional Cardiovascular Program and then Chair of Medicine. The search committee decided the ideal candidate would be a proven leader and an active and credible clinician; they would also have significant clinical research achievement and experience with a modern MD undergraduate curriculum. Cairns appeared to fill the bill.

In his first meeting of the Faculty Executive in October 1996, Cairns delineated what he saw to be some real strengths of the Faculty of Medicine, among them UBC's growing excellence, strong basic medical sciences departments, selected areas of excellence in clinical research (neurology, HIV/AIDS, infectious disease, medical genetics, ophthalmology, respirology, oncology), a tradition of innovation in the practicing medical community (cardiac surgery, nephrology, neurosurgery, orthopaedics, and minimally invasive general and thoracic surgery), substantial teaching hospital support for research (hospital-based research institutes, laboratory and office space, salary support of faculty members), the absence of competing medical schools in BC, private philanthropy, and a tradition at UBC of support for commercialization of intellectual property.

He also laid out his assessment of the challenges being faced by the FoM. Implementation of the new curriculum had been postponed until the autumn of 1997 because of significant resistance among faculty members and some of the leadership, and there were no new resources to allocate. During Cairns's recruitment, there had been occasional references to a FoM debt, but there was no precise estimate of its magnitude. Late in Hollenberg's term, UBC's finance department had revised their processes and came to recognize a huge disparity between the FoM's accessible assets and its liabilities. Hollenberg had persuaded the budget committee to allow the FoM to repay the debt by leaving open positions unfilled for a year, but by 1996 it was clear that the plan was insufficient to fully address it. Provincial university funding was steadily decreasing, relations with the provincial Ministry of Health were relatively minimal, and the FoM was immersed in the turbulence of health care reform. Despite its many strengths, UBC's Faculty of Medicine lagged behind other Canadian faculties in national and international stature—the road ahead was littered with obstacles.

Implementing the New Curriculum

Although Cairns had understood that a new curriculum was on track for implementation in autumn 1997, he soon realized that achieving this goal was far from a certainty, with significant resistance among some academic and many clinical faculty members. Implementation of the new curriculum with its nineteen new courses (none of them as

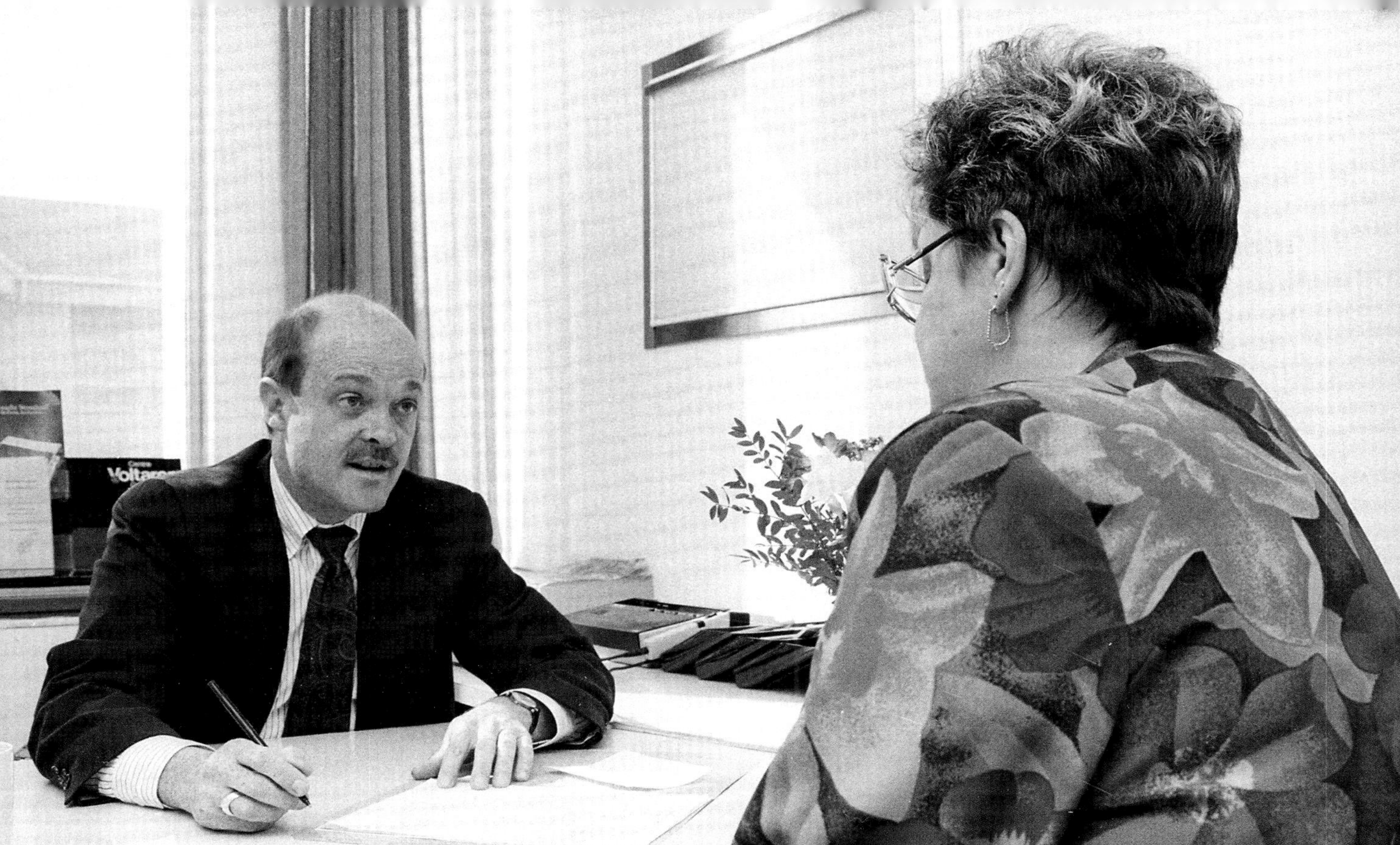

yet completely planned) would require not only approval by the Faculty Executive but the full faculty, wherein every faculty member has a vote. Both meetings had been scheduled for November 1996, within weeks of Cairns's arrival. More than 250 attended the full faculty meeting, far beyond the usual fifty or so, and the overall motion for approval passed by a vote of 153 to 69. Jubilation was tempered by the requirement for Senate approval, but it was duly granted in January 1997.

Cairns supported the new curriculum in every feasible manner, but resources were scarce. Full implementation of the most extensive education reform ever undertaken by the Faculty of Medicine initially fell to rheumatologist Andrew Chalmers, the Associate Dean of MD Undergraduate Curriculum. During four years of concerted effort, implementation was plagued by ongoing reservations and resistance. A few department heads were reluctant to yield department responsibilities for education to a more central authority and had reservations about the pedagogical soundness of the new curriculum. Clinical faculty wanted more academic and financial recognition for their teaching.

Cairns appointed an implementation task force under the chair of Bob Woollard (who later that year would also become Head of Family Practice) to focus directly on securing sufficient resources and gaining the buy-in of departments. The task force provided a sharp and task-oriented focus that had been missing in the early months of implementation. Persisting concerns about implementation led Cairns to commission an organizational review by outside experts who would work with David Ostrow, who had chaired the strategic planning committee from 1993 to '95. The external team concluded that

Carol-Ann Courneya and Heartfelt Images

Carol-Ann Courneya, a leader in the teaching of cardiovascular physiology, began encouraging students to conceptualize artistically their understanding of the cardiovascular system in 2001, referring to the initiative as "Heartfelt Images." Original student works were submitted in oils, watercolour, pastel, pen and ink, etching, or photographs and were judged on a combination of artistic merit and relevance to the cardiovascular system. An outstanding example by a non-Indigenous, former student Michiko Maruyama is shown in the illustrated figure below, reflecting her appreciation and the influence of Indigenous artists from the west coast of B.C.

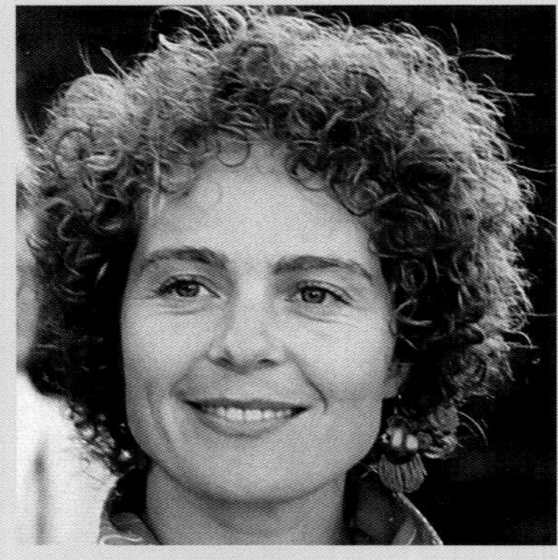

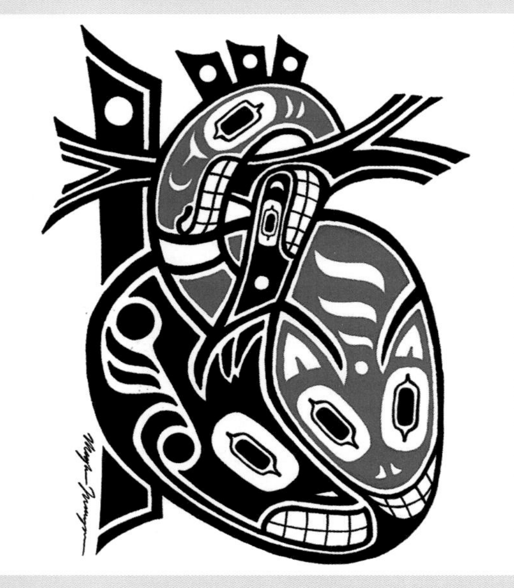

ABOVE Carol-Anne Courneya, cardiovascular physiologist, Assistant Dean Student Affairs (2013–20).

RIGHT "Spirit of the Heart" artist: Michiko Maruyama (UBC MD '15). In 2020, Dr. Maruyama was a cardiac surgery resident in Edmonton and a Master's in Industrial Design candidate.

the new curriculum was innovative and progressive, but it pointed out a number of weaknesses and provided extensive recommendations.

Although the first year of the new curriculum had been successfully completed and the new second year was nearing readiness for autumn 1998, the Dean established a search committee for the reconfigured role of Associate Dean of Curriculum. William "Wes" Schreiber, an anatomic pathologist who had also been a member of the strategic planning committee, accepted the new role. Schreiber was an accomplished teacher, disciplined and well organized, and knowledgeable about educational theory and innovation. He led the next stages of implementation of the new curriculum.

The curriculum was now more student focused rather than teacher focused. There were fewer formal lectures. Departments invested time and money in tutor training workshops to provide both basic science and clinical faculty with the skills to tutor small group sessions of eight students meeting for two hours two to three times a week for

Barry McBride, microbiologist, V.P. Academic and Provost, UBC (1998–2004).

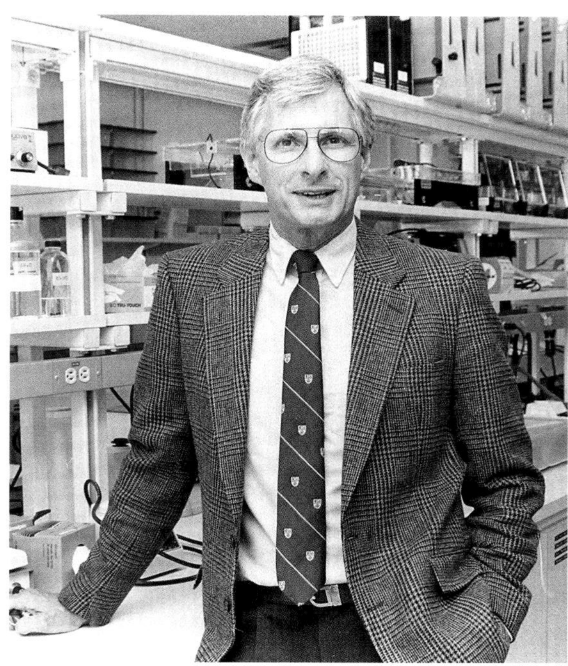

four-to-six-week system-based blocks. Many basic science faculty members encountered clinical-based problems for the first time. Large numbers of clinical faculty, many with no previous formal teaching experience but known for their problem-solving skills, were brought into the curriculum to assist with the small group tutorials. The new curriculum received approval at two special visits of the LCME and CACMS, beginning in 1999. The new curriculum proved to be robust.

The revolutionary curricular changes were enthusiastically received by students from the outset, and eventually by faculty as well. The new approaches came to have a profound effect on the medical school. The approach of practicing clinicians and basic scientists working together laid the foundations for the expansion of the school into non-traditional medical academic sites with the distributed curriculum which was to begin in 2004.

From the Faculty's earliest years, the student body has comprised mature self-starters who have characteristically created a network of clubs and support services. The Wellness Initiative Network is a student-run network of services for UBC medical students, which includes clubs for the arts, sports, different forms of dance, and student assistance. The network also advocates for students, developing absence policy recommendations, a wellness self-check tool for students to track their own mental and physical well-being, and a "wellness curriculum" which has become part of the undergraduate MD curriculum.

Crippling Debt and a New Strategy

Early in his term, Cairns realized the Faculty's finances would be a barrier not only to academic growth but to the very survival of the FoM. Extensive analysis revealed that the accumulated debt to UBC was approximately $6.5 million, arising primarily from multiyear financial commitments to high-profile recruits for leadership positions but also from the implementation (with no new funding) of a second year of family practice residency (obligatory for accreditation and Ministry of Health-funded in all other provinces). The new Provost, Barry McBride, former Dean of UBC's outstanding Faculty of Science, was emphatic that UBC would require repayment by the FoM and would hold the new dean responsible for a repayment plan.

Martha C. Piper, physiotherapist, eleventh President of UBC (1997–2006).

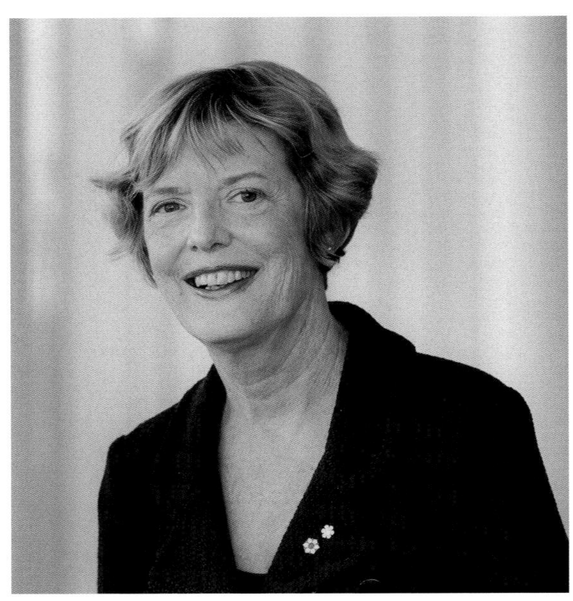

Debt was not the only financial problem. Annual reductions of the provincial operating grant to UBC and resulting annual reductions in UBC's allocations to the FoM had reached 4.5 percent by 1998–99. The cumulative effective reduction was estimated to reach twenty-two percent by the turn of the millennium. Cairns recognized there was no justification for inflicting the FoM's financial woes on other faculties, and that in the final analysis, it is the dean's responsibility to manage FoM financial challenges, whatever their origin. The debt was an albatross the Faculty bore throughout Cairns's time as Dean, but it served as a stimulus to begin exploring solutions that went beyond the university budget and ultimately proved highly successful.

To overcome the faculty's financial difficulties, Cairns explored new ways to engage with the BC government. In an early meeting, President Strangway had summarized his position in words to the effect of "Don't go near advanced education. That is the territory of the university president and his delegates. But the Ministry of Health, yes, if you can work with them, do so, and with my blessing." Cairns approached Minister of Health Joy McPhail, who seemed eager to hear about the Faculty and its impacts on the health care system, and when Cairns suggested that she pay a formal visit to the Faculty, she readily accepted.

The visit took place in March 1997 and was a great success. McPhail and Deputy Minister David Kelly stated that they were enormously impressed by the faculty, staff, students, and residents they had met in the Instructional Resources Centre and the adjacent UBC Hospital. McPhail was very interested in the capital facilities and the Faculty's educational and related missions. Follow-up communications established agreements for ongoing interactions between the Ministry of Health staffers and the FoM to go through the deputy minister. Cairns emphasized that close working relationships with the Ministry of Health were essential if the FoM was to assist the ministry in addressing issues of physician supply, quality and relevance of medical practice, and utilization of health care resources, drugs, and services.

David Strangway was a tough act to follow, but his successor, Martha Piper, was up to the task. A distinguished academic physiotherapist, she had led the School of Physical and Occupational Therapy at McGill, had been Vice-president of Research at University of Alberta, and in 1997 became UBC's eleventh President. She had considerable insight into health care delivery and the education of health professionals. Not long after

The Spring Galas

UBC medical students also tend to have a wide range of interests beyond medicine. Many have had an appreciation or talent for the arts. Associate Dean of Student Affairs Andrew Seal, a general surgeon who was also a talented artist and who attended the Medical School Ball in 1994, remarked: "The students' performances were however of such remarkable quality that it seemed to me they deserved an appropriate time and place for all to enjoy their amazing talents without distraction." He recruited Gordon Horner, a second-year student at the time, who then produced and brilliantly directed "The Spring Gala," which took place on April 12, 1995, in the Old Auditorium on the UBC campus. The performance was an outstanding success and was held again the next year at Centennial Theatre in North Vancouver, again a success. From then on, the performances have been held at the Chan Centre on the Point Grey Campus. Typical performances have included choral pieces, classical and pop music pieces by soloists and groups, piano, violin, and dance. The genres have ranged from the old classics to modern dance and Bhangra; the performances, all by students, have always been sold out.

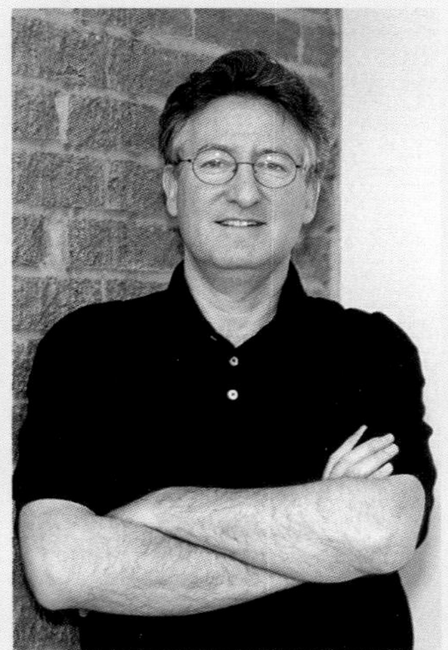

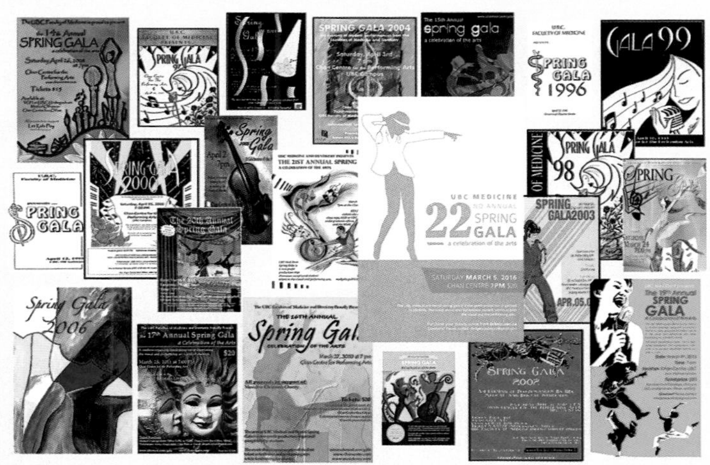

LEFT Andrew Seal, general surgeon, artist, Associate Dean of Student Affairs (1993–99).

RIGHT Collage of advertising posters for Spring Gala from 1995 onward.

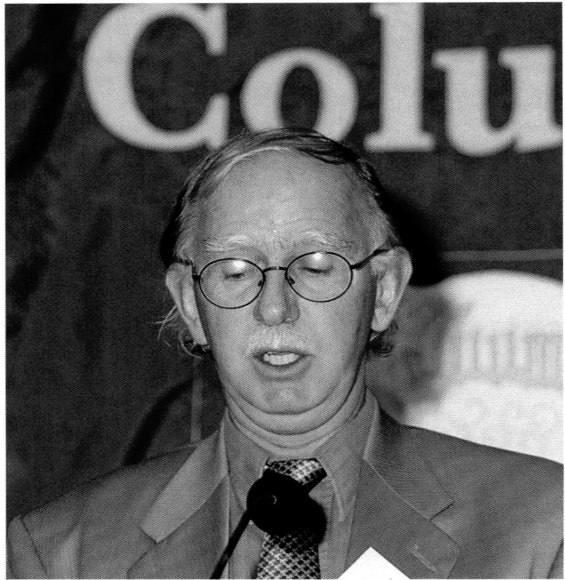

Derek Atkins, Associate V.P. Academic Planning, UBC (1999–2005).

her appointment, in October 1977, she arranged to meet with David Kelly. Cairns provided her with a detailed document which concluded by stating "the ultimate goal of the FoM is that of the optimal health of BC citizens, as well as making broader contributions to the health of citizens of Canada and beyond. These are achieved primarily by pursuing our threefold mission in education, research, and continuous quality improvement for the health care system." He asked her to stress to Kelly that the FoM could not fulfill provincial government expectations without financial support from the Ministry of Health, a common practice in other Canadian provinces.

Following his meeting with Piper, Kelly asked Cairns for data on funding of UBC's medical school and comparisons with other Canadian schools. Cairns's response included a proposal for a fully funded expansion of enrollment. Subsequent meetings with Kelly and staff in Victoria focused on details of potential direct funding from the Ministry of Health. Cairns was able to mobilize support from the CEOs and board chairs of Vancouver's four teaching hospitals, and when they met jointly with Piper, McBride, and UBC board chair Larry Bell, it was agreed to work together to support the requests for ministry funding.

McBride had already agreed with Cairns's proposal for an external funding analysis of the FoM, and it was decided to include representatives of the hospital CEOs on a provost's advisory committee to which the government appointed assistant deputy ministers from both health and advanced education. John Wade, former Dean of Medicine of University of Manitoba, was commissioned in early 1999 to review the Faculty's missions and finances and to prepare a formal report for UBC and the provincial government.

Ironically, despite the willingness of the Ministry of Health and the regional health board to support the FoM, the financial pressures from UBC had not let up. In March 1999, the UBC Board of Governors stated their requirement that the FoM meet strict financial targets for debt repayment and ongoing budget reductions. Provost Barry McBride and Associate VP, Academic Planning Derek Atkins were not satisfied with the lack of guarantees of new Ministry of Health funding and demanded from the FoM a set of firm plans to be presented to the Board of Governors in mid-July. Cairns froze all recruitment to the FoM and put all searches on hold. Cairns and Atkins worked out a detailed plan for using the salary funds saved by holding up recruitments following retirements or departures for the next one to three years, with the freed-up funds going to debt repayment rather than recruitment. Repayment of the full amount of the debt would require a plan extending over seven years and compromising recruitments across the entire FoM. Endowments were fully deployed, and tuition fee increases were drafted. The final plan with guaranteed milestones was presented to the Board of Governors in July 1999 and accepted.

By the summer of 1999, the FoM had been able to arrange with the Ministry of Health to provide an incremental $1.8 million per year directly to the Faculty to help in addressing immediate threats, beginning in 1999-2000 and continuing the next year. John Wade's detailed, hard-hitting report was delivered in October 1999, highlighting the need for substantial funding from the Ministry of Health for clinical education, the family practice residency, and compensation for medical administrative activities in association with clinical education. The report was constructively received by UBC and the relevant ministries. Deputy Minister of Health Leah Hollins stepped in to flow an additional $2 million a year to address shortfalls in funding of the residency programs.

Promptly following up on the recommendations of the Wade Report, in January 2000, Hollins appointed the Roles and Responsibilities Committee to move the financial proposals forward. Under the able chair of David Babiuk from the Ministry of Health; with Atkins, McBride, and Cairns from UBC; and representatives from the Ministry of Health and the Ministry of Advanced Education, the committee had by the spring of 2001 developed a detailed set of programs and requisite Ministry of Health funding was approved. The Faculty could finally see a glimmer of hope for financial stability fifty-one years after its founding.

Strategic Thinking and Plans

As the FoM worked through the spring of 1999 to manage its financial crisis, it had become apparent that a fundamental planning exercise and new initiatives were required. Strategic planning had already begun back in June 1997 with an externally facilitated retreat of Faculty leaders and innovators, followed that autumn by the creation of a Strategic Initiatives Advisory Group. Comprising eight wise and senior faculty members (David Hardwick, Aubrey Tingle, Richard Finley, George Mackie, Michael Hayden, John Mancini, Bruce McManus, and Carol Herbert), the advisory group had been convened by Cairns to help him understand key issues facing the FoM and to explore future directions. The stresses from inadequate UBC and provincial government funding, a new undergraduate curriculum, an overworked and somewhat resentful clinical faculty, constant churn in the health care system, and falling research performance were obvious–discussions focused on

LEFT Bruce McManus, cardiovascular pathologist, Head of Department of Pathology and Laboratory Medicine (1993–2000).

RIGHT Logo of the Golden Jubilee (2000) and subsequently adopted as Faculty of Medicine logo, created by Lyle Wilson, a Haisla artist.

FACING Golden Jubilee Program, November 2000.

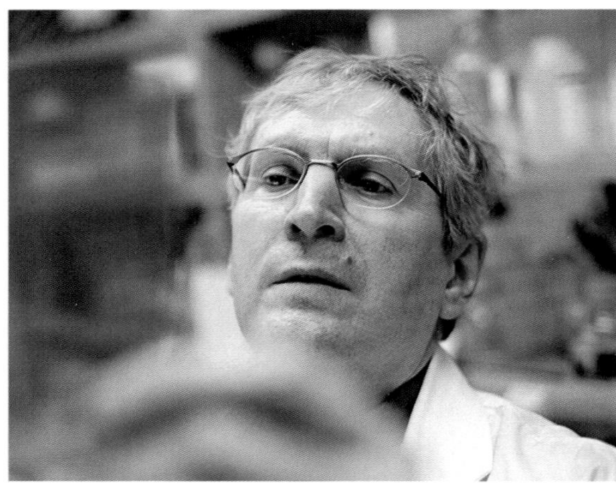

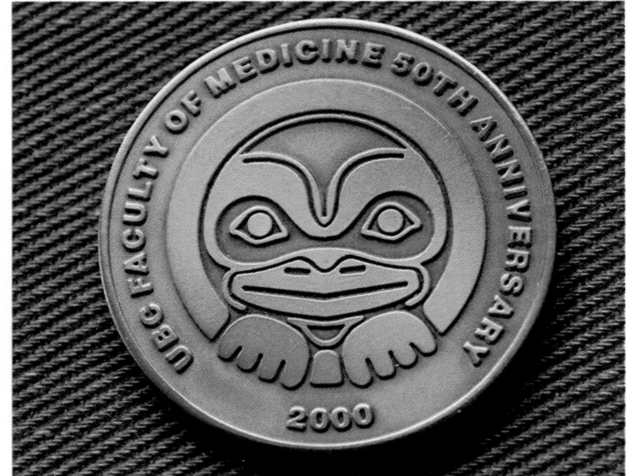

the generation of ideas for addressing them. An early insight developed by this group was that of the potential value of establishing closer working relationships with the Ministry of Health and help in addressing the FoM's financial exigencies.

Another insight from the advisory group was that their Faculty colleagues lacked the strong institutional culture and pride several of its members had experienced in other Canadian medical schools. In a move to strengthen awareness of and support for the FoM, a year-long celebration of the Faculty's Golden Jubilee was launched in 2000. Bob McGraw, inaugural Head of Orthopaedics, was asked to take on the role, and, after being assured by Cairns that the vision was indeed audacious and would be well funded, he accepted. He put together a large planning committee, a professional event planner was engaged, a Faculty logo was commissioned from Haisla artist Lyle Wilson, and the Vancouver Convention Centre was booked for two days of events to occur in November 2000. Student registration was funded by faculty endowments for student support and classes were cancelled. Distinguished guests spoke at the opening ceremonies, and the outstanding scientific program organized by Steve Tredwell drew large numbers of faculty and students. The social program included receptions, dinners, and a gala ball, all well attended. The November events capped a year-long celebration, which included hosting a successful ACMC meeting and several other national society meetings, a special issue of the *Alumni Chronicle* focused on the Faculty of Medicine, an article in the *Canadian Medical Association Journal*, and the eventual adoption of the fiftieth anniversary logo as the official logo of the FoM.

The idea and planning for the Golden Jubilee occurred in 1999, but facing challenges to its very existence, the FoM realized that a fundamental rethink and redirecting of its missions was required. At the recommendation of Bruce McManus, Head

FINAL PROGRAM AND ABSTRACT BOOK

UBC Faculty of Medicine

Golden Jubilee 2000

UBC FACULTY OF MEDICINE 50TH ANNIVERSARY

2000

November 3rd and 4th, 2000, Vancouver, British Columbia

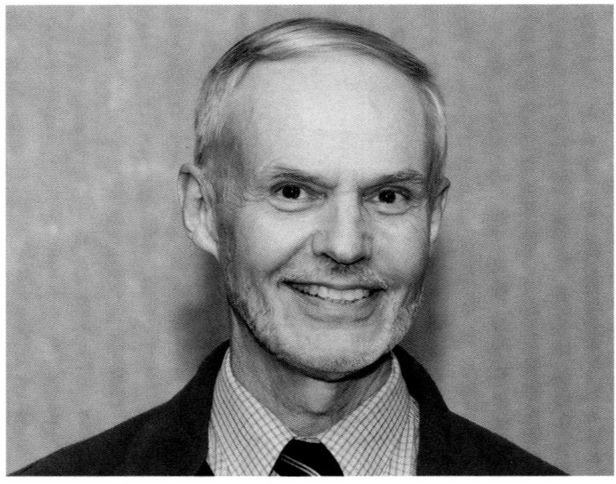

George Mackie, biochemist/molecular biologist, Head of Department of Biochemistry and Molecular Biology (1994–2004).

LEFT FACING Charles J. "Chuck" Jago, President of University of Northern BC (1997–2006).

RIGHT FACING On June 22, 2000, nearly 7,000 people attended a health care rally at the Multiplex (now the CN Centre) in Prince George to protest the state of health care in Northern BC. The event brought national attention to the local crisis and laid the groundwork for the Northern Medical Program.

of Pathology and Laboratory Medicine, the Faculty engaged an American management consultant to facilitate the Faculty's first formal strategic planning exercise. A group of faculty leaders, including all department heads, associate deans, and fresh blood from throughout the Faculty, assembled, and the consultant worked his magic. A group of seven heads of departments or schools coalesced–George Mackie (biochemistry and molecular biology), Bob Woollard (family practice), Bruce McManus, Rich Finley, Anne Carswell (rehabilitation sciences), Martin Schechter (health care and epidemiology) and Jan Friedman (medical genetics)–and agreed to take ongoing responsibility for working with the Dean to develop a formal strategic plan. Countless meetings at the end of long days followed, as the group met over many months, eventually crafting a green paper entitled "Strong Medicine."

The draft document was widely circulated, and the hundreds of responses were fed into the ongoing meetings of the planning group, eventually giving rise to a white paper ("Destination Health"). By September 2000, the final document ("The Best of Health") was complete, attractively printed, illustrated, and widely circulated, along with a detailed operational plan and timelines. The Faculty Executive (April 1999) had already accepted a wider health care system-based vision, which was embodied in the document's vision statement: "The Faculty of Medicine of the University of British Columbia aspires to internationally recognized achievement in education, research, and service that makes a vital contribution to the health of British Columbians." Very quickly, elements of the operational plan became manifest in the creation of a task force on integrating study and service (chaired by Bob Woollard and charged with developing a rationale for incremental funding from the Ministry of Health), a joint liaison committee with the Ministry of Health, an advisory committee to the provost from the FoM, a community advisory council, and the beginning of concerted efforts toward substantial expansion of the medical school.

A New Vision for Expansion

Integral to the evolving strategic plan was a growing realization that the future success of the Faculty lay in creating an ambitious plan for province-wide expansion of the medical school. As a first step, Cairns had visited Prince George in February 1998, together with Carol Herbert, Head of Family Practice. The visit was prompted in part by discussions Cairns had had with Deputy Minister David Kelly. In

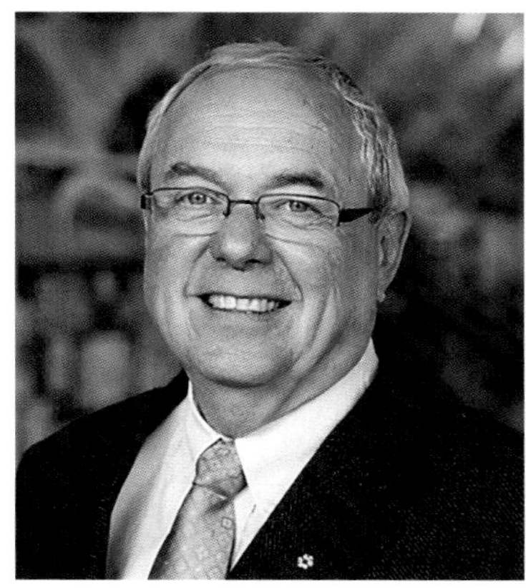

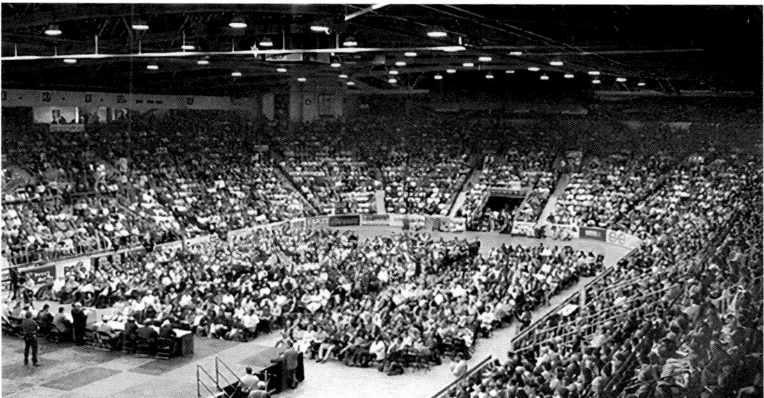

response to Kelly's concerns about northern physician supply, Cairns had raised the possibility of an expansion of enrollment with appropriate funding. It was widely reported that more than ten thousand people in Prince George could not find a family doctor. Cairns found fertile soil in Prince George. Most impressive were the programs and capital infrastructure of the new University of Northern BC (UNBC), its dynamic president, Charles "Chuck" Jago, who had begun to dream of medical education in the north centred on UNBC, and the recent rally in the Prince George arena of seven thousand members of the public and doctors to advocate for medical education in the north. The academic leadership of Galt Wilson, Bill Simpson, and Donald McRitchie pointed to the possibilities for more extensive FoM programming in Prince George.

Expansion of medical student enrollment had become a regular topic of discussion in the joint UBC-Government Roles and Responsibilities Committee, which had been charged by Deputy Minister Hollins with addressing the financial concerns of the FoM. The committee members became familiar with the data that BC's medical student to population ratio was by far the lowest of any Canadian province at 3.2 per 100,000, compared to a national mean of 6 per 100,000. Although the UBC entering class of 120 was exceeded only by the universities of Toronto (177) and Montreal (163), Ontario had five faculties of medicine, and Quebec had four, while BC had only one. To maintain its physician workforce, BC needed three hundred new practitioners each year. Only seventy-five of these were UBC graduates; the balance was drawn from elsewhere in Canada and from South Africa, Ireland, the UK, and other nations. At every opportunity Cairns had been placing these data before the BCMA, hospital boards, College of Physicians and Surgeons, local medical societies, Vancouver Board of Trade, business leaders, and the press. The focus of all previous governments had been on the expense of medical education and the idea that additional expenditures could not be justified when physician supply appeared to be adequate or even excessive. The flawed Barer-Stoddart report (1991) on physician human resources was used to justify their policies.

In June 2000, Minister of Health Mike Farnworth announced that the government recognized the need for BC to take increased responsibility for educating its own physicians and that it would be meeting with UBC to plan for expansion of the school. In July, together with President Piper and Provost McBride, Dean Cairns apprised Farnworth and David Babiuk of two fundamental requirements:

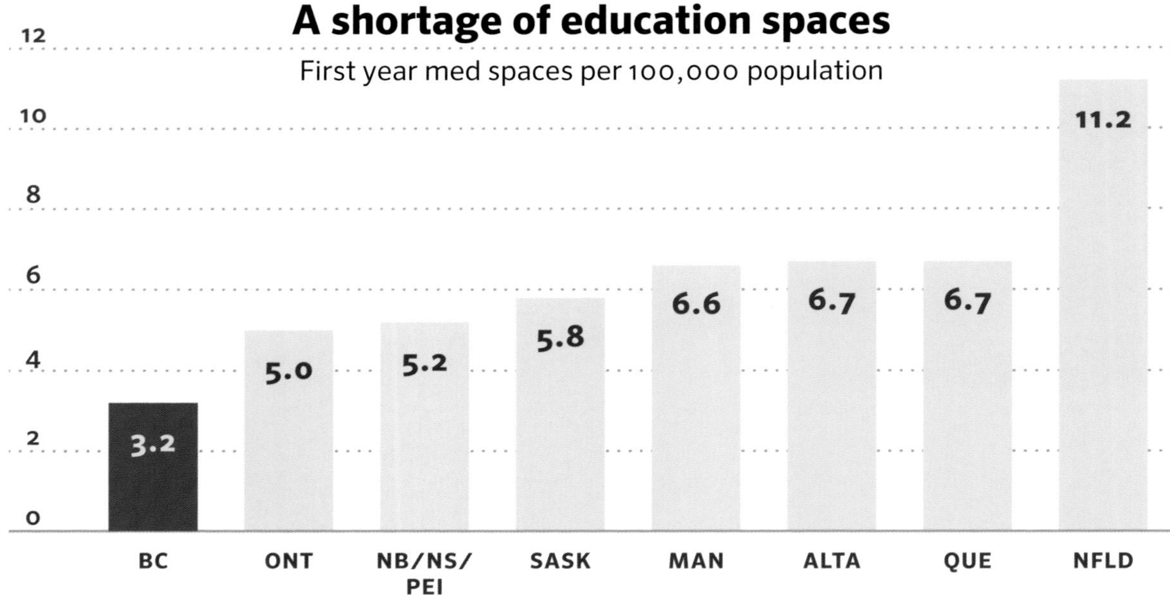

Source: Association of Canadian Medical Colleges (based on 1996 Canadian census)

1) appropriate funding of current medical education within the health care system (both residents and students), and 2) appropriate per-student and per-resident funding of expansion (at rates later to be negotiated). The Roles and Responsibilities Committee was directed to fast-track work on addressing currently unmet needs for clinical teaching and to begin planning for expansion of undergraduate and postgraduate programs; the committee delivered its report on September 19, 2000. The Provost's Advisory Committee on the FoM asked Bob Woollard, David McLean (Senior Associate Dean of Research, Planning, and Health Care System), and Derek Atkins to conduct final negotiations with the Ministry of Health and to prepare the case for the Treasury Board.

On December 5, 2000, Premier Ujjal Dosanjh announced the BC Health Action Plan, a $180-million commitment in new health investment, to provide "the funding to put more nurses, doctors, and other health care professionals into the system and improve access to hospital care and community care, so BC families can get the right care when they need it." Buried within the announcement was a final package of $9 million annually for the FoM beginning in fiscal year 2001-02. In parallel with the negotiations for the new Ministry of Health funding, the Integrating Study and Service Implementation Committee chaired by Bob Woollard had created the Strategic Teaching Initiative, to be the receptor site and vehicle for dispersion for the new ministry funding. The initiative was intended to consolidate clinical teaching in a distributed model to support a sustainable health professional workforce in BC.

The impacts of the Strategic Teaching Initiative were transformative and felt across the Faculty's clinical teaching missions. For the first time, there was funding for administrative stipends and support for residency program directors, clinical faculty teaching, planning and implementation, and a host

Hon. Gordon Campbell, Liberal, Premier of BC (2001–11).

FACING Graphic depiction of number of medical students per 100,000 provincial population in late 1990s – the ratio in BC was about half the national average.

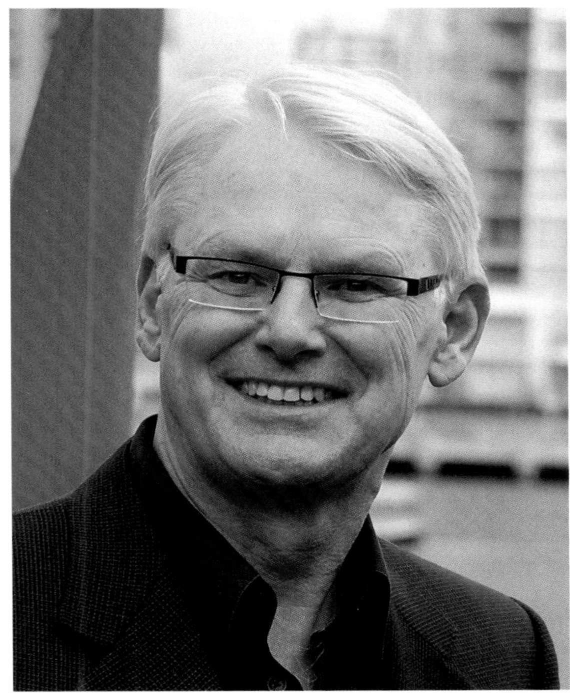

of other vital functions. In autumn 2001, the first increment of eight medical students enrolled (with the negotiated funding increment of $60,000 per year per student), and additional resident positions were also offered.

A long-delayed provincial election was announced for May 2001. Cairns had already met with the Leader of the Opposition Gordon Campbell and the Liberal health critic Colin Hanson to present the FoM's ideas about expansion. Campbell, the former mayor of Vancouver, had some familiarity with the school–his father was the much-loved Chargo Campbell, an internist who had been an associate dean in the 1970s. On the evening before the election campaign was to begin, Cairns received a phone call from Campbell, who was preparing his announcement of the Liberal platform the next morning and wanting to review details of the medical school expansion. He wished to confirm that the vision was a doubling of medical school enrollment, maintenance of a single medical school but with distributed sites in Prince George and Victoria (Kelowna to come later), and the creation of major new buildings at UBC, Prince George, and Victoria. Delighted to hear these elements of the UBC vision articulated by the likely premier-to-be, Cairns confirmed that these were his understandings and the next day, Campbell announced his explicit commitments. On May 16, 2001, the NDP government, compromised by two major scandals and nine years in power, was defeated in a Liberal landslide which captured seventy-seven of the seventy-nine seats.

Planning for a massive expansion in a distributed model began in earnest and accelerated rapidly. UBC leadership was key to the eventual success of this plan. Piper's strong and charismatic leadership of UBC, her vision for health professional education, and her skilled negotiations with both provincial and federal governments were critical factors. Derek Atkins had become very familiar with the FoM through overseeing its debt repayment plans and through increasing involvement in the conceptualization of the expansion. As Provost, Barry McBride was a champion in consolidating relationships with UNBC and the University of Victoria (UVic).

In addition to Dean Cairns, key faculty members during this intense planning were Joanna Bates, David McLean, and Alison Buchan. Bates, a family practitioner with a long educational pedigree,

LEFT FACING Joanna Bates, family physician, Associate Dean Admissions (1997–2001), Senior Associate Dean MD Undergraduate Education (2001–08), Inaugural Director of Centre for Health Education Scholarship.

RIGHT FACING Angela Towle, medical educator, Associate Dean MD Undergraduate Education, Curriculum, and Vancouver Fraser Medical Program (2002–10).

The conceptualization and functional planning of the massive expansion was substantial in itself, but being undertaken as a distributed program in partnership with two other universities added immeasurably to the complexity.

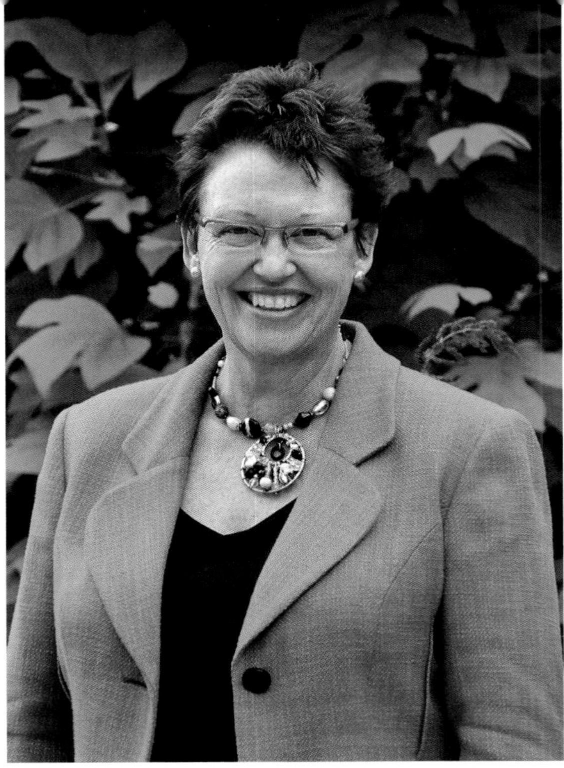

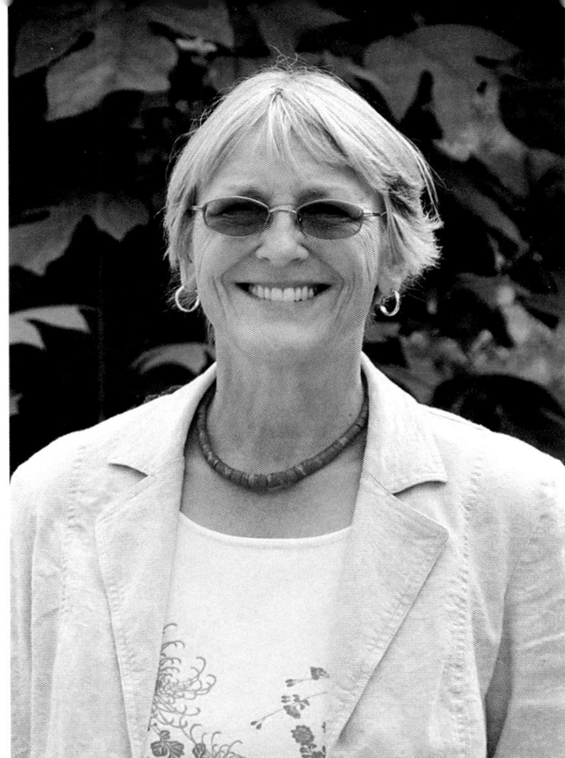

including being the daughter of former dean Bates, had moved from a clinical to a full-time faculty appointment only in 1997. First, as Associate Dean of MD Undergraduate Admissions, and then as the inaugural Senior Associate Dean, MD Undergraduate Education (2001), she played a major role. Her focus throughout the planning and implementation was on the creation of a distributed program of undergraduate medical education which would function effectively across the province and be respectful of the new university partners. Angela Towle, who had joined the MD undergraduate program in the mid-1990s as a medical education specialist, received a faculty appointment and eventually became Associate Dean of MD Undergraduate Education and Curriculum, reporting to Bates.

David McLean, a dermatologist and former Vice-president of Research of VHHSC, and now Senior Associate Dean, Research, Planning, and Health Care System, was aided by David Hardwick in providing strategic advice on new program development and took direct responsibility for the creation of new affiliation agreements and organizational frameworks for the interactions of UBC, FoM, UNBC, and UVic. The final affiliation structures were built on those developed earlier by Hardwick and implemented in agreements among the partner universities and the UBC president's legal group.

Alison Buchan, a physiologist who had been Assistant Dean of Research under McLean, became Associate Dean of Research and then assumed the role of co-director (along with Hugh Brock of the Faculty of Science) for the detailed conceptualization, planning, and commissioning of the jewel in the capital facilities' crown—the $110-million Life Sciences Centre on the UBC campus.

The conceptualization and functional planning of the massive expansion was substantial in itself, but being undertaken as a distributed program in partnership with two other universities added immeasurably to the complexity. In meetings of the Implementation Planning Subcommittee for Medical Expansion (IPSME), it was readily apparent that in a successful partnership, there was an

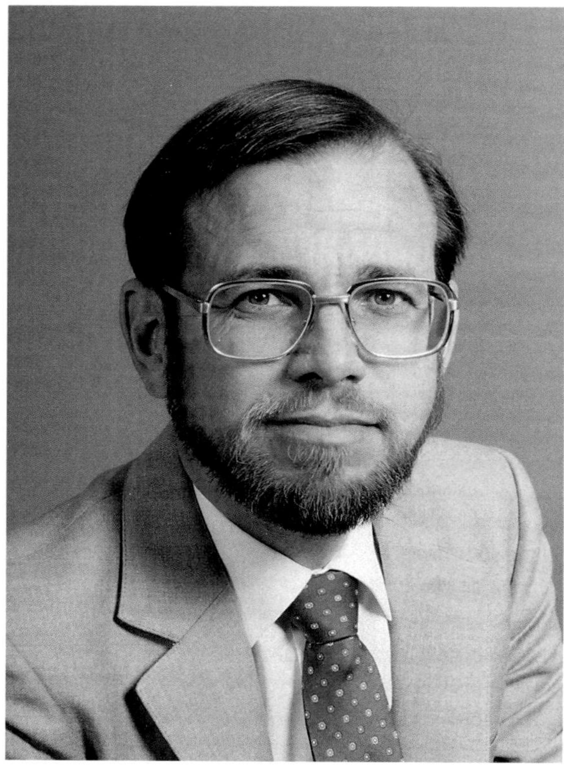

David McLean, dermatologist, Associate Dean of Research (2000–01), Senior Associate Dean Research, Planning and Health Care System (2001–03).

inherent need for give and take and compromise. UBC was represented by Cairns, Atkins, Bates, and Page; UNBC by VP, Academic and Provost Deborah Poff and Associate VP, Academic Max Blouw; and UVic by VP, Academic and Provost Jamie Cassels and Associate VP, Academic Valerie Kuehne. Although the fundamental expertise and credibility of the FoM was fully acknowledged, as was UBC as the lead institution and the MD degree-granting university, the representatives of the partner universities were forceful, articulate advocates for their institutions and for their fair share of funding, new faculty positions, and buildings as well as for autonomy within an overall framework. Atkins proved to be the ideal choice as chair of the committee, guiding it through countless meetings.

Reporting to a steering committee chaired by Dean Cairns were the MD Undergraduate Expansion Task Force (with Joanna Bates as chair), focused on the planning of the actual distributed education program; the Capital Project and Physical Infrastructure Task Force (with David McLean and later David Hardwick as chair); and the Postgraduate Expansion Task Force (with Associate Dean of Postgraduate Education Jody Wright as chair, followed by Kam Rungta and Kris Sivertz). Each of these committees had formally designated membership from the partner universities and was to seek regular input from them. The first flow of new operational funds for expansion was $5 million during the fiscal year 2003–04; this grew rapidly as planning accelerated toward enrollment of the first expanded class scheduled for August 2004.

Research and Clinical Faculty Initiatives

The financial constraints on the Faculty through the early 1990s had inevitably led to lower national ranking in peer review and overall research funding. When new federal resources became available in the late '90s, the FoM, desperately in need of stabilization and renewal, eagerly accessed them. The federal Liberal government had dramatically reduced the chronic budget deficits, freeing up resources for the creation of entirely new and visionary academic funding programs. These included

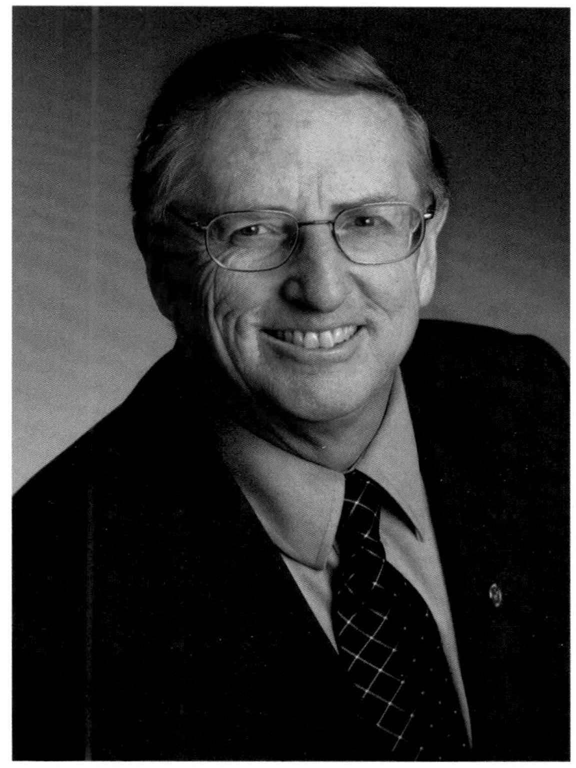

Aubrey Tingle, pediatric immunologist, inaugural President and CEO of Michael Smith Foundation for Health Research (2001–08).

the Canadian Institutes of Health Research (CIHR), Canada Foundation for Innovation (CFI), the Canada Research Chairs Program (CRCP), and the Canada Graduate Scholarships program. With the energetic leadership of President Piper and the commitment of Dean Cairns, the FoM was uniquely successful in securing funding and awards with these new opportunities. By 2002, the Faculty had reached second place in the national rankings.

The provincial government stepped forward in 2001 with the creation of the Michael Smith Foundation for Health Research (MSFHR). It began to provide the career salary support for FoM investigators which had been absent for many years and had compromised the Faculty's success with Medical Research Council applications. Its founding director was pediatrician-immunologist Aubrey Tingle, who had demonstrated his vision for research infrastructure and personnel as director of the BC Research Institute for Children's and Women's Health. Since 2001, the MSFHR has funded more than 1,700 individual researchers and 120 research teams. The naming of the new provincial health research foundation recognized Smith not only for his 1993 Nobel Prize but also for his deep and sustained legacy at UBC. In 1987, he had been appointed as the founding director of the interdepartmental UBC Biotechnology Laboratory (renamed the Michael Smith Laboratories in 2004) with a strong emphasis on interdisciplinary collaboration. He led efforts among UBC colleagues to play a role in the Human Genome Project, and with funding secured by the BC Cancer Agency from CFI and BC Knowledge Development Fund (BCKDF), he founded the Genome Sciences Centre in 1999. Unknown to all but a few of his confidants, Smith had been battling myelodysplastic syndrome and eventually died with acute myeloid leukemia in October 2000.

On the clinical faculty side of things, by the late 1990s there was growing dissatisfaction about increased requests for teaching (arising from the new undergraduate curriculum and the increasingly formalized Royal College of Physicians and Surgeons standards for resident education programs). A Clinical Faculty Affairs Committee had been created in 1980, and in the '90s the committee had become more active under the chair of Suzanne

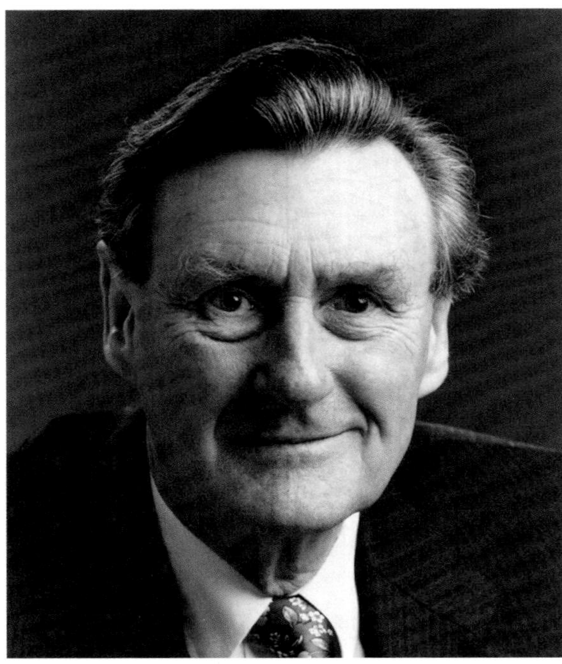

Angus Rae, nephrologist, inaugural President, University Clinical Faculty Association (1998–2001).

Lewis from the Department of Medical Genetics. Extensive work was done to develop a points-based system for quantifying teaching contributions. The FoM had only a modest budget for compensating clinical faculty for teaching. Payments were not directly linked to teaching contributions across the clinical departments, and clinical faculty in some departments were much more likely to receive compensation than those in other departments.

The University Clinical Faculty Association (UCFA) had been established in 1998 to create a formal voice for clinical faculty. The first president was nephrologist Angus Rae, noted for his fiery rhetoric and organizational skills. Soon thereafter, the FoM was confronted by strongly voiced demands for improved financial and academic recognition for clinical faculty. Suzanne Lewis was succeeded by gynecologist Monique Bertrand who became the chair of the Clinical Faculty Affairs Committee and was given increased status as director in the Office of Clinical Faculty Affairs. She had the unenviable task of leading a committee whose members were appointed by both the FoM and the UCFA. The committee was asked to document the extent of clinical faculty contributions to teaching and administration and to recommend improved recognition that would be feasible given the FoM's severe financial constraints.

The emergency Ministry of Health funding first flowed into the FoM in fiscal year 1999-2000; several hundred thousand dollars became available for increased stipendiary payments to clinical faculty for teaching and administrative contributions, but the hourly rates were low and were seen by the UCFA to be insulting. UBC legal staff advised Cairns that clinical faculty were independent contractors and under BC law were not allowed to band together to negotiate through the UCFA, and that the Dean was not permitted to negotiate with the UCFA. The Dean followed the advice, but the UCFA regarded it as a stalling tactic. Despite best efforts to discuss the issues and seek solutions, the UCFA decided to withdraw all teaching for a week. Although full-time faculty stepped in to teach as necessary and many clinical faculty members did not withdraw their teaching, significant numbers of planned clinical teaching activities did not happen during that tense week from February 26 through March 2, 2001. The strike was reported in the *Vancouver Sun* of March 7, 2001.

Although the strike added yet more stress to a Faculty just beginning to emerge from its darkest financial days, it led to several mediation sessions between faculty leaders and the UCFA. Fortunately, the first phase of the Strategic Teaching Initiative was ready for implementation in April 2001, and the Faculty was able to augment the hourly rate of compensation for teaching and to ensure that it was widely and evenly applied across all clinical departments. Compensation for administrative contributions was improved, a clinical faculty office was established at VGH (President Martha Piper attended the opening), and the role of associate dean, clinical faculty affairs was established.

Challenges lay ahead as the expansion planning progressed and the teaching role of clinical faculty became still larger. Emotions ran high and at times Dean Cairns and later his successor Dean Gavin Stuart came under strident and personal verbal attack. However, FoM financial planning for the expansion allocated major resources for clinical faculty compensation and the course to implementation of the expansion was reasonably smooth. The hourly levels of compensation remain at a fraction of what clinical faculty receive for patient care, and their teaching contributions are primarily altruistic, reflecting their ongoing appreciation for the clinical teaching they received during their own education.

Ready for a New Era

The much-feared global data meltdown of 2000 (the ominous "Y2K") never materialized, and instead the year marked the beginning of a great turnaround for the FoM. The Faculty's new curriculum had been implemented over the entire four-year program and had been strongly endorsed by renewed accreditation in May 2000. The Faculty debt restructuring and strict repayment schedule were constraining but did enable realistic planning. The FoM's desperate financial state had been eased by the dramatic new flows of funds from the Ministry of Health. Enrollment was also on a course to doubling, supported by new capital facilities at UBC and the partner universities; a major resurrection of research had begun; and relations with the clinical faculty had markedly improved.

The UBC leadership had made it clear in 2001 that they would not support a renewal of Cairns's term as dean, and he eventually stepped down in September 2003. Following a sabbatical during which he led the CIHR Clinical Research Initiative, he returned to his roots in the UBC Division of Cardiology, developing mentoring programs for early career faculty, engaging with the MD undergraduate curriculum planning, and reactivating his leadership of cardiovascular clinical trials. He received the Margolese National Heart Disorders Prize in 2012, was awarded the Order of BC in 2013 and served as President of the Canadian Academy of Health Sciences (2015-17).

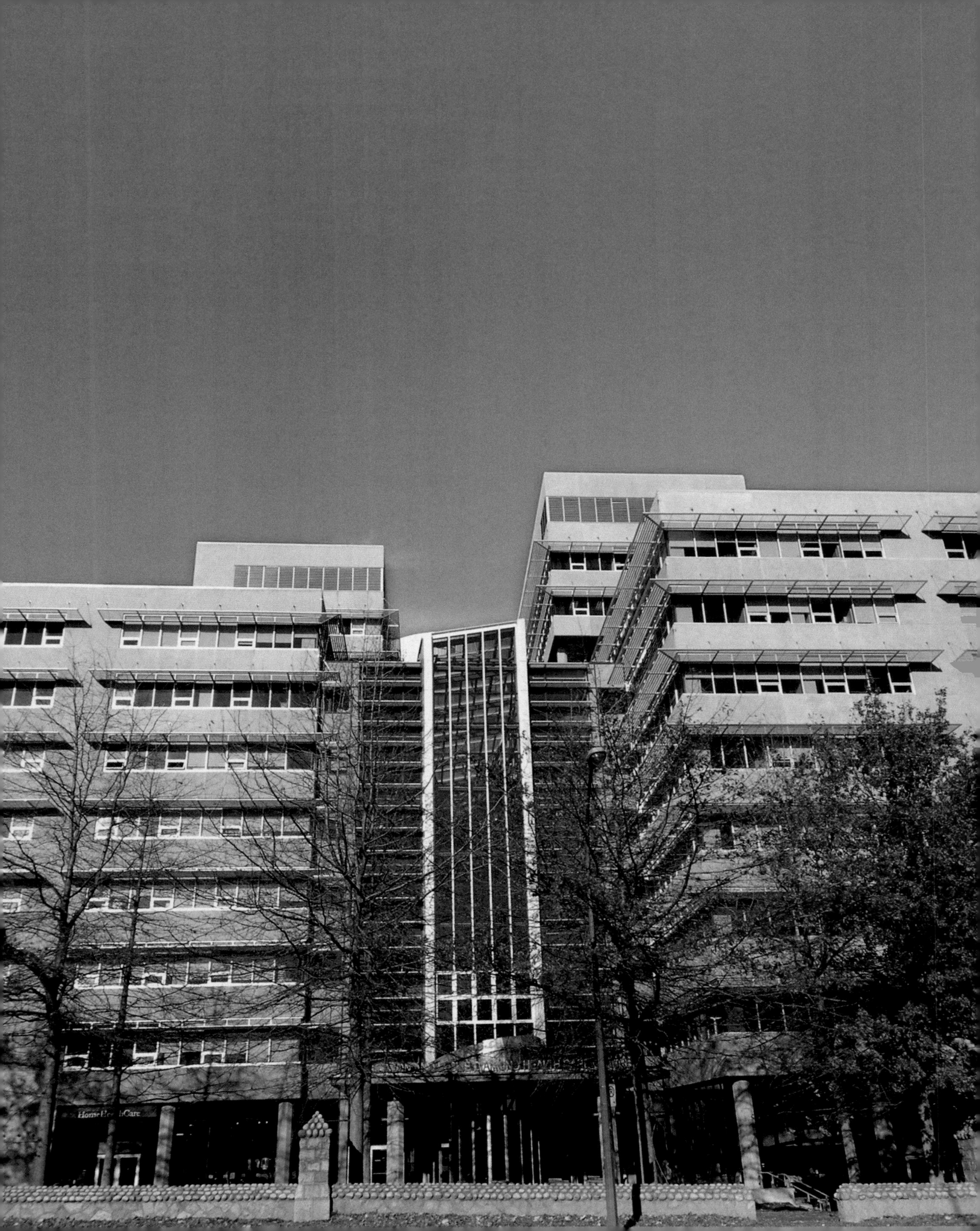

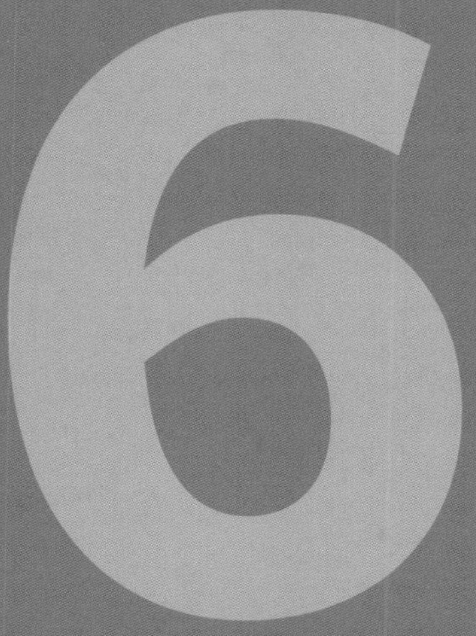

6 Canadian Best in Class

2003–15

FACING Gordon and Leslie Diamond Health Care Centre, VGH (opened 2005). Note original stone wall along north side of 12th Avenue, which enclosed the Fairview "Shacks" (page 9).

FACING Gavin Stuart, gynecologic oncologist, eighth Dean of Medicine (2003–15).

With Gavin Stuart's arrival at UBC, there was a sense amongst faculty and staff that expansion was going to be a success.

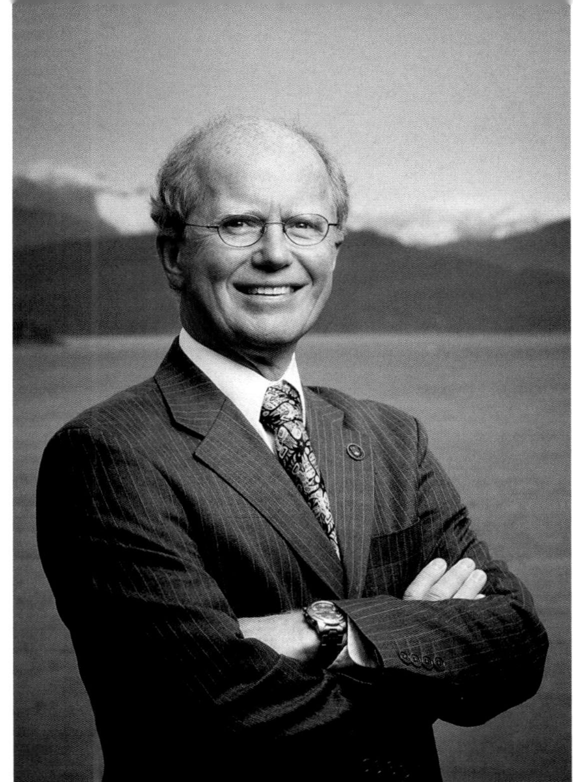

WHEN GAVIN STUART became Dean in October 2003, the energy was palpable. Stuart came from the University of Calgary where he had been Executive Director of the Tom Baker Cancer Centre and Vice-president of the Alberta Cancer Board. As a practicing academic gynecologic oncologist, he had also built a large new research-intensive Department of Oncology. His leadership experience both in the academic setting as well as the health services delivery sector would serve him well in his new role. He had a reputation for bringing diverse groups together around a common vision and building a program. He was attracted to UBC by the strong university leadership and the opportunity to be part of building a new model of medical education in the province. With his arrival at UBC, there was a sense amongst faculty and staff that expansion was going to be a success.

When Stuart arrived in 2003, Martha Piper had been very clear on what priorities faced the Faculty and required his attention. There were three: sustained growth of the research enterprise was non-negotiable; the implementation and nurturing of an expanded provincial model of distributed health education was paramount; and the integration of clinical faculty members as a valued and critically important component of a successful Faculty of Medicine was essential. Stuart readily agreed to these three priorities, and they helped shape his leadership for the next twelve years.

Growth of the Research Enterprise

A world-leading Faculty of Medicine does not wish to be known for education alone–it must also be a beacon of excellence in research. This has been enabled by at least five developments in the Faculty at UBC.

The first development was a renewed funding environment in BC. As the new millennium began, the construction of the Life Sciences Centre (LSC) on the Point Grey Campus was the most visible reflection of this. Funded initially through the provincial government, but then with substantial further federal investments in research, the LSC has become an icon of world-class research and internationally leading medical education. It became a key element of the distributed medical program, providing a 560,000-square-foot building that was home to the MD undergraduate program as well as the Life Sciences Institute.

The centre, opening in 2004, housed sufficient laboratory facilities (state-of-the-art gross anatomy and histology labs), tutorial rooms, study space, and

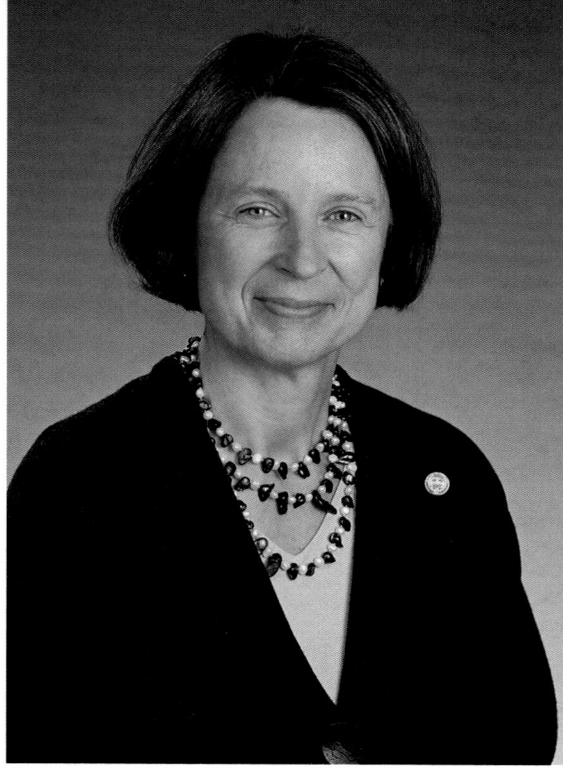

Allison Buchan, physiologist, Executive Associate Dean Research (2003–10).

administrative offices for an entry class of nearly three hundred medical students. It became the cornerstone for the entire provincial videoconferencing platform, which allowed for real-time high-fidelity connectivity across four or more sites. Students in Vancouver could ask questions directly of a lecturer in Prince George with both audio and video connection. Diagnostic images and other material could be shown in all sites simultaneously. Across the province, real-time "face-to-face" meetings occurred daily using this technology.

The LSC comprises five floors above ground and three floors below and offers more than 270,000 square feet of interdisciplinary research space. Included in the three lower floors are anatomy laboratories, animal facilities, and fully secure biosafety level 2 (BSL-2) and containment level 3 (CL-3) facilities. The planning and building of the LSC was a brilliant strategic move as it combined cutting-edge technology to support the distributed educational program with the best life sciences research space in Canada at the time.

The success of any physical plant is directly related to the people who fill it, and UBC researchers were uniquely successful in research-funding competitions from Canada Foundation for Innovation (CFI) and matching funds through the BC Knowledge and Development Fund (BCKDF). The leadership of Alison Buchan and Hugh Brock in coordinating this huge success was a critical factor. Research within the LSC is undertaken under the overall guidance of the Life Sciences Institute with a formal director and an organizational framework that has created a collaborative, multidisciplinary environment catalyzed by its organization into disease- or technology-focused research groups. Direct outcomes of this concept include numerous unique interdisciplinary collaborations and cross-sharing of ideas and resources. It has become the largest such entity in Canada.

The Centre for Blood Research, led by Ross MacGillivray, Dana Devine, Grant Mauk, Don Brooks, and Charles Haynes, has become an anchor of the Life Sciences Institute. The Centre for Disease Modeling includes exceptional BSL-3 facilities. Even outside of the LSC, CFI success enabled substantial research growth. The Centre for Drug Research and Development (CDRD) has evolved into a global life sciences venture. Phil Hieter, Brian Ellis, George Mackie, and Stephen Withers established the Centre for High-Throughput Biology (CHiBi) and Lawrence McIntosh led the CFI proposal for Advanced Structural Biology for Re-emerging Infectious Diseases (ASTRID). Collaborating closely with other

TOP Life Sciences Center (LSC), UBC (opened 2004).

BOTTOM LEFT LSC Atrium.

BOTTOM RIGHT Rix Lecture Hall, LSC.

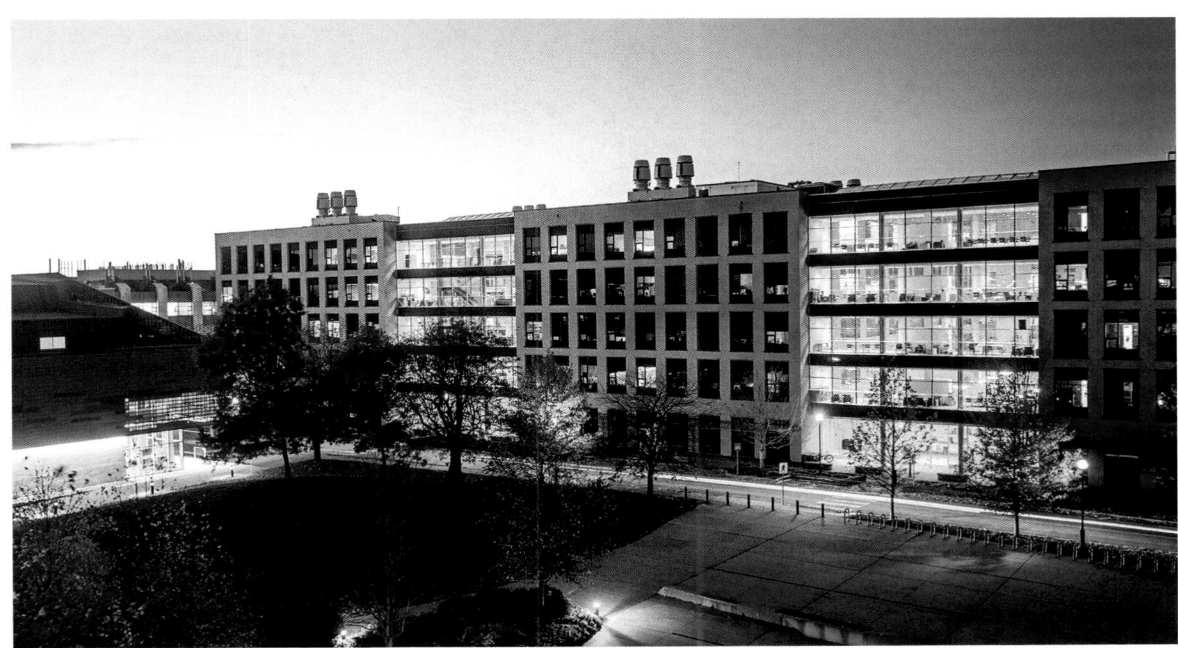

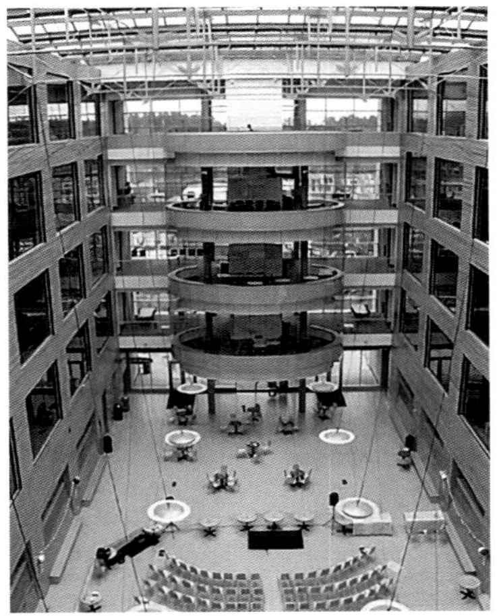

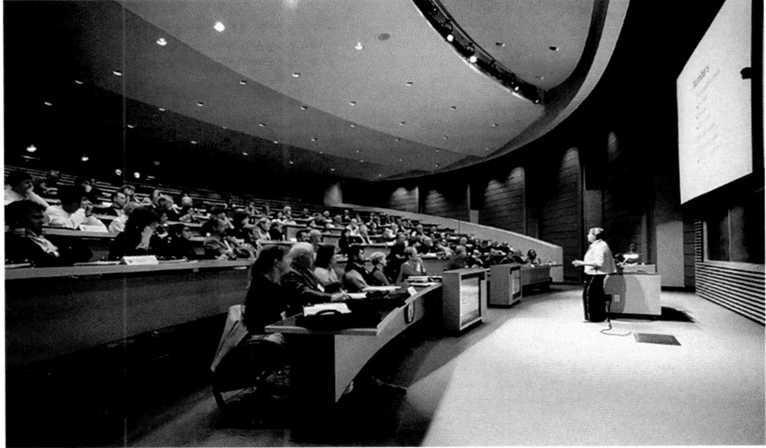

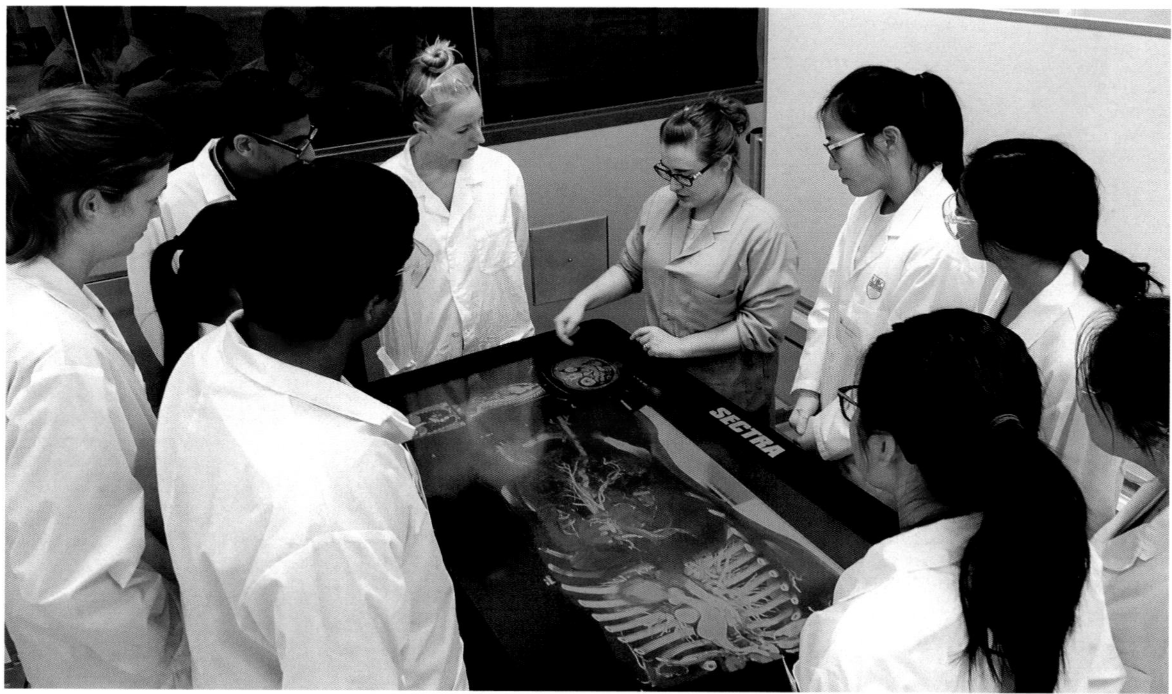

faculties on campus, Dr. Clyde Hertzman founded the Human Early Learning Partnership (HELP). All of these CFI-funded initiatives have become centres of scientific excellence.

Even though the LSC has now been operational for more than fifteen years, it continues to be a leader in both research and educational technology. Bruce Forster from the Department of Radiology and Claudia Krebs from the Department of Cellular and Physiological Sciences have come together to introduce the use of the Sectra Visualization Table into the teaching of gross anatomy and neuroanatomy. Using touch-screen technology and 3D CT scan reconstructions, the Sectra Visualization Table augments traditional anatomy teaching for medical students and all health professional learners.

The second development was the evolution from a focus on basic biomedical research to one that encompasses all four research pillars of the Canadian Institutes of Health Research (CIHR), including biomedical, clinical, health services, and population health. With a strong foundation in biochemistry and the neurosciences, the quality and quantity of research in the Faculty had increased through the late 1970s and '80s, much of it driven by faculty members in the basic sciences. New faculty leaders in the early 1990s set high expectations for faculty contribution to research at all levels. Research in health services exploded with the faculty in units such as the Centre for Health Services and Policy Research (CHSPR), the Centre for Health Evaluation and Outcome Sciences (CHEOS), and the Centre for Clinical Epidemiology and Evaluation (C2E2). The School of Population and Public Health started in 2008 and has made a major impact on research success in this domain.

Third, there has been a major shift of research from being sequestered on the university campus to being jointly conducted in many outstanding health authority-based research institutes. This synergy

BC Cancer Research Institute (opened 2005) on left with BC Cancer Vancouver Centre and cyclotron facility on right.

FACING Kathryn Darras, UBC Nuclear Medicine Fellow, and UBC Medical students using the Sectra table for anatomy learning.

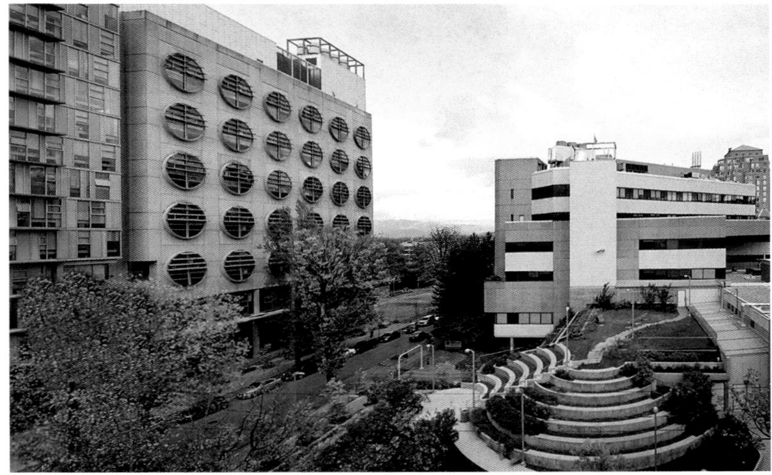

between UBC and outside health care institutions has enabled an environment in BC that is internationally acclaimed. The establishment of the Child and Family Research Institute at the BC Children's Hospital in 1995 provided a home to the Centre for Molecular Medicine and Therapeutics (CMMT) as well as for numerous other scientists, fueling a major growth in research. Over time, the Vancouver Coastal Health Research Institute (VCHRI) and the Providence Health Care Research Institute (PHCRI) have attracted a major proportion of research funds flowed through UBC.

One example of this shift from the Point Grey Campus was reflected when Michael Smith worked collaboratively in the 1990s with outstanding scientists such as Victor Ling, and later with Marco Marra, and Steve Jones to establish BC Cancer's Genome Sciences Centre (GSC) and to build the BC Cancer Research Centre (BCCRC) near the Vancouver General Hospital campus. Announced in 2001 by Don Carlow, CEO of the BC Cancer Agency (BCCA), and funded generously by the BC Cancer Foundation together with CFI and BCKDF funding, the GSC and the BCCRC have become some of the largest research facilities within UBC. Leadership of the BCCA, especially that of Dr. Simon Sutcliffe, was able to posit research as the only strategy capable of having a lasting impact on the burden of cancer. In 2020, the British Columbia Cancer Research Institute was established as an UBC Institute.

Further research success within the hospital environment is exemplified by the PHCRI Centre for Heart Lung Innovation (CHLI), among the most highly cited research groups in the world in pulmonary disease. This nexus of basic and translational research evolved from the original leadership and vision of Bruce McManus and others to create iCAPTURE, which would be renamed the James Hogg Research Centre and then, since 2013, the CHLI. Driven by the leadership of Larry Goldenberg, the Vancouver Prostate Centre is a world-renowned centre conducting cancer research across all pillars. Strategic recruitment has created a large team of excellent scientists now led by Martin Gleave. Similarly, the BC Professional Fire Fighters' Burn and Wound Healing Research Laboratory, established in 2005 at VCHRI and led by Aziz Ghahary, is a world leader in the pathophysiology of burn and wound healing.

The fourth development has been the emphasis on interdisciplinary and team-based research at UBC, which provided an exceptional platform for

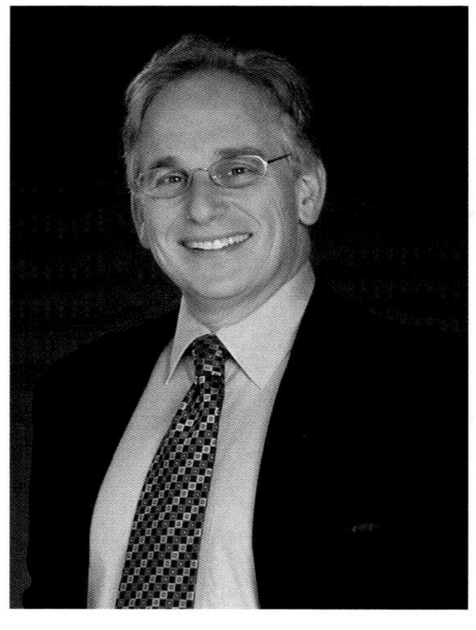

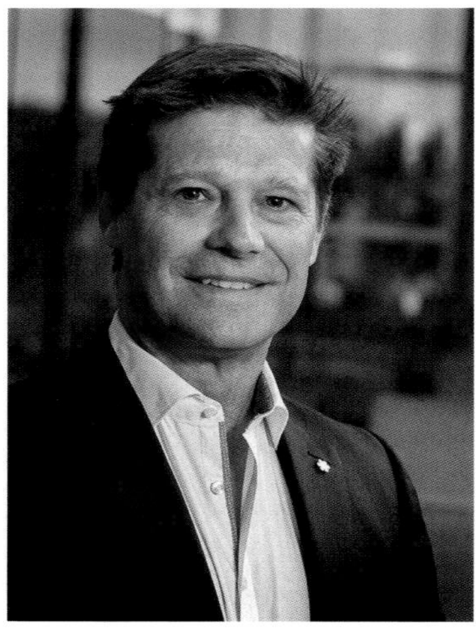

LEFT Larry Goldenberg, urologist, inaugural Director of Vancouver Prostate Centre, inaugural Head of Department of Urological Sciences (2006–15).

RIGHT Martin Gleave (UBC MD '84), urologist, Head of Department of Urological Sciences (2015–present).

FACING Djavad Mowafaghian Centre for Brain Health (opened 2014).

success. The incredible growth of research in the early part of this millennium was in large part due to funding of interdisciplinary and interdepartmental research centres. This same trend has continued with centres such as the Djavad Mowafaghian Centre for Brain Health, founded by Max Cynader and engaging the departments of Medicine, Psychiatry, Radiology, Physical Therapy, Ophthalmology and Visual Sciences as well as the schools of Population and Public Health and of Biomedical Engineering. These latter two schools exemplify the coalescence of scientific excellence to provide innovative teaching and outstanding research. The Centre for Hip Health and Mobility includes clinicians and scientists from Family Practice, Orthopaedics, Physical Therapy, Occupational Therapy and Occupational Sciences, as well as other faculties beyond Medicine. Other research centres follow similar pathways. Recognizing that the opportunities to address the health needs of the population we serve are dependent on the talents of scientists from many departments, current federal competitions fund team-based science and those groups that extend beyond traditional academic boundaries.

Finally, the substantial development and growth of research as a provincial opportunity beyond the cloistered halls of Vancouver alone has augmented the success of investigators at both UBC and its partner institutions. The defined structures of the health authorities, the distributed medical program, and the influence of the Michael Smith Foundation for Health Research and Genome BC have allowed for BC to become a "living laboratory" with a view to improving the health of the population. Biospecimens, population-level data, and genomic information now inform research province-wide.

In addition to these dynamics enabling success, strategic recruitment has been a focus. Dean Cairns's recruitment in 2001 of Garth Warnock as the new UBC and VCH Head of Surgery allowed the establishment of UBC's Ike Barber Human Islet Transplant Laboratory. Warnock and his team had recently performed Canada's first successful pancreatic islet cell transplantation at the University of Alberta. The Faculty has attracted two Canada Excellence Research Chairs (Matthew Farrer, 2010, and Sriram Subramaniam, 2019). Furthermore, Dean Kelleher recruited Josef Penninger in 2018 to UBC as director of the Life Sciences Institute and a Canada 150 Research Chair in functional genetics.

UBC's Faculty of Medicine has, in many instances, been able to translate this creation of new knowledge

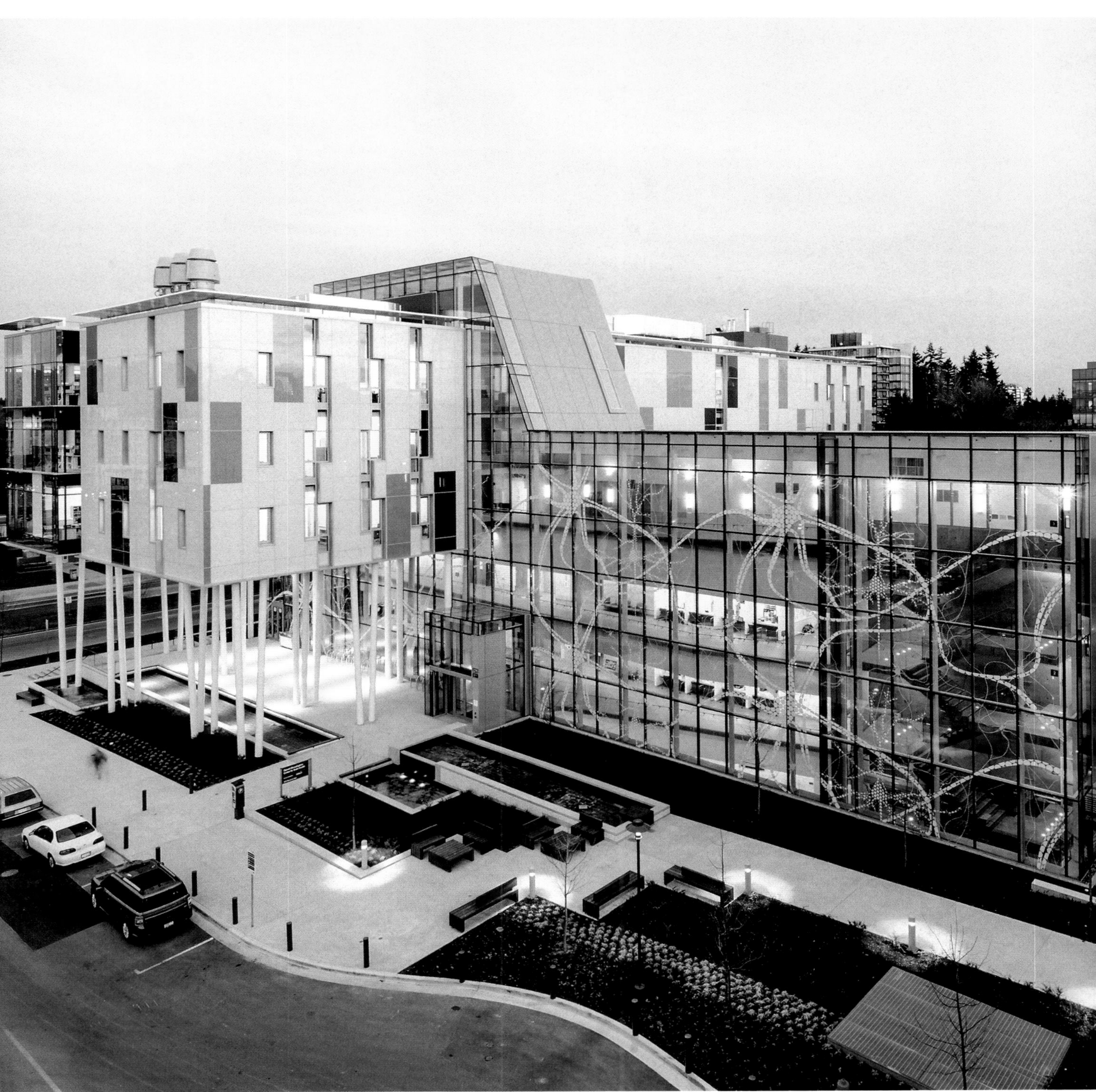

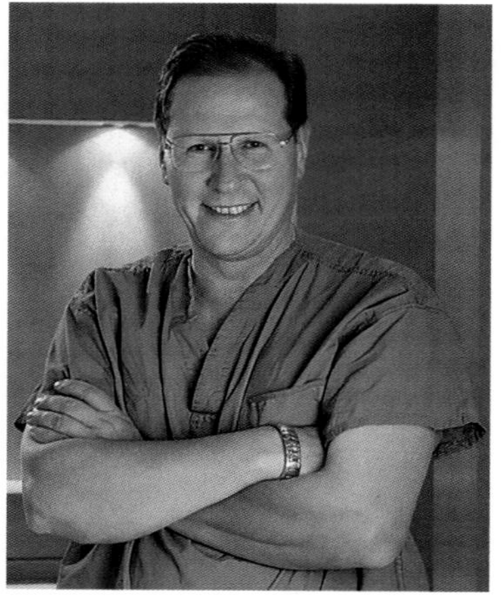

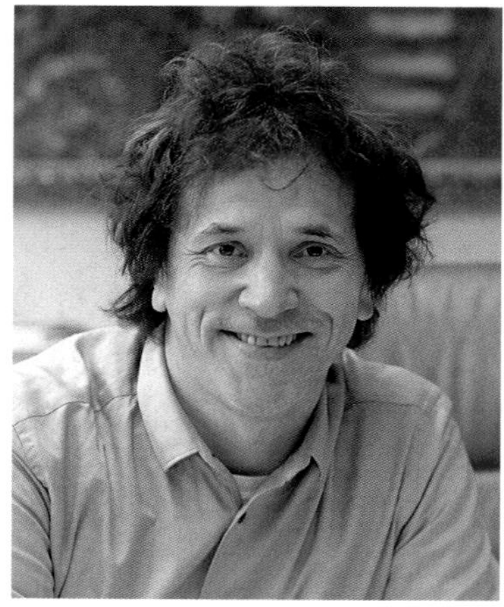

LEFT Garth Warnock, transplant surgeon, Head of Department of Surgery (2002–12).

RIGHT Josef Penninger, molecular immunologist, Canada 150 Research Chair in Functional Genetics, Director of the Life Sciences Institute (2018–present).

into economic success. Between 2005 and 2016, UBC spin-off companies attracted $540 million in investments and have created more than four hundred new jobs. Much of this is in the domain of health and life sciences.

A Provincial Model of Distributed Medical Education

Once the decision had been made to build an expanded and distributed model of education, several principles were enunciated as being foundational. They included commitments to social accountability in British Columbia, a single medical school on multiple sites, and partnerships among the community, the academy, the health system, and government.

Perhaps more than anywhere else in Canada, the planning, delivery, and evaluation of medical education in British Columbia has been grounded in the principles of social accountability. This much-used term is understood by medical schools to reflect the definition provided in a 1995 paper issued by the World Health Organization as "the obligation to direct their education, research, and service activities toward addressing the priority health concerns of the community, region, and/or nation they have a mandate to serve." Indeed, one could posit that the decades-long delay in starting a medical school in BC arose in part as a result of trying to broadly understand and address these health concerns. Fortunately, with only one medical school in the province, there is a clear vision of the population to be served. Since the release in 2001 of the Health Canada document entitled "Social Accountability: A Vision for Canadian Medical Schools," this level of accountability has guided and determined planning for UBC.

Social accountability is objectively reflected in at least three key aspects. First, the medical model must address the needs of the population being served. The establishment of the distributed sites reflected a thoughtful consideration of where health needs existed and not necessarily where the program could be most easily delivered. Within the bounds of a single accredited medical school, the programs have been able to provide a bespoke education and training focused on local needs. Additionally, this model has saved significant provincial resources to be expended on other important issues that may be critical social determinants of health. The fundamental vision from the beginning of this model was "to live where they learn and practice where they live."

Elaine Carty, midwife, inaugural Director of Faculty of Medicine Midwifery Program, (2001–06).

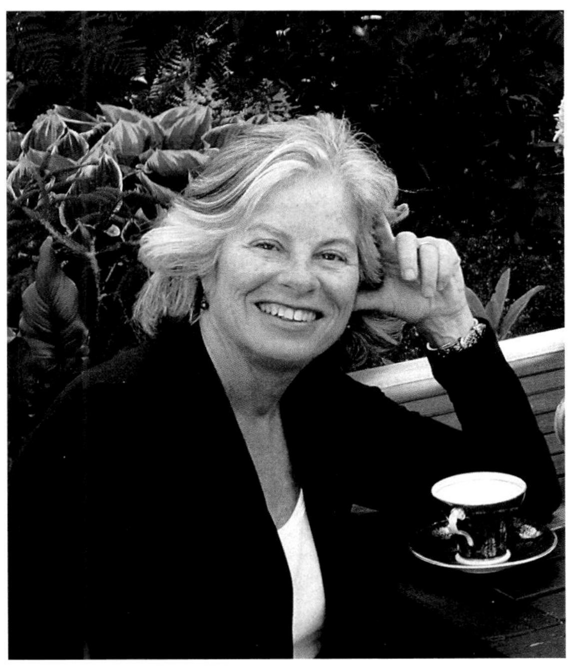

Beyond, medical practitioners, the Faculty has recognized the needs of the population and acted upon it by planning, implementing, and operating the UBC Midwifery Program, which is embedded in the Department of Family Practice. The first graduates entered practice in 2005. The leadership of Elaine Carty, the program's first director, was recognized by the awarding of an Order of BC in 2017.

A second facet of social accountability is the creation of a workforce that mirrors the society that it serves. This has been an uncompromising value of the Faculty of Medicine for many decades and was a priority in planning the distributed program. A balanced representation of learners addresses gender, race, ability/disability, and urban/rural geography. This includes the Indigenous populations of Status Indians under the Indian Act, Non-Status Indians, Metis, and Inuit. A target of five percent of the entry class has been in place since 2002 when the Aboriginal Admissions Policy was created. Application requirements remain similar to the general pathway, although if self-identified as Indigenous, the applicant must submit an additional essay and proof of ancestry. UBC has been uniquely successful in educating and graduating Indigenous students, in large part due to the efforts of Indigenous Student Initiatives Manager James Andrew, who has been working to enhance admission rates to medical school for Indigenous undergraduate students in health sciences. For the entire duration of the period of the expansion and distribution, James

Footballer Professors?

Dean Kelleher first met Josef Penninger while both were playing in the 2017 World Medical Football Championship (WMFC), in Leogang, Austria. The opening group game in the masters category between Austria and Ireland was won 3–2 by Austria. Kelleher was playing for Ireland and was taken down in the penalty area for a penalty kick which resulted in Ireland's second goal. Penninger was playing for Austria and scored a great goal in the first half. After the game, an energetic conversation ensued over refreshments and Kelleher told him about the Canada 150 Chair competition and raised the possibility of coming to UBC. Today, Penninger is a professor in the UBC Department of Medical Genetics, and both men still play soccer!

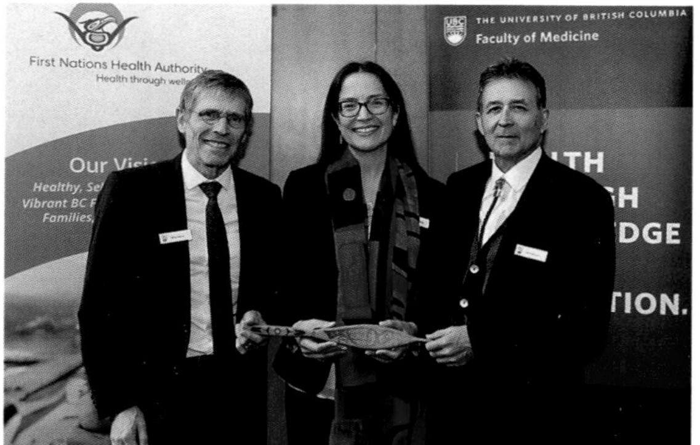

Mike Allard (UBC MD '81), pathologist, Vice-dean Health Engagement (2018–present); Nadine Caron (UBC MD '97), First Nations Health Authority Chair in Cancer and Wellness at UBC; Richard Jock, COO First Nations Health Authority.

has been fully committed to the Indigenous student admissions program as well as a program of support throughout their medical school years.

Thirdly, social accountability requires working with and within the health system. The UBC Faculty of Medicine and Vancouver General Hospital have had a cooperative relationship dating back to the planning of the medical school. As the major tertiary and quaternary institution in the province, VGH has enabled the educational programs of UBC as well as outstanding research. With time, St. Paul's Hospital, Women's and Children's, and BCCA have evolved into UBC partnerships based upon fulfilling the tripartite mission of education, research, and patient care. Most acute care institutions across BC now have "UBC Faculty of Medicine" on signage outside the facility. There are strong relationships between the Faculty and each of the seven health authorities in BC. Vice-Dean Health Engagement Mike Allard leads this intersection of the academy and the health system.

Resistance to a UBC School

The original model of distributed education included the Vancouver-Fraser Medical Program (VFMP) in the Lower Mainland; the Northern Medical Program (NMP), based in Prince George and partnered with University of Northern BC (UNBC); and the Island Medical Program (IMP), based in Victoria and partnered with the University of Victoria (UVic). From the beginning, the north of the province was excited to see the establishment of medical student education in Prince George. Soon after his arrival in BC, Stuart paid his first visit to Prince George. He learned from taxi drivers, health care professionals, civic leaders, and the community of the tremendous value and importance that Northern British Columbia placed on the new medical program-to-be as a means to improve the health of the population. This program was to be "owned" by the northern community.

This same dynamic did not initially exist in Victoria with the inception of the IMP. At first, the engagement of UVic did not engender the unbridled enthusiasm and support experienced at UNBC. Although the oldest established medical society in British Columbia is the New Westminster Medical Society, the history of the medical profession in BC is probably deepest in Victoria. Since its inception in 1895, the Victoria Medical Society had felt that a medical school would be started in Victoria, independent of any other that might be established in BC. When discussions about a distributed model of medical education began among UBC, UNBC, and UVic, there was some ambivalence amongst the UVic leadership and the medical community in Victoria. However, there was sufficient support to engage in the planning for the distributed model.

Indigenous MD Graduation Celebration, Class of 2019 at UBC's First Nations Longhouse. L-R: Meg Raymond, Taran Main, Deanna Kerrigan, Alan Rheaume, James Andrew, Dexter James, Cheryl Gascoyne, Zoe Friesen, Kelly Soros, Natalie Bjurman. (Missing: Kirsten Anderson, and Stephanie Zachary).

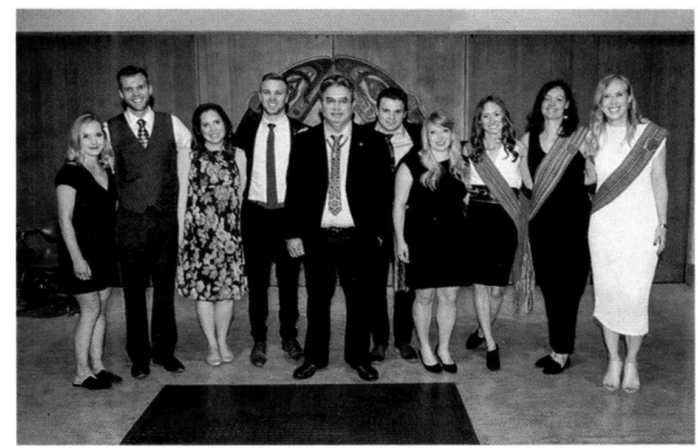

Certainly, UNBC did not view itself as establishing the entire infrastructure to support an independent school and agreed that a partnered model would be advantageous for all. The provincial government had no interest in creating new independent medical schools and found the proposed model was academically and financially attractive. The Victoria community gradually came to embrace this model.

The details of this distributed model for expansion became more relevant when Simon Fraser University (SFU) was considered as a potential partner. Though it was always clear to those leading the planning that any expansion of the medical program in Vancouver would have to engage with Surrey and the rapidly growing population in the Fraser Valley, the leadership of SFU at that time did not see themselves as becoming a "satellite" of the UBC medical school. They wanted an independent SFU medical school.

This disparate thinking about the evolving BC medical school model was unfortunate for both UBC and SFU, as at the level of senior administration it fueled a competitiveness that verged on animosity for several years following the establishment of the NMP and the IMP. Clear institutional boundaries were delineated, and several faculty members at each institution were recruited back and forth across the Lower Mainland as part of a "gown versus gown" rivalry. This may have advanced the careers of some faculty members but overall did little to grow the academic capital in British Columbia. Animosity became so intense that at one point, SFU considered launching their own private medical school, focusing on Canadians who were travelling internationally and paying handsomely in order to obtain their medical education and training. This model would engage the private sector and create new opportunities for those Canadians who were not able to gain admission into any one of the seventeen publicly funded Canadian medical schools. An underpinning objective was to repatriate not only these students but also the significant fees being paid to foreign medical schools only too willing to accept their cash. Although the premise had some traction, it was not seen as being socially acceptable in the system in BC that was generally publicly funded.

Thus, the government was drawn to a model that would continue to see UBC partner with other institutions to expand the capacity for medical education. The key premise was to educate learners where they lived, and that this would allow more of them to remain in this environment. With the passage of time, the Vancouver-Fraser Medical Program became more formalized, and by 2009 had faculty appointees, site coordinators, and student cohorts embedded across the facilities and programs of Fraser Health.

The Provincial Framework

In September 2004, when 196 new medical students arrived in Vancouver, the first four months of curricular study took place in Vancouver with the students from the NMP, the IMP, and the VFMP bonding together in the new LSC. The rationale was to create a cohesive class identity for all students entering their first year of medicine at UBC beyond that of the program in which they were enrolled. Then in January of their first year, the students relocated to their "home" program. This meant that for the first four months, the existing facilities of VGH and St. Paul's, together with a number of Vancouver-based primary care practices, would be insufficient to accommodate all needs for clinical placements even in the first year. There were multiple meetings in the Lower Mainland and into the Fraser Valley to reach out to colleagues and engage them in the educational mission in a manner they had not fully embraced previously. The Dean and others frequently had breakfast, lunch, or dinner meetings in hotels, hospital meeting rooms, or community offices. As the curriculum team led by Angela Towle revised and planned the curriculum to fit a distributed model, the faculty development team worked tirelessly with colleagues, and the facilities group documented needs and planned new initiatives.

For this model to be successful as a provincial program, there was a critical dependency on personal and institutional relationships. Stuart developed a strong, diverse leadership team that was bonded by a single vision for medical education that would benefit the population of BC. He himself travelled to attend meetings, functions, groundbreakings, openings, and other events across the province and regularly meet with the local health authority leadership, university leadership, and clinicians at each site in order to enhance the profile of a collaborative provincial program. These approaches were often enabled by his congenial approach and sense of humour. During his time as Dean, he ensured that, together with his wife and canine companions, he travelled to every community teaching site in the province at some point during the summer months. He remained strongly committed to ensuring that all the partners in the program enjoyed success in order for the entire model to succeed.

The model of distributed medical education depended on a clear delineation of the network of facilities. Each medical program was anchored to a University Academic Campus (UAC). These were

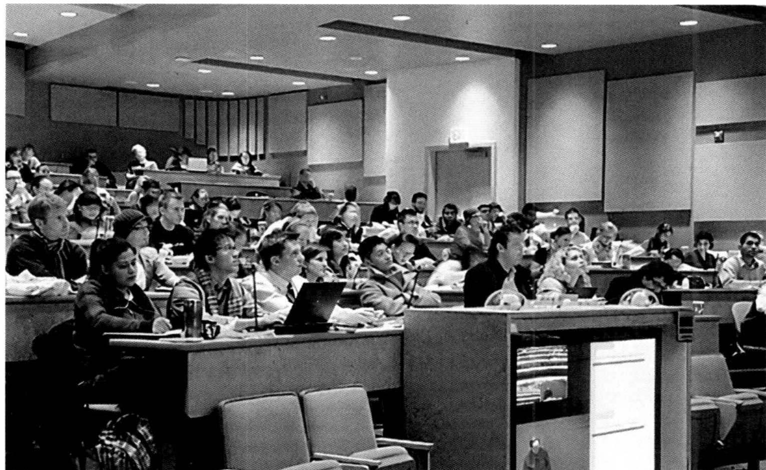

Robert and Greta Ho Auditorium, Gordon and Leslie Diamond Health Care Centre.

then aligned to one or more hospital-based Clinical Academic Campuses (CACs). Smaller hospitals would be designated as Affiliated Regional Centres (ARCs). Then for much of the ambulatory and primary care, there were designated Community Education Facilities (CEF) established at rural and remote sites across the province. This elaborate network of facilities is reflected in the figure on page 162.

These designations were very important as they allowed for planning and implementation of prerequisite infrastructure–space, technology, and personnel–to support the educational programs. For the most part, the educational programs mapped onto one of five regional health authorities. Considering that in the year 2000 the Faculty had 122 affiliation agreements with individual hospitals, interacting with the six health authorities established by the new government (later to become seven, with the inclusion of the First Nations Health Authority) was much easier.

In Vancouver, planning quickly began to build new facilities at VGH in the form of the new Gordon and Leslie Diamond Health Care Centre as the hub for the CAC at that site. New instructional facilities and support space for learners was either renovated or built at St. Paul's and BC Children's and BC Women's hospitals. This construction was to further reinforce the very positive impact of new major research facilities and buildings.

The Northern Medical Program

Prince George was the epicentre of the need and the catalyst for the distributed model of education in BC envisioned by FoM and government leaders beginning in 2000. Once the decision had been made in 2001 to implement this model, things happened quickly. The Northern Medical Society had been formed in 1999 by a group of physicians who were concerned by the shortage of qualified medical practitioners across the north. In 2003, they formed the Northern Medical Programs Trust with academic, community, and business leaders, establishing a platform for philanthropic support of what was to be called the NMP. The society brought together leaders from across the northern part of the province, representing many communities and Indigenous persons. All were bonded by a vision for better access to health care in the north.

A premier event of the society remains the annual Dr. Bob Ewert Memorial Dinner and Lecture which is now in its fifteenth year. Born in the north in 1927, Ewert established a general surgical

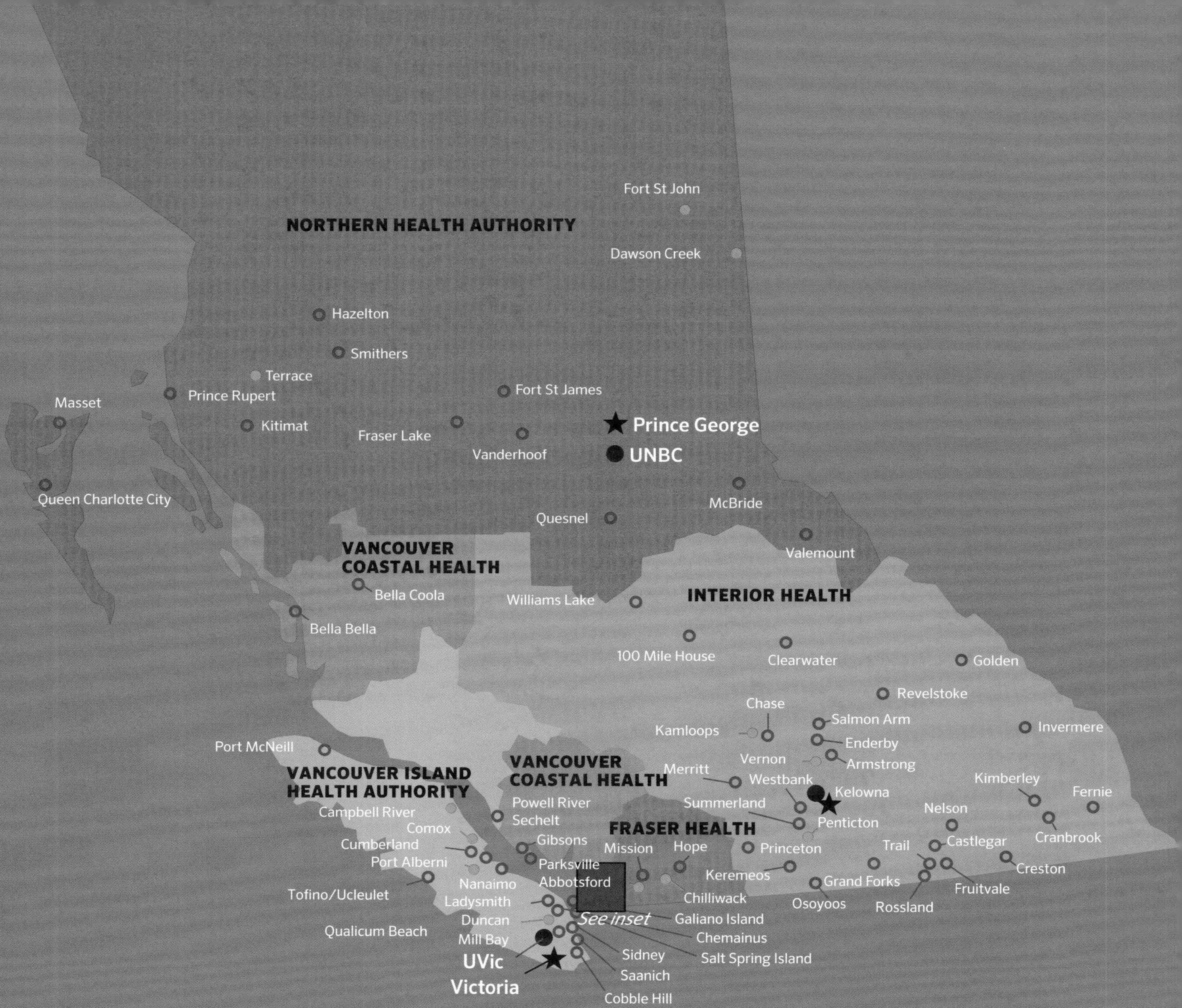

NORTHERN HEALTH AUTHORITY

Fort St John
Dawson Creek
Hazelton
Smithers
Terrace
Masset
Prince Rupert
Kitimat
Fort St James
Fraser Lake
Vanderhoof
Prince George
UNBC
Queen Charlotte City
McBride
Quesnel

VANCOUVER COASTAL HEALTH

Valemount
Bella Coola
Williams Lake

INTERIOR HEALTH

Bella Bella
100 Mile House
Clearwater
Golden
Revelstoke
Chase
Salmon Arm
Kamloops
Invermere
Enderby
Port McNeill
Vernon
Armstrong
Merritt

VANCOUVER ISLAND HEALTH AUTHORITY

VANCOUVER COASTAL HEALTH

Westbank
Kimberley
Kelowna
Fernie
Powell River
Summerland
Campbell River
Sechelt
Nelson
Penticton
Comox

FRASER HEALTH

Gibsons
Cranbrook
Cumberland
Castlegar
Trail
Mission
Hope
Princeton
Port Alberni
Parksville
Creston
Keremeos
Nanaimo
Abbotsford
Grand Forks
Tofino/Ucleulet
Fruitvale
Ladysmith
Chilliwack
Osoyoos
Rossland
Duncan
See inset
Galiano Island
Qualicum Beach
Mill Bay
Chemainus
UVic
Sidney
Salt Spring Island
Saanich
Victoria
Cobble Hill

GREATER VANCOUVER (inset from map)

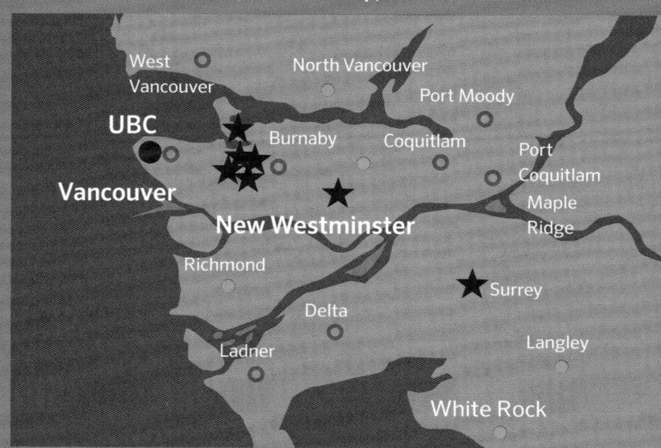

FACING UBC Faculty of Medicine network of health education and training sites across British Columbia

Legend

- ● University Academic Campus
- ★ Clinical Academic Campus
- ● Affiliated Regional Centre
- ○ Community Education Facility/ Rural and Remote Distributed Sites

● University Academic Campuses

University of British Columbia (UBC) Okanagan Campus

University of British Columbia (UBC) Vancouver Campus

University of Northern British Columbia (UNBC) in Prince George

University of Victoria (UVic) in Victoria

● Affiliated Regional Centres

Abbotsford Regional/Chilliwack General Hospitals

Burnaby/Langley Memorial/Peace Arch Hospitals

Ft. St. John General/Dawson Creek Hospitals

Lions Gate Hospital

Mills Memorial Hospital

Nanaimo Regional General Hospital

Richmond Hospital

Royal Inland Hospital

St. Joseph's General/Campbell River General/ Cowichan District Hospitals

Vernon Jubilee/Penticton Regional Hospitals

★ Clinical Academic Campuses

BC Cancer Agency

BC Children's Hospital

BC Women's Hospital and Health Centre

Kelowna General Hospital

Royal Columbian Hospital

Royal Jubilee Hospital

St. Paul's Hospital

Surrey Memorial Hospital

Vancouver General Hospital/UBC Hospital

Victoria General Hospital

University Hospital of Northern BC

○ Community Education Facilities, Rural and Remote Distributed Sites

Serving medical students and residents, student audiologists, speech language pathologists, occupational therapists, physical therapists and/ or midwives in the community.

Dave Snadden, rural family physician, inaugural Regional Associate Dean, NMP (2003–11), UBC Chair in Rural Health (2016–present).

FACING Dr. Donald Rix Northern Health Sciences Centre on the UNBC campus, home to the UBC Northern Medical Program (opened 2004).

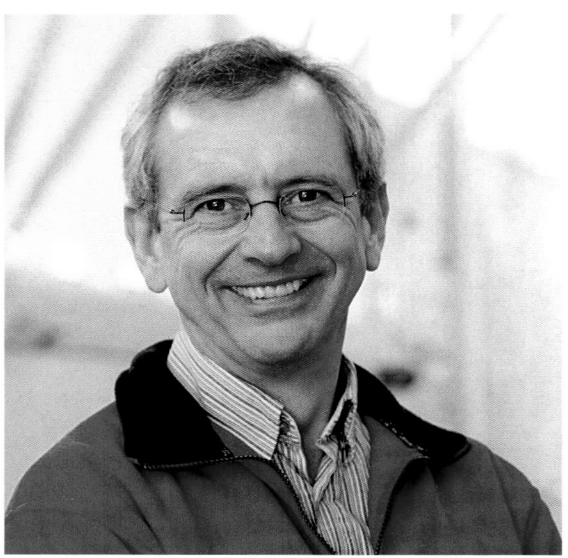

Northern Pioneers

After arriving in Canada from Dundee, Scotland, Dave Snadden, who was starting as the inaugural regional associate dean, NMP, and his wife, Moira, were ready to launch into their leadership role in the Northern BC health professional education space and thank all of those communities that helped to create the vision. Prior to his arrival, a trust fund with a goal of $6 million had been set up in the north to offset some of the expenses of medical students in the NMP. Nineteen northern communities had pledged to contribute, and the community of Tumbler Ridge was the first to make its donation of $65,000 to the trust. To celebrate this milestone, and perhaps because it could be done, Dave and Moira jumped on their yellow tandem bike and, over four days, rode from Prince George to Tumbler Ridge, a distance of some four hundred kilometres through mountainous passes and river valleys. The national media attention and the funds raised ensured that the NMP was "on the map." Snadden and his wife embraced the people, the mountains, the climate, the recreational opportunities, and the ethos of the northern part of BC—they were a perfect fit for the leadership of the NMP.

practice in Prince George in 1961. Charles Jago, President of UNBC, was a champion of the NMP, as were many prominent medical leaders including Bert Kelly, Bill Simpson, and Don McRitchie. Sadly, Dr. Kelly died in 2017, but he left a legacy of northern pride in and ownership of the NMP.

Dave Snadden was recruited in 2003 as the founding Associate Dean for the NMP as well as Vice-provost for UNBC.

Plans were quickly put in place to build the academic home of the NMP on the UNBC campus. The Northern Health Sciences Centre was completed in time for the arrival of the first students in 2004. It is a wonderful building that showcases the forestry sector, Indigenous Peoples, and the spirit of UNBC. This site provided student space for small group sessions and videoconferencing of large group lectures from anywhere in the province, laboratories, and faculty offices.

The clinical teaching space would be anchored at the Prince George Regional Hospital, later to be renamed the University Hospital of Northern British Columbia (UHNBC). Cathy Ulrich, the long-term CEO of Northern Health, never wavered on the value and

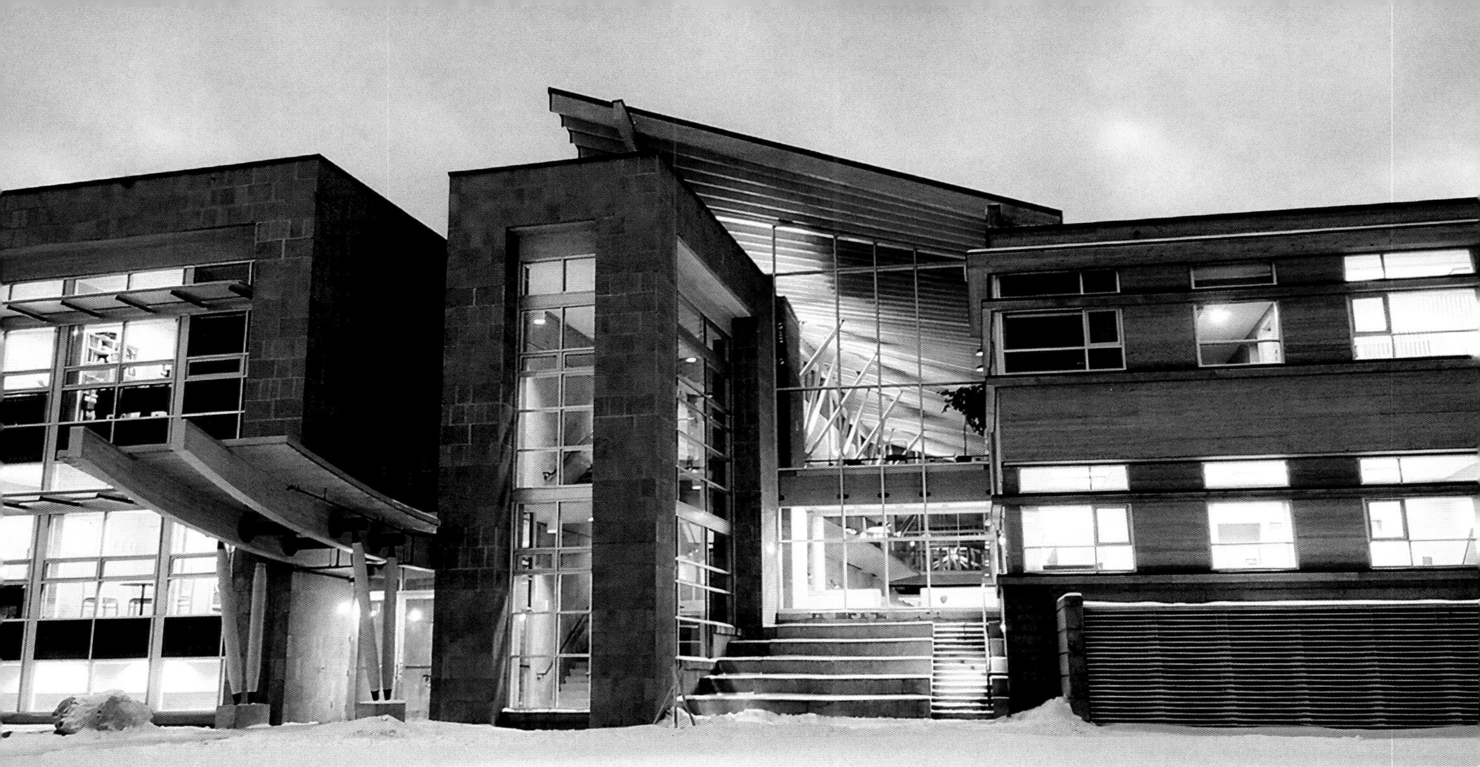

importance that the NMP brings to the health of the north. Space was designated on the fourth floor of the auxiliary building, and renovations created wonderful clinical teaching areas, on-call rooms, offices, and meeting space. A brand new four-storey, 120,000-square-foot addition to the hospital was completed in 2003 in preparation for the program.

Snadden quickly appreciated that if the full health benefits of the distributed model were to be realized, opportunities outside of the urban centre of Prince George would be required. He relentlessly visited and met with colleagues, administrators, community leaders, and others in Quesnel, Smithers, Terrace, Prince Rupert, Chetwynd, Dawson Creek, Fort St. John, and dozens of other communities. Family physicians and specialists embraced the teaching model in their practices and generously gave of their time and knowledge. Dean Stuart visited most of these communities with Snadden, and there are countless stories of the warmth and hospitality of colleagues and others throughout the north that are infused with humour and kindness.

All of this implementation required constant assessment, evaluation, and revision. To achieve this, there was a JAC formed among the Faculty, UNBC, and Northern Health. The JAC was a very important forum to ensure that the new program was fully implemented and operational. It benefitted from the participation of the Dean together with Joanna Bates, Kris Sivertz, Kam Rungta, and Dave Snadden from UBC, but also Chuck Jago, Howard Brunt, and Anne Maxwell from UNBC. Additionally, Michael McMillan, David Butcher, and Cathy Ulrich attended on behalf of Northern Health. For more than ten years, the JAC remained as a commitment for the very senior leadership of the partner institutions. This construct ensured that the three key partners were present and able to address any issues in a nimble and effective manner.

The NMP has deeply engaged the population of Northern BC and is celebrated by the communities, by UNBC, and by the provincial government. Since the first students and their families arrived in January 2005, Dave Snadden has ensured that rural

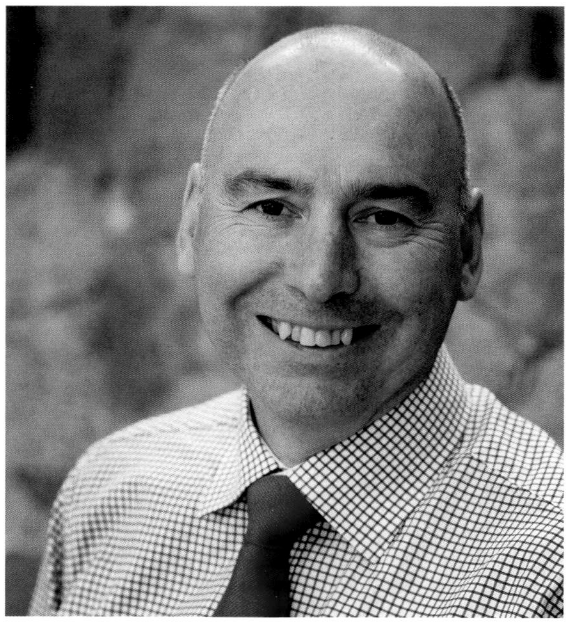

Paul Winwood, gastroenterologist, Regional Associate Dean NMP (2012–present).

medicine includes primary care, as well as access to secondary and tertiary care as required, for those who choose to live in the north. More than half of graduates of the NMP have entered into family practice. The program has built tremendous social capital and fundamentally changed the medical workforce in the north. Snadden was part of the leadership team that helped to build the BC Cancer Centre for the North, providing access for patients to high quality cancer care closer to home. In 2012, he took on a new role as Executive Associate Dean Education for the entire Faculty of Medicine. Paul Winwood succeeded him as Regional Associate Dean, continuing in this role to the present (2020).

The Island Medical Program

In 2002, when the IMP was agreed upon, the process of building and implementing began. In 2003, Oscar Casiro, the former Associate Dean of MD Undergraduate Education at the University of Manitoba, was attracted to BC. He arrived in September to new construction on the beautiful campus of UVic amongst colonies of feral rabbits and inquisitive students. Casiro was a perfect fit as leader of the IMP. His quiet, thoughtful approach to challenges allowed him to find solutions that others would not. The meaningful engagement of the clinicians in Victoria was not easy, yet Casiro established himself as a credible, trusted, and positive leader. The medical students in the IMP had the highest regard for him, possibly engendered by his occasional wake-up phone calls to students in the morning or his provision of donuts and coffee to start class.

The $12-million, 43,000-square-foot Medical Sciences Building was opened by Premier Gordon Campbell in December 2004 on the UVic campus. The Medical Sciences Building houses two state-of-the-art lecture theatres, anatomy and multipurpose research laboratories, eight problem-based learning rooms, a clinical skills teaching room, a computer lab, and administrative offices to support students during their four-year program. This building has become the anchor for IMP students in their first two years of medical education.

Within the environment of UVic, the new Division of Medical Sciences was created as a distinct academic unit reporting to the provost. Oscar Casiro was to become the first head of that division as well as the inaugural Regional Associate Dean of the IMP. The Division of Medical Sciences was a critical step toward success as it integrated the existing research excellence at UVic into the IMP and allowed the neuroscience graduate program to

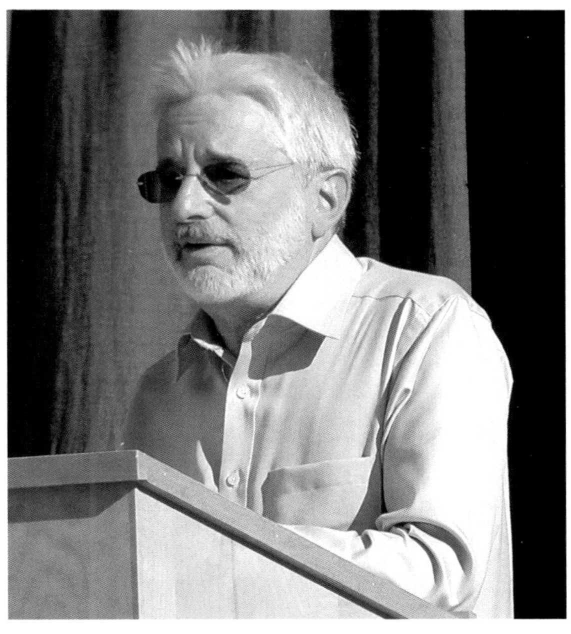

Oscar Casiro, neonatologist, inaugural Regional Associate Dean, IMP (2003–14).

flourish with outstanding faculty members from the UVic professoriate. There was a distinct synergy created as the resources provided to the IMP allowed for recruitment of new faculty who could contribute to undergraduate medical education while enhancing the research success of UVic. This also exposed numerous medical students to basic and translational science research within their school environment.

As in Prince George, there was a need for academic clinical space within the acute care facilities in Victoria and elsewhere across Vancouver Island. Island Health played a critical role as a supportive partner in these developments. At the Royal Jubilee Hospital (RJH) site, Begbie Hall was initially used for planning meetings and office space. However, a significant portion of the Coronation Annex was generously committed to develop the Clinical Academic Campus (CAC) for the IMP. Further clinical academic space was created at the Victoria General Hospital (VGH) site.

Casiro also identified the multidisciplinary champions, obtained the space, secured over $3 million in funding, and established agreements with UBC, UVic, and VIHA to build one multidisciplinary health simulation centre that would serve the needs of the island. Construction of the centre happened under the watch of Casiro, and it was officially opened in 2015, after Dermot Kelleher had become dean and Bruce Wright had become the regional associate dean for the IMP.

To develop this network of clinical teaching sites, Casiro worked diligently to engage teachers by travelling up and down Vancouver Island and using his personal attributes to ensure buy-in. When appropriate, Stuart would join him in these encounters. This was in an environment where physicians were threatening job action in Nanaimo and there was a furious public debate as to whether a new hospital should be built in Comox/Courtenay or Campbell River (eventually the "Canadian solution" was achieved by building a hospital in each site). Casiro made steady incremental gains first with the orthopaedics service in Duncan, then the internal medicine service in Nanaimo, and gradually the emergency medicine service in Victoria. He also leveraged the history and commitment of the Victoria Medical Society to the advantage of the IMP.

Similar to the NMP, the IMP benefitted from a JAC, including leadership from the Faculty, Island Health (IH), and UVic. The JAC was regularly attended by Howard Waldner and later Brendan Carr as CEO of IH, as well as Glen Lowther, Con Rusnak,

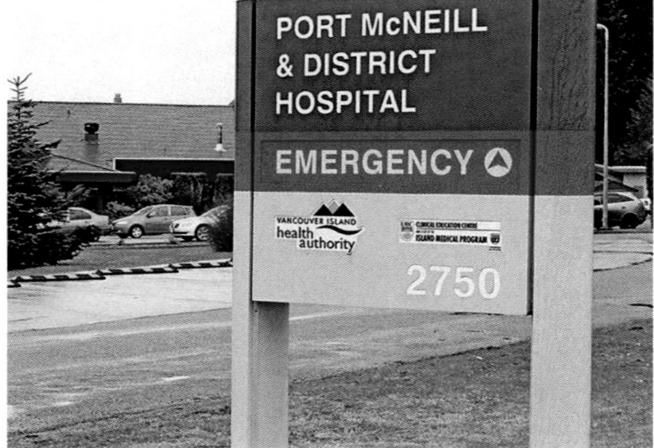

Entrance signage to the Port McNeill & District Hospital, a facility of Island Health.

FACING Medical Sciences Building, UVic, home to the UBC Island Medical Program (opened 2004).

Taj Baidwan, and Lynn Stevenson. Although UVic was fully committed to the IMP, in contrast to the north where the UNBC President attended, it was Provost Jamie Cassels and Valerie Kuehne who attended the JAC regularly. The same UBC leaders attended on behalf of the Faculty. Initially, less substantial issues such as an agreed-upon letterhead and logo size were items of discussion until the JAC members established trust and were able to reach a more strategic level when all major recruitments and program developments were discussed in this forum before proceeding.

Casiro completed ten years of leadership in the IMP in 2014. He had established the program as a unique educational, research, and service entity supported by a partnership among UVic, UBC Faculty of Medicine, Island Health, and the community. His legacy was celebrated in the publication of "The Island Medical Program: Celebrating the first 10 years." In July of 2014, Bruce Wright was recruited from the University of Calgary as the next Regional Associate Dean for the IMP. He was reappointed for a second term in 2019. He led the growth and further development of the Centre for Interprofessional Clinical Simulation Learning, co-governed by UVic, UBC, and Island Health, as well as the implementation of IMP master teachers and first patient program on the island.

The Southern Medical Program

UBC Okanagan (UBCO) had been announced as a new campus of UBC in Kelowna in 2004. The campus grew from the legacy of Okanagan University College with broad-based arts, humanities, and science programs. As Kelowna was one of the fastest growing communities in Canada, one could speculate that another medical campus might be needed in the future, considering population-based health needs. Premier Gordon Campbell had told Dean Cairns back in 2001 that it was then too early for a distributed site in the Okanagan, implying that it might be a future possibility. However, it was a political commitment that launched the program that came to be called the Southern Medical Program (SMP), named "south" despite Kelowna being north of Victoria in latitude.

One evening in March 2005, Dean Stuart received a call from President Martha Piper demanding to know what frivolous conversations had fueled speculation about a new medical campus in the Okanagan. As it transpired, neither Dean Stuart nor President Piper had any forewarning of the Premier's announcement at a dinner in Kelowna, that the province was now ready to fund another distributed medical campus based in the Okanagan. This announcement had roots in conversations between the Premier, MLA Brad Bennett from

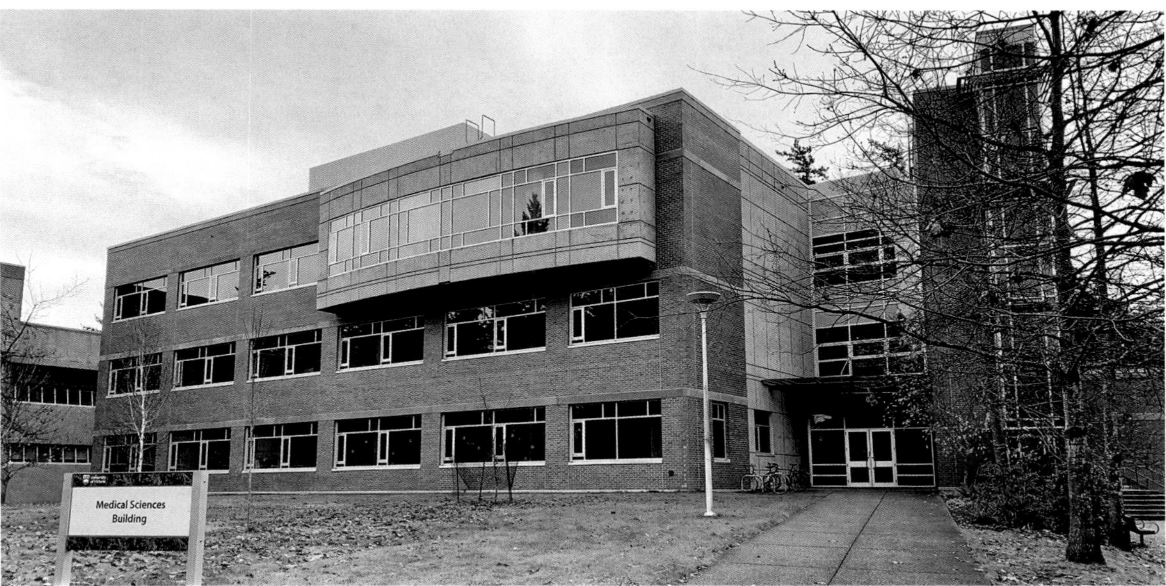

Kelowna, and the new Deputy Vice-chancellor at UBCO, Barry McBride, previously Provost at UBC Vancouver (UBCV).

This announcement surprised even the bureaucracies in the Ministries of Advanced Education and Health. The proposal seemed logical as a means to better meet the health needs of the population of the Interior, but its implementation as another distributed campus would be undertaken before a single doctor had graduated from the new programs in Prince George and Victoria. The exciting model had not yet been validated. There was much speculation about the risk of failing to gain approval of the educational program by the joint Canadian and US accrediting body. Nonetheless, the SMP was launched with strong political support and a commitment for funding. The SMP would eventually welcome medical students in 2011.

Planning began for new academic and clinical facilities in the valley. The target was to admit an additional cohort of thirty-two students to start in September 2011, only one year after the graduation of the first cohort of students in the expanded program from the other three sites and assessment of the success of the new model. There was no assurance that accreditation would be granted and allow such rapid growth. The Dean, the planning team, and the health authority leadership were subject to accreditation milestones almost every six months.

The dynamic in the Okanagan was very different from that in the other distributed sites. First, there were discussions as to whether Kamloops, with a long history of participation in medical education, or Kelowna, the rapidly growing "nexus" of the Okanagan valley, should be the epicentre of the new SMP. With the physical presence of a UBCO Kelowna campus, opened 2005, the debate was soon settled and this new campus, nearly fifteen kilometres from downtown Kelowna, was to be the home to the SMP. Many of the physicians in Kelowna had intentionally moved to practice there in a setting of boundless recreational opportunities. They had been completely unencumbered by the presence of a medical school and some had reservations about expectations for their participation in teaching and research.

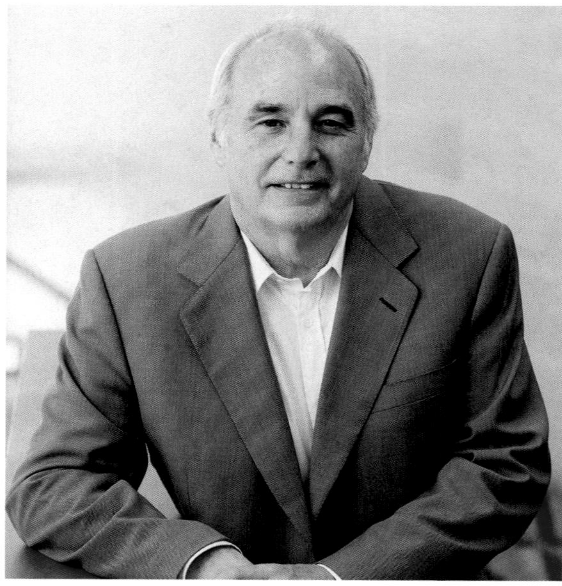

Allan Jones, hematologist, Inaugural Regional Associate Dean, SMP (2009–19).

FACING Reichwald Health Sciences Centre on the UBCO campus, home to the UBC Southern Medical Program (opened 2012).

There were also tensions on the new UBCO campus. The initial Deputy Vice-chancellor (DVC) at UBCO, Barry McBride, was a strong advocate for a provincial medical school. However, the next DVC, Doug Owram, who arrived from the University of Alberta in 2006, was not sure that he even wanted a medical school, never mind one that was a "satellite campus" of UBCV. The NMP and the IMP had been created in partnership with independent universities, whereas the SMP was to be established at the Okanagan campus of UBC. The SMP was a program of UBCV that happened to be located on the grounds of UBCO. In Alberta, Owram had been accustomed to a single medical school on the main university campus, one that was fully accountable to the University of Alberta. The SMP was to be an integral component of the Vancouver-based Faculty of Medicine, and it took some time for the new DVC to become comfortable with this.

Premier Campbell announced the formal funding plan for the program in 2007 and challenged the community to step forward to support the SMP. In September 2008, the premier attended the groundbreaking for what would become the Reichwald Health Sciences Centre on the UBCO campus. Klaus Reichwald was a gracious and committed local philanthropist who made a very generous gift to support the hub of the SMP.

Dr. Allan Jones was recruited in April 2009 as the inaugural Regional Associate Dean for the SMP. Jones came to the SMP with a rich experience as an associate dean at the University of Calgary. His thoughtful and personal style was a critical success factor in bringing together the community with the vision for the SMP. Jones's experience in Calgary had been the delivery of fairly traditional clinical clerkship experiences. This was usually in the senior year of medical school, when the medical student spent time on multiple different clinical services for prescribed periods of time. Jones arrived in BC just when the model of integrated community clerkships (ICC) was being developed by the MD undergraduate education leadership team. This changed the traditional model and now embedded third-year students in a community as a learning health system where they followed the health of a population for one year, working across disciplines rather than in truncated rotations on different medical disciplines. Jones was able to very effectively implement the ICC model in communities across the Interior, including Vernon and Trail. This model soon extended across the province. The first SMP class graduated with a UBC MD degree in 2015.

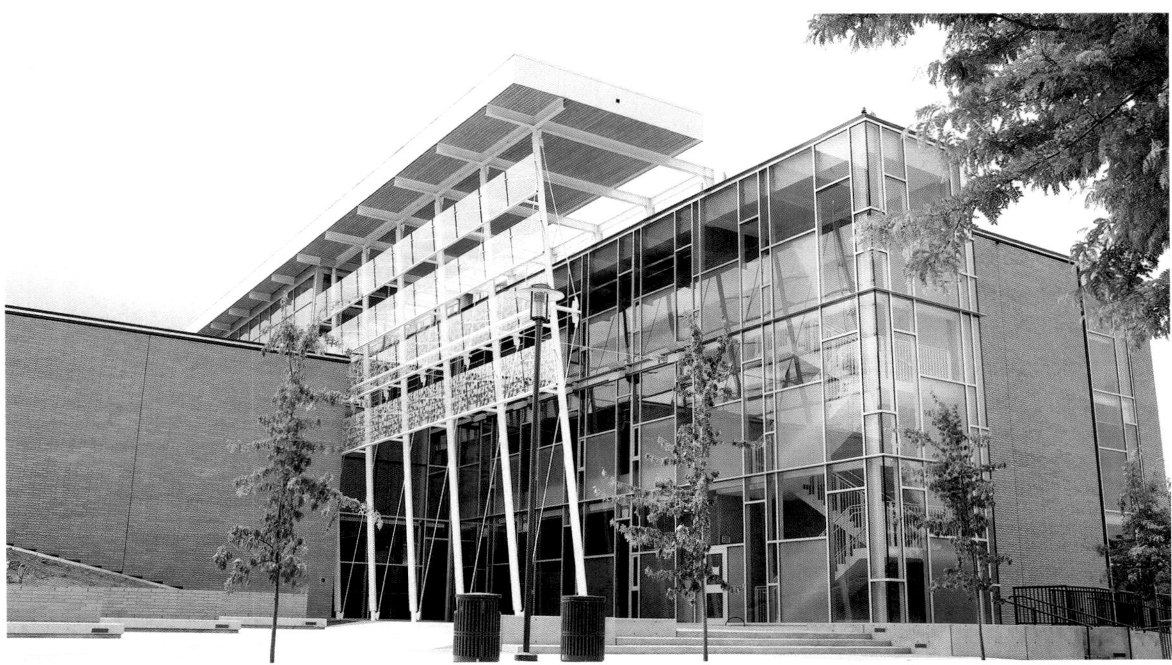

In the Okanagan, a structured joint advisory council supported the successful launch and operation of the program. The JAC benefitted from the active participation of the CEO of Interior Health (IH), Rob Halpenny and then Chris Mazurkewich, together with Jeremy Etherington and Susan Brown. This was particularly helpful in planning across the health authority in more rural and distributed communities such as Trail, Cranbrook, Vernon, and others. As noted earlier, the engagement of the leadership of UBCO was sporadic with the DVC Doug Owram and then Deborah Buzard as intermittent attendees. Fortunately, Dean of the UBCO Faculty of Health and Exercise Sciences Gordon Binsted was a strong supporter of the SMP. Although complex, these councils were critically important in providing a community network for the distributed programs to flourish as well as nurturing a sense of ownership.

In addition to the UBC Faculty leaders, Allan Jones was uniquely successful in recruiting available talent living in the Okanagan. Together with Executive Associate Dean Research Howard Feldman, he was able to attract Dr. Chris Fibiger, who had been a key part of the neurochemistry group at UBC several decades earlier, to serve as Assistant Dean of Research for the SMP, a role he held for eight years before stepping down in 2020. Jones also recruited Dr. Yvonne Lefebvre, previously VP of research for Providence Healthcare until 2014, to serve as scientific research director for the IH and the SMP. Engaging with persons who brought such a wealth of experience allowed the SMP to quickly build capacity for research and academic development.

In 2010, Premier Campbell opened the new Clinical Academic Campus at the Kelowna General Hospital. New or enhanced facilities were also created in Kamloops, Vernon, Penticton, and Trail. Undoubtedly, the facilities were critical components of success, but even more important was the engagement of hundreds of health care providers and community leaders across IH, a huge undertaking requiring the recruitment of many clinicians as leaders within the program. There were also many cultural and social contexts to be accommodated. The physicians in Cranbrook were very committed to the teaching enterprise but were also clear about the need to advise students coming from Vancouver in January to leave their bicycles and Birkenstocks at home for the duration of winter! However, it was becoming apparent that as the SMP matured alongside the NMP and the IMP, the province was becoming a living and learning health education resource. In 2003, there were 2,422 clinical faculty members with appointments in the Faculty. In 2019, this number exceeded nine thousand. Allan Jones completed ten years as the regional associate dean of the SMP in 2019. He had guided the program through the developmental stages into an evolving health learning system for Interior Health. His successor is Sarah Brears, who was appointed in 2020.

The different styles of leadership and priorities that each of the regional associate deans has brought to the entire UBC program were a significant factor in the sustainability and success of the medical program. Graduates from each of the four MD undergraduate programs are all highly educated and well-trained physicians, and each program has its distinctive attributes. Initially, there was a concern that students admitted to the NMP or IMP or SMP would be those who had not been successful in applying to the VFMP. It was also thought that it might be difficult to recruit talented students with an affinity for rural and remote lifestyles into the distributed programs. A unique Rural Remote Suitability Score (RRSS) was developed to help determine the suitability of applicants to placement in rural or remote areas. Applicants to the UBC MD undergraduate program were required to specify in rank order which program they were applying to. With time and demonstrated success, the data now show that the majority of students in all four programs have been accepted into their program of first choice.

Postgraduate Education

The next challenge in implementing expansion and distribution was to ensure that the number of postgraduate training positions available to UBC graduates would support the ultimate vision. Prior to 2000, there were fewer first-year postgraduate positions in BC than there were medical graduates from UBC. BC did not contribute fairly to the national pool of residency positions and relied to an unjustified extent upon programs elsewhere in Canada to provide postgraduate training to their graduates. Although Dean Cairns and Associate Dean Wright had secured an informal acknowledgement in 2002 by the Ministry of Health in BC to fund the same number of residency positions as there were graduates, or even slightly more, with the increasing number of UBC graduates in this new model, still more postgraduate positions were needed. By 2015, there were 288 new graduates per year from UBC. Graduates from other jurisdictions in Canada as well as international medical graduates also wished to apply for positions in BC, making it a highly competitive process. Furthermore, it was apparent that not all of these trainees could be accommodated in Vancouver.

Penny Ballem, Clinical Professor of Medicine, was also Deputy Minister of Health from 2001 to 2006. She was exceptionally helpful in providing support to Stuart in addressing these challenges. The Postgraduate Planning Task Force was convened, led by Dean Stuart and the Assistant Deputy Minister of Health and later became the Medical Human Resources Planning Task Force. After a few years of planning, negotiations, and innovation, a broader distributed model of postgraduate education evolved. The government agreed to fund at least 288 new postgraduate positions in BC each year, but in return mandated a focus on primary care providers and generalists (family practice, general internal medicine, pediatrics, general surgery, and psychiatry) rather than more focused specialties. Also new postgraduate clinical teaching sites would be developed across the province. Indeed, there was a strong logic that specialty training provided outside the Lower Mainland–for example, in Kelowna or elsewhere in BC–might be more likely to lead to the retention of those same trainees in smaller communities. Furthermore, it was always intended that undergraduate medical students should be exposed to and work with postgraduate trainees in clinical settings in all four programs to ensure a comparable environment for all learners. Again, Stuart very much benefitted from the support and understanding of Deputy Minister Stephen Brown in changing the model of clinical learning. The programs were starting to align with community needs in a manner that had not previously been considered.

Gradually, against some significant resistance from within and without, other specialties, including psychiatry, internal medicine, pediatrics, and emergency medicine, began to establish distributed programs of postgraduate education that in many ways were aligned with the undergraduate medical programs. Even today, there exists a sentiment that certain postgraduate specialty training programs cannot be delivered properly outside of the cloistered walls of large tertiary and quaternary institutions in urban settings. However, there are now Royal College program streams based in Prince George, Surrey, Kelowna, and Victoria.

With a program as large and bold as this, expectations were very high for improvements in physician supply throughout BC. When the early metrics demonstrated that the first graduates of the NMP were not all staying in Northern BC, though, there was much disappointment. There were some health planners who had expected that all of the first NMP class would remain in the north for postgraduate training. However, new graduates were pursuing

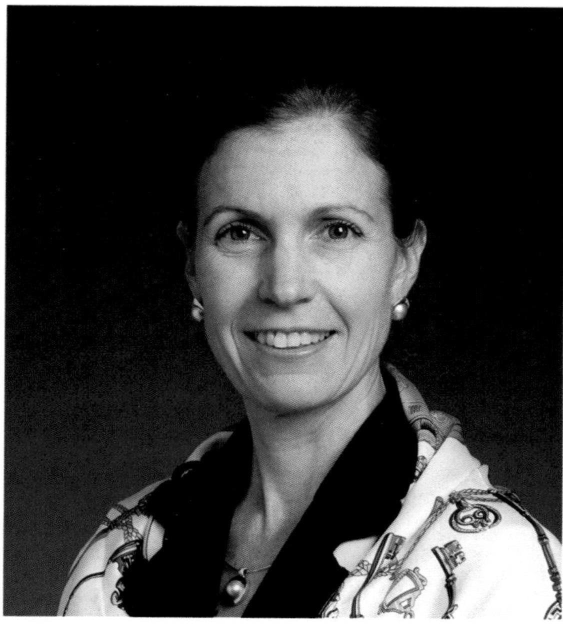

Katherine Paton, ophthalmologist and ocular oncologist, Executive Associate Dean Clinical Affairs (2006–12).

postgraduate training in the Lower Mainland, in other provinces, and often in rural programs outside of BC. Furthermore, some observers were dismayed that not all graduates chose to pursue family practice, even though Northern BC requires specialists in all disciplines as well as family practice.

Gradually, beginning in 2010, newly minted UBC family physicians, after two years of postgraduate training, started to take up practice positions outside of the Lower Mainland. Published results from UBC now demonstrate that students with a rural background who trained at a regional campus are highly likely to practice family medicine in a rural location. Beginning in 2013, after five years of specialty training, new urologists, neurologists, plastic surgeons, oncologists, and others who had graduated from UBC's distributed program, had started to practice in Northern BC and on Vancouver Island.

In order to ensure that the medical educational and training programs of this distributed model would continue to be aligned with the needs of the society that physicians serve, it became necessary to evaluate the quality and impact of these programs and to seek better and more innovative programs of pedagogy. In 2005, Joanna Bates had approached Dean Stuart to state that she was confident that her role in implementing the expansion and distribution of the program was now secondary to her zeal and commitment to teaching and innovation in medical education. With her characteristic passion, she shepherded the Centre for Health Education Scholarship (CHES) to its opening in 2008. With leadership from Bates and more recently Ian Scott, Kevin Eva, and Glenn Regehr, CHES has become internationally recognized as a beacon of pedagogical quality and innovation. This has been viewed as one of Joanna Bates's most significant legacies since her untimely death in 2020.

Clinical Faculty

The collective discontent of clinical faculty members had reached a zenith with the one-week strike in 2001. Additional funding from the Ministry of Health subsequently allowed Dean Cairns to implement increased compensation for clinical teaching and administrative responsibilities, and the planning group for the coming expansion ensured the allocation of substantial new resources for clinical teaching in the projected budgets. The stature of formal representation of clinical faculty was enhanced at the FoM level. Although the tensions

Graydon Meneilly, diabetologist and geriatrician, Head of Department of Medicine (2002–17).

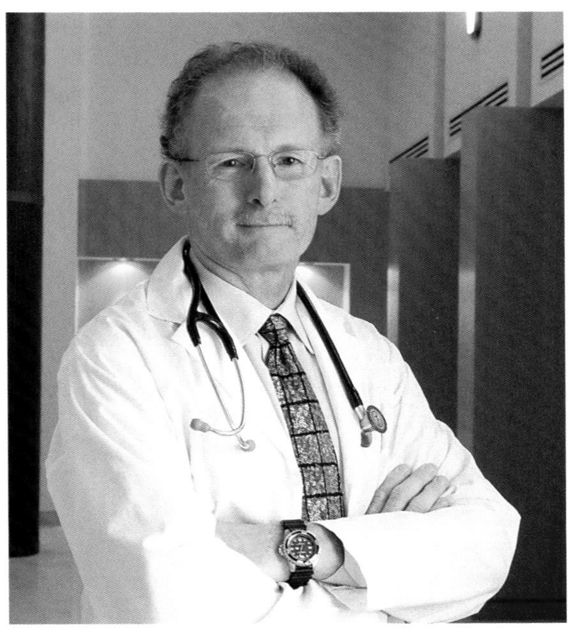

between the FoM and its clinical faculty had abated somewhat by the start of Stuart's term as Dean, they were far from completely resolved. There remained a pervasive discontent. In addition, expanding the medical program across the province in a distributed model was clearly going to require the majority of practicing clinicians to engage and participate if this was to be successful. Not only did this require valuing clinical teaching but it also required ensuring that the university and the academy recognized the essential value of all clinical facilities including hospitals, clinics, and community practices province-wide.

In part the challenge was to engage clinical colleagues across the province in the educational enterprise but at the same time provide them with the pedagogical tools to allow them to feel comfortable in their own clinical settings with learners. Many facilities and community settings had provided excellent patient care for decades but without the regular accommodation of learners. Starting in 2004, the leadership in the Faculty responsible for supporting clinical faculty members, including Katherine Paton, Dorothy Shaw, Gurdeep Parhar, and later Michael Nimmo, spent considerable time meeting with colleagues in diverse locations conducting needs assessments and attempting to provide them with the necessary tools to allow them to provide valuable educational experiences. Clinical care had to be seen as an integral component of the academic mission. When Stuart arrived in BC, he had made clear to everyone that in order to reflect this value, he intended to continue practicing clinically as a gynecologic oncologist. Throughout his term as Dean, he continued with a shared surgical practice with an outstanding group of colleagues and participated in the call roster and other clinical responsibilities. This had many collateral impacts amongst clinical colleagues who saw the dean in this role as a major positive.

This new distributed model also created unique challenges for the leadership of UBC clinical departments. From the original four clinical departments of Medicine, Surgery, Obstetrics/Gynecology, and Pediatrics, many other disciplines flourished and became formal departments over the next fifty years. In addition to Family Practice, the departments of Ophthalmology and Visual Sciences, Orthopaedics, Pathology and Laboratory Medicine, Psychiatry, and Radiology have long-standing histories. Within the term of Dean Stuart, the departments of Urologic Sciences, Dermatology and Skin Sciences, and

Emergency Medicine have been formalized, each achieving increased research productivity. Other departments have amalgamated around a common vision, such as the relatively new Department of Anesthesiology, Pharmacology and Therapeutics. The Anatomy and Physiology departments were amalgamated as the Department of Cellular and Physiological Sciences. The structure of departments within the school has evolved to keep pace with contemporary science and education. Excellence in other health disciplines is found in the School of Audiology and Speech Sciences, the Department of Physical Therapy, and the Department of Occupational Science and Occupational Therapy.

The new model required that department heads seek alignment with programs and departments within the health authorities. Where appropriate, the UBC head of department is usually the regional head in Vancouver. This model of "chair/chief" has been subjected to much discussion and continues to evolve. Furthermore, the chair of a clinical department at UBC has academic responsibilities not only in Vancouver but across the province and all four medical programs. This arrangement has made these leadership roles much more complex and challenging, but the aligned structure has ensured that the Faculty remains accountable to the society that it serves and is directly engaged within the health care system.

Even though the Department of Family Practice was formalized only in 1978, it has had the deepest and broadest provincial reach in its undergraduate and postgraduate programs. For other departments, this was a new challenge, one that for the Department of Medicine has been as complex as any. Since 2002, with the leadership of Dr. Graydon Meneilly as Head, the UBC Department of Medicine has had to evolve from being a large sophisticated university department based mainly at VGH and St. Paul's to being a diffuse multidisciplinary entity across the Lower Mainland, Vancouver Island, and throughout BC. For undergraduate and postgraduate teaching programs, Meneilly had to ensure that an academic framework was in place across the province. This required identifying local leadership, recruiting colleagues to engage in the teaching enterprise in settings that had not been accustomed to large numbers of learners, establishing comparable educational experiences across all sites, and still meeting all standards of accreditation. This included institutional and community settings. Concurrently, he had to ensure support and nurturing of the research programs across institutes, hospitals, clinical investigator programs, and other entities to ensure that the academic environment was provincial and not parochial. Enormous relationship building and goodwill were required to succeed.

Although the simultaneous appointment as Regional Head of Medicine for Vancouver Coastal and Physician-in-Chief at VGH was at times an advantage, it also added significant responsibility for financial, resource, and program management. Any influence within the departmental jurisdiction of other health authorities required a high degree of calm persuasion, diplomacy, and leadership. Meneilly was one of a stellar group of department leaders who held these same responsibilities and he was one of the longest serving heads of this era (2002–17). Bas Masri (Orthopaedics), Geoff Cundiff (Obstetrics and Gynecology), Garth Warnock (Surgery), Alison Eddy (Pediatrics), and Athanasios Zis and Bill Honer (Psychiatry) each spent considerable time and energy in developing a provincial framework for their departments. Academic leadership in BC has become uniquely challenging. However, with strong departmental leadership and support from the Faculty, the faculty ranks have grown tremendously.

When Stuart approached the end of his second term in 2015, UBC health and life sciences research was ranked number two in Canada, the distributed medical program graduated 287 new physicians from four programs in the province, and more than six thousand clinical faculty members were engaged in the academic program across the province. The previous estimate of need for the province of three hundred new physicians annually has now increased to four hundred annually but is now met by 288 UBC graduates and an ongoing immigration of roughly one hundred physicians per year from outside BC. After stepping down as Dean, Stuart continued as UBC Vice-provost of Health for an additional year. He remains as an active researcher, clinician, and educator at UBC. In 2020, he was appointed as Head of the UBC Department of Obstetrics and Gynecology on an interim basis.

In the years after 2015, in the Faculty of Medicine, UBC department heads have embraced their provincial roles and responsibilities. For many of the physicians who serve as clinical educators across BC, this has done much to create a sense of belonging to a provincial department and created some greater cohesion. Research opportunities and collaborations have grown throughout the province across communities and institutions. Graduates of the medical school are now recognized as UBC graduates and are not segregated by which program they trained in. This is a testament to the success of the distributed educational program.

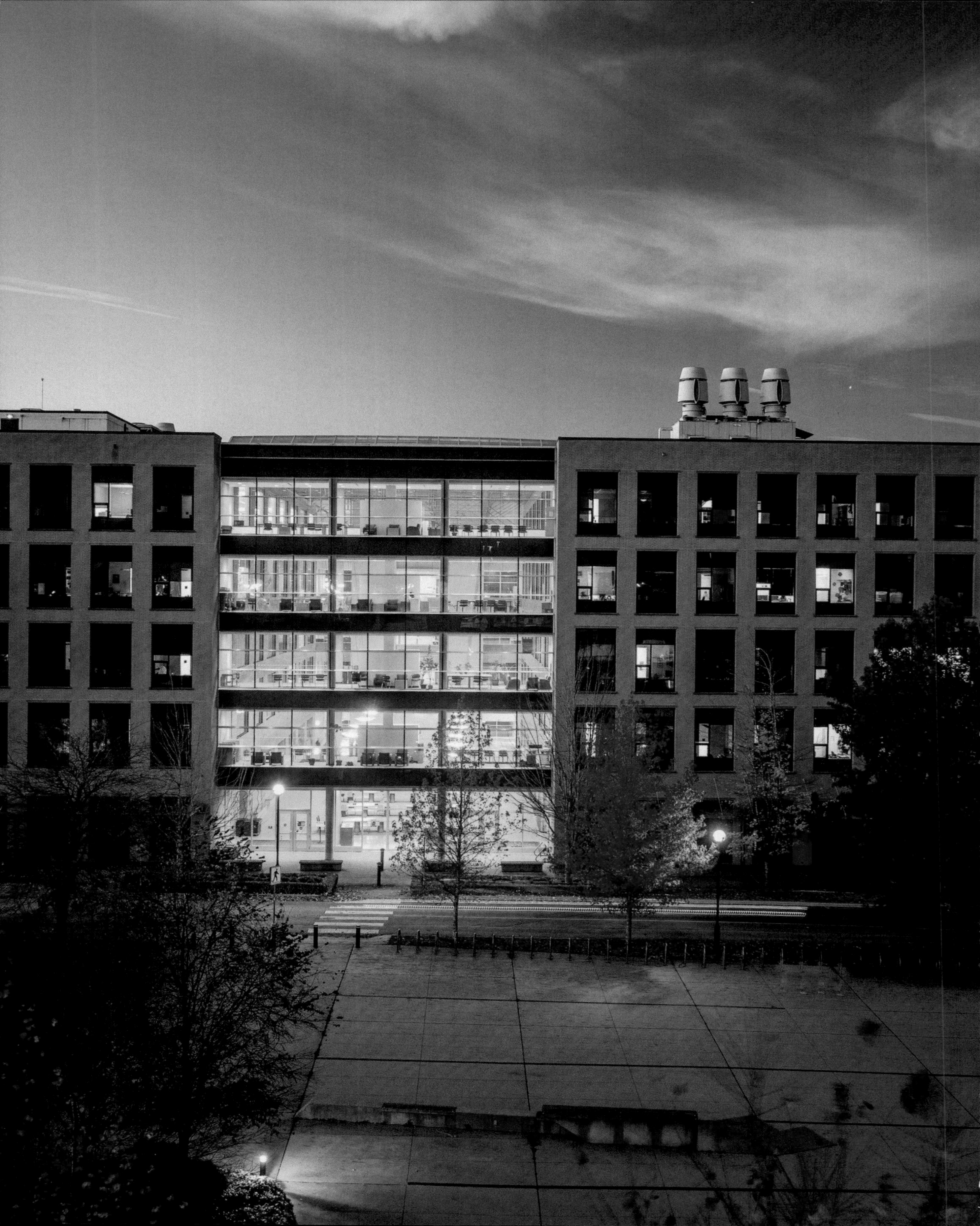

7

A World Class Medical School

2015 and Beyond

FACING Life Sciences Center, UBC.

FACING Dermot Kelleher, gastroenterologist, ninth Dean of Medicine (2015–present).

Kelleher saw no barriers to UBC's Faculty of Medicine becoming amongst the best in the world for its educational programs, outstanding research, and commitment to care and service.

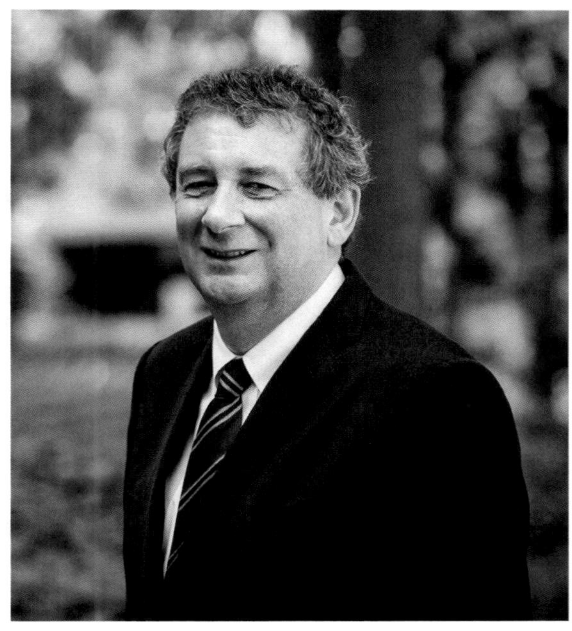

IN SEPTEMBER 2015, the University of British Columbia welcomed Dermot Kelleher as the new dean of the Faculty of Medicine. Substantial success had been achieved in recent decades, but the new dean would face challenges to sustain the momentum. He had graduated from the medical undergraduate program and completed his MD thesis at Trinity College, Dublin. He went on to serve as Head of the School of Medicine and Vice-provost for Medical Affairs at his alma mater. He came to UBC following his previous appointment as Dean of the Faculty of Medicine and Vice-president of Health, Imperial College London, UK, and a concurrent appointment as Dean of the Lee Kong Chian School of Medicine in Singapore. This latter experience as well as his time as a Fogarty Scholar at University of California San Diego provided him with a rich international view of academic health sciences.

The timing of his arrival was propitious. Coming from a different health care background than our completely publicly funded Canadian system, he was able to take a fresh look at the relationships between health authorities and the university in BC. He viewed the opportunity to profile British Columbia as a world-leading academic health sciences system as profound. Accordingly, Dean Kelleher started his term actively encouraging and, indeed, enabling UBC Faculty of Medicine to take its place on the world stage. He saw no barriers to UBC's FoM becoming amongst the best in the world for its educational programs, outstanding research, and commitment to care and service.

Accreditation

There were several critical steps to be reached in the medical program at the undergraduate and later at a postgraduate level. Four months after Kelleher's arrival, there was a full accreditation visit in February 2016 for the medical undergraduate program by both the Canadian and the US agencies. After all of the expansion and distribution in the preceding fifteen years, this was a seminal moment for the program. These agencies have the authority to severely limit change in a program or even to withdraw the approved status of an accredited school. There are twelve standards and ninety-five elements with which the MD undergraduate program must comply.

With outstanding leadership from Dave Snadden, Lua Lynch, and many, many others, the outcome

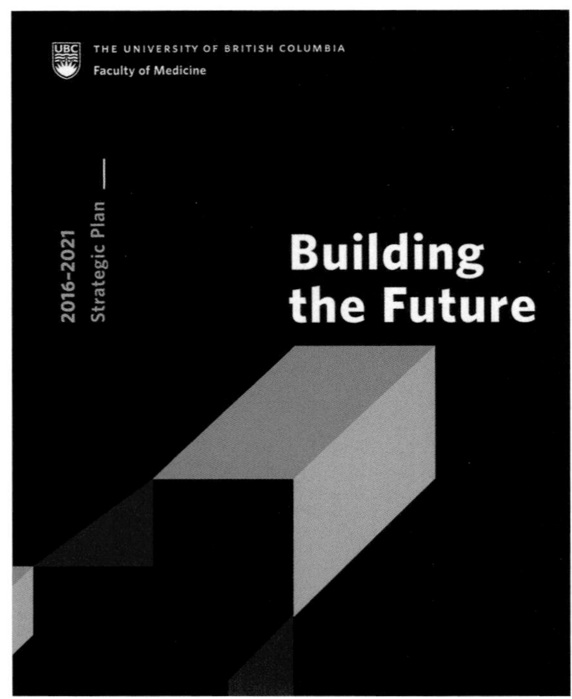

Building the Future, 2016–2021 Strategic Plan.

of the review process was deemed to be both very positive and constructive but with a list of elements that were either rated as "unsatisfactory" or "satisfactory but with monitoring." In response, the undergraduate program across the province worked to improve in all of these areas. In February 2019, a limited site visit took place by the accrediting agencies, and the decision rendered in August 2019 was to continue with full accreditation status for the program through to the 2023-24 academic year when the next full site visit will occur. This was a major accomplishment for the medical program at UBC given the pace of change over the preceding twenty-five years and reflected an accomplishment of which the Faculty of Medicine could be very proud.

A further testament to the success of the UBC model was the accreditation process of the Canadian Residency Accreditation Consortium (CanRAC). This is a consortium of the Royal College of Physicians and Surgeons of Canada and the College of Family Physicians of Canada to maintain national standards for the evaluation and accreditation of Canadian postgraduate medical training programs. In another major milestone, in March 2020, a team of approximately one hundred reviewers from CanRAC conducted an onsite accreditation review of each of the seventy-five UBC residency training programs and the Postgraduate Medical Education office. This process documented the excellence of the programs and the model that extends across the province. With leadership from Associate Dean Postgraduate Medical Education Ravi Sidhu and the team across all sites, the model of training physicians in the communities that they will serve appears to be successful.

The "Building the Future" Plan

Even though Dean Kelleher was very focused on ensuring successful accreditation of both the medical undergraduate and postgraduate programs, he also moved swiftly at a strategic level, beginning with the energetic development of a new Faculty strategic plan. "Building the Future" articulated the commitments, principles, and goals that would enable the Faculty to deepen and extend its leadership role in shaping British Columbia's health system and contributing to the knowledge economy of the province. Now that the FoM had stabilized its finances, it could move forward in meeting both internal and external demands for transformation and renewal.

The plan had four transformative goals:

1. Education: the teaching, development, and mentoring of practitioners and scientists who can work together effectively in an evolving system.
2. Research: knowledge creation, translation, and exchange to gain insight and promote improved outcomes in patient and public health.
3. Organization: creation of a working environment that inspires innovation, strengthens academic and operational affiliation, and fosters agility.
4. Partnership: collective system leadership to help shape practices and policies for improved care of the population across the province.

One outcome was a strategic investment fund that would enable the investment of $3.8 million across forty-one faculty- and staff-led projects. In response to the need to ensure that *people* are the drivers of change, a program of faculty renewal created thirty-six new junior faculty positions in the areas of critical succession and translational medicine and innovation, and three new senior faculty positions created through Canada Excellence Research Chairs, Canada 150 Chairs, and UBC President's Excellence Chairs. The focus on critical succession led to recruitments in the areas of sport and exercise medicine scholarship, cardiovascular pathology, and pharmacogenomics, amongst others. As of 2020, new recruitments were also underway within the translational medicine and innovation category in the areas of artificial intelligence in radiology and precision medicine, mental health systems and policy, bioinformatics and machine learning, as well as precision oncology in gynecology and other areas. Most of these new recruits will transcend traditional departments and bring a broad, cross-cutting context to new discoveries, reflecting Kelleher's commitment to a vision of excellence in research and education in the health sciences. A 2020 film entitled *The Vision* both reflects and celebrates the Faculty's impact across British Columbia.

From its inception, the Faculty has aspired to pursue science that leads to tangible health and economic benefits for society. Translational medicine seeks to translate discovery from the bench to the bedside to the community in order to realize these benefits more effectively. However, in the context of ever-changing paradigms and technologies, the systems, structures, and processes that support research have not generally been designed or optimized for this translational purpose. The Faculty has an ambitious plan to ameliorate these shortcomings in the immediate future. The goal is to re-engineer the approach with an explicit focus on getting better and safer drugs, diagnostics, and devices to people in a faster, cheaper, and more effective manner.

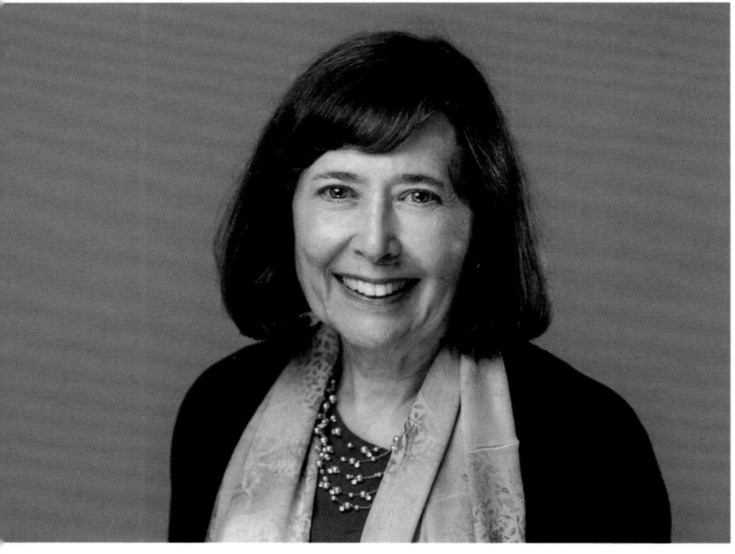

Connie Eaves, biologist, Department of Medical Genetics, Distinguished Scientist BC Cancer Research Centre, Terry Fox Laboratory.

The Faculty has defined those areas that are focused on translation and discovery science within academic settings as "pipelines." One of these pipelines is intimately linked to the new School of Biomedical Engineering, enabling a partnership with the Faculty of Applied Sciences. This initiative will also involve the development of new interactive spaces so clinicians, research scientists, engineers, and learners can seamlessly exchange ideas and disseminate information. Another example of this new strategic approach is the proposed Academy of Translational Medicine led by Professor Poul Sorensen. Development of these pipelines will require the recruitment of a cadre of translational research scientists and the development of innovative programs to educate undergraduates and postgraduates in translational science.

Celebrating Research and Innovation

Like his predecessors, Dean Kelleher continued to emphasize research. In 2020, UBC was ranked among the top thirty in the world by QS World University Rankings and the Times Higher Education World University Rankings in health and life sciences. Between 2015 and 2019, the Faculty of Medicine attracted more than $1.68 billion in research funding, of which more than $234 million came from outside of Canada.

As of 2020, the FoM held forty-four Tier 1 and 2 Canada Research Chairs. Three faculty members have received the Canada Gairdner Wightman Award (Michael Hayden, James Hogg, and Connie Eaves) and eight have been appointed to the prestigious Canadian Medical Hall of Fame (Harold Copp, Max Cynader, Julio Montaner, Judith Hall, Michael Hayden, Brett Finlay, Connie Eaves, and Marco Marra). The Faculty, uniquely positioned by generous philanthropy, also established three annual awards for Canadian scientists with demonstrated research excellence: the Dr. Chew Wei Memorial Prize in Cancer Research, the Margolese National Brain Disorders Prize, and the Margolese National Heart Disorders Prize now provide financial and reputational awards approaching those of the Gairdner Award.

As the home of the only faculty of medicine in the province, UBC is ideally positioned to host a coordinated translational medicine enterprise with provincial reach and end-to-end translational capabilities. The Faculty's major health research priorities–precision health, cancer, brain and mental health, heart and lung disease, population

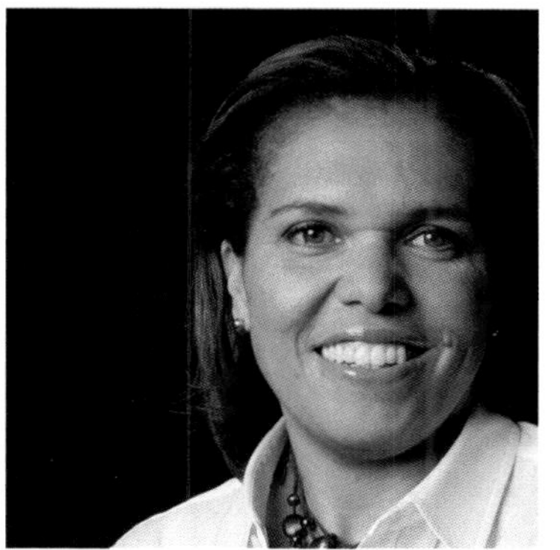

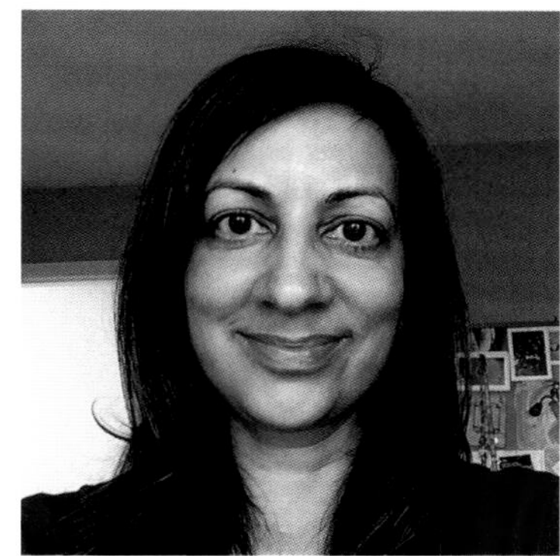

LEFT Gina Ogilvie, public health scientist, School of Population and Public Health, Tier 1 Canada research Chair in Global Control of HPV Related Diseases and Prevention.

RIGHT Videsh Kapoor (UBC MD '83), family physician, educator, global health leader.

health, and chronic disease–are pursued by a critical mass of globally respected experts with particular strengths in genomics and molecular pathology. The proposed model for the Academy of Translational Medicine embodies a unique combination of unparalleled strengths and partnerships. Nevertheless, there are gaps that must be filled to ensure a smooth, efficient translational pathway at UBC. The most common roadblocks faced by scientists in the translational process are specifically addressed in the FoM model.

Improving Access to Health Care for All British Columbians

Many medical schools are recognized globally for their innovation and leadership in medical education. Others are acclaimed as international leaders in health sciences research. Very few are able to achieve such recognition in both domains. There has been much written about bimodal medical schools, that is, those that are focused on educating and training excellent primary care and specialist practitioners but at the same time are ranked among the world leaders in groundbreaking research and the training of clinician-scientists. UBC's Faculty of Medicine is considered to be in this category. There are very few institutions renowned for innovation in rural health care concurrent with international leadership in genomic medicine. To maintain this bimodal excellence, Dean Kelleher created a strong leadership team to continue research growth and excellence as well as pedagogical innovation and leadership. As the Executive Vice-dean (2016–20), Deborah Money was a critical contributor to this success by supporting department heads and other faculty members in ensuring that the educational programs of the Faculty flourished as well as research.

The Faculty has achieved much recognition internationally for the excellence of its programs. However, it also has attempted to give back by establishing deep roots in global health. Most departments have leaders who have made an impact on continents other than North America. Within the medical undergraduate program, Videsh Kapoor has worked tirelessly to develop a curriculum for students in the Global Health Initiative (GHI) who may be travelling to other countries and wish to respect the local culture and ensure a lasting positive impact. The GHI has engaged in many countries in Asia and Africa. The School of Population and Public Health (SPPH) has an extensive cadre of faculty members contributing to the Health in Populations program. Annalee Yassi and Jerry Spiegel developed the Global Health Research Program nearly two decades ago. Many faculty members such as Gina Ogilvie have worked effectively across

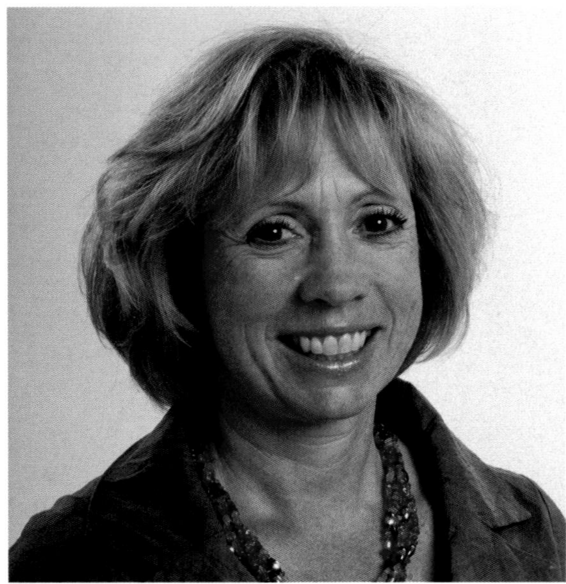

Deborah Money (UBC MD '85), obstetrician/gynecologist, Executive Vice-dean Faculty of Medicine (2016–20).

institutions such as SPPH, BC Women's Hospital, Women's Health Research Institute, and the BC Centre for Disease Control to develop programs of care, education, and research for populations of women in Uganda and elsewhere in Africa.

The vision of the distributed model of medical education has been to improve access to health care in BC by ensuring that there are adequate numbers of health practitioners embedded in those communities where the need exists. In 2003, 128 students comprised the entry MD undergraduate class. In 2019, 288 students were welcomed into the class with 196 in the Vancouver-Fraser Medical Program and 32 in each of the Island Medical Program, Northern Medical Program, and Southern Medical Program. UBC has consistently graduated approximately 288 new physicians annually since 2015. Every year across the province, more than 169 new doctors begin training in family practice and more than 177 in specialty practice.

Across all disciplines, the MD undergraduate program has been uniquely successful in graduating a diverse, representative workforce that seeks to meet the needs of BC, including those of the Indigenous communities and new Canadians. UBC's goal of graduating fifty Indigenous MDs by 2020 was surpassed in 2015, and to date there have been more than seventy Indigenous graduates from multiple First Nations in BC. UBC has had the highest rate of success in Canada over the past twenty years in accepting, educating, and graduating Indigenous learners. Our graduating class reflects the breadth and diversity of the population of BC. This has been underpinned by strong partnerships with University of Northern BC, University of Victoria, and UBC Okanagan, as well as all of the health authorities in BC.

As of 2019, ninety percent of trainees who completed their undergraduate and postgraduate training at UBC remain in BC. Of the graduates of the NMP who entered a residency in family practice, sixty-six now practice in rural areas. UBC's Department of Family Practice in 2020 had twenty training programs across many sites containing multiple streams. This provincial model for physician education and training is now being utilized in other disciplines including physiotherapy and occupational therapy.

Each program within the medical program has unique strengths. The NMP and IMP offer a much deeper understanding of Indigenous health issues. The SMP and the NMP focus on rural and remote populations. The VFMP is better able to spawn expertise in urban health issues and the conduct and commercialization of biomedical health research. All learners in the UBC medical school have a common

Rob McMaster, geneticist, Head of Department of Medical Genetics (2000–2010), Vice-dean Research (2016–present), Vice-president Research Vancouver Coastal Health (2008–present).

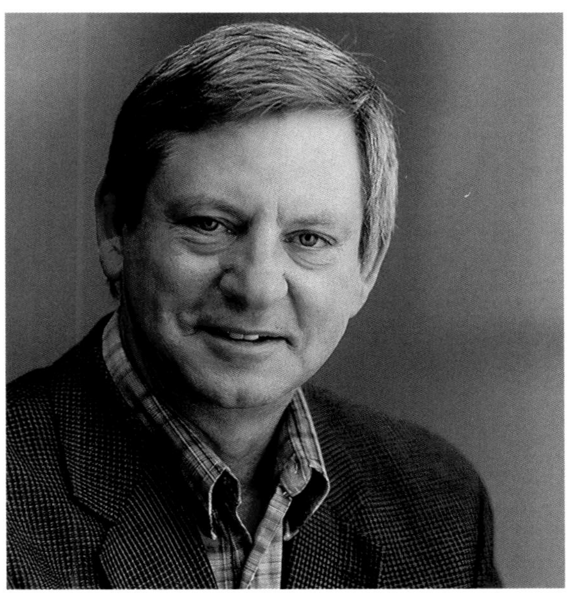

broad platform of education, while the commitment to social accountability is manifested differently in each program.

Within the distributed medical program, applicants are invited to complete a Rural Remote Suitability Score (RRSS) survey if they wish to be considered for the NMP. The RRSS tool is also used for up to ten positions in the SMP and up to two positions in the IMP. The proportion of first-year students from out of province is capped at ten percent. Entry through the Indigenous pathway has a target, but not a cap, of five percent of the class. The MD/PhD program is able to accept up to eight students per year, but this is largely limited by funding and there are usually about five students per year in this track. In 2017–18, the mean age of entering students was 24.1 years, with seventy percent aged twenty-three and above. In 2019, 57.5 percent of the total medical class at UBC was female.

The number of post-MD (residency) positions offered at UBC amounts to 10.2% of total Canadian positions (1,671 out of 16,458). In Canada, the majority (79.6%) are funded by governments. The sex distribution is similar to the Canadian average: 60.7% of residents in general internal medicine are female; 50% of residents in medical specialties are female. In the surgical specialties, 42.2% of the residents are women, up from 36% in 2008–09.

The optimal impact of the ambitious expansion and distribution of the medical program at UBC, embarked upon in 2004, was fully realized by 2020, when most members of the full expanded and distributed class had entered practice after completing either a two-year family practice residency or a five-year Royal College approved program. The vision became a reality with new oncologists in Prince George, new family physicians in Powell River, new emergency room physicians in New Westminster, and a new surgeon in Quesnel. They do indeed seem to "live where they learn and practice where they live."

COVID-19

Notwithstanding this trajectory of excellence and accomplishments, the year 2020 brought a challenge to the world with an order of magnitude not previously experienced. The COVID-19 pandemic has affected citizens, jurisdictions, and economies globally. It has also had a unique impact on the medical program and required the incredible agility, ingenuity, and resilience of all members of the Faculty. As noted throughout this book, the Faculty has endured financial hardship, the impact of

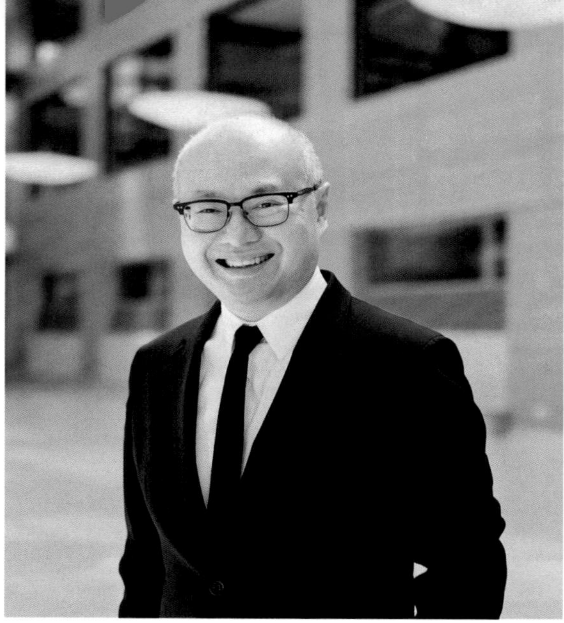

Roger Wong, geriatrician, Associate Dean Post Graduate Education (2012–16), Executive Associate, then Vice-dean Education (2016–present).

global conflict, political turmoil, and SARS. The SARS-CoV-2 virus presented an entirely new threat. As of March 2020, all educational and research programming changed. The Faculty placed a hold on all clinical experiences for medical students. All in-person classes were suspended. All research was suspended or curtailed, from on-campus basic science research to clinical trials. Exemptions were considered for critical research or maintaining critical research resources. Wherever possible, faculty and staff were encouraged to work remotely. For those faculty, residents, learners, and staff who continued to provide direct patient care, the need for appropriate personal protective equipment was preeminent and challenging. Personal safety became the priority.

Within British Columbia, it was remarkable that a faculty member from the School of Population and Public Health became a world leader in pandemic response and control. Provincial Health Officer Dr. Bonnie Henry, a clinical associate professor, very quickly became prominent as a wise, calm, informed voice that resonated internationally. Despite the personal, financial, and institutional impact, the entire Faculty responded quickly. Dean Kelleher was a vanguard among health leaders, successfully advocating for and accomplishing the move of all programs into a virtual online format within weeks while maintaining the integrity and continuity of the faculty operations. He was strident in ensuring the safety of the students, staff, and faculty as the number one priority. In the space of four months, all FoM educational programs were modified to be delivered mostly with remote instruction online and with very limited in-person delivery for hands-on instruction of curricular materials not amenable to online delivery. This included medical undergraduate, postgraduate, and research students. Learners on clinical rotations were gradually returned to the clinical interface in July 2020. The Continuing Professional Development team, led by Brenna Lynn, quickly developed and implemented programs to support faculty and staff now engaged in online teaching rather than the conventional face-to-face. The COVID-19 Resource Hub was developed. Additional resources quickly evolved, including the Centre for Health Education Scholarship, Continuing Professional Development, EdTech, Faculty Development, the HIVE (Hackspace for Innovation and Visualization in Education), and Woodward Library. The research enterprise has been both curtailed and enhanced by this crisis. Kelleher and the faculty leadership quickly brought together health sector leaders (academia, government, health authorities, industry) to scale up collaborative, critical COVID-19 research to compress timelines in delivery of new treatments and therapies. The COVID-19 Clinical Research Coordination Initiative of the Faculty of Medicine is aimed at creating innovative health systems and structures capable of capturing and collating collective input and feedback to enable the prioritization and coordination of COVID-19 translational research.

As of July 2020, there was a staged resumption of research. Hands-on laboratory-based research gradually returned, and dry-lab research continued remotely. Substantial new funding opportunities related to COVID-19 also stimulated the growth of existing and new programs. UBC researchers became international leaders in genotyping the virus, developing vaccines, and defining new preventive and therapeutic strategies. The pandemic fundamentally altered how the Faculty of Medicine functioned, and it met this change with incredible agility and creativity.

Moving Forward

In 2018, Dean Kelleher was concurrently appointed as Vice-president of Health for UBC. In 2020, he was appointed to a second five-year term as Dean of the Faculty of Medicine. The UBC Medicine program has been ranked consistently in the top thirty in the world for the past several years. The Faculty is committed to educational quality and research excellence, both of which are focused on improved health for the people it serves in British Columbia and beyond.

The Faculty of Medicine has come a long way from its primitive beginnings in 1950. As of 2020, there were more than nine thousand clinical faculty and more than six hundred full-time faculty as well as over two thousand staff. At the time of publication, there are 324 full professors, 159 associate professors, 62 assistant professors, 2 professors of teaching, and 27 instructors or senior instructors. Women constitute thirty-six percent of faculty and seventy-five percent of staff. There are two percent of staff who declare as Indigenous and an increasing number of faculty as well. People of colour constitute nineteen percent of faculty and thirty-nine percent of staff. At all faculty ranks–assistant, associate, and full professor–the mean salaries of women and men are similar.

Fulfillment of the mandate of the FoM, especially in its distributed model, has been possible only because of the enthusiastic engagement of the clinical and academic faculty based in communities, facilities, and the various teaching hospitals throughout the province. As evidenced by financial support, more research is conducted in the research institutes of the Vancouver teaching hospitals than on the UBC campus, and far more teaching of undergraduate and postgraduate students is conducted by faculty at the teaching hospitals. The mission of the Faculty of Medicine is being felt throughout British Columbia.

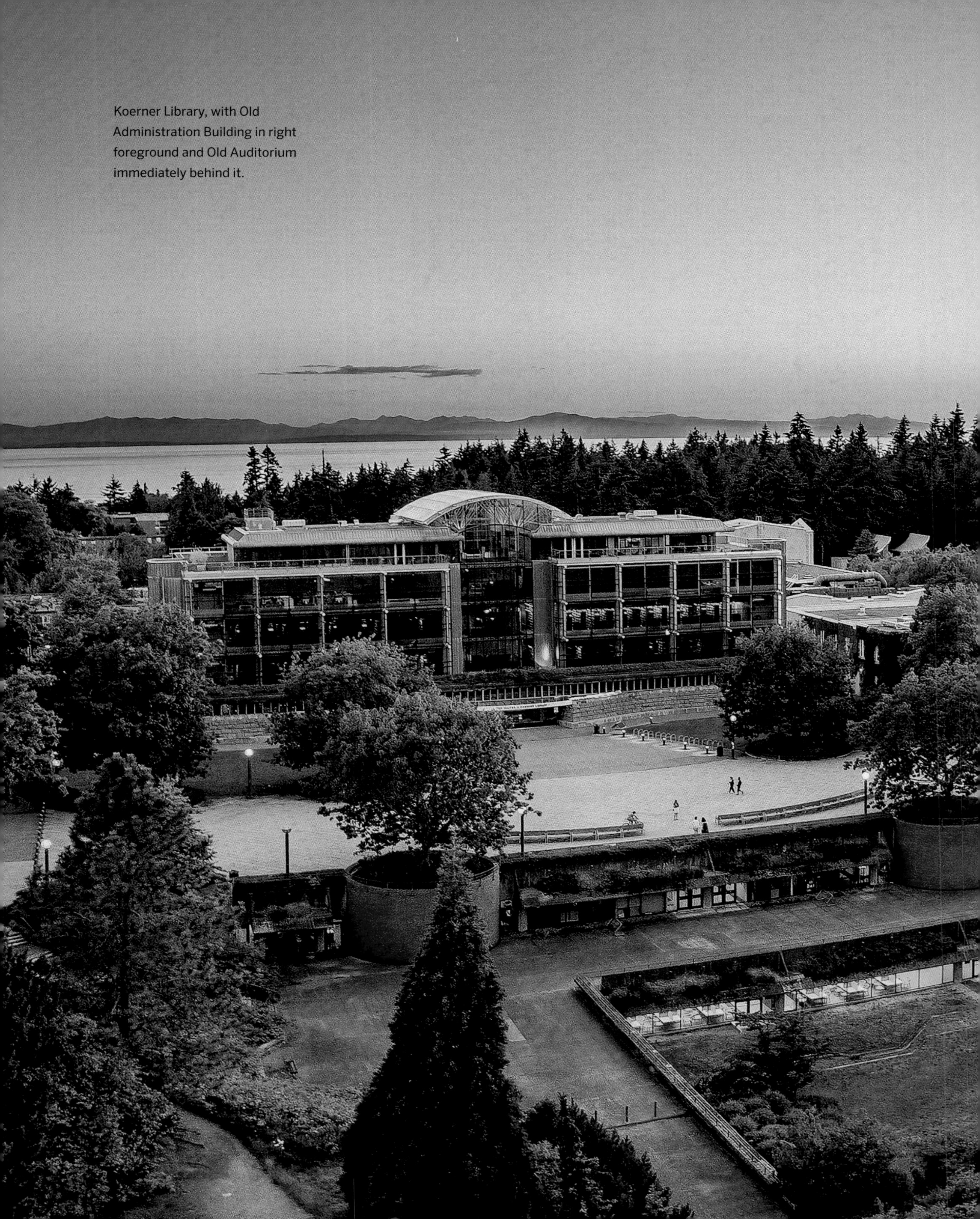

Koerner Library, with Old Administration Building in right foreground and Old Auditorium immediately behind it.

Acknowledgements

WE ARE GRATEFUL to many people for their assistance in the creation of this story. We acknowledge the Faculty's foresight in commissioning historical interviews (in 1984–85) with numerous individuals, including: Geoffrey Andrew, Alexander Boggie, Harold Copp, Albert Cox, Gordon Crossen, Claude Dolman, George Elliot, Sydney Friedman, William Gibson, Robert Kerr, Albert Knudsen, Norman MacKenzie, Rocke Robertson, William Webber, Donald Williams, and Sydney Zbarsky.

Setting out to write a history of the Faculty, Wendy Cairns conducted extensive research in the archives of UBC, the Faculty of Medicine, and the City of Vancouver. Between 1998 and 2002, she interviewed many key individuals, including: Patricia Baird, David Bates, Fred Bryans, William Cockroft, Max Cynader, John Dirks, Stephen Drance, Richard Finley, John Fleetham, Sydney and Constance Friedman, William Gibson, John Gilbert, Victor Gomel, David Hardwick, Carol Herbert, Martin Hollenberg, John Mancini, Pat and Edie McGeer, Robert McGraw, Donald Paty, Pauline Ranta (widow of Lawrence Ranta), John Ruedy, Charles Slonecker, Michael Smith, and Athanasios Zis.

Subsequent to our taking on the project, we conducted interviews with Al Boggie, Carol Anne Courneya, Peggy Cox, David Hardwick, Don Ricci, Andrew Seal, and John Wade. We are deeply appreciative to everyone interviewed in these three periods, who gave so generously of their time. Their recollections have provided personal perspectives on the events and have uncovered details of the Faculty of Medicine story not available in the various archives.

We are also grateful to those folks who reviewed an early version of the manuscript, correcting errors, contributing new information, and providing excellent feedback. These include: Jane Bryans, Oscar Casiro, Max Cynader, Richard Finley, Judy Hall, David Hardwick, Carol Herbert, John Mancini, David McLean, and Bob Meek.

We had help from many quarters for the compilation and preparation of photographs: Candice Bjur and John Moran from UBC Archives helped find and download high quality photos. Terry Lavender, Katie White, Bethany Saunders, Ali Liversage, Camilo Trujillo Sanchez, Stephanie Chow, Catherine Pang, John Hugh McNeill, Adele Aquino, Martin Dee, and Cindy Valensky provided help with photographs and with ferreting out other details that we have incorporated into the story. Sarah Burgess and Cecilia Tupper at St. Paul's Foundation, Shaf Hussain at Providence Health, Denise Flood and Cathy Helliwell at VGH + UBC Hospital Foundation, Cori Ross at Vancouver Coastal Health, Sarah Roth at BC Cancer Foundation, and Michelle Man at BC Children's also provided hard-to-find photographs. Candace Bjur accessed countless boxes of Faculty of Medicine files from the UBC Archives and copied numerous documents. Courtney Cousineau helped by arranging presentations to the UBC Medical Alumni Association executive and providing access to the Medical Student and Alumni Centre. John Dolman, Stephen Chung, and Jane Bryans provided us with unique family photographs. Eric Webber contributed really interesting background material for the "Webber Boot" sidebar.

We had outstanding professional support from the entire team at Page Two led by Trena White. Leslie Erickson helped us shape the manuscript with her excellent editing. Rachel Ironstone assisted with the detailed copy-editing and preparation for printing. Nadine Bachan provided us with the means to share, assess, and select the best photographs from the large numbers in our possession and to secure the permissions for use. Peter Cocking and his team (including Fiona Lee) were excellent in their creative layout and overall design of the book and in the processing of some of the difficult-to-use photographs. Caela Moffet kept us on track and on time and was a source of ideas for design and layout. We appreciate the expert advice of Megan O'Neill for marketing and Lorraine Toor for distribution.

We received generous financial support from Doctors of BC (Allan Seckel, CEO), the UBC Faculty of Medicine (Dermot Kelleher, Dean), and UBC (Santa Ono, President and Vice-chancellor), the Medical Alumni Association as well as from Jane Bryans (wife of Fred Bryans). These resources and their enthusiastic endorsement of our efforts made this book possible.

Finally, we need to acknowledge our respective families, who put up with the authors working on weekends, vacations, and evenings to meet the deadline to have this book published in the seventieth year of the Faculty.

Timeline

1866 Crown colony of British Columbia founded, New Westminster the capital

1871 BC joins Dominion of Canada, Victoria the capital

1887 Nine-bed hospital taken over from Canadian Pacific Railway (CPR) by the city of Vancouver, becomes "City Hospital"

1888 Smallpox hospital established on Deadman Island in Coal Harbour

1888 Vancouver City Hospital moves to new site at Pender and Cambie Streets

1894 Sisters of Providence open St. Paul's Hospital on Burrard Street

1899 Vancouver City Hospital Training School for Nurses opened

1900 St. Joseph's Hospital School of Nursing founded in Victoria

1900 BC Medical Association founded, Robert E. McKechnie first president

1906 Vancouver General Hospital (formerly City Hospital) moves to Heather Pavilion site at 10th Avenue

1907 St. Paul's Hospital opens School of Nursing

1911 University Endowment Lands secured with passing of University Site Act

1912 Flexner Report on medical education in North America published

1913 Frank Wesbrook appointed University of British Columbia's first president

1922 The Great Trek made to the Point Grey Campus

1927 Grace Hospital opens at Heather Street and 26th Avenue

1935 Claude E. Dolman becomes director of the division of laboratories of the department of health of British Columbia and UBC head of bacteriology and preventive medicine

1944 Joint Vancouver Medical Association/UBC committee under Dolman submits proposal for Faculty of Medicine

1946 Dolman's "Report on a Survey of Medical Education" delivered to UBC Board of Governors

1947 BC legislature votes for immediate organization of a Faculty of Medicine

1948 UBC Senate endorses development of FoM

1948 BC government announces it will establish a FoM and seven hundred new beds at VGH

1949 FoM established with Myron Weaver as first dean

1950 Quadrangle of huts for anatomy, physiology, and pharmacology and dean's office on UBC Main Mall

1950 First class of sixty students enter FoM

1951 Clinical wards along 10th Avenue open at VGH (floors A, B, and C)

1951 First Medical School Ball established by students

1955 Weaver steps down, Rocke Robertson becomes acting dean

1956 John Patterson becomes second dean

1957 UBC wing at VGH opens on Heather Street with lecture halls, offices, laboratories, and library

1958 Patterson steps down

1959 Jack McCreary becomes third dean; planning begins for a UBC-sited health sciences centre

1959 Centennial Pavilion opens at VGH

1961 Basic science buildings A, B, C open on Point Grey Campus

1961 School of Rehabilitation Medicine formed, Brock Fahrni first director

1964 Woodward Biomedical Library opens

1967 Detwiller Pavilion, psychiatry building on campus, opens

1970 McCreary appointed coordinator of health sciences

1972 McCreary steps down as dean, David Bates becomes fourth dean

1972 New Democratic Party government elected, abandons idea of acute care hospital on UBC campus

1972 Instructional Resources Centre opens on UBC campus

1972 First-year entry class expands to eighty

1974 British Columbia Medical Centre (BCMC) at Shaughnessy site concept announced

1975 Twenty-fifth anniversary of first medical students at UBC

1975 NDP defeated, new Social Credit government, Patrick McGeer is minister of education

1976 BCMC concept dropped but with government commitment to new beds and facilities

1977 Bates steps down, Bill Webber becomes fifth dean

1980 Koerner Pavilion opened at UBC

1980 First-year class size expands to 120

1982 BC Children's Hospital and new Grace Hospital (which becomes BC Women's Hospital and Health Centre in 1994) open on Oak Street

1983 Eye Care Centre opens at VGH

1990 Webber steps down, Martin Hollenberg becomes sixth dean

1990 Medical Student and Alumni Centre opens at Heather Street and 12th Avenue

1993 Founding director of UBC Biotechnology Laboratory, Michael Smith, awarded Nobel Prize in Chemistry

1994 Problem-based curriculum approved by Faculty Council

1996 New academic space opened at Jim Pattison North, VGH

1996 Hollenberg steps down, John Cairns becomes seventh dean

1998 New curriculum approved by UBC Senate for implementation

1999 "Wade Report" to UBC and Ministries of Health and Advanced Education

2000 FoM "The Best of Health" strategic plan published

2000 Golden Jubilee celebrations of the FoM

2000 NDP government announces BC Health Action Plan, including new FoM funding

2001 Liberal government announces plan for expansion of seats and distribution of medical school campuses

2001 First-year class size expands to 128

2003 Cairns steps down, Gavin Stuart becomes eighth dean

2003 Jim Pattison Pavilion at VGH opens

2004 First expanded class of 200 students in the Distributed Medical Educational Program begins in Vancouver-Fraser, Prince George (Northern Medical Program), and Victoria (Island Medical Program)

2004 Life Sciences Centre opens on UBC campus

2004 University Academic Campuses open at University of Victoria and University of Northern BC

2006 Gordon and Leslie Diamond Health Care Centre opens

2007 First-year class expands to 256 students

2010 Clinical Academic Campus opens in Kelowna

2011 First students start in Kelowna (first-year class now 288)

2014 Djavad Mowafaghian Centre for Brain Health opens at UBC Hospital

2015 Case-based learning curriculum instituted into MD undergraduate program

2015 New St. Paul's Hospital and integrated health campus at Station Street announced

2015 Stuart steps down, Dermot Kelleher becomes ninth dean

2016 "Building the Future — the Faculty of Medicine 2016–2021 Strategic Plan" released

2019 MD undergraduate program across all four campuses provided with full accreditation status until regular cycle of review in 2023–2024

2020 COVID-19 pandemic forces major reconfiguration of learning, research, and care programs

2020 Successful accreditation of all postgraduate programs by College of Family Physicians of Canada and Royal College of Physicians and Surgeons of Canada

Further Reading

Boggie, A. (2009). *Good friends, good family, a life story*. Vancouver, BC: Alexander Boggie.

Bryans, F.E. (2005). *The early years: The history of the University of British Columbia Department of Obstetrics and Gynecology, 1950-1980*. Vancouver, BC: UBC Department of Obstetrics and Gynecology.

Cambon, E.N. (2008). *Uppity women we are: 100-year history of medical women of British Columbia (1893-1993)*. Vancouver, BC: Vancouver Desktop Publishing Centre Ltd.

Damer, E., & Rosengarten, H. (2009). *UBC the First 100 years*. Vancouver, BC: University of British Columbia.

De Leeuw, S. & Swanky, T. (2011). *Front lines: Portraits of caregivers in Northern British Columbia*. Powell River, BC: Creekstone Press Ltd.

Gibson, W.C. (1975). *Health care, teaching and research: Prospect and retrospect*. Vancouver, BC: The UBC Alumni Association and the Faculty of Medicine UBC.

Gibson, W.C. (1996). *No time to slow down*. Vancouver, BC: University of British Columbia Alumni Association.

Hill, R. (1998). Paediatrics in BC: A history, with particular emphasis on the UBC Academic Department. *Canadian Medical Association Journal, 158*(10), 1355.

Hill, R. (2006). *Jack McCreary: Paediatrician, pedagogue, pragmatist, prophet*. Canada: Tantalus Research Limited.

Historical interviews (conducted by the FoM in 1984-85) are available in transcript form through the Woodward Biomedical Library at https://www.library.ubc.ca/woodward/memoroom/collection/oralhistory/pdf.

Patterson, F.P. (2000). *The cutting edge: Reminiscences of surgery at the Vancouver General Hospital and the University of British Columbia 1915-1985*. Vancouver, BC: Hatzic Publishing.

West Coast Editorial Associates. (2014). The Island Medical Program: Celebrating the first 10 years. Retrieved from issuu.com/ubc_medicine/docs/imp-10th-web-aug2014.

Index

Note: Page numbers in italics refer to photographs.

Photo credits

FRONT COVER: Paul H. Joseph / UBC Brand & Marketing.
BACK COVER: University of British Columbia Archives [UBC 1.1/2673].

Front Matter

PAGE II: © Geoff Lister, Photographer.
PAGE IX: Paul H. Joseph / UBC Brand & Marketing.
PAGE X: © Geoff Lister, Photographer.
PAGE XIV: University of British Columbia Archives [UBC 156.1/150].

Chapter 1

PAGE XVIII (TOP): City of Vancouver Archives, CVA 677-506.
PAGE XVIII (BOTTOM): University of British Columbia Archives, Photo by Royal Canadian Air Force [UBC 1.1/174].
PAGE 3: Image A-01351 courtesy of the Royal BC Museum.
PAGE 5 (TOP): City of Vancouver Archives, CVA 677-136, J. Wood Laing.
PAGE 5 (BOTTOM): City of Vancouver Archives, Bu P369, Major Matthews Collection.
PAGE 6: University of British Columbia Archives [UBC 1.1/13091].
PAGE 7: City of Vancouver Archives, CVA 677-140, Campbell Studio.
PAGE 9 (TOP): University of British Columbia Archives, Photo by Leonard Frank [UBC 1.1/144].
PAGE 9 (BOTTOM LEFT): University of British Columbia Archives, Photo by Bridgman Studio [UBC 1.1/1328].
PAGE 9 (BOTTOM RIGHT): University of British Columbia Archives, Photo by Hacking Photo Studio [UBC 1.1/1211].
PAGE 10: City of Vancouver Archives, Bu P483, Major Matthews Collection.
PAGE 11: Courtesy of the Dolman family.
PAGE 12: Courtesy of the GF Strong Rehabilitation Centre.
PAGE 13: University of British Columbia Archives [UBC 23.1/299.82].
PAGE 16: CE Dolman fonds, UBC. Report on a survey of medical education in Canada and the United States. 1946.
PAGE 21: Image B-08419 courtesy of the Royal BC Museum.

Chapter 2

PAGE 22: University of British Columbia, Main Mall, Point Grey Campus, circa 1950s. Photographer unknown.
PAGE 25: University of British Columbia Archives, Photo by White Studio [UBC 1.1/13051.2].
PAGE 26: University of British Columbia Archives [UBC 1.1/4306].
PAGE 29: University of British Columbia Archives [UBC 1.1/5355.2].
PAGE 30: Courtesy of the Department of Cellular and Physiological Sciences. Faculty of Medicine, UBC.
PAGE 31: University of British Columbia Archives [UBC 5.1/557].
PAGE 32: University of British Columbia Archives [UBC 1.1/5409.1].
PAGE 33 (LEFT): Photo by Rob Shaer, Mednet IT. Courtesy of the Faculty of Medicine, © University of British Columbia.
PAGE 33 (RIGHT): An original photo by Yousuf Karsh, taken on February 16 1949. Courtesy of the Estate of Yousuf Karsh.
PAGE 34: University of British Columbia Archives, Photo by David Margerison [UBC 41/2003.2].
PAGE 35: University of British Columbia Archives [UBC 5.2/2550].
PAGE 36 (LEFT): University of British Columbia Archives, Photo by Tony Archer [UBC 1.1/12884].
PAGE 36 (RIGHT): University of British Columbia Archives, Photo by Campbell Studios [UBC 53.1/9].
PAGE 38: Courtesy of Providence Health Care.
PAGE 39: University of British Columbia Archives [UBC 41.1/2627.1].
PAGE 40: Courtesy of Mrs. Jane Bryans and the Bryans family.
PAGE 41: University of British Columbia Archives [UBC 1.1/16559].

PAGE 44 (TOP): Courtesy of the Dolman family.
PAGE 44 (BOTTOM): University of British Columbia Archives [UBC 23.1/300.1a].
PAGE 46: University of British Columbia Archives [UBC 1.1/2673].
PAGE 47 (LEFT): UBC Wing, Vancouver General Hospital, circa late 1950s. Photographer unknown.
PAGE 47 (RIGHT): Courtesy of the Faculty of Medicine, © University of British Columbia.
PAGE 48: Courtesy of the VGH & UBC Hospital Foundation.
PAGE 51: Courtesy of Dr. Alexander Boggie.
PAGE 52: University of British Columbia Archives [UBC 3.1/991.5].
PAGE 54: Courtesy of Dr. Alexander Boggie.
PAGE 55: University of British Columbia Archives [UBC 3.1/991.6].

Chapter 3

PAGE 56: University of British Columbia Archives [UBC 3.1/746.8].
PAGE 59: University of British Columbia Archives [UBC 5.1/2369].
PAGE 60: University of British Columbia Archives [UBC 1.1/3103].
PAGE 62: Courtesy of the Faculty of Medicine, © University of British Columbia.
PAGE 63: Martin Dee / UBC.
PAGE 64: University of British Columbia Archives [UBC 40.1/12].
PAGE 67: University of British Columbia Archives, Photo by Michelle Cook [UBC 44.1/2091]. Used with permission of the photographer.
PAGE 68: Courtesy of Dr. David I. McLean, Department of Dermatology, UBC Faculty of Medicine.
PAGE 71: University of British Columbia Archives, Photo by Martin Dee [UBC 128.1/2].
PAGE 72 (TOP): University of British Columbia Archives [UBC 5.1/1461].
PAGE 72 (BOTTOM): University of British Columbia Archives [UBC 44.1/3038].
PAGE 74: Courtesy of the Faculty of Medicine, © University of British Columbia.
PAGE 75: University of British Columbia Archives [UBC 41.1/1493].

Chapter 4

PAGE 76: University of British Columbia Archives, Photo by Jim Banham [UBC 41.1/832-1].
PAGE 79: University of British Columbia Archives [UBC 85.1/20].
PAGE 80: University of British Columbia Archives [UBC 41.1/1947].
PAGE 82: University of British Columbia Archives, Photo by Dave Roels Photography [UBC 41.1/1798.2].
PAGE 84: University of British Columbia Archives [UBC 44.1/339].
PAGE 85 (LEFT): Brian K. Smith, Media Services Centre, Providence Health Care.
PAGE 85 (RIGHT): University of British Columbia Archives, Photo by Martin Dee and Don Erhardt [UBC 35.1/759].
PAGE 87: University of British Columbia Archives [UBC 41/20.35].
PAGE 88: Brian K. Smith, Media Services Centre, Providence Health Care.
PAGE 90: Courtesy of Vancouver Coastal Health.
PAGE 91: University of British Columbia Archives [UBC 5.1/4096].
PAGE 92: Courtesy of Dr. David Ostrow.
PAGE 93 (TOP): © 2020 2POS Canada.
PAGE 93 (BOTTOM): Courtesy of Dr. David Ostrow.
PAGE 94: Courtesy of the McCarthy family and BC Honours and Awards Secretariat.
PAGE 95 (LEFT): University of British Columbia Archives [UBC 5.1/4096].
PAGE 95 (RIGHT): University of British Columbia Archives, Photo by Jim Banham [UBC 41.1/507.2].
PAGE 96: Courtesy of Dr. Carol Herbert.
PAGE 97: University of British Columbia Archives, Photo by Jim Banham [UBC 41.1/703.1].
PAGE 98 (LEFT): Courtesy of the Faculty of Medicine, © University of British Columbia.
PAGE 98 (RIGHT): University of British Columbia Archives [UBC 44.1/3143].
PAGE 99: University of British Columbia Archives [UBC 41.1/1856].
PAGE 100: University of British Columbia Archives, Photo by Jim Banham [UBC 44.1/2613].
PAGE 101 (LEFT): University of British Columbia Archives, Photo by Kent Kallberg [UBC 44.1/2796].

PAGE 101 (RIGHT): Brian K. Smith, Media Services Centre, Providence Health Care.

PAGE 102 (LEFT): Courtesy of UBC Department of Surgery.

PAGE 102 (RIGHT): Courtesy of UBC Department of Surgery.

PAGE 104 (LEFT): UBC Photo / Kent Kallberg.

PAGE 104 (RIGHT): Courtesy of Dr. Robert McGraw.

PAGE 105: University of British Columbia Archives [UBC 44.1/1601].

PAGE 107 (LEFT): Courtesy of Dr. Jack Rootman.

PAGE 107 (RIGHT): University of British Columbia Archives, Photo by Kent Kallberg [UBC 44.1/3130].

PAGE 108 (TOP): Courtesy of the Faculty of Medicine, © University of British Columbia.

PAGE 108 (BOTTOM): Courtesy of the Faculty of Medicine, © University of British Columbia.

PAGE 110: Courtesy of the Faculty of Medicine, © University of British Columbia.

Chapter 5

PAGE 112: Photo by Dr. Gavin Stuart. Faculty of Medicine medallion, University of British Columbia.

PAGE 115: University of British Columbia Archives, Photo by Media Services [UBC 44.1/2957].

PAGE 116: University of British Columbia Archives, Photo by Kent Kallberg [UBC 44.1/2680].

PAGE 117: University of British Columbia Archives [UBC 44.1/1431].

PAGE 118: University of British Columbia Archives, Photo by Hilary Thomson [UBC 44.1/1105].

PAGE 119: Courtesy of Dr. John Mancini. Vancouver General Hospital Division of Cardiology Staff Photo, 2010.

PAGE 120 (LEFT): Courtesy of Dr. Richard Finley.

PAGE 120 (RIGHT): Courtesy of Dr. Felix Durity and BC Honours and Awards Secretariat.

PAGE 121: Courtesy of the Faculty of Medicine, © University of British Columbia.

PAGE 122: Courtesy of the Faculty of Medicine, © University of British Columbia.

PAGE 123: Courtesy of Dr. Robert Armstrong.

PAGE 124 (LEFT): Courtesy of Dr. David Ostrow.

PAGE 124 (RIGHT): Courtesy of the Faculty of Medicine, © University of British Columbia.

PAGE 125: Courtesy of the Faculty of Medicine, © University of British Columbia.

PAGE 127: University of British Columbia Archives, Photo by Martin Dee [UBC 44.1/2366].

PAGE 128 (LEFT): Courtesy of Dr. Carol-Ann Courneya.

PAGE 128 (RIGHT): Spirit of the Heart by Dr. Michiko Maruyama. Used by permission of the artist.

PAGE 129: University of British Columbia Archives, Photo by Martin Dee [UBC 41.1/2507].

PAGE 130: Martin Dee / UBC Brand & Marketing.

PAGE 131 (LEFT): Courtesy of the Faculty of Medicine, © University of British Columbia.

PAGE 131 (RIGHT): Photo collage by Dr. Andrew Seal.

PAGE 132: University of British Columbia Archives, Photo by John Chong [UBC 44.1/1325].

PAGE 134 (LEFT): University of British Columbia Archives, Photo by Martin Dee [UBC 44.1/1632].

PAGE 134 (RIGHT): Photo by Dr. Gavin Stuart. Faculty of Medicine medallion, University of British Columbia.

PAGE 135: Courtesy of the Faculty of Medicine, © University of British Columbia.

PAGE 136: Courtesy of the Faculty of Medicine, © University of British Columbia.

PAGE 137 (LEFT): Courtesy of Northern Health, External Relations & Communications.

PAGE 137 (RIGHT): Dave Milne / *Prince George Citizen*.

PAGE 138: Based upon data from the Association of Faculties of Medicine of Canada (formerly the Canadian Association of Medical Colleges) and 1996 Canadian census.

PAGE 139: Image courtesy of Mary McNeil, available under the Attribtution-ShareAlike 2.0 License (https://creativecommons.org/licenses/by-sa/2.0/).

PAGE 141 (LEFT): Courtesy of the Faculty of Medicine, © University of British Columbia.

PAGE 141 (RIGHT): Courtesy of the Faculty of Medicine, © University of British Columbia.

PAGE 142: University of British Columbia Archives [UBC 44.1/3189].

PAGE 143: Courtesy of the Faculty of Medicine, © University of British Columbia.

PAGE 144: Brian K. Smith, Media Services Centre, Providence Health Care.

Chapter 6

PAGE 146: Courtesy of the VGH & UBC Hospital Foundation.

PAGE 149: Courtesy of the Faculty of Medicine, © University of British Columbia.
PAGE 150: Courtesy of the Faculty of Medicine, © University of British Columbia.
PAGE 151 (TOP): Paul H. Joseph / UBC Brand & Marketing.
PAGE 151 (BOTTOM LEFT): Courtesy of the Faculty of Medicine, © University of British Columbia.
PAGE 151 (BOTTOM RIGHT): Courtesy of the Faculty of Medicine, © University of British Columbia.
PAGE 152: Courtesy of the Faculty of Medicine, © University of British Columbia.
PAGE 153: Courtesy of BC Cancer / Provincial Heath Services Authority.
PAGE 154 (LEFT): Courtesy of Dr. Larry Goldenberg.
PAGE 154 (RIGHT): Courtesy of Dr. Martin Gleave and the photographer Greg Morton. © Media Services/SPH/PHC.
PAGE 155: Don Erhardt / UBC Brand & Marketing.
PAGE 156 (LEFT): Courtesy of the Faculty of Medicine, © University of British Columbia.
PAGE 156 (RIGHT): Courtesy of the Faculty of Medicine, © University of British Columbia.
PAGE 157: Courtesy of the Faculty of Medicine, © University of British Columbia.
PAGE 158: Courtesy of the Faculty of Medicine, © University of British Columbia.
PAGE 159: Courtesy of the Faculty of Medicine, © University of British Columbia.
PAGE 161: Courtesy of the Faculty of Medicine, © University of British Columbia.
PAGE 162-163: Courtesy of the Faculty of Medicine, © University of British Columbia.
PAGE 164: Courtesy of the Faculty of Medicine, © University of British Columbia.
PAGE 165: Courtesy of the Faculty of Medicine, © University of British Columbia.
PAGE 166: Courtesy of the Faculty of Medicine, © University of British Columbia.
PAGE 167: Courtesy of the Faculty of Medicine, © University of British Columbia.
PAGE 168: Courtesy of the North Island Gazette & Publisher, Natasha Griffiths.
PAGE 169: Tloren5, CC BY-SA 4.0 <https://creativecommons.org/licenses/by-sa/4.0>, via Wikimedia Commons.
PAGE 170: Courtesy of UBC Okanagan.
PAGE 171: Courtesy of the Faculty of Medicine, © University of British Columbia.
PAGE 174: Courtesy of the Faculty of Medicine, © University of British Columbia.
PAGE 175: Courtesy of the Faculty of Medicine, © University of British Columbia.

Chapter 7

PAGE 178: Paul H. Joseph / UBC Brand & Marketing.
PAGE 181: Courtesy of the Faculty of Medicine, © University of British Columbia.
PAGE 182: Courtesy of the Faculty of Medicine, © University of British Columbia.
PAGE 184: Courtesy of Dr. Connie Eaves.
PAGE 185 (LEFT): Courtesy of Dr. Gina Ogilvie.
PAGE 186 (RIGHT): Courtesy of Dr. Videsh Kapoor, Clinical Assistant Professor, Department of Family Practice, Faculty of Medicine Family Physician.
PAGE 186: Courtesy of the Faculty of Medicine, © University of British Columbia.
PAGE 187: Courtesy of the Faculty of Medicine, © University of British Columbia.
PAGE 188: Courtesy of the Faculty of Medicine, © University of British Columbia.

PAGE 190: © Geoff Lister, Photographer.

Author photos (Page 211)

JOHN CAIRNS: Courtesy of MacGregor Studios.
WENDY CAIRNS: © Alastair Bird.
DAVID OSTROW: Courtesy of Dr. David Ostrow.
GAVIN STUART: Courtesy of Cameron Stuart.

PAGE 212-213: Djavad Mowafaghian Centre for Brain Health: Courtesy of Don Erhardt / UBC Brand & Marketing.

About the Authors

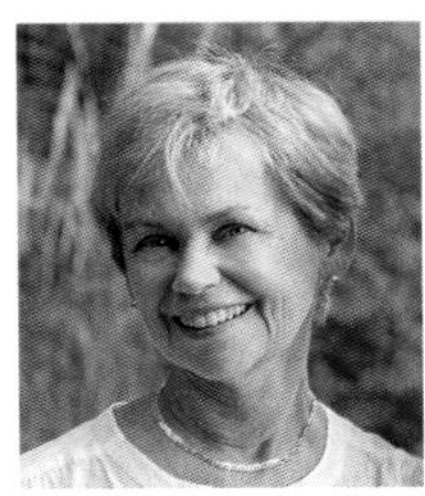

WENDY ELIZABETH CAIRNS was a UBC graduate who worked at the electronic library of the Canadian Centre for Occupational Health and Safety in Hamilton, Ontario. Returning to BC in 1997, she began a history of the Faculty of Medicine at UBC. Her extensive research, interviews, and eloquent prose languished following her premature death but were taken up and extended by Doctors Cairns, Stuart, and Ostrow, becoming the foundation of this book.

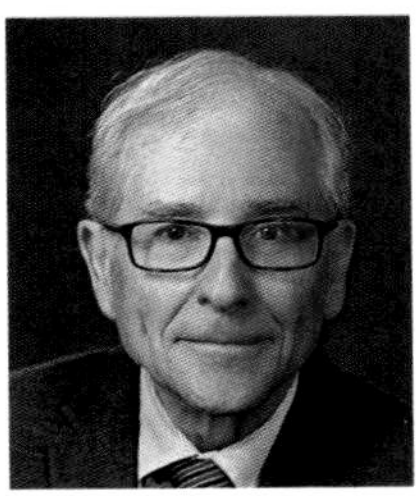

JOHN ALLAN CAIRNS is an extensively published clinical and academic cardiologist and was Dean of UBC's Faculty of Medicine from 1996 to 2003. He led efforts, in conjunction with UBC and two provincial governments, to conceptualize, secure the funding for, and establish university partnerships to enable the doubling of medical student enrollment centred at UBC but distributed throughout the province.

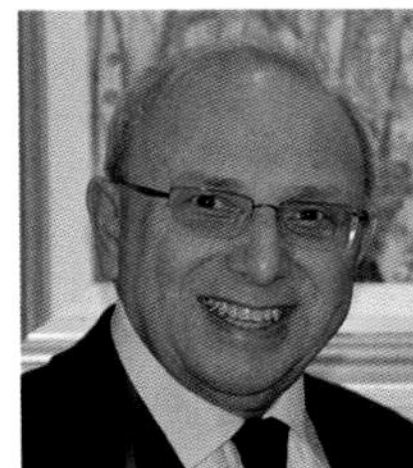

DAVID NEIL OSTROW is Emeritus Professor of Respiratory Medicine at the University of British Columbia. In 1995 he chaired the development of the Faculty of Medicine's problem-based curriculum. He was the President and Chief Executive Officer of Vancouver Coastal Health Authority from 2009 until his retirement, in April 2014.

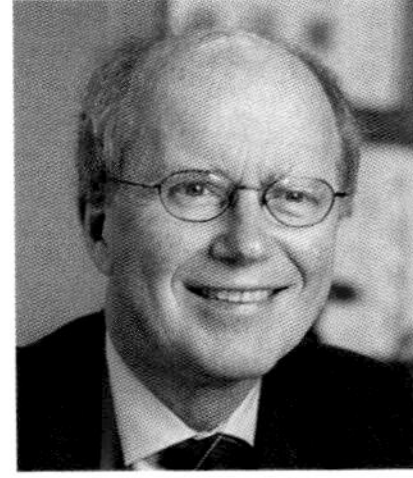

GAVIN CHARLES EDWARD STUART served as Dean of Medicine at UBC from 2003 to 2015 during which time he led the implementation of the distributed medical program across BC. He also held the role of UBC Vice-provost Health. Previously he was Vice-president of the Alberta Cancer Board. He is currently Professor and interim Head of the Department of Obstetrics and Gynecology and a practicing academic gynecologic oncologist in Vancouver.

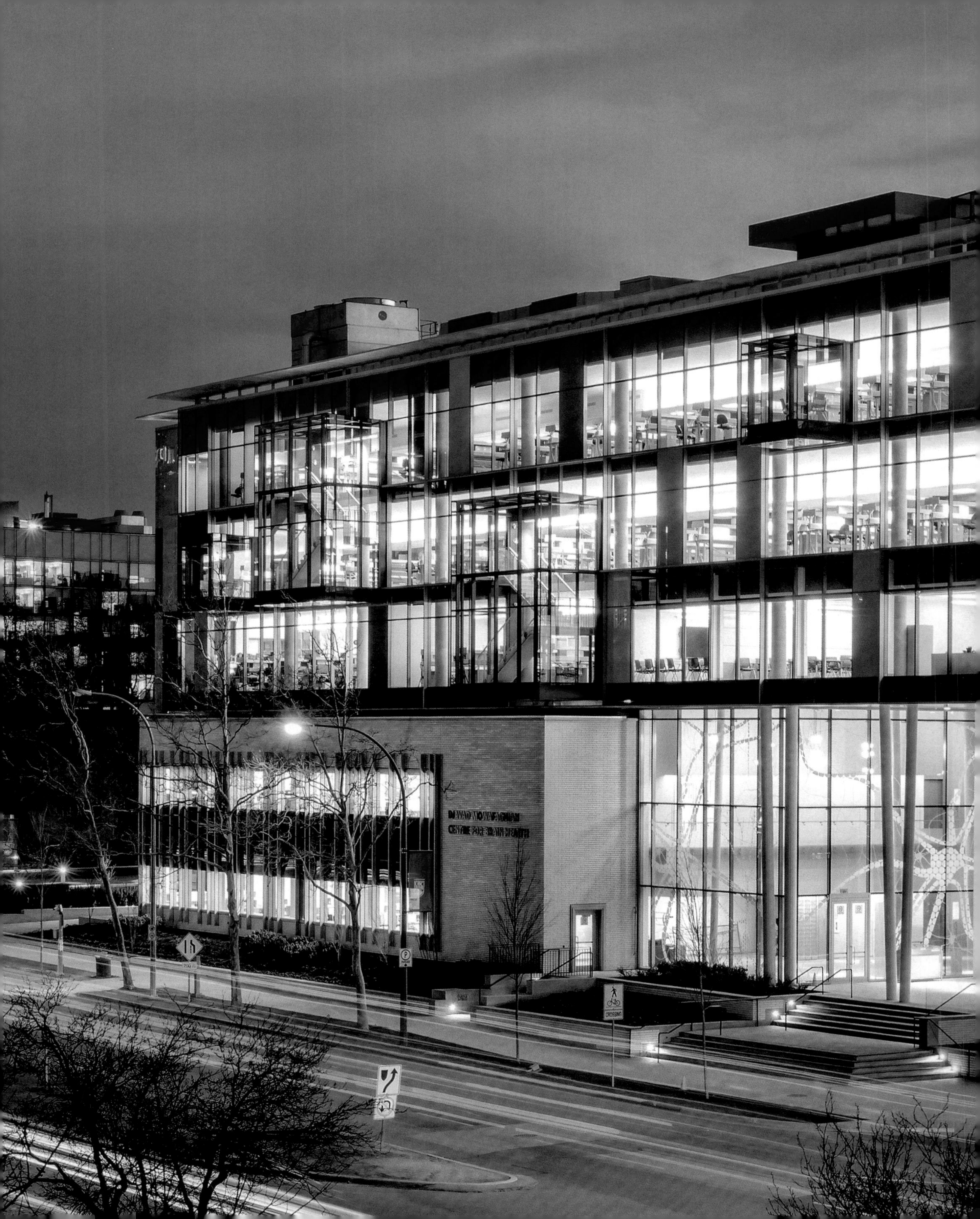

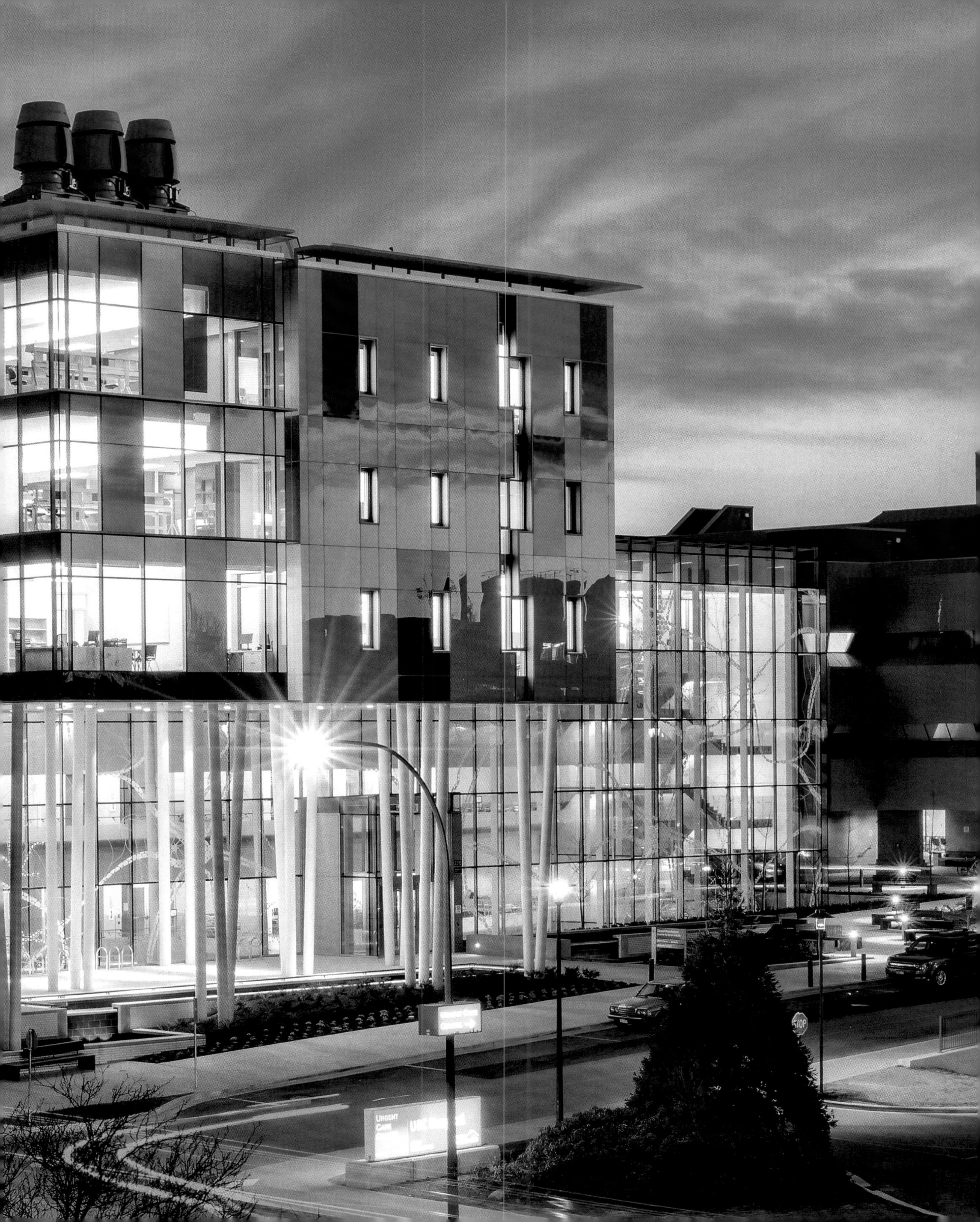
URGENT
CARE